BRODY'S HUMAN PHARMACOLOGY

MECHANISM-BASED THERAPEUTICS

BRODY'S HUMAN PHARMACOLOGY

MECHANISM-BASED THERAPEUTICS

SIXTH EDITION

Lynn Wecker, PhD

Distinguished University Professor
Department of Psychiatry and Behavioral Neurosciences
Department of Molecular Pharmacology and Physiology
University of South Florida Morsani College of Medicine
Tampa, Florida

With

David A. Taylor, PhD

Professor and Chair
Department of Pharmacology and Toxicology
Brody School of Medicine at East Carolina University
Greenville, North Carolina

Robert J. Theobald, Jr., PhD

Professor
Department of Pharmacology
A.T. Still University of Health Sciences
Kirksville, Missouri

ELSEVIER

ELSEVIER

1600 John F. Kennedy Blvd.
Ste 1800
Philadelphia, PA 19103-2899

BRODY'S HUMAN PHARMACOLOGY, SIXTH EDITION   ISBN: 978-0-323-47652-2

Notices

Knowledge and best practice in this field are constantly changing. As new research and experience broaden our understanding, changes in research methods, professional practices, or medical treatment may become necessary.

Practitioners and researchers must always rely on their own experience and knowledge in evaluating and using any information, methods, compounds, or experiments described herein. In using such information or methods they should be mindful of their own safety and the safety of others, including parties for whom they have a professional responsibility.

With respect to any drug or pharmaceutical products identified, readers are advised to check the most current information provided (i) on procedures featured or (ii) by the manufacturer of each product to be administered, to verify the recommended dose or formula, the method and duration of administration, and contraindications. It is the responsibility of practitioners, relying on their own experience and knowledge of their patients, to make diagnoses, to determine dosages and the best treatment for each individual patient, and to take all appropriate safety precautions.

To the fullest extent of the law, neither the Publisher nor the authors, contributors, or editors, assume any liability for any injury and/or damage to persons or property as a matter of products liability, negligence or otherwise, or from any use or operation of any methods, products, instructions, or ideas contained in the material herein.

Previous editions copyrighted in 2010, 2005, 1998, 1994, 1991

Library of Congress Cataloging-in-Publication Data
Names: Wecker, Lynn, editor. | Taylor, David A. (David Alan), 1948- editor. | Theobald, Robert James, Jr., editor.
Title: Brody's human pharmacology : molecular to clinical / [edited by] Lynn Wecker with David A. Taylor, Robert James Theobald, Jr.
Other titles: Human pharmacology
Description: Sixth edition. | Philadelphia, PA : Elsevier, Inc., [2019] | Includes bibliographical references and index.
Identifiers: LCCN 2018003347 | ISBN 9780323476522 (pbk. : alk. paper)
Subjects: | MESH: Pharmacology | Drug Therapy
Classification: LCC RM300 | NLM QV 4 | DDC 615.5/8–dc23 LC record available at https://lccn.loc.gov/2018003347

Content Strategist: Alexandra Mortimer
Content Development Manager: Laura Schmidt
Publishing Services Manager: Catherine Jackson
Senior Project Manager: Sharon Corell
Book Designer: Ryan Cook

Working together
to grow libraries in
developing countries

www.elsevier.com • www.bookaid.org

Printed in China.
Last digit is the print number: 9 8 7 6 5 4 3 2 1

Abdel A. Abdel-Rahman, MSc, PhD
Distinguished Professor and Vice Chair
Department of Pharmacology and
 Toxicology
Brody School of Medicine at East Carolina
 University
Greenville, North Carolina

Elena E. Bagley, BPharm, PhD
Associate Professor
Discipline of Pharmacology
Sydney Medical School
University of Sydney
Sydney, New South Wales
Australia

James E. Barrett, PhD
Professor
Departments of Neurology, Pharmacology,
 and Physiology
Drexel University College of Medicine
Philadelphia, Pennsylvania

Mary-Ann Bjornsti, PhD
Professor and Chair
Department of Pharmacology and
 Toxicology
University of Alabama at Birmingham
Birmingham, Alabama

Gerald B. Call, PhD
Professor of Pharmacology
Arizona College of Osteopathic Medicine
Midwestern University
Glendale, Arizona

Glenn Catalano, MD
Associate Chief of Staff
Mental Health and Behavioral Sciences
James A. Haley Veterans' Hospital
Professor
Department of Psychiatry and Behavioral
 Neurosciences
University of South Florida Morsani College
 of Medicine
Tampa, Florida

Briony Catlow, PhD
Grant Writer
Knoebel Insitute for Healthy Aging
University of Denver
Denver, Colorado

Larisa H. Cavallari, PharmD
Associate Professor
Department of Pharmacotherapy and
 Translational Research
Director
Center for Pharmacogenomics
Associate Director
Personalized Medicine Program
University of Florida
Gainesville, Florida

Julio A. Copello, PhD
Associate Professor
Department of Pharmacology
Southern Illinois University School of
 Medicine
Springfield, Illinois

Glenn W. Currier, MD, MPH
Professor and Chair
Department of Psychiatry and Behavioral
 Neurosciences
University of South Florida Morsani College
 of Medicine
Tampa, Florida

Javier Cuevas, PhD
Professor and Associate Chair
Department of Molecular Pharmacology
 and Physiology
University of South Florida Morsani College
 of Medicine
Tampa, Florida

Steven T. DeKosky, MD
Professor
Departments of Neurology, Neuroscience,
 and Aging and Geriatric Research
University of Florida College of Medicine
Gainesville, Florida

Kirk E. Dineley, PhD
Associate Professor
Department of Pharmacology
Midwestern University
Downers Grove, Illinois

Joshua R. Edwards, PhD
Professor
Department of Pharmacology
Midwestern University
Chicago College of Osteopathic Medicine
Downers Grove, Illinois

F.J. Ehlert, PhD
Professor
Departments of Pharmacology and
 Anatomy and Neurobiology
School of Medicine
University of California, Irvine
Irvine, California

Ahmed E.M. Elhassanny, PhD
Post-Doctoral Fellow
Department of Pharmacology and
 Toxicology
Brody School of Medicine at East Carolina
 University
Greenville, North Carolina

Keith S. Elmslie, BA, MS, PhD
Professor and Chair
Department of Pharmacology
Kirksville College of Osteopathic Medicine
A.T. Still University of Health Sciences
Kirksville, Missouri

Jill Fehrenbacher, PhD
Assistant Professor
Department of Pharmacology and
 Toxicology
Indiana University School of Medicine
Indianapolis, Indiana

Erin Foff, MD, PhD
Director
Clinical Research
ACADIA Pharmaceuticals Inc.
Princeton, New Jersey

James Carlton Garrison, II, PhD
Professor Emeritus
Department of Pharmacology
University of Virginia
Health Science Center
Charlottesville, Virignia

Kymberly Gowdy, MS, PhD
Assistant Professor
Department of Pharmacology and
 Toxicology
Brody School of Medicine at East Carolina
 University
Greenville, North Carolina

LaToya M. Griffin, PhD
Teaching Assistant Professor
Co-Director
Summer Biomedical Research Program
Department of Pharmacology and
    Toxicology
Brody School of Medicine at East Carolina
    University
Greenville, North Carolina

Robert W. Hadley, PhD
Associate Professor
Director of Education
Department of Pharmacology and
    Nutritional Sciences
University of Kentucky College of Medicine
Lexington, Kentucky

Frank Herrmann, BS, RPh
Clinical Pharmacist
Anticoagulation Clinic
Pennsylvania State Milton S. Hershey
    Medical Center
Hershey, Pennsylvania

Paul F. Hollenberg, MS, PhD
Professor Emeritus
Department of Pharmacology
University of Michigan Medical School
Ann Arbor, Michigan

Christian J. Hopfer, MD
Professor
Department of Psychiatry
University of Colorado
Aurora, Colorado

Susan L. Ingram, PhD
Associate Professor
Department of Neurological Surgery
Oregon Health and Science University
Portland, Oregon

Michael Jaffee, MD
Vice-Chair
Department of Neurology
Bob Paul Family Professor of Neurology
University of Florida College of Medicine
Gainesville, Florida

Julie A. Johnson, PharmD
Distinguished Professor
Department of Pharmacotherapy and
    Translational Research
Department of Medicine
Dean
College of Pharmacy
Director
Personalized Medicine Program
University of Florida
Gainesville, Florida

Peter W. Kalivas, PhD
Professor and Chair
Department of Neuroscience
Medical University of South Carolina
Charleston, South Carolina

Kelly D. Karpa, RPh, PhD
Professor
Department of Pharmacology
Pennsylvania State University College of
    Medicine
Hershey, Pennsylvania

Paul T. Kocis, PharmD
Clinical Pharmacist
Anticoagulation Clinic
Pennsylvania State Milton S. Hershey
    Medical Center
Hershey, Pennsylvania

Phillip Kopf, PhD
Associate Professor
Department of Pharmacology
Midwestern University
Downers Grove, Illinois

Daniel A. Ladin, PhD
Department of Pharmacology and
    Toxicology
Brody School of Medicine at East Carolina
    University
Greenville, North Carolina

John S. Lazo, PhD
Harrison Distinguished Teaching Professor
Department of Pharmacology
Associate Director for Basic Science
UVA Cancer Center
University of Virginia
Charlottesville, Virginia
Adjunct Professor
Virginia Tech Carilion Research Institute
Roanoke, Virginia

Latha Malaiyandi, PhD
Associate Professor
Department of Anatomy
Midwestern University
Downers Grove, Illinois

J. Scott McConnaughey, MD
Retired Deputy Director for Health Services
O'Berry Neuro-Medical Treatment Center
Goldsboro, North Carolina

Mona M. McConnaughey, PhD
Professor Emeritas
Department of Pharmacology and Toxicology
Brody School of Medicine at East Carolina
    University
Greenville, North Carolina

Adonis McQueen, BS, MS, PhD
IRACDA NY Postdoctoral Scholar
Stony Brook University
Stony Brook, New York

David S. Middlemas, PhD
Associate Professor
Department of Pharmacology
Kirksville College of Osteopathic Medicine
Kirksville, Missouri

Scott A. Mosley, PharmD
Postdoctoral Fellow
Center for Pharmacogenomics
Department of Pharmacotherapy and
    Translational Research
University of Florida College of Pharmacy
Gainesville, Florida

Margaret Nelson, BS
PhD Candidate
Department of Pharmacology and
    Toxicology
Brody School of Medicine at East Carolina
    University
Greenville, North Carolina

Julia Ousterhout, PhD
Assistant Professor
Department of Pharmacology
Kirksville College of Osteopathic Medicine
A.T. Still University of Health Sciences
Kirksville, Missouri

Jeffrey J. Pasternak, MS, MD
Assistant Professor
Department of Anesthesiology
Mayo Clinic
Rochester, Minnesota

J. West Paul, MD, PhD
Senior Vice President
Chief Quality and Medical Staff Officer
WakeMed Health and Hospitals
Raleigh, North Carolina

Rex M. Philpot, PhD
Assistant Professor
Department of Psychiatry and Behavioral
    Neurosciences
University of South Florida Morsani College
    of Medicine
Tampa, Florida

Michael T. Piascik, PhD
Assistant Dean for Foundational Sciences
Professor
Department of Pharmacology and
    Nutritional Sciences
University of Kentucky College of Medicine
Lexington, Kentucky

Pamela Potter, PhD
Professor and Chair
Department of Pharmacology
Arizona College of Osteopathic Medicine
Midwestern University
Glendale, Arizona

Walter Prozialeck, PhD
Professor and Chairman
Department of Pharmacology
Midwestern University
Downers Grove, Illinois

Gary Rankin, PhD
Professor and Chair
Department of Pharmacology, Physiology,
    and Toxicology
Marshall University
Huntington, West Virginia

**D. Samba Reddy, PhD, RPh, FAAPS,
FAAAS, FAES**
Professor
Department of Neuroscience and
    Experimental Therapeutics
College of Medicine
Texas A&M University Health Science
    Center
Bryan, Texas

Jennelle Durnett Richardson, PhD
Assistant Dean of Medical Student
    Education, Foundation Sciences
Assistant Professor of Clinical
    Pharmacology and Toxicology
Department of Pharmacology and
    Toxicology
Indiana University School of Medicine
Indianapolis, Indiana

Michael A. Rogawski, MD, PhD
Director
Center for Neurotherapeutics Discovery and
    Development
Professor
Departments of Neurology and
    Pharmacology
UC Davis Health
University of California, Davis
Sacramento, California

Charles Rudick, PhD
Assistant Clinical Professor
Department of Pharmacology and
    Toxicology
Indiana University School of Medicine
Indianapolis, Indiana
Adjunct Lecturer
School of Professional Studies
Northwestern University
Chicago, Illinois

Deborah L. Sanchez, MD, MPH
Chief of Psychiatry
James A. Haley Veterans' Hospital
Assistant Professor
Department of Psychiatry and Behavioral
    Neurosciences
University of South Florida Morsani College
    of Medicine
Tampa, Florida

Juan R. Sanchez-Ramos, PhD, MD
Helen Ellis Endowed Professor
Department of Neurology
Director
Huntington's Disease Center of Excellence
University of South Florida Morsani College
    of Medicine
Tampa, Florida

Michael Saulino, MD, PhD
Clinical Director of Intrathecal Therapy
    Services
MossRehab Physical Medicine Associates
Elkins Park, Pennsylvania
Associate Professor
Department of Rehabilitation Medicine
Sidney Kimmel Medical College at Thomas
    Jefferson University
Philadelphia, Pennsylvania

Jill Marie Siegfried, PhD
Professor and Head
Department of Pharmacology
University of Minnesota Medical School
Frederick and Alice Stark Endowed Chair
Associate Director for Translation
Masonic Cancer Center
Minneapolis, Minnesota

Eman Soliman, PhD
Post-Doctoral Fellow
Department of Pharmacology and
    Toxicology
Brody School of Medicine at East Carolina
    University
Greenville, North Carolina

Jack W. Strandhoy, PhD
Professor Emeritus
Physiology and Pharmacology
Wake Forest School of Medicine
Winston-Salem, North Carolina

David A. Taylor, PhD
Professor and Chair
Department of Pharmacology and
    Toxicology
Brody School of Medicine at East Carolina
    University
Greenville, North Carolina

Robert J. Theobald, Jr., PhD
Professor
Department of Pharmacology
A.T. Still University of Health Sciences
Kirksville, Missouri

Shelley Tischkau, PhD
Associate Professor
Department of Pharmacology
Southern Illinois University School of
    Medicine
Springfield, Illinois

David A. Tulis, MS, PhD, FAHA
Associate Professor
Department of Physiology
Brody School of Medicine at East Carolina
    University
Greenville, North Carolina

Monica Valentovic, PhD
Professor
Department of Biomedical Sciences
Toxicology Research Cluster Coordnator
Marshall University School of Medicine
Huntington, West Virginia

Rukiyah Van Dross-Anderson, PhD
Associate Professor
Department of Pharmacology and
    Toxicology
Brody School of Medicine at East Carolina
    University
Greenville, North Carolina

Kent E. Vrana, PhD, FAAAS
Elliot S. Vesell Professor and Chair of
    Pharmacology
Pennsylvania State University College of
    Medicine
Hershey, Pennsylvania

Stephanie W. Watts, PhD
Professor
Department of Pharmacology and
    Toxicology
Assistant Dean
The Graduate School
Michigan State University
East Lansing, Michigan

Amy Wecker, MD
Infectious Disease Physician
Community AIDS Network
Community Health–South Beach
Miami, Florida

Lynn Wecker, PhD
Distinguished Research Professor
Department of Psychiatry and Behavioral
  Neurosciences
Department of Molecular Pharmacology
  and Physiology
University of South Florida Morsani College
  of Medicine
Tampa, Florida

David R. Wetzel, MD
Senior Associate Consultant
Department of Anesthesiology
Division of Intensive Care and Respiratory
  Therapy
Mayo Clinic
Rochester, Minnesota

Charles A. Whitmore, MD, MPH
Resident Physician
Department of Psychiatry
University of Colorado
Aurora, Colorado

Meredith Wicklund, MD
Assistant Professor
Department of Neurology
University of Florida College of Medicine
Gainsville, Florida

The sixth edition of *Brody's Human Pharmacology* has been appropriately subtitled *Mechanism-Based Therapeutics* and has been designed to provide students in all health professions with pharmacological information and its clinical relevance.

A major goal of this edition has been to present information in the clearest and most concise manner, using prototypical drugs to illustrate basic mechanisms and boxes and tables to emphasize key points and relevant clinical information, with many new figures within each section.

Sections were created with a focus on therapeutics, and two new sections were added to this edition, including one on drug therapy for pain management and another on the treatment of inflammatory, allergic, and immunological disorders. In addition, several new chapters have been added to this edition including:

- A chapter on pharmacogenetics in the Therapeutic Principles Section, critical in this era of personalized medicine
- A chapter on the cannabinoids in the Pain Management Section, particularly important in light of the opioid crisis
- A chapter focused on drugs for the treatment of attention deficit hyperactivity disorder in the Central Nervous System Section, because these medications are being prescribed to an increasing number of children
- A chapter on drug treatment for human immunodeficiency virus and related opportunistic infections in the Chemotherapy Section, because millions of individuals are dying each year from AIDS-related illnesses.

Chapters were formatted using a consistent style and include the following section titles:
Therapeutic Overview
Mechanisms of Action
Relationship of Mechanisms of Action to Clinical Response
Pharmacokinetics
Pharmacovigilance: Adverse Effects and Drug Interactions

In addition, a chapter section titled New Developments presents the latest advancements in the field and may include discussions of drugs being investigated or developed as new information is gained. Another new section titled Clinical Relevance for Healthcare Professionals provides relevant information applicable to all professionals in the healthcare field, as well as clinically important information for specific professionals such as physical therapists, dentists, and nurses.

Many of the figures have been revised to more clearly illustrate the textual information and assist students in learning. As the number of drugs in each drug class has increased, an emphasis has been placed on major drug classes relevant to each chapter, with generic and trade-named materials presented at the end of each chapter.

As with prior editions, the multicolored figures explaining key concepts will be available on Student Consult.

I sincerely hope that the content revisions and additions, consistent organization, and new figures are helpful to both students and teachers of pharmacology in all health professions.

Lynn Wecker

DEDICATION AND ACKNOWLEDGMENTS

This book is dedicated to students and faculty in all basic and clinical sciences to facilitate their understanding and appreciation of the role and importance of pharmacology in our everyday lives. We are all exposed to many natural and synthetic compounds through our diets and the environment and from over-the-counter and prescription medications. As a consequence, it is imperative to understand the actions and inter-actions of these agents on our bodies and how they affect our health and well-being.

As an academic who has spent much time ensuring that students understand and keep abreast of basic concepts and developments in pharmacology, I am reminded of Albert Einstein who once said, "Wisdom is not a product of schooling but of the lifelong attempt to acquire it." This book is dedicated to all those with a thirst for knowledge.

This book is also dedicated to the many wonderful colleagues I have encountered throughout my career, some of whom are no longer with us, including Ted Brody, who laid the groundwork for others to follow.

I am very appreciative of the time, effort, and diligence devoted by my co-editors and all the authors and others who have contributed to this sixth edition of the book. I am especially thankful to Ms. Melanie Engberg who spent many hours reading chapters and providing the templates for many of the new figures in this edition.

Lynn Wecker

CONTENTS

xiii

Mechanisms of Drug Action and Therapeutic Principles

Introduction

Lynn Wecker

All health professionals certainly appreciate the fundamental importance of drug treatment as one of the primary means used for the prevention and alleviation of disease. The number of prescriptions dispensed in the United States has increased steadily during the past 10 years, with more than 4 billion prescriptions in 2015. Further, it is expected that this number will increase by 15% in 2021, reflecting several factors including:

- increased research translating into the development of new medications;
- increased life span, with elderly individuals commonly requiring multidrug treatment;
- changes in clinical guidelines and policies by professional medical organizations;
- an increased number of individuals with a prescription drug benefit plan.

In addition to prescription drugs, there are more than 80 classes of over-the-counter (OTC) preparations and thousands of herbal and dietary supplements. Both prescription and OTC compounds are widely used and have become part of daily life.

It is also important to mention that the term drug is used to refer to all agents that interact with the body. In the past, this included primarily synthetic chemicals, while recent developments in molecular biology have led to the introduction of molecular and cellular therapies for both preventing and treating disease. Indeed, the first monoclonal antibody for the treatment of transplant rejection was approved by the U.S. Food and Drug Administration 30 years ago, and since that time antibody development and therapeutic use, particularly for the treatment of cancer and autoimmune and inflammatory diseases, has grown tremendously. Concurrently, there have also been major developments in oligonucleotide therapeutics, including antisense therapies, gene silencing approaches through ribonucleic acid (RNA) interference, and most recently, oligonucleotides targeting microRNAs. Because all of these developments led to molecules that interact with cellular components, they are certainly considered drugs.

Every health professional must have an understanding of pharmacology, particularly in the era of personalized medicine. In its broadest sense, pharmacology is the study of all compounds (natural and synthetic, endogenous and exogenous) that interact with the body and includes knowledge of the interactions between these compounds and body constituents at all levels of organization. Pharmacology includes study of the therapeutic uses and effects of these compounds, as well as the adverse effects of these agents. The term *pharmacology* is derived from the Greek *pharmacos* (medicine or drug) + *logos* (study) and should not be confused with pharmacy, which is a professional field that trains individuals qualified to prepare and dispense drugs. Rather, pharmacology is a branch of medicine that trains individuals to study the action of drugs and encompasses pharmacodynamics, pharmacokinetics, and pharmacogenetics.

Pharmacodynamics can be thought of as what a drug does to the body, including the molecular mechanism(s) by which a drug acts. Most drugs interact with proteins, such as receptors or enzymes, to effect changes in the physiological or biochemical function of particular organs, while newly developed molecular therapeutics may target nucleic acids. Irrespective of the target, the goal of drug treatment is to alter pathology or abnormal biochemistry and physiology to benefit the patient. Although health professionals typically observe the obvious functional effects of drug administration, for example, an antihypertensive effect, the mechanism of drug action is less well recognized. With most drugs, outward effects provide little insight into the molecular events that occur following drug administration. Chapter 2 describes the principles governing how drugs interact with their targets to produce functional responses—that is, the mechanism(s) of action of drugs.

Pharmacokinetics can be thought of as what the body does to the drug. For almost all drugs, the magnitude of the induced pharmacological effect depends on the concentration of drug at its site(s) of action. The absorption, distribution, metabolism, and elimination of drugs and factors that influence these processes are all critical in determining the concentration of drug at its site(s) of action. Chapter 3 presents the dynamics of these processes that are fundamental to understanding the effects of any compound in the body. Temporal relationships between plasma concentrations of drugs and their pharmacological effects, including the concepts of half-life, steady-state, clearance, and bioavailability, are also discussed, as is how these parameters differ among children, adults, and the aged population.

Pharmacogenetics is the area of pharmacology concerned with how genetic differences among individuals may affect both the therapeutic and adverse effects of drugs. During the past 20 years, numerous advances have led to the identification of genetic differences in both pharmacokinetic parameters and pharmacodynamic targets and have provided valuable information that can explain why:

- some drugs are effective for some, but not all, patients.
- some, but not all, patients exhibit adverse reactions to the same dose of a drug.

It is important to note that the term pharmacogenomics is often used interchangeably with pharmacogenetics. However, these terms are not synonymous, as pharmacogenomics refers to the entire genome and typically involves the application of genomic technology to drug characterization and development, while pharmacogenetics often refers to clinical practice decisions based on knowledge of one or a few genetic variations, as discussed in Chapter 4. Nevertheless, both pharmacogenetics and pharmacogenomics fall within the field of personalized medicine, which utilizes genetic information for the prognosis and treatment of disease tailored for each individual patient.

The development and regulation of drugs is a complex process that takes many years, is quite costly, and involves a diverse group of professionals. An overview of drug discovery and development, including drug repurposing, is presented in Chapter 5, along with prescription writing.

An important aspect of drug therapy that often confounds both prescriber and patient is drug nomenclature. Serious errors in patient management can occur if this issue is not understood. It is critical to understand that a drug has three names:

1. The chemical name, which is often long and extremely complex, is of interest to chemists but of little concern to other medical professionals.

2. The generic, or nonproprietary, name is the name recognized internationally and used throughout this book. A drug has only one generic name, which often indicates that it is a member of a class of drugs having the same mechanism of action.

3. The proprietary, brand, or trade name is the patented exclusive property of the drug manufacturer. Trade names are often designed to be shorter and easier to remember than generic names, but they are often not helpful in identifying the pharmacological action or class of drug. In some instances, there may be as many as a dozen or more trade names for a single drug, marketed by different companies. Trade names in this book are used for recognition purposes only.

Last, to be able to evaluate drug responses and compare compounds, one must understand several terms, including potency, efficacy, and therapeutic index. Potency refers to the amount of drug necessary to elicit a response. Thus a drug that elicits a specific response at a dose of 1 mg is "more potent" than a drug that requires 10 mg to produce the same effect. Potency, however, is not always the most critical factor in the selection of a drug, particularly if adverse effects produced by less potent drugs are more tolerable that those produced by more potent drugs.

Efficacy, or effectiveness, is often confused with potency but has a very different meaning. The efficacy of a drug refers to its ability to produce the maximal desired response. For example, although morphine and codeine act through the same mu opioid receptors, no dose of codeine can produce the same degree of pain relief as morphine because morphine is more efficacious than codeine. In choosing a drug, efficacy is much more important than potency in determining whether a drug will be useful clinically because if a drug does not produce a desired outcome, its potency is irrelevant. On the other hand, if drugs have similar efficacies, the most potent one is often the most desirable.

The therapeutic index (TI), or margin of safety, of a drug is the ratio of the dose of drug producing undesirable effects to the dose producing the desired therapeutic response. Thus drugs with a large TI have a large margin of safety, whereas drugs with a low TI often need to be monitored in plasma because small increases in plasma levels of these compounds may lead to toxic side effects.

WEBSITES

https://www.cdc.gov/nchs/fastats/drug-use-therapeutic.htm
This website from the Centers for Disease Control and Prevention contains an overview of statistical information on therapeutic drug use in the United States compiled from several sources.

https://www.nlm.nih.gov/services/Subject_Guides/healthstatistics/pharmaceuticalstatistics/
The U.S. National Library of Medicine also has an excellent website with references to pharmaceutical statistics.

2

Pharmacodynamics: Receptors and Concentration-Response Relationships

James Carlton Garrison, II

Pharmacodynamics is the subject that describes the mechanisms used by drugs or other small molecules to affect human biology. While certain therapeutic molecules interact with nucleic acids, including ribonucleic acid (RNA) and deoxyribonucleic acid (DNA), the most common mechanism used by small molecules to affect physiological function is to bind to important regulatory proteins expressed widely or selectively in human cells. The biological response caused by the interaction of the small molecule and its target protein can be described mathematically when the drug dose or concentration is plotted against its biological effect. The resulting dose- or concentration-response curve is an important pharmacodynamic relationship that dictates how to administer the proper dosage of drug to achieve a therapeutic effect without untoward responses. This chapter expands on these important concepts.

BIOLOGICAL SITES AND SPECIFICITY OF DRUG ACTION

Most drugs are small molecules with a mass of 500–800 Da that interact with specific proteins in target cells to alter cell functions such as cell signaling events, enzymatic activity, or transcriptional- and translational-related processes. The term **drug target** is a general term that refers to any binding site (or sites) that interacts with a drug. Although drug targets may be classified into multiple categories of molecules, in general three types predominate:

- Biological molecules that have evolved specifically for intercellular communication, including **cell surface membrane receptors**, and/or enzymes involved in postreceptor signaling cascades. This category includes cell surface proteins that initiate physiological signaling cascades in response to neurotransmitters, hormones, cytokines, growth factors, autacoids, or other circulating signals.
- Membrane ion channels, including **ligand-gated ion channels** responding to neurotransmitters, and **transporters** that have evolved to regulate the traffic of ions and other molecules across the cell membrane.
- Macromolecules, such as enzymes, lipids, and nucleic acids essential for normal biological function and/or replication of cells.

The first two types of drug targets include molecules involved in neurotransmitter or hormone-initiated cell signaling and/or the regulation of the internal milieu of cells. These targets include molecules that detect chemical signals and initiate a cellular response via activation of signal transduction pathways. The third type of target is **generalized** and includes biological molecules with any function, often widely expressed in human cells; these targets provide more of a challenge in achieving **drug specificity**.

Drug specificity is a very important pharmacodynamic issue, with the most useful drugs affecting an intended specific cellular function

ABBREVIATIONS	
Ach	Acetylcholine
β-ARK	β-Adrenergic receptor kinase
cAMP	Cyclic adenosine monophosphate
DNA	Deoxyribonucleic acid
cGMP	Cyclic guanosine monophosphate
GABA	γ-Aminobutyric acid
GABA$_A$	γ-Aminobutyric acid type A receptor
GPCR	G-protein–coupled receptor
LGIC	Ligand-gated ion channel
NAM	Negative allosteric modulator
NE	Norepinephrine
NHR	Nuclear hormone receptor
NPR	Natriuretic peptide receptor
PAM	Positive allosteric modulator
RNA	Ribonucleic acid
RTK	Receptor tyrosine kinase

without eliciting untoward effects. A drug may achieve organ or tissue selectivity as a consequence of selective tissue expression of the drug target. Targets represented in the first two groups above regulate specific functions of particular cells and are expressed selectively in various organs, an advantage in achieving a selective response to drugs. These types of molecules represent the primary targets of many drugs in clinical use because the targets themselves have evolved for selective physiological functions. As an example, a limited number of cells in the body express the **β-adrenergic receptor**; thus, β-adrenergic receptor antagonists such as propranolol have relatively selective effects. An example of the selective expression of an intracellular enzyme as a target is **potassium/hydrogen adenosine triphosphate** (K$^+$/H$^+$-ATPase), which is selectively expressed by the parietal cells that line the gastric pits of the stomach and drives the secretion of H$^+$ ions into the stomach lumen. The **proton pump inhibitors**, such as esomeprazole, inhibit this enzyme by covalent modification of the protein and cause a large decrement in H$^+$ ion secretion. While a small number of drugs, such as osmotic diuretics (Chapter 38), do not work by interacting with macromolecules, the concept of receptors and intracellular enzymes as specific sites of drug action is essential to understanding pharmacology.

The specificity of such interactions introduces the concept of **molecular recognition**. Drug targets must have molecular domains that are spatially and energetically favorable for binding drug molecules with high affinity. It is not surprising that most drug targets are proteins because proteins fold to form three-dimensional structures that could easily be envisioned to complement the structures of drug molecules.

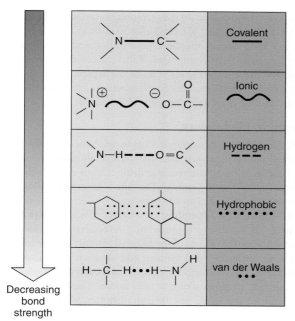

FIG. 2.1 The Nature of the Chemical Bonds and Attractive Forces Between Drugs and the Active Sites in Their Target Molecules.

Such molecules interact with their targets through chemical bonding; the principal types of chemical bonds between drugs and their macromolecular targets are depicted in Fig. 2.1. Covalent bonds require considerable energy to break and are often irreversible when formed in drug-receptor complexes. Ionic bonds are also strong but may be reversed by a change in the intracellular milieu or pH. Most drug-receptor interactions involve multiple weak bonds extended over the surface of a protein that lead to an affinity high enough to be clinically useful.

GENERAL PROPERTIES OF CELLULAR RECEPTORS

The concept of receptors was first proposed more than a century ago by the German chemist Paul Ehrlich, who was trying to develop specific drugs to treat parasitic infections. He proposed the idea of specific "side chains" on cells that would interact with a drug, based on mutually complementary structures. Each cell would have specific characteristics used to recognize particular molecules. He suggested that a drug binds to a receptor much like a key fits into a lock. While simplistic, this lock-and-key analogy still helps explain drug specificity because it emphasizes the idea that the drug and its target must be structurally complementary to recognize each other and allow the small molecule to bind to the macromolecule with high affinity.

Understanding the general properties of cellular receptors provides a foundation for an understanding of all drug-target interactions. The sequencing of the human genome has led to the identification of the amino acid sequences and the diversity of the many classes of cellular receptors, both those residing in the plasma membrane and in the cell cytoplasm. These advances have also revealed many new receptors that are potential targets for further pharmaceutical development. Parallel advances in understanding the many signaling systems activated by cell surface receptors have provided a more complete understanding of how a molecule acting at the surface of a cell can regulate cellular function. As many clinically useful drugs activate or inhibit these receptors and signaling systems, the large families of cellular receptors provide a foundation for understanding how drugs can act with biological precision.

BOX 2.1   General Features of Receptors

Many receptor molecules are membrane proteins, lipoproteins, and glycoproteins with one or more subunits

Molecular weights range from ~45 to 200 kDa

Receptors can have multiple subtypes with similar or different tissue distributions

Drug binding is usually reversible and stereoselective

Receptors are saturable because of their finite number

Specificity of drug binding is not absolute, leading to nonspecific effects

Agonist activation results in the generation of intracellular signals and cellular responses

May have allosteric mechanisms to amplify activation of the receptor

Magnitude of signal depends on degree of agonist binding

Receptor signal can be amplified by intracellular mechanisms

Drugs can enhance, diminish, or block signal generation or transmission

Receptor density may be up regulated or down regulated

Some general features of cellular receptors are listed in Box 2.1, and some important general concepts about drug targets can be gleaned from our current understanding of these molecules.

One concept is that there can be a quantitative relationship between the drug concentration in the fluid bathing the receptor and the subsequent physiological response. This response is determined both by the affinity of the drug for the receptor and the efficacy of the activation of the receptor's downstream signaling system. The affinity of a drug for its receptor is a measure of the binding constant of the drug for the receptor protein, and the efficacy of the response is a measure of the ability of the drug to activate the receptor and its signaling system. A high affinity means that low concentrations of drug are needed to occupy receptor sites, whereas a low affinity means that much higher concentrations of drug are needed. The concentration-response curve is also influenced by the number of receptors available for binding; in general, activating more receptors can produce a greater response (see Quantitative Relationships).

The size, shape, and charge of a drug binding site on a receptor determines its affinity for any of the vast array of chemically different hormones, neurotransmitters, or drug molecules it may encounter. If the structure of the drug changes even slightly, the drug's affinity for the specific receptor will also often change. Drug binding to receptors often exhibits stereoselectivity, in which stereoisomers of a drug that are chemically identical, but have different orientations around a single bond, can have very different affinities. For example, the L-isomers of opioid analgesics are approximately 1000 times more potent than the D-isomers, which are essentially inactive in relieving pain (Chapter 28).

A second key concept is that receptors and their distribution in the tissues of the body are a major determinant of the specificity of drug action. A corollary to this concept is that for a receptor to be physiologically relevant, it must receive a signal and be coupled to a downstream signaling system that regulates a key function of the tissue. As an example, histamine H_2 receptors can be found on many cells in the periphery, but only in the parietal cells in the stomach do they receive histamine as a signal to stimulate gastric acid secretion. Thus, histamine H_2 antagonists work very selectively to reduce acid secretion with few side effects (Chapter 71).

A third concept is that cellular receptors explain the importance of drugs that are pharmacological antagonists; i.e., drugs that interrupt the ability of the natural agonists to bind to and activate a receptor and its downstream signaling system. Administration of an antagonist will block tonic or stimulated activity of endogenous neurotransmitters and hormones, thus changing the normal physiological functions of a tissue. An example is metoprolol, which, by antagonizing β_1-adrenergic receptors, prevents the normal increase in heart rate caused by norepinephrine (NE) released via activation of the sympathetic nervous system (Chapters 6 and 12).

Finally, while a large number of receptors for therapeutically useful drugs are associated with the cell plasma membrane, not all receptors exist at this locale. The nuclear hormone receptors (NHR) are a large family of proteins in the cell cytoplasm that respond to the lipid-soluble steroid hormones such as androgens, estrogens, and glucocorticoids. These hormones easily cross the cell membrane to bind to their specific nuclear hormone receptors. When activated, these intracellular hormone-receptor complexes translocate to the nucleus where they interact with DNA to stimulate transcription, eventually leading to the increased synthesis of proteins (see Fig. 52.2). Although these receptors reside in a different locale within the cell, the general concepts about drug targets remain useful for understanding their pharmacology.

AGONISTS AND ANTAGONISTS

The physiological functions of most differentiated tissues are constantly regulated by neurotransmitters, hormones, or other signals through multiple types of cellular receptors. This fact leads to the very important concept that drugs acting on cellular receptors can have positive or negative actions. Thus, these drugs may be classified as agonists or antagonists.

Agonists

Our current understanding of receptor biology suggests that the structure of cell surface receptors allows them the flexibility to transition from a basal, inactive conformation to an active conformation. In some cases, this conformational change occurs in a single polypeptide chain, and in other cases, dimerization of receptor molecules is required. In either case, agonists bind to the receptor and have the proper structural features to generate the active conformation, leading to a greater number of receptors in the active conformation and the stimulation of one or more downstream signaling pathways. Any molecule that has the proper structural features to stabilize the active conformation of the receptor can be an agonist; the natural signal is one such molecule, as are many clinically useful drugs synthesized for this purpose. A simple example of the action of an agonist is the effect of the neurotransmitter acetylcholine (ACh) on the nicotinic cholinergic receptor in skeletal muscle. This receptor is a ligand-gated ion channel, and when ACh binds to its target sites on the external surface of the molecule, the ion channel opens and allows Na^+ to flow down its electrochemical gradient, depolarizing the muscle cell and leading to muscle contraction.

Antagonists

This term describes drugs that bind to the receptor but do not have the unique structural features necessary to generate the active conformation. Rather, antagonists stabilize the inactive conformation of the receptor and inhibit downstream signaling. Like agonists, antagonists bind to a specific site within the receptor. Most antagonists use the same binding domains within the receptor that are used by agonists and thus competitively inhibit the activation caused by agonists. However, some antagonists bind to different amino acids from those used by the agonist, often leading to the useful property of antagonists having a higher affinity for the receptor than the natural agonist (see Quantitative Relationships). In keeping with the skeletal muscle nicotinic cholinergic receptor example, the neuromuscular blocking drugs used routinely in the operating room to relax skeletal muscles during surgery are excellent examples of antagonists. Drugs such as rocuronium or

vecuronium bind to sites on the extracellular surface of the ion channel and block the ability of ACh or similar agonists to activate the channel. This blockade inhibits muscle depolarization and causes paralysis of skeletal muscle. The development of this class of drugs arose from the realization that curare, the active molecule in plant extracts historically used as arrow poisons by native South Americans, was a potent antagonist at the nicotinic cholinergic receptor (Chapter 10).

Allosteric Modulators

A third mechanism that drugs can use to affect the activity of receptors is termed allosteric modulation. Allosteric modulators are compounds that bind to a site on the receptor distinct from that which normally binds an agonist or antagonist. This site is termed an allosteric site. Occupation of this site can either increase or decrease the response to the natural agonist, depending on whether it is a positive (PAM) or negative (NAM) allosteric modulator, respectively. Because allosteric modulators bind to regions of the molecule distinct from where agonists bind, interactions between agonists and allosteric modulators are not competitive. The benzodiazepines are an excellent example of a class of drugs that act by an allosteric mechanism. These sedatives enhance the ability of the inhibitory neurotransmitter, γ-aminobutyric acid (GABA) to activate its receptor (the GABAA ligand-gated Cl⁻ ion channel) in the brain by binding to an allosteric site on the receptor (Chapter 17). The actions of agonists, antagonists, and allosteric modulators on an idealized cell surface receptor are shown in Fig. 2.2.

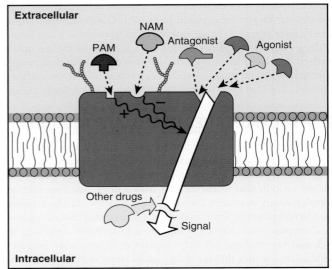

FIG. 2.2 Major Features of Cell Membrane Receptors Depicting Binding Sites for Agonists, an Antagonist, and Allosteric Modulators. Receptors are transmembrane proteins and have polypeptide chains that extend into the extracellular and intracellular regions near the membrane with carbohydrate (glycosylation) side chains often attached to these proteins on the extracellular side. Shown are sites on the extracellular side of the receptor for the binding of two molecules of an endogenous agonist transmitter *(dark blue icons)*, which activates the receptor to produce the signal *(white arrow)*. Agonist and antagonist drugs *(green icons)* can compete with the endogenous transmitter for binding sites. Positive (PAM) and negative (NAM) allosteric modulators *(purple icons)* enhance or block the signals, respectively, by binding to allosteric sites that stimulate (+) or inhibit (−) signal transmission *(wavy lines)*. Other drugs *(light blue icon)* can block signal transmission within the membrane or at intracellular sites. The white arrow indicates the direction of communication across the membrane.

RECEPTOR FAMILIES, SUBTYPES, AND SIGNALING CASCADES

Although it was first thought that a single receptor for each type of hormone, neurotransmitter, growth factor, or autacoid existed, it is now clear that in most cases, receptors belong to families of molecules with multiple subtypes. While the evolutionary pressure leading to the continued existence of so many receptors is not understood, it is clear that there can be complexity, redundancy, and multiplicity in the effects of a single agonist. Therefore understanding the tissue distribution and biology of different receptor isoforms is an important goal that may allow development of specific drugs for each novel target. This strategy may provide opportunities for obtaining specific therapeutic responses without unwanted side effects.

Receptor Nomenclature

Receptors are commonly named after the natural agonist that activates them. For example, ACh acts through cholinergic receptors, epinephrine (adrenaline) and NE (noradrenaline) act through adrenergic receptors, and serotonin acts through serotonergic receptors. Receptor activation is very specific, and natural agonists exhibit little cross-reactivity between their own and other receptors. For instance, ACh binds specifically to cholinergic receptors and not to adrenergic receptors or members of other receptor families. This type of selectivity is true for essentially all transmitters and hormones. However, a molecule like dopamine (the immediate precursor of NE in adrenergic neurons), which has its own family of dopaminergic receptors, can bind with low affinity to adrenergic receptors as a consequence of its structural similarity with NE. This property can be advantageous, as dopamine is used clinically to stimulate β_1-adrenergic receptors in cardiac failure (Chapter 44).

Receptor Selectivity

As mentioned, each receptor family typically contains multiple subtypes that may be characterized pharmacologically by the use of selective agonists and/or antagonists. For example, there are two major subfamilies of cholinergic receptors, nicotinic and muscarinic, that were originally named for the natural alkaloids extracted from plants that could activate them (nicotine and muscarine, respectively). Nicotinic cholinergic receptors are ligand-gated ion channels (LGICs) that are selectively activated by the agonist nicotine and selectively blocked by the neuromuscular blocking agents, such as curare (Chapters 9 and 10). In contrast, muscarinic cholinergic receptors are G-protein–coupled receptors (GPCRs) selectively activated by the agonist muscarine and selectively blocked by the antagonist atropine (Chapters 7 and 8). Nicotine and curare have essentially no effect on muscarinic cholinergic receptors, and muscarine and atropine have essentially no effect on nicotinic cholinergic receptors. In addition to family specificity, an additional level of specificity exists at the subtype level. Both the nicotinic and muscarinic cholinergic receptor subfamilies can consist of multiple subtypes, a situation common for most receptor families. Examples of receptor families, subfamilies, and subtypes for common signaling systems are shown in Table 2.1.

TABLE 2.1 Examples of Major Receptor Families, Subfamilies, and Subtypes and Their Associated Ligands

Receptor Type	Family	Subfamily/Subtype	Endogenous Ligand
LGICs			
	Cholinergic nicotinic	Neuromuscular, ganglionic, neuronal, immune	ACh
	GABAergic	GABAA, GABAC	GABA
	Ionotropic glutamate	NMDA, kainite, AMPA	Glutamate
	Serotonergic	5-HT$_3$	5-HT
GPCRs			
	Cholinergic muscarinic	M$_1$–M$_5$	ACh
	Dopaminergic	D$_1$–D$_5$	DA
	Adrenergic	α_1, α_2, β_1–β_3	NE and Epi
	GABAergic	GABAB	GABA
	Metabotropic glutamatergic	mglu$_{1-8}$	Glutamate
	Serotonergic	5-HT$_1$ family, 5-HT$_2$ family, 5-HT$_4$, 5-HT$_5$ family, 5-HT$_6$, 5-HT$_7$	5-HT
NHRs			
	Estrogen (3-hydroxy steroid)	α, β	Estrone, 17β-estradiol
	3-ketosteroid	Androgen	Testosterone, dihydrotestosterone
		Glucocorticoid	Cortisol, corticosterone
		Mineralocorticoid	Aldosterone
		Progesterone	Progesterone
Catalytic receptors			
	RTKs	Type I: EGF (EGFR, HER2-4)	EGF
		Type II: Insulin (InsR, IGF1R, IRR)	Insulin, IGFs
	NPRs	GC-A, GC-B	ANP, BNP, C-type
		GC-C	Guanylin, uroguanylin

Abbreviations: *AMPA*, α-Amino-3-hydroxy-5-methyl-4-isoxazoleproprionic acid; *ANP*, atrial natriuretic peptide; *BNP*, brain natriuretic peptide; *C-type*, C-type natriuretic peptide; *EGF*, epidermal growth factor; *IGF*, insulin-like growth factor; *GABA*, γ-aminobutyric acid; *GPCRs*, G-protein–coupled receptors; *LGICs*, ligand-gated ion channels; *NMDA*, N-methyl-D-aspartate; *NHRs*, nuclear hormone receptors; *NPRs*, natriuretic peptide receptors.

Further, multiple receptor subtypes for a single transmitter can coexist on a single cell, raising the possibility that one transmitter can deliver multiple opposing, complementary, or independent messages to the same cell. For example, the sympathetic nervous system uses NE to regulate both cardiac and vascular tissues. Thus, a cardiac or smooth muscle cell may express both α- and β-adrenergic receptors, each of which can respond to NE (Chapter 11). In this situation, NE may stimulate the β_1-adrenergic receptor to activate adenylyl cyclase through the G_s protein and stimulate the α_2-adrenergic receptor to inhibit adenylyl cyclase through the G_i protein. These opposing signals are integrated to produce a lower level of the messenger cyclic adenosine monophosphate (cAMP) within the cell than would be produced if there were no α_2-adrenergic receptor expressed by the cells (Fig. 2.3, top panel). In a like manner, additive signals can be generated by the presence of both the β_1 and the β_2 receptor (which also activates adenylyl cyclase through

G_s) in the same cell (see Fig. 2.3, middle panel). Alternatively, independent signals can be generated by the presence of the α_1 receptor, which couples to a different G protein, Gq, to activate phospholipase C and produce IP3 and DAG (see Fig. 2.3, bottom panel, and Chapter 6). Thus, the response of the cells in a given tissue to a single neurotransmitter (or a drug that mimics a neurotransmitter) depends on relative proportions of the specific subtypes of the receptor families expressed in the tissue.

Major Receptor Families

A very large number of therapeutically useful drugs target a small number of families of cell surface receptors and their intracellular signaling cascades. The major types of receptors and signaling cascades include **ligand-gated ion channels (LGICs)** that affect excitable tissue, GPCRs that regulate many types of signaling systems, **nuclear hormone receptors (NHRs)** that affect transcription, and **catalytic receptors**, including **receptor tyrosine kinases (RTKs)**, that mediate the effects of growth factors, **cytokine receptors** that affect the immune system and development, and **natriuretic peptide receptors (NPRs)** that increase intracellular **cyclic GMP (cGMP)**. Table 2.1 presents an overview of some of the receptors in these classes that are important for the actions of many therapeutically useful drugs.

Ligand-Gated Ion Channels

LGICs are expressed widely in the central and peripheral nervous systems, excitable tissues such as the heart, and the neuromuscular junction. LGICs are central to the regulation of these tissues by various branches of the nervous system. These molecules include nicotinic cholinergic receptors (Fig. 2.4) in autonomic ganglia and at the neuromuscular

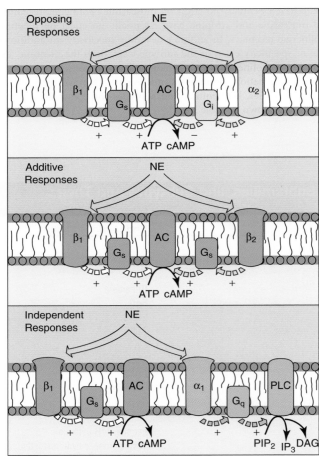

FIG. 2.3 Consequences of Activation of Multiple Receptors in a Cell by a Single Transmitter. Norepinephrine (NE) can activate multiple receptor subtypes including β_1-, β_2-, α_1-, and α_2-adrenergic receptors. β_1 and β_2 receptors both couple to the G_s protein and stimulate adenylyl cyclase (AC), catalyzing the conversion of adenosine triphosphate (ATP) to cAMP. α_2 Receptors couple to the G_i protein and inhibit AC, and α_1 receptors couple to the G_q protein and activate phospholipase C (PLC), producing inositol 1,4,5-triphosphate (IP_3) and 1,2-diacylglycerol (DAG) from phosphatidylinositol 4,5-bisphosphate (PIP_2). Activation of more than one receptor subtype for NE can result in opposing second messenger responses (*top panel,* less cAMP); additive second messenger responses (*middle panel,* more cAMP); or independent second messenger responses (*bottom panel,* other signals).

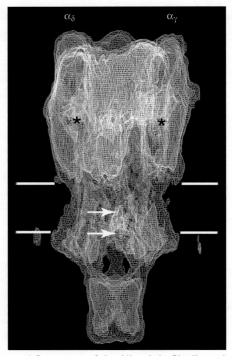

FIG. 2.4 Crystal Structure of the Nicotinic Cholinergic Receptor. Binding sites for acetylcholine are shown as black asterisks, with the gating portions of the channel indicated by white arrowheads. (From Unwin N. The Croonian Lecture 2000. Nicotinic acetylcholine receptor and the structural basis of fast synaptic transmission. *Philos Trans R Soc Lond B Biol Sci* 2000; 355:1813–1829.)

junction, many of the GABA and glutamate receptors in the brain, one type of serotonin receptor, and a number of other specialized channels that respond to signaling molecules. This type of receptor is usually responsible for fast synaptic transmission wherein release of a transmitter causes an electrical effect on the postsynaptic neuron by opening a specific ion channel, leading to a change in membrane potential. Typically, LGICs have two binding sites for agonists and may have additional binding sites for allosteric modulators, which increase or decrease the ability of the neurotransmitter to open the channel.

LGICs are macromolecular complexes with the complete molecule composed of four or five distinct subunits. The specific combinations of subunits expressed in various tissues are often different, which can lead to selectivity in the effects of drugs on the channels. This concept is exemplified when one considers nicotinic receptors at the neuromuscular junction versus those at autonomic ganglia. Although the responses to ACh and ion gating properties of these two channels are similar, their subunit composition differs, and as a consequence, these receptors are activated and antagonized by different drugs. Importantly, this property allows selective blockade of the neuromuscular junction by drugs that do not block the channel expressed in autonomic ganglia. Thus, skeletal muscle relaxation can be achieved without depressing overall autonomic function via the ganglia (Chapter 10).

G-Protein–Coupled Receptors

The GPCRs represent a true superfamily of proteins. Humans express over 800 of these receptors, representing about 2% of the genes in the human genome. Approximately half of this extravagant complement of GPCRs are odorant receptors, while the others respond to the signals

from neurotransmitters, multiple hormone families, autacoids such as histamine, cytokines, and other circulating signals. These receptors are composed of a single polypeptide chain that contains seven transmembrane spanning domains with varying numbers of amino acids at the N-terminal and C-terminal regions of the molecule (Fig. 2.5). Where available, the x-ray crystal structures of these receptors indicate the presence of a single ligand-binding site. Allosteric modulators are known to exist for a few GPCRs, but there are not yet drugs that exploit this property of the receptors. GPCRs activate signals by inducing a conformational change in the G-protein α subunit that initiates guanine nucleotide exchange, leading to activation of the G-protein heterotrimer, which, in turn, can activate many different signaling pathways. These signaling pathways often use protein kinases to propagate their effects and regulate a host of differentiated cellular functions (Box 2.2). Because receptors from this family have evolved for selective regulation of the function of many differentiated tissues, they are critically important targets for therapeutic entities. A very large number of diseases can be treated with drugs that target this receptor superfamily.

Nuclear Hormone Receptors

NHRs comprise a superfamily of 48 receptors, which reside in the cytoplasm of responsive cells. Unlike cell surface receptors, these molecules bind their ligand in the cytoplasm and translocate to the nucleus. These intracellular receptors respond to highly hydrophobic steroid ligands such as estrogens, androgens, and glucocorticoids, which regulate the differentiated functions of many endocrine cells. In addition to containing receptors that respond to steroidal hormones,

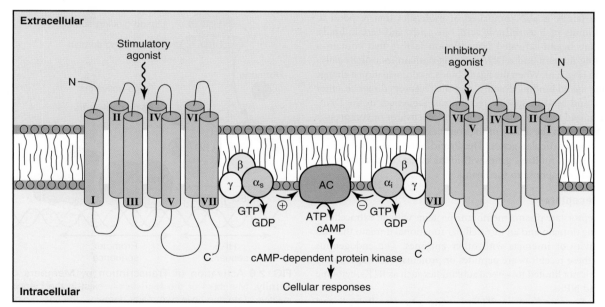

FIG. 2.5 GPCRs and the G-Protein Heterotrimer Involved in the Regulation of Adenylyl Cyclase (AC). Binding of an agonist ligand to a stimulatory receptor *(left)* produces a conformational change transmitted to the α subunit of G_s, initiating the exchange of bound guanosine 5'-diphosphate (GDP) with guanosine 5'-triphosphate (GTP) on the G-protein α_s subunit, causing it to dissociate from the $\beta\gamma$ subunits. Active $G\alpha_s$ binds to and activates AC to increase production of cAMP. The $\beta\gamma$ subunits are released from active $G\alpha_s$ and freed for other signaling functions. Activation of an inhibitory receptor *(right)* by an agonist causes activation of the inhibitory $G\alpha_i$ subunit via an analogous GDP-GTP exchange reaction. The $G\alpha_i$ subunit then binds to and inhibits AC. The cAMP produced activates cAMP-dependent protein kinase (PKA) to regulate cellular responses in differentiated tissues.

BOX 2.2   Details of G-Protein–Coupled Receptor (GPCR) Signaling

The binding of agonist to the receptor induces a conformational change that activates a family of heterotrimeric G proteins, which then regulate intracellular effector molecules such as enzymes and ion channels. All G proteins are located at the inner surface of the plasma membrane and consist of α, β, and γ subunits. The α subunit of the heterotrimer is an important component of the downstream signaling mechanisms because:

- It interacts specifically with receptors.
- Upon activation, it exchanges bound guanosine 5'-diphosphate (GDP) for guanosine 5'-triphosphate (GTP), undergoes a conformational change releasing the $\beta\gamma$ subunits, and can bind to and interact with effectors (enzymes or channels).
- It has an intrinsic ability to hydrolyze bound GTP, a process activated by a family of regulatory proteins (RGS proteins) that stimulate the formation of GDP, aiding in terminating the signal.
- α-GDP binds to and sequesters $\beta\gamma$ subunits, which exist as dimers and can also activate certain effectors such as channels.
- Activated α-GTP interacts directly with effectors such as adenylyl cyclase to stimulate activity and raise the concentration of cAMP.

Genes for 17 different Gα subunits have been identified, and the molecules have been grouped into four families. Although there is great structural homology between α subunits, each protein has unique regions that impart specificity to its interactions with receptors and effectors. The C-terminal region displays the most variability and interacts with receptors. Generally, members within a family have similar functional properties. The four families are:

- G_s, which activates adenylyl cyclase.
- G_i, which inhibits adenylyl cyclase; this family also includes G_o, which regulates ion channels, and G_t, which couples rhodopsin to a phosphodiesterase in the visual system.
- G_q, which activates phospholipase C-β.
- $G_{12/13}$, which binds to guanine exchange factors and activates small G proteins, such as *Rho*.

The β and γ subunits of G proteins form a tightly associated functional unit and are also characterized by multiple genes. Genes are known for seven β and 12 γ subunits. When $\beta\gamma$ is released from the α subunit following GTP binding, the freed $\beta\gamma$ subunits regulate effectors like ion channels and enzymes such as adenylyl cyclase or phospholipase C-β. $\beta\gamma$ is an important activator of K$^+$ channels in cardiac and neural cells and is an important inhibitor of L- and N-type Ca^{2+} channels in neurons.

Activation of G proteins raises the level of second messengers in target cells. Common second messengers are small molecules such as cAMP, inositol triphosphate (IP$_3$), or diacylglycerol (DAG) and ions such as Ca^{2+} or K$^+$. These messengers often activate protein kinases, which produce responses by phosphorylating other regulatory proteins. cAMP activates the cAMP-dependent protein kinase (PKA); IP$_3$ (by releasing Ca^{2+}) activates many Ca^{2+}/calmodulin-dependent protein kinases, and DAG and Ca^{2+} activate protein kinase C. The phosphorylation events mediated by these kinases lead to the activation or inhibition of downstream pathways and produces the characteristic responses of differentiated cells to receptor activation.

---

this receptor family is also comprised of molecules that respond to other compounds such as **retinoic acid**, bile acids, and certain lipids. The NHRs are ligand-activated transcription factors that contain a ligand-binding domain and a DNA-binding domain in a single polypeptide chain (Fig. 2.6). When the ligand binds, a conformational change occurs in the ligand binding domain, and the receptors dimerize, enter the nucleus, and bind to specific recognition sequences in the DNA. The ligand-bound receptor may also bind to coactivator or corepressor molecules that affect the ability of the complex to increase or decrease transcription of particular genes. The ligand-bound receptor affects the transcription of multiple genes within the target cell to achieve the complete cellular response to the ligand.

Catalytic Receptors

Catalytic receptors are plasma membrane proteins with an extracellular ligand binding domain and an intracellular functional domain that has catalytic activity or interacts with other enzymes. The endogenous agonists for these receptors are peptides or proteins. This superfamily includes, but is not limited to, several subfamilies such as RTKs, cytokine receptors, and NPRs.

Receptor Tyrosine Kinases. RTKs contain an extracellular ligand binding domain (LBD), one transmembrane-spanning segment, and an intracellular tyrosine kinase domain. Binding of a ligand to the extracellular domain causes dimerization of the receptor and stimulates the **tyrosine kinase** activity within the intracellular kinase domain (Fig. 2.7). RTKs include the insulin receptor and growth factor receptors such as epidermal growth factor and nerve growth factor receptors. When growth factors bind to these receptors, they lead to tyrosine phosphorylation of the receptor, other proteins, or both, activating

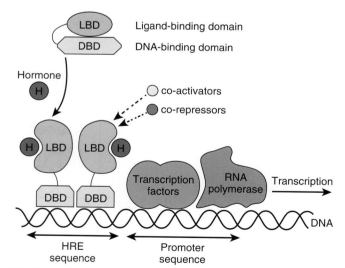

FIG. 2.6 Activation of Transcription by Members of the NHR Family. Members of the NHR family exist in the cytoplasm in their inactive state and have two major domains, the ligand-binding domain (LBD) and the DNA-binding domain (DBD). Binding of the hormone (H) to the LBD causes a conformational change in the receptor and dimerization of the receptors. The hormone-receptor complex translocates to the nucleus and binds to specific sequences of DNA in the promoter region of genes programmed to respond to the hormone (the hormone response element, HRE). The hormone-receptor complex also requires a member of a large family of accessory proteins (coactivators or corepressors, *blue and purple symbols*) for full activity. Once the complete complex is bound to the HRE, transcription is initiated and new proteins are synthesized.

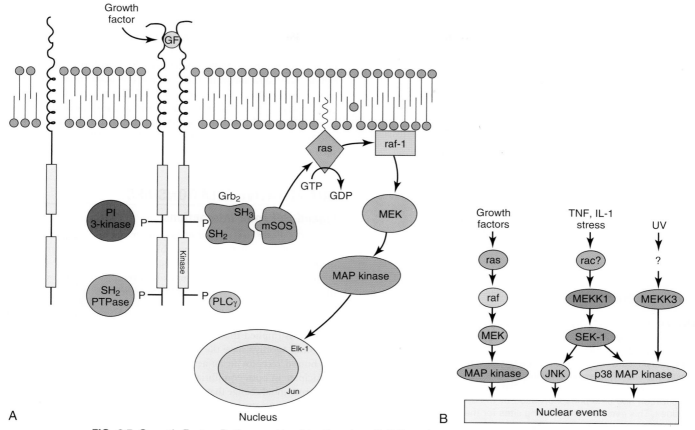

FIG. 2.7 Growth Factor Pathways Used to Regulate Cell Function. (A) Mechanism used by GFs to activate the mitogen-activated protein kinase (MAP kinase) signaling cascade. Binding of GF induces dimerization of the receptor, thereby activating its tyrosine kinase, leading to phosphorylation of the receptor (P) on tyrosine residues in specific intracellular domains of the receptor. This creates binding sites for the SH_2 domains (*src* homology domains) of multiple signaling proteins (PI 3-kinase, Grb_2, $PLC\gamma$, and an SH_2-containing tyrosine phosphatase [SH_2 PTPase] are shown). The specific interaction between Grb_2 and the mSOS protein activates ras (a low-molecular-weight GTP binding protein), which then activates the kinase raf-1, leading to activation of the other protein kinases in the MAP kinase cascade. (B) Similarity of the protein kinase cascades used by GF, tumor necrosis factor (TNF), interleukin-1 (IL-1), stressors, and ultraviolet radiation to activate MAP kinase and two related kinases, the Jun N-terminal kinase (JNK) and p38 MAP kinase. Other molecules shown in the cascades are Raf, a protein kinase that is activated by binding to ras; MEK, a kinase that can phosphorylate and activate MAP kinase; MEKK1 and MEKK3, two MEK kinases analogous in function to raf-1 but with differing substrate specificities; and SEK-1, a kinase analogous to MEK that phosphorylates and activates JNK. The MAP kinase cascade ultimately stimulates cell growth by activating nuclear events.

MAP kinase cascades and nuclear events. In spite of their complexity, RTKs are an increasingly important target for drugs treating **neoplastic diseases** in which cell growth is uncontrolled. There are small molecules that directly inhibit the tyrosine kinase activity of these receptors (e.g., gefitinib and erlotinib), but humanized monoclonal antibodies against the extracellular domains of the receptors achieve better therapeutic results in the treatment of cancer (Chapters 68 and 69).

Cytokine Receptors. **Cytokine receptors** have many features in common with the RTKs. However, instead of having an intrinsic tyrosine kinase domain within the receptor molecule, cytokine receptors have docking sites where cytoplasmic tyrosine kinases bind (Fig. 2.8). These receptors are activated by a variety of molecules such as **erythropoietin**, **interleukins**, and **growth hormone**. Cytokines are involved in inflammation, and humanized monoclonal antibodies against the receptors

or the cytokines themselves (e.g., adalimumab, which targets tumor necrosis factor-α) are effective for treatment of diseases such as arthritis and Crohn's disease (Chapters 35 and 71).

Natriuretic Peptide Receptors. NPRs bind a family of **natriuretic peptide hormones**, including **atrial natriuretic peptide (ANP)**, **brain natriuretic peptide (BNP)**, and **C-type natriuretic peptide (CNP)**, and are important for regulating production of the intracellular second messenger cGMP. These receptors consist of a single polypeptide chain containing three major domains, viz., an extracellular hormone-binding domain, a transmembrane domain, and an intracellular guanylyl cyclase domain (Fig. 2.9). Peptide hormone binding to the receptor leads to dimerization, activating the intracellular guanylyl cyclase domain to produce cGMP, which activates cGMP-dependent protein kinases and cGMP-dependent phosphodiesterases to produce its cellular effects.

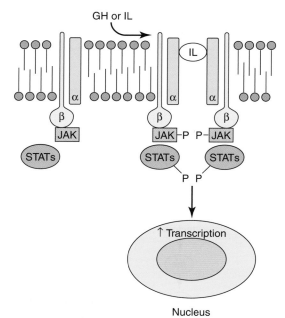

GH or IL

IL

FIG. 2.8 The JAK-STAT Pathway Used to Regulate Nuclear Events. The two subunits of a cytokine receptor, α and β are shown, with the cytoplasmic Janus tyrosine kinases (JAK) bound to the β form. The signal transducers and activators of transcription proteins (STAT proteins), which exist as cytoplasmic proteins, are shown as ovals. Activation of the receptor by growth hormone (GH) or interleukins (IL) leads to dimerization and auto-phosphorylation of the JAK kinases on tyrosine residues. This event creates binding sites for the STAT proteins, which also become phosphorylated on tyrosine residues. The phosphorylated STAT proteins translocate to the nucleus and activate transcription of certain genes.

It is important to note that activation of NPRs is not the only pathway for the synthesis of cGMP. Another guanylyl cyclase exists as a soluble protein found in most cells (see Fig. 2.9). This enzyme is activated by nitric oxide (NO), a labile gas produced from L-arginine by the enzyme nitric oxide synthase (NOS). NOS has multiple isoforms, one of which can be induced by inflammation, and all NOS isoforms are stimulated by Ca^{2+} ions via interaction with the Ca^{2+}/calmodulin complex. cGMP plays a very important role in the function of ocular, kidney, cardiac, lung, and vascular tissue; drugs that inhibit cGMP-dependent phosphodiesterases and increase the level of cGMP in vascular tissue, such as sildenafil, lead to vasodilation and are important for treating erectile dysfunction (Chapter 41).

QUANTITATIVE RELATIONSHIPS

Ligand-Receptor Interactions

Given the above description of how receptors and signaling systems regulate cellular function, it is possible to understand some important quantitative relationships underlying the actions of drugs.

In most cases, a drug (D) binds to a receptor (R) in a reversible bimolecular reaction, which can be described as:

$$D + R \rightleftarrows DR \rightleftarrows DR^* \rightarrow \rightarrow \rightarrow Response \qquad (2.1)$$

where it is implied that the drug is an agonist because it produces a response. Agonists have the appropriate structural features to stabilize the bound receptor in an active conformation (DR^*) and, therefore, participate in both equilibria, binding to the receptor and initiating a conformational change that produces a cellular response. It is important to note that occupancy of a receptor by a drug may or may not alter receptor conformation and produce a response. For example, antagonists participate only in the first equilibrium, as they bind to and occupy the receptor without producing a response (however, if a biological

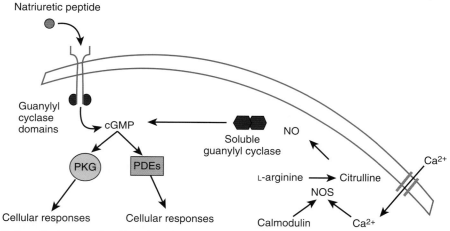

FIG. 2.9 Two Pathways Can Regulate the Level of cGMP in Cells. Natriuretic peptide hormones such as atrial natriuretic peptide (ANP), brain natriuretic peptide (BNP), and C-type natriuretic peptide (CNP) stimulate cell surface receptors that contain intracellular guanylyl cyclase domains. Binding of the ligand stimulates production of cGMP. Cells also contain a soluble guanylyl cyclase that can be activated by the labile gas nitric oxide (NO) formed locally by the enzyme nitric oxide synthase (NOS). NOS is activated by the Ca^{2+}/calmodulin complex to produce NO from L-arginine. Thus, a Ca^{2+} signal can also raise cGMP if the complement of enzymes needed to produce NO is present. Because NO rapidly diffuses through cell membranes, the NO signal may be generated by adjacent cells and diffuse to the site of action. The downstream effects of cGMP in differentiated tissues are mediated by the cGMP-dependent protein kinase (PKG) or a family of cGMP-dependent phosphodiesterases (PDEs).

system is under tonic stimulation by an agonist, the antagonist will produce a negative response). Nevertheless, it is important to remember that the equation for production of the DR complex is relevant for both agonists and antagonists, with some differences between synthetic drugs and the natural hormones or neurotransmitters.

As described in Eq. 2.1, the binding of a drug to a receptor is a reversible bimolecular interaction. This equation follows the **law of mass action**, which states that at equilibrium, the product of the active masses on one side of the equation divided by the product of active masses on the other side of the equation is a constant. Therefore, concentrations of both drug and receptor are important in determining the extent of receptor occupation and subsequent tissue response.

Quantification of the amount of drug necessary to produce a given response is referred to as a **concentration-response** relationship. Practically, one rarely knows the concentration of drug at the active site, so it is usually necessary to work with **dose-response relationships**. The dose of a drug is simply the amount administered (e.g., 10 mg), whereas the concentration is the amount per unit volume (e.g., mg/mL). To achieve similar concentrations in patients, it is often necessary to adjust the dose based on patient size, weight, and other factors (Chapter 3).

Dose-response curves are usually assumed to be at **equilibrium**, or steady state, when the rate of drug influx equals the rate of drug efflux, although this is an ideal that is not often achieved in practice. Once the drug reaches its receptors, many responses are **graded**; that is, they vary from a minimum to a maximum response. Most concentration- and dose-response curves are plotted on log scales rather than linear scales to make it easier to compare drug potencies; the linear scale yields a rectangular hyperbola, whereas the log scale yields an S-shaped curve, as shown in Fig. 2.10.

Quantal responses are all-or-none responses to a drug. For example, after the administration of a hypnotic drug, a patient is either asleep or not (if sleep is the end point). Construction of dose-response curves for quantal responses requires the use of populations of subjects who exhibit individual variability. A few subjects will demonstrate an initial response at a low dose, most subjects demonstrate an initial response

at an intermediate dose, and a few subjects demonstrate an initial response at a high dose, resulting in a bell-shaped "Gaussian" distribution of sensitivity (Fig. 2.11A). Quantal dose-response curves are often plotted in a cumulative manner, comparing the dose of drug on the x-axis with the cumulative percentage of subjects responding to that dose on the y-axis, yielding an S-shaped curve (see Fig. 2.11B).

Occupation of a receptor by a drug is derived from the law of mass action (see Eq. 2.1) and can be represented as:

$$\frac{[DR]}{[R_T]} = \frac{[D]}{[D]+K_D} \qquad (2.2)$$

where R_T represents the total number of receptors, and K_D is the equilibrium dissociation constant (or affinity constant) of the drug for the receptor. Therefore the proportion of drug bound, relative to the maximum proportion that could be bound, is equal to the concentration of drug divided by the concentration of drug plus its affinity constant. It is important to note that $[DR]/[R_T]$ describes the proportion of receptors bound, or **fractional occupancy**, which ranges from zero (0) when no drug is bound to one (1) when all receptors are occupied by drug. This equation can be used to calculate the *proportion* (not actual number) of receptors occupied at a particular concentration of drug, and it demonstrates that fractional occupancy depends only on the concentration of drug and its affinity constant, not on total receptor number.

The K_D value is a **fixed parameter** describing the affinity of a drug for a receptor-binding site. From Eq. 2.2, it is clear that when K_D equals $[D]$, half of the receptors are occupied; thus, K_D is the concentration of drug that achieves half maximal saturation of the receptor population. This means that drugs with a high K_D (low affinity) will require a high concentration for a given occupancy, whereas drugs with a low K_D (high affinity) require lower concentrations for the same occupancy. Thus, the K_D of a drug is a reflection of the affinity of the drug and its receptor or how tightly the drug binds to the receptor. The K_D is also equal to the ratio of the rate of dissociation of the [DR] complex divided by its

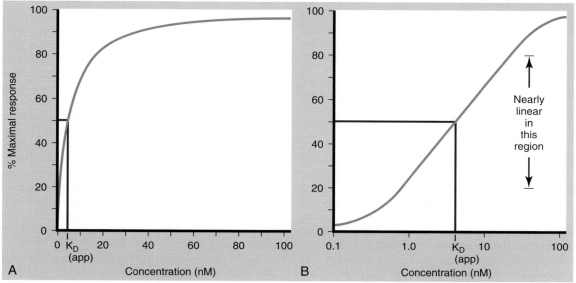

FIG. 2.10 A Concentration-Response Curve for Receptor Occupancy. (A) Arithmetic concentration scale. (B) Logarithmic concentration scale. K_D (app) is the concentration of drug occupying half of the available receptor pool in a situation where the response is directly proportional to receptor occupancy.

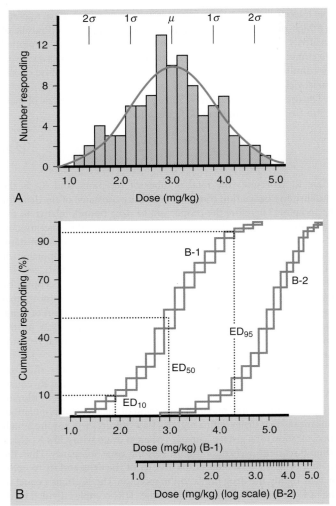

FIG. 2.11 Quantal Effects. A typical set of data obtained after administration of increasing doses of drug to a group of subjects followed by recording the minimum dose to which each subject responds. Data are from 100 subjects. The mean (μ) and median dose is 3.0 mg/kg; the standard deviation (σ) of the response is 0.8 mg/kg. (A) Results are plotted as a histogram (bar graph) showing the number responding at each dose; the smooth curve is a normal distribution function calculated for μ of 3.0 and σ of 0.8. (B) Data from A replotted as a cumulative percentage responding versus dose. The dose shown in *B-1* is on an arithmetic scale (as in A), and that in *B-2* is on a logarithmic scale (the separate line under the x-axis). The three ED (effective dose) values are shown for doses at which 10%, 50%, or 95% of subjects respond (on the arithmetic scale).

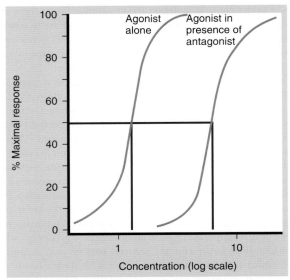

FIG. 2.12 Diagram Showing an Agonist Response Modified by Administration of a Competitive Antagonist. In this case, both the agonist and the antagonist compete for and bind reversibly to the same receptor site. The presence of the competitive antagonist causes a parallel right shift of the concentration-response curve for the agonist.

Antagonists

There are two major classes of antagonists, competitive and noncompetitive. Most antagonists are **competitive** antagonists. These drugs compete with agonists for the same binding site on a given receptor. If the receptor is occupied by a competitive antagonist, then agonist binding to the receptor is reduced. Likewise, if the receptor is bound by an agonist, antagonist binding will be diminished. When present alone, each drug will occupy the receptors in a concentration-dependent manner, as described in Eq. 2.2. However, when both drugs are present and competing for the same binding site, the equation describing agonist occupancy is:

$$\frac{[DR]}{[R_T]} = \frac{[D]}{[D] + K_D(1 + [B]/K_B)} \tag{2.3}$$

where D represents agonist concentration, B represents antagonist concentration, and K_D and K_B represent the relative affinity constants for agonist and antagonist, respectively. This equation demonstrates that in the presence of a competitive antagonist, the apparent affinity (K_D) of the agonist [D] for the receptor is altered by the factor (1 + [B]/K_B). Thus as the concentration of the antagonist increases, more agonist is required to cause an effect. Therefore, a competitive antagonist reduces the response to the agonist. However, if the concentration of the agonist is increased, it can overcome the receptor blockade caused by the competitive antagonist. In other words, blockade by competitive antagonists is **surmountable** by increasing the concentration of agonist. With two drugs competing for the same binding site, the drug with the higher concentration relative to its affinity constant can dominate. It is important to remember that the key factor is the ratio of the drug concentration **relative to** its affinity constant, not simply drug concentration.

Eq. 2.3 also demonstrates the very important point that the presence of a competitive antagonist causes a **parallel rightward shift** in the agonist dose-response curve (decreased apparent K_D) but no change in the shape of the curve such that every portion of the dose-response curve is shifted by exactly the same amount (Fig. 2.12). The magnitude

rate of formation (K_{off}/K_{on}). Because the rate of DR complex formation is usually determined by diffusion, the value of the K_D is determined by the rate of dissociation (K_{off}). Every drug-receptor combination will have a characteristic K_D, although these values can differ by many orders of magnitude. For example, glutamate has approximately millimolar affinity for its receptors, whereas some β-adrenergic antagonists have nanomolar affinities for their receptors. These different values are logical when one considers that a neurotransmitter can reach very high concentrations within the synapse and should dissociate quickly from its receptor for the repetitive function of the nervous system, whereas a therapeutic drug would be expected to have a higher affinity at its target.

of rightward shift depends on the concentration of antagonist (which is variable) divided by its affinity constant, which is fixed. Therefore, if the concentration of drug is known, measuring the magnitude of the rightward shift allows direct calculation of the value of K_B for the antagonist's affinity constant. This value is very useful because the affinity constant is essentially a molecular description of how well a drug binds to a particular receptor and is constant for any drug-receptor pair. Thus experimental comparison of affinity constants for antagonists at receptors in different tissues is one way to determine whether the binding sites (receptors) are the same or different. This fact makes antagonists useful in classifying the functions of receptor subtypes in vivo.

The second, much less common, type of antagonist is the **noncompetitive** antagonist. There are a number of different noncompetitive antagonists, but most drugs in this class are **irreversible alkylating** agents. An example of this type of drug is phenoxybenzamine, a drug that acts predominantly on α_1-adrenergic receptors and is used to mitigate the effects of circulating catecholamines secreted by tumors derived from adrenal chromaffin cells (Chapter 12). Drugs of this type contain highly reactive groups; when they bind to receptors they form covalent bonds within the binding site in an essentially irreversible manner. Because they decrease the number of available receptors, noncompetitive antagonists will usually decrease the maximum response to an agonist without affecting its EC_{50} (concentration causing half-maximal effect). The principal advantage of a noncompetitive antagonist is its long-lasting effect, as the inhibition lasts until new receptors are synthesized (Chapter 12).

Partial Agonists

As discussed, agonists can participate in both equilibria shown in Eq. 2.1, binding to and activating receptors to cause a conformational change and response. **Partial agonists** have a dual activity; that is, they act partially as agonists and partially as antagonists. When bound to their receptors, partial agonists are only partly able to shift the receptor to its activated conformational state. **Efficacy** is a term that describes the proportion of receptors that are stabilized in their active conformation when occupied by a particular drug. It can be used to describe the maximal effect of agonists in causing a receptor conformational change and can range from 0 to 1. Drugs with full efficacy (1.0) are termed **full agonists**, and drugs with some efficacy (>0 but <1.0) are **partial agonists**, whereas drugs with 0 efficacy are **antagonists**.

Partial agonists can also partially inhibit the response to full agonists acting at the same receptor type. If both full and partial agonists are present, as the concentration of partial agonist is increased, more receptors will be occupied by the partial agonist, thereby lowering the number of receptors available for activation by the full agonist. This will cause a decrease in response because some of the receptors will no longer be activated. At very high concentrations of the partial agonist relative to its affinity constant, all of the receptors will be occupied by the partial agonist, and the full agonist will not be effective. The magnitude of the cellular response will be determined by the response caused by the partial agonist alone. Therefore, a diagnostic feature of a partial agonist is that it inhibits the action of a full agonist to the level of the partial agonist's own maximal effect. Partial agonists are clinically very useful in treating opioid addiction. As shown in Fig. 2.13, the partial agonist buprenorphine blunts the effects of full opioid agonists such as oxycodone, morphine, or heroin (Chapter 28).

Signal Amplification

In some cases, the cellular response elicited by a drug is directly proportional to the fraction of receptors occupied by an agonist. However, more commonly, a maximal response can be achieved when only a small fraction of the total receptors available is occupied by an agonist.

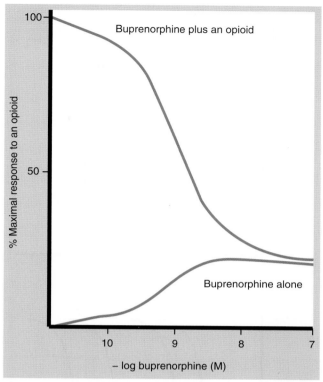

FIG. 2.13 Diagram Showing the Effect of a Partial Agonist on a Response to a Full Agonist. Buprenorphine is a mixed partial agonist used to treat opioid addiction. When buprenorphine is administered with an opioid such as morphine, oxycodone, or heroin, the effects of the opioid are reduced to the level caused by buprenorphine alone. (Modified from Romero, et al. Synapse. 1999;34:83–94.)

This phenomenon defines the concept that tissues express more receptors than are needed to elicit a maximal response. Thus, tissues contain a **receptor reserve** or **spare receptors**. This concept is based on the idea that downstream signaling cascades responding to activation of the receptor often provide amplification of the signal. As an example, consider the GPCRs and their downstream signaling cascades described in Box 2.2. Imagine a differentiated cell whose membrane contained 10,000 GPCRs and only 1000 G proteins that could couple to that receptor. In this cell, activation of all 1000 G proteins would lead to a full biological response. If there were a 1:1 stoichiometry between activation of receptors and activation of G proteins, only 10% of the receptors would need to be activated to cause a full response. Further receptor occupancy could not increase the magnitude of the response. When the signaling pathways involve amplification steps, the EC_{50} for an agonist may be much lower than the concentration needed to cause half-maximal receptor occupation (K_D), as shown in the top panel of Fig. 2.14.

Spare receptors are important in all-or-none responses, where it is biologically important that activation does not fail (e.g., the neuromuscular junction or the heart). The presence of these signal amplification mechanisms **shifts the agonist dose-response curve to the left** of the K_D for binding of agonist to receptor, and the degree of shift is proportional to the proportion of spare receptors, as shown in the bottom panel of Fig. 2.14. Thus, spare receptors render a tissue more sensitive to an agonist without having to change the affinity of the receptor. Because the existence of signal amplification is fairly common, the EC_{50} for agonist stimulation is usually smaller than its K_D for binding. For example, the β_1-adrenergic receptor has the same chemical and physical properties

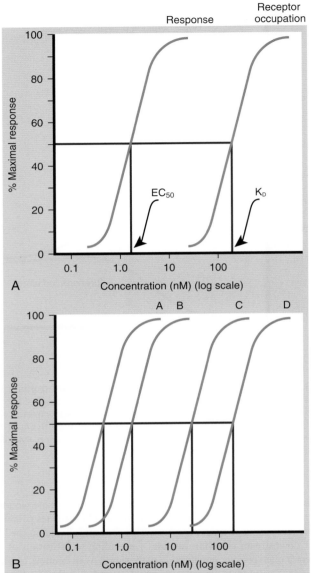

FIG. 2.14 Diagram Illustrating the Effect of a Contractile Agonist on Muscle Contraction in Vascular Tissues Expressing Different Levels of Signal Amplification. (A) Logarithmic concentration-response curves for contraction illustrating amplification between occupancy and response; note that the EC_{50} is to the left of the K_D. (B) Logarithmic concentration-response curves for contraction illustrating the effects of a single agonist acting on the same receptor subtype in different tissues with different proportions of receptor reserve (tissues A, B, C, and D); note that all tissues show the same maximum response as the concentration of the drug is increased (same intrinsic activity). The agonist exhibits its highest potency (lowest EC_{50}) in the tissue with greatest signal amplification (proportion of spare receptors) (tissue A), and its lowest potency in the tissue with the lowest proportion of spare receptors (tissue D).

in every tissue in which it is expressed. However, depending on the degree of receptor reserve in a given tissue, the EC_{50} for a particular β_1-agonist can vary markedly among tissues. A consequence of this situation is that if an agonist has a different EC_{50} in two different tissues in vivo, one cannot conclude that the receptors are different in the two tissues.

Spare receptors also complicate the analysis of partial agonists. If a drug is a partial agonist in one tissue, it may be a full agonist in another tissue, which has a higher proportion of spare receptors. In the GPCR example where only 10% of the receptor population must be activated to cause a full response, a weak partial agonist may activate this 10% and appear to be a full agonist. Because of this problem, a different term, **intrinsic activity**, is used to describe the ability of a given tissue to respond to agonist stimulation. **Efficacy**, which is the ability of the agonist to cause the receptor to assume an active conformation, is analogous to K_D in that both are constant for a given drug-receptor pair. It is an intrinsic property that depends on the structural complementarity of the drug and the receptor molecules. **Intrinsic activity**, however, is highly context dependent. It varies in different tissues because of the presence of different proportions of spare receptors and downstream amplification mechanisms. A drug can be a partial agonist in efficacy but a full agonist in intrinsic activity when spare receptors are present.

RECEPTOR REGULATION

Like other proteins in the cell, receptors themselves are subject to a variety of regulatory mechanisms. The overall response of any cell to hormones or neurotransmitters is tightly regulated and can vary depending on many different stimuli impinging on the cell. Very often, the number of receptors in the membrane of a cell or the responsiveness of the receptors themselves is regulated. One stimulus can **sensitize** a cell to the effects of another stimulus by up regulating or increasing the number of receptors. More commonly, when a cell is continuously stimulated by a transmitter or hormone, it may become **desensitized**. An example of the latter phenomenon is the loss of the ability of inhaled β_2-adrenergic agonists to dilate the bronchi of asthmatic patients after repeated use of the drug (Chapter 72). A hormone or agonist can affect the way a cell responds to itself (**homologous effects**) or how it responds to other hormones (**heterologous effects**). As an example of the latter phenomenon, exposure of a cell to estrogen sensitizes many cells to the effects of progesterone (Chapter 51).

Receptor Cycling

In the absence of a stimulus, most receptors are not localized to particular regions of the cell membrane. When a neurotransmitter or hormone binds, receptors rapidly migrate to coated pits. These are specialized invaginations of the membrane surrounded by an electron-dense cage formed by the protein **clathrin**; this is where receptor-mediated endocytosis occurs. As shown in Fig. 2.15, segments of membranes within coated pits rapidly pinch off to form intracellular vesicles rich in receptor-ligand complexes that fuse with tubular-reticular structures. In most cases, the dissociated neurotransmitter or hormone is incorporated into vesicles that fuse with lysosomes, with the ligand degraded by lysosomal enzymes. Dissociated receptors may recirculate to the cell surface or may be sequestered temporarily in an intracellular membrane compartment, the latter resulting in a decreased number of receptors in the membrane. Alternatively, receptors may be transported to lysosomes and degraded, again resulting in a net decrease in receptor number. A small fraction of internalized ligands bound to receptors may also be recirculated to the cell surface and then released, a process termed **retroendocytosis**.

Receptor Phosphorylation

Changes in receptor-binding affinity and signaling efficiency often occur rapidly. A common mechanism for regulating the responsiveness of GPCRs is the phosphorylation of serine or threonine residues in their C-terminal, intracellular tail by a family of **receptor kinases**. These

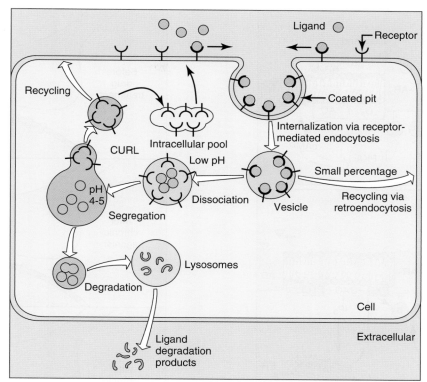

FIG. 2.15 Pathways for Receptor Internalization and Recycling. When ligands (neurotransmitter or hormone) bind to receptors, the receptors rapidly migrate to clathrin-coated pits, which are specialized invaginations of the membrane. Segments of membranes within the coated pits rapidly pinch off (receptor-mediated endocytosis) to form intracellular vesicles rich in receptor-ligand complexes. In most cases, the dissociated ligands are incorporated into vesicles that fuse with lysosomes followed by degradation. The dissociated receptors may recirculate to the cell surface, may be sequestered temporarily in an intracellular membrane compartment, or may be transported to lysosomes and degraded. A small fraction of internalized ligand bound to receptor may also be recirculated to the cell surface and then released by retroendocytosis. Abbreviations: *CURL*, Compartment in which uncoupling of receptor and ligand can occur.

phosphorylation events can rapidly change receptor affinity or signaling efficiency and can also direct receptors for internalization into coated pits, where they are ultimately degraded by proteases within the cell. The mechanisms involved in **homologous** and **heterologous desensitiza-tion** of the β-AR have been studied extensively and are well understood (Fig. 2.16). The phosphorylation of this receptor on serine or threonine residues by three different protein kinases plays a major role in the loss of receptor responsiveness. These kinases include the **β-adrenergic receptor kinase (β-ARK)**, which is a receptor-specific protein kinase; the multifunctional **cAMP-dependent protein kinase** (also known as protein kinase A); and protein kinase C, which also has a large number of substrates. Phosphorylation of the β-adrenergic receptor inhibits its ability to interact with G proteins and subsequently leads to its sequestra-tion or internalization in a compartment where it cannot interact with extracellular hormones. β-ARK is only capable of phosphorylating the active agonist-bound form of the receptor and is particularly important in **homologous desensitization**. Other protein kinases, such as the cAMP-dependent protein kinase, may also prefer the agonist-bound form of the receptor, but not to the same extent as β-ARK. Although β-ARK was originally described as kinase specific for the β-adrenergic receptor, its specificity is not unique, as a large family of related receptor protein kinases has been discovered that can phosphorylate many different GPCRs in their agonist-bound state.

Receptor Density

Finally, it is important to realize that the number of receptors in the plasma membrane of cells is not static and may be increased or decreased under the influence of hormonal mechanisms (Fig. 2.17). A decreased number of receptors (often referred to as **down regulation**) may result from increased internalization or degradation, processes with an intermediate time course, and typically manifest following continued receptor activation. In contrast, alterations in rates of receptor synthesis occur more slowly and may result in an increased number of receptors, often termed **up regulation** or **receptor supersensitivity**. Up regulation can occur as a consequence of the loss of the normal levels of transmitter stimulation (through disease) or after long-term exposure of the receptor to an antagonist. Moreover, the density of receptors in the plasma membrane may be regulated by unrelated hormones. For example, the number of β-adrenergic receptors in cardiac cells is regulated by thyroid hormone. Excessive production of thyroid hormone in Graves' disease increases the synthesis of β-adrenergic receptors in cardiac tissue, accounting for many of the cardiac symptoms of the disease (Chapter 54). In summary, the number of cell surface receptors is continuously regulated, thereby altering the sensitivity of a cell to endogenous or exogenous activation. This property of receptor biology is important to consider when using drugs acting as agonists on cell membrane receptors.

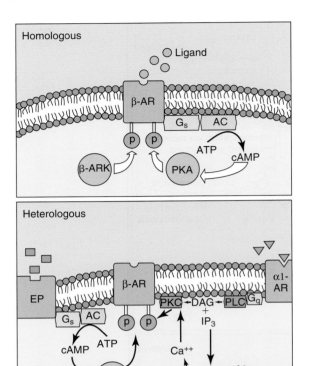

FIG. 2.16 Receptor Phosphorylation and Desensitization. The upper panel depicts homologous desensitization, which may occur when the β-adrenergic receptor (β-AR) is activated to produce cAMP. The ligand-activated receptor can be phosphorylated by either β-adrenergic receptor kinase (β-ARK) or cAMP-dependent protein kinase (PKA), leading to desensitization. The lower panel depicts heterologous desensitization of the β-adrenergic receptor in which the prostaglandin receptor (EP) stimulates cAMP production to activate the PKA, and the α₁-adrenergic receptor (α₁-AR) stimulates the production of 1,2-diacylglycerol (DAG), activating protein kinase C (PKC). Either kinase can phosphorylate the β-adrenergic receptor leading to desensitization. Abbreviations: *AC*, Adenylyl cyclase; *ER*, endoplasmic reticulum; *IP₃*, inositol triphosphate; *P*, phosphorylated state.

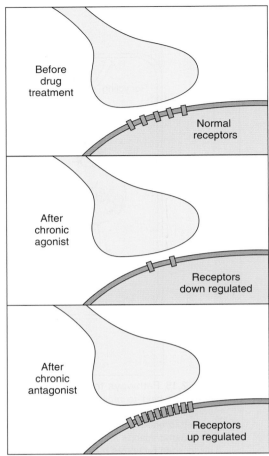

FIG. 2.17 Regulation of Receptor Density by Agonists and Antagonists. Continuous exposure of receptors to agonists often leads to a decreased number of receptors in the cell membrane (down regulation) as a result of increased internalization or degradation. Conversely, continuous exposure of receptors to antagonists often leads to an increased number of receptors in the cell membrane (up regulation) as a result of increased receptor synthesis.

SELF-ASSESSMENT QUESTIONS

1. Binding of a drug to its target most often:
   A. Involves covalent binding between the target and the drug.
   B. Involves more than one type of weak bond between the drug and its target.
   C. Requires long-lasting stable bonds between the drug and its target.
   D. Has a similar affinity for the several stereoisomers of the drug.
   E. Is characterized by high K_D values.

2. A patient was being maintained on a β-adrenergic receptor antagonist to control hypertension. The continuous exposure of receptor to this antagonist can:
   A. Result in supersensitivity.
   B. Desensitize the receptor.
   C. Produce tachyphylaxis.
   D. Cause down regulation of the receptor.
   E. B and C are correct.

3. Which of the following statements regarding drugs' action and cell surface receptors is not correct?
   A. By acting on receptors, drugs can enhance, diminish, or block generation or transmission of signals.
   B. The K_D of drug binding to receptors can vary widely.
   C. Agonist drugs are highly specific for each subtype of receptor in various classes of receptors.
   D. More than one drug molecule may be required to bind to a receptor and elicit a response.
   E. Receptors are frequently glycosylated.

4. Which of the following processes are involved in intracellular signaling cascades?
   A. Tyrosine phosphorylation.
   B. Receptor association with and stimulation of G proteins.
   C. Formation of second messengers, such as cAMP.
   D. Mobilization of Ca^{2+} from the endoplasmic reticulum.
   E. All of the above.

5. An in vitro experiment was performed that involved adding two different drugs to a solution bathing a strip of intestinal smooth muscle. Both drugs cause relaxation of the muscle but had very different EC_{50} values. Based on this single piece of information, which of the following statements is most correct?
   A. The two drugs have similar chemical structures.
   B. The two drugs have different potencies in causing relaxation.
   C. Both drugs activate the same receptor in the muscle.
   D. Both drugs are directly acting agonists.
   E. The maximum relaxation caused by the two different drugs will be similar.

6. The affinity constant of a drug for its target (K_D) is:
   A. An intrinsic property of the binding site of the target molecule for the drug and the drug itself.
   B. The ratio of the reverse to forward rate constants for the drug-target binding equation.
   C. Determined by the rate of diffusion of the drug in plasma.
   D. Characterized by A and B above.
   E. Characterized by C only.

WEBSITES

http://www.guidetopharmacology.org/
This website contains a database maintained by the International Union of Basic and Clinical Pharmacology and provides the latest information on receptor nomenclature, subtypes, and ligands.

3

Pharmacokinetics

Paul F. Hollenberg

Pharmacokinetics is the branch of pharmacology concerned with the movement and disposition of drugs within and by the body and includes drug absorption, distribution, metabolism, and elimination. Following administration, drugs are absorbed and distributed throughout the circulatory system to their sites of action. Most drugs are active in their administered form and are metabolized to inactive compounds, followed by elimination from the body; some drugs are metabolized to active compounds. Further, prodrugs are inactive in their administered forms and are metabolized to their active forms, typically followed by inactivation and elimination.

The rates of delivery and distribution of drugs to their sites of action, as well as their metabolism and elimination, are influenced by numerous variables depicted in Fig. 3.1. This chapter discusses the absorption, distribution, metabolism, and elimination of drugs and the diverse factors that affect these processes.

ABSORPTION AND DISTRIBUTION

Transport of Drugs Across Membranes

For all pharmacokinetic processes, drugs must be transported across biological membranes. Drugs administered orally, intramuscularly, or subcutaneously must cross membranes to be absorbed and enter the systemic circulation. Not all agents need to enter the systemic circulation, such as drugs given orally to treat gastrointestinal (GI) tract infections, stomach acidity, and other diseases within the GI tract; however, these agents often cross membranes and are absorbed into the general circulation. Drugs administered by intravenous injection must also cross capillary membranes to exit the systemic circulation and reach extracellular and intracellular sites of action. Even compounds whose actions are directed toward platelets or other blood-borne elements must cross membranes. Elimination also requires drugs or their metabolites to traverse membranes.

Membranes are composed of a lipid bilayer and are strongly hydrophobic. Drugs that are uncharged, nonpolar, and have low molecular weight and high lipid solubility are easily transported across membranes. In contrast, drugs that are ionized or in which the electronic distribution is distorted, so that there is a separation of positive and negative charge imparting polarity, are not compatible with the uncharged nonpolar lipid environment. In addition, the ordered lipid membrane does not allow for the existence of aqueous pores large enough (>0.4-nm diameter) to allow passage of most drugs (generally >1-nm diameter); thus only low-molecular-weight molecules can normally pass through membranes. Large-molecular-weight proteins cannot pass through many membranes, and often, transmembrane transport of these moieties is an active process requiring energy and a carrier molecule. Most high-molecular-weight polypeptides and proteins cannot be administered orally because there are no mechanisms for their absorption from the GI tract, even if they could survive the high acidity of the proteolytic enzymes in the stomach.

ABBREVIATIONS

AUC	Area under the drug plasma concentration-time curve
C_{ss}	Steady-state concentration of drug
C(t)	Concentration of drug in plasma at any time "t"
CL	Clearance
CL_h	Hepatic clearance
CL_p	Plasma clearance
CL_r	Renal clearance
CNS	Central nervous system
CSF	Cerebrospinal fluid
Da	Dalton
E	Hepatic extraction ratio
F	Bioavailability
GI	Gastrointestinal
IA	Intraarterial
IM	Intramuscular
IV	Intravenous
K_m	Michaelis constant
NAD(P)	Nicotinamide adenine dinucleotide (phosphate)
pH	Logarithm of the reciprocal of the hydrogen ion concentration
pK_a	Logarithm of the reciprocal of the dissociation constant
Q	Hepatic blood flow
SC	Subcutaneous
$t_{1/2}$	Half-life
T	Dosing interval
TI	Therapeutic index
UDP	Uridine diphosphate
UTP	Uridine triphosphate
V_d	Apparent volume of distribution
V_{max}	Maximum rate of reaction

In general, drugs that have high lipid solubility cross membranes better than those with low lipid solubility. Lipid solubility or hydrophobicity is expressed as the oil/water equilibrium partition coefficient of a compound and is measured by determining the amount of a compound in each phase of an oil-H_2O mixture following solubilization and attainment of equilibrium. The larger the partition coefficient, the greater the lipid solubility. This is exemplified in Fig. 3.2, which depicts the absorption of three different barbiturates from the stomach. In this example, the compounds selected all had a similar pK_a (i.e., the degree of ionization was similar for all compounds at the pH of the stomach). Thus differences in absorption could be attributed solely to lipid solubility, and absorption was greatest for the barbiturate with the largest lipid solubility.

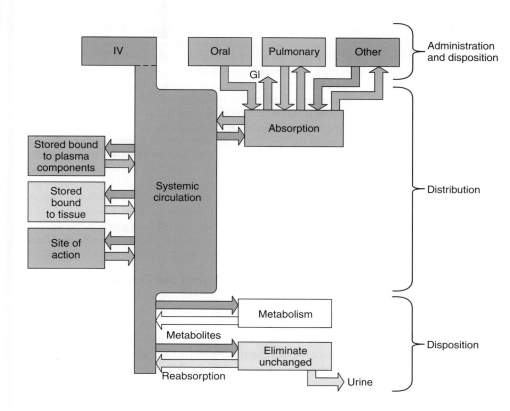

FIG. 3.1 Factors Influencing Drug Concentration at Its Site of Action and at Different Times After Administration. The circulatory system is the major pathway for drug delivery to its site of action. Possible entry routes and distribution and disposition sites are also shown.

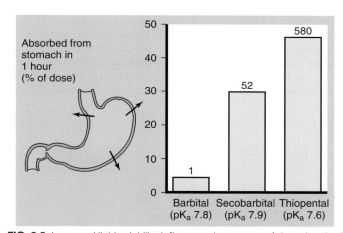

FIG. 3.2 Increased lipid solubility influences the amount of drug absorbed from the stomach for three different barbiturates. The number above each column is the oil/water equilibrium partition coefficient. The compounds have roughly equivalent pK_a values, so the degree of ionization is similar for all three drugs.

Influence of pH on Drug Absorption and Distribution

Many drugs are weak acids or bases and will be ionized in some pH ranges and unionized in others. An acid is defined as a compound that can dissociate and release a hydrogen ion, whereas a base can take up a hydrogen ion. By this definition, $RCOOH$ and RNH_3^+ are acids, and $RCOO^-$ and RNH_2 are bases. The equilibrium dissociation expression and the equilibrium dissociation constant (K_a) can be described for an acid HA or BH^+ and a base A^- or B, as shown below. The convention for K_a requires that the acid appear on the left, and the base appear on the right of the dissociation equation as:

$$HA \rightleftarrows A^- + H^+ \quad K_a = [A^-][H^+]/[HA] \tag{3.1}$$

$$BH^+ \rightleftarrows B + H^+ \quad K_a = [B][H^+]/[BH^+] \tag{3.2}$$

Taking the negative log of both sides yields:

$$-\log K_a = -\log[H^+] - \log[A^-]/[HA] \tag{3.3}$$

$$-\log K_a = -\log[H^+] - \log[B]/[BH^+] \tag{3.4}$$

By definition, the negative log of $[H^+]$ is pH, and the negative log of K_a is pK_a. Therefore Eqs. 3.3 and 3.4 can be simplified and rearranged to give:

$$pH = pK_a + \log[A^-]/[HA] \tag{3.5}$$

$$pH = pK_a + \log[B]/[BH^+] \tag{3.6}$$

Eqs. 3.5 and 3.6 are the acid and base forms, respectively, of the Henderson-Hasselbach equation, and they can be used to calculate the pH of the solution when the pK_a and the ratios of $[A^-]/[HA]$ or $[B]/[BH^+]$ are known. In pharmacology, it is often of interest to calculate the ratios of $[A^-]/[HA]$ or $[B]/[BH^+]$ when the pH and the pK_a are known. For this calculation, Eqs. 3.5 and 3.6 are rearranged to Eqs. 3.7 and 3.8 as follows:

$$pH-pK_a = \log[A^-]/[HA] \tag{3.7}$$

$$pH-pK_a = \log[B]/[BH^+] \tag{3.8}$$

Most drugs are transported across membranes by simple passive diffusion. The concentration gradient across the membrane is the driving force that establishes the rate of diffusion from high to low concentrations.

Passive diffusion of a drug that is a weak electrolyte is generally a function of the pK_a of the drug and the pH of the compartments across which the drug distributes because only the uncharged form of the drug can diffuse across membranes. From Eqs. 3.7 and 3.8, the degree of ionization of weak acids and bases across pHs can be determined; this is illustrated in Fig. 3.3, which depicts the fraction of the nonionized (HA or B) forms. When the pK_a equals the pH, the amounts of ionized and nonionized forms are equal.

The pH values of the major body fluids, which range from 1 to 8, are shown in Table 3.1. To predict how a drug will be distributed between gastric juice (pH 1.0) on one side of the membrane and blood (pH 7.4) on the other side, the degree of dissociation of the drug at each pH value is determined. Applying Eqs. 3.7 and 3.8 to an acidic drug with a pK_a of 6.0 enables one to calculate the degree of ionization for this drug in the stomach or blood (assuming the blood pH is 7.0 for ease of calculation), as follows:

Stomach: $1.0 - 6.0 = \log Y$; $\log Y = -5$, or $Y = 10^{-5}$; $Y = [A^-]/[HA] = 0.00001$; if [HA] is 1.0, then $[A^-]$ is 0.00001, and the compound is ionized to a very small extent.

Blood: $7.0 - 6.0 = \log Y$; $\log Y = +1$, or $Y = 10^{+1}$; $Y = [A^-]/[HA] = 10.0$; if [HA] is 1.0, then $[A^-]$ is 10.0, and the compound is ionized to a very large extent.

Thus because the drug is ionized slightly in the stomach and appreciably in the blood, it should cross easily from the stomach to the plasma but hardly at all in the reverse direction.

Another example is illustrated in Fig. 3.4 for a basic drug. This approach is particularly useful for predicting whether drugs can be absorbed in the stomach, the upper intestine, or not at all. Fig. 3.5 provides a summary of the effects of pH on drug absorption in the GI tract for several acidic and basic drugs. It also assists in predicting which drugs will undergo tubular reabsorption, which is discussed later.

In addition to simple passive diffusion, other mechanisms exist for transporting drugs across biological membranes, including active transport, facilitated diffusion, or pinocytosis. Active transport involves specific carrier molecules in the membrane that bind to and carry the drug across the lipid bilayer. Because there are a finite number of carrier molecules, they exhibit classical saturation kinetics. Drugs may also compete with a specific carrier molecule for transport, which can lead to drug-drug interactions that modify the time and intensity of action of a given drug. Further, because cellular energy is used to drive transport, an active transport system may concentrate a drug on one side of a membrane with no dependence on a concentration gradient. The primary active drug transport systems are present in renal tubule cells, the biliary tract, blood-brain barrier, and GI tract.

Distribution to Special Organs and Tissues

The rate of blood flow determines the maximum amount of drug that can be delivered per minute to specific organs and tissues at a given plasma concentration. Tissues that are highly perfused, such as the heart, receive a large quantity of drug, provided the drug can cross the membranes or other barriers present. Conversely, tissues that are poorly perfused, such as fat, receive drug at a slower rate; thus the concentration of drug in fat may still be increasing long after the concentration in plasma has started to decrease.

Two compartments of special importance are the brain and the fetus. Many drugs do not readily enter the brain. Capillaries in the brain differ structurally from those in other tissues, resulting in a barrier between blood within the brain capillaries and the extracellular fluid in brain tissue. This blood-brain barrier hinders the transport of drugs and other materials from the blood into the brain tissue. The blood-brain barrier exists throughout brain and spinal cord at all regions central to the arachnoid membrane, except for the floor of the hypothalamus and the area postrema. Structural differences between brain and nonbrain

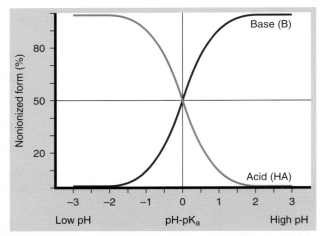

FIG. 3.3 Ionization of Acidic or Basic Drugs at Different pH Values, With pH Expressed Relative to the Drug pK_a. HA is the nonionized (uncharged) form of an acid, and B is the nonionized (uncharged) form of a base.

TABLE 3.1	pH of Selected Body Fluids
Fluids	**pH**
Gastric juice	1.0–3.0
Small intestine: duodenum	5.0–6.0
Small intestine: ileum	8
Large intestine	8
Plasma	7.4
Cerebrospinal fluid	7.3
Urine	4.0–8.0

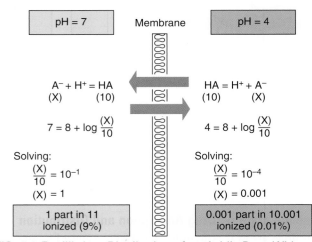

FIG. 3.4 Equilibrium Distribution of an Acidic Drug With a pK_a of 8.0 When the pH Is 4 on One Side and 7 on the Other Side of a Membrane. Nonionized form, HA, of the drug can readily cross the membrane. Thus HA has the same concentration on both sides of the membrane. The concentration of nonionized drug is arbitrarily set at 10 mg/mL, and the expressions are solved to determine the concentration of ionized species at equilibrium.

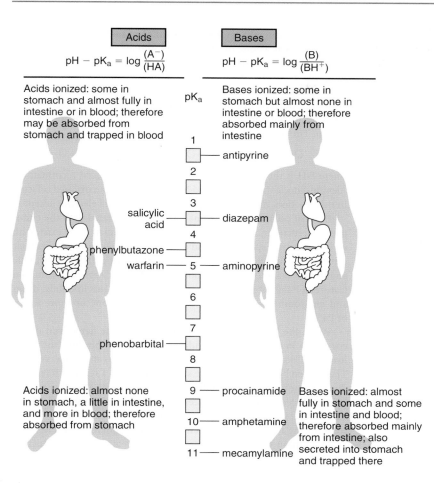

Acids	Bases
$pH - pK_a = \log \dfrac{(A^-)}{(HA)}$	$pH - pK_a = \log \dfrac{(B)}{(BH^+)}$

Acids ionized: some in stomach and almost fully in intestine or in blood; therefore may be absorbed from stomach and trapped in blood

Bases ionized: some in stomach but almost none in intestine or blood; therefore absorbed mainly from intestine

pK_a

1 — antipyrine

2

3 — diazepam
salicylic acid

4
phenylbutazone —

warfarin — 5 — aminopyrine

6

7

phenobarbital —

8

Acids ionized: almost none in stomach, a little in intestine, and more in blood; therefore absorbed from stomach

9 — procainamide

10 — amphetamine

11 — mecamylamine

Bases ionized: almost fully in stomach and some in intestine and blood; therefore absorbed mainly from intestine; also secreted into stomach and trapped there

FIG. 3.5 Summary of pH Effect on Degree of Ionization of Several Acidic and Basic Drugs. Statements refer to compounds with extremes of pK_a values and allow prediction of where drugs with various pK_as will be absorbed.

capillaries, and how these differences influence blood-brain transport of solutes, are illustrated in Fig. 3.6. Nonbrain capillaries have fenestrations (openings) between the endothelial cells through which solutes move readily by passive diffusion, with compounds having molecular weights greater than approximately 25,000 daltons (Da) undergoing transport by pinocytosis. Brain capillaries do not have fenestrations. Rather, tight junctions are present, and pinocytosis is greatly reduced. Special transport systems are available at brain capillaries for glucose, amino acids, amines, purines, nucleosides, and organic acids; all other materials must cross two endothelial membranes plus the endothelial cytoplasm to move from capillary blood to tissue extracellular fluid. Thus the main route of drug entry into central nervous system (CNS) tissue is by passive diffusion across membranes, restricting the available compounds used to treat brain disorders. At the same time, the potential deleterious effects of many compounds on the CNS are not realized because the blood-brain barrier acts as a safety buffer. Generally, only highly lipid-soluble drugs cross the blood-brain barrier, and thus for these drugs, no blood-brain barrier exists. In infants and the elderly, the blood-brain barrier may be compromised, and drugs may diffuse freely into the brain.

For the delivery of drugs that do not cross the blood-brain barrier, an alternative approach is by intrathecal injection into the subarachnoid space and the cerebrospinal fluid (CSF) using lumbar puncture. However, injection into the subarachnoid space can be difficult to perform safely because of the small volume of this region and the proximity to nerve, which can be easily damaged. In addition, drug distribution within the CSF and across the CSF-brain barrier can be slow and exhibit much variability; for some drugs, there may be no alternate route.

METABOLISM AND ELIMINATION OF DRUGS

The terms **metabolism** and **biotransformation** refer to the chemical alteration of a drug into other compounds called **metabolites**. As mentioned, most drugs are administered in their active forms, but several are prodrugs that are inactive when administered and must be metabolized to a pharmacologically active form. Drug metabolism occurs primarily in the liver, but almost all tissues and organs, especially the lung, can also metabolize drugs.

The term **elimination** refers to the removal of drug from the body. Some drugs are eliminated without being metabolized, but most drugs are eliminated following biotransformation to inactive metabolites. Elimination occurs primarily by renal mechanisms and excretion into the urine and to a lesser extent by mixing with bile salts for solubilization followed by transport into the intestinal tract. In many cases, drugs or their metabolites are reabsorbed from the intestine. A few drugs become essentially irreversibly bound to tissues and are metabolized or otherwise removed over long periods of time. Drugs may also be excreted in the feces or secreted through sweat or salivary glands; highly volatile or gaseous agents may be excreted by the lungs.

Metabolism of Drugs

Drug metabolism involves altering the chemical structure of a drug by an enzyme. When drugs are metabolized, the change generally involves conversion of a nonpolar, lipid-soluble compound to a more polar form that is more H_2O soluble and can be more readily excreted in the urine. Some drugs are administered as prodrugs in an inactive or less active form to promote absorption, to overcome potential destruction

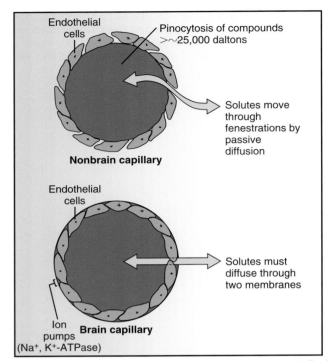

FIG. 3.6 Structural Differences Between Nonbrain and Brain Capillaries. In brain capillaries, lack of openings between endothelial cells in capillary wall requires drugs and other solutes to pass through two membranes to move from blood to tissue or the reverse. Ion pumps are mainly on the outer membrane of the brain endothelial cells and maintain a concentration difference between the two fluid regions.

by stomach acidity, to minimize exposure to highly reactive chemical species, or to allow for selective generation of pharmacologically active metabolites at specific target sites in vivo. In this case, drug-metabolizing systems convert the prodrug into a more active species following absorption. In other cases, drugs administered as the active species are biotransformed to active metabolites that produce pharmacological effects similar to or different from those generated by the parent drug. An example is diazepam, an antianxiety compound that is demethylated to an active metabolite. The half-life ($t_{1/2}$) of the parent drug (defined as the time it takes for the concentration of drug to decrease by half), is approximately 30 hours, while the $t_{1/2}$ of the metabolite averages approximately 70 hours. Thus the metabolite will be present long after the parent drug disappears. Although the pharmacological effects of this metabolite are much less than for the parent drug, the lingering presence of the active metabolite makes control of the intensity of pharmacological effects more difficult. This is not a problem with diazepam because the therapeutic index (TI; ratio of toxic to therapeutic dose) of the drug is large; however, it can present a problem for drugs with a low therapeutic index.

For most drugs, metabolism takes place primarily in liver, catalyzed by microsomal, and in some cases, nonmicrosomal, enzyme systems. However, drug-metabolizing enzymes are also present in other tissues, including the lung, kidney, GI tract, placenta, and GI tract bacteria.

Drug metabolism typically involves two sets of reactions—namely, phase I and phase II. Phase I reactions include oxidation, reduction, and hydrolysis, during which drugs are transformed to more polar moieties. The second set of reactions, termed phase II reactions, involves conjugation, during which the drug molecule is coupled to an endogenous substituent group, resulting in the formation of a product with greater H_2O solubility, leading to enhanced renal or biliary elimination.

Oxidation can take place at several different sites on a drug molecule and can appear as one of many chemical reactions. By definition, an oxidation reaction requires the transfer of one or more electrons to an acceptor. Typically, an oxygen atom may be inserted, resulting in hydroxylation of a carbon or a nitrogen atom, oxidation, N- or O-dealkylation, or deamination. Many drug-oxidation reactions are catalyzed by the cytochrome P450-dependent mixed-function oxidase system. The overall reaction can be summarized as:

$$DH + NAD(P)H + H^+ + O_2 = DOH + NAD(P)^+ + H_2O$$

where DH is the drug, NADH or NADPH is a reduced nicotinamide adenine dinucleotide cofactor, and NAD or $NADP^+$ is an oxidized cofactor. In this reaction, molecular oxygen serves as the final electron acceptor.

In most cells, the cytochrome P450s are associated with the endoplasmic reticulum. More than 50 isoforms of human P450 exist, with various substrate specificities and different mechanisms regulating their expression. This plethora of enzyme systems provides the body with the ability to metabolize large numbers of different drugs. The common feature of P450 substrates is their lipid solubility. Most lipophilic drugs and environmental chemicals are substrates for one or more forms of P450.

When the drug binds to cytochrome P450, the heme iron of the enzyme is in the ferric (+3) oxidation state. Upon binding, the heme iron is reduced to the ferrous (+2) state and binds molecular oxygen. The oxygen bound to the active site is reduced to a reactive form that donates one oxygen atom to the drug substrate, with the other oxygen being reduced to H_2O. This process restores the heme iron to the ferric state. Free radical or iron-radical groups are formed at one or more steps during this cycle. The reaction cycle is summarized in Fig. 3.7.

In addition to oxidation, phase I reactions also include reduction and hydrolysis, examples of which are depicted in Fig. 3.8.

Phase II, or conjugation reactions, require activation of the groups being coupled through the transfer of energy from high-energy phosphate compounds. The reaction sequence involved is shown in Fig. 3.9 for the formation of the ROH glucuronide of salicylic acid. Before conjugation can occur, glucuronic acid is activated by the reaction of glucose-1-phosphate with high-energy uridine triphosphate (UTP) to form uridine diphosphate (UDP)-glucose, which is oxidized to activated UDP-glucuronic acid. This active moiety can then conjugate salicylic acid, a reaction catalyzed by the enzyme UDP-glucuronosyltransferase. This sequence occurs for drugs of the general types ROH, RCOOH, RNH_2, or RSH, where R represents the remainder of the drug molecule.

Many drugs, as well as endogenous compounds including bilirubin, thyroxine, and steroids, also undergo conjugation with activated glucuronic acid in the presence of UDP-glucuronosyltransferase. Conjugation may also occur with activated moieties other than glucuronate, including glycine, acetate, sulfate, and other groups, leading to drug conjugates that are readily excreted.

Factors Regulating Rates of Drug Metabolism

The chemical reactions involved in drug metabolism are catalyzed by enzymes. Because these enzymes obey Michaelis-Menten kinetics, the rates of drug metabolism can be approximated by the relationship:

$$v = V_{max}[S]/K_m + [S] \qquad \textbf{(3.9)}$$

where v = rate of reaction; V_{max} = maximum rate of reaction; [S] = concentration of drug; and K_m = Michaelis constant.

The v is directly proportional to the concentration of the enzyme. If a change occurs in the concentration of enzyme, there should be a similar change in the rate of metabolism. Because different drugs may be substrates for the same metabolizing enzyme, they can competitively

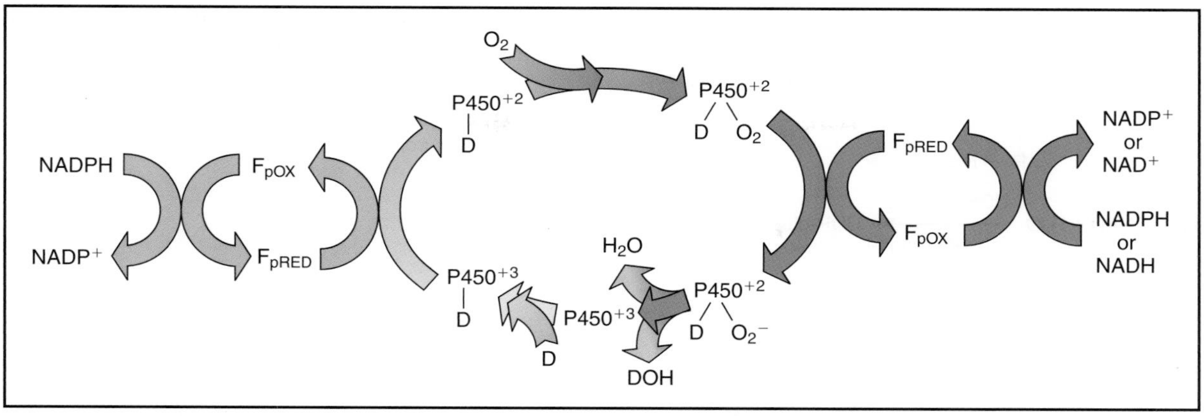

FIG. 3.7 Simplified Model of Cytochrome P450 Mixed-Function Oxidase Reaction Sequence. D is the drug undergoing oxidation to produce DOH. Molecular oxygen serves as the final electron acceptor. Flavin protein cofactor (F_p) systems are involved at several sites. The iron of the cytochrome P450 is involved in binding oxygen and electron transfer with changes in valence state.

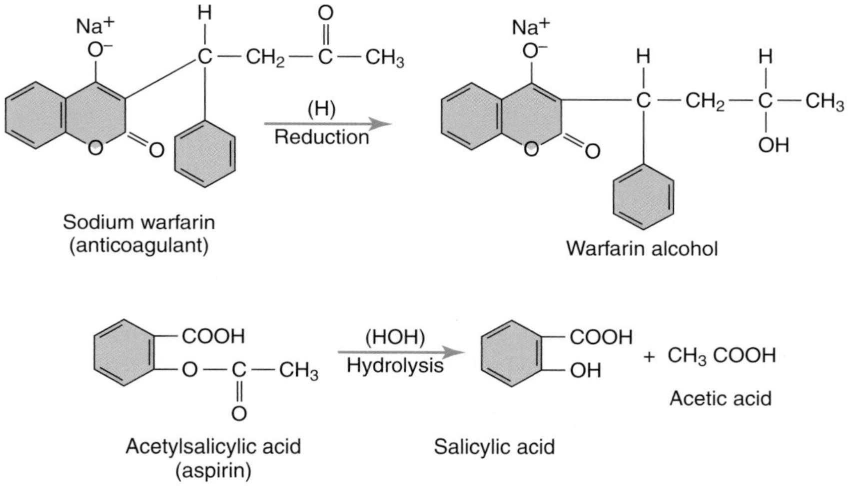

FIG. 3.8 Representative Reduction and Hydrolysis Reactions for Metabolism of Drugs.

inhibit the metabolism of each other. However, this is usually not a significant problem because the capacity of the metabolizing system is large, and drugs are usually present in concentrations less than their K_m.

Many drugs, environmental chemicals, air pollutants, and components of cigarette smoke stimulate the synthesis of drug-metabolizing enzymes. This process, termed enzyme induction, may elevate the level of hepatic drug-metabolizing enzymes. In most cases, the inducers are also substrates for the enzymes they induce. However, the induction is generally nonspecific and may result in increases in the metabolism of a variety of substrates. For example, phenobarbital and the highly reactive air pollutant 3,4-benzo[a]pyrene can increase the rate of oxidation of the CNS muscle relaxant zoxazolamine in animals, as depicted in Fig. 3.10. Because cigarette smoke contains compounds that can promote induction, chronic smokers have considerably higher levels of some hepatic and lung drug-metabolizing enzymes. Induction of P450 by polycyclic aromatic hydrocarbons in smoke causes female smokers to have lower circulating estrogen than nonsmokers.

For nearly all drugs, the normal therapeutic range of concentrations is much smaller than the K_m. Thus hepatic or other drug-metabolizing enzymes operate at substrate concentrations far below saturation, where Eq. 3.9 reduces to a first-order reaction—that is, typically following first-order kinetics. An exception is the metabolism of salicylic acid, in which enzyme saturation can occur at elevated drug concentrations. Aspirin (acetylsalicylic acid) is used extensively for the treatment of inflammatory diseases, with the optimum therapeutic concentration only slightly below that where signs of toxicity appear. Aspirin is hydrolyzed to salicylic acid, which, in turn, is metabolized by several routes before elimination (Fig. 3.11). Two of these pathways are subject to saturation in humans—namely, conjugation with glycine to form salicyluric acid and conjugation with glucuronic acid to form the salicyl phenolic glucuronide.

For enzyme saturation, the kinetics become zero order, and the rate of reaction becomes constant at V_{max}. This is consistent with Eq. 3.9, when [S] is much larger than K_m. Saturation of drug-metabolizing enzymes has a pronounced influence on drug-plateau concentrations. With zero-order kinetics, elimination rates no longer depend on dose or blood concentration.

Clearance of Drugs

Drug clearance, sometimes referred to as total body clearance, refers to the rate that an active drug is removed from the body—that is, the volume of blood cleared of drug per unit time. Knowledge of drug clearance is critical clinically for determining maintenance doses of drugs, and it represents the sum of drug removal by hepatic, renal, and other organs.

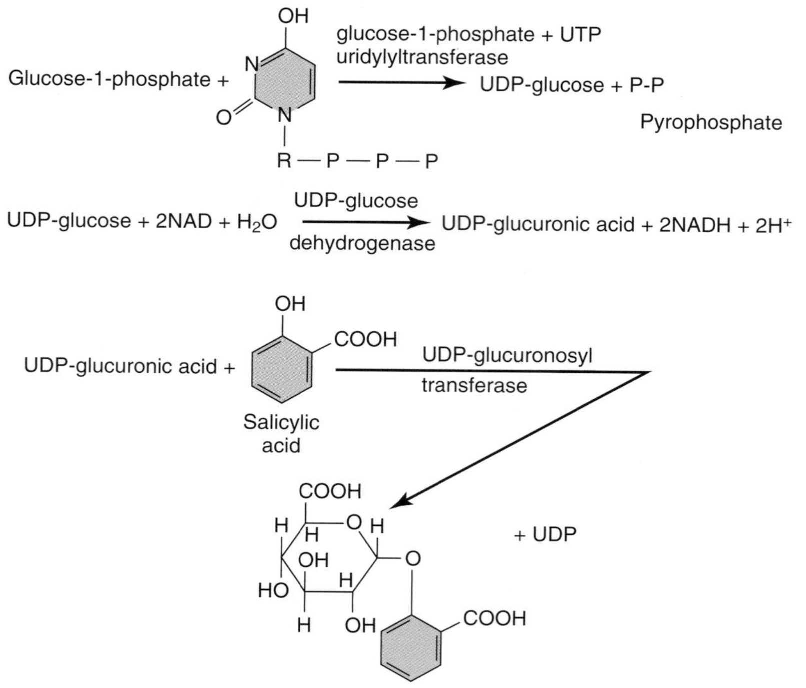

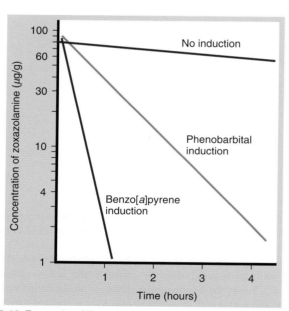

Glucose-1-phosphate + [uracil structure with R—P—P—P] $\xrightarrow{\text{glucose-1-phosphate + UTP uridylyltransferase}}$ UDP-glucose + P-P

Pyrophosphate

UDP-glucose + 2NAD + H_2O $\xrightarrow{\text{UDP-glucose dehydrogenase}}$ UDP-glucuronic acid + 2NADH + $2H^+$

UDP-glucuronic acid + [Salicylic acid structure] $\xrightarrow{\text{UDP-glucuronosyl transferase}}$ [glucuronide structure] + UDP

FIG. 3.9 Sequence of Reactions for Conjugation of Salicylic Acid to Form Salicyl Phenolic Glucuronide. The glucuronic acid must first be activated, with glucose-1-phosphate coupling with high-energy uridine triphosphate (UTP) to uridine diphosphate (UDP)-glucose followed by oxidation to UDP-glucuronic acid before conjugation can occur. *P*, Phosphate.

FIG. 3.10 Example of Enzyme Induction. Zoxazolamine administered by intraperitoneal injection to rats. For induction studies, phenobarbital or 3,4-benzo[a]pyrene was injected twice daily for 4 days before injection of zoxazolamine.

Hepatic and Biliary Clearance

Hepatic clearance (CL_h) is the apparent volume of plasma that is cleared of drug by the liver per unit time, has the units of volume/time, and can be defined as:

$$CL_h = \text{rate of drug removal by the liver/ concentration of drug in portal vein} \quad (3.10)$$

Biliary clearance can be similarly defined, with the bile flow rate times the drug concentration in bile a measure of the rate of biliary removal.

The direct measurement of hepatic or biliary clearance in humans is not practical because of the difficulty and risk in obtaining appropriate blood samples. Further, a confounding result of calculating the biliary elimination of a drug may occur when the drug is reabsorbed from the GI tract and returned to the systemic circulation. This is termed enterohepatic cycling and can result in a measurable increase in the plasma concentration of drug several half-lives after the drug was administered and will delay its eventual disposition. Nevertheless, the clinical significance of clearance and calculations used to determine maintenance doses of drugs are discussed later in this chapter.

Renal Elimination of Drugs

Renal clearance (CL_r) is defined similarly as:

$$CL_r = \text{rate of drug removal by the kidneys/ concentration of drug in renal artery} \quad (3.11)$$

For a drug removed entirely by renal elimination, such as the antibiotic cephalexin, renal clearance and total body clearance are equal. In this example, renal clearance can be determined from plasma data if one plots the log plasma concentration of cephalexin versus time after intravenous injection.

The mechanisms involved in the renal clearance of drugs are the same as those responsible for the renal elimination of endogenous substances and include glomerular filtration, tubular secretion, and tubular reabsorption, as depicted in Fig. 3.12. Molecules smaller than 15 Å readily pass through the glomeruli, with approximately 125 mL of plasma cleared each minute in a healthy adult. Because clearance is independent of the plasma concentration, removal by glomerular filtration (mg/min) increases linearly with increasing plasma drug concentrations in the renal artery. The glomerular filtration rate of 125 mL/min represents less than 20% of the total renal plasma flow of 650 to 750 mL/min, indicating that only a small fraction of the total renal plasma flow is cleared of drug on each pass through the kidneys. Because albumin and other plasma proteins normally do not pass through the glomeruli, drug molecules that are bound to these proteins are retained. Inulin and creatinine can be used to assess glomerular filtration capability in

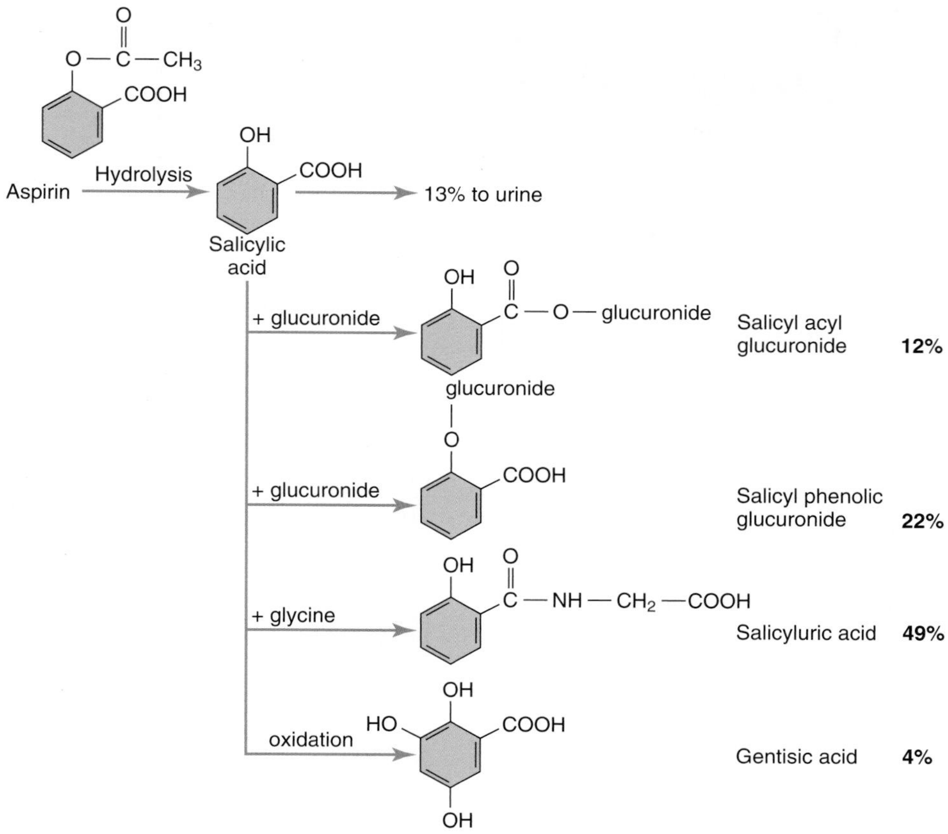

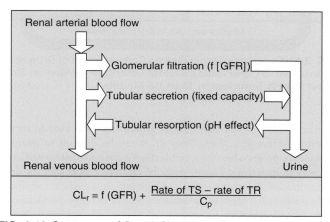

FIG. 3.11 Disposition of the Primary Metabolite of Aspirin, Salicylic Acid, at a Single Dose of 4 g (54 mg/kg of Body Weight) in a Healthy Adult. The percentage values refer to the dose. Oxidation produces a mixture of *ortho* and *para* (relative to original OH group) isomers.

FIG. 3.12 Summary of Renal Clearance (CL$_r$) Mechanisms. C_p, Renal arterial blood concentration of drug; *f*, fraction of drug in plasma not bound; *GFR*, glomerular filtration rate of drug; *TR*, tubular reabsorption of drug; *TS*, tubular secretion of drug.

$$CL_r = f\,(GFR) + \frac{\text{Rate of TS} - \text{rate of TR}}{C_p}$$

individual patients because these materials show very little binding to plasma proteins and do not undergo appreciable tubular secretion or reabsorption.

Following glomerular filtration, compounds may undergo tubular secretion; thus renal clearance represents the sum of both processes. Tubular secretion is an active process that occurs in the proximal tubule, with independent and relatively nonspecific carrier systems for the secretion of acids and bases. In addition, because tubular transit time can be sufficiently long such that dissociation from plasma proteins can take place, tubular secretion removes both bound and free drug. Tubular secretion involves active transport by a limited number of carriers, and thus the process can become saturated. The volume of plasma that can be cleared per unit time by tubular secretion varies with the concentration of drug in plasma. This is in contrast to glomerular filtration, where the volume filtered per unit time is independent of plasma concentration. At very low plasma concentrations, tubular secretion can operate at its maximum rate of approximately 650 mL/min. If the concentration of drug in arterial plasma is 4 ng/mL, clearing 650 mL/min removes 2600 ng each minute. If the concentration of the same drug increases to 200 ng/mL and tubular secretion is saturated at 4 ng/mL, the tubules will still remove only 2600 ng/min; thus the clearance by tubular secretion falls to 13 mL/min. If studies indicate that renal clearance is considerably greater than 125 mL/min, then tubular secretion must be involved because glomerular filtration cannot exceed that rate.

The third mechanism affecting renal clearance is tubular reabsorption of filtered or secreted drug back into the venous blood of the nephrons. Although this process may be either active or passive, for most drugs it occurs by passive diffusion. Drugs that are readily reabsorbed are characterized by high lipid solubility or by a significant fraction in a nonionized form at urine pH and in the ionized form at plasma pH. For example, salicylic acid (pK$_a$ = 3.0) is approximately 99.99% ionized at pH 7.4 (see Eq. 3.7) but only approximately 90% ionized at pH 4.0. Thus some reabsorption of salicylic acid could be expected from acidic urine. In drug overdose, the manipulation of urine pH is often used

TABLE 3.2 **Effect of Urine pH on Renal Clearance for Drugs That Undergo Tubular Resorption**	
Bases Cleared Rapidly by Making Urine More Acidic	**Acids Cleared Rapidly by Making Urine More Alkaline**
Amphetamine	Acetazolamide
Chloroquine	Nitrofurantoin
Imipramine	Phenobarbital
Levorphanol	Probenecid
Mecamylamine	Salicylates
Quinine	Sulfathiazole

to prevent reabsorption. Ammonium chloride administration leads to acidification of the urine; sodium bicarbonate administration leads to alkalinization of the urine. Some examples of drugs whose clearance can be increased following acidification or alkalinization of the urine are listed in Table 3.2.

Modified Renal Function and Drug Elimination

The renal clearance of drugs may be decreased in neonates, geriatric patients, and individuals with improperly functioning kidneys. The effect of patient age on renal clearance of drugs is discussed later in this chapter. In the case in which it is desirable to administer a drug that is disposed of primarily by renal elimination and the individual has impaired renal function, the extent of renal function must be determined. Creatinine clearance is the standard clinical determination used to obtain an approximate measure of renal function. To determine the rate of urinary excretion of creatinine, urine is collected over a known period (often 24 hours) and pooled, its volume is measured, and creatinine is measured. At the midpoint of the urine collection period, a serum sample is obtained and also assayed for creatinine. Creatinine clearance is calculated by dividing the rate of urinary excretion of creatinine (mg/min) by the serum concentration of creatinine (mg/mL), resulting in units of mL/min.

Creatinine clearance provides a measure of glomerular filtration. In addition, the relationship between creatinine clearance and the rate constant for renal elimination of unchanged drug must be demonstrated. For the usual case of first-order renal elimination, that relationship is linear; thus a creatinine clearance of 50% of normal means that renal elimination of this drug would be expected to operate at 50%, and the rate of drug input should be reduced accordingly. For example, if 100 mg of a drug was administered every 6 hours (400 mg in 24 hours) to a patient with normal creatinine clearance, then 40 mg of the drug should be administered every 12 hours (80 mg in 24 hours) to a patient with a creatinine clearance of only 20% of normal, assuming that other pathways for disappearance of this drug retained normal function.

CLINICAL CONSIDERATIONS

When planning drug therapy for a patient, deciding on the choice of drug and its dosing schedule is obviously critical. To make such decisions, an observable pharmacological effect is usually selected, and the dosing rate is manipulated until this effect is observed. This approach works quite well with some drugs. For example, blood pressure can be monitored in a hypertensive patient (Fig. 3.13, *Drug A*), and the dose of drug modified until blood pressure is reduced to the desired level. However, for other drugs, this approach is more problematic, usually because of the lack of an easily observable effect, a narrow TI, or changes in the condition of the patient that require modification of dosing rate.

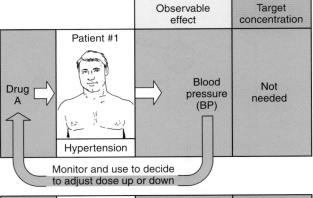

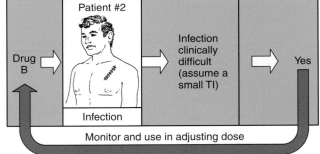

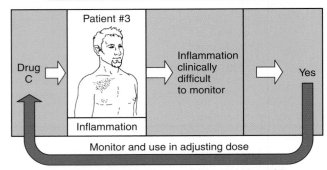

FIG. 3.13 Concept of Target Plasma Concentration of Drug as an Alternative to Observable Effect for Determining Whether Drug Input Rate Is Sufficient or Must Be Modified. For a discussion of target concentration, see the text.

For example, when an antibiotic with a low TI is used to treat a severe infection (Fig. 3.13, *Drug B*), it can be difficult to quantify therapeutic progress because a visible effect is not apparent immediately. Because of its narrow TI, care must be taken to ensure that the drug concentration does not become too high and cause toxicity. Similarly, if the desired effect is not easily visualized because of other considerations, such as inflammation in an internal organ, this approach is also problematic (Fig. 3.13, *Drug C*). Finally, changes in the condition of the patient can also necessitate adjustments in dose rates. For example, if a drug is eliminated through the kidneys, changes in renal function will be important. Without an observable effect that is easily monitored (as with drugs *B* and *C*), it is not always clear that such adjustments are beneficial.

An alternative approach is to define a target drug concentration in blood rather than an observable effect. The **plasma concentration** of a drug is usually chosen for simplicity and can be very useful in achieving therapeutic responses while minimizing undesirable side effects. In most clinical situations, it is important to maintain an appropriate response for prolonged periods. This requires maintaining a plasma concentration of drug over a specified time interval. Multiple doses or continuous administration is usually required, with dose size and frequency of administration constituting the dosing schedule or dosing regimen. In providing instructions for treatment of a patient, the choice of drug, the dosing schedule, and the mode and route of administration must be specified. Pharmacokinetic considerations have a major role in establishing the dosing schedule, or in adjusting an existing schedule, to increase effectiveness of the drug or to reduce symptoms of toxicity.

Dose Adjustments for Size of Patient

The average male adult weighs approximately 70 kg and has a body surface area of 1.7 m². The dose of drug is sometimes scaled to give a constant mg/kg body weight for persons of different sizes. For some drugs, especially with children, such scaling works better when based on body surface area because this correlates better with cardiac output and glomerular filtration rate. Body weight is favored by most clinicians because it is easily measured. Because therapeutic plasma concentrations of many drugs can cover a considerable range without evidence of toxicity, significant dose adjustments for patient size are required only in certain cases.

Routes of Drug Administration

Major routes of drug administration include enteral administration, which refers to drugs entering the body via the GI tract, and parenteral administration, which refers to drugs entering the body by injection; specific examples of each are presented in Box 3.1. The oral route of drug administration is most popular because it is most convenient. However, poor absorption in the GI tract, first-pass metabolism in the liver, delays in stomach emptying, degradation by stomach acidity, or forming complexes with food or food components may preclude this route; intramuscular (IM), subcutaneous (SC), and topical routes bypass these problems. In many cases, absorption into the blood is rapid for drugs given IM and only slightly slower after SC administration. The advantage of the intravenous (IV) route is a very rapid onset of action and a controlled rate of administration; however, this is countered by the disadvantages of possible infection, coagulation problems, and a greater incidence of allergic reactions. Also, most injected drugs, especially when given IV, require trained personnel.

Single IV Dose and Plasma Concentration

If a drug is injected into a vein as a single bolus over 5 to 30 seconds and blood samples are taken periodically and analyzed for the drug, the results appear as in Fig. 3.14, A, with the concentration of drug

BOX 3.1 Main Routes of Drug Administration

Per os (by mouth)
    Oral (swallowed)
    Sublingual (under the tongue)
    Buccal (in the cheek pouch)
Injection
    IV (intravenous)
    IM (intramuscular)
    SC (subcutaneous)
    IA (intraarterial)
    Intrathecal (into subarachnoid space)
Pulmonary
Rectal
Topical
    Transdermal patch
    Crème

greatest shortly after injection, when distribution of drug in the circulatory system has reached equilibrium. This initial mixing of drug and blood (red blood cells and plasma) is essentially complete after several passes through the heart. Drug leaves the plasma by several processes including:

- distribution across membranes to tissue or other body fluids;
- excretion of unchanged drug by renal or biliary routes;
- metabolism to other active or inactive compounds; and
- exhalation through the lungs, if the drug is volatile.

Some of the drug in plasma is bound to proteins or other plasma constituents; this binding occurs very rapidly and usually renders the bound portion of the drug inactive. Similarly, a considerable fraction of the injected dose may pass through capillary walls and bind to extravascular tissue, also rendering this fraction of drug inactive. The plasma concentrations of drug plotted on the y-axis in Fig. 3.14 represent the sum of unbound and bound drug. Note that the concentration-time profile shows continuous curvature.

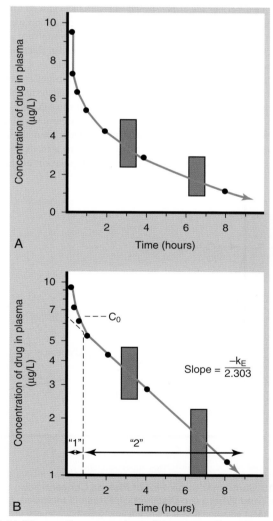

FIG. 3.14 Plasma Concentration of Drug as a Function of Time After IV Injection of a Single Bolus Over 5 to 30 Seconds. A, Arithmetic plot. B, Same data with concentrations plotted on a logarithmic scale. The 1 represents the distribution (or α) phase, and 2 represents the elimination (or β) phase. Fractional decrease in concentration is constant for a fixed time interval during the straight-line portion of B, shown here as an 18.6% decrease for any 1-hour period (shaded areas).

If concentrations are plotted on a logarithmic scale (Fig. 3.14, *B*), the terminal data points (after 1 hour) lie on a straight line. The section marked "1" on this graph represents the **distribution phase** (sometimes called **alpha phase**), representing the main process of drug distribution across membranes and into body regions that are not well perfused. Section "2" (**beta** or **elimination phase**) represents elimination of the drug, which gradually decreases plasma concentrations. In many clinical situations, the duration of the distribution phase is very short compared with that of the elimination phase.

If the distribution phase in Fig. 3.14 (*A* or *B*) is neglected, the equation of the line is:

$$C(t) = C_0 e^{-k_E t} \qquad (3.12)$$

where:

C(t) = concentration of drug in the plasma at any time
C_0 = concentration of drug in the plasma at time zero
e = base for natural logarithms
k_E = first-order rate constant for the elimination phase
t = time

Eq. 3.12 describes the curve shown in Fig. 3.14, *A* (on an arithmetic scale), that becomes a straight line in Fig. 3.14, *B* (on a semilogarithmic scale). In this case, the slope is $-k_E/2.303$, and the y-intercept is log C_0. A characteristic of this type of curve is that *a constant fraction of drug dose remaining in the body is eliminated per unit time.*

When elimination is rapid, the error describing C(t) becomes appreciable if the distribution phase is omitted. Although the mathematical derivation is beyond the scope of this text, such a situation is plotted in Fig. 3.15 to emphasize the importance of the distribution phase. For most drugs, distribution occurs much more rapidly than elimination, and therefore the distribution term becomes zero after only a small portion of the dose is eliminated. By back extrapolation of the linear

postdistribution data, the value of C_0 can be obtained, whereas k_E can be determined from the slope. The concentration component responsible for the distribution phase (shaded area in Fig. 3.15) is obtained as the difference between the actual concentration and the extrapolated elimination line. This difference can be used to calculate the rate constant for distribution (k_d) and the extrapolated time zero-concentration component for the distribution phase (C_0^d). However, this complexity is often ignored because the C(t) for many drugs can be described adequately in terms of the monoexponential Eq. 3.12. Therefore this chapter discusses only the postdistribution phase kinetics described by Eq. 3.12.

Single Oral Dose and Plasma Concentration

The plot of C(t) versus time after oral administration is different from that after IV injection only during the drug absorption phase, assuming equal bioavailability. The two plots become identical for the postabsorption or elimination phase. A typical plot of plasma concentration versus time after oral administration is shown in Fig. 3.16. Initially, there is no drug in the plasma because the preparation must be swallowed, undergo dissolution if administered as a tablet, await stomach emptying, and be absorbed, mainly in the small intestine. As the plasma concentration of drug increases as a result of rapid absorption, the rate of elimination also increases because elimination is usually a **first-order process**, where rate increases with increasing drug concentration. The peak concentration is reached when the rates of absorption and elimination are equal.

CALCULATION OF PHARMACOKINETIC PARAMETERS

As shown in Figs. 3.14 and 3.16, the concentration-time profile of a drug in plasma is different after IV and oral administration. The shape of the area under the concentration-time curve (AUC) is determined by several factors, including dose magnitude, route of administration, elimination capacity, and single or multiple dosing. The information derived from such profiles experimentally allows derivation of the important pharmacokinetic parameters of **clearance, volume of distribution, bioavailability**, and $t_{1/2}$. These terms are used to calculate drug dosing regimens.

Clearance

Drug clearance is defined as the volume of blood cleared of drug per unit time (e.g., mL/min) and describes the efficiency of elimination of a drug from the body. Clearance is an *independent* pharmacokinetic parameter; it does not depend on the volume of distribution, $t_{1/2}$, or bioavailability, and it is the most important pharmacokinetic parameter

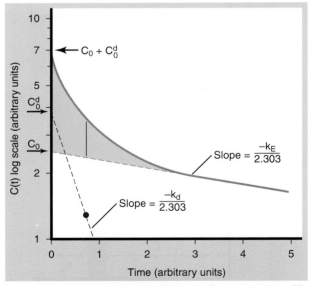

FIG. 3.15 Semilogarithmic Plot of Plasma Concentration of Drug Versus Time Where the Distribution Phase Is Included. Solid line represents an equation (not shown) governing distribution and elimination, which can be obtained using one of many available computer programs. This equation can also be obtained by graphical means in which extrapolation of the linear portion of the data (elimination phase) is used to obtain C_0 and k_E. The differences between the data points and the orange dotted extrapolated line in the distribution phase (vertical line at 0.65 time units and plotted as 1.3 concentration units shaded area) are plotted (blue dotted line) and extrapolated linearly to obtain C_0^d and k_d.

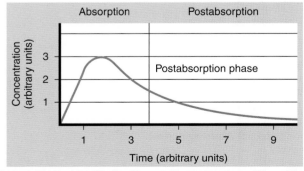

FIG. 3.16 Typical Profile for Plasma Concentration of Drug Versus Time After Oral Administration and With a Rate Constant for Drug Absorption of at Least 10 Times Larger Than That for Drug Elimination.

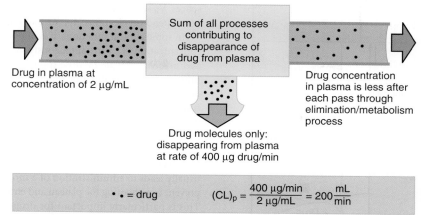

FIG. 3.17 Concept of Total Body Clearance of Drug From Plasma. Only some drug molecules disappear from plasma on each pass of blood through kidneys, liver, or other sites, contributing to drug disappearance (elimination). In this example, 200 mL of plasma was required to account for the amount of drug disappearance each minute (400 µg/min) at the concentration of 2 µg/mL. Total body clearance is thus 200 mL/min.

to know about any drug. It can be considered to be the volume of blood from which all drug molecules must be removed each minute to achieve such a rate of removal (Fig. 3.17). The mechanisms of clearance by renal, hepatic, and other organs have been described in this chapter. Total body clearance is the sum of all of these and is constant for a particular drug in a specific patient, assuming no change in patient status.

The plot of C(t) versus time (see Fig. 3.14) shows the concentration of drug decreasing with time. The corresponding elimination rate (e.g., mg/min) represents the quantity of drug being removed. The rate of removal is assumed to follow first-order kinetics, and total body clearance can be defined as follows:

$$CL_p = \text{rate of elimination of drug (mg/min)}/ \\ \text{plasma concentration of drug (mg/mL)} \quad \textbf{(3.13)}$$

where CL_p is plasma clearance and represents the total removal of drug from the plasma.

Clearance determines the maintenance dose rate required to achieve the target plasma concentration at steady state:

$$\text{Maintenance dose (mg/min)} = \text{target concentration (mg/mL)} \\ \times \text{clearance (mL/min)}$$

$$\textbf{(3.14)}$$

Thus for a given maintenance dose rate, steady-state drug concentration is inversely proportional to clearance.

Having determined that a drug is cleared mainly by hepatic mechanisms (metabolism) and having calculated a value for hepatic clearance (see Eq. 3.10), it is important to relate this to the functions (blood flow, enzyme activity) of liver. For example, if hepatic clearance of a drug is calculated to be 1000 mL/min and liver blood flow is 1500 mL/min, it does not mean that 1000 mL of blood going through liver is totally cleared of drug and the other 500 mL/min is not cleared of drug. It means that 1000/1500 (i.e., two-thirds) of the drug in blood entering liver is irreversibly removed (usually metabolized) by liver in one pass. The two-thirds refers to the **hepatic extraction ratio** (E), which is the fraction of the unbound dose of drug entering the liver from blood that is irreversibly eliminated (metabolized) during one pass through the liver.

$$\text{Extraction ratio (E)} = \text{rate of elimination/rate of entry} \quad \textbf{(3.15)}$$

Note that E can range from 0 (no extraction) to 1.0 (complete extraction). If Q is hepatic blood flow, then clearance by the liver can be described by the following equation:

$$CL = Q \times E \quad \textbf{(3.16)}$$

Thus clearance of a drug by any eliminating organ is a function of blood flow rate (rate of delivery) to the organ and the extraction ratio (efficiency of drug removal). It should now be clear that clearance of any drug cannot exceed the blood flow rate to its eliminating organ. In the case of drugs metabolized by liver, the maximum hepatic clearance value is approximately 1.5 L/min. For kidney, the maximum renal clearance value is 1.2 L/min (kidney blood flow).

For drugs cleared by the liver, hepatic clearance and bioavailability can be described in terms of three important physiologically based determinants: hepatic blood flow (Q), unbound fraction in plasma, and liver drug metabolizing activity.

Volume of Distribution

The actual volume in which drug molecules are distributed within the body cannot be measured. However, an apparent volume of distribution (V_d) can be obtained and is of some clinical utility. V_d is defined as the proportionality factor between the concentration of drug in blood or plasma and the total amount of drug in the body. Although it is a hypothetical term with no actual physical meaning, it can serve as an indicator of drug binding to plasma proteins or other tissue constituents. V_d can be calculated from the time zero concentration (C_0) after IV injection of a specified dose (D):

$$C_0 = D/V_d \quad \textbf{(3.17)}$$

If C_0 is in mg/L and D in mg, then V_d would be in L. In some cases, it is meaningful to compare the V_d with typical body H_2O volumes. The following volumes in liters and percentage of body weight apply to adult humans:

Body Weight	Body H₂O (percentage)	Volume (approx. liters)
Plasma	4	3
Extracellular	20	15
Total body	60	45

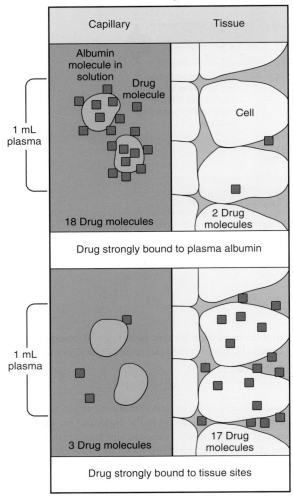

FIG. 3.18 Influence of Drug Binding to Plasma Protein Versus Tissue Sites on V_d. Numbers represent relative quantity of drug in 1 mL of plasma as compared with adjacent tissue. Only the plasma is sampled to determine V_d, and the albumin-bound drug is included in this sample.

Experimental values of V_d vary from 2 to 10 L for drugs, such as warfarin and furosemide, to 15,000 to 40,000 L for chloroquine and loratadine in a 70-kg adult. How can one have V_d values grossly in excess of the total body volume? This usually occurs as a result of different degrees of protein and tissue binding of drugs and using plasma as the sole sampling source for determination of V_d (Fig. 3.18). For a drug such as warfarin, which is 99% bound to plasma albumin at therapeutic concentrations, nearly all the initial dose is in the plasma; a plot of log $C(t)$ versus time, when extrapolated back to time zero, gives a large value for C_0 (for bound plus unbound drug). Using a rearranged Eq. 3.17, $V_d = D/C_0$, the resulting value of V_d is small (usually 2 to 10 L). At the other extreme is a drug such as chloroquine, which binds strongly to tissue sites but weakly to plasma proteins. Most of the initial dose is at tissue sites, thereby resulting in very small concentrations in plasma samples. In this case, a plot of log $C(t)$ versus time will give a small value for C_0 that can result in V_d values greatly in excess of total body volume.

V_d can serve as a guide in determining whether a drug is bound primarily to plasma or tissue sites or distributed in plasma or extracellular

spaces. V_d is also an *independent* pharmacokinetic parameter and does not depend on clearance, $t_{1/2}$, or bioavailability.

In some clinical situations, it is important to achieve the target drug concentration (C_{ss}) instantaneously. A **loading dose** is typically used and involves a single IV dose (bolus) before starting a continuous IV infusion, or a parenteral or oral dose at the start of discrete multiple dosing. Ideally, the loading dose is calculated to raise the plasma drug concentration immediately to the plateau target concentration. V_d determines the size of the loading dose as follows:

$$\text{Loading dose (mg)} = C_{ss}(\text{mg/L}) \times V_d(\text{L}) \qquad \textbf{(3.18)}$$

However, the uncertainty associated with V_d for individual patients usually leads to administration of a more conservative loading dose to prevent overshooting the plateau and encountering toxic concentrations. This is particularly important for drugs with a narrow TI.

Half-Life

Experimental data for many drugs demonstrate that the rates of drug absorption, distribution, and elimination are generally directly proportional to concentration. Such processes follow **first-order kinetics** because the rate varies with the first power of the concentration. This is shown quantitatively as:

$$dC(t)/dt = -k_E C(t) \qquad \textbf{(3.19)}$$

where $dC(t)/dt$ is the rate of change of drug concentration, and k_E is the **elimination rate constant**, which is negative because the concentration is being decreased by elimination.

Rate processes can also occur through **zero-order kinetics**, where the rate is independent of concentration. Two prominent examples are the metabolism of ethanol and phenytoin. Under such conditions, the process becomes saturated, and the rate of metabolism is independent of drug concentration.

The value of $t_{1/2}$ can be obtained directly from a graph of log $C(t)$ versus t (Fig. 3.14). Note that $t_{1/2}$ can be calculated following any route of administration (e.g., oral or SC). In practice, values of $t_{1/2}$ for the elimination phase range from several minutes to days or longer for different drugs.

Because the $t_{1/2}$ is a *dependent* pharmacokinetic parameter derived from the independent parameters of clearance (CL) and volume of distribution, it can be calculated as follows:

$$t_{1/2} = (0.693 \times V_d)/\text{CL} \qquad \textbf{(3.20)}$$

The $t_{1/2}$ determines how long it takes to reach steady state after multiple dosing or when dosage is altered and how long it takes to eliminate the drug from the body when dosing is ended. It is generally agreed that steady state is achieved after dosages of five half-lives. When dosing is terminated, most of the drug will have been eliminated after five half-lives (but could still exist as metabolites with longer half-lives).

Bioavailability and First-Pass Effect

Bioavailability (F) is defined as the fraction of the drug reaching the systemic circulation after administration. When a drug is administered by IV injection, the entire dose enters the circulation, and F is 100%. However, this is not true for most drugs administered by other routes, especially drugs given orally. Physical or chemical processes that account for reduced bioavailability include poor solubility, incomplete absorption in the GI tract, metabolism in the enterocytes lining the intestinal wall, efflux transport out of enterocytes back into the intestinal lumen, and rapid metabolism during the first pass of the drug through the liver. Processes involved in determining oral bioavailability are shown in Fig. 3.19.

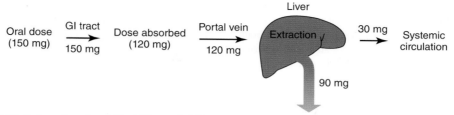

FIG. 3.19 Determinants of Oral Bioavailability. 150 mg of drug is swallowed, enters the lumen of the GI tract, and 120 mg is absorbed (30 mg is lost due to one or a combination of mechanisms) and enters the portal vein, which drains into the liver. The hepatic extraction ratio is 0.75, and the fraction escaping this first-pass loss is 0.25. Bioavailability is the fraction of the absorbed dose (0.8) entering the portal vein multiplied by the fraction escaping first-pass metabolism (0.25). In this example, bioavailability is 20% (or 30 mg/150 mg) (Modified from Birkett DJ: *Pharmacokinetics Made Easy*, McGraw-Hill Australia, 2002.)

Values of F can be determined by comparing the AUC for oral and IV doses:

$$F = (AUC)_{oral}/(AUC)_{IV} \times dose_{IV}/dose_{oral} \qquad (3.21)$$

In interpreting bioavailability, clearance is assumed to be independent of the route of administration. For drugs in which absorption from the GI tract is not always 100%, the drug formulations must now pass a stringent bioavailability test to verify that bioavailability is constant, within certain limits, among lots, and among generic formulations.

Low bioavailability can also result when the drug is well absorbed from the GI tract, but metabolism is high during its transit from the splanchnic capillary beds through the liver and into the systemic circulation. The drug concentration in the plasma is at its highest level during this first pass through the liver. Therefore drugs that are metabolized by the liver may encounter a very significant reduction in their plasma concentration during this first pass. For example, the first-pass effect of lidocaine is so large that this drug is not administered orally. Some drugs that show high first-pass effects include, but are not limited to, felodipine and propranolol (antihypertensives), isoproterenol (bronchodilator), methylphenidate (central nervous system stimulant), morphine and propoxyphene (analgesics), sumatriptan (antimigraine), and venlafaxine (antidepressant).

In summary, two calculations must be performed on plasma concentration-time data: the AUC and the terminal slope. These two calculations can then be used to calculate clearance, volume of distribution, $t_{1/2}$, and bioavailability.

Binding of Drug to Plasma Constituents

The degree of binding of a drug to plasma constituents is important because it helps with interpreting the mechanisms of clearance and volume of distribution. The free drug concentration is referred to as the unbound fraction. Some drugs, such as caffeine, have high unbound fractions (0.9), whereas other drugs, such as warfarin, have low unbound fractions (0.01).

The rates of drug disappearance and the concentration of free drug available to the site of action are altered substantially if a significant portion of the drug is bound to plasma constituents. Clinical tests for plasma drug concentrations are based on the total (bound plus unbound) concentration of drug and do not provide information about protein binding. A knowledge of the free drug concentration in plasma would be clinically useful because only the free drug is available to interact at its receptor(s); this information is rarely available.

The binding of drugs to plasma or serum constituents involves primarily albumin, α_1-acid glycoprotein, or lipoprotein (Table 3.3). Serum albumin is the most abundant protein in human plasma. It is

TABLE 3.3 **Drugs That Bind Appreciably to Serum or Plasma Constituents**		
Bind Primarily to Albumin	**Bind Primarily to α_1-Acid Glycoprotein**	**Bind Primarily to Lipoproteins**
Barbiturates	Alprenolol	Amphotericin B
Benzodiazepines	Bupivacaine	Cyclosporin
Bilirubin[a]	Dipyridamole	Tacrolimus
Digitoxin	Disopyramide	
Fatty acids[a]	Etidocaine	
Penicillins	Imipramine	
Phenylbutazone	Lidocaine[b]	
Phenytoin	Methadone	
Probenecid	Prazosin	
Streptomycin	Propranolol	
Sulfonamides	Quinidine	
Tetracycline	Sirolimus	
Tolbutamide	Verapamil	
Valproic acid		
Warfarin		

[a]May be displaced by drugs in some disease states.
[b]In the United Kingdom, the drug name is lignocaine.

synthesized in the liver at roughly 140 mg/kg of body weight/day under normal conditions, but this can change dramatically in certain disease states. Many acidic drugs bind strongly to albumin, but because of the normally high concentration of plasma albumin, drug binding does not saturate all the sites. Basic drugs bind primarily to α_1-acid glycoprotein, which is present in plasma at much lower concentrations than albumin but varies more widely between and within people as a result of disease. Less is known about drug binding to lipoproteins, although this is also often altered during disease.

MULTIPLE OR PROLONGED DOSING

As mentioned, most drugs require administration over a prolonged period to achieve the desired therapeutic effect. The two principal modes of administration used to achieve such prolonged effectiveness are continuous IV infusion or discrete multiple doses on a designated dosing schedule. The basic objective is to increase the plasma concentration of drug until a steady state is reached that produces the desired therapeutic effect with little or no toxicity. This steady-state concentration is then maintained for minutes, hours, days, weeks, or longer, as required.

Continuous Intravenous Infusion

Continuous IV infusion of a drug is used when it is necessary to obtain a rapid onset of action and maintain this action for an extended period under controlled conditions. This usually occurs in a hospital or emergency setting. During continuous infusion, the drug is administered at a fixed rate. The plasma concentration of a drug gradually increases and plateaus at a concentration where the rate of infusion equals the rate of elimination. A typical plasma concentration profile is shown in Fig. 3.20. The plateau is also known as the steady-state concentration (C_{ss}). Key points are:

- At steady state, the rate of drug input must equal the rate of drug disappearance.
- The input rate is the infusion rate (mg/min).
- Conversion of the steady-state concentration (mg/L) to the disappearance rate (mg/min) requires a knowledge of clearance (L/min).
- Thus at steady state, one calculates the maintenance dose rate = target concentration × clearance (see Eq. 3.14).

The plateau concentration is influenced by the infusion rate and the total body clearance. Of these factors, only the infusion rate can be easily modified. For example, if the plateau concentration is 2 ng/mL with an infusion rate of 16 µg/h, and it is determined that the concentration is too high such that 1.5 ng/mL would be better, this concentration can be achieved by decreasing the infusion rate by 25% to 12 µg/h, which should give a 25% decrease in the plateau concentration.

Dosing Schedule

Discrete multiple dosing is usually specified so that the size of the dose and T (the time between doses, or dosing interval) are fixed. Two considerations are important in selecting T. Smaller intervals result in minimal fluctuations in plasma drug concentration; however, the interval must be a relatively standard number of hours to ensure patient compliance. In addition, for oral dosing, the quantity must be compatible with the size of available preparations. Thus an oral dosing schedule of 28 mg every 2.8 hours is impractical because the drug is probably not available as a 28-mg tablet, and taking a tablet every 2.8 hours is completely impractical. More practical dosing intervals for patient compliance are every 6, 8, 12, or 24 hours.

Alterations in plasma concentration of drug versus time for multiple dosing by repeated IV injections is shown in Fig. 3.21. In *A*, T is selected so that all drug from the previous dose disappears before the next dose is injected, and there is no accumulation of drug; no plateau or steady state is reached. If a plateau concentration is desired, T must be short enough to ensure that some drug from the previous dose is still present when the next dose is administered. In this way, the plasma concentration gradually increases until the drug lost by elimination during T is equal to the dose of drug added at the start of T. When this is achieved, the mean concentration for each time period has reached a plateau. This stepwise accumulation is illustrated by *B* in Fig. 3.21, where a plot of plasma drug concentration versus time for multiple IV injections is shown, with T roughly equivalent to the $t_{1/2}$ of drug elimination. The average rate (over a dose interval) of drug input is constant at D/T (mg/min). The amount of drug eliminated is small during the first T but increases with drug concentration during subsequent intervals until the average rate of elimination and the average rate of input are equal. That is, the dose is eliminated during T. For significant accumulation, T must be at least as short as the $t_{1/2}$ and preferably shorter.

At the plateau, the C_{ss} is equal to the input dose rate divided by the clearance, just as for continuous infusion:

$$C_{ss} = (D/T)/CL_p \qquad (3.22)$$

This equation illustrates that the size of the dose or the duration of T can be changed to modify the mean plateau concentration of drug during multiple dosing regimens.

Duration of Time to Steady State

For a continuous IV infusion or a series of discrete multiple doses, the time to reach the plateau concentration or to move from one plateau concentration to another depends only on the $t_{1/2}$ of the drug. After 1 $t_{1/2}$, 50% of plateau steady-state concentration is achieved. In practice, steady state occurs when 95% of the plateau steady-state concentration has been achieved, which occurs after five $t_{1/2}$s. In summary, clearance determines the steady state concentrations, and $t_{1/2}$ determines when steady state has been achieved.

A practical example using these concepts and formulas is illustrated below.

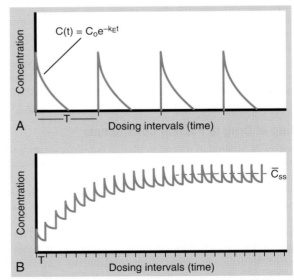

FIG. 3.21 Discrete Multiple-Dosing Profile of Plasma Concentration of Drug Given by IV Injections With the Same Dose Given Each Time. (A) Dosing interval (T) is long enough so that each dose completely disappears before administration of the next dose. (B) T is much shorter so that drug from previous injection is present before administration of the next dose. Accumulation results, with C_{ss} representing the mean concentration of drug at plateau level, where the mean rate of drug input equals the mean rate of drug elimination for each T. No loading dose is shown.

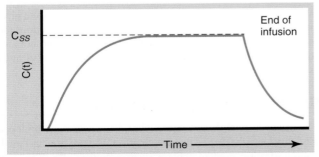

FIG. 3.20 Typical Profile Showing Drug Plasma Concentrations With Time for Continuous IV Injection (Infusion) at a Constant Rate and Without a Loading Dose. C_{ss} is the concentration at plateau, or steady state, where rate of drug input equals rate of drug elimination. At termination of infusion, decay in the concentration will be the same as for any acute IV injection, with C_o being equal to C_{ss}.

A patient received the cardiac drug digoxin orally at 0.25 mg (one tablet/day) for several weeks, and symptoms of toxicity have recently appeared. A blood sample was taken and indicated a plasma concentration of 3.2 ng/mL (in the toxic range). For therapeutic reasons, you do not want to drop the plasma concentration too low but decide to try to reduce it to 1.6 ng/mL. What new dosing schedule should be used, and how long will it take to reach the new plateau?

The once-a-day dosing interval is convenient, so you now specify 0.125 mg/day (one-half tablet/day); a 50% reduction in the plateau level requires a 50% decrease in dose. There are two options for reaching the lower plateau: (1) immediately switch to the 0.125-mg/day dosing rate and achieve the 1.6-ng/mL concentration in approximately five half-lives (you do not know what the $t_{1/2}$ for digoxin is in your patient), or (2) stop the digoxin dosing for an unknown number of days until the concentration reaches 1.6 ng/mL, and then begin again at a dosing schedule of 0.125 mg/day. The second procedure undoubtedly will be more rapid, but you must determine how many days to wait. You decide to stop all digoxin dosing, wait 24 hours from the previous 3.2 ng/mL sample, and get another blood sample. The concentration now has decreased to 2.7 ng/mL, or by approximately one-sixth in a day. From Eq. 3.12, the fractional decrease each day should remain constant. Therefore a decrease of one-sixth of the remaining concentration each day should result in 2.25 ng/mL after day 2, 1.85 ng/mL after day 3, and 1.55 ng/mL after day 4. Therefore by withholding drug for a total of 4 days, you can reduce the plasma concentration to 1.6 ng/mL. Because the $t_{1/2}$ is calculated to be 3.8 days in this patient, switching to the 0.125 mg/day dosing rate without withholding drug would have required 15 to 19 days to reach the 1.6-ng/mL concentration.

SPECIAL POPULATIONS AND DISEASE CONSIDERATIONS

Pharmacokinetic, pharmacodynamic, and pharmacological responses differ between young adults and infants and between young adults and the elderly. These differences are due to the many physiological changes that occur during the normal life span, but especially at the extremes—infants and the elderly (Fig. 3.22). In addition to age considerations, disease states, particularly those affecting the hepatic and renal systems, have significant effects on drug disposition and actions.

Neonates

The limited understanding of the clinical pharmacology of specific drugs in pediatric patients predisposes this population to problems in the course of drug treatment, particularly in younger children, such as newborns. The absence of specific FDA requirements for pediatric studies and the resulting reliance on pharmacological and efficacy data derived primarily from adults to determine doses for use of drugs in children calls for suboptimal drug therapy. The problems of establishing efficacy and dosing guidelines for infants are further complicated by the fact that the pharmacokinetics of many drugs change appreciably as an infant ages from birth (sometimes prematurely) to several months after birth. The dose-response relationships of some drugs may change markedly during the first few weeks after birth.

The physiological changes that occur during the first month include higher than normal gastric pH, prolonged gastric emptying (compounded by gastroesophageal reflux, respiratory distress syndrome, and congenital heart disease), lower adipose tissue and higher total body H_2O content, decreased plasma albumin, drug metabolizing activity, glomerular filtration, and tubular secretion. These result in decreased drug clearance and oral absorption and increased volume of distribution for H_2O-soluble drugs but decreased volume of distribution for lipid-soluble drugs.

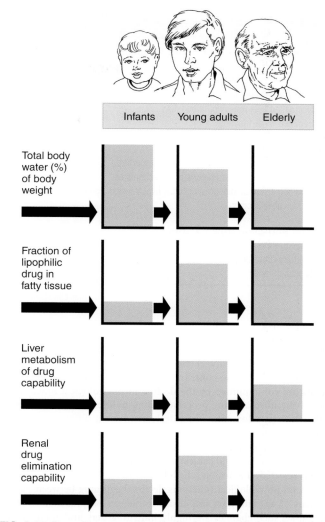

FIG. 3.22 Drug Pharmacokinetics Relative to Patient Age. Areas of boxes indicate the relative size or capability of function at each age.

Because of these dramatic and continuously changing parameters, dosing in neonates (<28 days) requires the advice of specialists.

Because of the often-compromised cardiac output and peripheral perfusion of seriously ill infants, IV drug administration is generally used to ensure adequate systemic delivery of the agent. The potential problems with such treatment can be serious, and minimizing such problems requires the dilution and timed administration of small dosage volumes, the maintenance of fluid balance, and consideration of the effect of the specific drug administration technique on resultant serum concentrations.

Certain drugs pose particular difficulties when used in neonates or during the perinatal period because of the unique characteristics of their distribution or elimination in patients in this age group or because of the unusual side effects they may cause. These drugs include antibiotics, digoxin, methylxanthine, and indomethacin.

The Aged Population

The rational use of drugs by the elderly population (>65 years) is a challenge for both patient and prescriber. Compared with young adults, the elderly have an increased incidence of chronic illness and multiple diseases, take more drugs (prescription and over-the-counter) and drug

BOX 3.2   Factors Contributing to Altered Drug Effects in the Elderly

Altered Drug Absorption and Disposition
Decreased gastric acid
Decreased lean body mass
Increased percentage of body fat
Decreased liver mass and blood flow
Reduced renal function

Altered Response to Drug
Altered receptor and/or postreceptor properties
Impaired sensitivity of homeostatic mechanisms
Common diseases: diabetes, arthritis, hypertension, coronary artery disease, cancer, glaucoma

Social and Economic Factors
Inadequate nutrition
Multiple-drug therapy
Noncompliance

combinations, and have more adverse drug reactions. Inadequate nutrition, decreased financial resources, and poor adherence to medication schedules may also contribute to inadequate drug therapy. These factors are compounded by the decline in physiological functions as part of the normal aging process, leading to altered drug disposition and sensitivity (Box 3.2). The elderly can have a different and more variable response to drugs compared with young adults. Drug selection and decisions about dosage in the elderly are largely based on trial and error, anecdotal data, and clinical impression. After the most appropriate drug is selected, the dosing schedule should be "start low, go slow."

Several physiological functions decline beginning between 30 and 45 years of age and have important influences on pharmacokinetics. Of course, such changes are highly individualized, and some elderly people show few changes compared with population means. Cardiac output decreases by approximately 1% a year beginning at 30 years of age and, in the elderly, is associated with a redistribution of blood flow favoring the brain, heart, and kidney and a reduction in hepatic blood flow. The percent of lean body mass also declines with age, whereas total body H_2O decreases by 10% to 15% between 20 and 80 years of age. Although plasma albumin concentrations are slightly lower in the elderly, chronically ill or poorly nourished individuals may have decreases of 10% to 20%. Concentrations of α_1-acid glycoprotein increase but do so more sharply in response to acute illness than simply aging. Glomerular filtration rate and effective renal plasma flow decline steadily with advancing age, although the serum creatinine concentration does not because of the smaller lean body mass. The tubular secretory capacity declines in parallel with the glomerular filtration rate.

Aging is also accompanied by impaired homeostatic mechanisms. Aging is often associated with decreased activity of aortic and carotid body chemoreceptors, reduced baroreceptor reflexes, impaired thermoregulation, inappropriate response of blood glucose and insulin to glucose, and altered neurological control of bowel and bladder. All of these may contribute to drug toxicity. The decreased baroreflex sensitivity may lead to an increased risk of orthostatic (postural) hypotension. This is a common problem in elderly patients taking some of the phenothiazines and antidepressants (those with significant α_1-adrenergic antagonist properties), nitrates, diuretics, and some antihypertensives, such as prazosin and α-methyldopa. Multiple mechanisms are implicated

in the impaired thermoregulation seen in many elderly people and include an absence of shivering, failure of metabolic rate to rise, poor vasoconstriction, and insensitivity to a low body temperature. Chlorpromazine and many other psychoactive drugs may cause hypothermia, and alcohol tends to augment this effect.

Drug Absorption, Distribution, and Metabolism

Several physiological alterations in GI function have been reported to occur with aging, although there is little clinically significant alteration in drug absorption in the elderly. One exception is a threefold increase in the bioavailability of L-DOPA, stemming from the reduced activity of dopa decarboxylase in the stomach wall.

The reduced lean body mass, reduced total body H_2O content, increased fat, and decreased plasma albumin concentration in the elderly can contribute to significant alterations in drug distribution, depending on the physiochemical properties of individual drugs. Lipid-soluble drugs, such as diazepam and lidocaine, have a larger V_d in the elderly, whereas H_2O-soluble drugs, such as acetaminophen and ethanol, have a smaller V_d. Digoxin also has a lower V_d in the elderly, and therefore loading doses must be reduced.

The decline in the ability of the elderly to metabolize most drugs is relatively small and difficult to predict. In general, phase I metabolic reactions decrease slightly with aging, whereas conjugation reactions, such as glucuronidation, are not greatly affected. The effects of cigarette smoking, diet, and alcohol consumption may be more important than physiological changes. For example, decreased dietary protein intake or reduction in cigarette smoking may lead to decreased liver microsomal enzyme activity. Whereas hepatic enzyme inhibition by drugs is similar in the elderly compared with young adults, the response to enzyme inducers (cigarette smoke, drugs, etc.) is more variable.

Drug Clearance and Elimination

For drugs with a high hepatic clearance, the age-related decline in total liver blood flow of approximately 40% results in a similar reduction in total body clearance. The effect on first-pass hepatic extraction (and hence bioavailability) is complicated by potential alterations in other physiological variables such as protein binding and enzyme activity. In healthy elderly subjects, first-pass metabolism and bioavailability are generally not markedly altered. However, on chronic oral dosing, the higher plasma concentrations often observed in the elderly are the result of reduced phase I metabolism, irrespective of whether the drug has a high or low hepatic clearance.

Most hepatically eliminated drugs are classified as being either of low or high (hepatic) clearance. This makes it possible to predict the influence of altered liver function or drug interactions on plasma concentrations and pharmacological response. For example, metabolism of a drug is often reduced in patients with liver disease or when a second drug inhibits its metabolic enzyme. For a high-clearance drug, this results in no change in the plasma concentration-time profile after IV dosing because blood flow is the sole determinant of clearance (whereas plasma and tissue binding are determinants of V_d). However, when the drug is administered orally, a decrease in metabolism will result in a small reduction in E and therefore a large increase in bioavailability, resulting in substantially increased plasma concentrations. For a low hepatic clearance drug, a decrease in metabolism will cause increased concentrations after IV dosing because metabolism is a determinant of clearance. There will be no change in bioavailability, however, because that is already close to 100%. On the other hand, concentrations after oral dosing will be raised because clearance has decreased. The outcome of this scenario is that for a low-clearance drug, both the oral and IV dose may need to be reduced to avoid toxicity, but for a high-clearance drug, only the oral dose may need adjustment.

Consistent with the physiological decline in renal function that occurs with aging, the rate of elimination of drugs excreted by the kidney is reduced. Such drugs include aminoglycosides, lithium carbonate, metformin, allopurinol (due to its active metabolite), and digoxin. To prevent drug toxicity, renal function must be estimated and downward adjustments in dosage made accordingly. Although there are no absolute guidelines, two general principles apply. First, most elderly patients do not have "normal" renal function even though serum creatinine appears "normal." Second, most elderly patients require adjustments in dosage for drugs (or drugs with active metabolites) eliminated primarily by the kidneys.

Thus it is important to know which drugs are eliminated via renal or hepatic mechanisms. If the latter is the case, then it is important to characterize the drug as being of low or high clearance. If low, enzyme activity and binding are determinants of clearance, and bioavailability is unchanged. If high, liver blood flow is the sole determinant of clearance, and blood flow, binding, and enzyme activity all affect bioavailability. From these parameters, it is then often possible to predict the effect of disease (e.g., liver, cardiac) and administration of other drugs on the resultant pharmacokinetics of the drug, which helps in designing a rational dosage regimen.

The decreased rate of elimination of inhalation anesthetics, resulting from declining pulmonary function with aging, is another important consideration for elderly patients receiving general anesthesia.

Disease-Induced Changes

It is common for elderly patients to have multiple chronic diseases such as diabetes, glaucoma, hypertension, coronary artery disease, and arthritis. The presence of multiple diseases leads to the use of multiple medications. Many elderly patients receive as many as 12 drugs concurrently, resulting in many opportunities for drug-drug interactions and adverse drug reactions (Table 3.4).

A drug interaction refers to a change in magnitude or duration of the pharmacological response of one drug because of the presence of another drug. Drug interactions can cause either more rapid or slower elimination, with plasma concentrations increasing or decreasing above or below minimum effective values. There are many mechanisms by which drugs interact, including acceleration or inhibition of metabolism, displacement

TABLE 3.4 **Drug-Disease Interactions**	
Drug	**Disease**
Ibuprofen, other NSAIDs	GI tract hemorrhage, increased blood pressure, renal impairment
Digoxin	Dysrhythmias
Levothyroxine	Coronary artery disease
Prednisone, other glucocorticoids	Peptic ulcer disease
Verapamil, diltiazem	Congestive heart failure
Propranolol, other β-adrenergic antagonists	Congestive heart failure, chronic obstructive pulmonary disease

NSAIDs, Nonsteroidal antiinflammatory drugs; GI, gastrointestinal.

of plasma protein binding, impaired absorption, altered renal clearance, modifications in receptors, and changes in electrolyte balance, body fluid pH, or rates of protein synthesis. Many drug interactions are well documented in the literature, and these potential interactions should be taken into account when multiple drugs are prescribed.

Moreover, a disease may increase the risk of adverse drug reactions or preclude the use of the otherwise most effective or safest drug for treatment of another problem. For example, anticholinergic drugs may cause urinary retention in men with enlarged prostate glands or precipitate glaucoma, and drug-induced hypotension may cause ischemic events in patients with vascular disease.

It is critical to appreciate that many drugs exhibit narrower therapeutic indexes when used in the elderly. The impact of the physiological changes that occur with aging alter the pharmacokinetics and pharmacodynamics of drugs and predispose the elderly to adverse drug effects. This is amplified by their reduced physiological compensatory capacity. Practical considerations when prescribing for the elderly include (1) use nonpharmacological approaches when possible; (2) use the lowest possible dose and the smallest dose increment ("start low, go slow"); (3) use the smallest number of medications; (4) regularly review drug treatments and potential interactions; and (5) recognize that any new symptoms may be caused by the drugs prescribed and not by the aging process.

SUMMARY

Understanding the major routes of disposition of a drug and the factors that influence the functionality and capacity of each route can aid profoundly in the safe and effective use of drugs, especially in patients in whom the state of the disease has compromised one or more of the main drug disposition routes.

Pharmacokinetics provides a firm basis for the design of dosing regimens and characterization of the kinetics of drug disposition, although many parameters must be taken into account for such rational design, particularly at the extremes of age. The major points include:
- clearance;
- bioavailability and first-pass metabolism;
- half-life;
- the effects of plasma protein binding;
- the concept of the V_d;
- the exponential disposition of drug (first-order decline), in which a constant fraction of drug is disposed of per unit time;

- the concept that the rates of drug input and elimination are equal at the steady-state or plateau concentrations;
- how to modify a dosing regimen to achieve a desired change in plateau concentration;
- the concept that the time to reach plateau depends only on the elimination $t_{1/2}$ of the drug, and the plateau concentration is determined by clearance;
- the use of a loading dose to accelerate the onset of the desired therapeutic effect;
- the requirement for special expertise in determining drug dosage in neonates;
- changes in pharmacodynamic and pharmacokinetic parameters associated with aging; and
- simultaneous administration of multiple drugs can alter their disposition and bioavailability.

SELF-ASSESSMENT QUESTIONS

1. Cell membranes are composed of:
   A. Phospholipids.
   B. Receptor proteins.
   C. DNA.
   D. *A* and *B*.
   E. All of the above are correct.

2. The plasma concentration of drug in a 40-year-old male would be increased by which of the following mechanisms?
   A. Metabolic biotransformation.
   B. Renal tubular reabsorption.
   C. Binding to plasma proteins.
   D. Renal secretion.
   E. Biliary excretion.

3. Drugs A, B, C, and D have lipid:water partition coefficients of 0.1, 1.0, 10, and 100, respectively. Which of these drugs will cross membranes the fastest?
   A. A.
   B. B.
   C. C.
   D. D.
   E. Cannot be determined based on the information provided.

4. The percent of the unionized (HA) form of a weak acid with a pK_a greater than 7 will be greatest in which body compartment?
   A. The gastric juice with a pH of 2.
   B. The duodenum with a pH of 5.5.
   C. The cerebrospinal fluid (CSF) with a pH of 7.3.
   D. The ileum and large intestine with a pH of 8.
   E. The urine with a pH of 4-8.

5. Drugs A, B, C, D, and E have therapeutic indices of 2, 5, 15, 20, and 50, respectively. Based on this, which drug has the lowest potential to have adverse or toxic effects?
   A. A.
   B. B.
   C. C.
   D. D.
   E. E.

6. The time it takes for the body to decrease the levels of drug in the circulation by half is known as:
   A. Clearance.
   B. Bioavailability.
   C. Time of distribution.
   D. Half-life.
   E. First pass

FURTHER READING

Bartelink IH, Rademaker CM, Schobben AF, van den Anker JN. Guidelines on paediatric dosing on the basis of developmental physiology and pharmacokinetic considerations. *Clin Pharmacokinet.* 2006;45:1077–1097.

Bauer LA. *Applied Clinical Pharmacokinetics.* New York: McGraw Hill; 2001.

Birkett DJ. *Pharmacokinetics Made Easy.* Sydney: McGraw Hill; 2002.

Guengerich FP. Mechanisms of cytochrome P450 substrate oxidation: MiniReview. *J Biochem Mol Toxicol.* 2007;21:163–168.

Tompkins LM, Wallace AD. Mechanisms of cytochrome P450 induction. *J Biochem Mol Toxicol.* 2007;21:176–181.

Pharmacogenetics

Larisa H. Cavallari, Scott A. Mosley, and Julie A. Johnson

The term **pharmacogenetics** was first coined in the 1950s when it was recognized that toxicities to certain drugs showed inheritance patterns among families and/or were more common in individuals from one continental population than others. However, advances in the 1990s in molecular genetic tools facilitated discovery of the molecular genetic basis for these differences, after which the field of pharmacogenetics progressed. Since that time, there has been extensive work investigating genetic variations that influence drug efficacy, toxicity, and dose requirements. As molecular genetic technologies advanced, it became possible to study the entire genome, and thus the term **pharmacogenomics** began to enter common usage in the early 2000s. In fact, most discovery work at present takes a genome-wide pharmacogenomics approach. In this chapter, the term *pharmacogenetics* is used because at the clinical practice level, it is typically one or a few genes that guide treatment decisions.

Advances in pharmacogenetics during the past two decades have led to clinically actionable examples in which genetic variation provides sufficient predictive value to be useful in the clinical setting and help guide decisions about drug therapy. Several variations affecting both the capacity of individuals to transport and metabolize drugs (**pharmacokinetics**) and the effect of drugs at target sites (**pharmacodynamics**) have been identified to determine:

- why some drugs are effective for specific conditions in some patients, but not others; and
- why some individuals exhibit marked adverse reactions to a particular drug while others do not.

One important advance for translating pharmacogenetic research findings to clinical practice was the formation of the **Clinical Pharmacogenetics Implementation Consortium (CPIC)** in 2009. The CPIC is an international collaboration of experts in pharmacogenetics with clinicians, regulatory scientists, and others interested in advancing the field. The objective of the CPIC is to provide a robust review of the literature on a given drug and relevant genes that may be useful to guide drug selection or dosing in clinical practice. The CPIC uses a standardized process for literature query, with a grading system of individual studies and a systematic approach to grading recommendations. The purpose of the CPIC is not to make recommendations on whether a pharmacogenetic test should be ordered but what to do with the information if it is available on a patient. The philosophy that underpins this approach is the expectation that sometime in the near future, genetic information will be widely available on patients and in the electronic health record, and the clinician will need to know when and how to use that information. At present, the CPIC does not provide guidelines for the use of **somatic** (tumor) variations to guide drug therapy but rather focuses on **germline** (inherited) genetic variations.

It is anticipated that use of pharmacogenetic information to guide clinical decisions about drugs will become increasingly common, and practicing clinicians will need to be prepared to add this knowledge to their clinical toolkit. This chapter provides context for the general principles underlying pharmacogenetics and focuses on examples currently being employed in healthcare settings for which there are CPIC guidelines. In addition, information on cancer drugs that are guided based on somatic mutations is also included.

ABBREVIATIONS

ALL	Acute lymphoblastic leukemia
ALK	Anaplastic lymphoma kinase
ATP	Adenosine triphosphate
BCR-ABL	Breakpoint cluster region-Abelson murine leukemia
BRAF	v-Raf murine sarcoma viral oncogene homolog B
CML	Chronic myelogenous leukemia
CPIC	Clinical Pharmacogenetics Implementation Consortium
CRC	Colorectal cancer
CYP	Cytochrome P450 enzyme
DPD	Dihydropyrimidine dehydrogenase
DPYD	Dihydropyrimidine dehydrogenase gene
EGFR	Epidermal growth factor receptor
ER	Estrogen receptor
5-FU	5-Fluorouracil
FDA	United States Food and Drug Administration
HER2	Human epidermal growth factor receptor 2
HLA-B	Human leukocyte antigen-B
IM	Intermediate metabolizer
INR	International normalized ratio
KRAS	Kirsten rat sarcoma viral oncogene homolog
MHC	Major histocompatibility complex
NCCN	National Comprehensive Cancer Network
NM	Normal metabolizer
NSCLC	Non–small cell lung cancer
OATP	Organic anion transporting polypeptide
PM	Poor metabolizer
PPI	Proton pump inhibitor
PR	Progesterone receptor
RM	Rapid metabolizer
SSRI	Selective serotonin reuptake inhibitor
TCA	Tricyclic antidepressant
TGMP	Thioguanosine monophosphate
TKI	Tyrosine kinase inhibitor
TPMT	Thiopurine *S*-methyltransferase
UM	Ultra-rapid metabolizer
VKOR	Vitamin K epoxide reductase

GENES AFFECTING PHARMACOKINETICS: DRUG METABOLISM AND DRUG TRANSPORTERS

Genetic variations affecting drug-metabolizing enzymes and drug transporters are important sources of variability in drug pharmacokinetics and can lead to increased or decreased enzyme or transporter function. In cases where a drug is metabolized to an inactive form, genetic variation resulting in reduced metabolizing enzyme activity can lead to increased drug plasma concentrations with the potential for increased efficacy and/or an increased risk for toxicity. Alternatively, in cases where a metabolizing enzyme converts a prodrug to its pharmacologically active form, genetic variations resulting in reduced enzyme activity may lead to subtherapeutic drug concentrations and increased risk for treatment failure. Genetic polymorphisms in *CYP* genes confer four to five major CYP phenotypes: poor metabolizer (PM), intermediate metabolizer (IM), normal metabolizer (NM), rapid metabolizer (RM), and ultrarapid metabolizer (UM), as shown in Table 4.1.

Similarly, genotypes for drug transporter proteins can influence the distribution of drugs and drug concentrations at their site of action, influencing the risk for adverse effects or treatment failure.

Cytochrome 450s (CYPs)

The *CYP2D6*, *CYP2C19*, *CYP2C9*, and *CYP3A5* genes have common genetic variations that lead to significant effects on enzyme function, leading to significant implications for drug safety and efficacy. It should be noted that throughout this chapter, by convention, genes will be italicized while enzymes will not.

CYP2D6

The CYP2D6 enzyme metabolizes approximately 25% of medications, including some opioid analgesics and most antidepressants. More than 130 known variants with 75 formally recognized alleles have been reported, with several leading to decreased or no enzyme function (*3, *4, *9, and *17) and others (*1 or *2 duplications) leading to increased enzyme function. The implication of *CYP2D6* genetic variations on drug response depends on whether the drug substrate is a prodrug that requires enzyme-mediated activation or an active drug that relies on the enzyme for conversion to inactive metabolites (Fig. 4.1). In the case of the opioid analgesics codeine and tramadol, CYP2D6 is required to convert these drugs to their more active metabolites, morphine and O-desmethyltramadol, respectively. PMs cannot activate codeine or tramadol and thus will derive little to no analgesic effects from these drugs. On the other hand, UMs can rapidly convert codeine and tramadol to their active forms, potentially leading to toxic plasma concentrations of the active metabolites and increasing the risk for opioid toxicity. Incidents of serious toxicity, especially in children, have been reported following exposure of individuals with the UM phenotype to codeine or tramadol. This prompted the FDA to issue a safety communication regarding the increased risk of life-threatening adverse effects in children with the UM phenotype treated with codeine after tonsillectomy or adenoidectomy for obstructive sleep apnea syndrome. Guidelines from the CPIC recommend the use of analgesics that do not depend on CYP2D6 for bioactivation for both PMs and UMs.

In the case of selective serotonin reuptake inhibitors (SSRIs) and tricyclic antidepressants (TCAs), which are administered in their active forms, the CYP2D6 PM phenotype can lead to greater drug exposure and an increased risk for adverse effects. The CPIC guidelines for SSRIs focus on paroxetine and fluvoxamine, for which the largest amount of data has accumulated. The recommendation is for clinicians to consider lower starting doses or an alternative SSRI not predominantly metabolized by CYP2D6 for PMs. Similarly, the CPIC guidelines recommend lower doses of TCAs for IMs and either avoidance of TCAs or use of lower

TABLE 4.1	The Major CYP Phenotypes
Phenotype	**Characterization**
Poor metabolizer (PM) (individuals with little to no enzyme function)	Homozygous for two no-function alleles (e.g., *CYP2C19*2/*2*, or *CYP2D6 *4/*5*) or, in the case of *CYP2C9*, combination of two decreased function alleles (e.g., *CYP2C9*2/*3*)
Intermediate metabolizer (IM) (individuals with reduced enzyme decreased enzyme function)	One normal function and one no-function allele (e.g., *CYP2C19*1/*2*), one normal function and one decreased function allele (e.g., *CYP2C9*1/*2* or one no function and one decreased function allele (*CYP2D6*4/*10*)
Normal (extensive) metabolizer (NM) (individuals with normal, fully functional enzyme function)	Two normal function alleles (e.g., *CYP2C19*1/*1*) or, in the case of *CYP2D6*, one functional allele and one no-function allele (*CYP2D6*1/*4*) or two decreased function alleles (*CYP2D6*10/*10*)
Rapid metabolizer (RM) (individuals with increased enzyme function compared to normal metabolizers)	One normal function and one increased function allele (e.g., *CYP2C19*1/*17*)
Ultra-rapid metabolizer (UM) (individuals with increased enzyme function compared to rapid metabolizers)	Two increased function alleles (e.g., *CYP2C19*17/*17*) or multiple (>2) copies of normal function alleles (*CYP2D6*1/*2xN*)

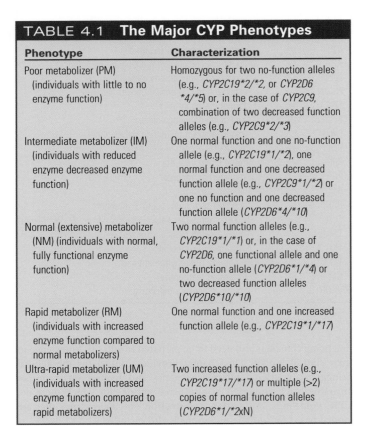

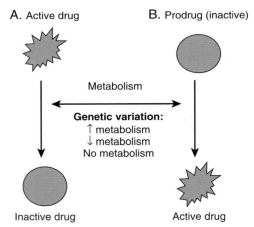

FIG. 4.1 The effect of genetic variation for drug-metabolizing enzymes on drug response depends on (1) whether the drug is a prodrug, requiring biotransformation, or administered in its active form; and (2) whether the variation leads to decreased or increased enzyme function. (A) For active drugs, genotypes conferring reduced or absent enzyme function can result in supratherapeutic drug plasma concentrations and increased risk for toxicity. Genotypes conferring increased enzyme activity can result in subtherapeutic drug concentrations and treatment failure. (B) For prodrugs that require enzymatic bioactivation, genotypes conferring reduced or absent enzyme function can result in subtherapeutic concentrations of the active drug and treatment failure. Genotypes conferring increased enzyme function can lead to supratherapeutic concentrations of the active drug and increased risk for toxicity.

TABLE 4.2 CYP2D6 and CYP2C19 Phenotypes and Their Prevalence Across Populations

Enzyme	Phenotype[a]	PREVALENCE		
		Whites	Blacks	East Asians
CYP2D6	PM	5%	2%–3%	0.5%
	IM	5%	10%–11%	5%
	NM	87%	82%–84%	94%
	UM	3%	4%	1%
CYP2C19	PM	2%	4%	15%
	IM	25%	30%	50%
	NM	33%	21%	30%–35%
	RM or UM	40%	45%	<5%

[a]For definition of phenotypes, see Table 4.1.

doses with therapeutic drug monitoring for PMs because of increased risk for toxicity. In contrast, the UM phenotype is associated with very low concentrations of SSRIs and TCAs and increased risk for drug ineffectiveness with usual doses. CPIC guidelines recommend avoiding paroxetine and TCAs in UMs or the use of higher TCA doses because of the potential lack of efficacy.

In addition to the drug groups mentioned, other drugs metabolized by CYP2D6 include the commonly prescribed β-blockers metoprolol and carvedilol, as well as the estrogen-receptor modulator tamoxifen, used to treat estrogen receptor–positive breast cancer.

The implications for *CYP2D6* gene variations noted above are significant when considering drug dosing for individuals from diverse populations. The frequencies of CYP2D6 phenotypes across populations are shown in Table 4.2. From this information, one might expect that the incidence of adverse effects associated with the administration of drugs inactivated by CYP2D6 would be greatest in the black population, in which the percent of individuals with poor or intermediate metabolism is greatest relative to whites or East Asians.

CYP2C19

Approximately 10% of drugs, including **clopidogrel** and **proton pump inhibitors (PPIs)**, are metabolized by CYP2C19. Similar to *CYP2D6*, 31 known variants of *CYP2C19* have been identified with 21 recognized alleles, whose frequency varies across racial and ethnic groups. Alleles *2 through *8 render nonfunctional enzymes, while *17 results in increased enzyme function.

The *CYP2C19* genotype significantly impacts the efficacy of clopidogrel in patients who undergo percutaneous coronary intervention. Clopidogrel is commonly prescribed in this population to prevent cardiovascular events such as myocardial infarction, stroke, and stent thrombosis. Clopidogrel is a prodrug that requires hepatic bioactivation to the pharmacologically active metabolite that inhibits platelet aggregation. The CYP2C19 enzyme has a major role in clopidogrel bioactivation, as shown in Fig. 4.2. Individuals with the PM or IM phenotype have a reduced ability to activate clopidogrel and are at increased risk for cardiovascular events and stent thrombosis after percutaneous coronary intervention. As a consequence of this finding, in 2010, the FDA approved a **boxed warning** on the clopidogrel labeling, the most serious kind of warning, regarding the likelihood for reduced drug effectiveness in PMs. CPIC guidelines recommend the use of alternative antiplatelet agents that are not affected by the *CYP2C19* genotype for PMs and IMs; tests are available to determine a patient's *CYP2C19* genotype.

The *CYP2C19* genotype may also influence the effectiveness of PPIs such as omeprazole, lansoprazole, and pantoprazole, which are commonly

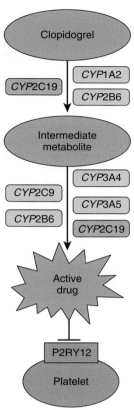

FIG. 4.2 Clopidogrel Metabolism. Clopidogrel is a prodrug that requires activation via a two-step process. CYP2C19 is involved in both steps.

prescribed for treatment of *Helicobacter pylori* infection, gastroesophageal reflux disease, and other indications. In this case, CYP2C19 metabolizes PPIs to their inactive forms, and reduced function is associated with increased plasma drug levels and effectiveness. Specifically, higher eradication rates of *H. pylori* have been reported in PMs and IMs compared to NMs; PMs and IMs may also be at increased risk for toxicity compared to NMs. Higher PPI doses may be needed for RMs and UMs to achieve response rates with PPIs that are similar to those achieved with usual doses for PMs and IMs.

Other drugs metabolized by CYP2C19 include the SSRIs citalopram, escitalopram, and sertraline and the anticonvulsants diazepam, phenytoin, and phenobarbital. The CPIC recommendations on dosing citalopram, escitalopram, and sertraline incorporate information based on genotype.

The prevalence of CYP2C19 phenotypes across different populations is shown in Table 4.2 and indicates that phenotype prevalence distributes very differently across populations. Asians have a higher prevalence of the PM and IM phenotypes (>60%) and a lower prevalence of the RM and UM phenotypes as compared to whites and blacks, with implications as discussed.

CYP2C9

Over 35 functionally relevant genetic polymorphisms have been identified in the gene for *CYP2C9*, which metabolizes approximately 15% of drugs, including the narrow therapeutic index drugs, warfarin and phenytoin. By far, the most commonly described *CYP2C9* alleles are *2 and *3, which result from nonsynonymous single-nucleotide polymorphisms that change an encoded amino acid and lead to decreased enzyme function. Approximately 30% of whites have a *2 or *3 allele compared to approximately 6% of blacks. About 6%–8% of Asians carry the *3 allele, but the *2 allele is rare to absent in this population. Additional decreased function alleles include *5, *6, *8, and *11, which occur almost exclusively in individuals of African ancestry. The *8 allele is the most common decreased function allele in African Americans, occurring in approximately 10%–12% of the population; when all decreased function alleles are considered, about 25% of African Americans have at least one decreased function allele.

The CYP2C9 genotype has important relevance for dosing warfarin, a commonly prescribed oral anticoagulant. Warfarin is a racemic mixture, and the more potent S-enantiomer is biotransformed by CYP2C9 to inactive metabolites. CYP2C9 decreased function alleles have been associated with reduced clearance of S-warfarin, reduced warfarin dose requirements, and an increased risk for bleeding. In fact, doses of warfarin 5- to 10-fold lower than usual may be required in patients homozygous for decreased function alleles (e.g., *2/*3 or *3/*3). The FDA-approved labeling for warfarin includes dosing recommendations based on CYP2C9 genotype (in addition to the VKORC1 genotype discussed below), and CPIC guidelines are available to further assist with genotype-guided warfarin dosing. Similarly, per the CPIC guidelines, at least a 25% reduction in the starting dose of the anticonvulsant phenytoin is recommended for patients with the heterozygous genotype (e.g., *1/*3), and at least a 50% dose reduction should be considered in homozygotes to reduce the risk for drug toxicity.

CYP3A5

The CYP3A family (CYP3A4/3A5) is responsible for metabolism of the largest number of drugs, and the CYP3A5 enzyme contains a common inactivating polymorphism. The CYP3A5*3 allele occurs secondary to an aberrant splice site in intron 3. The CYP3A5 *3/*3 genotype is associated with complete loss of CYP3A5 expression and enzyme function and is the most common genotype observed across populations. Individuals with the *3/*3 genotype are termed nonexpressors, meaning they do not express a functional protein, whereas those with the *1/*1 or *1/*3 genotype are termed expressors. Most whites are nonexpressors, with only about 15%–20% being expressors. In contrast, about 50% of blacks and 30%–40% of Asians are CYP3A5 expressors. CYP3A5 is involved in the metabolism of tacrolimus, an immunosuppressant frequently used after solid organ transplantation to prevent rejection. Expressors are at risk for subtherapeutic plasma concentrations of tacrolimus with usual doses, placing them at increased risk for organ rejection. The CPIC guidelines recommend initiating tacrolimus for CYP3A5 expressors at doses that are 1.5 to 2 times higher than usually prescribed.

Non-CYP450 Enzymes
Thiopurine S-Methyltransferase (TPMT)

Thiopurines are a class of antimetabolite prodrugs used for their antineoplastic and immunosuppressive properties and include azathioprine, thioguanine, and 6-mercaptopurine. Azathioprine is a prodrug metabolized to mercaptopurine and indicated for renal transplantation and rheumatoid arthritis; off-label uses include multiple sclerosis, Crohn disease, and ulcerative colitis. Thioguanine and mercaptopurine are an integral part of treatment for acute lymphoblastic leukemia (ALL) and lymphomas. These compounds are biotransformed by separate pathways to form thioguanosine monophosphate (TGMP), which is further metabolized to thioguanine nucleotides that are incorporated, as false metabolites, into DNA and RNA, leading to cell death. Just as the efficacy of thiopurine drugs is dependent on biotransformation, so is the toxicity. The enzyme TPMT is essential for metabolizing TGMP and mercaptopurine to inactive metabolites that are eliminated from the body. Clinically relevant gene alleles include TPMT *2 and *3, which code

for an enzyme with decreased function and account for over 90% of variant TPMT alleles. Decreased TPMT activity shunts the metabolic pathway to produce greater amounts of the cytotoxic thioguanine nucleotides. Approximately 11% of the population in the United States carries a single defective allele, while 1 in 300 are homozygous with no TPMT enzyme function. The risk of myelosuppression, a dose-limiting toxicity of thiopurines, is significantly greater in patients with defective TPMT function. When treated with conventional thiopurine doses, 35% of patients with the heterozygous genotype and 100% of homozygotes will require dose reductions, compared with only 7% of patients without mutations.

The drug labeling for thiopurine warns that there are individuals with a TPMT deficiency who may be prone to developing myelosuppression, but no recommendations for dose adjustments based on genotype are included. The National Comprehensive Cancer Network (NCCN) for ALL advocates for preemptive TPMT genotyping before initiating mercaptopurine or thioguanine as a safety precaution. The CPIC recommends 30%–70% dose reduction of thiopurines in heterozygotes and a 90% dose reduction in homozygotes.

DPYD

5-Fluorouracil (5-FU) and capecitabine, an oral prodrug metabolized to 5-FU, are pyrimidine antimetabolites used for the treatment of several malignancies, including colon, rectal, and breast cancers. Dihydropyrimidine dehydrogenase (DPD, encoded by the DPYD gene) is the rate-limiting enzyme responsible for inactivating >80% of 5-FU doses. Several DPYD nonfunctional alleles, *2A (rs3918290), *13 (rs55886062), and rs67376798, have been described, with approximately 3%–5% of patients heterozygous for these alleles and less than 0.5% homozygous. Patients with nonfunctional DYPD variants are at an increased risk for potentially life-threatening toxicities with 5-FU or capecitabine, including myelosuppression, gastrointestinal toxicities, mucositis, and hand-foot syndrome. Labeling for these drugs warns that, rarely, severe toxicity associated with 5-FU is attributed to DPD deficiency but provide no recommendations for testing or dose modifications based on genotype. The CPIC recommends alternative therapy for patients who are homozygous for DPYD nonfunctional alleles and a 50% dose reduction in 5-FU or capecitabine in heterozygotes.

Drug Transporter Genotypes

Drug transporter proteins mediate the transport of many medications across cell membranes, including the gastrointestinal tract, blood-brain barrier, and into the bile and urine. The organic anion transporting polypeptide (OATP) 1B1, which is encoded by the solute carrier organic anion transporter family member 1B1 gene (SLCO1B1), is an example of a drug transporter protein that exhibits clinically relevant genetic polymorphism. OAT1B1 transports most HMG-CoA reductase inhibitors, or statins, from the circulation to the liver. Statins are commonly prescribed to lower LDL cholesterol and reduce the risk for cardiovascular events in patients with coronary heart disease. However, their use is associated with an increased risk for myopathy, which is more likely to occur with higher statin plasma concentrations. Symptoms of myopathy range from mild myalgia, which can threaten adherence to statin therapy, to, rarely, rhabdomyolysis, which can have life-threatening consequences. Deficiency in OAT1B1, secondary to a SLCO1B1 Val174Ala polymorphism, leads to reduced statin transport to the liver; the greatest effects are for simvastatin. By contributing to higher simvastatin plasma concentrations, the SLCO1B1 Val174Ala genotype influences the risk for simvastatin-induced myopathy. The CPIC guidelines recommend simvastatin doses no higher than 20 mg per day or use of an alternative statin in variant allele carriers to reduce this risk.

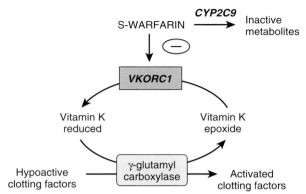

FIG. 4.3 Genes Involved in Warfarin Pharmacokinetics *(CYP2C9)* and Pharmacodynamics *(VKORC1)*.

GENES AFFECTING PHARMACODYNAMICS

VKORC1

Vitamin K epoxide reductase (VKOR) is the target protein for warfarin. Specifically, warfarin inhibits VKOR, inhibiting the formation of a reduced form of vitamin K needed for carboxylation and activation of vitamin K–dependent clotting factors 2, 7, 9, and 10 as depicted in Fig. 4.3. Warfarin is dosed according to a measure of anticoagulation called the international normalized ratio (INR). For most indications, the target INR is 2–3. The risk for bleeding increases with an INR above 3, and especially above 4, while the risk of thrombosis increases with an INR below 2. The dose necessary to achieve target anticoagulation (i.e., an INR = 2–3) varies significantly among patients. The VKOR complex 1 gene *(VKORC1)* encodes the warfarin-sensitive component of VKOR and significantly contributes to warfarin dose requirements. A single-nucleotide polymorphism in the *VKORC1* regulatory region (c.-1693G>A) reduces gene expression and increases warfarin sensitivity, with high, intermediate, and low sensitivity with the AA, AG, and GG genotypes, respectively. This coincides with low ($\leq$3 mg/day), intermediate (4–6 mg/day), and high ($\geq$6 mg/day) dose requirements for warfarin. There are marked ethnic differences in *VKORC1* genotype frequencies. The AG (intermediate sensitivity) genotype is the most common in whites, whereas the AA (high sensitivity) and GG (low sensitivity) genotypes are most common in Asians and blacks, respectively. This explains why, on average, the warfarin dose requirements are higher for blacks and lower for Asians than for whites. Together, the *CYP2C9* and *VKORC1* genotypes explain 40%–60% of the interpatient variability in warfarin dose requirements.

HLA-B

Human leukocyte antigen-B *(HLA-B)* is a member of the major histocompatibility complex (MHC) gene family, which functions to trigger an immune response to proteins/substances recognized as foreign. As such, the HLA complex has been linked to drug hypersensitivity reactions that were previously described as idiosyncratic. In particular, these include the serious cutaneous reactions Stevens-Johnsons syndrome and toxic epidermal necrolysis; there is some evidence for a role of HLA in severe hepatotoxicity reactions. The *HLA* genes are considered among the most complex in the human genome, and several different genetic polymorphisms have been linked specifically to severe adverse effects for certain drugs, including abacavir, used for the treatment of HIV, the immunosuppressant allopurinol, and the anticonvulsants carbamazepine and phenytoin. CPIC guidelines exist for all of these drugs relative to specific *HLA-B* genotypes, and in all cases, alternative therapy is recommended when the genotype is present.

CANCER PHARMACOGENETICS

Pharmacogenetics continues to shift and shape the cancer treatment paradigm from site-specific cytotoxic treatment to molecularly targeted treatment, making precision medicine the standard of care in several cancer types, including breast cancer, non–small cell lung cancer (NSCLC), and melanoma. Choosing the most appropriate therapy is complicated because there are two relevant genomes that require consideration—namely, the patient's genome (germline) that influences drug exposure and toxicity and the tumor genome (somatic) that helps determine prognosis and effectiveness of therapy. A revolutionary realization in cancer drug development was that the same somatic mutations causing, or "driving," the disease may also provide an actionable drug target. Somatic DNA variations can be a prognostic tool (BRCA), which provides information about disease outcome, regardless of the treatment, or a predictive tool (EGFR), which helps predict the effectiveness of a given drug. Either way, somatic biomarkers help clinicians and patients make more informed decisions regarding cancer chemotherapy options.

BCR-ABL

The Philadelphia chromosome, formed by a translocation between chromosomes 9 and 22 fusing the breakpoint cluster region *(BCR)* with the c-Abelson murine leukemia *(ABL)* oncogene, is associated with >95% of chronic myelogenous leukemia (CML) cases. Imatinib is a tyrosine kinase inhibitor (TKI) approved as first-line treatment for *BCR-ABL*–positive CML. Approximately, 10%–15% of CML patients present with resistance to imatinib, and another 20%–25% develop resistance through additional mutations acquired during treatment. Nilotinib and dasatinib, second-generation TKIs, were developed to address resistance to imatinib therapy. In addition to guiding initial therapy, pharmacogenetic findings can help direct subsequent therapies based on the resistance mutation. For example, nilotinib is the preferred choice for mutations at positions F317L/V/I/C, T315A, and V299L, and dasatinib is preferred for mutations at positions Y253H, E255K/V, and F359V/C/I.

EML4-ALK

Several fusion mutations involving anaplastic lymphoma kinase (ALK), resulting in constitutive activation that inhibits apoptosis, have been identified. Echinoderm microtubule-associated protein–like 4 *(EML4-ALK)* is most common fusion, occurring in approximately 5% of all NSCLC cases. Early research trials for crizotinib, an oral adenosine triphosphate (ATP)-competitive selective inhibitor of the ALK and MET tyrosine kinases, enrolled patients with any solid tumor refractory to standard therapy. *ALK* rearrangements were identified in two NSCLC patients who showed good response during the Phase 1 trial. Subsequent studies enrolled patients with *ALK*-positive mutations in NSCLC, and the drug was approved for this indication. The unexpected discovery of ALK rearrangements during clinical studies of crizotinib highlights a valuable benefit of integrating pharmacogenomics throughout the drug development process to help identify the patients most likely to benefit from a therapy while reducing unnecessary treatment and potential toxicity in patients who will not respond.

BRAF

The median survival for advanced melanoma is approximately 6–10 months. About 50% of metastatic melanoma cases and 7%–8% of all cancers carry mutations in the v-raf murine sarcoma viral oncogene homolog B *(BRAF)*. *BRAF* mutations lead to cell proliferation, invasion, and survival of tumor cells. The primary mutation results in glutamic acid substituted for valine at codon 600, termed V600E. Vemurafenib, an ATP inhibitor, was discovered using a high-throughput screening approach to identify candidate drugs that would specifically inhibit the BRAF V600E-mutant enzyme. After exhibiting superiority to standard chemotherapy, vemurafenib was approved for initial therapy for patients with unresectable melanoma that harbors a BRAF V600E mutation.

Human Epidermal Growth Factor Receptor 2 (HER2)

Breast cancer tumors are classified by their expression of the estrogen receptor (ER), progesterone receptor (PR), and human epidermal growth factor receptor 2 (HER2). About 75% of all breast cancers are ER positive, 60% are PR positive, and 15%–20% present with *HER2* amplification. Further, about 30% of metastatic breast cancers display *HER2* gene amplification and protein overexpression. *HER2* is an oncogene that stimulates cell proliferation, migration, and invasion, primarily in breast cancer cells, but it has been identified in other tumors, including lung cancer. While PR status serves primarily as a prognostic marker with PR-positive having a better prognosis than PR-negative tumors, ER and

HER2 are both prognostic and predictive of response to targeted therapies. For example, the ER antagonist tamoxifen and aromatase inhibitors anastrozole, letrozole, and exemestane are only indicated to treat tumors that express ER. Similarly, trastuzumab and pertuzumab are humanized monoclonal antibodies that specifically bind to HER2, decreasing downstream signaling and inducing antibody-related cytotoxic effects. ER and *HER2* testing is required before using any of these agents.

Epidermal Growth Factor Receptor (EGFR)

Lung cancer is the leading cause of cancer death for both men and women in the United States, and NSCLC makes up approximately 85% of lung cancer cases. Activating EGFR mutations are present in about 20% of advanced NSCLC tumors and in more than half of East Asians, women, and nonsmokers with adenocarcinomas. Erlotinib and gefitinib are reversible TKIs that were initially approved for treatment of NSCLC in an unselected population (Fig. 4.4). Retrospective analysis revealed that almost all of the benefit with drug therapy was observed

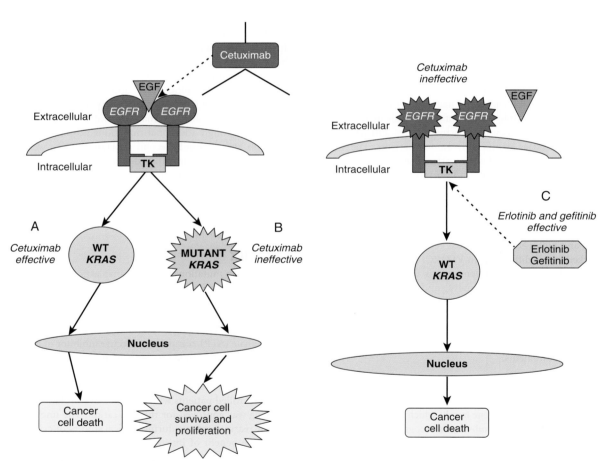

FIG. 4.4 Epidermal Growth Factor Receptor (EGFR) Signaling Pathway and Drug Actions in Cancer Cell. (A) Cetuximab is an EGFR antibody that inhibits extracellular signaling of EGFR and induces cell death only in cancer cells expressing wild-type (WT) *KRAS*. (B) Cetuximab is ineffective in cancer cells expressing mutant *KRAS*. Mutant *KRAS* is permanently activated, and downstream signaling to the nucleus continues, even if upstream signaling is blocked. Cancer cell survival, proliferation, and metastasis occur when activating signals are transmitted to the nucleus. (C) Activating *EGFR* mutations continuously signal downstream, even in the absence of epidermal growth factor (EGF). This inappropriate signaling is blocked by EGFR-tyrosine kinase inhibitors (erlotinib, gefitinib) but not cetuximab. Erlotinib and gefitinib inhibit intracellular signaling mediated by EGFR-tyrosine kinase (TK) and are indicated for cancer cells with activating *EGFR* mutations. Whether or not erlotinib and gefitinib are effective for cancer cells expressing mutant *KRAS* is under investigation.

in NSCLC patients with an activating EGFR mutation, and prospective trials confirmed the observation. Currently, erlotinib is first-line therapy in patients with an activating EGFR mutation, replacing the more toxic and less efficacious platinum-based chemotherapy. Afatinib, a second-generation irreversible EGFR inhibitor, is also considered first-line treatment and is active against resistant tumors that have progressed on erlotinib or gefitinib. Although EGFR inhibitors are less toxic and are associated with longer progression-free survival, when compared to standard chemotherapy, there is no difference in overall survival.

Kirsten Rat Sarcoma Viral Oncogene Homolog (KRAS)

KRAS is a downstream signaling protein in the EGFR pathway that increases cell proliferation when activated (Fig. 4.4). Cetuximab, an EGFR monoclonal antibody, inhibits EGFR downstream signaling, including KRAS, and was initially indicated for metastatic colorectal cancer (CRC). However, only a subset of patients responded to treatment. Analysis of the tumor samples from cetuximab-treated patients revealed that only tumors with wild-type KRAS status responded, and those with KRAS mutations (about 40% of CRC) did not respond to therapy. In fact, patients with mutant KRAS tumors may be at risk for increased toxicity with cetuximab without deriving any benefit. Professional guidelines and the FDA recommend KRAS testing prior to initiation of cetuximab therapy.

Future Directions of Pharmacogenetics in Oncology

The current approach of using pharmacogenetics to identify extreme responders for tumor genotyping will continue to play an important role in detecting "driver" mutations, which may serve as drug targets for therapy. NCI-Molecular Analysis for Therapy Choice (NCI-MATCH) is an ongoing prospective clinical trial that analyzes patients' tumors to detect "actionable mutations," meaning the mutation has an FDA-approved targeted therapy, and assigns them to targeted treatment specific for the mutation rather than tumor type (breast, colon, lung, etc.). This trial and other research efforts are putting pharmacogenetics at the forefront of therapeutic decisions by treating cancers according to their molecular abnormalities, regardless of tumor tissue or location.

SUMMARY

Pharmacogenetics began as a research field that sought to provide understanding for the genetic contributions to clinically observed differences among individuals in efficacy, toxicity, and dose requirements for drugs. Research in the field continues, but some examples have now advanced to a stage where the genetic information can be useful in guiding clinical decisions about the use of a drug or the appropriate dose for an individual patient. As a result, in recent years, numerous healthcare institutions have begun adopting pharmacogenetic approaches, and clinicians are increasingly interested in learning about how to use this tool to improve treatment decisions for their patients. This personalized approach to care is expected to increase, and it will be increasingly important for clinicians to understand how and when to use these tools when making drug therapy decisions about their patients.

SELF-ASSESSMENT QUESTIONS

1. A patient has to undergo a percutaneous coronary intervention to alleviate stenosis of his or her coronary artery. Which phenotype is predictive of reduced clopidogrel effectiveness for this individual?
   A. CYP2C19 Poor metabolizer.
   B. CYP2D6 Ultra-rapid metabolizer.
   C. CYP3A4 Poor metabolizer.
   D. CYP2C9 Rapid metabolizer.
2. Carbamazepine is prescribed to control seizures in individuals with simple or complex partial seizures. Which gene is predictive for these individuals developing severe cutaneous reactions with carbamazepine?
   A. *CYP3A4*.
   B. *TPMT*.
   C. *HLA-B*.
   D. *CYP2C9*.
3. The *SLCO1B1* genotype influences the risk for adverse reactions to:
   A. Warfarin.
   B. Simvastatin.
   C. Codeine.
   D. Paroxetine.

4. What is an appropriate initial therapy for patients with unresectable melanoma that harbor a BRAF V600E mutation?
   A. Trastuzumab.
   B. Imatinib.
   C. Vemurafenib.
   D. Cetuximab.
5. Patients with nonfunctional *DYPD* variants that are exposed to 5-FU or capecitabine are at increased risk for all of the following potentially life-threatening toxicities EXCEPT:
   A. Peripheral neuropathy.
   B. Myelosuppression.
   C. Hand-foot syndrome.
   D. Mucositis.

FURTHER READING

Johnson JA, Ellingrod VL, Kroetz DL, Kuo GM, eds. *Pharmacogenomics: Applications to Patient Care.* 3rd ed. Lenexa: American College of Clinical Pharmacy; 2015:79–101.

Relling MV, Evans WE. Pharmacogenomics in the clinic. *Nature.* 2015;526:343–350.

Relling MV, Klein TE. CPIC: Clinical Pharmacogenetics Implementation Consortium of the Pharmacogenomics Research Network. *Clin Pharmacol Ther.* 2011;89:464–467.

WEBSITES

https://cpicpgx.org/

The Clinical Pharmacogenetics Implementation Consortium, a comprehensive website with complete guidelines containing concise recommendations and comprehensive supplemental information that underpins the recommendations. Included is a continuously updated list of drugs for which genetic guidance is possible.

https://www.pharmgkb.org/

The Pharmacogenomics Knowledgebase website is a comprehensive resource providing knowledge on the impact of genetic variations on drug responses for clinicians and researchers. The site includes the CPIC guidelines, information on cancer drugs that are guided based on somatic mutations, and more.

Drug Discovery, Development, and Regulation

James E. Barrett

The discovery and development of new therapeutics, followed by their regulatory approval for commercial use, is a lengthy, highly regulated, and complex process. The sequence of activities required to bring a new therapeutic to market can take as many as 15 years and cost upward of US$2.6 billion. The lengthy processes of drug discovery and development involve multiple disciplines that interact in a highly coordinated manner over this extended period of time. It has been estimated that by the time a drug is approved for human use, approximately 2000 individuals with wide-ranging expertise have participated at various stages. Unfortunately, the vast amount of time, effort, and cost typically results in a success rate of approximately 10% for drugs that enter clinical development. This low probability of success is frequently due to unanticipated toxicity or insufficient efficacy. The pharmaceutical industry and academic scientists continue to analyze the complex processes of drug discovery and development to improve analytic techniques and develop more effective predictive tools to curtail cost and minimize failures. In the early phases of drug discovery, this includes the development of methods to detect potential signs of organ toxicity and the identification of critical aspects of the pharmaceutical properties of a compound, such as bioavailability and drug metabolism, before advancing compounds further in development that might eventually fail at later stages and at a higher cost. Because drug discovery and development are lengthy, cumulative processes, it is exceedingly important that a high level of confidence surrounds each step in the decision to move forward. An overview of the processes involved in drug discovery and development is presented in Fig. 5.1.

DRUG DISCOVERY AND DEVELOPMENT

The Introduction of New Drugs

Most drug development begins with the identification of a **drug target**, which is a native protein or nucleic acid in the body that has been identified to be involved in the pathophysiology of a particular disorder, and which, when modified by a drug, produces a therapeutically relevant response. Although the most frequent approach over decades has been on identifying a single target—the concept of a "magic bullet"—recently, it has been recognized that many complex disorders, such as cancer and several neurodegenerative and psychiatric disorders, require a **multitargeted** or polypharmacological approach. Typically, these conditions are not static and are often regulated by a number of genes. For example, cancer is a heterogeneous, highly adaptive, and constantly evolving disease, driven in large part by the targeted therapeutic agents designed specifically to suppress it. The challenges of therapeutic intervention at any stage of the disease necessitate a strategy not only directed toward the existing target(s) but also toward target(s) that

ABBREVIATIONS	
ADME	Absorption, distribution, metabolism, and excretion
ANDA	Abbreviated new drug application
BLA	Biologics license application
CFDA	China Food and Drug Administration
CMC	Chemistry, manufacturing, and control
EMA	European Medicines Agency
FDA	United States Food and Drug Administration
GLP	Good laboratory practice
GMP	Good manufacturing practices
IND	Investigational new drug
NDA	New drug application
NIH	National Institutes of Health

emerge following mutations or the development of resistance. Similarly, neurodegenerative disorders such as Alzheimer or Parkinson diseases are progressively debilitating conditions for which treatments differ during the early and later stages of the diseases. While the development of a multitargeted single drug directed at an optimal array of targets poses several challenges, informed drug combinations have the potential to interact with several sites within a network of both static and emerging targets.

Once a target has been identified, it must be validated. **Target validation** represents a critical step in the drug discovery process and can include the use of cellular assays, genetically modified animals, or animal models of a particular disorder to provide verification for further development. Although these are important early assessments that aid in the confidence that modulation of a target will produce a therapeutic effect, a target can only be fully validated in a clinical study. Once a target has been validated in preclinical assays, a small-molecule or biologic that engages the target and produces the desired therapeutic activity will be developed and optimized, and its pharmacological properties will be determined. The **pharmacokinetic** (absorption, distribution, metabolism, and elimination) and **pharmacodynamic** properties of the compound will be determined to ensure that the drug, if it is to be orally administered, has good **bioavailability**, an accepted duration of action, and actually engages the target identified during the earlier phases of the discovery process. Once a candidate drug is selected, a detailed evaluation of its **toxicology** will be initiated, a step that is critically important for establishing the preclinical safety profile prior to use in humans. These studies vary in duration according to the intended clinical use of the drug and proposed length of time it

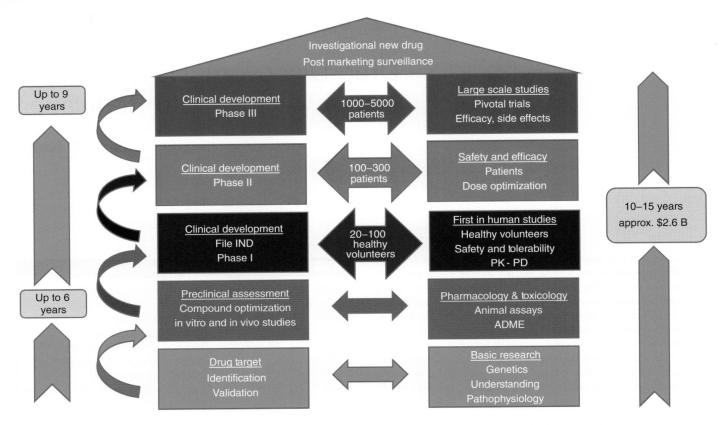

FIG. 5.1 Overview of the Drug Discovery and Development Process. *IND,* Investigational new drug; *PD,* pharmacodynamics; *PK,* pharmacokinetics.

will be prescribed and typically involve repeated administration of a wide range of doses and an assessment of organ, genetic, and possible reproductive toxicity. A considerable effort is directed toward providing a strong basis and rationale for establishing the initial starting dose when the compound moves into the first in-human studies. It is crucially important to initially identify a therapeutic index to ensure safety when the compound is first administered to healthy volunteers.

At selected points in this process, usually when the lead compound has been identified, large-scale quantities of the substance will have to be produced to enable extensive safety and pharmacology studies. This phase of the process, often designated as chemistry, manufacturing, and control (CMC), is a key component of the information used to establish the basis for eventual product manufacturing that is evaluated by the regulatory authorities. The guidelines for the conduct of early phase laboratory studies are embodied in a system of laboratory management controls published by the United States Food and Drug Administration (FDA) and known as "good laboratory practice" (GLP), whereas the manufacturing guidelines are governed by "good manufacturing practices" (GMP). Both GLP and GMP guidelines are designed to ensure the reliability and integrity of the manufactured substance, as well as provide quality assurance in both the preclinical and developmental phases leading to regulatory approval.

Clinical Evaluation of New Drugs

Once preclinical studies are completed and the drug is considered ready for evaluation in humans, the sponsor of the potential product files an investigational new drug (IND) application with the FDA. In other countries, these are filed with comparable regulatory authorities such as the European Medicines Agency (EMA) or the China Food and Drug Administration (CFDA). There are nearly 225,000 clinical studies registered on the National Institutes of Health (NIH) Clinical Trials website, which was made publicly available in 2000 and is now the largest trial registry in the world, with a rich database of ongoing and completed studies, and including clinical trial results for approximately 10% of the completed studies.

When the FDA approves the IND application to proceed to development with humans, the drug enters the first phase of a three-phase process. Phase I studies are designed to determine drug safety and tolerability and involve the exposure of approximately 20–100 healthy volunteers to different single and multiple drug doses to establish a range of pharmacological activity and determine a maximal tolerated dose. During Phase I studies, drug metabolism, distribution, and other clinical features, including side effects, are evaluated. Phase II studies follow the successful completion of Phase I and are designed to assess efficacy, as well as to continue to evaluate safety and tolerability. This is generally the first time the compound will be evaluated in patients with the disorder for which the drug is being developed, and it involves 100–300 patients. Typically, only two or three doses of drug are selected for this phase based on the single- and multiple-dose results acquired during Phase I. If efficacy is demonstrated during Phase II and the compound continues to be safe and well tolerated, much larger Phase III studies will be initiated involving thousands of individuals. The goals of the first two phases of clinical development are to establish safety and tolerability and determine the effective dose(s) that can be more fully evaluated during Phase III. In most cases, only a single dose is carried into Phase III, although there are exceptions where additional doses may be incorporated. If this last phase is completed successfully, it will result in the filing of a new drug application (NDA) or a biologics license application (BLA) with the FDA or comparable regulatory authorities in other countries. These agencies will determine whether the compound will be reviewed by an advisory committee, an independent panel of experts, prior to making a recommendation for approved commercial use. Some drugs approved for marketing are followed during an additional phase called Phase IV, postmarketing surveillance, during which additional safety information on the drug following its entrance into the market will be obtained by the manufacturer.

After the NDA has been approved, the drug manufacturer will develop the label with the FDA that describes how the drug can be marketed and prescribed. This also includes the development of the package insert that accompanies the product and contains all of the information pertinent to the drug, including its clinical pharmacology, indications and usage, dosages, and contraindications. Although there are strict regulations associated with drug development and commercialization, it is important to note that the FDA does not restrict the use of approved drugs to those conditions described in the label, and a physician is permitted to use the drug off-label for conditions other than those for which the drug was approved. The decision to pursue other uses or indications must be made ethically and responsibly and based on compelling scientific evidence.

In general, most drugs are developed and approved for use in adults, and, after approval, companies may often conduct pediatric clinical studies to seek approval to extend their use to children. There are often considerable differences in the metabolism of drugs between adults and children, as well as differences depending on the children's age that require special caution and consideration. A number of FDA initiatives have been implemented that address problems of inadequate testing of drugs in pediatric populations. The FDA has issued specific guidance and general requirements for developing drugs for pediatric use under the Pediatric Research Equity Act or the Best Pharmaceuticals for Children Act. One feature of these provisions is the possibility of obtaining an additional 6 months of market exclusivity for a patented drug that has been evaluated for use in children.

Generic Drug Development

Most drugs approved by the regulatory authorities have a period of market exclusivity related to the patent filed originally by the company or by the inventor of that drug. The lifetime of a patent is 20 years in the United States, and during that time, the owner of the patent, typically a pharmaceutical company, has exclusive rights to market the drug. Because the drug development and approval process is lengthy, provisions can be made for extending the life of the patent. However, once the patent has expired, other companies may file an abbreviated new drug application (ANDA) to develop and manufacture a generic version of that drug. The primary requirement for approval is demonstration that the generic preparation is pharmaceutically equivalent to the reference drug. The generic version must have the same active ingredient, dosage form and strength, and must be administered by the same route as the reference drug. In addition, the generic version must not differ from the reference drug in the rate and extent of absorption and distribution of the active pharmaceutical ingredient. These requirements are characterized as establishing bioequivalence between the reference drug and the generic version. Generic products tested by the FDA and determined to be therapeutic equivalents are listed by the FDA in the publication *Approved Drug Products with Therapeutic Equivalence Evaluations* (commonly known as the Orange Book). This book identifies drug products approved on the basis of safety and effectiveness by the FDA under the Federal Food, Drug, and Cosmetic Act (the Act) and also contains related patent and exclusivity information. The generic drug is typically not manufactured or distributed by the company that developed and marketed the original drug, and the cost to consumers is considerably less than that of the original drug; thus the commercial impact of the generic version on the organization that developed and marketed the drug is significant.

Natural Products

Although many small-molecule compounds are derived synthetically through medicinal chemistry or as biologics such as monoclonal antibodies, historically many therapeutic agents were derived from natural products extracted from plants, fungi, and marine organisms. Most natural products are complex, chemically diverse molecules that have multiple components and physicochemical features, making it necessary to isolate the active ingredient(s) to ensure uniformity and be able to manufacture the therapeutic substance on a large scale. It has been estimated that approximately one-half of the small-molecule drugs currently on the market are based on structures derived from natural products. These drugs include morphine, the first pharmacologically active compound isolated from a plant more than 200 years ago, antibiotics such as penicillin isolated from microorganisms, the antimalarial drug quinine, the immunosuppressant rapamycin, the lipid-lowering agents such as several of the statins, and numerous anticancer drugs such as taxol.

Orphan Drugs

There has been an emerging interest in the discovery and development of drugs that may benefit only a small number of patients with rare diseases, defined in the United States as affecting fewer than 200,000 individuals. The Orphan Drug Act of 1983 provides special incentives such as tax advantages and marketing exclusivity for pharmaceutical companies for the development of such orphan drugs. Further, the path to marketing approval is also easier because demonstration of a potential therapeutic effect involves a limited number of individuals with the disorder and not several thousand patients. The FDA has approved over 500 drugs and biologic products for rare diseases since the Orphan Drug Act was implemented, with orphan drugs accounting for nearly one-half (21 of 45) of all new drugs approved in 2015. The EMA has designated over 1500 products as orphan, with over 120 approvals since legislation similar to the Orphan Drug Act was approved in 2000. Although the costs for the development of orphan drugs is less, particularly in the clinical development phases, the cost of orphan drugs is considerably higher than those without orphan drug status due to the limited number of patients for whom the drug is prescribed.

Repurposing

Recently, and in part due to the high failure rate of developing new drugs, a growing interest has emerged in discovering new therapeutic uses for drugs that have been on the market or have failed in their intended or primary indication. The repurposing or repositioning of existing drugs is now an active area of research that promises to greatly expand treatment options. The advantage of this approach is that safety and tolerability profiles for these agents through Phase I or Phase II clinical studies have already been established, permitting substantial time and expense savings in evaluating the compounds for new therapeutic indications. The interest in repositioning or repurposing drugs has arisen from clinical observations of a beneficial side effect or from basic research indicating that the molecular target of a compound may play a role in an illness other than that of the original indication. Insight into possible repurposing or repositioning might also derive from pharmacoepidemiologic studies in which it may be discovered that patients treated with a drug for one indication have a lower incidence of a seemingly unrelated disorder. This is the case with metformin, commonly used to treat type 2 diabetes, for which studies have shown that patients treated with metformin have a lower risk of cancer or an improved prognosis when treated for cancer. In some instances, repositioning or repurposing is similar to developing extensions for a drug, such as the use of the anticonvulsant gabapentin or the antidepressant duloxetine for the treatment of pain. Increasingly, sophisticated computational approaches are being used to screen known compounds for off-target activities and discover new uses for drugs that have been on the market for several years. This approach has yielded several drugs that, when used in combination with another drug, allow for the targeting of multiple receptors or pathways.

New Approaches to Drug Discovery and Development

Although the failure rate for drug development differs across various therapeutic areas, in general it is unacceptably high, and considerable efforts have been expended to increase the percentage of drugs reaching the market. Several developments hold promise for increasing confidence in moving compounds through the various stages of development, including a focus on elucidating appropriate biomarkers designed to provide early predictability of therapeutic activity and efficacy. These biomarkers may include measures of a pathogenic process or a pharmacological response related to the potential efficacy of the compound, such as visualization that the compound under investigation actually reaches the intended target. The use of biomarkers to detect whether a compound has an action on processes associated with a particular disease may provide early insight into the potential efficacy of new compounds. Further, incorporating pharmacogenomic/pharmacogenetic knowledge (Chapter 4) and biomarker identification into the drug evaluation process will identify individuals likely to respond to a particular drug. These individuals can be stratified according to biomarker and genomic profiles, contributing to the concept of an evolving approach described as precision medicine in which patients can be prescribed medication based on their genotype, metabolic profile, or metabolome, and other relevant characteristics that determine efficacy and safety. Last, the sophisticated integration of microfluidic devices and cellular physiology to construct organs-on-a-chip that can capture the physiology and pharmacology of the lung, heart, and other organs will enable early assessments of both drug toxicity and the metabolic profile before compounds are administered in vivo. Thus drug discovery and development are dynamic fields, relying heavily on principles of pharmacology throughout the entire process and integrating those principles with emerging technologies.

In addition to efforts focused on predicting therapeutic activity and efficacy early in the development process, there has also been considerable effort to develop more robust and faster means of assessing clinical efficacy without compromising patient safety through modifications of the design of clinical trials. Traditionally, clinical trials have been designed, submitted to, and approved by regulatory agencies prior to being initiated, and once approved, they proceed without modification until the study is completed and the outcome analyzed. The clinical trial may be placed on hold or terminated if adverse events occur during any of the phases, but otherwise, the initial trial design is executed until completed. This means that for the duration of the study, some patients may be exposed to noneffective doses of drug. In addition, many clinical studies are plagued by high rates of placebo responders, making a drug effect difficult to establish. As a consequence of these limitations, adaptive clinical trials have been proposed and conducted in which a treatment is evaluated by observing results (e.g., efficacy, side effects) on a predefined schedule proposed and accepted by the regulatory authorities. This approach permits modification of the conduct of the trial at interim evaluation points and may involve dropping a noneffective dose, thereby shifting patients from a noneffective dose to

another treatment arm. In attempts to minimize the impact of placebo responders, all patients may be started on a placebo initially, and following a period of time, placebo responders may be dropped from the study before investigating the actual effects of a drug. Major objectives of the adaptive trial are to identify therapeutic activity more quickly, eliminate unnecessary exposure to noneffective doses, and curtail some of the expense associated with the most expensive part of drug development. As per the FDA, it is essential that an adaptive trial design adhere to the more traditional design of clinical trials—that is, being "adequate and well controlled" while also ensuring that false positive results and the introduction of bias are avoided. A major consideration is that pertinent personnel involved in making decisions while the study is ongoing are "blinded"— that is, the treatment group assignments of study subjects are unknown.

PRESCRIPTION WRITING AND REGULATION

Prescriptions are written by a prescriber to instruct the pharmacist to dispense a specific medication for a specific patient. Many prescriptions are now computer based (e-prescribing) and involve the electronic generation, transmission, and filling of a prescription, but the essential information required is the same whether handwritten or computer generated (Fig. 5.2). It is vitally important that a prescription communicate clearly to the pharmacist the exact medication needed and how this medication is to be used by the patient. Patient compliance is often related to the clarity of the directions on the prescription, and terms such as "take as directed" should be avoided. Equally important is the necessity for clarity when using proprietary drug names because

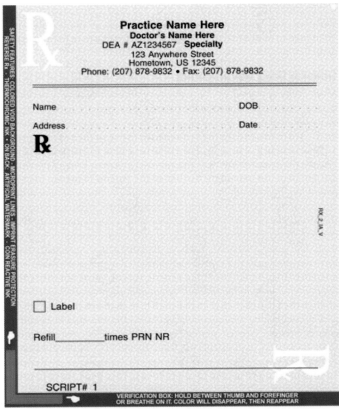

FIG. 5.2 Sample Prescription Form.

of the similarities for many drugs. In these instances, the physician should designate the generic name (if a generic version is available) and the brand name to avoid confusion. Prior to actually preparing the prescription, it is important to have carefully evaluated the patient's medical history (e.g., any renal or hepatic dysfunction that might alter the pharmacokinetic properties of the drug being prescribed) and also to consider any concomitant medications that might result in drug-drug interactions.

Prescriptions for most drugs are not subject to restrictions. The exception is drugs with a potential for abuse—that is, scheduled drugs are prescribed with specific limitations depending on schedule. As part of the United States Comprehensive Drug Abuse Prevention and Control Act of 1970, the Controlled Substances Act established drug policy under which the manufacture, importation, possession, use, and distribution of certain drugs is regulated. The legislation created five schedules, or classifications, by which drugs with a potential for abuse are designated, as shown in Table 5.1. These controlled drugs are classified according to their potential for abuse and include a wide variety of compounds ranging from opioids, stimulants, and sedative-hypnotics to anticonvulsants and cough medicine. Schedule I drugs have a high abuse potential and no currently accepted medical use in the United States, whereas Schedule II drugs, which include some opioids and stimulants, also have a high abuse potential but have an accepted medical use. Schedule II drugs may not be refilled or prescribed by telephone. Schedule III drugs include preparations with low doses of opioids, as well as the anabolic steroids and testosterone, while Schedule IV drugs, which

have low to moderate abuse potential, include the benzodiazepines. Schedule III and IV drugs have a five-refill maximum, with the prescription invalid 6 months from the date of issue. Drugs in Schedule V have the lowest potential for abuse and include some anticonvulsants such as pregabalin and antidiarrheal drugs such as diphenoxylate. These drugs may be dispensed by a pharmacist in a limited quantity without a prescription if the patient is at least 18 years old.

For both written and computer-based prescriptions, the following information is essential:
- physician's name, address, and office telephone number
- date of the prescription
- patient's full name and date of birth
- address
- how the prescription is to be taken
- the ages of children under 12 and adults over 60
- refill and any safety cap information
- DEA number of the physician required for controlled substances.

Because both the apothecary and metric systems are in use in the United States, it is important that prescribers become familiar with conversion units. Table 5.2 lists commonly used equivalents with household units also noted where applicable.

Patient instructions (signature) on a prescription are sometimes written using Latin abbreviations as a shortcut for prescribers, giving concise directions to the pharmacist on how and when a patient should take the medication. Although instructions written in English are preferred, some common Latin abbreviations are as follows:

po: by mouth
ac: before meals
pc: after meals
qd: every day
b.i.d.: twice a day
t.i.d.: three times a day
q.i.d.: four times a day
hs: at bedtime
prn: as needed

Additional instructions may be added to the prescription to instruct the pharmacist to place an additional label on the prescription container (e.g., take with food). When a prescriber intends to use a drug for an unauthorized indication, or when two drugs have been prescribed that may cause a clinically significant drug interaction, the prescriber should communicate to the patient and pharmacist that this is indeed the intended therapy.

TABLE 5.1	Controlled Substance Schedules	
Schedule	Definition	Examples
I	Compounds with no currently accepted medical use, a lack of accepted safety, and a high potential for abuse	Heroin, lysergic acid diethylamide (LSD), marijuana (cannabis), 3,4-methylenedioxymethamphetamine (ecstasy), methaqualone, and peyote
II/IIN	Compounds with a high potential for abuse, leading to severe psychological or physical dependence	Cocaine, methamphetamine, methadone, hydromorphone, meperidine, oxycodone, fentanyl, morphine, opium, codeine, hydrocodone, amphetamine
III/IIIN	Compounds with a moderate to low potential for physical and psychological dependence	Products containing <90 mg codeine per dosage unit, buprenorphine, ketamine, benzphetamine, anabolic steroids, testosterone
IV	Compounds with a low potential for abuse and low risk of dependence	Carisoprodol, benzodiazepines
V	Compounds with a low potential for abuse	Cough preparations containing <200 mg codeine/100 mL or 100 g

Adapted from the US Department of Justice, Drug Enforcement Administration, Diversion Control Division, https://www.deadiversion.usdoj.gov/schedules/#define.

TABLE 5.2	Common Apothecary, Metric, and Household Equivalents		
	Metric	**Apothecary**	**Household**
Volume	1 mL	20 drops	20 drops
	5 mL	1 fl dm	1 tsp
	15 mL	4 fl dm	1 tbsp
	30 mL	1 oz	2 tbsp
	240 mL	8 oz	½ pt (1 cup)
	480 mL	16 oz	1 pt
	960 mL	32 oz	1 qt
Weight	454 g	1 lb	
	1 kg	2.2 lb	

dm, Dram; *g*, grams; *kg*, kilogram; *lb*, pound; *mL*, milliliter; *oz*, fluid ounce; *pt*, pint; *qt*, quart; *tbsp*, tablespoonful; *tsp*, teaspoonful.

SUMMARY

Drug discovery and development are clearly essential parts of the life sciences and of the overall healthcare system. There have been tremendous advances in clinical care, attributed largely to the development of drugs for the treatment of several conditions, including cardiovascular diseases, infectious diseases, and cancer. These advances have been led by increased knowledge of fundamental principles of pharmacology coupled to an abiding commitment to research on pathophysiology and mechanisms. Progress is being made in many spheres that intersect in the process of discovering new drugs, including more robust assessments of targets, improved techniques to assess metabolism, safety, and toxicology, proceeding to improvements in the manner in which clinical trials are conducted. The focus on developing an increased understanding of complex disorders requiring polypharmacological approaches that incorporate computational modeling and repurposing drugs is an innovative means of addressing many unmet medical needs and of improving treatment outcomes. Drug discovery and development represent a risky, lengthy, and costly endeavor, but despite the formidable obstacles, the benefit to society has been and will continue to be tremendous.

SELF-ASSESSMENT QUESTIONS

1. You have been asked to volunteer for a Phase I clinical trial for a new antihypertensive medication. Phase I studies are important to:
   A. Demonstrate the potential of genetic factors contributing to the effects of a new drug in humans.
   B. Determine the efficacy of a new drug in a specific disease or disorder.
   C. Determine the safety and tolerability of a range of doses for a new drug in humans.
   D. Indicate the effectiveness of a new drug in an animal model of the disease.

2. Which of the following controlled drug schedules contains drugs that have no accepted medical use in the United States?
   A. Schedule I.
   B. Schedule II.
   C. Schedule III.
   D. Schedule IV.
   E. Schedule V.

3. Target validation refers to:
   A. The identification of a therapeutically relevant drug target.
   B. Finding a genetic linkage to a pathological disorder.
   C. The finding that modulating the target with a drug produces the desired therapeutic effect.
   D. The idea that the target is safe and modulating it will be nontoxic.

4. A generic drug is one that:
   A. Has been demonstrated in clinical studies to have the same therapeutic effect as the reference drug.
   B. Is bioequivalent to the reference drug.
   C. Can be approved by the FDA, but the sponsor must demonstrate a different route of administration for efficacy.
   D. Must be evaluated for possible toxicological effects, just like the reference drug.

5. A patient received a new prescription from his or her physician that indicated the drug should be taken q.i.d. This Latin abbreviation means that the drug should be taken:
   A. Twice a day.
   B. Four times a day.
   C. Whenever needed.
   D. Every day.
   E. Every other day.

FURTHER READING

Chae YK, Arya A, Malecek MK, et al. Repurposing metformin for cancer treatment: current clinical studies. *Oncotarget.* 2016;7:40767–40780.

Esch EW, Bahinski A, Huh D. Organs-on-chips at the frontiers of drug discovery. *Nat Rev Drug Discov.* 2015;14:248260.

Gautam A. The changing model of big pharma: impact of key trends. *Drug Discov Today.* 2016;21:379–384.

Hay M, Thomas DW, Craighead JL, et al. Clinical development success rates for investigational drugs. *Nat Biotechnol.* 2014;32:40–51.

Issa NT, Byers SW, Dakshanamurthy S. Drug repurposing: translational pharmacology, chemistry, computers and the clinic. *Curr Top Med Chem.* 2013;13:2328–2336.

Johnson JA, Weitzel KW. Advancing pharmacogenomics as a component of precision medicine: how, where and who? *Clin Pharmacol Ther.* 2016;99:154–156.

Lai TL, Lavori PW, Shih M-C. Adaptive trial designs. *Annu Rev Pharmacol Toxicol.* 2012;52:101–110.

Lancaster MA, Knoblich JA. Organogenesis in a dish: modeling development and disease using organoid technologies. *Science.* 2014;345:6194.

Li YY, Jones SJ. Drug repositioning for personalized medicine. *Genome Med.* 2012;4:27.

Scannell JW, Blanckley A, Boldon H, Warrington B. Diagnosing the decline in pharmaceutical R & D efficiency. *Nat Rev Drug Discov.* 2012;11:191–200.

WEBSITES

https://clinicaltrials.gov
This website is sponsored by the US NIH and contains a database of more than 200,000 clinical trials (and results where applicable) being conducted in the United States and nearly 200 countries around the world.

www.fda.gov
This website is maintained by the US FDA and contains information for industry, physicians, and consumers. It includes information on the drug development and approval process; guidance, compliance, and regulatory information; drug approval databases; and information on drug safety and availability.

Chemical Mediators and Drugs Affecting Autonomic and Neuromuscular Synapses

Introduction to the Autonomic Nervous System

Lynn Wecker and Robert J. Theobald, Jr.

ABBREVIATIONS

ACh	Acetylcholine
AChE	Acetylcholinesterase
ANS	Autonomic nervous system
cAMP	Cyclic adenosine monophosphate
CNS	Central nervous system
COMT	Catechol-O-methyltransferase
DA	Dopamine
L-DOPA	Dihydroxyphenylalanine
Epi	Epinephrine
GI	Gastrointestinal
MAO	Monoamine oxidase
NE	Norepinephrine
PNS	Peripheral nervous system

The human nervous system is the most complex of all systems in the body and is responsible for perceiving, processing, and transmitting information throughout the organism and generating responses to the information. The nervous system is divided into the peripheral nervous system (PNS) and the central nervous system (CNS) (Fig. 6.1). The PNS is subdivided into the autonomic nervous system (ANS), which controls automatic functioning like breathing and heart rate, and the somatic or somatosensory nervous system, which is composed of both sensory and motor nerves and is involved in voluntary movement. The CNS is comprised of the brain and spinal cord and integrates and controls all bodily functions as well as thought processes. All these systems are interconnected and work together.

The ANS innervates the heart, blood vessels, visceral organs, exocrine glands, and virtually all other organs that contain smooth muscle. Although the ANS regulates the function of these tissues, the organs innervated by the ANS have intrinsic activity independent of intact innervation, and thus denervation does not lead to a loss of function. Smooth muscle function is also controlled by chemical substances released locally or systemically. The ANS controls key visceral processes, including cardiac output, blood flow to specific organs, glandular secretions, waste removal, and activities related to reproduction. Regulation of the functions of these organs is generally not under conscious control, which is why the ANS is often referred to as the "involuntary" nervous system.

In contrast, skeletal muscle is under the voluntary control of higher centers in the CNS. Nerves that innervate and regulate the contraction of skeletal muscle are called somatic motor nerves and are functionally and anatomically different from autonomic nerves. Somatic motor nerves are myelinated and do not form networks, and their excision leads to paralysis and atrophy of skeletal muscle. Sensory nerves are afferent fibers located throughout the body that convey information to the CNS related to the senses, including touch, temperature, position in space, and pain.

DIVISIONS OF THE AUTONOMIC NERVOUS SYSTEM

The two major divisions of the ANS, the parasympathetic and sympathetic systems, function in parallel to maintain homeostasis by regulating bodily functions. Stimulation of the sympathetic system expends energy and leads to "flight, fright, or fight" responses characterized by increased heart rate, blood pressure, and respiration; increased blood flow to skeletal muscles; and dilation of the pupil (mydriasis). In contrast, stimulation of the parasympathetic system conserves energy ("rest and digest") and leads to responses characterized by decreased heart rate, blood pressure, and respiration; increased secretions; and constriction of the pupil (miosis).

Although the parasympathetic and sympathetic systems differ both anatomically and functionally, they also share some features. The outflow of both divisions from the CNS consists of two neuron relays named after their anatomical location relative to the autonomic ganglia, or relay centers. Preganglionic neurons have their cell bodies in the spinal cord and the brainstem and their nerve terminals at autonomic ganglia, where they relay information to postganglionic neurons. Postganglionic neurons send their axons directly to effector organs (heart, blood vessels, visceral organs, and glands), where they relay information to cells; these synapses are often referred to as neuroeffector junctions. Thus the preganglionic fibers of both the sympathetic and parasympathetic systems synapse with postganglionic fibers at autonomic ganglia, the location of which differs for the two systems.

Parasympathetic neurons arise from the brainstem and sacral region of the spinal cord, whereas sympathetic neurons arise from thoracic and lumbar regions of the spinal cord.

Both parasympathetic and sympathetic preganglionic neurons are myelinated and release acetylcholine (ACh) as the neurotransmitter. Postganglionic parasympathetic and sympathetic neurons are unmyelinated, with parasympathetic neurons also releasing ACh at the neuroeffector junction, whereas most sympathetic postganglionic fibers release norepinephrine (NE, also called noradrenaline). Sympathetic fibers that innervate some sweat glands release ACh rather than NE but are still considered sympathetic because these neurons are defined anatomically and not by the neurotransmitter released.

As shown in Fig. 6.2, the cranial portion of the parasympathetic outflow includes cranial nerves III, VII, IX, and X and innervates structures in the head, neck, thorax, and abdomen, while the sacral portion forms the pelvic nerve and innervates portions of the

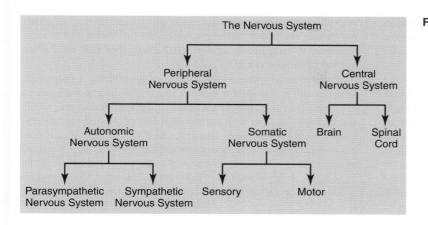

FIG. 6.1 Divisions of the Nervous System.

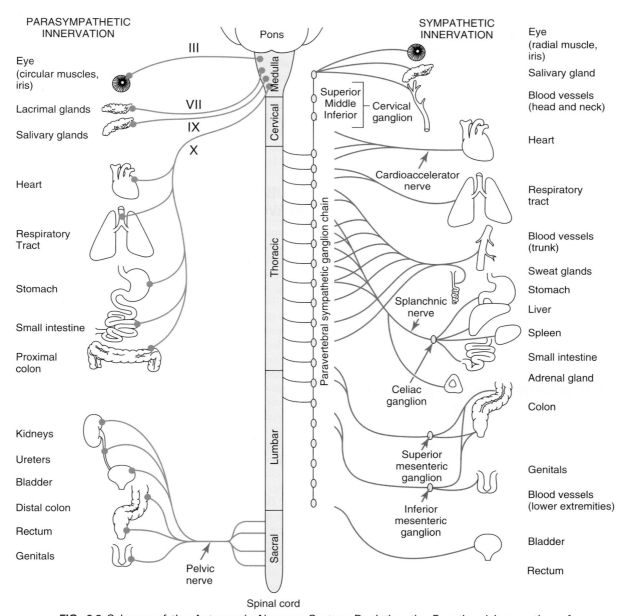

FIG. 6.2 Schema of the Autonomic Nervous System Depicting the Functional Innervation of Peripheral Effector Organs and the Anatomical Origin of Peripheral Autonomic Nerves From the Spinal Cord. The Roman numerals on nerves originating in the tectal region of the brainstem refer to the cranial nerves that provide parasympathetic outflow to the effector organs of the head, neck, and trunk.

gastrointestinal (GI) tract and the pelvic viscera, including the bladder and reproductive organs. In contrast, preganglionic sympathetic neurons originate in the intermediolateral cell column of the spinal cord at the thoracic and lumbar levels from T1 to L2.

Parasympathetic ganglia are located close to the organ innervated, while most sympathetic ganglia are located outside the spinal vertebrae. Most of these neurons synapse in the 22 segmentally arranged ganglia that form two chains located bilaterally adjacent to the spinal cord and are often called the paravertebral chain. Although most preganglionic sympathetic neurons synapse in the paravertebral sympathetic ganglia, several are prevertebral and lie near the bony vertebral column in the abdomen and pelvis (celiac, superior and inferior mesenteric, and aorticorenal), while a few (cervical ganglia and ganglia connected to urinary bladder and rectum) lie near the organs innervated.

As a consequence of the different locations of parasympathetic and sympathetic ganglia, the lengths of the preganglionic fibers relative to the postganglionic fibers differ between the systems. Preganglionic parasympathetic neurons are longer than postganglionic parasympathetic neurons, whereas preganglionic sympathetic neurons are of approximately equal length or shorter than postganglionic sympathetic neurons.

The adrenal medulla is also a part of the sympathetic nervous system. It contains chromaffin cells that are embryologically and anatomically similar to sympathetic ganglia and are innervated by typical preganglionic sympathetic nerves. These cells synthesize and secrete epinephrine (Epi, also called adrenaline), which is a catecholamine like NE, into the blood, analogous to postganglionic sympathetic neurons, which release NE. Some chromaffin cells also release small amounts of NE.

Although many consider the ANS to be an efferent system, almost all peripheral nerves (both autonomic and somatic) have afferent sensory fibers. These visceral afferent fibers have their cell bodies in the dorsal root ganglia of the spinal nerves and in cranial nerve ganglia and function as a feedback system to autonomic efferent control centers in the CNS, mediating sensation and vasomotor, respiratory, and viscerosomatic outflow.

The enteric nervous system is often considered to be a third division of the ANS. This system is composed of a meshwork of fibers innervating the GI tract, pancreas, and gallbladder. The enteric nervous system is independent of CNS control and releases a variety of neurotransmitters. Although components of the enteric system are innervated by parasympathetic preganglionic fibers, local control appears to dominate function.

FUNCTIONAL RESPONSES MEDIATED BY THE AUTONOMIC NERVOUS SYSTEM

The responses to parasympathetic and sympathetic stimulation that occur in many important organs of the body are presented in Table 6.1. Most organs of the body are innervated by both parasympathetic and sympathetic nerves, which generally, but not always, produce opposing responses in effector organs such that inhibition of one system often leads to an increase in the response mediated by the other. Often an organ is under the predominant control of a single division of the ANS, although both components are usually present and can influence any given response. Organs innervated by both sympathetic and parasympathetic nerves include the heart, eye, bronchial tree, GI tract, urinary bladder, and reproductive organs. Some structures, such as blood vessels, the spleen, and piloerector muscles, receive only a single type of innervation, generally sympathetic.

It is important to note that the responses listed in Table 6.1 represent only those mediated by stimulation of nerves in innervated tissues and that activation of autonomic receptors located in tissues lacking nerve innervation can also lead to responses. For example, although vascular

smooth muscle has no parasympathetic innervation, it expresses muscarinic cholinergic receptors, which are functional and mediate responses to exogenously administered drugs; they play little or no normal physiological role.

Parasympathetic preganglionic neurons generally form only single synapses with postganglionic neurons, resulting in discrete and localized responses. In contrast, one sympathetic preganglionic neuron may ramify and ultimately synapse with many postganglionic sympathetic neurons, leading to diffuse responses. This anatomical distinction has profound physiological significance. Activation of sympathetic outflow, triggered by anger, fear, or stress, causes a state of activation characteristic of the fight, flight, or fright response. Heart rate is accelerated, blood pressure is increased, perfusion to skeletal muscle is augmented as blood flow is redirected from the skin and splanchnic region, the blood glucose concentration is elevated, bronchioles and pupils are dilated, and piloerection occurs.

In contrast, activation of parasympathetic outflow is associated with conservation of energy and maintenance of function during periods of lesser activity, hence "rest and digest" functions. Activation of parasympathetic outflow reduces heart rate and blood pressure, activates GI movements, and results in emptying of the urinary bladder and rectum. Furthermore, lacrimal, salivary, and mucous cells are activated, and the smooth muscle of the bronchial tree is contracted.

Although the parasympathetic nervous system is essential for life, the sympathetic nervous system is not. Animals completely deprived of their sympathetic nervous system can survive in a controlled environment but have difficulty responding to stressful conditions.

NEUROTRANSMISSION IN THE AUTONOMIC NERVOUS SYSTEM

Communication between neurons in the ANS is mediated by chemical neurotransmission, which involves the Ca^{++}-mediated release of neurotransmitter into the synapse, receptor activation, and transduction of the signal, leading to functional alterations in the cell. As depicted in Fig. 6.3, depolarization of a presynaptic nerve terminal leads to a large influx of Ca^{++} caused by opening voltage-dependent Ca^{++} channels in the membrane. This influx leads to alterations in cytoplasmic proteins surrounding the transmitter-containing synaptic vesicles, leading to translocation of the vesicles toward the plasma membrane and resulting in fusion of the vesicles with the membrane, releasing neurotransmitter into the synapse, a process termed exocytosis. After exocytosis, the voltage-dependent Ca^{++} channels inactivate rapidly, and the intracellular Ca^{++} concentration returns to normal by sequestration into intracellular compartments and active extrusion from the cell.

It is important to understand that voltage-dependent Ca^{++} channels in nerve terminals differ from those in other tissues. The Ca^{++} channel antagonists are an important class of drugs that block voltage-dependent Ca^{++} channels in cardiac and smooth muscle (Chapter 40). However, distinct subtypes of these channels exist that can be distinguished by their electrical and pharmacological properties. The Ca^{++} channel antagonists block the channels most often found in cardiac and smooth muscle, which are L-type Ca^{++} channels and have no effect on most of the voltage-dependent Ca^{++} channels in nerve terminals, which are N-type channels. This is fortunate, because if Ca^{++} channel antagonists also blocked neurotransmitter release, their toxicity would undoubtedly prevent them from being useful therapeutically.

After release, neurotransmitter diffuses across the synaptic cleft to interact with specific receptors on the dendrites and cell body of the postganglionic neuron or on cells of the effector organ, leading to a response. Efficient mechanisms for terminating the action of the neurotransmitter ensure that the system returns to baseline.

TABLE 6.1 Responses Elicited in Effector Organs by Stimulation of Sympathetic and Parasympathetic Nerves

Effector Organ	SYMPATHETIC (ADRENERGIC) RESPONSE		PARASYMPATHETIC (CHOLINERGIC) RESPONSE		Dominant Response
	Response	Receptor	Response	Receptor	
Heart					
Rate of contraction	Increase	β_1	Decrease	M_2	C
Force of contraction	Increase	β_1	Decrease	M_2	C
Blood Vessels					
Arteries (most)	Vasoconstriction	$\alpha_1\,(\alpha_2)^a$	–	–	A
Skeletal muscle	Vasodilation	β_2^b	–	–	A
Veins	Vasoconstriction	$\alpha_2\,(\alpha_1)$	–	–	A
Bronchial tree	Bronchodilation	β_2^b	Bronchoconstriction	M_3	C
Splenic capsule	Contraction	α_1	–	–	A
Uterus	Contraction	α_1	Variable	–	A
Vas deferens	Contraction	α_1	–	–	A
Gastrointestinal tract	Relaxation	α_2	Contraction	M_3	C
Eye					
Radial muscle, iris	Contraction (mydriasis)	α_1	–	–	A
Circular muscle, iris	–	–	Contraction (miosis)	M_3	C
Ciliary muscle	Relaxation	β_2^b	Contraction (accommodation)	M_3	C
Kidney	Renin secretion	β_1	–	–	A
Urinary Bladder					
Detrusor	Relaxation	β_2^b	Contraction	M_3	C
Trigone and sphincter	Contraction	α_1	Relaxation	M_3	A, C
Ureter	Contraction	α_1	–	–	A
Insulin release from pancreas	Decrease	α_2	–	–	A
Fat cells	Lipolysis	$\beta_1\,(\beta_3)$	–	–	A
Liver glycogenolysis	Increase	$\alpha_1\,(\beta_2)$	–	–	A
Hair follicles, smooth muscle	Contraction (piloerection)	α_1	–	–	A
Nasal secretion	Decrease	$\alpha_1\,(\alpha_2)^a$	Increase	–	C
Salivary glands	Increase secretion	α_1	Increase secretion	–	C
Sweat glands	Increase secretion	α_1	Increase secretion	–	C

[a]In general, postjunctional α_2-receptors are located outside synapses (extrajunctional) and are activated by circulating Epi.
[b]β_2 receptors are poorly activated by NE and tend to be located outside synapses; receptor activation may be in response to circulating Epi.
A, Adrenergic; *C*, cholinergic; *M*, muscarinic.

Neurotransmission at autonomic ganglia and neuroeffector junctions is illustrated in Fig. 6.4. In both sympathetic and parasympathetic ganglia and in the adrenal medulla, preganglionic stimulation leads to the release of ACh, which activates postjunctional nicotinic acetylcholine receptors, leading to a fast excitatory postsynaptic potential (EPSP) in postganglionic neurons, corresponding to the influx of cations through the nicotinic receptor ion channel. This EPSP may result in the generation of an action potential in postganglionic neurons or the release of Epi and NE from adrenal chromaffin cells. When the impulse reaches the neuroeffector junction, either ACh or NE is released to activate muscarinic cholinergic or adrenergic receptors, respectively, on cells of the effector organ to produce an appropriate response.

NEUROTRANSMITTERS IN THE AUTONOMIC NERVOUS SYSTEM

Acetylcholine

ACh is synthesized in cholinergic nerve terminals by the acetylation of choline, a process catalyzed by the enzyme choline acetyltransferase

(ChAT). As shown in Fig. 6.5, acetyl coenzyme A provided by mitochondria serves as the acetyl donor; choline is provided by both high-affinity uptake after ACh hydrolysis and phospholipid hydrolysis within the neuron.

Following ACh synthesis, the neurotransmitter is transported actively into vesicles by the vesicular ACh transporter (VAChT) and stored in vesicles from which ACh is released by exocytosis to interact with cholinergic muscarinic or nicotinic receptors. The action of ACh is terminated by the enzyme acetylcholinesterase (AChE), which hydrolyzes ACh rapidly, producing acetic acid and choline. The acetic acid diffuses from the synaptic cleft, whereas most (>50%) of the choline is taken back up into the nerve terminal by the Na^+-dependent high-affinity choline transporter (HAChT). Once inside the nerve terminal, choline can be reused for ACh synthesis.

Norepinephrine and Epinephrine

NE is synthesized in adrenergic nerve terminals by a series of enzymatic reactions beginning with the precursor tyrosine, as shown in Fig. 6.6. Tyrosine is transported into the neuron, followed by its hydroxylation

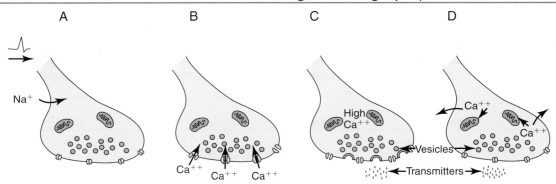

FIG. 6.3 Sequence of Events Linking Nerve Terminal Depolarization to Release of Neurotransmitter.
(A) The action potential arrives at the nerve terminal and depolarizes the membrane. (B) Voltage-gated Ca^{++} channels open, allowing the influx of Ca^{++} down its concentration gradient. (C) The increased intracellular Ca^{++} concentration affects cytoplasmic proteins interacting with transmitter-containing synaptic vesicles and promotes the translocation of vesicles to the plasma membrane, resulting in membrane fusion and exocytotic neurotransmitter release. (D) The Ca^{++} channels inactivate rapidly, and the intracellular Ca^{++} concentration returns to baseline by both sequestration into mitochondria and active extrusion from the cell.

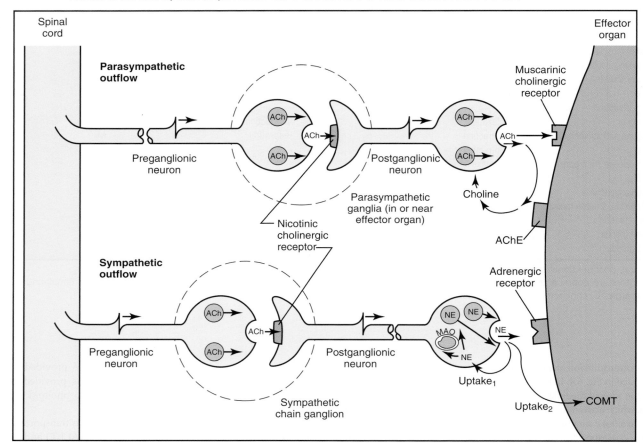

FIG. 6.4 Neurochemical Transmission in the Parasympathetic and Sympathetic Divisions of the ANS. Upon the arrival of an action potential at the preganglionic nerve terminal, the neurotransmitter acetylcholine (ACh) is released by both parasympathetic and sympathetic ganglia. ACh diffuses across the synaptic cleft to interact with nicotinic cholinergic receptors on postganglionic neurons (often referred to as ganglionic receptors). This interaction results in the generation of postsynaptic potentials that may lead to the generation and propagation of action potentials down postganglionic neurons to elicit the release of neurotransmitter at the postganglionic neuroeffector junction. The neurotransmitter released from postganglionic parasympathetic nerves is ACh, which activates muscarinic cholinergic receptors on the effector organ. The liberated ACh is metabolized rapidly by acetylcholinesterase (AChE) to acetic acid and choline; the latter is transported into the parasympathetic nerve terminal and is used to resynthesize ACh. At the postganglionic sympathetic neuroeffector junction, the neurotransmitter released is norepinephrine (NE), which stimulates adrenergic receptors to elicit the end-organ response. Most of the liberated NE is actively transported back into the sympathetic nerve terminal (Uptake$_1$) where it can be either transported back into vesicles or metabolized by monoamine oxidase (MAO) located in the mitochondria membrane. A smaller amount of the liberated NE may be taken up by extraneuronal cells (Uptake$_2$), after which it may be metabolized by catechol-O-methyltransferase (COMT).

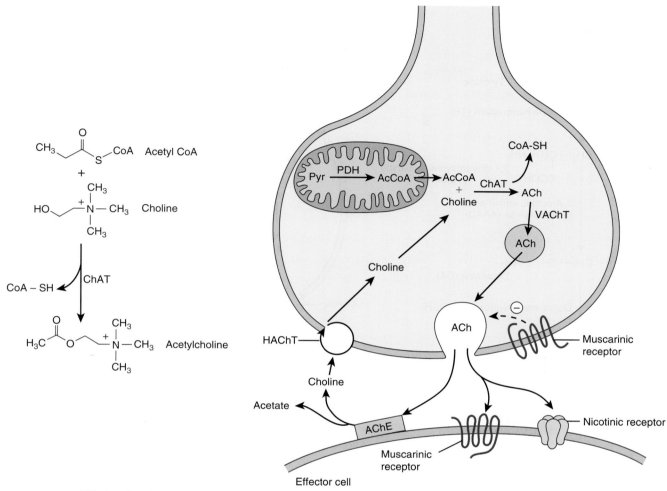

FIG. 6.5 Synthesis, Storage, and Inactivation of Acetylcholine (ACh). ACh is synthesized in cholinergic nerve terminals from acetyl coenzyme A (AcCoA), provided by mitochondria, and choline, provided by both high-affinity choline uptake (HAChT) and phospholipid hydrolysis within the neurons, through a reaction catalyzed by the enzyme choline acetyltransferase (ChAT). The ACh is transported actively into synaptic vesicles via the vesicular ACh transporter (VAChT). Upon the arrival of an action potential, the vesicles translocate to the plasma membrane, and through exocytosis, release ACh, which can interact with muscarinic or nicotinic cholinergic receptors. Following interaction with its receptors, the ACh is hydrolyzed by acetylcholinesterase (AChE) to acetate and choline; the latter is taken back up into the nerve terminal by the HAChT and is reused for ACh synthesis.

in the meta position by the rate-limiting enzyme **tyrosine hydroxylase** to form the catechol 3,4-dihydroxyphenylalanine (L-DOPA). L-DOPA is rapidly decarboxylated to DA by L-aromatic amino acid decarboxylase (AAAD), also known as DOPA decarboxylase. The DA is transported into the synaptic vesicles by the vesicular monoamine transporter (VMAT2 in neurons or VMAT1 in adrenal chromaffin cells). Within the vesicle of NE neurons, the enzyme dopamine β-hydroxylase (DBH) adds a hydroxyl group to DA to form NE, which is retained in the vesicle associated with ATP until the arrival of an action potential, leading to exocytosis. In some adrenergic neurons in the CNS and in some chromaffin cells of the adrenal medulla, an additional enzyme is present within the vesicles, phenylethanolamine-*N*-methyltransferase (PNMT), which methylates NE to Epi.

Following the interaction of released NE with **adrenergic α- or β-receptors**, its action is terminated primarily by the neuronal NE transporter (NET or Uptake₁), a Na⁺- and Ca⁺⁺-dependent high-affinity carrier that transports NE back into the sympathetic neuron for repackaging and eventual rerelease (Fig. 6.6). A small fraction of the NE in the synapse is taken up by a Na⁺- and Ca⁺⁺-independent lower affinity extraneuronal monoamine transporter present in myocardial, smooth muscle, or glandular cells (Uptake₂). Some of the NE taken back into sympathetic neurons is oxidatively deaminated by **monoamine oxidase (MAO)** located on the external mitochondrial membrane, followed by further metabolism in the blood by **catechol-*O*-methyltransferase (COMT)**, with excretion in the urine (Fig. 6.7). Similarly, the NE that is transported into postjunctional cells can be metabolized by COMT, followed by further metabolism in the blood by MAO, with excretion in the urine. It is critical to remember that the high-affinity transport of NE back into presynaptic terminals by NET represents the major mechanism terminating the actions of NE, with COMT and MAO important in metabolizing circulating catecholamines and some exogenously administered sympathomimetic amines.

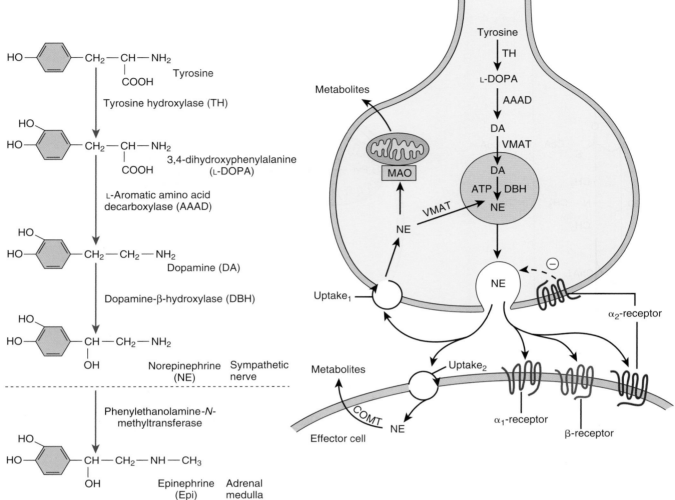

FIG. 6.6 Synthesis, Storage, and Termination of the Action of Norepinephrine (NE). NE is synthesized in adrenergic nerve terminals by a sequence of reactions beginning with the hydroxylation of tyrosine to 3,4-dihydroxyphenylalanine (L-DOPA), a rate-limiting reaction catalyzed by the enzyme tyrosine hydroxylase. The L-DOPA formed is decarboxylated to dopamine (DA) by the action of L-aromatic amino acid decarboxylase (AAAD) in the cytoplasm, followed by the active transport of DA into synaptic vesicles via the vesicular monoamine transporter (VMAT2 in neurons or VMAT1 in adrenal chromaffin cells), where it is hydroxylated to NE in a reaction catalyzed by the enzyme dopamine β-hydroxylase. The NE is stored with adenosine triphosphate (ATP), and upon the arrival of an action potential, the vesicles translocate to the plasma membrane, and through exocytosis, release NE, which can interact with α- or β-adrenergic receptors. The action of NE is terminated by reuptake (Uptake₁) back into the nerve terminal, where NE can be transported into the vesicle. Some of the NE taken back into sympathetic neurons can be oxidatively deaminated by monoamine oxidase (MAO) located on the external mitochondrial membrane, followed by further metabolism in the blood by catechol-O-methyltransferase (COMT), with excretion in the urine. Some NE may be taken up by a Na⁺- and Ca⁺⁺-independent lower affinity extraneuronal monoamine transporter present in myocardial, smooth muscle, or glandular cells (Uptake₂), and can be metabolized by COMT, followed by further metabolism in the blood by MAO, with excretion in the urine.

NEUROTRANSMITTER RECEPTORS IN THE AUTONOMIC NERVOUS SYSTEM

The receptor families and subtypes mediating the actions of ACh and NE are listed in Fig. 6.8.

Cholinergic Receptors

The action of ACh leads to different effects at various sites throughout the body, typically resulting from differences in the types and subtypes of cholinergic receptors activated. The actions of ACh are mediated by nicotinic or muscarinic receptors, the former ligand-gated ion channels, and the latter, G-protein–coupled receptors (Chapter 2).

The primary actions of ACh at both parasympathetic and sympathetic ganglia are mediated by activation of ganglionic nicotinic cholinergic receptors. These receptors are structurally and functionally similar to nicotinic receptors in the CNS and on immune cells but differ from those in skeletal muscle. Drugs affecting ganglionic and skeletal muscle nicotinic receptors are discussed in Chapters 9 and 10.

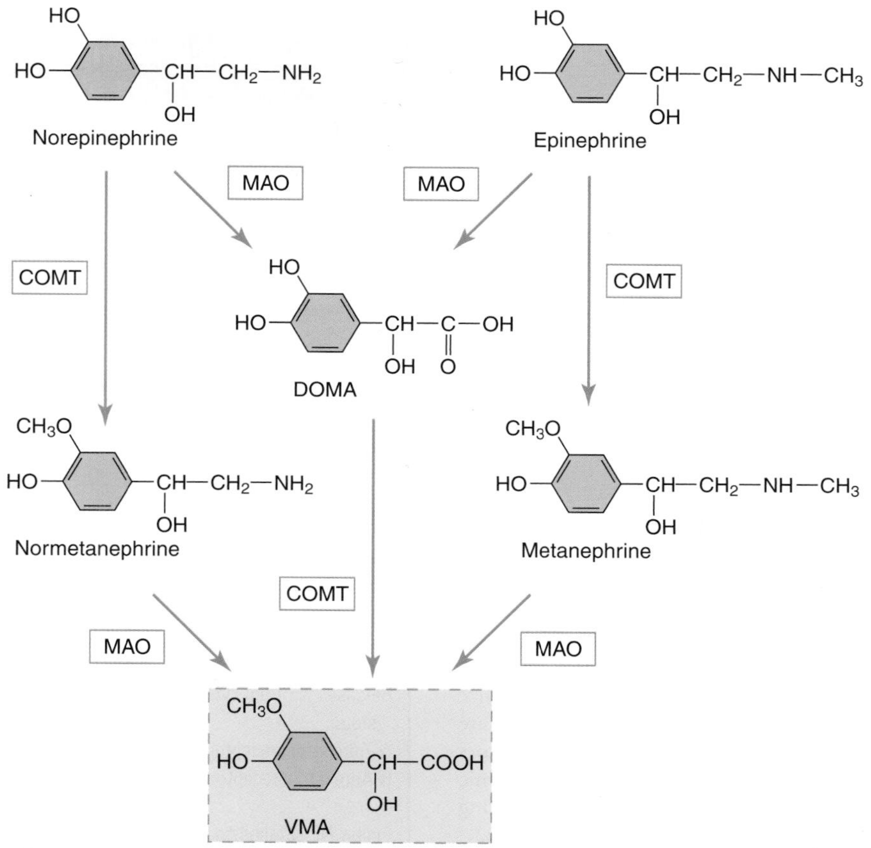

FIG. 6.7 Major Catabolic Pathways for Norepinephrine and Epinephrine. Both norepinephrine and epinephrine can be metabolized by monoamine oxidase (MAO) to dihydroxymandelic acid (DOMA), which is then converted by catechol-O-methyltransferase (COMT) to 3-methoxy-4-hydroxymandelic acid (VMA). Alternatively, norepinephrine may be metabolized to normetanephrine by COMT, followed by metabolism to VMA by MAO, whereas epinephrine may be metabolized to metanephrine by COMT, followed by metabolism to VMA by MAO. VMA is the final common metabolite for each of these catecholamines.

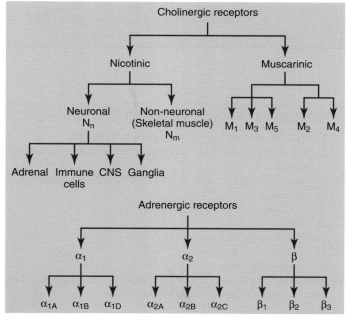

FIG. 6.8 Classification of Cholinergic and Adrenergic Receptor Types and Subtypes.

The receptors mediating responses to ACh at parasympathetic neuroeffector junctions are muscarinic and consist of five subtypes (M_1 to M_5) based on their pharmacological specificities, amino acid sequences, and genes. Stimulation of M_1, M_3, and M_5 receptors leads to activation of G_q and the phospholipase C–mediated generation of diacylglycerol and inositol-1,4,5-trisphosphate. Stimulation of M_2 and M_4 receptors activates $G_{i/o}$, decreasing adenylyl cyclase and neuronal Ca^{++} channels and activating inwardly rectified K^+ channels. Drugs affecting muscarinic receptors are discussed in Chapters 7 and 8.

Adrenergic Receptors

There is a total of nine adrenergic receptors, subdivided into three subfamilies (α_1, α_2, and β), each of which contains three distinct subtypes encoded by separate genes with amino acid sequences very similar among the subtypes within a given subfamily, and all of which are **G-protein–coupled receptors** (Fig. 6.8). The α_1-adrenergic receptors produce their effects via activation of G_q and phospholipase C–mediated generation of diacylglycerol and inositol-1,4,5-trisphosphate. The α_2-adrenergic receptors usually produce their effects by inhibiting adenylyl cyclase through $G_{i/o}$ and decreasing intracellular cyclic adenosine monophosphate (cAMP). However, α_2-adrenergic receptors may also use other mechanisms of signal transduction. For example, in blood vessels, α_2-receptor stimulation leads to the activation of a membrane Ca^{++} channel, resulting in Ca^{++} influx. The β-adrenergic receptors are all coupled to G_s, with activation leading to increased adenylyl cyclase and activation of cAMP-dependent protein kinases, leading to the phosphorylation of various intracellular proteins.

NE released from sympathetic neurons activates α_1-, α_2-, β_1-, and β_3- (low potency at β_2) adrenergic receptors on exocrine glands, fat cells, smooth muscle, and cardiac muscle to produce sympathetic responses. In addition, Epi released from the adrenal gland activates all adrenergic receptor subtypes.

Although adrenergic receptors mediating the actions of NE at sympathetic neuroeffector junctions are located postsynaptically on the organ innervated, prejunctional $\alpha2$-receptors have been identified on adrenergic nerve terminals. Activation of these receptors by released NE or by α_2-adrenergic receptor agonists decreases further release of neurotransmitter. This presynaptic inhibitory "autoreceptor" mechanism may be involved in the normal regulation of neurotransmitter release because blockade of prejunctional α_2-receptors leads to enhanced NE release.

DRUGS AFFECTING THE AUTONOMIC NERVOUS SYSTEM

Drugs can affect all processes involved in the functioning of the ANS and either enhance or inhibit cholinergic or adrenergic transmission. Drugs can act presynaptically to affect the synthesis, storage, release, reuptake, and degradation of ACh or NE. Drugs can also stimulate or antagonize cholinergic or adrenergic receptors. Examples of such compounds are listed in Table 6.2. Drugs affecting cholinergic muscarinic receptors are discussed in Chapters 7 and 8, those affecting cholinergic nicotinic receptors are discussed in Chapters 9 and 10, while drugs affecting adrenergic α- and β-receptors are discussed in Chapters 11 and 12.

NEW DEVELOPMENTS

Pharmacogenomic differences in several proteins involved with both cholinergic and noradrenergic systems have been observed, including both muscarinic and adrenergic receptor variants. In addition, single-nucleotide polymorphisms have been found to be associated with certain abnormal phenotypes (e.g., cardiovascular abnormalities). The area of personalized medicine as it applies to autonomic pharmacology has embarked on a new wave of discovery, with the goal of ensuring that all patients receive safer and more effective drugs through personalized medicine approaches (Chapter 4).

TABLE 6.2 Mechanisms of Action of Pharmacological Compounds Affecting the Autonomic Nervous System (ANS)

Cellular Mechanism	Example
Agents That Enhance Cholinergic Neurotransmission	
Releases ACh from vesicles	Black widow spider venom (latrotoxins)
Inhibition of ACh hydrolysis (AChE inhibitors)	Physostigmine, neostigmine
Nicotinic receptor agonist	Nicotine, varenicline
Muscarinic receptor agonist	Methacholine, bethanechol
Agents That Inhibit Cholinergic Neurotransmission	
Inhibition of high-affinity choline uptake	Hemicholinium-3
Inhibition of exocytosis	Botulinum toxin
Inhibition of vesicular ACh transport (VAChT)	Vesamicol
Ganglionic blockers	Hexamethonium, mecamylamine
Nicotinic receptor blockers	D-Tubocurarine
Muscarinic receptor blockers	Atropine
Agents That Enhance Adrenergic Neurotransmission	
Releases NE from cytoplasmic stores	Tyramine, amphetamine
α-Adrenergic receptor agonists	Phenylephrine (α_1), clonidine (α_2)
β-Adrenergic receptor agonists	Isoproterenol (β), dobutamine (β_1), terbutaline (β_2)
Inhibit NE catabolism	Pargyline (inhibits MAO), Tolcapone (inhibits COMT)
Agents That Inhibit Adrenergic Neurotransmission	
Inhibit NE biosynthesis	α-Methyltyrosine (inhibits tyrosine hydroxylase)
Inhibits NE release	Guanethidine
Inhibits vesicular NE transport	Reserpine
Inhibits uptake$_1$	Cocaine
α-Adrenergic receptor antagonists	Phentolamine (α_1 and α_2), prazosin (α_1), yohimbine (α_2)
β-Adrenergic receptor antagonists	Propranolol (nonselective)

■ SELF-ASSESSMENT QUESTIONS

1. Which one of the following is a characteristic of the parasympathetic nervous system?
   A. NE is the neurotransmitter at parasympathetic ganglia.
   B. ACh is the neurotransmitter at autonomic ganglia.
   C. Postganglionic neurons are long and myelinated.
   D. Cell bodies for preganglionic neurons originate in the lumbar and thoracic regions of the spinal cord.
   E. Parasympathetic neurons innervating the respiratory system mediate bronchodilation.

2. The sympathetic nervous system is characterized by which one of the following?
   A. Ganglia are located close to the organ innervated.
   B. The neurotransmitter at postganglionic sympathetic neuroeffector junctions is NE.
   C. Postganglionic sympathetic neurons are short.

   D. NE is the neurotransmitter at sympathetic ganglia.
   E. The absence of nicotinic cholinergic receptors at the paravertebral ganglia.

3. Which one of the following autonomic receptors are ligand-gated ion channels?
   A. Nicotinic.
   B. Muscarinic.
   C. α_1-Adrenergic receptor.
   D. α_2-Adrenergic receptor.
   E. β_1-Adrenergic receptor.

4. Stimulation of prejunctional or presynaptic α_2-adrenergic receptors on postganglionic sympathetic neurons causes:
   A. Inhibition of ACh release.
   B. Stimulation of Epi release.
   C. Stimulation of NE release.

D. Inhibition of NE release.

E. Inhibition of Epi release.

5. Activation of the parasympathetic nervous system results in which of the following responses?

A. An increase in heart rate.

B. Vasoconstriction.

C. Bronchoconstriction.

D. Renin secretion.

E. Relaxation of the GI tract.

FURTHER READING

Goldstein DS, Kopin IJ. Homeostatic systems, biocybernetics, and autonomic neuroscience. *Auton Neurosci.* 2017;208:15–28.

Gourine AV, Machhada A, Trapp S, Spyer KM. Cardiac vagal preganglionic neurons: an update. *Auton Neurosci.* 2016;199:24–28.

Lieve KV, van der Werf C, Wilde AA. Catecholaminergic polymorphic ventricular tachycardia. *Circ J.* 2016;80:1285–1291.

WEBSITES

http://www.merckmanuals.com/home/brain,-spinal-cord,-and-nerve-disorders/autonomic-nervous-system-disorders/overview-of-the-autonomic-nervous-system

An excellent overview of the autonomic nervous system is presented on this site from the Merck Manual.

http://www.guidetopharmacology.org

This is the International Union of Basic and Clinical Pharmacology (IUPHAR) receptor website with excellent information on autonomic receptors.

7

Muscarinic Agonists, Cholinesterase Inhibitors, and Their Clinical Uses

F.J. Ehlert

THERAPEUTIC OVERVIEW

Muscarinic receptors are expressed in brain and peripheral tissues and can be activated either directly by **muscarinic agonists** or indirectly by prolonging acetylcholine (ACh)-mediated activation with **cholinesterase (ChE) inhibitors**. Both classes of agents have effects on peripheral tissues that are similar to those elicited by stimulation of parasympathetic nerves (Chapter 6). Inducing this **parasympathomimetic** action in specific tissues is therapeutic for several clinical situations. For example, in the treatment of **glaucoma**, muscarinic agonists are applied topically to the eye to reduce intraocular pressure by facilitating the drainage of aqueous humor. Muscarinic agonists are also administered orally for the treatment of **xerostomia**, particularly in Sjögren syndrome, because of their ability to stimulate secretions from salivary glands. Finally, muscarinic agonists stimulate smooth muscle contractions and hence are useful in the treatment of **gastroparesis**, urinary retention, and decreased bowel motility. The choice of drug and the route of administration depend on pharmacokinetics and the intended site of action. A list of these uses is presented in the Therapeutic Overview Box. The use of ChE inhibitors for the treatment of Alzheimer's disease is discussed in Chapter 14 and for the treatment of neuromuscular disorders in Chapter 9.

MECHANISMS OF ACTION

Muscarinic Receptors

Muscarinic cholinergic receptors are selectively activated by the fungal alkaloid **muscarine** and inhibited by **atropine**, the prototypical muscarinic antagonist. Muscarinic receptors mediate cellular responses by

THERAPEUTIC OVERVIEW

Muscarinic Receptor Agonists
   Glaucoma
   Postoperative ileus, congenital megacolon, urinary retention
   Xerostomia, Sjögren syndrome

Cholinesterase (ChE) Inhibitors
   Glaucoma
   Postoperative ileus, congenital megacolon, urinary retention

interacting with heterotrimeric G-proteins to affect ionic conductances and the cytosolic concentration of second messengers (Chapter 2). The active state of the agonist-receptor complex is steadily phosphorylated by a receptor kinase, with the phosphoryl residues providing docking sites for β-arrestin. The binding of β-arrestin to the receptor prevents G-protein signaling but also establishes β-arrestin signaling platforms that mediate a variety of cellular responses.

There are five muscarinic receptor subtypes (M_1–M_5), with M_1, M_3, and M_5 receptors coupled to G_q-proteins and M_2 and M_4 receptors coupled to $G_{i/o}$. Thus stimulation of M_1, M_3, or M_5 receptors activates phospholipase C-β (PLC-β), leading to increased phosphoinositide hydrolysis, the release of intracellular Ca^{2+}, and the suppression of a noninactivating K^+ conductance, termed the *M current*. In contrast, M_2 and M_4 receptor activation leads to inhibition of adenylyl cyclase and neuronal Ca^{2+} channels and an activation of inwardly rectified K^+ channels.

In the heart, M_2 muscarinic receptors are expressed in conducting tissue, pacemaker cells, and the myocardium of the ventricles and atria, where they mediate an increase in atrioventricular conduction time and a decrease in heart rate (**negative chronotropic**) and force of contraction (**negative inotropic**), respectively. The signaling mechanisms mediating these effects are depicted in Fig. 7.1.

Both M_2 and M_3 muscarinic receptors are expressed on smooth muscle, where they mediate contraction. The signaling pathways mediating the contraction of smooth muscle upon activation of M_2 and M_3 receptors are depicted in Fig. 7.2A. Activation of M_3 receptors causes smooth muscle contraction directly, whereas activation of M_2 receptors promotes contraction indirectly by suppressing Ca^{2+}-activated K^+ channels, enhancing a cation conductance and suppressing β-adrenergic receptor–mediated relaxation of smooth muscle. Thus activation of these receptors in the airways of the lung, gastrointestinal (GI) tract,

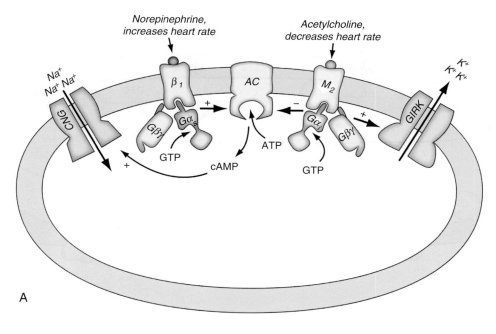

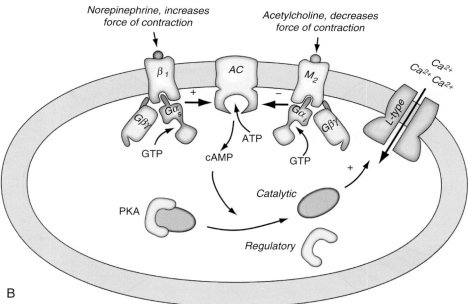

FIG. 7.1 Signaling Mechanisms of the M$_2$ Muscarinic Receptor in Cardiac Tissue. (A) In pacemaker cells, β$_1$-adrenergic receptors signal through the heterotrimeric G$_s$-protein, which activates adenylyl cyclase (AC) and increases intracellular levels of cyclic adenosine monophosphate (cAMP). cAMP binds to and opens a cyclic nucleotide-gated cation channel (CNG) that depolarizes pacemaker cells and increases their firing rate, which increases heart rate. M$_2$ muscarinic receptor activation opposes this effect by activating G$_i$, which inhibits adenylyl cyclase. The M$_2$ muscarinic receptor also directly slows heart rate through the βγ subunits that are released upon activation of G$_i$. These stimulate an inwardly rectified K$^+$ conductance (GIRK) at resting membrane potentials, which slows the rate of depolarization of pacemaker cells, resulting in decreased heart rate. (B) In the ventricular myocardium, the β$_1$-adrenergic and M$_2$ muscarinic receptors also have opposing effects on adenylyl cyclase. cAMP binds to the regulatory subunit of protein kinase A (PKA), releasing the catalytic subunit, which phosphorylates voltage-sensitive Ca^{2+} channels. This phosphorylation increases Ca^{2+} influx and ultimately the force of contraction. β$_1$-adrenergic (stimulatory) and M$_2$ muscarinic (inhibitory) receptors have opposing effects on contractility through regulation of adenylyl cyclase.

Smooth muscle cell

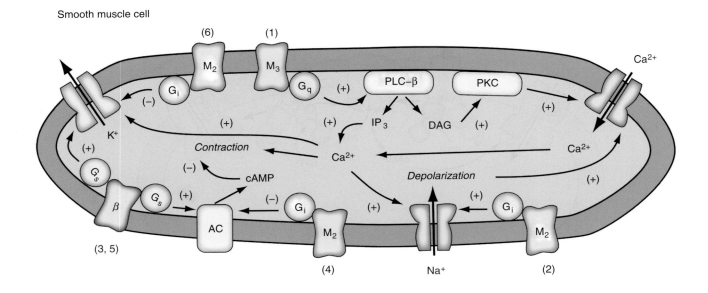

Blood vessel

Gastrointestinal sphincter

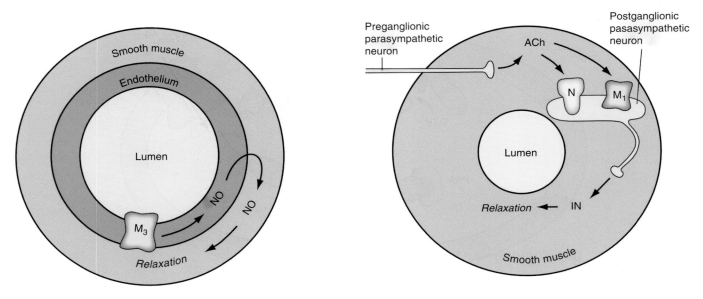

FIG. 7.2 Muscarinic Receptor-Mediated Contraction and Relaxation in Different Types of Smooth Muscle. (A) Most smooth muscle cells express M_2 and M_3 receptors that cause contraction. *(1)* Activation of M_3 receptors elicits contraction through stimulation of phospholipase C-β (PLC-β), which cleaves phosphatidylinositol-4,5-bisphosphate to diacylglycerol (DAG) and inositol-1,4,5-trisphosphate (IP_3). The IP_3 mobilizes Ca^{2+} and triggers contraction. *(2)* Activation of the M_2 receptor mediates a Ca^{2+}-dependent cation influx (mainly Na^+) that causes depolarization and activation of voltage-sensitive Ca^{2+} channels. The Ca^{2+}-dependency of this influx is satisfied by simultaneous activation of the M_3 receptor. *(3)* β-adrenergic receptors stimulate adenylyl cyclase *(AC)* activity, causing an increase in cyclic adenosine monophosphate *(cAMP)* accumulation, which mediates relaxation. *(4)* M_2 receptor activation opposes β-adrenergic receptor-mediated relaxation through inhibition of AC. *(5)* β-adrenergic receptors activate large conductance, Ca^{2+}-activated K^+ channels, causing hyperpolarization and relaxation. *(6)* Activation of the M_2 receptor inhibits large conductance Ca^{2+}-activated K^+ channels, which promotes contraction. (B) Most peripheral blood vessels express M_3 receptors on their endothelium, which trigger the synthesis of nitric oxide (NO). The NO diffuses into the smooth muscle, where it mediates relaxation through the production of cyclic guanosine monophosphate (cGMP). (C) Activation of M_1 receptors and nicotinic receptors (N) in parasympathetic ganglia causes the release of an inhibitory neurotransmitter (IN) from postganglionic neurons in gastrointestinal sphincters. This inhibitory neurotransmitter is usually ATP, NO, or VIP and causes relaxation of the sphincter smooth muscle.

and urinary bladder causes bronchoconstriction, an increase in motility, and micturition, respectively.

Despite their lack of innervation by cholinergic nerves, many peripheral blood vessels express M_3 muscarinic receptors on their endothelium. Activation of these receptors by an administered muscarinic agonist increases the production of nitric oxide (NO), which diffuses to the muscle and causes relaxation of the underlying smooth muscle and ultimately vasodilatation (Fig. 7.2B). Similarly, activation of M_1 receptors in parasympathetic ganglia releases an inhibitory neurotransmitter such as adenosine triphosphate (ATP), NO, or vasoactive intestinal peptide (VIP) to relax smooth muscle sphincters (Fig. 7.2C).

In the anterior chamber of the eye, muscarinic agonists constrict the iris sphincter, causing miosis, and contract the circular ciliary muscle, causing accommodation of the lens.

The M_3 receptor, and to a lesser extent the M_1 receptor, are expressed in exocrine glands, where they mediate secretion. Thus muscarinic agonists increase secretions of sweat, salivary and lacrimal glands, and the glands of the trachea and GI mucosa. The M_3 receptor is also expressed on gastric parietal cells, where it mediates gastric acid secretion.

Muscarinic agonists also activate receptors throughout the CNS, where they play a role in numerous functions, including learning, memory, movement, control of posture, and temperature regulation. Excessive activation of central muscarinic receptors causes tremor, convulsions, and hypothermia.

Drugs Activating Muscarinic Receptors

Drugs activate muscarinic receptors either directly or indirectly, the former termed muscarinic agonists, and the latter ChE inhibitors, producing their effects by inhibiting ACh hydrolysis, thereby increasing the concentration and prolonging the action of ACh at cholinergic synapses.

Muscarinic Receptor Agonists

The structures of several direct-acting cholinergic agonists are shown in Fig. 7.3. Introduction of a methyl group in the β position of ACh yields methacholine and bethanechol, agonists selective for muscarinic receptors. The substitution of an amino group for the terminal methyl group yields corresponding carbamic acid ester derivatives (i.e., carbachol and bethanechol), which are resistant to hydrolysis by acetylcholinesterase (AChE) and consequently have a longer duration of action than the

corresponding acetic acid esters. The structures of the selective muscarinic agonists, pilocarpine and cevimeline, are also shown in Fig. 7.3.

Cholinesterase Inhibitors

Two types of ChE enzymes are expressed in the body, AChE and butyrylcholinesterase (BuChE, also called plasma ChE or pseudo-ChE), each with a different distribution and substrate specificity. AChE is located at synapses throughout the nervous system and is responsible for terminating the action of ACh. BuChE is located at nonneuronal sites, including plasma and liver, and is responsible for the metabolism of certain drugs, including ester-type local anesthetics (Chapter 27) and succinylcholine (Chapter 10). Most enzyme inhibitors used clinically do not discriminate between the two types of ChEs.

The mechanism involved in the hydrolysis of ACh is shown in Fig. 7.4. AChE is a member of the serine hydrolase family of enzymes and contains a serine (Ser)-histidine (His)-glutamate (Glu) triad at the active site. When ACh binds to AChE, the quaternary nitrogen of ACh binds to the choline subsite, positioning the ester group near the catalytic site. The ester moiety undergoes a nucleophilic attack by the serine of the catalytic site, resulting in the hydrolysis of ACh and binding of acetate to the serine of the catalytic domain (acetylation). The acetylated serine is rapidly hydrolyzed, and the free enzyme is regenerated. This enzymatic reaction is one of the fastest known; approximately 10^4 molecules of ACh are hydrolyzed per second by a single AChE molecule.

ChE inhibitors are divided into two main types, reversible and irreversible. Reversible inhibitors are further subdivided into noncovalent and covalent enzyme inhibitors. Noncovalent inhibitors, such as edrophonium, bind reversibly to the anionic domain of AChE. The duration of action is determined in part by the way in which the inhibitor binds. Edrophonium binds weakly and has a rapid renal clearance, resulting in a brief duration of action (approximately 10 minutes). Tacrine and donepezil are also noncovalent ChE inhibitors used to treat Alzheimer's disease (Chapter 14); they have higher affinities and partition into lipids, providing for longer durations of action.

Covalent reversible ChE inhibitors, such as physostigmine and neostigmine, are carbamic acid ester derivatives and are sometimes referred to as carbamate inhibitors. These compounds bind to AChE and are hydrolyzed, resulting in carbamylation of the serine in the active site (Fig. 7.5). Hydrolysis of the carbamylated enzyme requires 2–4 hours,

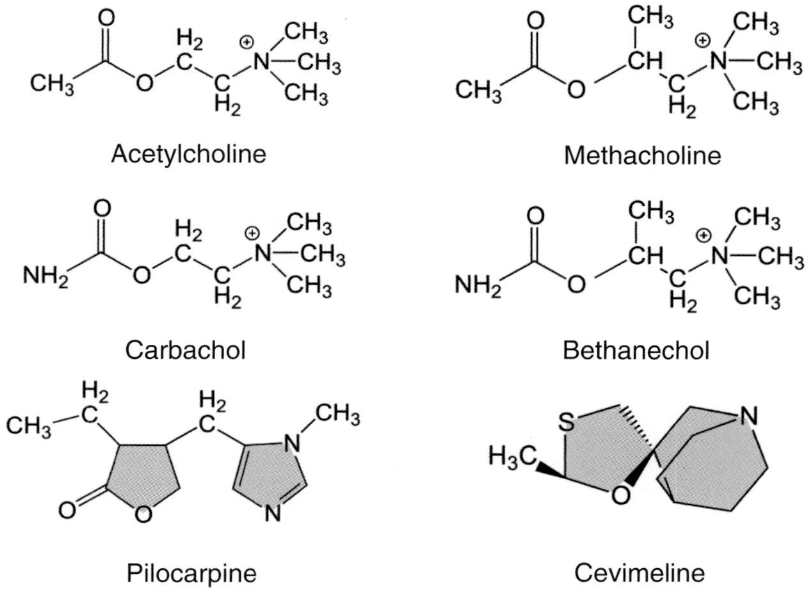

Acetylcholine

Methacholine

Carbachol

Bethanechol

Pilocarpine

Cevimeline

FIG. 7.3 Structures of Some Direct-Acting Cholinergic Agonists.

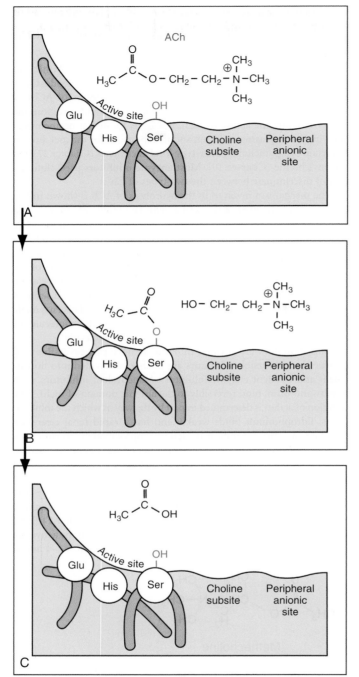

FIG. 7.4 Hydrolysis of Acetylcholine (ACh) by Acetylcholinesterase (AChE). The active site of the AChE enzyme contains an amino acid triad consisting of serine (Ser), histidine (His), and glutamate (Glu). In addition, there are two aromatic cages that interact with the positive charge of choline (choline subsite) and of some cholinesterase inhibitors (peripheral anionic site), respectively. (A) The quaternary (+) nitrogen of the choline portion of the ACh molecule is attracted to the choline subsite, positioning the ester portion of ACh in close proximity to the catalytic site. (B) The ester bond on ACh is cleaved, the enzyme is acetylated, and choline is released. (C) Hydrolysis of the acetylated enzyme **rapidly** liberates the acetate, and the free enzyme can hydrolyze another ACh molecule.

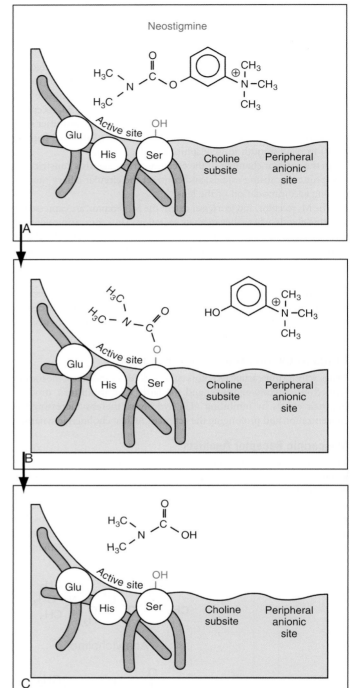

FIG. 7.5 The Interaction of a Reversible Acetylcholinesterase (AChE) Inhibitor, Neostigmine, With AChE. The active site of the AChE enzyme contains an amino acid triad consisting of serine (Ser), histidine (His), and glutamate (Glu). (A) The quaternary (+) nitrogen of neostigmine is attracted to the peripheral anionic site, positioning the ester portion of the molecule in close proximity to the catalytic site. (B) The carbamic acid ester bond on neostigmine is cleaved, the enzyme is carbamylated, preventing the enzyme from interacting with ACh, and the remainder of the neostigmine molecule is released. (C) Hydrolysis of carbamylated enzyme occurs **slowly**, causing reversible inhibition of the enzyme.

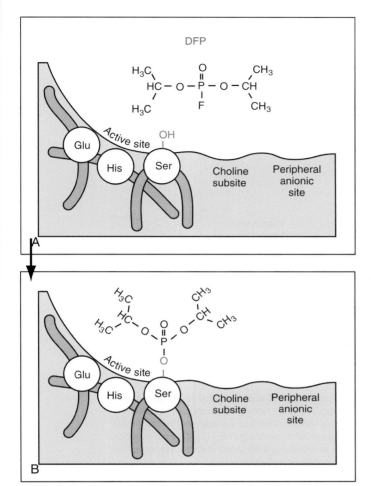

FIG. 7.6 The Interaction of an Irreversible Acetylcholinesterase (AChE) Inhibitor, Isoflurophate (*DFP*, or Diisopropyl Flurophosphate), With AChE. The active site of the AChE enzyme contains an amino acid triad consisting of serine (Ser), histidine (His), and glutamate (Glu). (A) The phosphate portion of DFP aligns with the catalytic site of the enzyme. (B) The enzyme is phosphorylated, representing a very stable moiety. Enzyme inhibition is considered **irreversible**; dephosphorylation, if it occurs, takes hours. With the passage of time, the phosphorylated enzyme undergoes a process termed *aging*, which involves hydrolysis of one of the isopropyl groups of the inhibitor, rendering the complex unable to dissociate. Note: An oxime such as 2-PAM, if administered before aging occurs, can bind to and release the phosphate moiety attached to the enzyme; this process reverses the enzyme inhibition.

TABLE 7.1 Direct- and Indirect-Acting Cholinomimetic Drugs and Their Uses

Action	Agent	Use
Direct-Acting (Muscarinic Receptor Agonists)		
	Pilocarpine	Glaucoma
	Carbachol	Glaucoma
	Bethanechol	Postoperative ileus, congenital megacolon, urinary retention
Indirect-Acting (ChE Inhibitors[a])		
	Physostigmine	Glaucoma
	Demecarium	Glaucoma
	Echothiophate	Glaucoma
	Isoflurophate	Glaucoma
	Neostigmine	Postoperative ileus, congenital megacolon, urinary retention, reversal of neuromuscular blockade
	Edrophonium	Diagnosis of myasthenia gravis, reversal of neuromuscular blockade, supraventricular tachyarrhythmias
	Ambenonium	Treatment of myasthenia gravis
	Pyridostigmine	Treatment of myasthenia gravis, reversal of neuromuscular blockade

[a]ChE inhibitors used for Alzheimer disease are discussed in Chapter 14.

inactivate other serine hydrolases, including trypsin and chymotrypsin. Enzyme reactivation with **oximes**, such as **pralidoxime** (**2-PAM**), is used in conjunction with respiratory support and muscarinic receptor antagonists to treat poisoning from organophosphorus ChE inhibitors.

ChE inhibitors amplify the effects of ACh at all sites throughout the nervous system, which results in both therapeutic and adverse effects. Thus ChE inhibitors indirectly activate both nicotinic and muscarinic receptors throughout the brain and peripheral nervous system, including receptors at the neuromuscular junction, sympathetic and parasympathetic ganglia, and peripheral tissues innervated by parasympathetic nerves.

RELATIONSHIP OF MECHANISMS OF ACTION TO CLINICAL RESPONSE

The muscarinic agonists and ChE inhibitors are used primarily for the treatment of glaucoma, to stimulate smooth muscle contraction, and to promote secretions. Specific agents used for these indications are listed in Table 7.1.

Ophthalmology

If untreated, high intraocular pressure (glaucoma) damages the optic nerve and retina, resulting in blindness. Usually, glaucoma is caused by impaired drainage of aqueous humor, which is produced by the ciliary epithelium in the posterior chamber of the eye. Normally, aqueous humor flows into the anterior chamber by first passing between the lens and iris and then out through the pupil (Fig. 7.7A). It leaves the anterior chamber by flowing through the fenestrated trabecular meshwork and into the canal of Schlemm, which lies at the vertex of the angle formed by the intersection of the cornea and the iris. This region is known as the ocular angle. In primary **closed-angle glaucoma**, pressure from the posterior chamber pushes the iris forward, closing the ocular angle and preventing the drainage of aqueous humor (Fig. 7.7B). People with narrow angles are predisposed to closed-angle glaucoma. In primary

contributing to the moderate duration of action of these compounds. By contrast, the acetylated enzyme produced during the hydrolysis of ACh decays within seconds to yield the free enzyme.

Irreversible ChE inhibitors phosphorylate the serine in the active site of AChE (Fig. 7.6). These compounds include the toxic nerve gases **sarin**, **soman**, and **tabun**; the insecticides **parathion** and **malathion**; and the therapeutic agents **echothiophate** and **isoflurophate**. Collectively, these compounds are termed **organophosphorus** or **organophosphate** ChE inhibitors. The phosphorylated enzyme formed with these compounds is extremely stable. Dephosphorylation of the phosphorylated enzyme takes hours, if it occurs at all. In the case of secondary (isoflurophate) and tertiary (soman) alkyl-substituted phosphates, the phosphorylated enzyme is so stable that it is not dephosphorylated, and new enzyme molecules must be synthesized for enzyme activity to recover. Many organophosphorus ChE inhibitors also irreversibly phosphorylate and

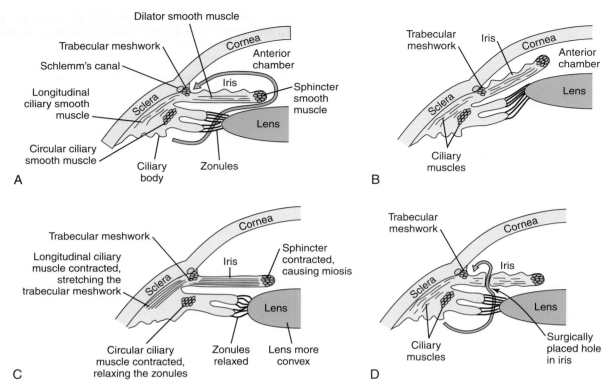

FIG. 7.7 **The Anterior Chamber of the Eye and the Pharmacological and Surgical Measures Used to Treat Glaucoma.** (A) The flow of aqueous humor *(arrow)* from the ciliary body to the trabecular meshwork. (B) In closed-angle glaucoma, pressure from the posterior chamber pushes the iris against the trabecular meshwork, closing the ocular angle and preventing the drainage of aqueous humor. (C) Cholinomimetics constrict the iris sphincter, thereby opening up the ocular angle and causing a decrease in intraocular pressure in closed-angle glaucoma. Cholinomimetics also elicit contraction of the longitudinal and circular ciliary muscles. Contraction of the longitudinal ciliary muscle stretches open the trabecular meshwork and facilitates the drainage of aqueous humor, particularly in open-angle glaucoma. The circular ciliary muscle forms a sphincter-like ring around the lens, into which the zonules are attached. Constriction of the circular muscle relaxes the tension on the zonules and allows the lens to relax into a more convex shape, which increases its refractive power and enables near vision. (D) The surgical treatment of closed-angle glaucoma entails the placement of a hole in the peripheral iris, either surgically or with a laser. The procedure provides a pathway for drainage of aqueous humor *(arrow)* and thus reduces intraocular pressure.

open-angle glaucoma, the ocular angle remains open, but abnormalities in the trabecular meshwork cause the outflow of aqueous humor to be impeded. In secondary glaucoma, inflammation, trauma, or various ocular diseases can cause intraocular pressure to increase.

Glaucoma is treated with both direct-acting muscarinic agonists and ChE inhibitors. Open-angle glaucoma is also treated with carbonic anhydrase inhibitors, β-adrenergic receptor antagonists, and epinephrine (Epi).

When applied topically to the eye, cholinomimetics constrict the pupil, contract the longitudinal and circular ciliary muscles, and decrease intraocular pressure. In open-angle glaucoma, the contraction of the longitudinal ciliary muscle decreases intraocular pressure by stretching the trabecular meshwork and opening its tubules. In closed-angle glaucoma, pupillary constriction lowers the intraocular pressure by pulling the iris away from the trabeculum and opening the angle (Fig. 7.7C). Closed-angle glaucoma is a medical emergency that is corrected surgically by cutting a drainage pathway in the peripheral portion of the iris to release pressure in the posterior chamber (Fig. 7.7D). Cholinomimetics are used acutely to treat closed-angle glaucoma until surgery can be performed. Occasionally, patients with closed-angle glaucoma exhibit a paradoxical increase in intraocular pressure in response to cholinomimetics because constriction of the pupil causes

the iris to be pressed against the lens, thereby blocking the flow of aqueous humor into the anterior chamber. Cholinomimetics are also used to treat a variety of noninflammatory secondary glaucomas.

Among the cholinomimetics, pilocarpine is most commonly used. Because its duration of action is approximately 6 hours, it must be administered topically approximately four times a day. Pilocarpine can also be delivered in a reservoir. Although pilocarpine can cause local irritation, it is better tolerated than other cholinomimetics. Other short-acting cholinomimetics used in the treatment of glaucoma are carbachol and physostigmine. The long-acting organophosphorus ChE inhibitor, echothiophate, is sometimes used to treat glaucoma; however, it can lead to cataracts with long-term use. Thus it is used only in patients with artificial lenses or in those cases in which other agents are ineffective.

Gastrointestinal and Urinary Tracts

The muscarinic agonist bethanechol and the ChE inhibitor neostigmine are used to treat congenital megacolon, urinary retention, and decreased stomach and bowel motility when there is no obstruction (e.g., postoperatively). When administered orally, these drugs primarily affect the GI tract by stimulating muscarinic receptors on smooth muscle and promoting micturition and GI motility.

The muscarinic agonists pilocarpine and cevimeline are used in the symptomatic treatment of Sjögren syndrome, a chronic autoimmune inflammatory condition of the exocrine glands, including the lacrimal and salivary glands. Patients suffering from this condition have dry eyes and mouth and have difficulty swallowing food. Pilocarpine and cevimeline are administered to promote the flow of saliva and facilitate swallowing and ingestion of food. These agents exhibit selectivity for M_3 and M_1 muscarinic receptors, the major and minor muscarinic receptor subtypes expressed in salivary glands, respectively.

Other Uses of Cholinesterase Inhibitors

Neuromuscular blocking agents are often administered as adjuncts during general anesthesia (Chapter 10) and are sometimes useful to rapidly reverse neuromuscular blockade after surgery. The reversible quaternary ChE inhibitors, such as neostigmine and pyridostigmine, are used for this purpose to enable ACh to more effectively compete with nondepolarizing neuromuscular blockers and restore function at the neuromuscular junction. Atropine is often used in combination with the ChE inhibitors to counteract the muscarinic effects of ChE inhibition.

PHARMACOKINETICS

Many drugs used clinically to enhance cholinergic function lack prominent selectivity for receptor subtypes. Nevertheless, a degree of selectivity can be achieved in vivo, depending on the route of administration and tissue distribution of the drug. The extent of ionization of a drug has an influence on its absorption and penetration into brain because permanently charged quaternary ammonium compounds do not cross the blood-brain barrier (Chapter 2), whereas tertiary amines often do.

The rapid hydrolysis of ACh obviates its clinical utility. Among the ChE-resistant muscarinic receptor agonists, lipid solubility is important in influencing absorption and distribution. Quaternary ammonium agonists such as bethanechol do not penetrate into the brain and are poorly absorbed orally. Consequently, oral administration confines their action to the GI tract, making them useful for enhancing GI motility.

The tertiary amines pilocarpine and physostigmine are well absorbed from the GI tract and penetrate readily into the brain. They are administered topically (eye drops) to treat glaucoma. Pilocarpine is available in a reservoir-type diffusional device, which is placed behind the lower eyelid to deliver the drug at a constant rate for up to 1 week. Pilocarpine is also used to stimulate salivary secretion in Sjögren syndrome and in patients after laryngeal surgery.

Highly lipophilic organophosphorus ChE inhibitors are well absorbed from the GI tract, lung, eye, and skin, making these compounds extremely dangerous and accounting for their use as nerve gases. The carbamate insecticides are not highly absorbed transdermally. The organophosphorus insecticides malathion and parathion are inactive in their parent state but can be metabolized to the active ChE inhibitors malaoxon and paraoxon, respectively. Malathion is relatively safe in mammals because it is hydrolyzed rapidly by plasma carboxylesterases. This detoxification occurs much more rapidly in birds and mammals than in insects. Malathion is available outside the United States in the form of a lotion or shampoo for the treatment of head lice.

PHARMACOVIGILANCE: ADVERSE EFFECTS AND DRUG INTERACTIONS

Muscarinic Receptor Agonists

The side effects of muscarinic receptor agonists are an extension of their parasympathomimetic actions and include miosis, blurred vision, lacrimation, excessive salivation and bronchial secretions, sweating, bronchoconstriction, bradycardia, abdominal cramping, increased gastric acid secretion, diarrhea, and polyuria. Muscarinic receptor agonists that can penetrate into the brain also cause tremor, hypothermia, and convulsions. Although most peripheral blood vessels lack cholinergic innervation, they express muscarinic receptors on the endothelium that trigger vasodilation and a decrease in blood pressure. Similarly, cardiac ventricles receive little parasympathetic innervation, yet they express muscarinic receptors that decrease the force of contraction. If given in sufficient doses or administered parenterally, muscarinic receptor agonists can trigger acute circulatory failure with cardiac arrest. Atropine antagonizes all of these effects and is a useful antidote to poisoning with muscarinic receptor agonists (Chapter 8).

Muscarinic receptor agonists are contraindicated in patients with specific conditions, such as chronic obstructive pulmonary disease (COPD) and asthma that are exacerbated by parasympathetic stimulation. The bronchoconstriction induced by muscarinic receptor agonists can have disastrous consequences in patients with COPD or asthma. Similarly, these agents are contraindicated in patients with peptic ulcer disease because they stimulate gastric acid secretion, as well as in patients with GI or urinary tract obstructions because the stimulatory effect exacerbates the blockage, causing pressure to build up that may lead to perforation.

Mushrooms of the genera *Inocybe* and *Clitocybe* contain appreciable amounts of muscarine, which can cause rapid-type mushroom poisoning. Signs and symptoms occur within 30–60 minutes after ingestion of these mushrooms and are similar to the peripheral muscarinic effects described. Again, the muscarinic antagonist, atropine, is administered as an antidote.

Cholinesterase Inhibitors

The side effects of the ChE inhibitors are similar to those of the muscarinic receptor agonists but also include toxic effects at nicotinic receptors. For quaternary ammonium compounds, the cholinergic symptoms are confined to the peripheral nervous system, whereas for tertiary compounds, symptoms include actions on the brain. These agents are contraindicated in patients with asthma, COPD, peptic ulcer disease, or GI or urinary tract obstructions for the same reasons that muscarinic receptor agonists are contraindicated in these patients.

Organophosphorus ChE inhibitors are particularly dangerous because they are readily absorbed through the skin, lungs, and conjunctiva.

People can be exposed to irreversible ChE inhibitors accidentally when these agents are used as insecticides or deliberately when these agents are used as poison gas in terror or battlefield attacks. Individuals exposed to these organophosphorus compounds experience miosis, blurred vision, profuse salivation, sweating, bronchoconstriction, difficulty breathing, bradycardia, abdominal cramping, diarrhea, polyuria, tremor, and muscle fasciculations. Convulsions may also be manifest as a result of effects on the brain. With increased exposure, blood pressure decreases, and skeletal muscles weaken as a result of depolarization blockade at the neuromuscular junction, causing paralysis of the diaphragm and respiratory failure, exacerbated by increased bronchial secretions and pulmonary edema. Death usually results from respiratory failure.

ChE inhibitor poisoning is diagnosed on the basis of the signs and symptoms and the patient's history. Diagnosis can be verified by plasma or erythrocyte ChE determinations, if time permits. Atropine is used to reverse the effects of ACh at muscarinic synapses and must be continually administered as long as ChE is inhibited. With several organophosphorus ChE inhibitors, following phosphorylation of the serine hydroxyl group in the active site of the enzyme (Fig. 7.6), which results in excessive accumulation of ACh, an additional reaction occurs called "aging." This mechanism involves the elimination of an alkyl or alkoxy group from the ChE inhibitor molecule, resulting in a complex that is resistant to spontaneous hydrolysis or reactivation.

Oxime compounds such as 2-PAM can be used to reactivate the ChE and treat the adverse effects of organophosphorus ChE inhibitor poisoning. 2-PAM is a site-directed nucleophile that reacts with the phosphorylated-ChE complex to regenerate the free enzyme. To be effective, the oxime must be administered before the enzyme ages and, hence, as soon as possible after organophosphorus exposure. 2-PAM does not penetrate the blood-brain barrier and is ineffective against the toxicity caused by carbamate inhibitors. In the United States, 2-PAM is the only nucleophile available as a fixed combination with atropine in an injectable form known as ATNAA (antidote treatment-nerve agent, auto-injector).

Reversible cholinesterase inhibitors, such as pyridostigmine, protect against subsequent poisoning by organophosphorus inhibitors, and there is considerable interest in administering reversible ChE inhibitors prophylactically in battlefield situations where exposure to nerve gas is possible; the efficacy of this approach is unclear. Benzodiazepines, including diazepam (Chapter 17), are used to treat the seizures caused by the ChE inhibitors. Supportive therapy is also important, including airway maintenance, ventilatory support, and O_2 administration.

Clinical problems associated with the use of these agents are summarized in the Clinical Problems Box.

CLINICAL PROBLEMS

Cholinomimetics

Excessive parasympathetic activity: decreased blood pressure, bronchoconstriction, salivation, miosis, sweating, and gastrointestinal discomfort

Contraindicated in patients with asthma, chronic obstructive pulmonary disease, peptic ulcer, and obstruction of the urinary or gastrointestinal tract

NEW DEVELOPMENTS

Pharmacogenomic research indicates that genetic polymorphisms occur in the AChE enzyme. These include 13 single-nucleotide polymorphisms (SNPs) in the human gene. Several of these alleles are associated with different ethnic/national groups. Although some of these are unlikely to affect the catalytic properties of AChE, they could have antigenic consequences. These SNPs suggest the possible association of AChE with deleterious phenotypes, which could lead to increased adverse drug responses to AChE inhibitors.

ACh is synthesized and secreted by nonneuronal cells and by neurons. This nonneuronal cholinergic system is present in airway inflammatory cells, and ACh is either proinflammatory or antiinflammatory, depending on the type of white blood cell. Expression and function of the nonneuronal cholinergic system can be modified by the inflammation of asthma and COPD and represents a possible target for drugs to treat these lung disorders.

Muscarinic receptors have an allosteric site that exhibits substantial variation among receptor subtypes. Numerous muscarinic allosteric ligands have been identified, including allosteric agonists with substantial receptor subtype selectivity. The latter may find clinical usefulness, given their greater selectivity as compared to conventional agonists that bind to the acetylcholine site.

CLINICAL RELEVANCE FOR HEALTHCARE PROFESSIONALS

Because the muscarinic agonists and ChE inhibitors have negative chronotropic and inotropic actions, caution must be used if these agents are given to individuals with compromised cardiovascular function. In addition, all healthcare professionals need to be aware of the adverse effects of these compounds, particularly the bronchoconstrictor and vasodilator actions that may affect any exercise program requiring exertion.

Because the organophosphorus ChE inhibitors are used as insecticides, they can be dangerous to livestock agricultural workers and farmers who use these agents on their crops. In addition, several of these agents are sprayed from trucks in municipalities throughout the United States to control for mosquitoes, putting many individuals at risk. Thus it is imperative for healthcare workers in these municipalities to be aware of and recognize the symptoms resulting from exposure to these agents and be able to administer atropine and other compounds to treat toxicity.

TRADE NAMES

In addition to generic and fixed-combination preparations, the following trade-named materials are some of the important compounds available in the United States.

Cholinomimetic Agonists

Acetylcholine (Miochol)
Bethanechol (Myotonachol, Urecholine)
Carbachol (Miostat)
Cevimeline (Evoxac)
Methacholine (Provocholine)
Pilocarpine (Akarpine, Isopto Carpine, Ocusert Pilo, Pilagan, Pilocar, Salagen)

Cholinesterase (ChE) Inhibitors

Ambenonium (Mytelase)
Demecarium (Humorsol)
Donepezil (Aricept)
Echothiophate (Phospholine Iodide)
Edrophonium (Enlon, Reversol, Tensilon)
Galantamine (Razadyne, Reminyl)
Neostigmine (Prostigmin)
Physostigmine (Antilirium)
Pyridostigmine (Mestinon, Regonol)
Rivastigmine (Exelon)
Tacrine (Cognex)

Cholinesterase Reactivator

Pralidoxime (Protopam, 2-PAM) (available in combination with atropine)

SELF-ASSESSMENT QUESTIONS

1. An elderly woman with elevated intraocular pressure is diagnosed with open-angle glaucoma. Her physician prescribes instillation of pilocarpine ophthalmic solution into the eye every 6 hours. The anticipated effect of pilocarpine eye drops would be to:
   A. Relax the ciliary muscles.
   B. Constrict the pupil.
   C. Relax the sphincter muscle of the iris.
   D. Inhibit the production of aqueous humor.
   E. Increase the intraocular pressure.

2. An agricultural worker is accidentally sprayed with an insecticide and is brought to the local emergency department. He complains of tightness in the chest and difficulty with vision and was observed to have pinpoint pupils and to be profusely salivating. Assuming he has been exposed to a cholinesterase inhibitor, the most appropriate medication for treating his condition would be:
   A. Atropine.
   B. Physostigmine.
   C. Edrophonium.
   D. Propantheline.
   E. Pilocarpine.

3. What is the most severe and potentially lethal symptom that the agricultural worker in question 2 may exhibit?
   A. Hypertension
   B. Hypotension
   C. Respiratory insufficiency
   D. Congestive heart failure
   E. Hyperthermia

4. Bethanechol is administered subcutaneously to a patient with post-operative abdominal distention and gastric atony. The subcutaneous route of administration is chosen over the oral route because gastric retention is complete and there is no passage of gastric contents into the duodenum. Which of the following effects is likely to be observed after the subcutaneous administration of bethanechol?
   A. Skeletal muscle paralysis.
   B. Increase in heart rate.
   C. Peripheral vasoconstriction.
   D. Bronchoconstriction.
   E. Dry mouth.

5. Several teenagers were brought to the emergency department at a local hospital with miosis, bradycardia, salivation, abdominal cramping, and diarrhea. Upon questioning, it was determined that they ate some mushrooms they found in a local forest. Which of the following medications should be administered to these individuals to counteract their symptoms?
   A. Physostigmine.
   B. Diazepam.
   C. Atropine.
   D. 2-PAM.
   E. ATNAA.

FURTHER READING

Eglen RM. Muscarinic receptor subtypes in neuronal and non-neuronal cholinergic function. *Auton Autacoid Pharmacol.* 2006;26:219–233.

Ehlert FJ, Pak KJ, Griffin MT. Muscarinic agonists and antagonists: effects on gastrointestinal function. *Handb Exp Pharmacol.* 2012;208:343–374.

Gwilt CR, Donnelly LE, Rogers DF. The non-neuronal cholinergic system in the airways: an unappreciated regulatory role in pulmonary inflammation? *Pharmacol Ther.* 2007;115:208–222.

Kruse AC, Kobilka BK, Gautam D, et al. Muscarinic acetylcholine receptors: novel opportunities for drug development. *Nat Rev Drug Discov.* 2014;13:549–560.

WEBSITES

https://nei.nih.gov/health/glaucoma/glaucoma_facts
This website is maintained by the National Eye Institute and is an excellent resource on glaucoma and its treatment.

http://www.idph.state.il.us/bioterrorism/factsheets/organophosphate.htm
This website is maintained by the Illinois Department of Public Health and provides an overview of organophosphate toxicity and its treatment.

Muscarinic Antagonists and Their Clinical Uses

F.J. Ehlert

THERAPEUTIC OVERVIEW

Muscarinic receptors are distributed in autonomic ganglia, various regions of the brain, and peripheral tissues innervated by parasympathetic nerves (Chapters 6 and 7). There are several clinical situations for which antagonizing the effect of acetylcholine (ACh) on muscarinic receptors can be therapeutic. When applied topically to the eye, muscarinic antagonists relax the circular ciliary and pupillary constrictor muscles, causing accommodation and dilation of the pupil, respectively, enabling the clinician to view the retina more readily and to measure refractive errors of the lens during eye exams. Muscarinic antagonists counteract the constricting effect of vagal tone on the pulmonary airways, an action useful for the treatment of chronic obstructive pulmonary disease (COPD) and, to a lesser extent, asthma. Muscarinic antagonists also reduce gastrointestinal (GI) tract motility and are sometimes used for the treatment of diarrhea associated with dysenteries and inflammatory bowel conditions. Muscarinic antagonists reduce micturition frequency and an unstable bladder and are used in the treatment of urge incontinence and overactive bladder. Muscarinic antagonists have the potential to reduce motion sickness due to inhibition of the vestibular apparatus of the inner ear, with the free base form of scopolamine available as a patch applied to the skin behind the ear over the mastoid process to treat this condition prophylactically. Muscarinic antagonists are also used as antidotes to poisoning by mushrooms containing muscarine and by insecticides and war gases containing cholinesterase (ChE) inhibitors. The choice of muscarinic antagonist for these various clinical applications depends on the route of administration and the pharmacokinetic properties of the specific antagonist. A summary of the primary uses of muscarinic antagonists are listed in the Therapeutic Overview Box.

THERAPEUTIC OVERVIEW

Muscarinic Receptor Antagonists

Examination of the retina and measurement of refraction; inflammatory uveitis

Excessive motility of GI and urinary tract; urinary incontinence; irritable bowel syndrome

Chronic obstructive pulmonary disease

Motion sickness

Antidotes to cholinesterase inhibitors and mushrooms containing muscarine

---

MECHANISMS OF ACTION

The structures of representative muscarinic antagonists that have been isolated or synthesized are illustrated in Fig. 8.1. The prototypical compound is the alkaloid atropine, which has been used for many years to define muscarinic responses. Scopolamine differs from atropine by the addition of an epoxide group that reduces the basicity of the tertiary nitrogen and enables scopolamine to penetrate into the brain more readily. Ipratropium is a quaternary ammonium derivative of atropine used in the treatment of COPD. A number of antagonists have been described that show little structural resemblance to atropine including tolterodine, pirenzepine, and darifenacin. The latter two agents have marked selectivity for M_1 and M_3 receptors, respectively. Other drugs, including some antihistamines, tricyclic antidepressants, and antipsychotics, are structurally similar to the muscarinic receptor antagonists and have prominent antimuscarinic side effects. The anticholinergic effects of these compounds are presented in chapters discussing these drugs.

Muscarinic antagonists mediate their effects by opposing the stimulation of muscarinic receptors elicited by ACh throughout the body, with specific actions explained on the basis of the distribution of the five subtypes of muscarinic receptors (Chapters 6 and 7).

In the anterior segment of the eye, muscarinic receptor antagonists relax the iris sphincter and circular ciliary muscles, causing pupillary dilation (mydriasis) and paralysis of the accommodation reflex (cycloplegia), respectively, the latter resulting in blurred vision. Muscarinic antagonists also relax nonvascular smooth muscle, including the GI tract, urinary bladder, and pulmonary airways. Muscarinic antagonists inhibit the secretion of substances from sweat, salivary, and lacrimal glands, as well as from the mucosa of the trachea and GI tract. In moderate to high doses, muscarinic receptor antagonists block the effects of ACh on the heart, resulting in an increased heart rate (tachycardia).

Muscarinic antagonists that reach the brain (e.g., atropine and scopolamine) interfere with short-term memory and in moderately high doses cause delirium, excitement, agitation, and toxic psychosis. Quaternary ammonium versions of these compounds are available, but they do not penetrate the blood-brain barrier very well and hence have little effect on the central nervous system (CNS).

Atropine and other muscarinic receptor antagonists produce moderately selective dose-related effects after systemic administration. Low doses of scopolamine are more sedative than low doses of atropine. Low doses of atropine cause dry mouth, whereas high doses cause tachycardia and blockade of acid secretion by gastric parietal cells. These selective actions are attributed to the differential release of ACh at various synapses and junctions. Atropine antagonizes the effects of ACh more readily at sites where less neurotransmitter is released (e.g., salivary glands) than at sites where more is released (e.g., sinoatrial node).

Neurotransmission in sympathetic and parasympathetic ganglia and in the adrenal medulla is mediated primarily by ganglionic nicotinic receptors, whose activation leads to a fast excitatory postsynaptic potential (EPSP) in postganglionic neurons corresponding to the influx of cations

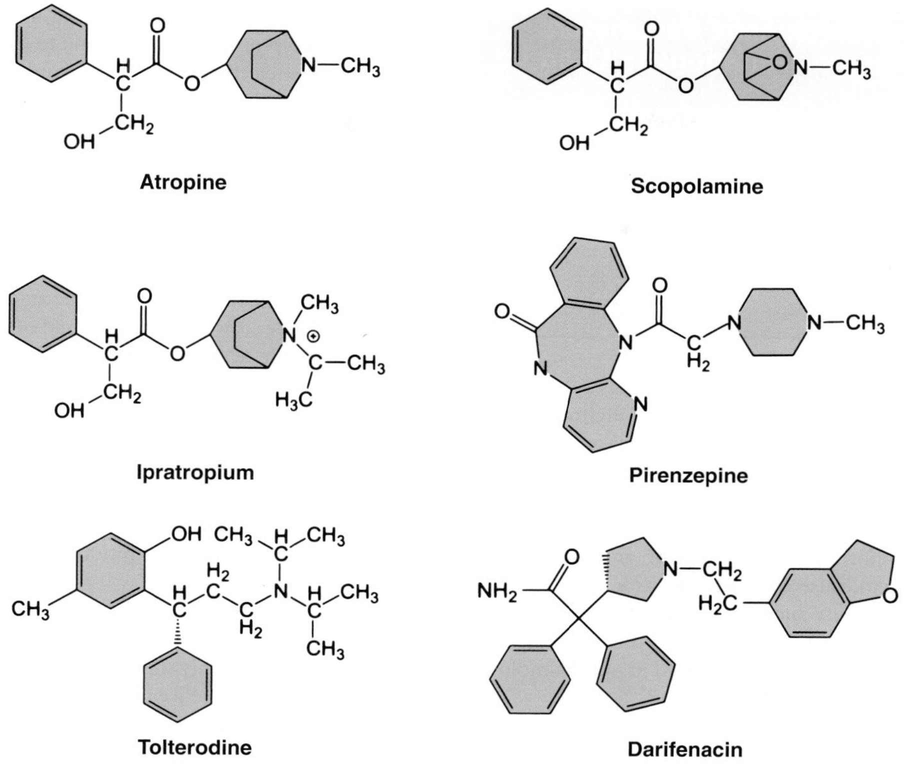

FIG. 8.1 The Structures of Some Muscarinic Antagonists.

through the nicotinic receptor ion channel (Chapters 6 and 9). Some postganglionic neurons also express M_1 muscarinic receptors that mediate a slow EPSP that increases excitability. Thus in the presence of both nicotinic and M_1 muscarinic receptor stimulation, greater postganglionic responses are elicited as compared to that caused by nicotinic stimulation alone. Pirenzepine selectively antagonizes the M_1 receptor–induced slow EPSP, and antagonism of this current in the parasympathetic ganglia of the stomach wall is thought to mediate the blockade of gastric acid secretion by pirenzepine.

RELATIONSHIP OF MECHANISMS OF ACTION TO CLINICAL RESPONSE

Commonly used muscarinic receptor antagonists and their clinical indications are presented in Table 8.1.

Central Nervous System

Scopolamine is effective for preventing motion sickness through an inhibitory effect on the vestibular apparatus. Scopolamine base is available in a transdermal patch placed behind the ear that delivers scopolamine for approximately 3 days. When administered in this fashion, scopolamine is effective against motion sickness without causing substantial anticholinergic side effects. It is more effective when administered prophylactically.

Muscarinic antagonists such as trihexyphenidyl and benztropine are used in the treatment of both Parkinson and Huntington diseases. They are commonly used to alleviate the tremor in Parkinson disease but are also useful for the dystonia. They are also used to alleviate both the spasticity and dystonia associated with Huntington disease. Their use for these disorders is discussed in Chapter 15.

TABLE 8.1 Muscarinic Receptor Antagonists and Their Uses

Agent	Use
Tertiary Amines	
Atropine	Treatment of anti-ChE poisoning
Scopolamine	Treatment of motion sickness
Homatropine	Mydriatic and cycloplegic; for mild uveitis
Dicyclomine	Alleviates GI spasms, pylorospasm, and biliary distention
Darifenacin	Treatment of urinary incontinence
Fesoterodine	Treatment of urinary incontinence
Oxybutynin	Treatment of urinary incontinence
Tolterodine	Treatment of urinary incontinence
Oxyphencyclimine	Antisecretory agent for peptic ulcer
Cyclopentolate	Mydriatic and cycloplegic
Tropicamide	Mydriatic and cycloplegic
Benztropine	Treatment of Parkinson and Huntington diseases
Trihexyphenidyl	Treatment of Parkinson and Huntington diseases
Pirenzepine	Antisecretory agent for peptic ulcer
Quaternary Ammonium Derivatives	
Methylatropine	Mydriatic, cycloplegic and antispasmodic
Methylscopolamine	Antisecretory agent for peptic ulcer, antispasmodic
Ipratropium	Aerosol for COPD
Glycopyrrolate	Antisecretory agent for peptic ulcer, antispasmodic
Tolterodine	Treatment of urinary incontinence
Propantheline	GI antispasmodic
Tiotropium	Aerosol for COPD

TABLE 8.2 Pharmacokinetic Parameters for Muscarinic Receptor Antagonists Used in Ophthalmology

Antagonist	Duration of Cycloplegia	Duration of Mydriasis
Atropine	6–12 days	7–10 days
Scopolamine	3–7 days	3–7 days
Homatropine	1–3 days	1–3 days
Cyclopentolate	6 hr–1 day	1 day
Tropicamide	6 hr	6 hr

Ophthalmology

Muscarinic antagonists dilate the pupil and relax the longitudinal and circular ciliary muscles, useful for examination of the retina and measurement of refractive errors of the lens, which often requires complete paralysis of the ciliary muscles. Choice of a mydriatic depends on its effectiveness and duration of action. Young children have a powerful accommodation reflex, requiring a highly potent and long-acting mydriatic such as atropine to cause complete blockade (cycloplegia). In contrast, shorter-acting agents such as tropicamide are used in older children and adults. The durations of action of the mydriasis and cycloplegia of muscarinic receptor antagonists used in ophthalmology are presented in Table 8.2.

Muscarinic antagonists are also used in the treatment of inflammatory uveitis and its associated glaucoma. Although the mechanism is not completely understood, these agents reduce the pain and photophobia associated with inflammation by paralyzing the eye muscles. Muscarinic antagonists are also useful for breaking adhesions (synechiae) between the lens and iris that may be produced by inflammation. When treating uveitis, it is desirable to achieve a continuous relaxation of the eye muscles. Consequently, the long-acting agents atropine and scopolamine are frequently used.

Gastrointestinal and Urinary Tracts

Muscarinic antagonists are used to treat conditions of the GI and genitourinary tracts that would benefit from an inhibition of smooth muscle tone, such as irritable bowel syndrome. This condition is associated with abdominal pain and a change in bowel habit, including constipation or diarrhea. The underlying etiology may involve inflammation of the bowel and aberrant autonomic function. The two most commonly used muscarinic antagonists to treat this condition are atropine and dicyclomine. Both compounds improve conditions in irritable bowel syndrome but are accompanied by anticholinergic side effects in other tissues, including dry mouth, dizziness, and blurred vision.

Several muscarinic antagonists are used to treat urge incontinence and overactive bladder, including oxybutynin, trospium, tolterodine, darifenacin, solifenacin, and fesoterodine. Side effects vary with each agent and include dry mouth, dizziness, blurred vision, constipation, and dyspepsia. These unwanted effects are more often reported with oxybutynin than with the other agents. Oxybutynin, trospium, and tolterodine lack selectivity for muscarinic receptor subtypes, yet tolterodine exhibits moderate selectivity for the bladder relative to the GI tract and salivary glands. Tolterodine is metabolized to a more potent muscarinic antagonist, 5-methoxytolterodine, which also lacks selectivity for muscarinic receptor subtypes but nonetheless exhibits bladder selectivity. The 5-methoxy metabolite of tolterodine is not readily absorbed from the GI tract when administered orally, but acetylation of its 5-methoxy hydroxyl group yields the drug fesoterodine, which does have good oral bioavailability. Following oral administration, fesoterodine is metabolized to 5-methoxytolterodine, which presumably is responsible for its therapeutic utility in urinary incontinence.

Darifenacin and solifenacin exhibit marked selectivity for the M_3 muscarinic receptor relative to M_2, and to a lesser extent, M_1 receptors. These subtype-selective receptor antagonists relieve the symptoms of urgency, frequency, and incontinence and exhibit reduced inhibitory effects on salivation and GI motility. While M_2 receptors have an important role in enhancing M_3 receptor–mediated contraction of bladder smooth muscle, their signaling mechanisms are contingent upon M_3 receptor activation (Chapter 7, Fig. 7.2A), and consequently, selective inhibition of the M_3 receptor also interrupts M_2 receptor signaling in the bladder.

The therapeutic utility of muscarinic antagonists in the treatment of overactive bladder is well established and often attributed to a decrease in the contractile activity of the bladder smooth muscle (detrusor) during micturition. The effect of muscarinic antagonists on bladder function, however, can be attributed to an increase in the micturition interval without an effect on the strength of the voiding response. Consequently, several investigators have suggested that the mechanism for muscarinic antagonists in alleviating the symptoms of overactive bladder involves antagonism of afferent sensory nerve pathways from the bladder rather than an inhibition of muscarinic receptor-mediated contraction of the bladder.

Nonselective muscarinic receptor antagonists were occasionally used to inhibit gastric acid secretion in peptic ulcer disease but have now been supplanted by the histamine receptor antagonists and proton pump inhibitors (Chapter 71). Pirenzepine, a selective M_1 receptor antagonist that causes fewer side effects, is used in Europe to treat peptic ulcer disease but is not currently available in the United States.

Respiratory Tract

COPD is characterized by a persistent narrowing of the airways and excessive vagal tone contributing to bronchoconstriction. Muscarinic receptor antagonists are useful in the treatment of COPD. The quaternary antagonists ipratropium and tiotropium are administered as aerosols with the use of an inhaler (Chapter 72). Because systemic absorption of these compounds by the lung is poor, their muscarinic receptor–blocking effects are usually confined to the lung. Tiotropium has a much longer duration of action than ipratropium. In addition, neither ipratropium nor tiotropium has inhibitory effects on mucociliary clearance, unlike most other muscarinic receptor antagonists such as atropine, which typically inhibit this function.

Other Uses of Muscarinic Antagonists

Atropine is used to counteract the effects of muscarinic agonists and ChE inhibitors. Excessive muscarinic receptor stimulation can occur: following accidental exposure to insecticides containing ChE inhibitors; in clinical situations, such as when a ChE inhibitor is administered to reverse the effects of neuromuscular blocking agents; or when organophosphorus ChE inhibitors are used as nerve gases. Similarly, atropine is administered as an antidote following the ingestion of mushrooms of the *Inocybe* and *Clitocybe* genera, which contain substantial amounts of the muscarinic agonist muscarine.

PHARMACOKINETICS

Many of the muscarinic antagonists used clinically lack prominent selectivity for receptor subtypes. Nevertheless, modest selectivity can be achieved in vivo, depending on the route of administration and tissue distribution of the drug. The degree of ionization influences penetration into the brain because partially charged tertiary amines readily cross the blood-brain barrier, whereas permanently charged quaternary ammonium compounds do not.

The lipophilicity and degree of ionization of muscarinic antagonists also influence their absorption and distribution. Quaternary ammonium antagonists are poorly absorbed from the lungs and GI tract and do not penetrate readily into the CNS. The passage of these agents across the blood-brain barrier is strongly influenced by their degree of ionization, even among the tertiary amines. Although atropine and scopolamine have a similar affinity for muscarinic receptors, scopolamine is approximately 10 times more potent at producing CNS effects. This is attributed to its weaker base strength (pK_a = 7.53) relative to that of atropine (pK_a = 9.65). Hence, a greater fraction of scopolamine is present in the unionized form at physiological pH relative to that of atropine (Chapter 3). The somewhat low pK_a of scopolamine enhances its absorption through the skin; this characteristic led to the development of the transdermal patch containing the free base for the treatment of motion sickness. The selective M_1 receptor antagonist pirenzepine contains three tertiary amine groups, which enhances its ionization and prevents its entry into brain.

PHARMACOVIGILANCE: ADVERSE EFFECTS AND DRUG INTERACTIONS

The side effects associated with the use of muscarinic antagonists can be attributed to blockade of muscarinic receptors throughout the CNS and peripheral nervous system. These agents cause mydriasis, cycloplegia, blurred vision, dry mouth, tachycardia, urinary retention, cutaneous vasodilation, and decreased motility of the stomach and intestines with constipation. The cutaneous vasodilatation is particularly evident in the blush area of the face. In low doses, muscarinic antagonists that enter the brain cause sedation and interfere with memory. Sedation is a prominent side effect of scopolamine, for example. In moderate to high doses, however, centrally active muscarinic receptor antagonists cause excitation, hallucinations, delirium, stupor, toxic psychosis, and convulsions, which may lead to respiratory depression and death.

The ophthalmological use of muscarinic receptor antagonists is contraindicated in the elderly and in patients with narrow ocular angles. In the latter, topical application of muscarinic receptor antagonists to the eye can trigger acute angle-closure glaucoma. Muscarinic receptor antagonists are also contraindicated in patients with reduced bowel motility, urinary retention, or prostatic hypertrophy. They are also contraindicated in patients receiving other drugs with prominent anticholinergic side effects.

Clinical problems associated with the use of muscarinic antagonists are summarized in the Clinical Problems Box.

CLINICAL PROBLEMS

Muscarinic Receptor Antagonists

Urinary retention, constipation, tachycardia, dry mouth, mydriasis, blurred vision, inhibition of sweating, toxic psychosis

Contraindicated in patients with reduced bowel motility, urinary retention, or prostatic hypertrophy

Ophthalmological use contraindicated in the elderly and in patients with narrow ocular angles

---

NEW DEVELOPMENTS

Muscarinic receptors have an allosteric site that has been well studied. Various positive and negative allosteric modulators have been identified that alter the responses elicited by ACh. The allosteric site is less conserved across muscarinic receptor subtypes, and several allosteric ligands with marked selectivity for muscarinic receptor subtypes have been identified. Negative allosteric modulators have an advantage over competitive muscarinic antagonists because there is a limit to their inhibitory effect at high concentrations, depending on the amount of

negative cooperativity. Hence allosterism provides a mechanism for protection against overdose. It is possible that suitable subtype-selective negative allosteric modulators can be developed that have fewer side effects than the currently used muscarinic antagonists. In addition, the use of long-acting muscarinic antagonists for the treatment of asthma is in the early stages of clinical development.

CLINICAL RELEVANCE FOR HEALTHCARE PROFESSIONALS

All healthcare professionals should be aware of the common side effects associated with the use of drugs with muscarinic receptor antagonist activity, including the commonly used antidepressants. The presence of dry mouth is particularly bothersome for many individuals, especially the elderly, and is a major reason underlying drug noncompliance. In addition, because muscarinic antagonists may compromise cognitive function, their use in the elderly population should be limited. Last, all healthcare professionals should be aware of the use of muscarinic antagonists for accidental poisonings.

MAJOR DRUG CLASSES

Muscarinic receptor antagonists

ABBREVIATIONS

ACh	Acetylcholine
AChE	Acetylcholinesterase
ChE	Cholinesterase
CNS	Central nervous system
COPD	Chronic obstructive pulmonary disease
EPSP	Excitatory postsynaptic potential
GI	Gastrointestinal

TRADE NAMES

In addition to generic and fixed-combination preparations, the following trade-named materials are some of the important compounds available in the United States.

Muscarinic Receptor Antagonists

Atropine (Isopto Atropine, Atreza, Atropisol)
Benztropine mesylate (Cogentin)
Biperiden (Akineton)
Darifenacin (Enablex)
Fesoterodine (Toviaz)
Glycopyrrolate (Robinul)
Homatropine methylbromide (Homapin)
L-Hyoscyamine (Anaspaz, Cystospaz-M, Levsinex)
Ipratropium (Atrovent)
Methscopolamine (Pamine)
Oxybutynin (Ditropan, Oxytrol)
Procyclidine (Kemadrin)
Propantheline (Pro-Banthine)
Scopolamine (Maldemar, Transderm Scop)
Solifenacin (VESIcare)
Tiotropium (Spiriva)
Tolterodine (Detrol)
Trihexyphenidyl (Artane)
Trospium (Sanctura)

SELF-ASSESSMENT QUESTIONS

1. You plan to prescribe transdermal scopolamine (scopolamine skin patch) for a patient susceptible to motion sickness who is leaving on a 5-day sport-fishing trip off the coast of California. What preexisting condition would make prescribing scopolamine inappropriate?
   A. Asthma.
   B. Urinary incontinence.
   C. Bradycardia.
   D. Irritable bowel syndrome.
   E. Diabetic neuropathy with urinary retention.

2. An overly curious ethnobotanist ingested some plant material and developed signs of intoxication. Upon delivery to a hospital emergency department, the patient presents with bizarre behavior and delirium, facial flushing, high heart rate, distended abdomen and full bladder, high fever, dilated pupils, dry mouth, clear lungs, and absence of bowel sounds. Which of the following alkaloids is the most likely cause of these symptoms?
   A. Physostigmine.
   B. Reserpine.
   C. Atropine.
   D. Pilocarpine.
   E. Nicotine.

3. Among the following, which is most useful in the treatment of chronic obstructive pulmonary disease?
   A. Atropine.
   B. Ipratropium.
   C. Bethanechol.
   D. Pilocarpine.
   E. Neostigmine.

4. An elderly woman receives the antimuscarinic agent cyclopentolate topically as eye drops for refraction during an eye exam. Which of the following represents a contraindication for this procedure?
   A. Bradycardia
   B. Urinary incontinence
   C. Asthma
   D. Narrow ocular angles
   E. Peptic ulcer

5. When atropine is used as an antidote to organophosphate insecticides, against which of the following symptoms is it least effective?
   A. Salivation
   B. Skeletal muscle fasiculations
   C. Bronchoconstriction
   D. Diarrhea
   E. Miosis

FURTHER READING

Abrams P, Andersson KE. Muscarinic receptor antagonists for overactive bladder. *BJU Int.* 2007;100:987–1006.

Eglen RM, Hegde SS, Watson N. Muscarinic receptor subtypes and smooth muscle function. *Pharmacol Rev.* 1996;48:531–565.

May LT, Leach K, Sexton PM, Christopoulos A. Allosteric modulation of G protein-coupled receptors. *Annu Rev Pharmacol Toxicol.* 2007;47:1–51.

Wess J, Eglen RM, Gautam D. Muscarinic acetylcholine receptors: mutant mice provide new insights for drug development. *Nat Rev Drug Discov.* 2007;6:721–733.

WEBSITES

http://www.arhp.org/Publications-and-Resources/Quick-Reference-Guide-for-Clinicians/OAB/Pharmacologic-Treatment

This website is maintained by the Association of Reproductive Health Professionals and contains excellent information and guidelines on the use of muscarnic antagonists for overactive bladder.

Nicotinic Agonists and Their Clinical Uses

Lynn Wecker and Robert J. Theobald, Jr.

MAJOR DRUG CLASSES

Plant alkaloid agonists
Synthetic partial agonists

ABBREVIATIONS

ACh	Acetylcholine
CNS	Central nervous system
GI	Gastrointestinal

THERAPEUTIC OVERVIEW

Nicotinic receptors are ligand-gated ion channels that mediate the actions of acetylcholine (ACh) at numerous synapses in both the peripheral and central nervous systems (CNS). In the peripheral nervous system, activation of nicotinic receptors mediates cholinergic neurotransmission at both parasympathetic and sympathetic ganglia and at the skeletal neuromuscular junction and mediates the sympathetically mediated release of epinephrine and norepinephrine from the adrenal medulla. Nicotinic receptors are also abundant in the brain and present on immune cells. The receptors at ganglia and in the brain and immune system are referred to as neuronal nicotinic receptors and differ markedly from the receptors at the neuromuscular junction, which are often referred to as muscle-type nicotinic receptors.

Neuronal nicotinic receptor agonists that activate receptors in the brain are used currently for smoking cessation therapy but are being investigated actively for their use in disorders involving impaired cognition, including Alzheimer disease (Chapter 14) and schizophrenia (Chapter 16), for the relief of pain, and for the treatment of motor disorders such as Parkinson disease and some ataxias. Agonists that directly stimulate ganglionic or neuromuscular nicotinic receptors have limited therapeutic application. However, these actions can explain the effects of nicotine on the nervous system.

The primary therapeutic uses of nicotinic agonists are presented in the Therapeutic Overview Box.

THERAPEUTIC OVERVIEW

Smoking Cessation
Replacement therapy: nicotine and lobeline
Antagonism: varenicline via partial agonism

Possible Other Indications
Cognitive deficits associated with Alzheimer disease and schizophrenia
Pain
Motor disorders (Parkinson disease and ataxia)

MECHANISMS OF ACTION

Nicotinic Receptors

Nicotinic cholinergic receptors represent a diverse family of pentameric proteins that mediate the effects of ACh at many peripheral and central synapses. Neuronal receptors in autonomic ganglia, the adrenal gland, the brain, and immune cells are composed of α or α and β subunits. The genes have been cloned for nine α ($\alpha2$–$\alpha10$) and three β ($\beta2$–$\beta4$) subunits, with heteromeric receptors typically containing a stoichiometry of 2α and 3β subunits. Homomeric receptors contain only α subunits and can be formed from $\alpha7$, $\alpha8$, and $\alpha9$ subunits. Autonomic ganglia express $\alpha3$, $\alpha4$, $\alpha5$, $\alpha7$, $\beta2$, and $\beta4$ subunits, with the number of cells expressing α subunits in sympathetic ganglia approximately three times more than in parasympathetic ganglia. Receptors containing the combination $\alpha3\beta4$ followed by $\alpha3\beta2$ are prevalent in autonomic ganglia, with the pentamers also containing $\alpha5$ or $\alpha7$ subunits.

In contrast to neuronal nicotinic receptors, receptors at the skeletal neuromuscular junction are composed of $\alpha1$, $\beta1$, δ, and ϵ (γ during development) subunits. Furthermore, the activation of muscle-type receptors leads to a five to six times greater increase in Na^+ permeability relative to Ca^{++}, whereas activation of neuronal receptors leads primarily to increased (1.5 times for heteromeric receptors and 6–20 times for homomeric receptors) Ca^{++} permeability relative to Na^+. Differences in the subunit composition of neuronal and muscle receptors, which are illustrated in Fig. 9.1, underlie differences in the responses of these receptors to pharmacological agents.

Both neuronal and muscle-type receptors exhibit desensitization or inactivation following sustained exposure to nicotinic agonists. This phenomenon is of critical pharmacological relevance and underlies the complex time- and dose-dependent changes observed following the administration of nicotinic receptor agonists, as well as that following the administration of the depolarizing neuromuscular blocking agent succinylcholine (Chapter 10).

Nicotinic Receptor Agonists

The structures of the current clinically relevant nicotinic agonists are shown in Fig. 9.2. Nicotine and lobeline are naturally occurring plant alkaloids with similar actions, albeit lobeline is less potent than nicotine. These compounds are full agonists at most, if not all, nicotinic receptors and activate receptors at sympathetic and parasympathetic ganglia, at the adrenal medulla, on immune cells, and in the brain, leading to a wide range of physiological effects.

Cytisine is a plant alkaloid, whereas varenicline is a synthetic compound. Both of these agents are full agonists at some ($\alpha3\beta4$ and $\alpha7$) and partial agonists at other ($\alpha4\beta2$) nicotinic receptors.

Muscle-type nicotinic receptor

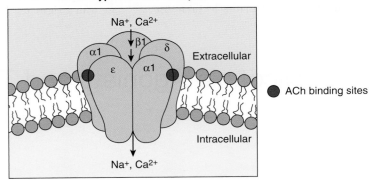

Neuronal nicotinic receptors

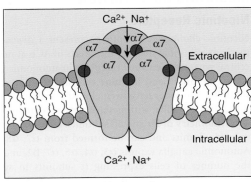 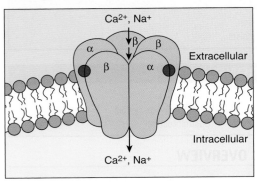

Homomeric   Heteromeric

FIG. 9.1 Nicotinic Receptor Structures. The subunit compositions of muscle-type and neuronal nicotinic receptors are shown. For neuronal receptors, representative examples of both homomeric and heteromeric pentamers are shown. Binding sites for agonists are noted at subunit interfaces, and the predominant cation whose permeability increases following agonist-induced activation is listed first—that is, either Na$^+$ for muscle-type receptors or Ca^{2+} for neuronal receptors.

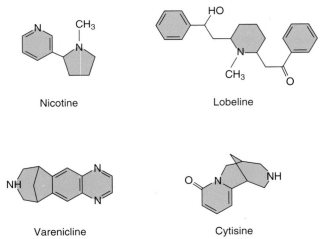

FIG. 9.2 Structures of Clinically Relevant Nicotinic Receptor Agonists.

RELATIONSHIP OF MECHANISMS OF ACTION TO CLINICAL RESPONSE

The acute administration of nicotine increases the activity of the cardiovascular and gastrointestinal (GI) systems, resulting in tachycardia, hypertension, and increased gastrointestinal motility and secretions.

The cardiovascular effects of nicotine represent both activation of sympathetic ganglionic activity and stimulation of nicotinic receptors at the adrenal medulla, leading to increased release of circulating catecholamines. The GI and urinary tract effects reflect activation of parasympathetic ganglia, increasing both the tone and motility of GI smooth muscle.

High doses of nicotine, or prolonged exposure of receptors to agonist, lead to **desensitization** of nicotinic receptors, which depresses ganglionic transmission and the splanchnic nerve–induced release of catecholamines from the adrenal medulla; thus resultant effects resemble the actions of ganglionic blockers (Chapter 10). Similarly, nicotinic receptors at the skeletal neuromuscular junction rapidly desensitize in response to nicotine, leading to depolarization blockade, resembling the paralytic actions of succinylcholine (Chapter 10).

Nicotine induces nausea and vomiting through activation of the chemoreceptor trigger zone in the area postrema, and low doses stimulate respiratory centers, while high doses depress respiration through both blockade of the diaphragm and intercostal muscles and central paralysis.

Nicotine readily enters the brain to activate neuronal receptors, leading to a multitude of effects, including the release of several neurotransmitters, particularly dopamine from the ventral tegmental–nucleus accumbens pathway, which regulates reward and is involved in the addictive process (Chapter 24).

Nicotine in gum, patches, and other smoking cessation delivery devices is used in smoking cessation programs as nicotine replacement therapy (NRT) to minimize withdrawal symptoms associated with decreased smoking. NRT increases the rate of quitting by 50%–70% in individuals with a desire to quit smoking. In contrast, lobeline, which is also available in several commercial preparations for this purpose, has not been shown to increase quit rate.

Varenicline was developed as a partial agonist at $\alpha 4\beta 2$ neuronal nicotinic receptors for use in smoking cessation regimens. As such, varenicline leads to limited activation of $\alpha 4\beta 2$ receptors and functions like an antagonist to block the ability of nicotine to elicit its response (Chapter 2). Cytisine has a similar action, has been used in Central and Eastern Europe for many years as a smoking cessation drug, and was approved by the Food and Drug Administration in 2017 for development as a smoking cessation treatment in the United States.

PHARMACOKINETICS

Nicotine is well absorbed from many routes of administration, including mucous membranes, skin, and the lungs; it has limited GI absorption. More than 75% of absorbed nicotine is metabolized primarily by the liver but also by the lungs and kidneys. The primary (70%–80%) metabolite of nicotine in mammals is cotinine, which is formed in a two-step sequence catalyzed by the enzyme CYP2A6 followed by the action of cytoplasmic aldehyde oxidase. About 5% of nicotine is converted to nicotine N'-oxide by a flavin monooxygenase and the remainder methylated and glucuronidated. Nicotine metabolism is highly determined by genetics and affected by numerous factors, including the environment, diet, age, gender, other drugs, and smoking itself. Nicotine has a half-life of about 2 hours following inhalation, and both nicotine and its metabolites are eliminated by the kidneys. Limited information is available on the pharmacokinetics of lobeline in humans.

Varenicline is well absorbed following oral administration and exhibits low (<20%) plasma protein binding. It is minimally metabolized and has an elimination half-life of about 24 hours. More than 90% of the drug is eliminated unchanged via the kidneys through glomerular filtration and active tubular secretion. Varenicline has been shown to be successful in smoking cessation programs. Limited information is available on the pharmacokinetics of cytisine in humans.

PHARMACOVIGILANCE: ADVERSE EFFECTS AND DRUG INTERACTIONS

Nicotine poisoning results from the ingestion of tobacco products or exposure to nicotine-containing insecticides. A major source of nicotine poisoning in children is concentrated nicotine solutions packaged for use with e-cigarettes. Hallmark effects of toxicity include GI upset, diarrhea, emesis, abdominal pain, perturbed vision, and mental confusion. At very high concentrations, tremors, and convulsions ensue, followed by depression and coma. Death is attributed to respiratory failure as a consequence of paralysis of the diaphragm and intercostal muscles.

Varenicline leads to nausea and GI discomfort as the most common adverse effects. It can also cause weakness, dry mouth, headache, and sleep problems, with vivid and unusual dreams very troublesome for some individuals. Effects on the GI system include stomach pain, indigestion, constipation, and gas. In 2009, 3 years after varenicline became available in the United States, several incidences of serious neuropsychiatric symptoms were reported, including agitation, depressed mood, suicidal ideations and suicidal behavior, and a boxed warning concerning this effect was mandated by the FDA. However, in 2016, in consideration of more postmarketing data, this warning was discontinued.

Clinical problems associated with the use of nicotine and varenicline are summarized in the Clinical Problems Box.

CLINICAL RELEVANCE FOR HEALTHCARE PROFESSIONALS

All healthcare professionals should encourage their patients to quit smoking and help these individuals identify the best treatment program for them. Research demonstrates that agents used in cessation programs are more successful when counseling accompanies drug therapy, and all efforts should be made to provide patients access to these resources.

NEW DEVELOPMENTS

Understanding the role and regulation of nicotinic receptors throughout the body represents a major area of research. The role of nicotinic receptors in several neuropsychiatric disorders is being studied actively and may lead to new treatments for pain, Alzheimer disease, schizophrenia, and motor disorders. Further, studies on the role of nicotinic receptors in regulating the enteric nervous system has led to understanding the potential benefit of nicotinic agonists in restoring bowel function in opioid-induced constipation (OIC). Thus we are just beginning to understand the role of specific members of this diverse receptor family, and research efforts may lead to new treatment regimens for several disorders.

SELF-ASSESSMENT QUESTIONS

1. Prolonged exposure of ganglionic nicotinic receptors to nicotine may be expected to lead to:
   A. Tachycardia.
   B. Hypertension.
   C. Increased gastrointestinal motility.
   D. Increased catecholamine release from the adrenal medulla.
   E. Ganglionic blockade.
2. A patient interested in participating in a smoking cessation program would likely achieve the best results if he or she had:
   A. Counseling and lobeline.
   B. Nicotine.
   C. Counseling and nicotine.
   D. Varenicline.
   E. None of the above is effective.
3. A major difference between neuronal and muscle-type nicotinic receptors is that neuronal receptors:
   A. Contain γ subunits, while muscle-type receptors do not.
   B. Are pentamers, while muscle receptors are monomers.
   C. Contain α and β subunits, while muscle-type receptors do not.
   D. Are only permeable to NA$^+$, while muscle-type receptors are not.
   E. Only contain α and/or β subunits, while muscle-type receptors contain α, β, and other subunits.

CLINICAL PROBLEMS

Nicotine	Gastrointestinal distress, nausea, vomiting, respiratory distress and failure, muscle weakness and fatigue, confusion, tremor and convulsions
Varenicline	Nausea, gastrointestinal discomfort, headache, vivid and unusual dreams

TRADE NAMES

In addition to generic and fixed-combination preparations, the following trade-named materials are some of the important compounds available in the United States.

Lobeline

Nicotine (Nicorette, Nicotrol)

Varenicline (Chantix)

FURTHER READING

Albuquerque EX, Pereira EFR, Alkondon M, Rogers SW. Mammalian nicotinic acetylcholine receptors: from structure to function. *Physiol Rev.* 2009;89:73–120.

Benowitz NL, Hukkanen J, Jacob P. Nicotine chemistry, metabolism, kinetics and biomarkers. *Handb Exp Pharmacol.* 2009;192:29–60.

Skok VI. Nicotinic acetylcholine receptors in autonomic ganglia. *Auton Neurosci.* 2002;97:1–11.

WEBSITES

http://www.guidetopharmacology.org/GRAC/FamilyDisplayForward?familyId=76

This is the International Union of Basic and Clinical Pharmacology (IUPHAR) receptor website with excellent information on nicotinic receptors.

Neuromuscular Blocking Drugs and Nicotinic Antagonists

Lynn Wecker and Robert J. Theobald, Jr.

THERAPEUTIC OVERVIEW

In the peripheral nervous system, nicotinic receptor antagonists block the actions of acetylcholine (ACh) at the neuromuscular junction, autonomic ganglia, and the adrenal medulla. These agents can be classified as **neuromuscular blockers** or **ganglionic blockers**, the former acting at muscle-type nicotinic receptors and the latter at neuronal ganglionic nicotinic receptors (Chapter 9). Further, the **neuromuscular blockers** may be categorized according to their use and mechanisms of action as either **depolarizing** or **nondepolarizing** agents. These drugs are useful in several clinical situations when skeletal muscle relaxation can be beneficial, including use as a surgical adjunct and for orthopedic procedures, endotracheal intubation, scoping procedures, and electroconvulsive therapy (ECT). The **ganglionic blockers** can be used to treat hypertensive emergencies or for producing controlled hypotension during surgery.

Clinical uses of the neuromuscular and ganglionic blockers are listed in the Therapeutic Overview Box.

THERAPEUTIC OVERVIEW

Neuromuscular Blocking Drugs
Surgery, orthopedic procedures, endotracheal intubation, electroconvulsive therapy

Ganglionic Blocking Drugs
Hypertensive emergencies, controlled hypotension during surgery

MECHANISMS OF ACTION

Neuromuscular Transmission

Skeletal muscles are innervated by somatic motor nerves, which originate in the spinal cord and release ACh as their neurotransmitter (Chapter 6). Following release, ACh interacts with nicotinic receptors located at the end plates of adult muscle to initiate an excitatory endplate potential (EPP). When the potential reaches sufficient amplitude, a muscle action potential ensues, leading to Ca^{++} influx, the release of Ca^{++} from the sarcoplasmic reticulum via the ryanodine receptor 1 (Chapter 22, Fig. 22.3), and contraction of skeletal muscle. Pharmacological compounds can interfere with transmission at the neuromuscular junction by affecting numerous processes, including inhibition of the action potential by local anesthetics (Chapter 27), blocking ACh release with botulinum toxin (Chapter 22), inhibiting acetylcholinesterase (AChE) to prolong the actions of ACh leading to depolarization blockade (Chapter 7), inhibiting Ca^{++} release with dantrolene (Chapter 22), or antagonizing neuromuscular nicotinic receptors with the depolarizing or nondepolarizing neuromuscular blockers. These processes are depicted in Fig. 10.1.

Neuromuscular Blocking Drugs

The nondepolarizing neuromuscular blockers include the natural alkaloid **d-tubocurarine**, the aminosteroids **pancuronium**, **pipecuronium**, **rocuronium**, and **vecuronium**, and the benzylisoquinolines **atracurium**, **doxacurium**, **mivacurium**, and related compounds (Fig. 10.2). All of the compounds contain multiple rings and are relatively large, bulky molecules that hinder ACh from binding to the receptor. These compounds are pure competitive antagonists and do not activate the receptor, producing a flaccid paralysis. Because these agents are competitive, their action can be reversed with an AChE inhibitor, increasing synaptic concentrations of ACh.

In contrast, the depolarizing agent **succinylcholine** is a flexible molecule whose structure represents two ACh molecules attached at the methyl ends (noncharged). Succinylcholine binds to and activates the receptor, producing muscle contraction that may lead to transient fasciculations followed by a flaccid paralysis. However, because succinylcholine is relatively resistant to hydrolysis by AChE, it remains bound to the receptor for a prolonged period of time, longer than ACh, leading to blockade. This action, referred to as **phase I block**, is attributed to the failure of perijunctional Na^+ channels to reopen until repolarization of the endplate. During this time, the membrane is unresponsive to further stimuli, and thus the blockade cannot be reversed by AChE inhibitors. Rather, it may be potentiated by these compounds.

Upon continued exposure to succinylcholine, the depolarization block may convert to a nondepolarizing block, referred to as **phase II block**, during which time the blockade appears similar to that produced by nondepolarizing agents, that is, it becomes responsive to high concentrations of ACh and may be reversed by AChE inhibitors. The development of a phase II block following succinylcholine depends highly on the general anesthetic used.

83

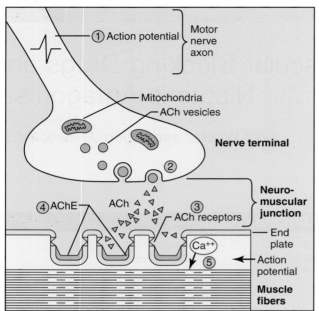

FIG. 10.1 Neuromuscular Transmission and Sites of Drug Action.
(1) The action potential conducted down the motor nerve axon can be blocked by Na^+ channel blockers, such as local anesthetics or tetrodotoxin. (2) When the action potential reaches the nerve terminal, the Ca^{++}-mediated exocytotic release of vesicular acetylcholine *(ACh)* occurs, a process that can be blocked by botulinum toxin. (3) Following release, ACh diffuses across the synaptic cleft and binds to nicotinic receptors in the motor endplate. Binding can be blocked competitively by nondepolarizing neuromuscular blockers such as d-tubocurarine or noncompetitively by the depolarizing neuromuscular blocker succinylcholine. (4) ACh is rapidly hydrolyzed by acetylcholinesterase *(AChE)*, which can be inhibited by AChE inhibitors, such as neostigmine. (5) ACh-activated nicotinic receptors in the motor endplate generate a muscle action potential, which leads to Ca^{++} release from the sarcoplasmic reticulum, mediated by ryanodine receptors, initiating excitation-contraction coupling and muscle contraction; this release can be blocked by the antispasticity drug dantrolene.

Ganglionic Blocking Drugs

Both sympathetic and parasympathetic ganglia use ACh as a neurotransmitter. ACh, released from preganglionic fibers, activates neuronal nicotinic receptors on the postganglionic neuron, leading to an excitatory postsynaptic potential (EPSP), which can generate an action potential (Fig. 10.3). The ganglionic blockers, which include mecamylamine and trimethaphan, are structurally dissimilar compounds (see Fig. 10.2) with different mechanisms. Mecamylamine appears to be a voltage-dependent noncompetitive antagonist that penetrates and blocks the open cation channel, thereby preventing further activation. In contrast, trimethaphan competes with ACh for receptor binding.

RELATIONSHIP OF MECHANISMS OF ACTION TO CLINICAL RESPONSE

Neuromuscular Blocking Drugs

Muscle contraction is partially impaired when 75%–80% of receptors are occupied and inhibited totally when 90%–95% are occupied. Required concentrations vary with the drug, the muscle and its location, and the patient. Because nondepolarizing blockers compete with ACh, the blockade can be reversed by the AChE inhibitors neostigmine, edrophonium, and pyridostigmine, all of which are used clinically.

Because of its rapid onset and short duration of action, succinylcholine is used primarily for facilitation of endotracheal intubation and for relaxation during extremely short surgical procedures, while the nondepolarizing agents are more frequently used when a longer procedure is being performed. Spontaneous respiration is usually inhibited, and respiratory support must be available.

The rate of neuromuscular block and recovery varies with different muscles. Small muscles of the face are affected prior to large muscles of the limbs and trunk, with muscles of respiration, the intercostal muscles, and the diaphragm usually among the last to be paralyzed and the first to recover. It is not practical to attempt selective blockade of one anatomical area for prolonged periods because of the widespread distribution of these drugs.

It is noteworthy to mention that sugammadex, which was approved in 2015, is available to reverse the neuromuscular blockade produced by rocuronium and vecuronium. This drug forms water soluble complexes with the neuromuscular blocking agents, creating a concentration gradient favoring their movement from the neuromuscular junction back into the plasma, resulting in recovery of function and reversing deep blockade without muscle weakness. The drug is administered intravenously, and most patients recover within 5 minutes of administration.

Ganglionic Blocking Drugs

Irrespective of mechanism, the results of ganglionic blockade by mecamylamine and trimethaphan depend on the predominant tone of a specific organ. As discussed in Chapter 6, most organs in the body receive both parasympathetic and sympathetic innervation. Further, each organ is under the predominant tone of one system, as shown in Table 10.1. Therefore interruption of ganglionic transmission selectively eliminates the dominant component. For example, in the heart, the cholinergic system generally dominates at the level of the sinoatrial (SA) node. When a ganglionic blocker is administered, its greatest effect is on this cholinergic component, resulting in an apparent adrenergic effect (tachycardia).

PHARMACOKINETICS

Neuromuscular Blocking Drugs

Selected pharmacokinetic parameters for representative neuromuscular blocking agents are shown in Table 10.2. These agents differ considerably in many pharmacokinetic properties, particularly in duration of action, which is a major consideration for the choice of a particular compound and is partly determined by redistribution of the drug. In most surgical procedures in which neuromuscular blocking agents are used, the drugs enter the systemic circulation and are distributed widely. Many of these compounds are metabolized by the liver and excreted by the kidneys, and thus liver or renal disease will have a marked effect on the duration of action of these agents. Relative potency is not a principal consideration, despite a 100-fold variation in the doses of different drugs needed to attain 95% neuromuscular blockade.

The aminosteroids pancuronium, pipecuronium, rocuronium, and vecuronium are metabolized by the liver to active compounds that have about 50% of the activity of the parent compound. In contrast, atracurium is metabolized by plasma carboxylesterase and spontaneous degradation, with minimal renal elimination, and is a drug of choice for patients with renal or hepatic dysfunction. Succinylcholine, mivacurium, and doxacurium are metabolized by plasma butyrylcholinesterase, which is synthesized in the liver, and thus patients with hepatic disease may exhibit decreased enzyme production, prolonging the effects of these agents. Allelic variations in this enzyme may also account for prolonged actions.

Neuromuscular blockers

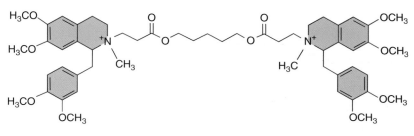

Succinylcholine

d-Tubocurarine

Pancuronium

Atracurium

Ganglionic blockers

Mecamylamine

Trimethaphan

FIG. 10.2 Structures of Representative Neuromuscular and Ganglionic Blocking Drugs.

Ganglionic Blocking Drugs

Mecamylamine and trimethaphan are erratically absorbed following oral administration, and both compounds are excreted mostly unchanged by the kidneys.

PHARMACOVIGILANCE: ADVERSE EFFECTS AND DRUG INTERACTIONS

Neuromuscular Blocking Drugs

The major side effects of the neuromuscular blocking drugs are cardiovascular effects and histamine release, with the older compounds exhibiting greater effects and the newer drugs having fewer effects. Histamine release from mast cells, which can lead to bronchospasm, excessive bronchial and salivary secretions, and hypotension, is a major problem with tubocurarine, but a lesser problem with succinylcholine and mivacurium, and an even smaller problem with the aminosteroids. Approximately 30% of patients receiving atracurium experience significant histamine release, while pancuronium, doxacurium, rocuronium,

and vecuronium are devoid of this action and free of cardiovascular effects. Histamine release may also occur with cisatracurium and mivacurium, but no cardiovascular effects are observed at clinical doses. Pancuronium can cause moderate increases in heart rate, blood pressure, and cardiac output as a consequence of sympathomimetic and anticholinergic effects. Dysrhythmias can be induced with the older agents, but the newer agents have greater cardiac safety margins, reducing their cardiac effects.

Although nondepolarizing neuromuscular blocking drugs are generally selective for nicotinic cholinergic receptors in skeletal muscle, parasympathetic and sympathetic ganglia can be affected if drug concentrations are sufficiently high. At normal doses, most agents do not exhibit these effects except for tubocurarine, which produces a significant degree of ganglionic blockade. Succinylcholine may stimulate ganglia, resulting in alterations in heart rate and hypertension. Muscarinic effects can be evoked with pancuronium at doses used to produce neuromuscular blockade and with tubocurarine and atracurium at higher doses.

Adverse effects of the neuromuscular blocking agents may lead to prolonged apnea and cardiovascular collapse, often exaggerated in

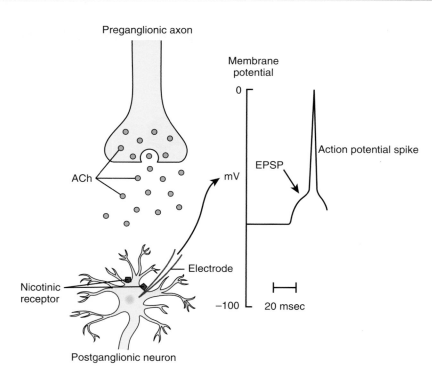

Preganglionic axon

Membrane potential

ACh

mV

EPSP

Action potential spike

Electrode

Nicotinic receptor

−100

20 msec

Postganglionic neuron

FIG. 10.3 The Role of Nicotinic Receptor Activation at Ganglia. Acetylcholine *(ACh)* released from preganglionic fibers activates neuronal ganglionic nicotinic receptors on postganglionic neurons, leading to the generation of an excitatory postsynaptic potential *(EPSP)*, that can lead to an action potential within milliseconds. Not shown are downstream events involving muscarinic M_2 and M_1 receptors that lead to a sequential inhibitory postsynaptic potential, followed by a slow EPSP in seconds, and a peptidergic receptor–mediated late, slow EPSP that occurs in minutes.

TABLE 10.1	Effects of Ganglionic Blockade on Major Organ Systems	
Predominant Tone	**Site**	**Consequences of Ganglionic Blockade**
Sympathetic	Arterioles and veins	Vasodilation, decreased venous return, hypotension
	Ventricle	Reduced force of contraction
Parasympathetic	Atria; SA node	Tachycardia
	Iris of the eye	Mydriasis
	Ciliary muscle	Cycloplegia (loss of accommodation)
	Gastrointestinal tract	Decreased tone, motility, and secretions
	Pancreas	Decreased secretions
	Urinary bladder	Urinary retention
	Salivary glands	Xerostomia (dry mouth)
Sympathetic (cholinergic)	Sweat glands	Anhidrosis (decreased sweat)

patients with comorbid conditions, such as burns, soft tissue damage, spinal cord injury, or other trauma. Further, the electrolyte content of body fluids can have a major influence on the degree of blockade and consequent adverse effects of succinylcholine, which can release K^+ rapidly from many cells. This may pose an unacceptable risk in patients with extensive soft tissue injury because the prolonged depolarization can lead to severe hyperkalemia and result in prolonged apnea or cardiac arrhythmias and arrest if plasma K^+ concentrations ≥ 13 mM.

Drug interactions are known to occur between neuromuscular blockers, anesthetics, Ca^{++} channel blockers, and some antibiotics. Many volatile anesthetic agents enhance the action of the nondepolarizing neuromuscular blockers by decreasing the open time of the nicotinic receptor. Enflurane has the strongest effect, followed by halothane. The local anesthetic bupivacaine potentiates blockade by nondepolarizing and depolarizing agents, and lidocaine and procaine prolong the duration of action of succinylcholine by inhibiting butyrylcholinesterase.

The administration of succinylcholine with halogenated inhalational anesthetics can precipitate malignant hyperthermia in genetically susceptible patients. This reaction, which is manifest by sustained muscle contraction, an increased O_2 consumption, and an increased body temperature, is a pharmacogenetic disorder and results from the failure of the sarcoplasmic reticulum to resequester Ca^{++}. Malignant hyperthermia is rare, with the highest incidence following the combined use of halothane and succinylcholine (Chapter 26). However, it is a potentially life-threatening situation and, if untreated, may prove fatal. Treatment involves cessation of drug administration, rapid cooling, and administration of dantrolene.

Ca^{++} channel blockers, many antibiotics, and, to a lesser extent, β-adrenergic receptor blockers potentiate neuromuscular blocking drugs. The duration of action of vecuronium, pancuronium, doxacurium, and pipecuronium is reduced in patients taking the anticonvulsants phenytoin or carbamazepine because these agents decrease the affinity of nicotinic receptors for neuromuscular blockers and increase the number of receptors on muscle fibers. In addition, the duration of action of vecuronium is prolonged in patients treated with cimetidine.

Naturally, neuromuscular blocking agents must be used with caution in patients with neuromuscular disorders, such as myasthenia gravis or Lambert-Eaton myasthenic syndrome. These individuals may require adjusted dosing to assure patient safety.

Genetic variations in butyrylcholinesterase activity, resulting in either lower concentrations of normal enzyme or an abnormal enzyme, may also lead to prolonged actions of succinylcholine. A clinically effective dose of succinylcholine in healthy patients produces neuromuscular blockade lasting <15 minutes; in a patient with a variant of this enzyme with decreased effectiveness, the same dose may last much longer. This is illustrated in Fig. 10.4, with block defined as the duration of apnea. Trauma, alcoholism, pregnancy, use of oral contraceptives, and other

TABLE 10.2 Selected Pharmacokinetic Parameters

Compound	Onset (min)	Duration of Action (min)[a]	Plasma Protein Binding (%)	Metabolism	Elimination
Atracurium	3–6	Intermediate	80	Carboxylesterase and nonenzymatic	R (6%–10%)
Cisatracurium	5–7	Intermediate	nd	Carboxylesterase and nonenzymatic	R (<10%), B (<10%)
Doxacurium	4–6	Long	30–35	Butyrylcholinesterase (75%)	R (25%–50%)
Mivacurium	2–4	Short	nd	Butyrylcholinesterase (100%)	R (<10%)
Pancuronium	4–6	Long	85	Hepatic (35%)	R (40%–60%), B (10%–20%)
Pipecuronium	3–6	Long	nd	Hepatic (20%)	R (40%–60%), B (10%–20%)
Rocuronium	2–4	Intermediate	nd	Hepatic (35%)	R (20%–30%), B (50%–60%)
Succinylcholine	1–2	Ultrashort	nd	Butyrylcholinesterase (100%)	R (<10%)
Tubocurarine	4–6	Long	35–55	Hepatic (50%)	R (45%–60%), B (10%–40%)
Vecuronium	2–4	Intermediate	70	Hepatic (35%)	R (20%–30%), B (50%–60%)

[a]Duration: Ultrashort ≤10 min; Short = 10–30 min; Intermediate = 30–90 min; Long ≥90 min.
B, Biliary; nd, not determined due to rapid metabolism in plasma; R, renal.

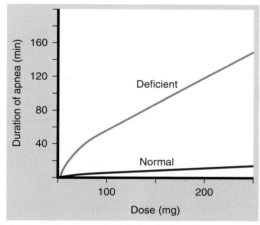

FIG. 10.4 Dose-related succinylcholine-induced neuromuscular block (duration of apnea) after intravenous administration to a normal individual and an individual with a genetic variant in plasma butyrylcholinesterase activity, leading to decreased enzyme activity.

conditions in which butyrylcholinesterase activity is changed can alter the duration of neuromuscular block produced by succinylcholine.

Ganglionic Blocking Drugs

The adverse effects of the ganglionic blocking agents represent an extension of their pharmacological actions and include dry mouth, tachycardia, constipation, and urinary retention, as well as excessive hypotension and impotence.

The major adverse effects associated with the use of the neuromuscular and ganglionic blocking agents are summarized in the Clinical Problems Box.

NEW DEVELOPMENTS

Neuromuscular blocking drugs are commonly used acutely during anesthesia for surgical procedures and chronically in patients in intensive care units to allow controlled ventilation, a practice that is not without problems, including prolonged muscle paralysis after termination of treatment. In recent years, the search for new neuromuscular relaxants has concentrated on developing drugs with a rapid onset and shorter and more predictable duration of action with minimal side effects. In

CLINICAL PROBLEMS

Neuromuscular blocking drugs	Prolonged apnea, hyperkalemia, malignant hyperthermia, histamine release, cardiovascular collapse
Ganglionic blocking drugs	Hypotension, tachycardia, mydriasis, dry mouth, constipation

TRADE NAMES

In addition to generic and fixed-combination preparations, the following trade-named materials are some of the important compounds available in the United States.

Neuromuscular Blocking Drugs
Atracurium (Tracrium)
Cisatracurium (Nimbex)
Doxacurium (Nuromax)
Mivacurium (Mivacron)
Pancuronium (Pavulon)
Rocuronium (Zemuron)
Succinylcholine (Anectine)
Tubocurarine
Vecuronium (Norcuron)

Ganglionic Blocking Drugs
Mecamylamine (Inversine)
Trimethaphan (Arfonad)

addition, agents are being sought to reverse the actions of currently available drugs.

CLINICAL RELEVANCE FOR HEALTHCARE PROFESSIONALS

Although the neuromuscular blocking agents are used typically in a controlled environment, all healthcare professionals should be aware of their mechanisms of action and possible life-threatening adverse effects. These drugs can produce effects that may impact nursing care or physical or occupational therapy in certain settings. Understanding the actions of these agents will help provide awareness of the potential impact of these agents on the care provided.

SELF ASSESSMENT QUESTIONS

1. The general anesthetic halothane was administered with succinylcholine to a surgical patient, and shortly thereafter the patient exhibited sustained muscle contractions, an elevated temperature, and tachycardia. This situation likely arose because:
   A. The amount of succinylcholine administered was too high.
   B. The patient has a butyrylcholinesterase mutation leading to decreased enzyme activity.
   C. The halothane was contaminated.
   D. The time interval between administration of the two drugs was insufficient.
   E. The patient was female, and this drug combination can be toxic to females.

2. What would you expect to see in an individual given the ganglionic blocker mecamylamine?
   A. Vasoconstriction.
   B. Bradycardia.
   C. Urinary retention.
   D. Increase gastrointestinal motility and secretion.
   E. Miosis.

3. Potential therapeutic uses of neuromuscular blockers include:
   A. The diagnosis of myasthenia gravis.
   B. The control of ventilation during surgery.
   C. The control of spasticity associated with cerebral palsy.
   D. The production of high airway pressures in intensive care.
   E. Blockade of muscle contractions during electroconvulsive therapy.

4. At low doses, tubocurarine blocks only nicotinic receptors at the neuromuscular junction, whereas mecamylamine blocks only nicotinic receptors at autonomic ganglia because:
   A. Ganglionic nicotinic receptors are different from skeletal muscle nicotinic receptors.
   B. Mecamylamine rapidly penetrates the blood-brain barrier.
   C. Mecamylamine is very bulky and charged and cannot access muscle receptors.
   D. Tubocurarine is a slender and flexible molecule.
   E. None of the above.

FURTHER READING

Bowman WC. Neuromuscular block. *Br J Pharmacol.* 2006;147(suppl 1):S277–S286.

deBacker J, Hart N, Fan E. Neuromuscular blockade in the 21st century management of the critically ill patient. *Chest.* 2017;151:697–706.

Gamboa A, Okamoto LE, Arnold AC, et al. Autonomic blockade improves insulin sensitivity in obese subjects. *Hypertension.* 2014;64(4):867–874.

WEBSITES

https://sccm.org/News/Pages/SCCM-Releases-Neuromuscular-Blockade-in-the-Adult-Critically-Ill-Patient-Guidelines.aspx

This website is maintained by the Society of Critical Care Medicine and has a link to Guidelines for Neuromuscular Blockade in the Adult Critically Ill Patient.

11

Adrenergic Agonists and Their Clinical Uses

Javier Cuevas

MAJOR DRUG CLASSES

Endogenous catecholamines
α-Adrenergic receptor agonists
β-Adrenergic receptor agonists
Indirect-acting sympathomimetics
Mixed-action sympathomimetics

ABBREVIATIONS

AAAD	Aromatic L-amino acid decarboxylase
CNS	Central nervous system
COMT	Catechol-*O*-methyltransferase
DA	Dopamine
Epi	Epinephrine
GI	Gastrointestinal
L-DOPA	3,4-Dihydroxyphenylalanine
MAO	Monoamine oxidase
NE	Norepinephrine
ISO	Isoproterenol

THERAPEUTIC OVERVIEW

The sympathetic nervous system is responsible for helping preserve homeostasis in peripheral organs and tissues and is an **ergotropic**, or energy-expending, system. The consequences of activation of the sympathetic nervous system are best characterized by the phrase "**flight-or-fight**" response, which helps predict the types of physiological responses caused by both stimulation of this system and the use of **sympathomimetic** (mimicking sympathetic responses) pharmacological interventions. The physiological consequences of sympathetic activation include increasing heart rate and cardiac contractility to elevate cardiac output, shifting blood flow from internal organs not critical for fight or flight (e.g., intestines) to skeletal muscle, and providing energy via lipolysis, glycogenolysis, and gluconeogenesis. Additional relevant physiological changes include bronchodilation to increase airflow and consequently enhanced gas exchange (i.e., increased O_2 uptake and CO_2 excretion), mydriasis to increase light entry and allow greater focus, activation of sudomotor pathways to facilitate thermoregulation, and stimulation of the central nervous system (CNS) for heightened alertness and memory consolidation.

Almost all postganglionic sympathetic neurons release **norepinephrine (NE)** as their neurotransmitter; minor exceptions include a small number of anatomically sympathetic neurons projecting to sweat glands and a few blood vessels that release acetylcholine, and sympathetic neurons innervating renal medullary blood vessels that release **dopamine (DA)**, which is the precursor for NE (Chapter 6). NE released from sympathetic neurons activates α_1-, α_2-, β_1-, and β_3- (low potency at β_2) **adrenergic receptors** on exocrine glands, fat cells, smooth muscle, and cardiac muscle to produce sympathetic responses. In addition, activation of sympathetic outflow also causes the secretion of **epinephrine (Epi)** and NE from the adrenal medulla into the blood to cause a global sympathetic effect. Epi itself is considered the fight-or-flight hormone and activates all adrenergic receptor subtypes—that is, α_1, α_2, β_1, β_2,

and β_3. Epi is synthesized from NE and, along with DA, represents the endogenous catecholamines. Outside the United States, Epi and NE are referred to as adrenaline and noradrenaline, respectively, from which the adjectives "adrenergic" and "noradrenergic" are derived.

Drugs that facilitate or mimic the actions of the sympathetic nervous system are called **sympathomimetics**, **adrenomimetics**, or **adrenergic agonists**. Sympathomimetics may exert their effects by binding directly to adrenergic receptors (direct-acting agonists), by elevating endogenous catecholamines (indirect-acting agents), or via both mechanisms (mixed-action agents). In general, these drugs are used clinically for disorders in which mimicking the fight-or-flight response helps improve or provide relief from the underlying disease. Many of these agents are also relevant drugs of abuse (Chapter 24).

Most adrenergic receptor agonists, with the exception of α_2 agonists, function as sympathomimetics. The therapeutic use of these agents is dictated primarily by the specific receptor subtype(s) with which they interact. Clinically important sympathomimetic effects in a specific organ or tissue can be achieved without a major disruption in the function of other organs or tissues because the distribution of adrenergic receptor subtypes varies by organ and tissue. For example, α_1-adrenergic receptor agonists, such as **phenylephrine**, are useful for promoting vasoconstriction to decrease nasal congestion without direct effects on the heart. In contrast, β-selective agonists, such as **isoproterenol**, are preferred when increased cardiac contractility is desired and vasoconstriction would be detrimental, such as ionotropic support in heart failure. Similarly, due to the distribution of β_2-adrenergic receptors, drugs that selectively activate these receptors, such as **albuterol**, promote bronchodilation without having significant cardiovascular effects. Finally, agents with broader effects, such as NE, can be used when it is desirable to produce a sympathomimetic effect in multiple organs and tissues—for example, to both increase cardiac output and vasoconstrict during septic shock.

Unlike drugs that activate α_1- and β-adrenergic receptors, agonists at α_2-adrenergic receptors reduce sympathetic tone and are **sympatholytic**. Drugs that activate α_2-adrenergic receptors, such as **clonidine** and **guanfacine**, are beneficial when a reduction in the fight-or-flight response is warranted. Thus activation of α_2-adrenergic receptors reduces heart rate and promotes vasodilation, beneficial for the management of hypertension.

A summary of the primary uses of different classes of compounds that affect the sympathetic nervous system is presented in the Therapeutic Overview Box.

THERAPEUTIC OVERVIEW

Endogenous Catecholamines
Hypotension
Shock (cardiogenic and septic)
Anaphylaxis
Bradycardia

α_1-Adrenergic Receptor Agonists
Nasal congestion
Hypotension
Mydriasis induction
Hemorrhoids

α_2-Adrenergic Receptor Agonists
Hypertension
Attention deficit-hyperactivity disorder (ADHD)
Neuropathic pain

Nonselective β-Adrenergic Receptor Agonists
Heart block
Cardiac arrest
Bradycardia[a]
Torsades de pointes[a]

β_1-Adrenergic Receptor Agonists
Cardiogenic shock

β_2-Adrenergic Receptor Agonists
Asthma/Bronchospasm
Chronic obstructive pulmonary disease

[a]Off-label.

MECHANISMS OF ACTION

The biochemistry and physiology of the autonomic nervous system, including a discussion of NE metabolism and release and an overview of adrenergic receptors, are presented in Chapter 6. Additional information on receptors and signaling pathways is in Chapter 2. The noradrenergic system can be activated by either stimulating postsynaptic adrenergic receptors directly with α or β agonists, facilitating the release of NE from adrenergic neurons, or blocking the neuronal reuptake of NE following its release to prolong its actions at receptors. Conversely, the noradrenergic system can be inhibited by directly stimulating presynaptic feedback receptors with α_2 agonists.

Adrenergic receptors are grouped into three major families (α_1, α_2, and β), each containing three different members (Chapter 6). Of these, only four receptors (α_1, α_2, β_1, and β_2) are important in current clinical pharmacology. Both NE and Epi activate α_1, α_2, and β_1 receptors with similar potencies, with Epi exhibiting greater potency at β_2 receptors, while the synthetic catecholamine **isoproterenol (ISO)** exhibits greater potency than either Epi or NE at β_1 receptors and similar potency to Epi at β_2 receptors, illustrated in Fig. 11.1. The presence of different receptor subtypes in these tissues is further supported by comparing the effects of selective antagonists, as shown in Fig. 11.2. **Phentolamine**, a competitive antagonist at α_1 receptors, causes a parallel shift to the right of NE-induced contractions of arterial strips but does not affect NE-induced contraction of the heart or ISO-induced relaxation of bronchial smooth muscle. In contrast, **propranolol**, a competitive antagonist at both β_1 and β_2 receptors, causes a parallel shift to the right of responses mediated by both cardiac β_1 receptors and bronchial β_2 receptors without affecting the α_1 receptor response.

Direct-Acting Adrenergic Receptor Agonists

The structures of representative α and β receptor agonists are shown in Fig. 11.3. Direct-acting adrenergic receptor agonists mimic some of the effects of sympathetic nervous system activation by binding to and activating specific receptor subtypes. Agonists selective for α_1 receptors include **phenylephrine** and **methoxamine**, while agonists selective for α_2 receptors include **clonidine** and **guanfacine**. Selective agonism of α_2 receptors can also be achieved with **α-methyldopa**, an analogue of L-DOPA that is transported into NE neurons, where it is converted to **α-methyl-NE**, which is transported into synaptic vesicles and released in place of NE, functioning as a false neurotransmitter (Fig. 11.4).

As mentioned, ISO activates all β receptors; **dobutamine** exerts a combination of actions with primarily agonist activity at β_1 receptors, while **albuterol**, **bitolterol**, **formoterol**, **metaproterenol**, **pirbuterol**, **salmeterol**, and **terbutaline** are all specific for β_2 receptors.

Indirect-Acting Sympathomimetics

Indirect-acting sympathomimetics stimulate or enhance adrenergic transmission by affecting the transport of NE at the plasma membrane and/or the synaptic vesicle. **Amphetamine** and related drugs are taken up into presynaptic nerve terminals by the **plasma membrane transporter (uptake1)** and transported into synaptic vesicles via the **vesicular monoamine transporter (VMAT2)**. This latter action displaces NE from the vesicles, leading to an increase in cytoplasmic neurotransmitter. Because amphetamines also reverse the direction of the plasma membrane transporter, the release of this cytoplasmic NE is enhanced, producing a sympathomimetic effect. **Amphetamine** exists as D- and L-optical isomers, which are equipotent at peripheral sympathetic neurons, but not in the CNS, where the D-isomer is three to four times more potent than the L-isomer.

The related dietary compound **tyramine** is also taken up by and reverses the direction of the plasma membrane transporter, similar to amphetamine; it is unclear whether it affects VMAT2. In contrast, other compounds, such as **cocaine**, also produce a sympathomimetic effect by inhibiting the plasma membrane transporter, preventing the clearance of NE from the synapse, thus prolonging its action at adrenergic receptors.

Mixed-Action Sympathomimetics

Drugs flike **ephedrine** and **pseudoephedrine** evoke sympathomimetic effects by both reversing the plasma membrane NE transporter and directly activating adrenergic receptors. Ephedrine has two asymmetric carbons and thus represents a racemic mixture of D- and L-ephedrine

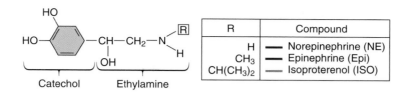

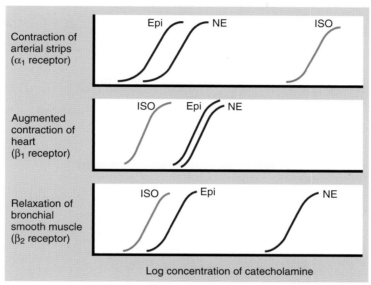

FIG. 11.1 Concentration-Response Curves (Arbitrary Scales) for Epinephrine (Epi), Norepinephrine (NE), and Isoproterenol (ISO). Muscles were incubated with progressively increasing concentrations of each compound, and changes in the force of contraction (arterial and heart muscle) or relaxation (bronchial muscle) were measured. Shown is an arbitrary scale.

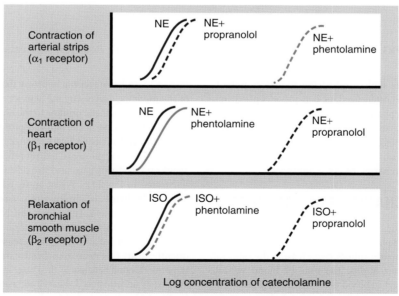

FIG. 11.2 Effects of Antagonists on the Concentration-Response Curves for Norepinephrine (NE) and Isoproterenol (ISO). Muscles were incubated with progressively increasing concentrations of each compound in the absence or presence of a fixed concentration of the α-receptor antagonist phentolamine or the β-receptor antagonist propranolol. Changes in the force of contraction (arterial and heart muscle) or relaxation (bronchial muscle) were measured. Shown is an arbitrary scale.

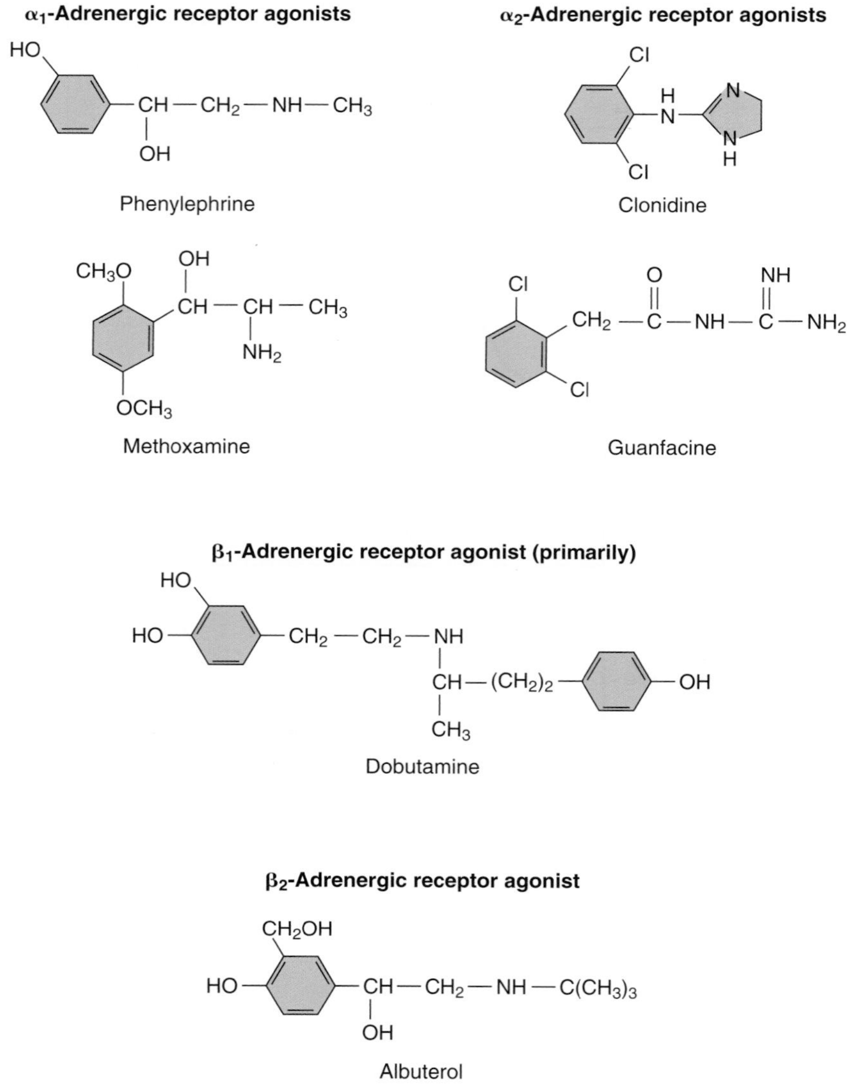

α₁-Adrenergic receptor agonists

Phenylephrine

Methoxamine

α₂-Adrenergic receptor agonists

Clonidine

Guanfacine

β₁-Adrenergic receptor agonist (primarily)

Dobutamine

β₂-Adrenergic receptor agonist

Albuterol

FIG. 11.3 Structures of Some Direct-Acting Adrenergic Receptor Agonists.

and D- and L-pseudoephedrine, with L-ephedrine the most potent, although the racemic mixture is often used, as is D-pseudoephedrine. Both ephedrine and pseudoephedrine promote the cytoplasmic release of NE, but the specific adrenergic receptor subtype(s) they activate is controversial. Data suggest that ephedrine likely activates only β-adrenergic receptors in humans, while pseudoephedrine may be activating both α- and β-adrenergic receptor subtypes.

RELATIONSHIP OF MECHANISMS OF ACTION TO CLINICAL RESPONSE

The sympathetic nervous system plays an important role regulating the cardiovascular system, with sympathomimetics increasing the rate and force of contraction of the heart and/or the tone of blood vessels, increasing blood pressure. Changes in blood pressure trigger compensatory adjustments via the baroreceptor reflex to maintain homeostasis, and thus mean arterial blood pressure does not fluctuate widely (Fig. 11.5). Baroreceptors are mechanosensors that respond to stretch and are located in the walls of the heart (atria and right ventricle), blood vessels (pulmonary vessels, carotid sinus, aortic arch), and the juxtaglomerular apparatus. An elevation in blood pressure increases the firing

rate of these baroreceptor neurons that project to vasomotor centers in the medulla, decreasing the activity of these cells and concomitantly decreasing sympathetic outflow to the heart and blood vessels. In addition, the increased firing of the baroreceptor neurons increases vagal activity to the heart, decreasing heart rate.

The clinical response to a drug reflects both the direct effects of the agent on effector organs and the reflex response. This phenomenon is illustrated in Fig. 11.6. When an α₁-adrenergic receptor agonist, such as **phenylephrine**, is administered, vascular smooth muscle contracts, increasing peripheral resistance and blood pressure. This increase in pressure elevates afferent baroreceptor neuronal activity, thereby reducing sympathetic nerve activity and increasing vagal nerve activity. Consequently, heart rate decreases (bradycardia), while peripheral resistance remains elevated because of the drug. In contrast, if a pure β₁-adrenergic agonist is administered, heart rate and cardiac contractility increase, leading to an elevation in blood pressure. Activation of the baroreceptor reflex reduces sympathetic output, which decreases peripheral resistance. Thus while an increase in heart rate and cardiac contractility persist because of the drug, blood pressure decreases as the sympathetic tone to blood vessels is diminished. Further, as shown in Fig. 11.6, if a vasodilator such as **histamine** is applied, the resulting decrease in blood

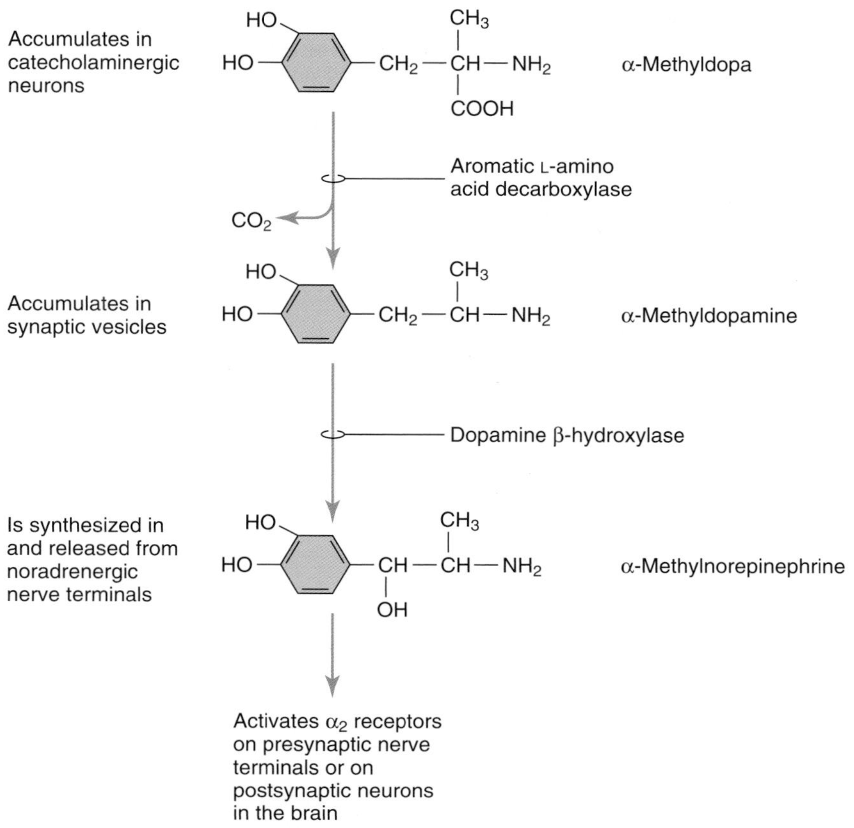

FIG. 11.4 Metabolism of α-Methyldopa in Central Noradrenergic Nerve Terminals.

pressure triggers a systemic elevation in sympathetic nerve activity (i.e., to heart and blood vessels) and a decrease in parasympathetic (vagal nerve) activity in the heart, resulting in an increased heart rate and cardiac contractility in an attempt to elevate blood pressure. Thus drugs causing vasoconstriction will cause reflex slowing of the heart, whereas drugs increasing heart rate and contractility will promote a reflex vasodilation.

Epinephrine
The Cardiovascular System

Epi is the prototype direct-acting sympathomimetic because it activates all known adrenergic receptors. By activating **cardiac β₁ receptors**, Epi increases the strength, rate, and rhythm of cardiac contractions, actions that may be either desirable or undesirable. Epi increases the force of contraction (**positive inotropic effect**) by activating β₁ receptors on cardiomyocytes and increases the rate of contraction (**positive chronotropic effect**) by activating β₁ receptors on pacemaker cells in the sinoatrial node. Epi also accelerates the rate of myocardial relaxation (**positive lusitropic effects**) to shorten systole more than diastole. Thus the fraction of time spent in diastole is increased, allowing for increased filling of the heart. The combination of an increased diastolic filling time, more forceful ejection of blood, and increased rates of contraction and relaxation of the heart results in increased cardiac output.

Epi also activates conducting tissues, increasing conduction velocity and reducing the refractory period in the atrioventricular node, the bundle of His, Purkinje fibers, and ventricular muscle. These changes and the activation of latent pacemaker cells may lead to alterations in heart rhythm. Large doses of Epi may cause tachycardia, increased cardiac muscle excitability, premature ventricular contractions, and ventricular

fibrillation. These effects are more likely to occur in hearts that are diseased or have been sensitized by halogenated hydrocarbon anesthetics (Chapter 26).

Vascular smooth muscle is regulated primarily by α₁ and/or β₂ receptors, depending on the location of the vascular bed. Epi is a powerful vasoconstrictor in vascular beds expressing primarily α₁-adrenergic receptors, including arteries and arterioles in the skin, mucosa, brain, lungs, and abdominal viscera. However, it is a vasodilator in resistance vessels expressing primarily β₂ receptors, particularly those in skeletal muscle. In veins, vascular beds such as those of the kidney and coronary arteries express both α₁ and β₂ receptors, and Epi leads to a mixed effect. Thus Epi increases blood flow in skeletal muscle but reduces flow in most other organs, consistent with the endogenous fight-or-flight function of Epi.

While the vascular effects of Epi have a major impact on blood flow in organs, other factors also influence the clinical effect. For example, systemic administration of Epi alters cerebral and coronary blood flow, but the changes do not result primarily from direct actions of Epi on vascular smooth muscle. Rather, changes in cerebral blood flow reflect changes in systemic blood pressure, and increased coronary blood flow results from a greater duration of diastole and production of vasodilator metabolites (e.g., adenosine) secondary to the increased work of the heart.

Other Smooth Muscle

Epi is a potent bronchodilator, relaxing bronchial smooth muscle by activating β₂ receptors. It dramatically reduces responses to endogenous bronchoconstrictors and can be lifesaving in acute asthmatic attacks (Chapter 72). Epi also relaxes smooth muscle in other organs, also

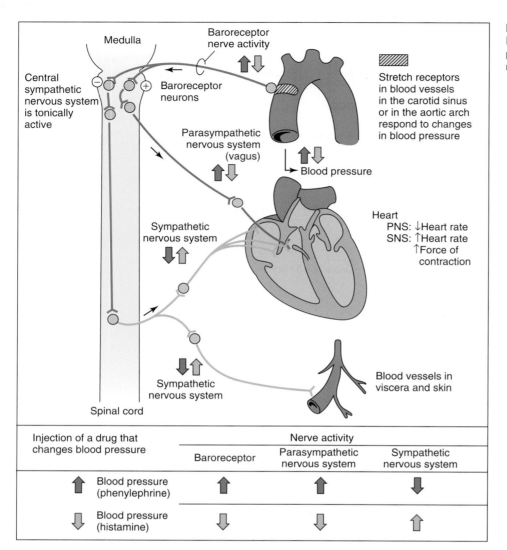

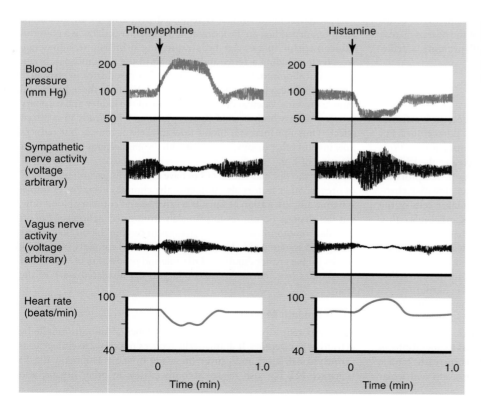

FIG. 11.5 Baroreceptor Control of Blood Pressure and Heart Rate. *PNS*, Parasympathetic nervous system; *SNS*, sympathetic nervous system.

FIG. 11.6 Cardiovascular Responses to a Vasoconstrictor and a Vasodilator. The vasoconstrictor phenylephrine or the vasodilator histamine was administered intravenously and responses measured.

through activation of β₂ receptors. It reduces the frequency and amplitude of gastrointestinal (GI) contractions, decreases the tone and contractions of the pregnant uterus, and relaxes the detrusor muscle of the urinary bladder. In contrast, Epi causes the smooth muscle of the prostate and splenic capsule and of the GI and urinary sphincters to contract by activating α₁ receptors. Epi can foster urinary retention by relaxing the detrusor muscle and contracting the trigone and sphincter of the urinary bladder.

The radial pupillary dilator muscle of the iris contains α₁ receptors and contracts in response to activation of sympathetic neurons, causing mydriasis. However, such a response is not observed when Epi is applied topically onto the conjunctival sac of a normal eye. The primary effect of instilling Epi onto the eye is a decrease in intraocular pressure. The ocular hypotensive mechanism appears to involve multiple actions of Epi due to activation of α₂-adrenergic receptors, including a reduction in aqueous humor formation and an increase in aqueous humor outflow via the trabecular meshwork.

Metabolic Effects

Epi exerts many metabolic effects, some of which are the result of its action on the secretion of insulin and glucagon. The predominant action of Epi is inhibition of insulin secretion from pancreatic β cells through activation of α₂ receptors. However, activation of β₂ receptors on these cells stimulates insulin release to a lesser extent, providing some counterbalance to the α₂ receptor–mediated response. Similarly, activation of β₂ receptors elicits glucagon secretion from pancreatic α cells.

The major metabolic effects of Epi are increased circulating concentrations of glucose, lactic acid, and free fatty acids. In humans, these effects are attributable to the activation of β receptors at liver, skeletal muscle, heart, and adipose cells (Fig. 11.7). Activation of β receptors results in Gₛ-protein–mediated activation of adenylyl cyclase, increasing cyclic adenosine monophosphate (cAMP), culminating in activation of phosphorylase and lipase. In fat, lipase catalyzes the metabolism of triglycerides to free fatty acids. The characteristic "calorigenic action" of Epi, which is reflected in a 20%–30% increase in O₂ consumption, is caused partly by the breakdown of triglycerides in brown adipose tissue and subsequent oxidation of the resulting fatty acids. In liver, phosphorylase catalyzes the conversion of glycogen to glucose. The release of glucose from the liver is accompanied by K⁺ efflux, resulting in both a hyperglycemia and a brief period of hyperkalemia due to activation of hepatic α receptors. The hyperkalemia is followed by a

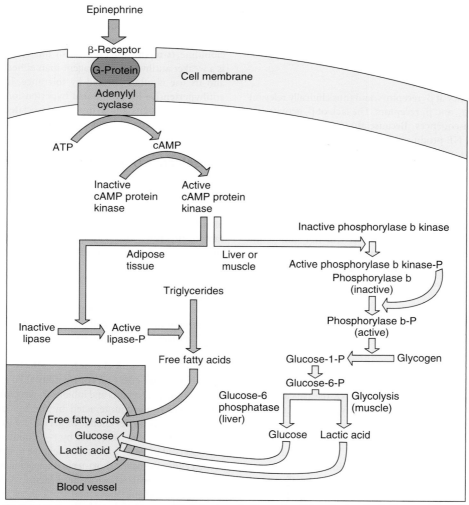

FIG. 11.7 Metabolic Consequences of β-Adrenergic Receptor Stimulation in Adipose, Liver, Heart, and Skeletal Muscle Cells.

more pronounced hypokalemia, as the K^+ released from the liver is taken up by skeletal muscle as a result of activation of muscle β_2 receptors. In muscle, glycogenolysis and glycolysis produce lactic acid, which is released into the blood.

Other Actions

The secretion of sweat from glands located on the palms of the hands and forehead is increased during psychological stress, an effect mediated by α_1 receptors. Epi activates these glands when injected locally but not when administered systemically. Epi also causes the release of renin from the juxtaglomerular apparatus in the kidney by acting on β_1 receptors.

Because Epi has a broad range of action, systemic application will affect adrenergic receptors in the heart, blood vessels, and lungs, particularly useful for the treatment of hypersensitivity reactions. Epi can reduce both the bronchospasm associated with anaphylaxis and counter the hypotension of anaphylactic shock by promoting vasoconstriction in some vascular beds and increasing cardiac output. Similarly, Epi may be used to treat hypotension associated with septic shock or shock unresponsive to volume resuscitation. The ability of Epi to constrict blood vessels has also been employed to promote hemostasis to reduce local bleeding and to limit the systemic absorption of drugs such as the local anesthetics. Due to the effects on cardiac muscle and conduction, Epi may facilitate restoration of regular rhythm with shock/defibrillation in patients with asystole/pulseless arrest, ventricular fibrillation, or pulseless ventricular tachycardia. Moreover, Epi is also recommended following cardiac arrest because it can increase coronary and cerebral perfusion during cardiopulmonary resuscitation. Epi may also help resolve bradycardia unresponsive to atropine or pacing.

Norepinephrine

NE has relatively low potency at β_2 receptors, and thus clinically relevant doses stimulate only α_1, α_2, and β_1 receptors. The lack of β_2 activity has clinically significant consequences. Because there is no appreciable β_2-induced vasodilation, NE produces only vasoconstriction, evoking a significant elevation in total peripheral resistance and a more robust increase in diastolic blood pressure than Epi. This pressor response evokes a reflex slowing of heart rate. Thus NE is superior to Epi and is considered the first-choice vasopressor for the treatment of septic shock. However, because NE does not relax bronchial smooth muscle, an effect dependent on activation of β_2 receptors, it is not useful for the treatment of anaphylactic shock because it will not inhibit the bronchospasms observed in this condition. Lastly, because the metabolic effects of sympathetic activation, such as hyperglycemia, involve primarily β_2 receptors, these effects are also much less for NE than those produced by Epi.

Dopamine

DA produces complex dose-dependent peripheral actions. Low doses of DA (0.5–2 mg/kg/min) relax smooth muscle in various vascular beds, including renal, mesenteric, and coronary. These effects are due to a combination of direct vascular smooth muscle relaxation caused by D_1 receptor activation and decreased NE release caused by presynaptic D_2 receptor activation. In the kidney, DA also increases glomerular filtration rate, Na^+ excretion, and urinary output, effects mediated primarily by D_1 receptors in the renal vasculature that can be blocked by many antipsychotic drugs (Chapter 16). Moderate doses of DA (2–10 mg/kg/min) activate β_1 receptors in addition to DA receptors and thus elicit positive chronotropic and inotropic effects. DA has actions similar to dobutamine at these doses. High doses of DA (>10 mg/kg/min) activate α_1 receptors in addition to β_1 and cognate

DA receptors. Thus the receptor activation profile of DA is similar to NE when administered at high doses, and it may be used therapeutically like NE.

Selective α₁-Adrenergic Receptor Agonists

Phenylephrine and methoxamine are selective α_1-receptor agonists and primarily act on vascular smooth muscle, with little or no direct effects on the heart and other organs, such as the lungs. Activation of α_1 receptors increases total peripheral resistance by causing vasoconstriction in most vascular beds. Consequently, these drugs produce a reflex slowing of the heart that can be blocked by atropine. This reflex response is greater than for NE because of the lack of direct β_1 receptor stimulation produced by NE. Phenylephrine and methoxamine are less potent but longer acting than NE and have been used to treat hypotension and shock. Phenylephrine is also used in topical preparations as a mydriatic, as a nasal decongestant and for the treatment of hemorrhoids.

Selective α₂-Adrenergic Receptor Agonists

Clonidine, guanfacine, and methyldopa are selective α_2-adrenergic receptor agonists, evoking a sympatholytic response. Clonidine and guanfacine are lipid soluble and penetrate the blood-brain barrier to activate α_2 receptors in the medulla, resulting in diminished sympathetic outflow. In peripheral sympathetic neurons, these agents activate presynaptic α_2 receptors, which enhances negative feedback and reduces NE release. The net effect of clonidine and guanfacine is a reduction in blood pressure due to decreased total peripheral resistance, heart rate, and cardiac output. Accordingly, these agents are used to lower blood pressure in patients with moderate to severe hypertension. Like clonidine, α-methyldopa is used for the treatment of hypertension but is a weaker antihypertensive agent than either clonidine or guanfacine, and its use is often affected by tolerance. It is, however, a first-line antihypertensive for gestational hypertension. Clonidine is also used to ameliorate signs and symptoms associated with increased activity of the sympathetic nervous system that accompany withdrawal from long-term opioid use.

Nonselective β-Adrenergic Receptor Agonists

ISO is a potent agonist at all β receptor subtypes and differs from Epi because it does not activate α receptors. ISO reduces total peripheral resistance through β_2 receptors, resulting in a reduction in diastolic blood pressure. It has a strong stimulatory effect on the heart, increasing rate, contractility, and pulse pressure. Tachycardia may result from a combination of direct stimulation of cardiac β_1 receptors and a reflex response produced by the drop in peripheral vascular resistance. Like Epi, ISO relaxes bronchial smooth muscle and induces metabolic effects. Therapeutically, ISO may be used to relieve bronchoconstriction; however, clinical use of the drug has been significantly reduced due to side effects.

Dobutamine is a sympathomimetic with complex effects, attributable to differences in receptor selectivity of the (+) and (−) enantiomers. The (+) enantiomer activates β_1 receptors in the heart, leading to both positive inotropic and chronotropic effects. However, relative to ISO, there is a greater effect on contractility than rate. The (+) enantiomer also activates β_2 receptors and inhibits α_1 receptors, leading to vasodilatory effects, which are counteracted by the (−) isomer, an agonist at α_1 receptors. Thus no net change in peripheral vascular resistance occurs. The activation of α_1 receptors by (−) dobutamine may contribute to the observed increase in inotropy relative to chronotropy. Dobutamine is used clinically for the short-term management of cardiac decompensation in patients with refractory heart failure (American Heart Association Stage D), cardiogenic shock, and septic shock who have been adequately fluid resuscitated but have low cardiac output.

Selective β₂-Adrenergic Receptor Agonists

Albuterol, bitolterol, formoterol, metaproterenol, pirbuterol, salmeterol, and terbutaline are relatively specific agonists at β₂ receptors. Because these drugs have lower affinity for β₁ receptors, they are less likely to produce direct effects on the heart (i.e., chronotropic and inotropic effects). Nevertheless, their selectivity for β₂ receptors is not absolute, and at higher doses, these drugs stimulate the heart directly. These drugs differ from ISO because they are effective orally and have a longer duration of action. Selective β₂-receptor agonists relax vascular smooth muscle in skeletal muscle and in bronchi and the uterus. Although the pharmacological properties of all β₂-receptor agonists are similar, ritodrine is marketed as a tocolytic agent—that is, it relaxes uterine smooth muscle and thereby arrests premature labor. By activating β₂ receptors, these drugs cause bronchodilation and may inhibit the release of inflammatory and bronchoconstrictor mediators (histamine, leukotrienes, and prostaglandins) from mast cells in the lungs. The compounds are most effective when delivered by inhalation and are used for the treatment of asthma and chronic obstructive pulmonary disease (COPD). When used orally, selective β₂-receptor agonists have an advantage over ephedrine because they lack CNS stimulant properties.

Indirect-Acting Sympathomimetics

The clinical use of amphetamine compounds for the treatment of attention deficit-hyperactivity disorder is discussed in Chapter 18.

Because ephedrine exerts a direct action on β₂ receptors, it has some limited usefulness as a bronchodilator. It also readily crosses the blood-brain barrier. Pseudoephedrine has fewer central stimulant actions than ephedrine and is widely available as a component of over-the-counter preparations used as a decongestant for relief of upper respiratory tract conditions that accompany the common cold. The decongestant activity of pseudoephedrine has been attributed to both NE release and activation of α receptors, constricting nasal blood vessels. The use of pseudoephedrine has been subject to legal restrictions because it can be modified chemically to yield an abused substance (methamphetamine). It is often combined with analgesics, anticholinergics, antihistaminics, and caffeine.

PHARMACOKINETICS

Epi is administered intravenously (IV), by inhalation, or topical application and not given orally because it is oxidized by the GI mucosa and liver by monoamine oxidase (MAO) and catechol-O-methyltransferase (COMT), as detailed in Chapter 6. NE is administered only IV, with similar metabolism, while ISO is administered IV or by inhalation and is metabolized primarily by COMT. These agents have a half-life of 1–2 minutes following injection.

Phenylephrine is administered IV, orally, and topically with complete absorption after oral administration. It is 95% bound to plasma proteins and undergoes extensive first-pass metabolism by MAO in the intestinal epithelium. Both parent and metabolites are excreted in the urine.

Clonidine is administered both orally and IV and exhibits dose-dependent pharmacokinetics. It exhibits low protein binding (20%–40%) and limited metabolism by the liver, with the parent compound excreted primarily unchanged in the urine (40%–60%) and bile (20%).

Guanfacine is administered orally with moderate (70%) plasma protein binding. It is metabolized in the liver, and both parent and glucuronidated metabolites are excreted primarily by the kidneys.

Methyldopa exhibits variable absorption after oral administration, with limited (20%) plasma protein binding. It is extensively metabolized by the liver, and parent and metabolites are excreted in the urine.

Ephedrine is administered IV, IM, or subcutaneously (SC). It exhibits limited metabolism and is excreted primarily unchanged in the urine.

Pseudoephedrine is administered orally, completely absorbed from the GI tract, and not bound appreciably to plasma proteins. It is metabolized to a limited extent in the liver and is excreted primarily (70%–90%) unchanged in the urine.

Dobutamine is administered IV, has a very short half-life (2 minutes), and is excreted as conjugates in the urine.

The β₂-receptor agonists have been classified according to their bronchodilator duration of action with albuterol, levalbuterol, metaproterenol, pirbuterol, and terbutaline classified as short-acting β₂ agonists (SABAs) and formoterol and salmeterol as long-acting β₂ agonists (LABAs). The SABAs can be taken orally or by inhalation and generally have a duration of action of 2–8 hours, with the exception of sustained-release albuterol, which can last up to 12 hours. In contrast, the LABAs have a duration of action of 12 hours or more. These drugs are metabolized to a variable extent, with both parent and metabolites excreted in the urine. Known pharmacokinetic parameters for major drugs are summarized in Table 11.1.

PHARMACOVIGILANCE: ADVERSE EFFECTS AND DRUG INTERACTIONS

The systemic administration of Epi can cause anxiety, restlessness, and headache. The most significant adverse effects relate to the cardiovascular system. The increased cardiac output and vasoconstriction may result in hypertension, the increased heart rate and cardiac muscle excitability may result in arrhythmias, and the elevation in cardiac muscle O₂ demand may precipitate angina. Prolonged local hemostasis can result in tissue necrosis due to inadequate perfusion. The adverse effects of NE are similar to those of Epi, but there is a more pronounced hypertension due to α₁ stimulation without β₂ offset. The adverse effects of high doses of DA are similar to those of NE.

The adverse effects of α₁ receptor agonists include angina due to coronary vasoconstriction and increased O₂ demand produced by elevated afterload, hypertension, tissue necrosis, and reflex bradycardia.

The side effects of clonidine may include dry mouth, sedation, dizziness, nightmares, anxiety, and mental depression. Various signs and symptoms related to sympathetic nervous system overactivity (hypertension, tachycardia, sweating) may occur after withdrawal of long-term therapy; thus the dose of clonidine should be reduced gradually. Guanfacine is less likely to reduce cardiac output and is less sedating than clonidine.

ISO commonly leads to tachycardia, headache, and flushing and may lead to arrhythmias in patients with underlying coronary artery disease. The usefulness of dobutamine is particularly limited by its proarrhythmogenic properties, including premature ventricular contractions, ventricular ectopy, ventricular tachycardia, and supraventricular arrhythmias.

The β₂ receptor agonists all lead to nervousness, restlessness, tremor, headache, and insomnia. They also cause angina, hypertension, tachycardia, and hyperglycemia. The chronic use of albuterol and metaproterenol inhalers has been reported to cause a paradoxical bronchospasm. Concurrent use of these compounds with other adrenergic agents can lead to additive effects. Further, these agents should not be used with MAO inhibitors, as they may precipitate a hypertensive crisis.

Tyramine, which is an indirect-acting sympathomimetic, is present in a variety of foods (e.g., ripened cheese, fermented sausage, wines) and is also formed in the liver and GI tract by the decarboxylation of tyrosine. Normally, significant quantities of tyramine are not present

TABLE 11.1	Selected Pharmacokinetic Parameters for Representative Agents			
Drug	Route of Administration	Elimination $t_{1/2}$ (hours)	Disposition	Duration of Action (hours)
Selective α_1-Adrenergic Receptor Agonists				
Phenylephrine	Oral, topical	2.1–3.4	M, R	
Methoxamine	IV, IM	1	M, R	
Selective α_2-Adrenergic Receptor Agonists				
Clonidine	Oral, IV	~12	M, R (50%), B (20%)	
Guanfacine	Oral	4–6	M	
α-methyldopa	Oral	17	M, R	
Mixed-Action Sympathomimetics				
Ephedrine	IV, IM, SC	3–6	R	
Pseudoephedrine	Oral	9–16	M, R	
Selective β_1-Adrenergic Receptor Agonist				
Dobutamine	IV	2 min	M, R	
Selective Short-Acting β_2-Adrenergic Receptor Agonists				
Albuterol	Oral, inhalation	2.7–5 (oral) 3.8 (inhalation)	M, R	4–6 (oral) 3–6 (inhalation) 12 (SR)
Metaproterenol	Oral, inhalation	~6	M	1–5 (oral) 2–6 (inhalation)
Terbutaline	Oral, SC	5.5–6	M, R	4–8 (oral) 1.5–4 (SC)
Selective Long-Acting β_2-Adrenergic Receptor Agonists				
Formoterol	Oral, inhalation	10	M, R	12
Salmeterol	Inhalation	5.5	M, R	>12

IM, Intramuscular; *IV,* intravenous; *M,* metabolism; *R,* renal; *SC,* subcutaneous; *SR,* sustained release.

in blood or tissues because tyramine is rapidly metabolized by MAO in the GI tract, liver, and other tissues, including sympathetic neurons. However, in patients treated with MAO inhibitors for depression, increased circulating concentrations of tyramine may be achieved, particularly after the ingestion of foods containing large concentrations of tyramine. This can lead to the massive release of NE from sympathetic nerve endings, resulting in a severe hypertensive response. Thus patients treated with MAO inhibitors should avoid eating foods containing tyramine (Chapter 17).

Major clinical problems associated with the use of the sympathomimetics are summarized in the Clinical Problems Box.

NEW DEVELOPMENTS

The selective agonists and antagonists for adrenergic α_1-, α_2-, β_1-, and β_2-adrenergic receptor subtypes have led to fewer and less severe side effects than those used previously, and several additional adrenergic receptor subtypes and new drugs with greater selectivity continue to be tested for their therapeutic potential. Pharmacogenomic studies indicate that β_2-receptor polymorphisms occur in association with asthma severity. Such genetic polymorphisms may also contribute to variability in responses to β-receptor agonists. Human genotyping has indicated that polymorphic differences exist in the genes encoding both α and β receptors of human populations based on ethnic or national origin. These genetic variations include changes in expression at transcriptional or translational levels and modification of coupling to heterotrimeric G-proteins, resulting in gain or loss in function and altered susceptibility to down regulation.

CLINICAL PROBLEMS

Selective α_1 receptor agonists	Angina, anxiety, bradycardia, hypertension, tissue necrosis
Selective α_2 receptor agonists	Dry mouth, sedation, depression, bradycardia, edema, orthostatic hypotension, rebound hypertension
Nonselective β receptor agonists	Angina, dizziness, hypertension, nervousness/restlessness, palpitations, premature ventricular contractions, sinus tachycardia, ventricular tachycardia
Selective β_2 receptor agonists	Tremors, CNS stimulation, palpitations, tachycardia (direct and reflex)

CLINICAL RELEVANCE FOR HEALTHCARE PROFESSIONALS

Because the use of the β_2-adrenergic receptor agonists for asthma and other respiratory conditions is so common, all healthcare professionals need to be aware of the adverse effects associated with the use of these agents. These effects are more common in children than adults, who may also use inhalers more frequently, leading to both tolerance and paradoxical bronchospasm. Parents should be advised of the long-term effects of these agents and be urged to limit use by their children to only when necessary.

TRADE NAMES

In addition to generic and fixed-combination preparations, the following trade-named materials are some of the important compounds available in the United States.

Endogenous Catecholamines
Dopamine (Intropin)
Epinephrine (Medihaler, EpiPen)
Norepinephrine (Levophed)

Selective α₁-Adrenergic Receptor Agonists
Methoxamine (Vasoxyl)
Phenylephrine (Neo-Synephrine)

Selective α₂-Adrenergic Receptor Agonists
Clonidine (Catapres)
Guanfacine (Intuniv)
Methyldopa (Aldomet)

Nonselective β-Adrenergic Receptor Agonists
Isoproterenol (Isuprel)
Dobutamine (Dobutrex)

Selective β₂-Adrenergic Receptor Agonists
Albuterol (Proventil)
Bitolterol (Tornalate)
Metaproterenol (Alupent, Metaprel)
Ritodrine (Yutopar)
Salmeterol (Serevent)
Terbutaline (Brethine, Brethaire)

SELF-ASSESSMENT QUESTIONS

1. A patient with cardiogenic shock is administered dopamine at a rapid rate, but no improvement was observed, and the patient decompensates. Upon examination, it was determined that the patient was given 1/10 of the dose ordered by the attending physician. Which of the following events is likely to have resulted in the patient's deterioration?
   A. Arrhythmias due to activation of β_1-adrenergic receptors causing sudden cardiac death.
   B. Decrease in total peripheral resistance due to activation of D_1 receptors and a lack of β_1 and α_1 stimulation.
   C. Pronounced vasoconstriction due to activation of α_1-adrenergic receptors causing elevated afterload and cardiogenic shock.
   D. Spike in blood pressure caused by fluid retention resulting in elevated preload and heart failure.
   E. Sudden drop in peripheral vascular resistance due to activation of presynaptic α_2 receptors.

2. A 27-year-old man with a history of severe shellfish allergies is brought to the emergency department after eating a fish stew that contained shrimp. Immediately after entering the emergency department, the patient starts to have difficulty breathing. His pulse becomes weak, and he loses consciousness. Which of the following is the most appropriate medication to administer at this time?

   A. Albuterol.
   B. Epinephrine.
   C. High-dose dopamine.
   D. Isoproterenol.
   E. Norepinephrine.

3. A 69-year-old man with refractory congestive heart failure is admitted into the emergency department. The patient is dyspneic, pale, and diaphoretic and has severe pulmonary and peripheral edema. His blood pressure is 86/40 mm Hg. Which of the following medications would be most appropriate to administer at this time?
   A. Clonidine.
   B. Albuterol.
   C. Dobutamine.
   D. Low-dose dopamine.
   E. Phenylephrine.

FURTHER READING

Chowdhurn BA, DalPan G. The FDA and safe use of long-acting β-agonists in the treatment of asthma. *N Engl J Med.* 2010;362:1169–1171.

Schaak S, Mialet-Perez J, Flordellis C, Paris H. Genetic variation of human adrenergic receptors: from molecular and functional properties to clinical and pharmacogenetic implications. *Curr Top Med Chem.* 2007;7:217–231.

Shin J, Johnson JA. Pharmacogenetics of β-blockers. *Pharmacotherapy.* 2007;27:874–887.

WEBSITES

https://www.nhlbi.nih.gov/health/health-topics/topics/copd/

https://www.nhlbi.nih.gov/health-pro/resources/lung/naci/asthma-info/asthma-guidelines.htm

https://www.nhlbi.nih.gov/health-pro/guidelines/current/asthma-guidelines

These websites maintained by the National Heart, Lung, and Blood Institute have information and links to multiple resources useful for both professionals and patients on the use of bronchodilators for the treatment of asthma and COPD.

Adrenergic Antagonists and Their Clinical Uses

Javier Cuevas

THERAPEUTIC OVERVIEW

The ability of the sympathetic nervous system to influence the function of many organs, often in ways that contribute to pathophysiological conditions, makes this branch of the autonomic nervous system an important target for pharmacological intervention in various disease states. Drugs that block or reduce the actions of epinephrine (Epi) or norepinephrine (NE) are called sympatholytics or adrenergic receptor antagonists. By disrupting sympathetic input to organs, these agents can alter function and oppose the "flight-or-fight" response. The sympatholytics decrease cardiovascular demand, thus reducing tissue O_2 and energy requirements. These drugs decrease heart rate, cardiac contractility, and cardiac output; lead to vasodilation of most vessels; and cause bronchoconstriction. Energy is conserved, and lipolysis, glycogenolysis, and gluconeogenesis are all reduced.

Due to the widespread distribution of sympathetic nerves throughout the body and the different types and subtypes of adrenergic receptors (Chapter 6), drugs that modify the actions of sympathetic neurons produce many different clinically important responses. Based on receptor subtype selectivity, α_1-adrenergic receptor antagonists are useful to promote vasorelaxation and, while not first-line antihypertensives, are frequently used in antihypertensive combinations. Similarly, by promoting relaxation of the prostate, these agents are also useful for treating symptoms associated with benign prostatic hyperplasia. In contrast, β_1-adrenergic receptor antagonists are useful for decreasing blood pressure via actions on both the heart (decreasing cardiac output) and kidney (decreasing renin production and ultimately fluid retention). These cardiac effects are also important for decreasing O_2 demand for the treatment of angina, reducing arrhythmias, and disrupting cardiac remodeling following myocardial infarction and in heart failure.

A summary of the primary uses of the sympatholytics is presented in the Therapeutic Overview Box.

MECHANISMS OF ACTION

The specific effects of the sympatholytics, including both desired and unwanted effects, are determined by both the receptor selectivity of these compounds and the distribution of receptors that they target. Table 12.1 lists the clinically relevant distribution of adrenergic receptors and the consequences of antagonizing these receptors. Structures of representative compounds are shown in Fig. 12.1.

Nonselective α-Adrenergic Receptor Antagonists

Phentolamine is a prototypical competitive antagonist at both α_1- and α_2-adrenergic receptors. As a competitive antagonist, the antagonism can be overcome by increasing the concentration of agonist, as shown in Fig. 12.2. In contrast, phenoxybenzamine binds covalently to both α_1- and α_2-adrenergic receptors and produces an irreversible blockade that cannot be overcome by addition of more agonist (see Fig. 12.2). Both phentolamine and phenoxybenzamine block the sympathetic input to effector targets mediated by α-adrenergic receptors. Thus they inhibit sympathetic tone affecting splanchnic blood vessels and promote vasodilation because sympathetic constriction of these vessels is dependent on activation of α_1-adrenergic receptors. It is important to note that the magnitude of this effect will be proportional to the degree of sympathetic tone. In a normal individual without hypertension, α-adrenergic receptor antagonists cause only small decreases in recumbent blood pressure but can produce a sharp decrease during the compensatory vasoconstriction that occurs upon standing because reflex sympathetic control of capacitance vessels is lost. This can result in orthostatic or postural hypotension accompanied by reflex tachycardia.

In addition to antagonizing α_1 receptors, as their name implies, the mixed α_1/α_2-adrenergic receptor antagonists will alter sympathetic input to organs via antagonism of presynaptic α_2 receptors. The consequences of combined α_1/α_2 receptor antagonism in peripheral synapses are depicted in Fig. 12.3. In the absence of drug, released NE can activate postsynaptic

TABLE 12.1 Distribution of Adrenergic Receptors and Consequences of Receptor Antagonism

Receptor	Location	Effect of Receptor Antagonism
α_1	Most vascular smooth muscle	Relaxation
	Heart	Decreased force[a]
	Prostate	Relaxation
	Radial and sphincter muscles of iris	Relaxation (miosis)
α_2	Presynaptic (autonomic nervous system)	Increased neurotransmitter release
	Postsynaptic (autonomic nervous system)	Tissue dependent
	Some vascular smooth muscle	Relaxation
β_1	Heart	Decreased force and rate
	Juxtaglomerular cells	Decreased renin release
β_2	Skeletal muscle blood vessels	Contraction
	Bronchial smooth muscle	Contraction
	Liver	Inhibition of glycogenolysis and gluconeogenesis

[a]Less important effect.

α_1 receptors, with NE release regulated by presynaptic α_2 autoreceptor feedback inhibition (Fig. 12.3A). A mixed α_1/α_2-adrenergic receptor antagonist like phentolamine will block both postsynaptic α_1 receptors, decreasing sympathetic input, and presynaptic α_2 receptors, blocking the negative feedback inhibition of NE release and increasing release (Fig. 12.3B).

Selective α_1-Adrenergic Receptor Antagonists

Drugs such as doxazosin and prazosin selectively inhibit α_1-adrenergic receptors, with little or no effects on the α_2-adrenergic receptor subtype. Therefore unlike mixed α_1/α_2 receptor antagonists, these drugs do not block the negative feedback provided by α_2 receptors, and there is no concomitant increase in NE release (Fig. 12.3C).

Nonselective β-Adrenergic Receptor Antagonists

Propranolol is the prototypical nonselective β receptor antagonist and is a competitive antagonist at both β_1- and β_2-adrenergic receptors. Like all adrenergic receptor–blocking drugs, its pharmacological effects depend on the activity of the sympathetic system. When impulse traffic in sympathetic neurons and circulating concentrations of NE and Epi are high (e.g., during exercise), the effects of the drugs are more pronounced. Propranolol, but not all β receptor antagonists, also has a direct membrane-stabilizing action (local anesthetic action), which may contribute to its cardiac antiarrhythmic effect.

Selective β_1-Adrenergic Receptor Antagonists

At low doses, acebutolol, atenolol, metoprolol, and esmolol are more selective in blocking β_1 receptors than β_2 receptors. Thus these agents are more likely to have effects on cardiac muscle and the conduction system than on bronchial smooth muscle.

Mixed-Action α_1/β-Adrenergic Receptor Antagonists

Drugs like labetalol and carvedilol are competitive antagonists of α_1, β_1, and β_2 receptors. Consequently, they have effects similar to those of a combination of propranolol (β_1- and β_2-adrenergic receptor blockade) and prazosin (α_1-adrenergic receptor blockade).

RELATIONSHIP OF MECHANISMS OF ACTION TO CLINICAL RESPONSE

Nonselective α-Adrenergic Receptor Antagonists

The effects of α receptor blockade on mean blood pressure and heart rate in response to NE and Epi are illustrated in Fig. 12.4. The intravenous injection of NE and Epi produces a brief increase in blood pressure by activating α_1-adrenergic receptors in blood vessels. A reflex decrease in sympathetic and increase in vagal tone to the heart occurs, but reflex bradycardia may be masked by direct activation of cardiac β_1 receptors; bradycardia is often seen with NE because systolic and diastolic pressure both increase.

Blockade of α receptors with phentolamine lowers blood pressure and leads to a reflex increase in heart rate. The tachycardia that occurs after administration of α receptor antagonists is attributable in part to blockade of presynaptic α_2 receptors on sympathetic neurons (see Fig. 12.2B). Activation of these receptors inhibits NE release, and this feedback inhibition is disrupted when α_2 receptors are blocked.

In the presence of phentolamine, NE has little effect on blood pressure, but increases heart rate as a consequence of stimulation of cardiac β_1-adrenergic receptors. When Epi is administered in the presence of phentolamine, the former pressor response becomes a strong depressor response because the vasodilatation as a consequence of β_2-adrenergic receptor activation is unmasked. Epi also causes pronounced tachycardia by direct activation of cardiac β_1 receptors, as well as a reflex in response to the decreased blood pressure. Thus effects of sympathetic activation are enhanced when α_2 receptors are blocked, increasing NE release and enhancing reflex tachycardia (see Fig. 12.2B). When α-adrenergic receptors are blocked, the actions of Epi resemble those of the pure β receptor agonist isoproterenol (Chapter 11).

The use of these compounds is limited because of the adverse effects resulting from α_2-adrenergic receptor blockade. However, phenoxybenzamine and phentolamine are useful for the management of hypertensive episodes caused by pheochromocytoma and are preferred over selective α_1 receptor blocking agents. Phenoxybenzamine is particularly useful because of the irreversible block of α_1-adrenergic receptors providing longer blood pressure control. Phentolamine is also approved for uses in which inhibition of α_1-adrenergic receptors overcome vasoconstriction caused by exogenous NE and Epi application, in particular for the management of NE extravasation and reversal of local anesthesia containing a vasoconstrictor.

Selective α_1-Adrenergic Receptor Antagonists

Prazosin, terazosin, doxazosin, tamsulosin, and alfuzosin are selective α_1-adrenergic receptor antagonists with similar pharmacological profiles but some differences in pharmacokinetics. Like the mixed α_1/α_2 receptor antagonists, by blocking α_1 receptors in arterioles and veins, these drugs reduce peripheral vascular resistance and lower blood pressure. However, these selective α_1 receptor antagonists cause less reflex tachycardia than nonselective α receptor antagonists because the α_2 receptors, including those that reduce NE release onto the heart, are not blocked by these drugs (see Fig. 12.3C). While these drugs effectively reduce blood pressure, current guidelines for the management of hypertension, such as those of the Canadian Hypertension Education Program, do not include these drugs as first-line antihypertensives because they fail to improve long-term cardiovascular outcomes. These drugs, however, may be used as add-on therapy when combinations of first-line drugs do not provide effective blood pressure control.

Adrenergic α_1 receptor antagonists also relax smooth muscle in the prostate and bladder neck and thereby relieve urinary retention and

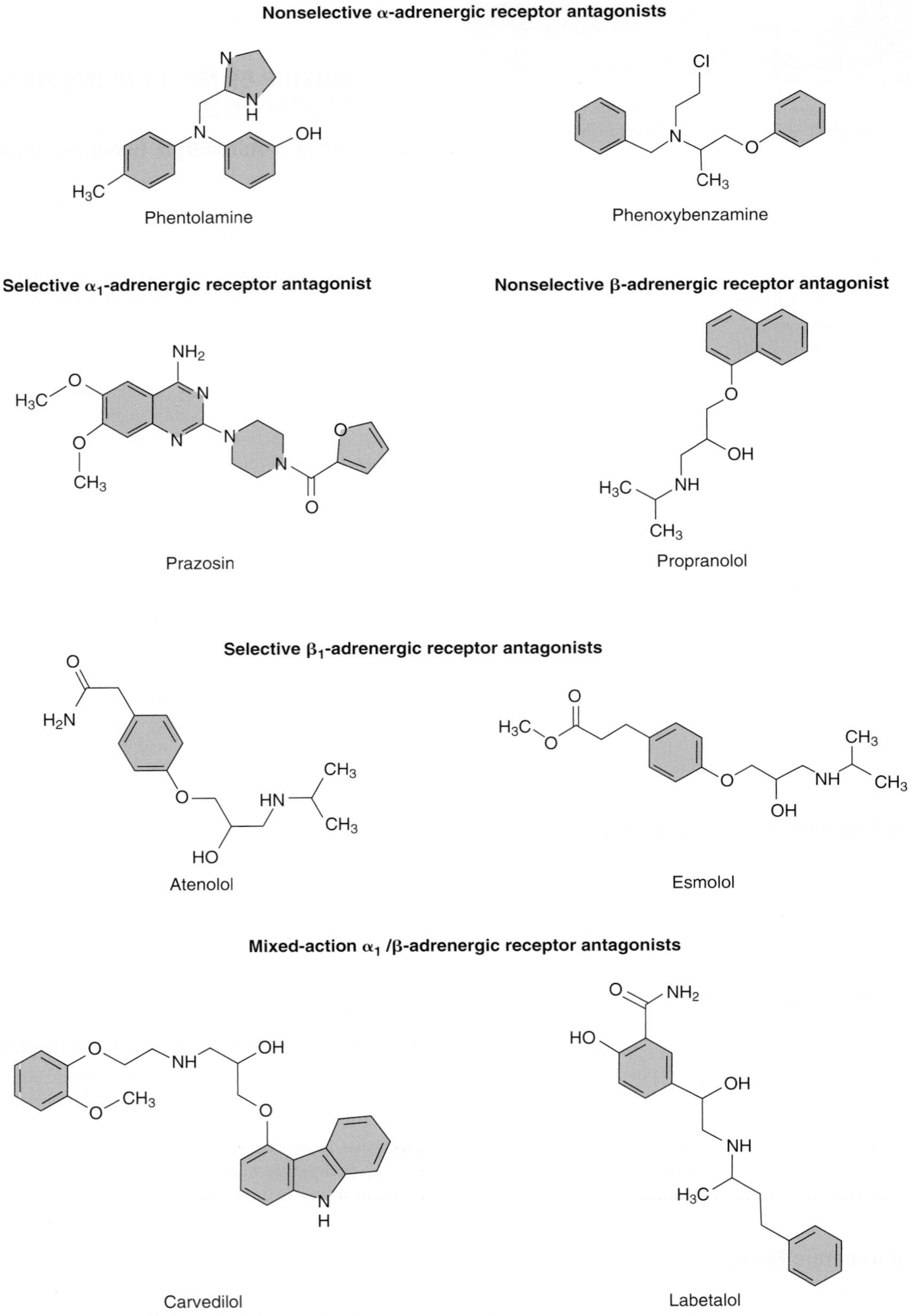

Nonselective α-adrenergic receptor antagonists

Phentolamine

Phenoxybenzamine

Selective α₁-adrenergic receptor antagonist

Prazosin

Nonselective β-adrenergic receptor antagonist

Propranolol

Selective β₁-adrenergic receptor antagonists

Atenolol

Esmolol

Mixed-action α₁/β-adrenergic receptor antagonists

Carvedilol

Labetalol

FIG. 12.1 Structures of Representative Adrenergic Receptor Antagonists.

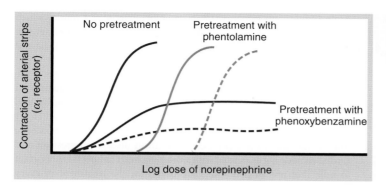

FIG. 12.2 Comparison of the Effects of a Reversible (Phentolamine) and an Irreversible (Phenoxybenzamine) α-Adrenergic Receptor Antagonist. Changes in the force of contraction of arterial strips were recorded after addition of increasing concentrations of NE in the absence and presence of low and high concentrations of phentolamine and low and high concentrations of phenoxybenzamine. The broken lines represent responses to larger doses of the antagonist.

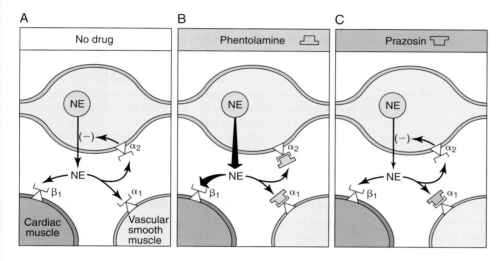

FIG. 12.3 Comparison of the Actions of Phentolamine (Nonselective α-Adrenergic Receptor Antagonist) and Prazosin (Selective α₁-Adrenergic Receptor Antagonist) at Noradrenergic Neuroeffector Junctions in Cardiac Muscle (β_1 Receptors) and Vascular Smooth Muscle (α_1 Receptors). *NE*, Norepinephrine.

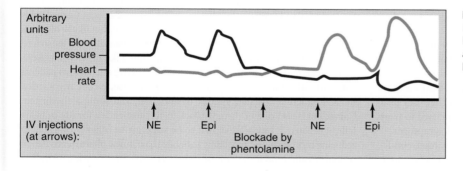

FIG. 12.4 Effects of Intravenous Injections of Norepinephrine *(NE)* and Epinephrine *(Epi)* on Mean Blood Pressure and Heart Rate Before and After Blockade of α-Adrenergic Receptors by Phentolamine.

other symptoms associated with benign prostatic hyperplasia (Chapter 52). Tamsulosin, terazosin, doxazosin, and alfuzosin are commonly prescribed for this condition. Table 12.2 lists the most common clinical applications of α-adrenergic receptor antagonists.

Nonselective β₁-Adrenergic Receptor Antagonists

The first-generation and prototypical β-adrenergic receptor blocker propranolol exerts its clinically relevant effects via the inhibition of both β_1 and β_2 receptors. Newer compounds differ primarily in their duration of action and subtype selectivity. As indicated in Table 12.1, the heart is a major site of β_1-adrenergic receptor expression and thus the target of propranolol. Propranolol blocks the positive chronotropic, dromotropic, and inotropic responses to β receptor agonists and to sympathetic activation. It reduces the rate, conduction velocity, and contractility of the heart at rest, but these effects are more dramatic during exercise or in pathophysiological conditions in which there is elevated sympathetic tone, such as heart failure. In addition to these effects on the heart, propranolol reduces renin secretion and consequently activation of the renin-angiotensin-aldosterone system (Chapter 39), and has anxiolytic properties (Chapter 17). All of these effects of propranolol, and β-blockers in general, are believed to contribute to the antihypertensive properties of these drugs, which are effective for the treatment of systolic-diastolic hypertension. There is some controversy as to whether β-blockers should be considered first-line antihypertensives, and guidelines vary by organization. There is some evidence suggesting that β-blockers are not as effective at reducing the risk of stroke relative to other antihypertensives. However, consensus exists that β-blockers should not be considered as first-line therapy for individuals over 60 years of age. Because β-blockers lower both systolic and diastolic blood pressure to a similar extent, these drugs are less

TABLE 12.2 Most Common Clinical Applications of Specific α-Adrenergic Receptor Antagonists

Drug Class	Drug Name	Clinical Use
Nonselective α-adrenergic receptor antagonist	Phentolamine	Anesthesia reversal, extravasation of α-agonist, pheochromocytoma
	Phenoxybenzamine	Pheochromocytoma
Selective α$_1$-adrenergic receptor antagonist	Prazosin, doxazosin	Hypertension,[a] benign prostatic hyperplasia (BPH)

[a]Not first line. Increased risk of heart failure compared to diuretics. The Antihypertensive and Lipid-Lowering Treatment to Prevent Heart Attack (ALLHAT) Trial had an arm with an α-adrenergic blocker stopped early due to poor outcomes.

useful than angiotensin receptor blockers (Chapter 39) or calcium-channel blockers (Chapter 40) for the treatment of isolated systolic hypertension. However, because of some of their benefits, such as decreasing cardiac remodeling, the β-blockers are first-line antihypertensives for individuals with both systolic-diastolic hypertension and ischemic heart disease, a recent history of myocardial infarction, left ventricular systolic dysfunction, and some types of arrhythmias.

Due to significant effects on the heart, nonselective β-blockers such as propranolol are also useful for the treatment of other cardiovascular diseases and are frequently used in patients with angina pectoris, following myocardial infarction, or with various types of arrhythmias. By lowering O_2 demand, propranolol helps prevent angina and decreases injury following myocardial infarction. Similarly, the negative chronotropic effects of propranolol are useful in the management of supraventricular arrhythmias.

Nadolol is a nonselective β-adrenergic receptor blocking drug that is less lipid soluble than propranolol and less likely to cause central nervous system (CNS) effects. Carteolol, pindolol, and penbutolol are nonselective β-adrenergic receptor antagonists that have modest intrinsic sympathomimetic properties. These drugs cause less slowing of resting heart rate and fewer abnormalities of serum lipid concentrations than other β receptor antagonists, and it has been suggested that they also produce less up regulation of β receptors. These drugs are used to treat hypertension and generally cause less severe withdrawal symptoms.

Nonselective β-blockers are also used for several noncardiac conditions. For example, timolol may be used for the treatment of glaucoma. Inhibition of β-adrenergic receptors in the ciliary epithelium of the eye by timolol reduces aqueous humor production and lessens intraocular pressure. Likewise, propranolol is approved for the treatment of essential tremor, which likely depends on the central depressant effects of propranolol via inhibition of β-adrenergic receptors.

Selective β$_1$-Adrenergic Receptor Antagonists

Like nonselective β-blockers, β$_1$-adrenergic receptor antagonists such as atenolol and metoprolol are useful for the treatment of systolic-diastolic hypertension and angina pectoris. By selectively blocking β$_1$ receptors, these drugs decrease cardiac output, reduce renin release, and have effects in the CNS that together help lower blood pressure. Like the nonselective blockers, there is controversy as to the appropriateness of these compounds as first-line antihypertensives, as there is concern about increased risk for adverse cardiovascular events relative to some other classes of antihypertensives. However, selective β$_1$-adrenergic antagonists are preferred agents in the treatment of hypertension with coronary artery disease and other

comorbidities similar to mixed β$_1$/β$_2$ receptor antagonists. Esmolol, which has a very short half-life, is administered intravenously for hypertensive emergencies and for the emergency treatment of sinus tachycardia and atrial flutter or fibrillation.

One important use for members of this class of β-blockers is the treatment of heart failure. Bisoprolol and long-acting metoprolol (metoprolol succinate) have been shown to reduce morbidity and mortality significantly in patients with symptomatic (American Heart Association Stage C) heart failure (Chapter 44). By reducing sympathetic tone to the heart, these β-blockers diminish disease progression and cardiac remodeling associated with worsening heart failure. It is important to note that not all β-blockers are useful for the treatment of every condition (i.e., there is generally not a drug class effect), and use of specific agents often depends on factors such as pharmacokinetics of the drug. Agents with longer half-lives, for example, have been shown to be of greater benefit in heart failure.

The selective β$_1$ antagonists have several advantages for some patient populations relative to the nonselective antagonists that also block β$_2$ receptors. Receptor selectivity lessens the likelihood of increasing bronchoconstriction, advantageous for patients with asthma. Similarly, the lack of β$_2$ receptor antagonism tempers disruption in the recovery from hypoglycemia caused by nonselective β-blockers in patients with diabetes and is preferred in patients with peripheral vascular disease because the selective β$_1$ agents do not inhibit β$_2$-mediated dilation of skeletal muscle blood vessels.

Table 12.3 lists the most common clinical uses for selective and nonselective β-adrenergic receptor antagonists.

Mixed-Action α$_1$/β-Adrenergic Receptor Antagonists

Agents with combined α$_1$/β$_1$/β$_2$ receptor antagonism, such as carvedilol, have pronounced effects on both the heart and vascular beds by inhibiting a broad population of adrenergic receptor types. Thus these drugs can affect blood pressure by an even greater number of mechanisms than selective β-blockers and can prevent some of the reflex responses that contribute to the loss of blood pressure regulation and/or adverse effects. Carvedilol is used for the control of systolic-diastolic hypertension, but like β-blockers of other classes, the use of carvedilol as a first-line antihypertensive in uncomplicated hypertension remains debatable. Like other β-blockers, carvedilol is particularly useful for the treatment of hypertension in patients with comorbidities such as ischemic heart disease, recent myocardial infarction, left ventricular systolic dysfunction, and some arrhythmias. Carvedilol is also one of three β-blockers recommended for use in heart failure because it has been shown to be superior to other β-blockers in reducing morbidity and mortality. Labetalol has similar pharmacodynamic properties and is preferred for use in hypertensive emergencies, including hypertensive emergencies in pregnancy. Due to a relatively safe profile in pregnancy, labetalol is considered a first-line antihypertensive in pronounced gestational hypertension, preeclampsia, and eclampsia.

The common clinical uses of these agents are listed in Table 12.3.

PHARMACOKINETICS

Most adrenergic receptor antagonists are administered orally; some are available for oral and intravenous administration, while esmolol is available only for intravenous administration. Pharmacokinetic parameters, including bioavailability, plasma protein binding, and half-lives, differ markedly among the agents. Metoprolol exhibits the lowest protein binding (12%) and carvedilol the highest (98%). The half-life of esmolol is very short (approximately 10 minutes), while that of nadolol is approximately 22 hours and is significantly longer than most other β-adrenergic receptor antagonists. Most compounds are metabolized in the liver and excreted by the kidneys.

TABLE 12.3 Most Common Clinical Applications of β-Adrenergic Receptor and Combination Antagonists

Drug Class	Drug Name	Clinical Use
Nonselective β-adrenergic receptor antagonist	Propranolol	Angina, cardiac arrhythmias, hypertension, migraine prophylaxis, myocardial infarction prophylaxis, pheochromocytoma, post–myocardial infarction, thyrotoxicosis, essential tremor
	Timolol	Glaucoma, hypertension, migraine prophylaxis, myocardial infarction prophylaxis, post–myocardial infarction
	Sotalol	Cardiac arrhythmias
Selective β1-adrenergic receptor antagonist	Atenolol	Acute myocardial infarction, angina, hypertension, cardiac arrhythmias,[a] migraine prophylaxis[a]
	Bisoprolol	Angina,[a] heart failure[a] (one of three recommended), hypertension
	Esmolol	Peri/postoperative hypertension, cardiac arrhythmias (supraventricular tachycardia), arrhythmia/rate control during acute myocardial infarction[a]
	Metoprolol	Same as atenolol, heart failure (one of three recommended) (long-acting form: succinate for SUCCESS)
Mixed-action α1/β-adrenergic receptor antagonist	Carvedilol	Acute myocardial infarction, angina, cardiomyopathy, heart failure (one of three recommended), hypertension, post–myocardial infarction
	Labetalol	Hypertension, hypertensive emergency (intravenous), hypertensive emergency in pregnancy[a]

[a]non–FDA-approved indication.

Selected pharmacokinetic parameters of representative adrenergic receptor antagonists are shown in Table 12.4.

PHARMACOVIGILANCE: ADVERSE EFFECTS AND DRUG INTERACTIONS

The major side effects of α-adrenergic receptor antagonists are related to a reduced sympathetic tone at α receptors and include orthostatic hypotension, tachycardia (less common with selective α1 receptor antagonists), inhibition of ejaculation, and nasal congestion.

The adverse effects of propranolol and other nonselective β-blockers stem from receptor inhibition, blocking activation of the sympathoadrenal system. The agents inhibit increases in plasma free fatty acids and glucose from lipolysis in fat and glycogenolysis in liver, heart, and skeletal muscle, which can pose a problem for diabetics by augmenting insulin-induced hypoglycemia. These antagonists also reduce the premonitory tachycardia associated with insulin-induced hypoglycemia, requiring that diabetic patients taking these agents learn to recognize sweating (induced by activation of cholinergic sympathetic neurons) as a symptom of low blood glucose.

Propranolol causes few serious side effects in healthy people but can lead to or exacerbate heart failure in patients with various diseases. Propranolol is usually contraindicated in patients with sinus bradycardia or partial heart block. Caution should always be used when treating patients with congestive heart failure with β-blockers because they suppress contractility and decrease cardiac output. While β-blockers are a useful tool in the management of heart failure, these drugs should be titrated up slowly to prevent heart failure exacerbation.

Sudden withdrawal of propranolol from patients who have received this drug over the long term can cause withdrawal symptoms such as angina, myocardial infarction, tachycardia, dysrhythmias, and anxiety. Rebound hypertension may occur in such patients taking propranolol to control blood pressure. These symptoms likely result from the functional up regulation of β-adrenergic receptors and can be minimized by gradually reducing the dose of the drug. Replacing a centrally acting adrenergic antagonist, such as clonidine, with a β-blocker may cause pronounced peripheral vasoconstriction due to unopposed stimulation of α-adrenergic receptors.

The ability of propranolol to increase airway resistance is of little clinical importance in healthy people but can be very hazardous in patients with obstructive pulmonary disease or asthma because nonselective antagonism of β receptors increases the risk of bronchospasms. Selective β1-adrenergic receptor antagonists should be used in these patients, although even these drugs should be used with caution because they are not completely inactive at β2 receptors. The selective β1-adrenergic agents are also preferred in patients with peripheral vascular disease since these agents do not inhibit β2-mediated dilation of skeletal muscle blood vessels.

Major clinical problems associated with the use of these compounds are summarized in the Clinical Problems Box.

NEW DEVELOPMENTS

The development of selective agonists and antagonists for adrenergic α1, α2, β1, and β2 receptor subtypes have led to fewer and less severe side effects than those used previously, and several additional adrenergic receptor subtypes and new drugs with greater selectivity continue to be tested for their therapeutic potential. Pharmacogenomic studies indicate that β2-adrenergic receptor polymorphisms occur in association with asthma severity, likely contributing to variability in responses to β receptor antagonists. Human genotyping indicates that polymorphic differences in the genes encoding both α and β receptors of human populations are present based on ethnic or national origin. These genetic variations include changes in expression at transcriptional or translational levels, modification of coupling to heterotrimeric G-proteins, which can result in gain or loss in function, and altered susceptibility to down regulation. Knowledge of these alterations may lead to the development of even more selective compounds.

CLINICAL RELEVANCE FOR HEALTHCARE PROFESSIONALS

All healthcare professionals should be aware of the exercise intolerance that develops from the chronic administration of β-adrenergic receptor antagonists and caution patients about this effect. It is also critical to monitor closely the status of specific patient populations taking these drugs, including people with diabetes and individuals with asthma.

TABLE 12.4   Selected Pharmacokinetic Parameters of Adrenergic Receptor Antagonists

Drug	Route of Administration	Protein Binding (%)	$t_{1/2}$ (hrs)	Disposition
α-Adrenergic Receptor Antagonists				
Phentolamine	IV, IM		19 min	R (13%), M
Prazosin	Oral	>90	2.5	M (main), B
Terazosin	Oral	>90	~12	M
Doxazosin	Oral		10–20	M
β-Adrenergic Receptor Antagonists				
Propranolol	Oral	90	4	M
Nadolol	Oral	30	22	R (90%)
Pindolol	Oral	40	3.5	M (60%), R (40%)
			7 (aged)	
Atenolol	Oral	10	6.5	R (90%)
Metoprolol	IV, oral, aerosol	12	5	M (90%), R (50%)
Esmolol	IV	55	10 min	M (98%), R
Mixed-Action α₁/β-Adrenergic Receptor Antagonists				
Carvedilol[a]	oral	98	7–10	M
Labetalol	IV, oral	50	5	M (65%)

[a]Active metabolite 13 times more potent than carvedilol.
B, Biliary; *IM*, intramuscular; *IV*, intravenous; *M*, metabolism; *R*, renal, unchanged drug.

CLINICAL PROBLEMS

α-Adrenergic receptor antagonists	Orthostatic hypotension, hypotension, miosis, tachycardia, nasal congestion, impairment of ejaculation, Na^+ and H_2O retention
Nonselective β-adrenergic receptor antagonists	Heart failure in patients with cardiac disease; sinus bradycardia; increased airway resistance; exacerbation of asthma, fatigue, and depression; rebound hypertension; augmented hypoglycemia; hypertriglyceridemia; and decreased plasma high-density lipoproteins
Selective β₁-adrenergic receptor antagonists	Similar to the nonselective β-blockers, but with lower risks for bronchospasms and hypoglycemia than nonselective β-blockers
Mixed-action α₁/β-adrenergic receptor antagonists	Similar to the nonselective β-blockers (e.g., bronchospasms), similar to α₁ antagonists (e.g., postural hypotension), less reflex tachycardia than α₁ antagonists, less peripheral vasoconstriction than with other classes of β-blockers

TRADE NAMES

In addition to generic and fixed-combination preparations, the following trade-named materials are some of the important compounds available in the United States.

Nonselective α-Adrenergic Receptor Antagonists
  Phentolamine (Regitine)

Selective α₁-Adrenergic Receptor Antagonists
  Doxazosin (Cardura)
  Prazosin (Minipress)
  Tamsulosin (Flomax)
  Terazosin (Hytrin)

Nonselective β-Adrenergic Receptor Antagonists
  Carteolol (Cartrol, Ocupress)
  Nadolol (Corgard)
  Pindolol (Visken)
  Propranolol (Inderal, Innopran, Pronol)
  Timolol (Blocadren, Timoptic)

Selective β₁-Adrenergic Receptor Antagonists
  Atenolol (Tenormin)
  Betaxolol (Kerlone, Betoptic)
  Esmolol (Brevibloc)
  Metoprolol (Lopressor, Toprol-XL)

Mixed-Action α₁/β-Adrenergic Receptor Antagonists
  Carvedilol (Coreg)
  Labetalol (Normodyne, Trandate)

SELF-ASSESSMENT QUESTIONS

1. A 54-year-old man presents to a free clinic after using up all of his carvedilol. Several adrenergic drugs are available in the clinic's pharmacy but no carvedilol. Which of the following combinations would most closely mimic the effects of carvedilol and could replace the drug with minimal adverse effects?
   - **A.** Atenolol and phentolamine.
   - **B.** Metoprolol and prazosin.
   - **C.** Propranolol and doxazosin.
   - **D.** Atenolol and prazosin.
   - **E.** Phentolamine and prazosin.

2. The cardiovascular effects of epinephrine in a person treated with phentolamine will most closely resemble the responses after the administration of:
   - **A.** Isoproterenol.
   - **B.** Norepinephrine.
   - **C.** Labetalol.
   - **D.** Prazosin.
   - **E.** None of the above.

3. Metoprolol would be most effective in blocking the ability of epinephrine to:
   - **A.** Reduce insulin secretion from the pancreas.
   - **B.** Increase the release of renin from the juxtaglomerular apparatus.
   - **C.** Increase glucagon secretion from the pancreas.
   - **D.** Dilate the pupil, leading to mydriasis.
   - **E.** Increase secretions from the salivary glands.

FURTHER READING

Schaak S, Mialet-Perez J, Flordellis C, Paris H. Genetic variation of human adrenergic receptors: from molecular and functional properties to clinical and pharmacogenetic implications. *Curr Top Med Chem.* 2007;7:217–231.

Shin J, Johnson JA. Pharmacogenetics of β-blockers. *Pharmacotherapy.* 2007;27:874–887.

WEBSITES

http://www.acc.org/tools-and-practice-support/clinical-toolkits/heart-failure-practice-solutions/beta-blocker-therapy
This website is maintained by the American College of Cardiology and contains guidelines for the use of β-blockers.

https://www.ncbi.nlm.nih.gov/books/NBK47172/
This is a link to Drug Class Reviews for β-blockers from the Oregon Health and Science University, published in 2009.

http://www.auanet.org/guidelines/benign-prostatic-hyperplasia-(2010-reviewed-and-validity-confirmed-2014)
This is the American Urological Association website on the management of benign prostatic hyperplasia.

Drug Treatment for Disorders Affecting the Central Nervous System

The Central Nervous System

Lynn Wecker

ABBREVIATIONS

ACh	Acetylcholine
BBB	Blood-brain barrier
CNS	Central nervous system
CO	Carbon monoxide
DA	Dopamine
Epi	Epinephrine
GABA	γ-Aminobutyric acid
Glu	Glutamate
5-HT	Serotonin
L-DOPA	3,4-dihydroxy-phenylalanine
NE	Norepinephrine
NMDA	N-methyl-D-aspartate
NO	Nitric oxide

INTRODUCTION

Drugs acting on the central nervous system (CNS) are among the most widely used of all drugs. Humankind has experienced the effects of mind-altering drugs throughout history, and many compounds with specific and useful effects on brain and behavior have been discovered. Drugs used for therapeutic purposes have improved the quality of life dramatically for people with diverse illnesses, whereas illicit drugs have altered the lives of many others, often in detrimental ways.

Discovery of the general anesthetics was essential for the development of surgery, and continued advances in the development of anesthetics, sedatives, muscle relaxants, and pain relievers have made possible the complex microsurgical procedures in use today. Discovery of the typical antipsychotics and tricyclic antidepressants in the 1950s and the introduction of the atypical antipsychotics and new classes of antidepressants within the past 25 years have revolutionized psychiatry and enabled many individuals afflicted with these mind-paralyzing diseases to begin to lead productive lives and contribute to society. Similarly, the introduction of 3,4-dihydroxy-phenylalanine (L-DOPA) for the treatment of Parkinson disease in 1970 was a milestone in neurology and allowed many people who had been immobilized for years the ability to move and interact with their environment. Other advances led to the development of drugs to reduce pain or fever, relieve seizures and other movement disorders associated with neurological diseases, and alleviate the incapacitating effects associated with psychiatric illnesses, including bipolar disorder and anxiety.

The nonmedical use of drugs affecting the CNS has also increased dramatically. Alcohol, hallucinogens, caffeine, nicotine, and other compounds were used historically to alter mood and behavior and are still in common use. In addition, many stimulants, depressants, and antianxiety agents intended for medical use are obtained illicitly and used for their mood-altering effects. Although the short-term effects of these drugs may be exciting or pleasurable, excessive use often leads to physical dependence or toxic effects that result in long-term alterations in the brain. Drug dependence is a major problem in the United States, as we are currently experiencing an opioid crisis, with drug overdoses escalating exponentially in the past 25 years. Approximately 60,000 people died in the United States in 2016 from drug overdoses, and the numbers continue to climb.

Although tremendous advances have been made, our knowledge of the brain and how it functions is incomplete, as is an understanding of the molecular entities underlying neuropsychiatric disorders and the molecular targets through which drugs alter brain function. In addition, although many compounds have been developed with beneficial therapeutic effects for countless patients, many patients do not respond to any available medications, underscoring the need for further research and development.

Understanding the actions of drugs on the CNS and their rational use for the treatment of brain diseases requires knowledge of the organization and component parts of the brain. Most drugs interact with specific proteins at defined sites associated with specific neurotransmitter pathways. These interactions are responsible for the primary therapeutic actions of drugs as well as many of their unwanted side effects.

To induce CNS effects, drugs must obviously be able to reach their targets in the brain. Because the brain is protected from many harmful and foreign blood-borne substances by the blood-brain barrier (BBB), the entry of many drugs is restricted. Therefore it is important to understand the characteristics of drugs that enable them to enter the CNS. This chapter covers basic aspects of CNS function, with a focus on the cellular and molecular processes and neurotransmitters thought to underlie many CNS disorders. The mechanisms through which drugs act to alleviate the symptoms of these disorders are emphasized.

NEUROTRANSMISSION IN THE CENTRAL NERVOUS SYSTEM

Cells in the Central Nervous System: Neurons and Glia

The CNS is composed of two predominant cell types, neurons and glia, each of which has morphologically and functionally diverse subclasses. For many years, it was believed that glial cells functioned primarily as "support" cells and outnumbered neurons by 10:1, with 1 trillion glia and 100 billion neurons in the human brain. We know now, however, that glial cells express many proteins and play a key role in neurotransmission, depending on specific glial cell type, and that the number of glial cells varies dramatically across brain regions and

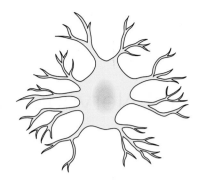

Astrocyte

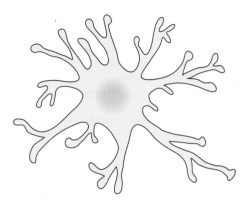

Oligodendrocyte

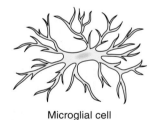

Microglial cell

FIG. 13.1 Types of Glia in the CNS.

may actually be less than the number of neurons, with recent estimates of 40–130 billion glia in the human brain.

There are three types of glial cells: astrocytes, oligodendrocytes, and microglia (Fig. 13.1). **Astrocytes** physically separate neurons and multineuronal pathways, assist in repairing nerve injury, and modulate the metabolic and ionic microenvironment. These cells also express ion channels and neurotransmitter transport proteins and play an active role in modulating synaptic function. **Oligodendrocytes** form the myelin sheath around axons and play a critical role in maintaining transmission as signals proceed down axons. Interestingly, polymorphisms in the genes encoding several myelin proteins have been identified in tissues from patients with both schizophrenia and bipolar disorder and may contribute to the underlying etiology of these disorders. **Microglia** proliferate after injury or degeneration, move to sites of injury, and transform into large macrophages (phagocytes) to remove cellular debris. These antigen-presenting cells

with innate immune function also appear to play a role in endocrine development.

Neurons are the major cells involved in intercellular communication because of their ability to conduct impulses and transmit information. They are structurally different from other cells, with four distinct features (Fig. 13.2, top):

- **Dendrites**, characterized by multiple spiny projections, that contain numerous neurotransmitter receptors to receive information, as well as sites for neurotransmitter release;
- A **perikaryon** (cell body or soma) containing the nucleus, rough endoplasmic reticulum, ribosomes, Golgi apparatus, mitochondria, lysosomes, and cytoskeletal elements responsible for protein synthesis, cell maintenance, and information integration, as well as neurotransmitter receptors to receive information;
- An **axon** containing neurofilaments and microtubules responsible for the **axonal transport** of proteins and peptides, organelles, and cytoskeletal components, as well as ion channels and receptors for propagating impulses to nerve terminals. The axon maintains ionic concentrations of Na^+ and K^+ to ensure a transmembrane potential of −65 mV. In response to an appropriate stimulus, ion channels open and allow Na^+ influx, causing depolarization toward the Na^+ equilibrium potential (+30 mV). This causes opening of neighboring channels, resulting in unidirectional propagation of the action potential. When it reaches the nerve terminal, depolarization causes release of chemical messengers to transmit information to nearby cells; and
- A **nerve terminal** with vesicles containing neurotransmitters and cellular components and proteins (enzymes) that support classical neurotransmitter synthesis and release, autoreceptors for feedback regulation, and transport proteins to regulate neurotransmitter reuptake and storage. They may also contain proteolytic enzymes important in the final processing of peptide neurotransmitters.

Neurons are often shaped according to their function. **Unipolar** or pseudounipolar neurons have a single axon, which bifurcates close to the cell body, with one end typically extending centrally and the other peripherally (Fig. 13.2, bottom). Unipolar neurons tend to serve sensory functions. **Bipolar** neurons have two extensions and are associated with the retina, vestibular cochlear system, and olfactory epithelium; they are commonly interneurons. Finally, **multipolar** neurons have many processes, but only one axon extending from the cell body. Multipolar neurons are the most numerous types of neurons in the CNS and represent a heterogeneous group, including spinal motor, pyramidal, and Purkinje neurons.

Neurons may also be classified by the neurotransmitter they release and the response they produce. For example, neurons that release γ-aminobutyric acid (GABA) generally hyperpolarize postsynaptic cells; thus GABAergic neurons are generally inhibitory. In contrast, neurons that release glutamate (Glu) depolarize postsynaptic cells and are excitatory.

The Synapse

The effective transfer and integration of information in the CNS requires passage of information between neurons or other target cells. The nerve terminal is usually separated from adjacent cells by a gap of 20 nm or more; therefore signals must cross this gap. This is accomplished by specialized areas of communication, referred to as **synapses**. The synapse is the junction between a nerve terminal and a postsynaptic specialization on an adjacent cell where information is received.

Most neurotransmission involves communication between nerve terminals and dendrites or perikarya on the postsynaptic cell, called **axodendritic** or **axosomatic synapses**, respectively. However, other areas of the neuron may also be involved in both sending and receiving

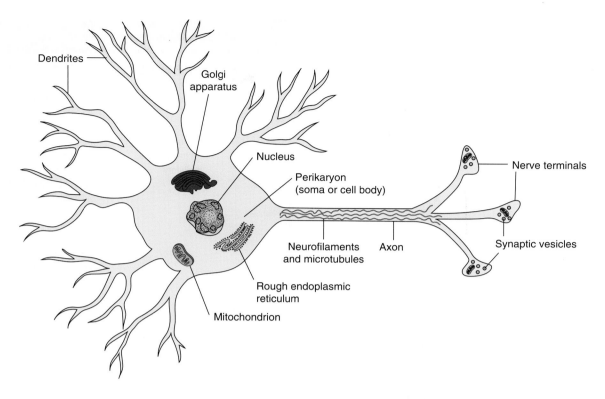

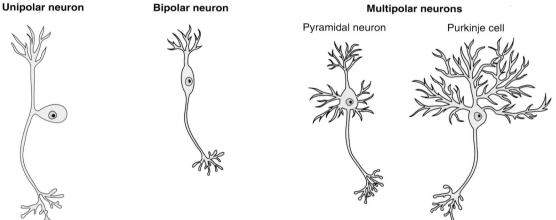

FIG. 13.2 Structural Components and Types of Nerve Cells.

information. Neurotransmitter receptors are often spread diffusely over the dendrites, perikarya, and nerve terminals but are also commonly found on glial cells, where they likely serve a functional role. In addition, transmitters can be stored in and released from dendrites. Thus transmitters released from nerve terminals may interact with receptors on other axons at axoaxonic synapses, while transmitters released from dendrites can interact with receptors on either "postsynaptic" dendrites or perikarya, referred to as dendrodendritic or dendrosomatic synapses, respectively (Fig. 13.3A).

In addition, released neurotransmitters may diffuse from the synapse to act at receptors in extrasynaptic regions or on other neurons or glia distant from the site of release. This process is referred to as volume transmission (Fig. 13.3B). Although the significance of volume transmission is not well understood, it may play an important role in the actions of neurotransmitters in brain regions where primary inactivation mechanisms are absent or dysfunctional.

The Life Cycle of Neurotransmitters

Neurotransmitters are any chemical messengers released from neurons. They represent a highly diverse group of compounds including amines, amino acids, peptides, purines, gases, and growth factors (Table 13.1). The amine neurotransmitters include acetylcholine (ACh), dopamine (DA), norepinephrine (NE), epinephrine (Epi), serotonin (5-HT), and histamine (Hist); the amino acid neurotransmitters include the excitatory compounds Glu and aspartate (Asp) and the inhibitory compounds GABA and glycine. The amine and amino acid neurotransmitters are synthesized in nerve terminals and are generally stored in and released from small vesicles (Fig. 13.4). Following interaction with their postsynaptic receptors, these molecules are inactivated by reuptake into nerve terminals or astrocytes, or in the case of ACh, by the enzyme acetylcholinesterase (AChE).

In contrast to the amine neurotransmitters, the peptide neurotransmitters, which are 3–30 amino acids in length, are synthesized and

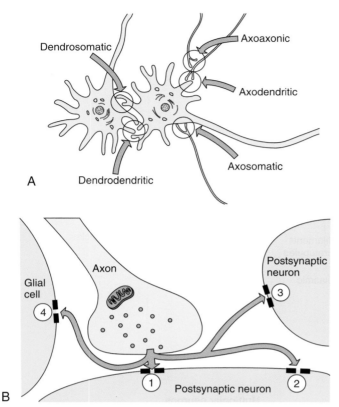

FIG. 13.3 Types of Synaptic Connections and Neurotransmission in the CNS. (A) Transmitters released from nerve terminals can interact with receptors on other axons via axoaxonic synapses, dendrites via classical axodendritic synapses, or the soma via axosomatic synapses. In addition, transmitters released from dendrites can interact with receptors on dendrites or the soma of other neurons, termed *dendrodendritic* and *dendrosomatic* synapses, respectively. (B) Transmitter released from nerve terminals can interact with receptors on an adjacent postsynaptic neuron at a site close to the release site (1) or at an extrajunctional site (2). Transmitter can also interact with receptors on a postsynaptic neuron distant to the release site (3) or on a distant glial cell (4).

TABLE 13.1	Representative Neurotransmitters in the CNS	
Category	**Subcategory**	**Neurotransmitter**
Primary amines	Quaternary amines	Acetylcholine
	Catecholamines	Dopamine, norepinephrine, epinephrine
	Indoleamines and related compounds	Serotonin, histamine
Amino acids	Excitatory	Glutamate, aspartate
	Inhibitory	γ-Aminobutyric acid, glycine
Purines		Adenosine triphosphate, adenosine
Peptides		Cholecystokinin, dynorphin, β-endorphin, enkephalins, neuropeptide Y, neurotensin, somatostatin, substance P, vasoactive intestinal peptide, vasopressin
Gases		Nitric oxide, carbon monoxide
Growth factors		Brain-derived neurotrophic factor, nerve growth factor

processed from larger precursors by proteolytic enzymes in neuronal perikarya, where they are also packaged into large vesicles that are transported down the axon to the nerve terminal. These compounds are inactivated by enzymes or diffusion and include somatostatin, substance P, and vasoactive intestinal peptide, to name a few.

Often, these peptides are coreleased with amine neurotransmitters and interact with specific postsynaptic receptors. For many years, it was assumed that a single neuron synthesized and released only *one* neurotransmitter. We know now that many classical neurotransmitters coexist with peptide neurotransmitters in neurons, and both are released in response to depolarization. ACh coexists with enkephalin, vasoactive intestinal peptide, and substance P, whereas DA coexists with cholecystokinin and enkephalin. In some cases, both substances cause physiological effects on postsynaptic cells, suggesting the possibility of multiple signals carrying independent, complementary, or mutually reinforcing messages.

The **purines** adenosine and ATP function as both neurotransmitters and neuromodulators in the CNS. These compounds are synthesized in nerve terminals and stored in large vesicles, either alone or with an amine neurotransmitter such as NE, from which they are released and interact with purinoceptors. ATP is catabolized to adenosine, which

can either be further metabolized or taken back up into the nerve terminal much like the amine neurotransmitters.

The **gas neurotransmitters** include **nitric oxide (NO)** and **carbon monoxide (CO)**. These compounds are not stored in vesicles or nerve terminals but rather are synthesized and released upon demand. NO is synthesized from arginine via the enzyme nitric oxide synthase (NOS), while CO is generated from the conversion of heme to biliverdin and catalyzed by heme oxygenase (HO). Upon their synthesis and release, the gases complex the iron of guanylyl cyclase to increase cGMP, activating cGMP-dependent protein kinases and leading to the phosphorylation of several substrates.

Several neurotrophic factors, including **brain-derived neurotrophic factor (BDNF)** and **nerve growth factor (NGF)**, are now recognized as both neurotransmitters and growth factors. These proteins are stored in vesicles and released constitutively from both perikarya and dendrites. Their signaling is mediated by interactions with both high- and low-affinity neurotropin receptors and is involved with activating major pathways affecting cell survival.

Because many centrally acting drugs act by altering the synthesis, storage, release, or inactivation of specific neurotransmitters, it is critical to understand these processes. For neurons to fire rapidly and repetitively, they must maintain sufficient supplies of neurotransmitter. The classical neurotransmitters are synthesized locally in the nerve terminal and have complex mechanisms for regulating this process. Synthesis is usually controlled by either the amount and activity of synthetic enzymes or the availability of substrates and cofactors. For example, ACh synthesis is regulated primarily by substrate availability, whereas the synthesis of DA, NE, and Epi is regulated primarily by the activity of the synthetic enzyme tyrosine hydroxylase (Chapter 6); 5-HT synthesis is regulated similarly by the enzyme.

After synthesis, neurotransmitters are concentrated in vesicles by carrier proteins through an energy-dependent process (see Fig. 13.4). This mechanism transports neurotransmitters into vesicles at concentrations 10–100 times higher than in the cytoplasm. Several families of **vesicular transporters** have been identified, including ones that transport monoamines (VMATs), ACh (VAChT), GABA (VGAT), and Glu (VGLUTs). Vesicular storage protects neurotransmitters from

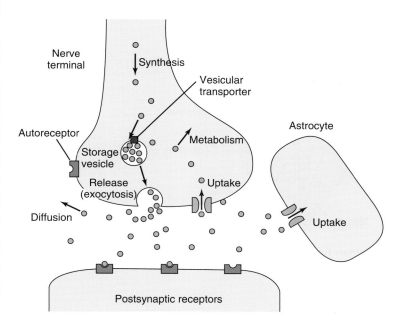

FIG. 13.4 Life Cycle of a Neurotransmitter.

catabolism by intracellular enzymes and maintains a ready supply of neurotransmitters for release.

The arrival of an action potential causes the nerve terminal membrane to depolarize, resulting in release of neurotransmitter into the synaptic cleft. This process is initiated by opening voltage-dependent Ca^{++} channels in the membrane, enabling Ca^{++} to enter the cell. Ca^{++} influx leads to a complex sequence of events resulting in translocation and fusion of vesicles with the plasma membrane, releasing their contents into the synaptic cleft by exocytosis (Fig. 13.4).

After receptor activation, neurotransmitters must be inactivated to terminate their actions and allow for further information transfer. Rapid enzymatic hydrolysis of ACh terminates its action, while the actions of biogenic amines are terminated primarily by reuptake into presynaptic terminals by specific energy-dependent transporters (Chapter 6). The amino acid neurotransmitters are taken up primarily by astrocytes, and recent data suggest that biogenic amines may also be taken up by these cells, a process that may play an important role in some disease states and in the action of the antidepressant agents. Inside the terminal, neurotransmitters can be repackaged into vesicles and rereleased. All inactivation processes are important targets for drug action.

The action of any transmitter may also be terminated by simple diffusion or nonspecific (energy-independent) absorption into surrounding tissues. These processes are effective and more important in terminating the actions of peptides and gaseous neurotransmitters than in inactivating classical small molecule neurotransmitters.

Neurotransmitter Receptors

As discussed in Chapter 2, receptors are sensors by which cells detect incoming messages. Many different types of receptors can coexist on cells, including receptors for different transmitters and multiple subtypes for a single transmitter. The response of a particular neuron to a neurotransmitter depends as much on the types of receptors present as on the type of transmitter released. Because each transmitter can activate a receptor family composed of different receptor subtypes associated with distinct signal transduction mechanisms, a single transmitter may cause completely different effects on different cells (Chapter 2). The function of the neuron is to integrate these multiple messages, from a single transmitter or from multiple transmitters, to control the impulse activity of its own axon.

ORGANIZATION OF THE CENTRAL NERVOUS SYSTEM

An understanding of the effects and side effects of drugs affecting the CNS requires a basic understanding of CNS organization. This organization can be viewed from anatomical, functional, or chemical perspectives.

Gross Anatomical and Functional Organization

The gross anatomy of the brain includes the cerebrum or cerebral hemispheres, subcortical structures including the **thalamus** and **hypothalamus** (the diencephalon), the midbrain, and the hindbrain, composed of the **pons**, **medulla**, and **cerebellum** (Fig. 13.5). The cerebrum, or cerebral cortex, is the largest part of the human brain and is divided into apparently symmetrical left and right hemispheres, which have different functions. The right hemisphere is associated with creativity and the left with logic and reasoning. The cerebral cortex processes most sensory, motor, and associational information and integrates many somatic and vegetative functions.

The cerebral cortex contains four regions, the frontal, parietal, occipital, and temporal lobes (Fig. 13.6). The frontal lobe extends anterior from the central sulcus and contains the motor and prefrontal cortices. It is associated with higher cognitive functions and long-term memory storage; the posterior portion is the primary motor cortex and controls fine movements. The parietal lobe, between the occipital lobe and central sulcus, is associated with sensorimotor integration and processes information from touch, muscle stretch receptors, and joint receptors. This area contains the primary somatosensory cortex. The temporal lobe is located laterally in each hemisphere and is the primary cortical target for information originating in the ears and vestibular organs; it is involved in vision and language. The occipital lobe is located in the posterior cortex and is involved in visual processing. It is the main target for axons from thalamic nuclei that receive inputs from the visual pathways and contains the primary visual cortex.

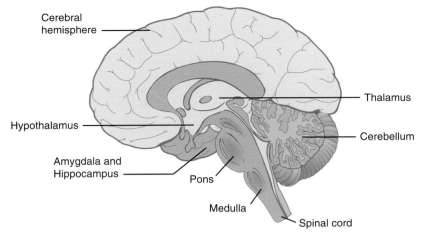

FIG. 13.5 Gross Anatomical Structures in the Human Brain. Shown is a sagittal section through the brain illustrating several major anatomical structures.

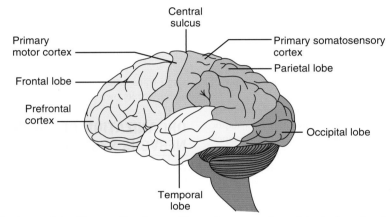

FIG. 13.6 Regions of the Human Cerebrum. Shown is a gross view of the brain noting the major lobes and cortical regions.

The thalamus and hypothalamus are part of the diencephalon. The thalamus has both sensory and motor functions. Sensory information enters the thalamus and is transmitted to the cortex. The hypothalamus is involved in homeostasis, emotion, thirst, hunger, circadian rhythms, and control of the autonomic nervous system. It also controls the pituitary gland. The limbic system, often referred to as the emotional brain, consists of several structures beneath the cerebral cortex that integrate emotional state with motor and visceral activities. The hippocampus is involved in learning and memory; the amygdala in memory, emotion, and fear; and the ventral tegmental area/nucleus accumbens septi in addiction.

The medulla, pons, and often midbrain are referred to as the brainstem and are involved in vision, hearing, and body movement. The medulla regulates vital functions such as breathing and heart rate, while the pons is involved in motor control and sensory analysis and is important in consciousness and sleep. The cerebellum is associated with the regulation and coordination of movement, posture, and balance. The cerebellum and brainstem relay information from the cerebral hemispheres and limbic system to the spinal cord for integration of essential reflexes. The spinal cord receives, sends, and integrates sensory and motor information.

Chemical Functional Anatomy

The effects of drugs are determined primarily by the types and activities of cells in which their molecular targets are located and the types of neural circuits in which those cells participate. Thus an understanding of the chemical organization of the brain is particularly useful in pharmacology. CNS diseases often affect neurons containing specific neurotransmitters, and drugs often activate or inhibit the synthesis, storage, release, or inactivation of these neurotransmitters. Many neurotransmitter systems arise from relatively small populations of neurons localized in discrete nuclei in the brain that project widely through the brain and spinal cord.

Dopaminergic Systems

Neurons synthesizing DA have their cell bodies primarily in two brain regions, the midbrain, containing the substantia nigra and adjacent ventral tegmental area, and the arcuate nucleus of the hypothalamus (Fig. 13.7). Nigrostriatal DA neurons project to the striatum (caudate nucleus and putamen) and are involved in the control of posture and movement; these neurons degenerate in Parkinson disease. The ventral tegmental neurons extend to the cortex and limbic system, referred to as the mesocortical and mesolimbic pathways, respectively, and are important for complex target-oriented behaviors, including psychotic behaviors. Those neurons projecting from the ventral tegmental area to the nucleus accumbens septi are believed to be involved in addiction. DA is also synthesized by much shorter neurons originating in the arcuate and periventricular nuclei of the hypothalamus that extend to the intermediate lobe of the pituitary and into the median eminence, known as the tuberoinfundibular pathway. These neurons regulate

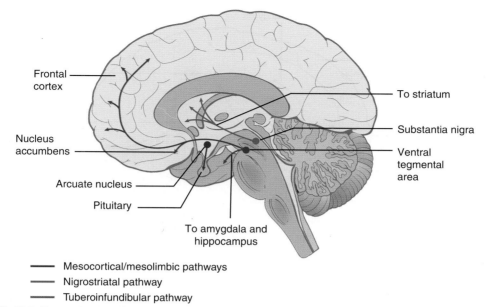

Mesocortical/mesolimbic pathways
Nigrostriatal pathway
Tuberoinfundibular pathway

FIG. 13.7 **Dopaminergic Systems in the Human Brain.** A sagittal section through the midline is shown, with the three major dopaminergic pathways of pharmacological importance noted.

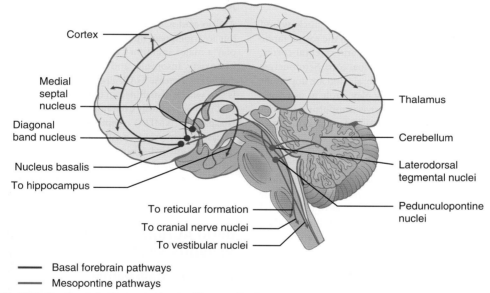

Basal forebrain pathways
Mesopontine pathways

FIG. 13.8 **Cholinergic Systems in the Human Brain.** A sagittal section through the midline is shown, with the two major cholinergic projections of pharmacological importance from the basal forebrain (medial septa nucleus, diagonal band nucleus, and nucleus basalis) and midbrain (laterodorsal tegmental and pedunculopontine nuclei) noted.

pituitary function and decrease prolactin secretion. Drugs used for the treatment of Parkinson disease (Chapter 15) stimulate these DA systems, whereas drugs used for the treatment of psychotic disorders, such as schizophrenia (Chapter 16), block them.

Cholinergic Systems

Three primary groups of cholinergic neurons are located in the brain: those originating in ventral areas of the forebrain (nucleus basalis and nuclei of the diagonal band and medial septum) and the pons (Fig. 13.8) and small interneurons in the striatum. Neurons from the **nucleus basalis** project to large areas of the cerebral cortex, while **septal and**

diagonal band neurons project largely to the hippocampus. These pathways are important in learning and memory and degenerate in Alzheimer disease. Thus treatment of this disorder involves the use of acetylcholinesterase (AChE) inhibitors in attempts to alleviate this cholinergic deficit (Chapter 14). Neurons originating in the pons project to the thalamus and basal forebrain and have descending pathways to the reticular formation, cerebellum, vestibular nuclei, and cranial nerve nuclei; they are involved in arousal and REM sleep. Finally, there are small cholinergic interneurons in the striatum that are inhibited by nigrostriatal DA neurons, forming the basis for the use of muscarinic receptor antagonists in treating Parkinson disease (Chapter 15).

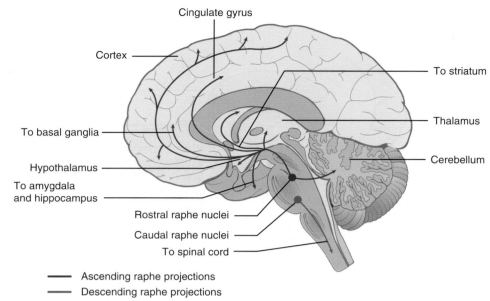

FIG. 13.9 Serotonergic Systems in the Human Brain. A sagittal section through the midline is shown, with the major serotonergic projections of pharmacological importance from the raphe nucleus noted.

Serotonergic Systems

Serotonergic neurons originate primarily in the raphe nucleus and have widespread projections (Fig. 13.9). Neurons from the rostral raphe project to the limbic system, thalamus, striatum, and cerebral cortex, whereas caudal raphe neurons descend to the spinal cord. Serotonergic pathways have broad influences throughout the brain and are important for sensory processing and homeostasis. They play a role in psychotic behaviors (Chapter 16), depression and obsessive-compulsive disorder (Chapter 17), and eating behavior (Chapter 20) and are major targets for drugs used to treat these diseases.

Noradrenergic Systems

Neurons synthesizing NE have their cell bodies primarily in the locus coeruleus and lateral tegmental region in the pons (Fig. 13.10). The locus coeruleus neurons project anteriorly to large areas of the cerebral cortex, thalamus, hypothalamus, and olfactory bulb, with descending projections to the spinal cord. The lateral tegmental neurons have ascending pathways to the limbic system and descending projections to the cerebellum and spinal cord, with fibers passing in the ventrolateral column. Noradrenergic pathways are involved in controlling responses to external sensory and motor stimuli, arousal and attention, and learning and memory and may be important in major depression (Chapter 17). Midbrain neurons also play important roles in the control of autonomic and neuroendocrine function.

Histaminergic Systems

All known histaminergic neurons originate in magnocellular neurons in the posterior hypothalamus, referred to as the tuberomammillary nucleus (Fig. 13.11). These neurons form long ascending connections to many telencephalic areas, including all areas of the cerebral cortex, the limbic system, caudate putamen, nucleus accumbens septi, and globus pallidus. Also, long descending neurons project to mesencephalic and brainstem structures, including cranial nerve nuclei, the substantia nigra, locus coeruleus, mesopontine tegmentum, dorsal raphe, cerebellum, and spinal cord. Histaminergic neurons play a major role in arousal, in coupling neuronal activity with cerebral metabolism, and in neuroendocrine regulation.

Amino Acid Neurotransmitter Systems

Amino acid neurotransmitters are not restricted to specific pathways but are widespread throughout the brain and spinal cord. GABA neurons play a major inhibitory role in most brain regions and are important in anxiety, insomnia, and seizure disorders. Drugs for treating these disorders increase GABAergic activity (Chapters 17, 19, and 21). Glu is also widely distributed in the brain and functions opposite to GABA; that is, it is primarily excitatory. An antagonist of glutamate N-methyl-D-aspartate (NMDA) receptors is used for the treatment of Alzheimer disease (Chapter 14), while an antagonist of glutamate α-amino-3-hydroxy-5-methyl-4-isoxazole-propionic acid (AMPA) receptors is used for the treatment of seizures (Chapter 21).

A summary of major neurotransmitter pathways and the specific brain disorders in which they play important roles is presented in Table 13.2.

DRUG ACTION IN THE CENTRAL NERVOUS SYSTEM

The Blood-Brain Barrier

As mentioned, drugs acting on the brain must be able to gain access to their targets. Because of its unique importance, the brain is "protected" by a specialized system of capillary endothelial cells known as the BBB. Unlike peripheral capillaries that allow relatively free exchange of substances between cells, the BBB limits transport through both physical (tight junctions) and metabolic (enzymes) barriers (Chapter 3, Fig. 3.6). The primary BBB is formed by firmly connected endothelial cells with tight junctions lining cerebral capillaries. The secondary BBB surrounds the cerebral capillaries and is composed of glial cells.

There are several areas of the brain where the BBB is relatively weak, allowing substances to cross. These circumventricular organs include the pineal gland, area postrema, subfornical organ, vascular organ of the lamina terminalis, and median eminence.

Factors that influence the ability of drugs to cross the BBB include size, flexibility and molecular conformation, lipophilicity and charge, enzymatic stability, affinity for transport carriers, and plasma protein binding. In general, large polar molecules do not pass easily through

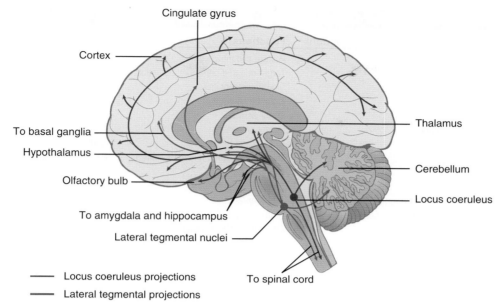

FIG. 13.10 **Noradrenergic Systems in the Human Brain.** A sagittal section through the midline is shown, with the major noradrenergic projections of pharmacological importance from the lateral tegmental nuclei and locus coeruleus noted.

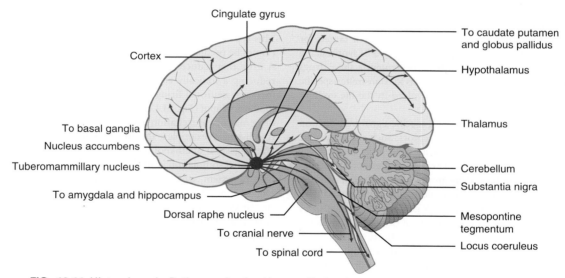

FIG. 13.11 **Histaminergic Pathways in the Human Brain.** A sagittal section through the midline is shown, with the major histaminergic projections of pharmacological importance from the tuberomammillary nucleus noted.

the BBB, whereas small, lipid-soluble molecules, such as barbiturates, cross easily. Most charged molecules cross slowly, if at all. It is clear that the BBB is the rate-limiting factor for drug entry into the CNS.

The BBB is not formed fully at birth, and drugs that may have restricted access in the adult may enter the newborn brain readily. Similarly, the BBB can be compromised in conditions such as hypertension, inflammation, trauma, and infection. Exposure to microwaves or radiation has also been reported to open the BBB.

Although the action of many CNS-active drugs is based on their ability to cross the BBB, it may also be advantageous for a drug to be restricted from entering the brain. For example, L-DOPA, used for the treatment of Parkinson disease, must enter the brain to be effective. When administered alone, only 1%–3% of the dose reaches the brain;

the rest is metabolized by plasma DOPA decarboxylase to DA, which cannot cross the BBB. Thus L-DOPA is administered in combination with carbidopa, which inhibits DOPA decarboxylase in the plasma and does not itself cross the BBB, thereby increasing the amount of L-DOPA available in the circulation to enter the brain (Chapter 15).

Target Molecules

Most centrally acting drugs produce their effects by modifying cellular and molecular events involved in synaptic transmission. The distribution of these targets determines which cells are affected by a particular drug and is the primary determinant of the specificity of drug action. Drugs acting on the CNS can be classified into several major groups, based on the distribution of their specific target molecules. Drugs that act on

TABLE 13.2   Neurotransmitter Pathways and Associated Disorders

Neurotransmitter	Associated Pathways/Projections	Functions	Associated Disorders
DA	Nigrostriatal	Posture and movement	Parkinson disease
	Mesolimbic/mesocortical	Target-oriented behaviors, addiction, reinforcement	Psychoses, drug abuse
	Tuberoinfundibular	Prolactin secretion	Hyperprolactinemia/hypoprolactinemia
ACh	Intrastriatal	Motor activity	Parkinson disease
	Basal forebrain	Learning/memory	Alzheimer disease
	Mesopontine	Arousal and REM sleep	Narcolepsy (?)
5-HT	Raphe-telencephalic and diencephalic	Broad homeostatic functions, sensory processing	Depression/suicide, psychoses, obsessive compulsive disorder, anxiety
NE	Locus coeruleus	Learning/memory	Depression
	Midbrain reticular formation	Attention/arousal	Narcolepsy
Hist	Tuberomammillary projections	Arousal, cerebral metabolism	Insomnia (?)
GABA	Widespread	Anxiolytic, anticonvulsant	Anxiety, seizures
Glu	Widespread	Proconvulsant, synaptic plasticity (LTP)	Seizures, Alzheimer and Parkinson diseases (?)

molecules expressed by all types of cells (DNA, lipids, and structural proteins) have "general" actions. Other drugs act on molecules that are expressed specifically in neurons and not on other cell types. These drugs are neuron specific and interact with the transporters and channels that maintain the electrical properties of neurons.

Many drugs interact specifically with the macromolecules involved in the synthesis, storage, release, receptor interaction, and inactivation processes associated with particular neurotransmitters. The targets for these transmitter-specific drugs are expressed only by cells synthesizing or responding to specific neurotransmitters; consequently, these drugs have more discrete and limited actions. The targets for transmitter-specific drugs can be any of the macromolecules involved in the life cycle of specific transmitter molecules.

Last, some drugs mimic or interfere with specific signal transduction systems shared by a variety of different receptors. Such signal-specific drugs affect responses to activation of various receptors that use the same pathway for initiating signals. The transmitter-specific drugs represent the largest class of these drug groups used in clinical practice. Because the distribution of their target molecules is more limited than that of the general, neuron-specific, or even signal-specific classes, these compounds often result in a greater specificity of drug action, reflected clinically by a lower incidence of unwanted side effects.

It is important to remember that all drugs have multiple actions. No drug causes only a single effect because few, if any, drugs bind to only a single target. At higher concentrations, most drugs can interact with a wide variety of molecules, often resulting in cellular alterations. Some drugs have potent actions on so many different processes in the CNS that it is difficult to identify their primary targets. Although some drugs may cause their therapeutic effects by combinations of specific actions, others may exert their primary effects through their interaction with a single cellular target. The window of selectivity of any particular drug will dramatically influence its incidence of unwanted side effects.

Levels of Neuronal Activity

Drug actions on neuronal systems in the CNS are largely dependent on the level of tonic activity. In the absence of synaptic input, neurons can exist in either of two states. They can be relatively quiescent by maintaining a constant and uniform hyperpolarization of their cell membrane, or they can initiate action potentials at uniform intervals by spontaneous graded depolarizations. A system with intrinsic spontaneous activity has different characteristics than those of a quiescent system. Although both can be activated, only a spontaneously active system

can be inhibited. Drugs that inhibit neuronal function (CNS depressants) may have quite different effects depending on the activity of the neuronal system involved. Systems with tonic activity (either intrinsic or externally driven) are inhibited by CNS depressants, whereas quiescent systems are relatively unaffected.

The activity of a tonically active neural network can be increased or decreased by excitatory or inhibitory control systems, respectively. This type of bidirectional regulation implies that the effect of a drug cannot be predicted solely on the basis of its effect on isolated neurons. A drug that reduces neuronal firing can activate a neural system by reducing a tonically active inhibitory input. Conversely, a drug that increases neuronal firing can inhibit a neural system by activating an inhibitory input (Fig. 13.12). Thus in some circumstances, a "depressant" drug may cause excitation, and a "stimulant" drug may cause sedation. A well-known example is the stimulant phase that is observed frequently after ingestion of ethanol (Chapter 23), a general neuronal depressant. The initial stimulation is attributable to the depression of an inhibitory control system, which occurs only at low concentrations of ethanol. Higher concentrations cause a uniform depression of nerve activity. A similar stage of excitement can be observed during induction of general anesthesia, which is also caused by the removal of tonically active inhibitory control systems (Chapter 26).

Normal physiological variations in neuronal activity can also alter the effects of centrally acting drugs. For example, anesthetics are generally less effective in hyperexcitable patients, and stimulants are less effective in more sedate patients. This is attributable to the presence of varying levels of excitatory and inhibitory control systems, which alter sensitivity to drugs. Other stimulant and depressant drugs administered concurrently also alter responses to centrally acting drugs. Depressants are generally additive with other depressants, and stimulants are additive with stimulants. For example, ethanol potentiates the depression caused by barbiturates, and the result can be fatal. However, the interactions between stimulant and depressant drugs are more variable. Stimulant drugs usually antagonize the effects of depressant drugs, and vice versa. Because such antagonism is caused by activating or inhibiting competing control systems and not by neutralizing the effect of the drugs on their target molecules, concurrently administered stimulants and depressants typically do not completely cancel the effects of each other.

Adaptive Responses

Adaptive mechanisms exist in all cells to control signaling. Adaptation can occur at several levels, predominantly at the receptors themselves.

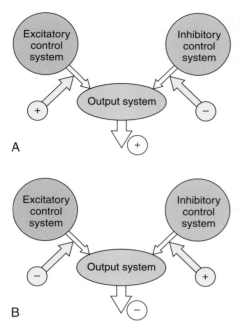

FIG. 13.12 Hierarchical Control Systems in the CNS. (A) Neuronal output can be increased by increasing tonic excitatory control or decreasing tonic inhibitory control. (B) Output can be reduced by decreasing tonic excitatory control or increasing tonic inhibitory control.

Two mechanisms are involved, sensitization and desensitization. As discussed in Chapter 2, sensitization is a process whereby a cell becomes more responsive to a given concentration of compound, whereas desensitization is a process whereby a cell becomes less responsive.

Receptor sensitization and desensitization play a major role in the action of drugs in the CNS in terms of both therapeutic effects and side effects.

Chronic activation of receptors, as occurs typically after long-term agonist administration, decreases the density of receptors in the postsynaptic cell membrane, whereas sustained decreases in synaptic activation, as a result of long-term antagonist administration, increases receptor density (Chapter 2, Fig. 2.17). Such changes occur slowly and are only slowly reversible because increasing receptor density requires synthesis of new receptors, and reversing such an increase requires degrading these new receptors. Thus changing receptor density usually represents a long-term (days to weeks) adaptive response to changes in synaptic input.

Postsynaptic cells can also regulate the efficiency with which receptor activation is coupled to changes in cell physiology. These changes usually occur at the level of the coupling of a receptor to channel opening or second messenger production and can be extremely rapid in onset. Often, a change in coupling efficiency results from increases or decreases in covalent modifications of the receptors, G-proteins, channels, or enzymes responsible for signal transduction (Chapter 2).

Overall, it is clear that determining the mechanisms by which drugs affect CNS function is challenging. Clearly, the mechanisms by which psychoactive drugs exert their effects at a molecular level are only beginning to be understood. Manipulating brain chemistry and physiology with specific drugs and observing the effects on integrated behavioral parameters are two of the few approaches available currently for relating the function of brain cells with complex integrated behaviors. Such information will be useful in the future for the rational design of drugs for the treatment of various CNS diseases. It will also be satisfying to understand more about the genesis and control of human thought and emotion. Although understanding the actions of drugs on the CNS poses a great challenge, it also promises great rewards.

SELF-ASSESSMENT QUESTIONS

1. The mechanism of action of which of the following neurotransmitters is terminated by enzymatic degradation?
   A. ACh.
   B. NE.
   C. DA.
   D. Serotonin.
   E. Epi.
2. Which of the following is true concerning the synthesis and storage of biogenic amine neurotransmitters?
   A. They are stored in and released from vesicles in nerve terminals.
   B. They are synthesized in perikarya.
   C. Their concentration in the presynaptic cytosol is greater than in the vesicles.
   D. They are passively transported into vesicles.
   E. They are transported down axons by anterograde transport.
3. Which of the following represents an adaptive response to the long-term use of agonists?
   A. Increased synthesis of receptors.
   B. Decreased degradation of receptors.
   C. Decreased density of postsynaptic receptors.
   D. Increased density of postsynaptic receptors.
   E. None of the above.

4. Which types of neurons originate primarily in the substantia nigra and hypothalamus?
   A. Noradrenergic.
   B. Serotoninergic.
   C. Dopaminergic.
   D. GABAergic.
   E. Histaminergic.
5. What characteristics increase the likelihood that a drug will penetrate the blood-brain barrier and enter the CNS?
   A. Negative charge.
   B. High degree of lipophilicity.
   C. High molecular weight.
   D. Positive charge.
   E. High degree of binding to plasma proteins.
6. Why does ethanol, a CNS depressant, cause an initial phase of excitation following ingestion?
   A. It activates excitatory glutamate receptors.
   B. It inhibits GABAergic inhibition.
   C. It reduces activity of a tonically active inhibitory system.
   D. It blocks serotonin reuptake.
   E. It is metabolized to aspartate, an excitatory compound.

FURTHER READING

Fuxe K, Borroto-Escuela DO. Volume transmission and receptor-receptor interactions in heteroreceptor complexes: understanding the role of new concepts for brain communication. *Neural Regen Res.* 2016;11:1220–1223.

von Bartheld CS, Bahney J, Herculano-Houzel S. The search for true numbers of neurons and glial cells in the human brain: a review of 150 years of cell counting. *J Comp Neurol.* 2016;524:3865–3895.

WEBSITES

http://www.brainfacts.org/

This is a public information website sponsored by several global nonprofit organizations dedicated to advancing research on the brain and is a valuable resource for everything about the brain.

Drug Therapy for Alzheimer Disease and Other Cognitive Disorders/Dementias

Michael Jaffee, Meredith Wicklund, Erin Foff, and Steven T. DeKosky

MAJOR DRUG CLASSES

Acetylcholinesterase inhibitors
NMDA receptor antagonists

ABBREVIATIONS

Aβ	Beta amyloid
ACh	Acetylcholine
AChE	Acetylcholinesterase
AChEI	Acetylcholinesterase inhibitor
AD	Alzheimer disease
APP	Amyloid precursor protein
BuChE	Butyrylcholinesterase or cholinesterase
DLB	Dementia with Lewy bodies
MCI	Mild cognitive impairment
NMDA	*N*-Methyl-D-aspartate

THERAPEUTIC OVERVIEW

Alzheimer disease (AD) is the most common cause of dementia in the elderly and is characterized by both behavioral and pathological alterations. AD progresses in three stages, from an early preclinical stage with no apparent cognitive alterations, to a middle stage characterized by mild cognitive impairment (MCI), to the final stage of dementia, with impaired judgment and memory that disrupts daily living.

AD results from the widespread degeneration of synapses and neurons in the cerebral cortex and hippocampus, as well as in some subcortical structures. The defining pathological characteristics of AD are the presence of extracellular senile/amyloid plaques and intracellular neurofibrillary tangles. The plaques in the AD brain consist of an amyloid core surrounded by dystrophic (swollen, distorted) neurites and activated glia secreting a number of inflammatory mediators. The amyloid core consists of aggregates of a polymerized 40– to 42–amino acid peptide termed beta amyloid (Aβ) that is an alternate processing product of the transmembrane amyloid precursor protein (APP) and several accessory proteins. The neurofibrillary tangles are intracellular filaments composed of the microtubule associated protein tau, which is highly phosphorylated at multiple sites.

AD may be early onset, occurring prior to 65 years of age, or may occur later in life. The former is rare and may be linked to mutations in the genes coding for APP or presenilins, which are proteins involved in APP processing. The latter, or more common form of AD, is referred to as sporadic AD, and approximately 50% of individuals with sporadic AD also exhibit a genetic link. In particular, studies indicate that the risk of developing sporadic AD is more than threefold higher in individuals carrying the ε4 allele of the *APOE* gene, which encodes the lipid carrier protein, apolipoprotein E (apo E). These individuals may also exhibit a different response to drug therapy than those who do not express this allele.

Pathophysiology

Though controversial, the production and accumulation of amyloid plaques appears to be the critical event in the initiation and pathogenesis of AD and occurs when the patient is still cognitively normal. Neurofibrillary tangles more closely relate to cognitive symptoms than does plaque formation. However, the most direct correlation of clinical symptoms is neurodegeneration, which manifests as synaptic and neuronal loss, atrophy, and gliosis.

Neurotoxic Aβ, which aggregates into oligomers and then plaques, is formed from the proteolytic degradation of APP (Fig. 14.1). APP is a transmembrane protein that can undergo nonamyloidogenic (does not form amyloid plaques) or amyloidogenic processing. For the former, APP is first cleaved in its extracellular domain by either α-secretase or β-secretase. Products of α-secretase cleavage are nonamyloidogenic, whereas the transmembrane peptide remaining from β-secretase cleavage can be further degraded by γ-secretase to form Aβ, leading to plaque formation.

Coincident to the synaptic and neuronal loss in AD is the deterioration of several neurotransmitter systems. AD results in a profound loss of cholinergic activity due to the loss of acetylcholine (ACh) projections from the nucleus basalis of Meynert, located in the basal forebrain, to the hippocampus and cerebral cortex (Chapter 13). Thus there is a marked loss of the synthetic enzyme choline acetyltransferase in the areas innervated by these neurons. The intrinsic striatal cholinergic system and muscarinic cholinergic receptors remain largely intact in AD. Because central cholinergic neurotransmission is critical for attention, learning, and memory, loss of these neurons leads to cognitive impairment.

The glutamatergic system has also been implicated in AD. *N*-Methyl-D-aspartate (NMDA) glutamate receptors, which are ligand-gated ion channels, are critical to learning and memory and neural plasticity in the brain. The excessive opening of these channels has been shown to be associated with excitotoxicity in neurons, and it has been hypothesized that increased glutamatergic activity mediated by NMDA receptors may contribute to the neurodegeneration in AD.

Thus current treatment strategies for AD target cholinergic and glutamatergic neurotransmission in the brain. Strategies to increase cholinergic transmission involve the use of the acetylcholinesterase (AChE) inhibitors (AChEIs) donepezil, galantamine, and rivastigmine, while inhibition of the excitotoxic effects of glutamate may be achieved by the NMDA receptor antagonist memantine. A summary of the cognitive and pathological changes in AD and drug treatment are presented in the Therapeutic Overview Box.

THERAPEUTIC OVERVIEW

Alzheimer Disease
Behavioral Alterations
    memory loss that disrupts daily living activities
    judgmental alterations and inability to plan or solve problems
    difficulty completing familiar tasks
    confusion with place or time
    inability to recognize visual objects or relationships
    problems with writing or speaking
    misplacing objects
    social withdrawal
    mood and personality changes
Pathology
    degeneration of basal forebrain cholinergic neurons
    presence of amyloid plaques and neurofibrillary tangles
    neuron and synapse loss in cerebral cortex and hippocampus
Treatment
    AChE inhibitors
    NMDA receptor antagonists

MECHANISMS OF ACTION

AChE Inhibitors

Following the release of ACh from nerve terminals and receptor interactions, the action of this neurotransmitter at cholinergic synapses is terminated by rapid hydrolysis by the enzyme AChE (Chapters 6 and 7). Thus drugs for the treatment of AD include the AChEIs that prevent the hydrolysis of ACh, thereby prolonging the duration of action of neurotransmitter released from remaining cholinergic terminals (Chapter 7). These drugs include donepezil, galantamine, and rivastigmine; their structures are shown in Fig. 14.2.

These drugs are all reversible AChEIs that cross the blood-brain barrier. Donepezil and galantamine are specific for AChE, whereas rivastigmine inhibits both AChE and butyrylcholinesterase (BuChE). In addition, galantamine is a positive allosteric modulator at several types of neuronal nicotinic ACh receptors that enhance ACh release.

Because the AChEIs inhibit the catabolism of ACh released from nerve terminals, their effects are more pronounced on active than on quiescent cholinergic neurons. This state dependency helps retain the spatial and temporal patterning of cholinergic activity in the brain, unlike directly acting receptor agonists, which would tonically activate all receptors, contributing to adverse side effects.

NMDA Receptor Antagonists

Memantine is an uncompetitive, low-affinity, voltage-dependent NMDA receptor antagonist that binds to the open state of the glutamate NMDA receptor to inhibit Ca^{2+} influx through this channel. It is hypothesized that this action prevents tonic activation while still permitting opening of the channel during periods of elevated activity critical for memory formation. In addition to its actions at the NMDA receptor, memantine also noncompetitively antagonizes serotonin type 3 and neuronal nicotinic α7–containing receptors and has agonist activity at dopamine type 2 receptors, perhaps contributing to its side effect profile.

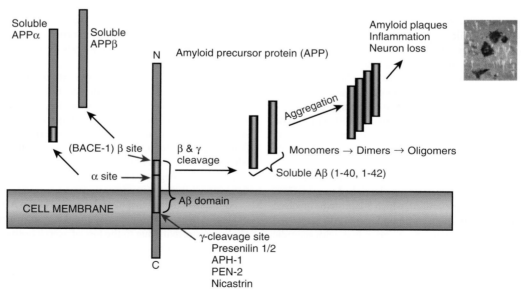

FIG. 14.1 Processing of Amyloid Precursor Protein (APP). The extracellular domain of APP is a substrate for both α-secretase and β-secretase. The proteolytic degradation of APP by α-secretase results in the formation of soluble APP, which is nonamyloidogenic. In contrast, the action of β-secretase yields a shorter soluble APP, with a membrane residue that can be cleaved within the transmembrane domain by γ-secretase to yield the 1-40 or 1-42 soluble Aβ. These proteins may fold and aggregate, forming sticky oligomers that associate with other proteins to form a plaque, which is neurotoxic. APH-1, Anterior pharynx defective -1; PEN-2, presenilin enhancer-2; BACE-1, β-site amyloid precursor protein cleaving enzyme 1.

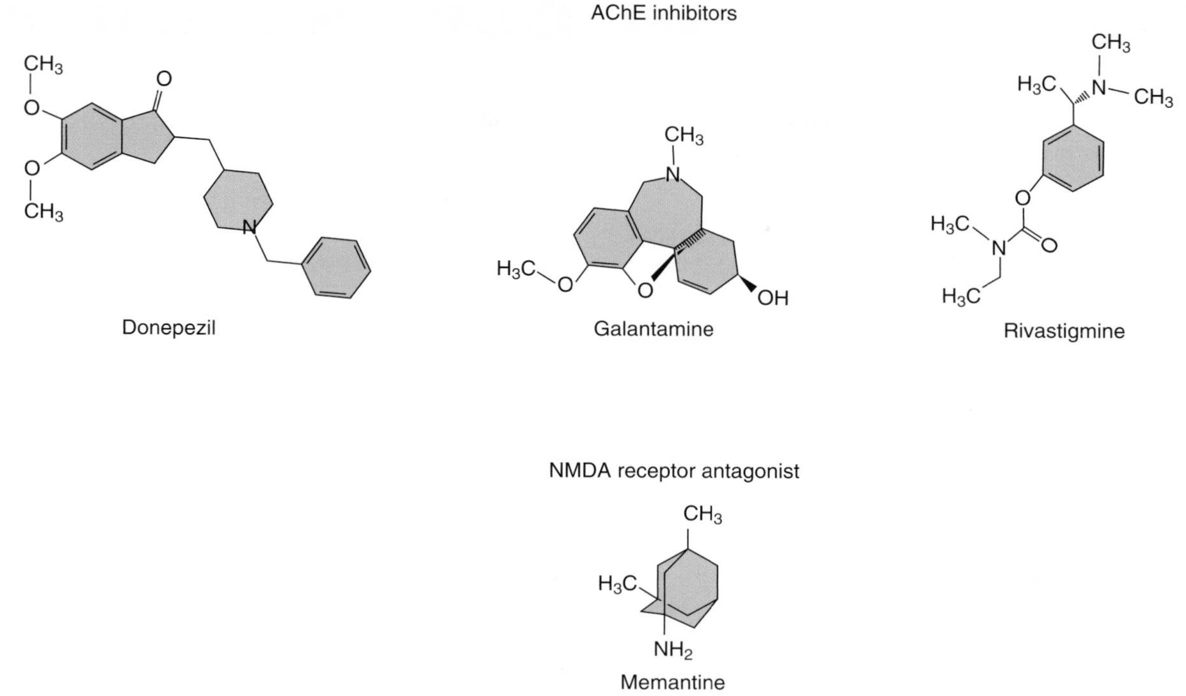

FIG. 14.2 Chemical Structures of Drugs for the Treatment of Alzheimer Disease.

RELATIONSHIP OF MECHANISMS OF ACTION TO CLINICAL RESPONSE

AChE Inhibitors

The cognitive benefits of the AChEIs, although statistically significant, are clinically modest. Not all patients benefit, and those who do typically show only a slight improvement in functional ability (daily activities), cognitive function (6- to 12-month reversal of cognitive impairments), and possibly some neuropsychiatric symptoms. This initial improvement is followed by subsequent decline, albeit from an elevated level of performance. AChEIs do not slow the progression of AD. It is not clear if these drugs improve long-term outcomes significantly, such as delay in institutionalization, which may have the most benefit from both a pharmacoeconomic and quality-of-life perspective.

The efficacy of the AChEIs, albeit modest, has been established for mild to moderate dementia of AD. The AChEIs do not prevent progression of MCI to dementia or improve cognition in MCI. Donepezil and rivastigmine are approved by the United States Food and Drug Administration for the treatment of all stages of dementia due to AD, while galantamine is approved for the treatment of only mild to moderate dementia due to AD. Significant clinical differences among these medications have not been demonstrated.

These drugs may also benefit dementias resulting from other causes, notably dementia with Lewy bodies (DLB), vascular dementias, or mixed dementias. The effect of the AChEIs may be greatest in DLB, with reported benefits in cognition, hallucinations, and parkinsonian symptoms, likely because of significant cholinergic deficits in this disorder.

NMDA Receptor Antagonists

Memantine was approved for use in the United States in 2003 but had been available in Europe for several years before. Memantine improves daily activities and cognitive function scores in moderate to severe cases of AD, but like the AChEIs, these effects are modest. Individuals with milder AD have not been shown to have significant benefit from

TABLE 14.1 Selected Pharmacokinetic Parameters			
Drug	**$t_{1/2}$ (hrs)**	**Plasma Protein Binding (%)**	**Disposition/ Excretion**
Donepezil	70	96	M, R
Galantamine	7	18	M, R
Rivastigmine	1.5	40	Plasma BuChE, R
Memantine	70	45	R

B, Biliary; *BuChE*, butyrylcholinesterase; *M*, metabolized; *R*, renal; $t_{1/2}$, half-life.

memantine. Importantly, patients taking donepezil benefit significantly from memantine, indicating that these two drugs acting through different mechanisms are additive in improving cognitive function. A combination capsule containing these drugs is now available.

PHARMACOKINETICS

All drugs used to treat AD have good oral bioavailability but differ widely in their pharmacokinetic profiles, which are shown in Table 14.1.

AChE Inhibitors

Donepezil, which has a very long half-life, is highly bound to plasma proteins and is metabolized in the liver by CYP2D6 and CYP3A4 followed by glucuronidation. Two of its four metabolites are active, with one as effective as the parent compound in inhibiting AChE activity. Approximately 20% of a dose of donepezil is excreted unchanged, and its hepatic metabolism does not appear to lead to drug interactions or limitations in special populations, other than cautions for subjects with cardiac disease, especially arrhythmias and bradycardia.

Galantamine, which is available in immediate-release and extended-release formulations, is also metabolized by CYP2D6 and CYP3A4, but its metabolites are inactive. Inhibitors of both of these metabolic pathways increase the bioavailability of galantamine, and poor metabolizers (7% of the population with a genetic variation with decreased CYP2D6 activity) exhibit a significant reduction in galantamine clearance.

Rivastigmine is available in oral and transdermal formulations. The absorption of rivastigmine is delayed by food, and unlike the other AChEIs, rivastigmine is metabolized rapidly by plasma BuChE with a half-life of 1.5 hours; the metabolite is excreted via the kidneys.

NMDA Receptor Antagonists

Memantine has a long half-life, with approximately 50% of an administered dose metabolized to three polar compounds, all of which are inactive and excreted in the urine. The other 50% is excreted unchanged in the urine.

PHARMACOVIGILANCE: ADVERSE EFFECTS AND DRUG INTERACTIONS

AChE Inhibitors

All AChEIs currently available are relatively free of serious side effects. As expected, these compounds have a high incidence of peripheral cholinergic effects such as nausea, vomiting, anorexia, and diarrhea (Chapter 7). Rivastigmine is associated with a greater incidence of these effects than the other drugs; it is uncertain if inhibition of BuChE activity is responsible. Use of the transdermal formulation of rivastigmine reduces these side effects without compromising efficacy. Fortunately, many of these effects demonstrate tolerance, and slow, gradual dosage escalation permits many patients to tolerate their full therapeutic doses.

Use of the AChEIs is associated with an increased incidence of insomnia and abnormal dreams due to effects of the cholinergic system on the regulation of rapid eye movement (REM) sleep. Caution should be used in administering AChEIs to individuals with serious arrhythmias or at risk of bradycardia or heart block, as these drugs may potentiate vagal activity (Chapter 6). However, the incidence of clinically significant bradycardia in the controlled trials was similar to placebo.

NMDA Receptor Antagonists

Adverse events reported for memantine were low in clinical trials, with none exceeding twice the placebo values in 5% or more of patients. Dizziness is the most common reported side effect. High doses can produce dissociative anesthetic-type effects similar to ketamine, including confusion, hallucination, and stupor.

The renal clearance of memantine involves active tubular secretion that may be altered by pH-dependent reabsorption, indicating that memantine clearance can be decreased by alkalinization of the urine. Hence, the use of carbonic anhydrase inhibitors or bicarbonate increases plasma concentrations of memantine and elevates the risk of adverse responses.

The adverse effects of drugs for the treatment of AD are listed in the Clinical Problems Box.

NEW DEVELOPMENTS

Research efforts of the past two decades have led to a wealth of knowledge about the structural and biochemical changes in the brain in AD. Since memantine was approved in 2003, no new drugs for AD have been approved, despite assessment of many compounds. Potential therapies continue to emerge based on our increasing knowledge of the disease. New imaging techniques have enabled identification of early, even asymptomatic, AD by the presence of amyloid plaques in the brain. These approaches will allow therapeutic intervention earlier in the course of the disease when there may be less brain damage and a greater chance for a clinical benefit.

Similarly, the ability to directly measure the presence of the AD-associated proteins, amyloid and tau, has improved diagnosis of the disease and will enable assessment of responses to antiamyloid or antitau drugs. Research trials of antiamyloid therapeutics have indicated a measurable decrease in amyloid burden in some studies, though the effects on cognition were not significant. Since tau deposition more closely aligns with cognitive impairment than do amyloid plaques, reliable and accurate tau tracers have the potential to revolutionize both AD diagnostics and therapeutic development.

Enzymatic inhibitors of β-secretase and/or γ-secretase, tipping the balance to favor the nonamyloidogenic α-secretase pathway and preventing the aggregation of Aβ into plaques (see Fig. 14.1), have all been proposed as potential therapies for AD. The ability to prevent or slow the progression of the disease by targeting the underlying pathophysiology represents a highly active area of research, as is the use of antioxidant or antiinflammatory agents. These latter approaches are based on evidence that Aβ accumulation may be promoted by increasing reactive oxygen species, and thus inhibiting their synthesis may slow down the buildup of Aβ.

Last, immunotherapeutic approaches have been tried, but none has been successful to date. Both active and passive immunizations have been tested, with serious adverse effects. Nevertheless, several monoclonal antibodies to human Aβ have been developed (aducanumab, gantenerumab, and crenezumab) and are in various stages of clinical trials. The search continues for more effective treatment of the cognitive and neuropsychiatric symptoms of people with mild, moderate, and severe AD.

CLINICAL RELEVANCE FOR HEALTHCARE PROFESSIONALS

AD is a devastating disorder for both patients and their caregivers. All healthcare professionals need to be aware of the signs and symptoms of this disorder, particularly at its earliest stages when these alterations might be barely recognizable. In addition, all healthcare professionals need to be cognizant of the new guidelines for the clinical diagnostic criteria for AD and the new approaches for treatment that have been developed. Last, it is critical that dementia not associated with AD be recognized to ensure that an accurate diagnosis is made and appropriate therapy is initiated.

SELF-ASSESSMENT QUESTIONS

1. A caretaker drives an 82-year-old patient to his physical therapy session in the morning. When therapy is complete, the patient walks out the door, and you find him still sitting on the bench waiting for a ride home when you are leaving. When you ask him where he lives, he tells you that he "gets all turned around and can't remember." Which of the following drugs is commonly prescribed to treat this condition?
   A. Donepezil.
   B. Fluoxetine.
   C. Selegiline.
   D. Alprazolam.
   E. Haloperidol.

2. Most drugs used for the treatment of Alzheimer disease are directed toward increasing the amount of which neurotransmitter in the brain?
   A. Norepinephrine.
   B. Dopamine.
   C. Serotonin.
   D. Glutamate.
   E. Acetylcholine.

3. The severe cognitive impairments manifested by a 52-year-old may be attributed to:
   A. Sporadic Alzheimer disease.
   B. Abnormal apolipoprotein E.
   C. Mutations in the gene coding for amyloid precursor protein.
   D. Mutations in acetylcholinesterase.
   E. Altered glutamate NMDA receptors.

4. What would you expect when comparing brain images of a 72-year-old woman when she was first diagnosed with Alzheimer disease with those 15 years later after taking donepezil daily?
   A. The images would be about the same.
   B. The images after 15 years on the drug would show less atrophy.
   C. The images after 15 years on the drug would likely show more atrophy.

5. The children of an 82-year-old man recently diagnosed with Alzheimer disease sought advice from their physician about whether a drug could help their father. It is likely that the physician told them that:
   A. The use of memantine would cure their father's cognitive issues.
   B. Their father may or may not respond to the drugs currently available.
   C. Galantamine would have the greatest benefit in a man with advanced disease.
   D. Donepezil would definitely help their father improve.

6. The cholinesterase inhibitor approved for the treatment of Alzheimer disease that has a dual mechanism of action is:
   A. Donepezil.
   B. Galantamine.
   C. Memantine.
   D. Rivastigmine.

FURTHER READING

Cummings J, Aisen PS, DuBois B, et al. Drug development in Alzheimer's disease: the path to 2025. *Alzheimers Res Ther*. 2016;8:39. doi:10.1186/s13195-016-0207-9.

Khanna MR, Kovalevich J, Lee VM, et al. Therapeutic strategies for the treatment of tauopathies: hopes and challenges. *Alzheimers Dement*. 2016;12(10):1051–1065. doi:10.1016/j.jalz.2016.06.006.

Loveman E, Green C, Kirby J, et al. The clinical and cost-effectiveness of donepezil, rivastigmine, galantamine and memantine for Alzheimer's disease. *Health Technol Assess*. 2006;10(1):iii–iv, ix–xi, 1–160.

MacLeod R, Hillert EK, Cameron RT, Baillie GS. The role and therapeutic targeting of α-, β- and γ-secretase in Alzheimer's disease. *Future Sci OA*. 2015;1(3):FSO11. doi:10.4155/fso.15.9. eCollection 2015.

Ruthirakuhan M, Herrmann N, Suridjan I, et al. Beyond immunotherapy: new approaches for disease modifying treatments for early Alzheimer's disease. *Expert Opin Pharmacother*. 2016;17(18):2417–2429. [Epub 2016 Nov 22].

WEBSITES

https://www.nia.nih.gov/alzheimers
This site is maintained by the National Institute on Aging and contains information for both caregivers and patients and for healthcare professionals on all aspects of AD.

http://www.alz.org/about_us_about_us_.asp
The Alzheimer's Association is a well-recognized resource for both healthcare professionals and patients and their caregivers.

Pharmacotherapy of Basal Ganglia Disorders: Parkinson Disease and Huntington Disease

Juan R. Sanchez-Ramos and Briony Catlow

MAJOR DRUG CLASSES

Drugs for Parkinson disease
   L-DOPA/carbidopa
   Monoamine oxidase inhibitors
   Catechol *O*-methyl transferase inhibitors
   Dopamine receptor agonists
Drugs for Huntington disease
   Vesicular monoamine transporter 2 inhibitors
   Dopamine receptor antagonists

ABBREVIATIONS

AAAD	Aromatic L-amino acid decarboxylase
BBB	Blood-brain barrier
COMT	Catechol *O*-methyl transferase
DA	Dopamine
DOPAC	3,4-Dihydroxyphenylacetic acid
5-HT	Serotonin
GABA	γ-Aminobutyric acid
HD	Huntington disease
L-DOPA	3,4-Dihydroxyphenylalanine
MAO	Monoamine oxidase
NMDA	*N*-methyl-D-aspartate
PD	Parkinson disease
VMAT2	Vesicular monoamine transporter 2

THERAPEUTIC OVERVIEW

Parkinson Disease

Parkinson disease (PD) is a progressive neurodegenerative disorder caused by a loss of dopamine (DA) neurons in the substantia nigra and the presence of Lewy bodies (eosinophilic cytoplasmic inclusions) in surviving DA neurons. Traditionally, PD was considered a primary motor disorder characterized by resting tremor, bradykinesia (slowness), rigidity, and postural instability (impaired balance), the latter appearing late in the course of the disease. Recently, the nonmotor features of PD have come to the forefront, including depression, cognitive impairments, and autonomic nervous system dysfunction, the latter involving delayed gastric emptying and constipation. Long-term disability is related to both motor and nonmotor features with worsening of motor fluctuations, dyskinesias, and imbalance, as well as depression, dementia, and psychoses, with death resulting from the complications of immobility, including pulmonary embolism, or aspiration pneumonia.

Current evidence implicates environmental and genetic factors in PD, as well as the possible overexpression and accumulation of the α-synuclein protein. This protein accumulates in the colon and skin of PD patients, as well as in the brain, where it is a major component of Lewy bodies. Studies have suggested that too much α-synuclein interferes with the vesicular release of neurotransmitters, including DA.

While the term *Parkinson disease* refers to the idiopathic disease, parkinsonism refers to disorders that resemble PD but have a known cause and variable rates of progression and responses to drug therapy. These include encephalitis lethargica, multiple small strokes, and traumatic brain injury (pugilistic parkinsonism). In addition, parkinsonism can be induced by the long-term use of typical antipsychotic drugs and results from poisoning by manganese, carbon monoxide, or cyanide.

PD is one of the few neurodegenerative diseases whose symptoms can be improved with drugs. Primary treatments for the motor effects of PD include drugs that increase DA synthesis, decrease DA catabolism, and stimulate DA receptors; secondary compounds antagonize muscarinic cholinergic receptors, enhance DA release, and may antagonize *N*-methyl-D-aspartate (NMDA) glutamate receptors. Depression associated with PD is best treated with the serotonin selective reuptake inhibitors (SSRIs) (Chapter 17), the psychoses with pimavanserin or clozapine (Chapter 16), and the dementia with rivastigmine (Chapter 14).

Huntington Disease

Huntington disease (HD) is a hereditary neurodegenerative disease that results from a mutation of the Huntington gene *htt*. Symptoms and signs of HD include motor, cognitive, and psychiatric disturbances. The most common motor manifestation in adult-onset HD is chorea. As the disease progresses, dystonic features take over as the chorea "burns out," leaving the end-stage patient in a rigid, akinetic state. Other features of the disease include weight loss, sleep and circadian rhythm disturbances, and autonomic nervous system dysfunction. The mean age at onset is between 30 and 50 years, and the duration of the disease is 17–20 years. The progression of the disease leads to more dependency in daily life and finally death, typically associated with pulmonary embolism or aspiration pneumonia. The second most common cause of death is suicide.

The pattern of inheritance is autosomal dominant, meaning that only one *htt* allele needs to be abnormal to express the disease. Hence, each child of an affected parent has a 50% probability of inheriting the disease. The mutation involves an abnormal expansion of a trinucleotide repeat sequence CAG (cytosine-adenine-guanosine) of *htt*, leading to the expression of an aberrant huntingtin protein that folds abnormally and accumulates in both the nuclei and cytoplasm of neurons and astrocytes, leading to cell degeneration. Striatal projection neurons are lost early in the disease, resulting in involuntary movements known as chorea. As the disease progresses, neuronal populations degenerate in the cerebral cortex and brainstem, resulting in the clinical spectrum of motor, cognitive, and behavioral (emotional) problems.

Current drug treatments to decrease the chorea include vesicular monoamine transport 2 (VMAT2) inhibitors such as tetrabenazine that deplete DA, or DA receptor antagonists (Chapter 16). When HD manifests at a young age (<20 years), patients may never exhibit chorea but instead manifest a Parkinson-like condition with rigidity, slowness, and resting tremor. Childhood onset of the disease manifests with a disorder that resembles cerebral palsy with dystonia, spasticity, and developmental delay. In these cases, muscarinic receptor antagonists, such as trihexyphenidyl (Chapter 8) can be used to lessen the dystonia, while the γ-aminobutyric acid (GABA) receptor agonist baclofen (Chapter 22) can be used to lessen spastic rigidity. Neuropsychiatric disturbances manifest as a result of HD can be treated with the atypical antipsychotics, antidepressants, and anxiolytics (Chapters 16 and 17).

A summary of the pathology and treatment of PD and HD is provided in the Therapeutic Overview Box.

THERAPEUTIC OVERVIEW

Parkinson Disease
Pathology
   Degeneration of nigrostriatal DA neurons and presence of Lewy bodies in
      surviving neurons
Treatment
   L-DOPA, MAO, and COMT inhibitors; DA agonists; muscarinic receptor
      agonists; NMDA receptor antagonists

Huntington Disease
Pathology
   Degeneration of neurons and synaptic loss, presence of huntingtin protein
      inclusions in nuclei and cytoplasm, early degeneration of striatal projection
      neurons
Treatment
   VMAT2 inhibitors, DA receptor antagonists, muscarinic receptor antagonists,
      GABA receptor agonists

MECHANISMS OF ACTION

Treatment of Parkinson Disease

Current strategies for the treatment of PD are directed at increasing dopaminergic activity in the striatum to compensate for the loss of nigrostriatal DA neurons. The major drugs used include compounds that increase the synthesis and decrease the catabolism of DA or directly stimulate DA receptors; secondary compounds block muscarinic cholinergic receptors, enhance DA release, and perhaps antagonize NMDA receptors.

Drugs That Increase Dopamine Synthesis

The reactions involved in the synthesis of DA from tyrosine are depicted chemically in Chapter 6 (see Fig. 6.6). Tyrosine is hydroxylated to 3,4-dihydroxyphenylalanine (L-DOPA), which is the immediate precursor of DA. Because DA does not cross the blood-brain barrier (BBB), L-DOPA is used to increase DA synthesis. When given alone, only 1%–3% of an administered dose of L-DOPA reaches the brain; the rest is metabolized peripherally by aromatic L-amino acid decarboxylase (AAAD) and catechol O-methyl transferase (COMT), as shown in Fig. 15.1. To prevent the peripheral metabolism of L-DOPA and increase its availability to the brain, L-DOPA is administered with carbidopa, an AAAD inhibitor that does not cross the BBB. Carbidopa does not have any therapeutic benefit when used alone but increases the amount of L-DOPA available to the brain. However, the peripheral inhibition of AAAD also provides more L-DOPA for metabolism by plasma COMT, producing 3-O-methyldopa. To overcome this, the COMT inhibitors tolcapone or entacapone are used in combination with L-DOPA/carbidopa. These compounds prolong the plasma half-life of L-DOPA, increasing the time the drug is available to cross the BBB, and prevent the buildup of 3-O-methyldopa, which competitively inhibits L-DOPA transport across the BBB. Entacapone does not cross the BBB, and its actions are limited to the periphery. In contrast, tolcapone does cross the BBB and prevents the formation of 3-O-methyldopa in both the plasma and brain.

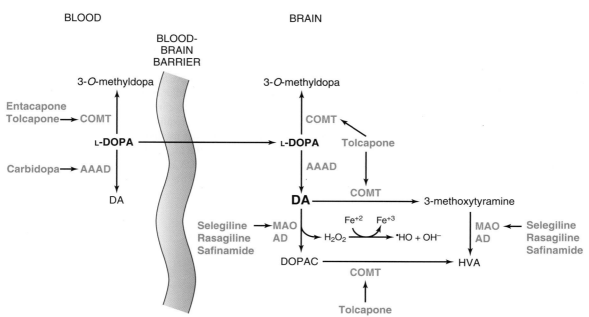

FIG. 15.1 Peripheral and Central Metabolism of L-DOPA and DA, Depicting the Sites of Action of Enzyme Inhibitors. *AAAD*, Aromatic L-amino acid decarboxylase; *AD*, aldehyde dehydrogenase; *COMT*, catechol O-methyltransferase; *DA*, dopamine; *DOPAC*, 3, 4-dihydroxyphenylacetic acid; *HVA*, homovanillic acid; *MAO*, monoamine oxidase.

Drugs That Decrease Dopamine Catabolism

Another approach to increase brain DA levels involves the use of the monoamine oxidase (MAO) type B (MAO-B) inhibitors, as shown in Fig. 15.1. The irreversible inhibitors selegiline and rasagiline or the newly available reversible inhibitor safinamide all inhibit the catabolism of DA in the brain. In addition, by inhibiting the catabolism of DA to 3,4-dihydroxyphenylacetic acid (DOPAC), these compounds decrease the production of hydrogen peroxide (H_2O_2), limiting the possible formation of free radicals that form when the peroxide reacts with ferrous iron.

Dopamine Receptor Agonists

As their name implies, DA receptor agonists directly stimulate DA receptors. Bromocriptine, the only ergot derivative DA agonist still marketed in the United States, has agonist activity at D_2 receptors and partial agonist activity at D_1 receptors. Ropinirole and pramipexole are non–ergot derivatives that selectively activate D_2 and D_3 receptors, whereas the newer non–ergot agent rotigotine, which is available as a transdermal preparation, activates D_1, D_2, and D_3 receptors. The non–ergot DA agonist apomorphine, which is approved as an injectable drug for patients with advanced disease, is an agonist at D_1 and D_2 receptors.

Other Compounds

The antimuscarinic compounds trihexyphenidyl and benztropine inhibit muscarinic cholinergic receptors in the striatum. Normally, nigrostriatal DA neurons inhibit ACh release from striatal interneurons. In PD, the loss of nigrostriatal DA neurons leads to increased firing of striatal cholinergic neurons, with a consequent increased stimulation of muscarinic receptors. The muscarinic cholinergic receptor antagonists block this effect.

The antiviral drug amantadine, which is used for the treatment and prophylaxis of influenza, has several actions that appear beneficial in PD. Amantadine moderately increases DA release and has antimuscarinic activity. In addition, although the role of glutamate in PD is unclear, amantadine antagonizes glutamate NMDA receptors, possibly protecting neurons from the excitotoxic actions of excessive glutamate.

Pimavanserin is a serotonin type 2A ($5\text{-}HT_{2A}$) inverse agonist approved specifically for the treatment of the delusions and hallucinations manifest by some PD patients. The atypical antipsychotics clozapine and quetiapine, which block both D_2 and $5\text{-}HT_{2A}$ receptors (Chapter 16), are also beneficial for psychotic manifestations.

Treatment of Huntington Disease

Current treatment for the chorea of HD is directed primarily at decreasing activity of the nigrostriatal dopaminergic system, a key component of the neural network responsible for automatic execution of motor programs. This can be achieved with agents that either deplete DA or block DA receptors (antipsychotics). Tetrabenazine and deutetrabenazine are the only currently approved drugs for the treatment of chorea in HD; deutetrabenazine is an analogue of tetrabenazine that contains two deuterium atoms in place of hydrogens (Fig. 15.2). These agents are reversible inhibitors of VMAT2 and prevent the uptake of DA into vesicles in the presynaptic neuron. As a consequence, the DA in the cytoplasm is catabolized by monoamine oxidase B (MAO-B) on the outer mitochondrial membrane, depleting the cell of DA, as shown in Fig. 15.3.

Chorea may also be treated with both typical (haloperidol and chlorpromazine) and atypical (olanzapine, risperidone, quetiapine, and aripiprazole) antipsychotic agents that block DA receptors in both the nigrostriatal and mesolimbic DA systems (Chapter 16).

Young-onset patients with prominent dystonia can benefit from the administration of antimuscarinic receptor antagonists such as trihexyphenidyl and benztropine. These agents block overactive cholinergic neurotransmission in basal ganglia responsible for the progressive dystonia. The spasticity associated with young-onset HD can be improved with the GABA-B agonist baclofen, which activates receptors within the brainstem, the dorsal horn of the spinal cord, and other pre- and postsynaptic sites, leading to inhibition of voltage-gated Ca^{2+} channels that decrease glutamate release, and activation of inwardly rectifying K^+ channels, all of which result in decreased neuromuscular rigidity.

RELATIONSHIP OF MECHANISMS OF ACTION TO CLINICAL RESPONSE

Treatment of Parkinson Disease

The combination of L-DOPA/carbidopa remains the most effective symptomatic treatment for PD to date, and both immediate- and controlled-release formulations are available, the latter of benefit for patients exhibiting wearing-off effects. The COMT inhibitors do not provide any therapeutic benefit when used alone, but may increase a patient's responses to L-DOPA, especially by reducing motor fluctuations in patients with advanced disease. However, there may be an increased incidence of dyskinesia requiring decreased doses of L-DOPA. L-DOPA does not stop progression of the disease.

Selegiline, rasagiline, and safinamide enhance clinical responses to L-DOPA and are approved as adjuncts for patients experiencing clinical deterioration and motor fluctuations during L-DOPA therapy.

The DA receptor agonists are effective as monotherapy early in the disease or as an adjunct to L-DOPA/carbidopa in later stages. These compounds are not as efficacious as L-DOPA and have a lower propensity to cause dyskinesias or motor fluctuations. As monotherapy, these compounds are effective for 3–5 years, at which time L-DOPA/carbidopa must be initiated. As adjunctive therapy in advanced disease, DA receptor agonists contribute to clinical improvement and allow a reduction in the dose of L-DOPA required. Although the ergot derivatives were used for many years, their use has declined in favor of the non–ergot compounds because the former led to several serious adverse effects.

The non–ergot DA agonist apomorphine is approved as an injectable drug for use in patients with advanced disease, particularly for patients

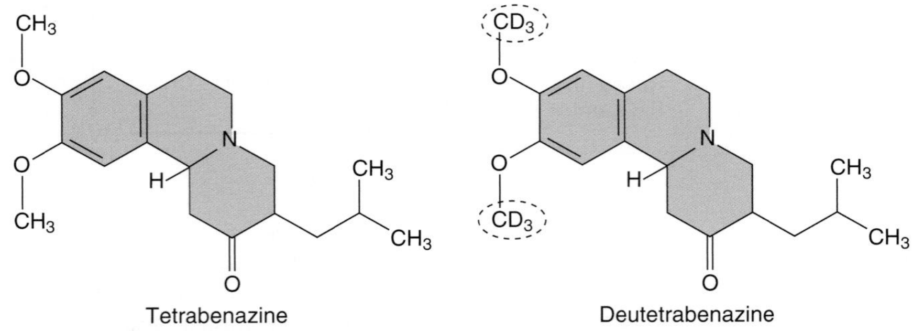

Tetrabenazine   Deutetrabenazine

FIG. 15.2 Structures of Tetrabenazine and Deutetrabenazine.

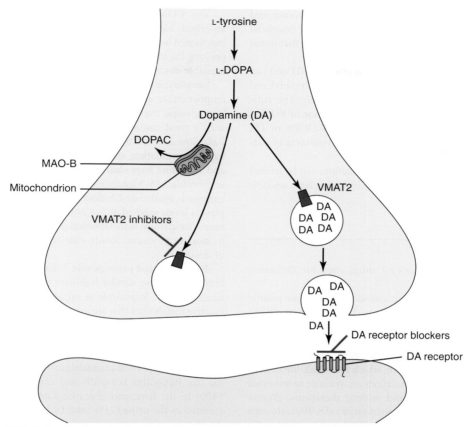

FIG. 15.3 A Dopaminergic Synapse Illustrating the Sites of Action of VMAT2 Inhibitors and DA Receptor Blockers. In the normal situation, DA synthesized in the presynaptic nerve terminal is transported into the synaptic vesicle from which it is released upon nerve terminal depolarization to activate postsynaptic DA receptors. In the presence of a VMAT2 inhibitor, the DA cannot be transported into the vesicle and thus is subject to catabolism by mitochondrial MAO-B to DOPAC, resulting in the depletion of DA in the nerve terminal. *DA*, Dopamine; *DOPAC*, 3,4-dihydroxyphenylacetic acid; *MAO-B*, monoamine oxidase type B; *VMAT2*, vesicular monoamine transporter type 2.

who experience episodes of immobility ("off" times) despite L-DOPA therapy. However, apomorphine has strong emetic effects, and an antiemetic such as trimethobenzamide must be administered prophylactically, typically for 3 days, before initiating therapy with apomorphine.

Antimuscarinics are useful in some patients for controlling tremor and drooling and may have additive therapeutic effects at any stage in the disease. They may be used for short-term monotherapy in tremor-predominant disease, but have little value for akinesia or impaired postural reflexes. In contrast, amantadine helps alleviate mild akinesia and rigidity, but does not alter tremor. Like the antimuscarinics, it may be useful for short-term monotherapy in patients with mild to moderate disease before initiation of L-DOPA.

Pimavanserin, clozapine, and quetiapine are all beneficial for psychotic manifestations of PD without exacerbating the motor symptoms of the disorder.

Treatment of Huntington Disease

Tetrabenazine and deutetrabenazine result in depletion of DA from vesicular storage sites in both the nigrostriatal and mesolimbic DA systems. Interventions that diminish nigrostriatal dopaminergic neurotransmission decrease spontaneous normal movement and attenuate or eliminate choreiform movements. Tetrabenazine also depletes brain levels of 5-HT and norepinephrine, leading to serious depression in

some patients. These agents are also used to treat other hyperkinetic movement disorders, including tic disorders and tardive dyskinesia. Valbenazine is another VMAT2 inhibitor approved currently only for the treatment of tardive dyskinesia.

Classical antipsychotics block D_2 dopamine receptors of the nigrostriatal and mesolimbic dopaminergic systems, while the atypical compounds also block 5-HT_{2A} receptors. Diminished dopaminergic transmission in the nigrostriatal system is responsible for the attenuation of chorea. However, excessive blockade can diminish normal, spontaneous movement and result in parkinsonism (slowness, rigidity, rest tremor). The appearance of antipsychotic-induced dyskinetic movements in patients being treated for psychoses (Chapter 16) can be mistaken as the onset of chorea in persons who carry the HD gene.

Few high-quality clinical studies evaluating the efficacy and safety of these agents for the control of HD chorea have been published because these agents produce a dose-dependent akinetic state as a side effect of their actions. The atypical antipsychotics have been used to control chorea with varying degrees of success. Olanzapine has been investigated in small, open-label studies to treat the motor symptoms of HD, with variable effects on chorea, ranging from a 66% reduction to no reduction at all. There are no clinical trials of risperidone for HD, but several reports indicate a positive effect on the disease with a tolerable adverse effect profile. Quetiapine has been tried in multiple, small, uncontrolled, nonrandomized trials for HD, with some success on both motor and psychiatric symptoms. Aripiprazole has been shown to be beneficial in a few small trials with a reduction in chorea equivalent to that noted with tetrabenazine.

Dystonia and spasticity are common in young-onset HD and can be treated with muscarinic receptor antagonists (trihexyphenidyl and benztropine) and GABA agonists (baclofen), respectively. The anticholinergics are more commonly used to treat the tremor of PD, but are also useful for dystonia. Dopaminergic agents (L-DOPA or DA agonists) are not effective in treating the signs and symptoms of parkinsonism manifested in young-onset HD.

Depression, highly prevalent in the HD population, can be treated with antidepressant amine reuptake inhibitors, including both selective and nonselective agents.

PHARMACOKINETICS

Drugs for Parkinson Disease

Selected pharmacokinetic parameters for drugs used for Parkinson disease are listed in Table 15.1.

L-DOPA is always administered with carbidopa to increase plasma levels and the half-life of L-DOPA and to ensure that sufficient L-DOPA is available to cross the BBB. L-DOPA/carbidopa is rapidly absorbed by the gastrointestinal tract but competes with dietary protein for both intestinal absorption and transport across the BBB. L-DOPA/carbidopa is available in an immediate-release form, which has a half-life of only 60–90 minutes. Controlled-release formulations are available to minimize the number of daily doses required and prolong therapeutic plasma concentrations. A rapidly dissolving formulation of L-DOPA/carbidopa that dissolves on the tongue is available for Parkinson patients who have difficulty swallowing. This preparation dissolves immediately and releases the active drugs within 30 minutes, with other pharmacokinetic parameters similar to the oral preparations.

The COMT inhibitors entacapone and tolcapone are rapidly absorbed, highly bound to plasma proteins, and almost completely inactivated before excretion. Like carbidopa, the COMT inhibitors also prolong the half-life of L-DOPA approximately twofold; entacapone is available in combination with L-DOPA/carbidopa.

Selegiline is rapidly absorbed and metabolized to N-desmethylselegiline, amphetamine, and methamphetamine with half-lives of 2, 18, and 20 hours, respectively. Rasagiline is also rapidly absorbed, but if taken with a meal containing high fat, absorption decreases substantially. Rasagiline is almost totally metabolized in the liver by CYP1A2, followed by glucuronidation and urinary excretion. Although both selegiline and rasagiline have short to intermediate half-lives, because they are irreversible MAO inhibitors, their effects will be manifest until new enzyme is synthesized. Safinamide is also rapidly absorbed, with peak plasma levels reached at 2–4 hours and a half-life of approximately 22 hours. Safinamide is metabolized primarily by nonmicrosomal enzymes to inactive products. Steady-state levels are achieved within 5–6 days of dosing.

Ropinirole and pramipexole differ markedly in their plasma protein binding but have similar half-lives and must be taken orally several times per day. Ropinirole is metabolized extensively by CYP1A2 to inactive metabolites that are excreted in the urine, whereas pramipexole does not appear to be metabolized, with 90% of an administered dose excreted unchanged in the urine. The transdermal rotigotine patch releases drug continuously over 24 hours and, in contrast to the other DA agonists, appears to maintain fairly constant plasma levels throughout the day. Rotigotine is rapidly and extensively metabolized by several P450s in the liver, and glucuronidated and sulfated metabolites are excreted in the urine (71%) and feces (23%).

Drugs for Huntington Disease

Tetrabenazine is moderately absorbed (75%) following oral administration, with no effect of food. It is 83%–88% bound to plasma proteins

TABLE 15.1	**Selected Pharmacokinetic Parameters**		
Drug	**$t_{1/2}$ (hours)**	**Plasma Protein Binding (%)**	**Disposition/Excretion**
Parkinson Disease Drugs			
Bromocriptine	5–7	90–96	B
Entacapone	0.4–0.7; 2.4 (biphasic)	98	B
Pramipexole	8 (young) 12 (aged)	15	R
Rasagiline	3	88–94	R, B
Ropinirole	6	40	M, R
Rotigotine	5–7 (after patch removal)	—	M, R, B
Selegiline	7–9	—	R
Tolcapone	2–3	>99.9	R
L-DOPA/carbidopa	1.5–2	L-DOPA: 10–30 Carbidopa: 36	M, R
Huntington Disease Drugs			
Tetrabenazine	10	83–88	M, R
α-Dihydrotetrabenazine (active metabolite)	4–8	60–68	M, R
Risperidone	3–20	90	M, R
Haloperidol	14–26	90–92	M, B
Quetiapine	7	83	M, B
Olanzapine	21–54	93	M, B
Baclofen	1.5–4	35	R

B, Biliary; *M*, metabolized; *R*, renal.

and has a low bioavailability (approximately 0.05), as it is metabolized rapidly by carbonyl reductase in the liver to α- and β-dihydrotetrabenazine, the former an active metabolite, followed by further metabolism primarily by CYP2D6, and to a lesser extent by CYP1A2 and CYP3A4/5. Tetrabenazine has a half-life of 10 hours, with the half-life of the active metabolite 4–8 hours, requiring that the drug be taken 2–3 times per day. The pharmacokinetic profile of deutetrabenazine is identical to that of tetrabenazine.

The pharmacokinetics of the antipsychotics are discussed in Chapter 16.

PHARMACOVIGILANCE: ADVERSE EFFECTS AND DRUG INTERACTIONS

Drugs for Parkinson Disease

The peripheral side effects of L-DOPA include actions on the gastrointestinal and cardiovascular systems. Vomiting may be caused by stimulation of DA neurons in the area postrema, which is outside the BBB. The peripheral decarboxylation of L-DOPA to DA in plasma can activate vascular DA receptors and produce orthostatic hypotension, while the stimulation of both α- and β-adrenergic receptors by DA can lead to cardiac arrhythmias, especially in patients with preexisting conditions. L-DOPA is contraindicated for individuals taking MAO inhibitors, as severe hypertension may ensue.

Central nervous system effects include depression, anxiety, agitation, insomnia, hallucinations, and confusion, particularly in the aged, and may be attributed to enhanced mesolimbic and mesocortical dopaminergic activity. The tricyclic antidepressants or serotonin selective reuptake inhibitors (Chapter 17) may be used for depression, but the latter may worsen motor symptoms.

Although L-DOPA/carbidopa remains the most effective treatment for PD to date, for most patients it is effective for only 3–5 years. As the disease progresses, even with continued treatment, the duration of therapeutic activity from each dose decreases. This is known as the "wearing-off" effect, and many patients fluctuate in their response between mobility and immobility, known as the "on-off" effect. In addition, after 5 years of continued drug treatment, as many as 75% of patients experience dose-related dyskinesias, characterized by chorea and dystonia, inadequate therapeutic responses, and toxicity at subtherapeutic doses. These effects may represent an adaptive process to alterations in plasma and brain levels of L-DOPA and involve alterations in expression of DA and NMDA receptors.

The COMT inhibitors can lead to dyskinesias, nausea, discoloration of the urine, and increased daytime sleepiness and sleep attacks. Tolcapone has been taken off the market in Canada, but not the United States, as a consequence of induced fatal hepatotoxicity. Because of this risk, tolcapone should be used only in patients who have failed to respond to other drugs and who are experiencing motor fluctuations. Baseline liver function tests should be performed before starting tolcapone and should be repeated for the duration of therapy. If patients do not demonstrate a clinical response within 3 weeks, the drug should be withdrawn. Tolcapone is contraindicated in patients with compromised liver function.

The MAO-B inhibitors can cause nausea and orthostatic hypotension. At doses recommended for PD, which inhibit MAO-B, but not MAO-A, these agents are unlikely to induce a tyramine interaction (Chapters 11 and 17). Selegiline, rasagiline and safinamide may cause rare toxic interactions with meperidine and can increase the adverse effects of L-DOPA, particularly dyskinesias and psychoses in the aged population. Rasagiline has been reported to increase the incidence of melanoma, and because rasagiline is metabolized by CYP1A2, plasma concentrations may increase in the presence of CYP1A2 inhibitors such as ciprofloxacin

and fluvoxamine. MAO inhibitors must be used with caution in patients taking any drug enhancing serotonergic activity, including the antidepressants, dextromethorphan, and tryptophan (Chapter 17). Combinations of these compounds could induce "serotonin syndrome," a serious condition characterized by confusion, agitation, rigidity, shivering, autonomic instability, myoclonus, coma, nausea, diarrhea, diaphoresis, flushing, and even death.

DA receptor agonists cause side effects similar to those with L-DOPA, including nausea and postural hypotension. These compounds cause more central nervous system–related effects than L-DOPA, including hallucinations, confusion, cognitive dysfunction, and sleepiness. They should not be used in patients with dementia.

The DA agonists are also known to induce impulse control disorders such as pathological gambling, hypersexuality, uncontrollable spending, and excessive computer use. The compulsive behaviors may reflect stimulation of the midbrain dopaminergic ventral tegmental-nucleus accumbens pathway thought to mediate addictive behaviors (Chapter 13). When these symptoms become apparent, the DA agonists should be tapered and stopped, and L-DOPA initiated.

The muscarinic receptor antagonists all cause typical anticholinergic effects, as discussed in Chapter 8. Because PD is predominantly an age-related disorder, and aged individuals show increased vulnerability to other dysfunctions including dementia and glaucoma, anticholinergics must be used with caution in the aged, because these drugs impair memory, exacerbate glaucoma, and may cause urinary retention.

Amantadine may produce hallucinations and confusion, nausea, dizziness, dry mouth, and an erythematous rash of the lower extremities. Symptoms may worsen dramatically if it is discontinued, and amantadine should be used with caution in patients with congestive heart disease or acute angle-closure glaucoma.

Drugs for Huntington Disease

The primary adverse effect of the VMAT2 inhibitor tetrabenazine is an increased risk of worsening depression and suicidality. HD patients with a serious history of depression or prior suicide attempts should not be treated with tetrabenazine, and there is a boxed warning about these effects. In addition to depression and anxiety, the most commonly reported adverse effects included sedation and somnolence, insomnia, fatigue, and diarrhea. Tetrabenazine can also lead to extrapyramidal symptoms of parkinsonism and akathisia and has been shown to lead to a small prolongation of the QT interval. Because tetrabenazine is metabolized by CYP2D6, drug interactions may ensue with inhibitors or inducers of this enzyme, and patients should be genotyped for the presence of CYP2D6 polymorphisms before initiating therapy with this drug.

Deutetrabenazine has been reported to have a more favorable profile than tetrabenazine, with a lower risk of adverse effects, including less sedation or insomnia, depression, akathisia, and extrapyramidal symptoms.

The adverse effects of the antipsychotics are discussed in Chapter 16. Common side effects associated with drugs used for PD and HD are listed in the Clinical Problems Box.

NEW DEVELOPMENTS

The treatment of PD has focused largely on drugs that slow or ameliorate symptoms of this disorder, but recent studies have begun to focus on developing compounds with neuroprotective, as well as restorative actions, to perhaps slow down or stop the progression of disease. Based on evidence that α-synuclein plays a major role in the neurodegenerative process, early clinical trials have begun to investigate possible therapeutic strategies to block or inhibit the actions of this protein. Additionally,

CLINICAL PROBLEMS

Parkinson Disease

L-DOPA	Nausea and vomiting, orthostatic hypotension, cardiac arrhythmias, depression, anxiety, hallucinations, sleepiness, limited effectiveness, fluctuations in response, and dyskinesias after 3 to 5 years of treatment
DA Receptor Agonists	Nausea and vomiting, orthostatic hypotension, cardiac arrhythmias, marked depression, confusion, hallucinations, sleepiness, impulsivity

Huntington Disease

VMAT2 Inhibitors	Dizziness, drowsiness, nausea, tiredness, trouble sleeping, parkinsonism (slowness, rigidity, rest tremor), depression, tardive akathisia (restlessness)

TRADE NAMES

In addition to generic and fixed-combination preparations, the following trade-named materials are some of the important compounds available in the United States.

Parkinson Disease Drugs
Drugs That Increase DA Synthesis
Entacapone (Comtan)
Entacapone/L-DOPA/carbidopa (Stalevo)
L-DOPA (Larodopa)
L-DOPA/carbidopa (Sinemet, Parcopa)
Tolcapone (Tasmar)

Drugs That Decrease DA Catabolism
Rasagiline (Azilect)
Selegiline (Eldepryl, Zelapar)

DA Receptor Agonists
Apomorphine (Apokyn)
Bromocriptine (Parlodel)
Pramipexole (Mirapex)
Ropinirole (Requip)
Rotigotine (Neupro)

Huntington Disease Drugs
Tetrabenazine (Xenazine)
Deutetrabenazine (Austedo)

antiinflammatory agents and neuroimmunophilin ligands that have been shown to promote regeneration in animal models are being tested in humans. With the success, albeit somewhat limited, of tetrabenazine and deutetrabenazine for HD, additional VMAT2 inhibitors are actively being studied for the treatment of several hyperkinetic disorders. Lastly, attention is focusing on gene-silencing technology using small interfering RNA (siRNA) or antisense oligonucleotides (ASO). Based on evidence of significant downregulation of *htt* expression following treatment with siRNA in rodent models of HD, clinical trials are being conducted in HD subjects.

CLINICAL RELEVANCE FOR HEALTHCARE PROFESSIONALS

Although neurodegenerative disorders are typically thought of as affecting only the aged population, both PD and HD can be manifest in children. Thus it is important for all healthcare professionals to be aware of this and have children with abnormal movements tested for possible genetic mutations. For PD, novel related mutations are being identified in families, and as more is known about specific genetic alterations, new agents to target these proteins will be developed. The past few years have seen major advances in our knowledge of movement disorders that need to be appreciated by all those involved in the healthcare of these individuals. Of particular importance are the nonmotor symptoms associated with PD that may become apparent much earlier than the tremor and postural instability. If these symptoms were recognized before 70%–75% of nigrostriatal neurons degenerated, perhaps neuroprotective strategies could be implemented, halting the progression of the disorder.

SELF-ASSESSMENT QUESTIONS

1. A 72-year-old man with Parkinson disease is being treated with L-DOPA/carbidopa. The beneficial effect of carbidopa may be attributed to which of the following actions?
   A. Its conversion to L-DOPA.
   B. Its conversion to dopamine.
   C. Its inability to cross the blood-brain barrier.
   D. Inhibition of COMT.
   E. Inhibition of MAO.

2. An 82-year-old woman with Parkinson disease has been taking L-DOPA/carbidopa for 7 years. She has recently noticed that some abnormal choreiform-like movements have developed in her arms and legs. These movements are a typical example of which of the following?
   A. L-DOPA-induced psychosis.
   B. L-DOPA-induced dyskinesia.
   C. "On-off" effects of L-DOPA.
   D. Toxicity of L-DOPA.
   E. "Wearing-off" effects of L-DOPA.

3. A 68-year-old woman with advanced Parkinson disease waiting at the bus is unable to get up from the bench. Her young companion reaches into her purse and administers a drug subcutaneously that enables the woman to get up. Which of the following is the most likely drug used in this patient?
   A. Amantadine.
   B. Apomorphine.
   C. Entacapone.
   D. Ropinirole.
   E. Selegiline.

4. The choreiform movements exhibited by a 50-year-old man with Huntington disease were alleviated by a drug that depleted DA from presynaptic nerve terminals. This drug was likely:
   A. Selegiline.
   B. Entacapone.
   C. Tetrabenazine.
   D. Amantadine.
   E. Trihexyphenidyl.

FURTHER READING

Connolly BS, Lang AE. Pharmacological treatment of Parkinson disease: a review. *JAMA*. 2014;311(16):1670–1683.

Frank S. Treatment of Huntington's disease. *Neurotherapeutics*. 2014;11(1): 153–160.

WEBSITES

https://www.ninds.nih.gov/Disorders/All-Disorders/Parkinsons-Disease-Information-Page

https://www.ninds.nih.gov/Disorders/All-Disorders/Huntingtons-Disease-Information-Page

These websites are maintained by the National Institute of Neurological Disorders and Stroke and are valuable for both healthcare professionals and patients, with numerous links to resources for Parkinson disease and Huntington disease.

https://www.aan.com/Guidelines/Home/ByTopic?topicId=17

This website, maintained by the American Academy of Neurology, has practice guidelines for the treatment of movement disorders.

16

Drug Therapy for Psychoses and Bipolar Disorder

Lynn Wecker, Glenn W. Currier, and Glenn Catalano

MAJOR DRUG CLASSES

Typical antipsychotics
    Phenothiazines
    Thioxanthines
    Butyrophenones
Atypical antipsychotics
Lithium

ABBREVIATIONS

D_2	Dopamine receptor type 2
DA	Dopamine
H_1	Histamine receptor type 1
5-HT	Serotonin
$5\text{-}HT_2$	Serotonin receptor type 2
NMDA	*N*-methyl-D-aspartate

THERAPEUTIC OVERVIEW

Psychoses

Psychotic behaviors are characterized by impaired cognitive functioning, distortions of reality and perception, and disturbances of affect (mood). Psychotic disorders may have an organic basis (disease induced, such as occurs in systemic lupus erythematosus), may be drug induced (such as occurs with the hallucinogen phencyclidine), or may be idiopathic (schizophrenia). Schizophrenia is the most common psychotic disorder, which affects 2.2 million Americans (1% of the population) and typically develops between 16 and 30 years of age. Schizophrenia interferes with a person's ability to think clearly, manage emotions, make decisions, and relate to others. The symptoms of schizophrenia fall into three clusters.

- Alterations in cognitive control represent the core domain of dysfunction, with the lack of ability to adjust thoughts or behaviors to achieve goals, manifest by attentional and short-term memory deficits.
- Positive symptoms are reality distortions characterized by delusions, hallucinations, and, often, agitated behaviors.
- Negative symptoms include a flattened affect and apathy, with emotional and social withdrawal or detachment.

Although schizophrenia is of unknown etiology, evidence supports a role for genetic and environmental factors, including neurodevelopmental abnormalities. Evidence supporting a role for genetic factors includes findings that relatives of schizophrenics have a higher risk of illness as compared with the general population and that there is a higher concordance of schizophrenia in monozygotic (40%–50%) as compared with dizygotic (15%) twins. In fact, a child born to two schizophrenic parents has a 40 times greater risk of developing the illness than the general population.

Structural studies have demonstrated that the brains of individuals with schizophrenia have enlarged cerebral ventricles, atrophy of cerebral cortical layers, a decreased number of synaptic connections in the prefrontal cortex, and alterations in neocortical, limbic, and subcortical structures. Functional abnormalities include reduced cerebral blood flow and reduced glucose use in the prefrontal cortex.

Although neurochemical alterations in schizophrenia have been inconsistent, studies have implicated changes in the expression or function of several neurotransmitter-associated proteins such as those for the type 4 dopamine receptor and the synthetic enzyme catechol-O-methyltransferase. Other studies have suggested that schizophrenia may involve alterations in signaling pathways, particularly those involving the scaffolding protein disrupted-in-schizophrenia 1 (DISC1), the transcription factor c-Fos, the cell signaling protein neuregulin, and oligodendrocyte-associated proteins, including proteolipid protein, the most abundant myelin-related protein.

Psychotic behaviors are treated pharmacologically with typical (first-generation or traditional) or atypical (second-generation or novel) antipsychotic drugs, classes that differ with respect to mechanisms of action, side effect profiles, and patient responses. The typical antipsychotics include the prototypes chlorpromazine and haloperidol, which were introduced in the 1950s. The atypical antipsychotics appeared in the 1990s and represented a more heterogeneous group, including compounds such as clozapine, olanzapine, risperidone, and others.

Bipolar Disorder

Bipolar disorder (manic-depressive disease) is characterized by depressive cycles with manic episodes interspersed with periods of normal mood. Bipolar disorder type 1 involves periods of severe mood alterations ranging from depression to full mania, while bipolar disorder type 2 involves severe depression alternating with hypomania, which is less severe. The characteristics of the depressive phase resemble those of unipolar depression (Chapter 17), whereas the manic phase manifests as increased psychomotor activity and grandiosity, feelings of euphoria, poor judgment and recklessness, extreme irritability, a decreased need for sleep, and symptoms sometimes resembling psychotic behavior. Bipolar disorder affects 2 million people in the United States, often begins in adolescence or early adulthood, and may persist for life. Evidence suggests a role for genetic factors because the concordance rate in identical twins is 61%–75%. However, the disorder cannot be attributed to a single major gene, suggesting multifactorial inheritance.

Lithium has been, and remains, the mainstay of treatment to control manic episodes. Several anticonvulsants are also frequently used,

134

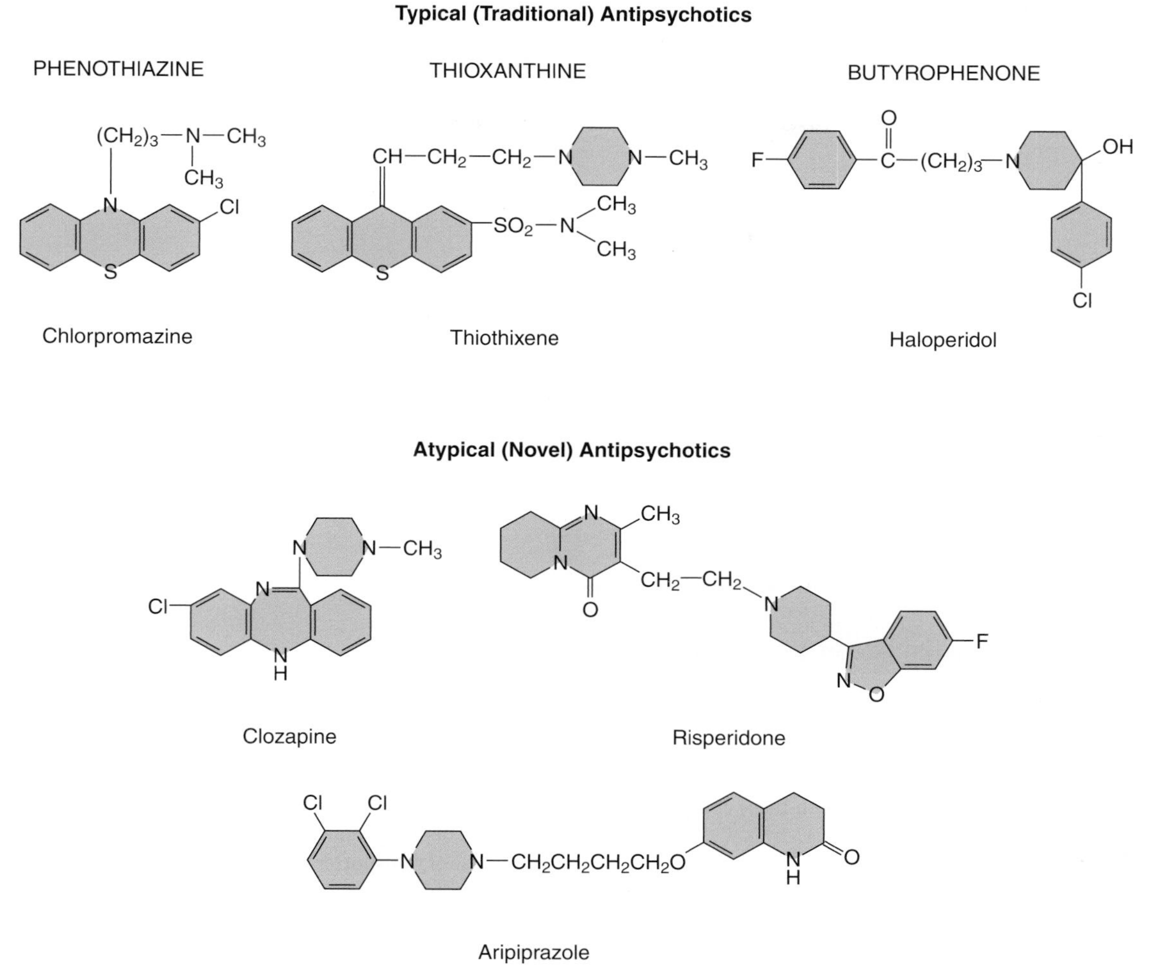

Typical (Traditional) Antipsychotics

PHENOTHIAZINE

Chlorpromazine

THIOXANTHINE

Thiothixene

BUTYROPHENONE

Haloperidol

Atypical (Novel) Antipsychotics

Clozapine

Risperidone

Aripiprazole

FIG. 16.1 Structures of Various Antipsychotic Agents.

including **valproic acid**, **lamotrigine**, and **carbamazepine** (Chapter 21), as are many **atypical antipsychotics**.

The characteristics and treatment of psychotic and bipolar disorders are summarized in the Therapeutic Overview Box.

THERAPEUTIC OVERVIEW

Psychoses
Characterized by alterations in cognitive control, reality distortions (positive symptoms), flattened affect with detachment (negative symptoms)
Typical antipsychotics may alleviate positive symptoms
Atypical antipsychotics may alleviate positive and improve negative symptoms

Bipolar Disorder
Characterized by depressive cycles with manic episodes
Lithium, several atypical antipsychotics, and several anticonvulsants may temper the manic phase
Antidepressants may be used with a mood stabilizer to avoid "manic overshoot"

MECHANISMS OF ACTION

Typical Antipsychotics

The typical antipsychotics were the first group of compounds developed for the treatment of schizophrenia, and based on chemical structure, these compounds were classified as phenothiazines or thioxanthines,

which have a characteristic three-ring structure, or butyrophenones, which were unrelated chemically (Fig. 16.1).

The effects of the typical antipsychotics have been attributed to blockade of 70%–75% of postsynaptic dopamine (DA) type 2 (D_2) receptors. Indeed, a positive linear correlation exists between the therapeutic potency of the typical antipsychotics and their ability to bind to and block D_2-receptors (Fig. 16.2). Inhibition of these receptors in mesolimbic and mesocortical regions (Chapter 13) is believed to mediate the ability of these compounds to relieve some behavioral manifestations of schizophrenia. On the other hand, blockade of greater than 70%–75% of these receptors in the basal ganglia underlies the motor side effects of these compounds, and inhibition of these receptors in the tuberoinfundibular pathway in the hypothalamus leads to increased prolactin secretion from the pituitary gland.

Acute administration of the typical antipsychotics increases the firing rate of both mesolimbic and nigrostriatal DA neurons as a compensatory response to D_2-receptor blockade. However, long-term administration inactivates these pathways via **depolarization blockade**. Because the therapeutic effects of the typical antipsychotics may require several weeks to become apparent, it is believed that this inactivation of mesolimbic DA transmission mediates the time-dependent amelioration of some symptoms.

In addition to blocking D_2-receptors, the typical antipsychotics may also block muscarinic cholinergic receptors, α_1- and α_2-adrenergic receptors, histamine type 1 (H_1) receptors, and serotonin type 2 (5-HT_2)

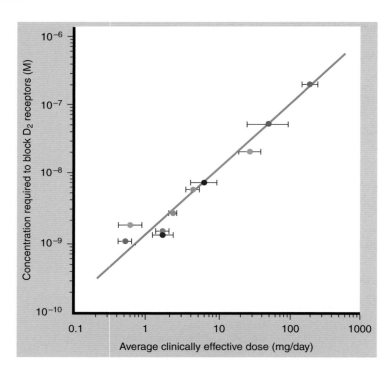

FIG. 16.2 Correlation Between the Therapeutic Dose of Typical Antipsychotics and the Concentration to Block D_2 Receptors.

receptors. Although blockade of 5-HT_2 receptors may contribute to the antipsychotic efficacy of these agents, blockade of other receptors underlies many of the side effects associated with these compounds.

Atypical Antipsychotics

The atypical antipsychotics represent a heterogeneous group of compounds with differences in chemical structure (see Fig. 16.1). These agents occupy and block D_2-receptors, albeit fewer than the typical antipsychotics (50%–60% compared with >70%). However, they also block a preponderance (75%–95%) of 5-HT_{2A} receptors. Because of their lower occupancy of D_2-receptors, the atypical antipsychotics have a lower propensity than the typical compounds to induce motor side effects. They also have an increased ability to decrease the rate of relapse after drug administration relative to the typical antipsychotics.

Clozapine and other atypical antipsychotics also have actions at muscarinic cholinergic, α_1-and α_2-adrenergic, H_1, 5-HT_{1A}, 5-HT_{2C}, and D_4-receptors, although the nature of the effects (agonism versus antagonism) and contribution of these actions to antipsychotic efficacy remains unknown. In addition to actions at these receptors, clozapine, olanzapine, and several other agents increase regional blood flow in the cerebral cortex through an undefined mechanism, an action that may contribute to the beneficial effects of these compounds on cognitive functions such as working memory and attention.

Aripiprazole is a unique atypical antipsychotic because, unlike all the other agents in this group, it is a partial agonist at D_2- and 5-HT_{1A} receptors and a full antagonist at 5-HT_{2A} receptors. Similarly, pimavanserin is a 5-HT_{2A} inverse agonist devoid of DA receptor–blocking activity. Thus the therapeutic and side effect profile for these agents differs somewhat from other atypical antipsychotics.

Lithium

Although lithium has been the standard prophylactic agent for the treatment of bipolar disorder for decades, its cellular mechanisms of action remain unclear. Currently, several cellular actions of lithium have been postulated to mediate its clinical efficacy. Lithium affects several signaling systems in the brain (Fig. 16.3). It interferes with

receptor-activated phosphatidylinositol turnover by blocking the hydrolysis of inositol bisphosphate to inositol monophosphate to free inositol, decreasing free inositol concentrations and depleting the further formation of phosphatidylinositol (Chapter 2). It also inhibits the sodium/myo-inositol transporter (SMIT), contributing to the reduction in free inositol. Lithium directly inhibits protein kinase C, glycogen synthesis kinase-3β (GSK-3β), and myristoylated alanine-rich protein kinase C substrate (MARCKS), all of which play a role in cell survival/death. Lithium activates both β-catenin, which regulates the integrity of the cytoskeleton, and the extracellular signal–regulated kinase/mitogen-activated protein kinase (ERK/MAPK) cascade, promoting cell survival and proliferation and preserving synaptic plasticity and morphology, which may be required for mood stabilization. Thus lithium has multiple effects on several signaling systems. Most interestingly, most of these actions are shared by the anticonvulsant valproic acid, which is also used to treat the manic phase of bipolar disorder.

Lithium has also been shown to inhibit 5-HT_{1A} and 5-HT_{1B} autoreceptors on serotonergic dendrites and nerve terminals, thereby preventing feedback inhibition of 5-HT release. Last, sustained lithium exposure enhances glutamate reuptake by glutamatergic neurons, thereby decreasing the time glutamate is present at synapses and dampening the ability of glutamate to stimulate its receptors. Clearly, additional studies are needed to elucidate the actions of lithium that underlie its unique efficacy in bipolar disorder.

The mechanisms of action of the anticonvulsants are discussed in Chapter 21.

RELATIONSHIP OF MECHANISMS OF ACTION TO CLINICAL RESPONSE

Schizophrenia

The intensity of positive (hallucinations, delusions, and paranoia) and negative (blunted affect, poverty of speech and thought, apathy) symptoms and cognitive impairments characteristic of schizophrenia varies among patients and, importantly, in patients over time, such that a patient may exhibit predominantly one set of symptoms at any

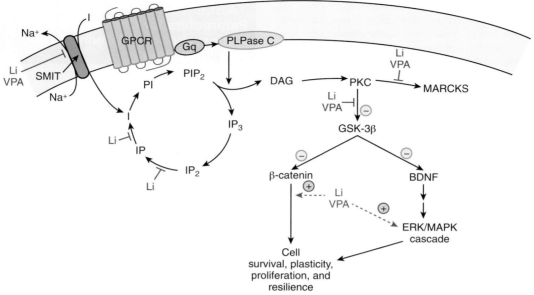

FIG. 16.3 Postulated Sites of Action of Lithium. Depicted are several signaling systems regulating cell survival, proliferation, plasticity, and resilience. The sites of action of lithium (Li) and the anticonvulsant valproic acid (VPA) are shown. Abbreviations: *BDNF*, Brain-derived neurotrophic factor; *DAG*, diacylglycerol; *ERK/ MAPK*, extracellular signal–regulated kinase/mitogen-activated protein kinase; *GPCR*, G-protein–coupled receptor; *GSK-3β*, glycogen synthase kinase-3β; *I*, inositol; *IP*, inositol monophosphate; *IP₂*, inositol 1,4-bisphosphate; *IP₃*, inositol 1,4,5-triphosphate; *MARCKS*, myristoylated alanine-rich protein kinase C substrate; *PI*, phosphatidylinositol; *PIP₂*, phosphatidylinositol 4,5-biphosphate; *PKC*, protein kinase C; *PLPase C*, phospholipase C; *SMIT*, sodium/myo-inositol transporter.

particular time. In general, the positive symptoms of schizophrenia respond better to the antipsychotics than the negative symptoms or cognitive impairments. It is critical to understand that within the schizophrenic population, few patients achieve full recovery with or without medication, with approximately 30%–35% exhibiting good responses, 30%–35% demonstrating partial improvement, and 20%–30% resistant to all drugs, underscoring the heterogeneity of the disorder.

The choice of antipsychotic drug is based on the particular symptoms manifested by the patient, as well as on sensitivity to undesirable side effects and previous therapeutic response to a particular agent. Although the typical antipsychotics were first-line compounds, the use of the atypicals is increasing because of their better tolerated side effect profile, leading to better compliance. Further, although clozapine has not been considered a first-line drug because of multiple significant side effects (including agranulocytosis, seizures, and myocarditis), it is clearly of tremendous benefit for patients who fail to respond to other antipsychotics.

The short-term goal of the management of a psychotic episode is to reduce positive symptoms. To this end, there appears to be an "optimal" level of mesolimbic D₂-receptor block required to achieve this effect. Further, transient receptor antagonism, such as occurs with clozapine and several other atypical compounds, is sufficient to achieve this effect without a large increase in the risk of adverse reactions mediated by blockade of striatal receptors. This is in contrast to the persistent receptor blockade produced by the typical antipsychotics. Although persistent receptor blockade alleviates positive symptoms, it also leads to deteriorating clinical responses in some patients, as well as an increased risk of extrapyramidal effects. Interestingly, aripiprazole, which is a partial agonist atypical agent, maintains both optimal blockade of mesolimbic D₂-receptors while maintaining the function of striatal receptors.

The long-term goal for the management of schizophrenic patients includes the prevention of relapse because it is believed that multiple psychotic episodes negatively affect long-term outcome. Relapse is the result of noncompliance and not the development of drug tolerance and is best prevented by the continuous rather than intermittent use of atypical antipsychotic agents.

It is critical to understand that D₂-receptor blockade occurs rapidly after initial antipsychotic treatment, whereas a maximal therapeutic response is not observed for several weeks and correlates with the induction of depolarization blockade of mesolimbic DA neurons. The long-term consequences of 5-HT₂A receptor blockade are less well understood, as are the roles of other neurotransmitter receptors. Based on the ability of the antipsychotics to block D₂- and 5-HT₂A receptors, enhanced DA and 5-HT activity clearly plays a role in the positive symptoms of schizophrenia. Further, based on findings that the glutamate *N*-methyl-ᴅ-aspartate (NMDA) receptor antagonist phencyclidine leads to psychotic behaviors in humans, evidence also supports a role for glutamate in the positive manifestations of schizophrenia.

The negative and cognitive symptoms have been suggested to reflect reductions in prefrontal cortical metabolic activity, which has been ascribed to impaired perfusion. Indeed, several atypical antipsychotics increase cerebral cortical blood flow, perhaps contributing to their beneficial effects on working memory and attention. Concomitantly, studies have shown that these agents enhance the release of acetylcholine (ACh) and have suggested a role for altered cholinergic systems in the cognitive impairment in psychotic behavior. This idea is underscored by the vast literature supporting a role for ACh in learning and memory and the role of impaired cholinergic activity in Alzheimer disease (Chapter 14).

In addition to their use in schizophrenia, several antipsychotics have been of therapeutic benefit in other neuropsychiatric disorders. Many of the atypical antipsychotics (including risperidone, quetiapine, and olanzapine) are effective as primary monotherapy or as an augmenting agent with mood stabilizers in the treatment of bipolar disorder, regardless of whether psychotic features were present at the time, and are often prescribed concomitantly with antidepressants and mood stabilizers for schizoaffective disorder. Haloperidol and pimozide are approved, and risperidone is gaining use off-label to treat behavioral syndromes accompanied by motor disturbances, specifically Gilles de la Tourette syndrome. In addition, many atypicals, such as risperidone and aripiprazole, are approved for irritability associated with pervasive developmental disorders such as autism, Asperger syndrome, and Rett syndrome. Pimavanserin is approved specifically for the treatment of psychoses associated with Parkinson disease (Chapter 15).

Although antipsychotic drug therapy greatly improves the clinical outcome in patients with schizophrenia and other disorders, improvement in the quality of life of these individuals requires the use of psychosocial interventions. Clinical outcomes appear to be more positive in patients who can engage in an occupation, maintain family contact, and function in a social environment, all of which benefit from appropriate psychosocial interventions.

Bipolar Disorder

Lithium continues to be the standard treatment for bipolar disorder and is the drug of choice for maintenance treatment. It can be used as monotherapy or in combination with atypical antipsychotics or anticonvulsants for the treatment of an acute manic episode. For patients who either do not respond to lithium or cannot tolerate its adverse effects, the anticonvulsants valproate, carbamazepine, and lamotrigine are widely used. Lamotrigine has been shown to be effective for the prevention of recurrent depressive episodes. Further, several atypical antipsychotics are approved for the treatment of both acute mania and mixed episodes, while olanzapine and aripiprazole are approved for maintenance therapy.

Because the use of an antidepressant in a patient with bipolar depression may destabilize the underlying bipolar disorder, the concomitant use of an antidepressant with a mood stabilizer is no longer first-line treatment. At this time, the atypical antipsychotics quetiapine and lurasidone, along with the combination preparation olanzapine/fluoxetine, are the only medications approved for the treatment of bipolar depression. If these drugs are ineffective, the clinician may need to consider using a regimen that includes both a mood stabilizer and an antidepressant.

PHARMACOKINETICS

The antipsychotics are readily but erratically absorbed after oral administration, and most undergo significant first-pass metabolism. Most of these compounds are highly lipophilic and protein bound, have variable half-lives after oral administration, are oxidized by hepatic microsomal enzymes, and are excreted as glucuronides. Several agents have active metabolites with potencies equal to or greater than the parent compound, viz., thioridazine is metabolized to mesoridazine, which is more potent than the parent compound, and risperidone is metabolized to paliperidone (9-hydroxyrisperidone), another prescribed atypical agent.

Most antipsychotics are metabolized by CYP2D6 and/or CYP3A4. Chlorpromazine is both a substrate and inhibitor of CYP2D6 and induces its own metabolism, while haloperidol is metabolized by both CYP2D6 and CYP3A4, as are aripiprazole and iloperidone. Quetiapine is metabolized by CYP3A4, whereas risperidone is metabolized by CYP2D6, both to active compounds. Ziprasidone is mainly reduced by aldehyde oxidase but is also oxidized by CYP3A4. Clozapine is

TABLE 16.1 Selected Pharmacokinetic Parameters for Commonly Used Antipsychotics Following Oral Administration

Drug	$t_{1/2}$ (hrs)	Plasma Protein Binding (%)	Active Metabolites	Disposition/ Excretion
Typical Antipsychotics				
Chlorpromazine	8–35	>90		M, R
Fluphenazine	14–24	>90		M, R, B
Haloperidol	12–36	92		M, R, B
Pimozide	50–60	>90		M, R
Thioridazine	6–40	>90	Y	M, R
Thiothixene	30–40	>90		M, R
Atypical Antipsychotics				
Aripiprazole	75–94	>99	Y	M, R, B
Clozapine	4–66	97	Y	M, R, B
Lurasidone	18	>99	Y	M, R, B
Olanzapine	21–54	93		M, R, B
Quetiapine	5–10	83	Y	M, R, B
Risperidone	20–24	90	Y	M, R
Ziprasidone	5–10	>99		M, R, B

B, Biliary; *M*, metabolism; *R*, renal; *Y*, yes.

metabolized primarily by CYPs 1A2, 2C9, and 3A4 and to a lesser extent by CYPs 2C9 and 2D6, with N-desmethylclozapine, an active metabolite. Olanzapine is inactivated by CYP1A2. The half-lives, percent plasma protein binding, active metabolites, and routes of elimination of commonly used antipsychotics following oral administration are shown in Table 16.1.

Depot formulations of some antipsychotics (e.g., aripiprazole, fluphenazine, haloperidol, olanzapine, paliperidone, and risperidone) are available and can be used for maintenance therapy administered intramuscularly at 2- to 4-week intervals. In addition, for patients who have difficulty taking oral medications, risperidone and olanzapine are available as rapidly dissolving oral wafers. Both the risperidone-dissolving wafer and the oral solution provide rapid relief of acute psychotic episodes, as does the intramuscular administration of aripiprazole, ziprasidone, and olanzapine, which are currently the only atypical antipsychotics available in this formulation.

Haloperidol is available in an intravenous form, which is commonly used in intensive care settings. However, because intravenous haloperidol bypasses first-pass metabolism, it is effectively twice as potent as oral haloperidol. In general, once an effective dose is established, a regimen of single-daily oral dosing is effective for symptomatic treatment.

Lithium is most often administered as a carbonate salt but is also administered as a citrate salt. Orally administered lithium is rapidly absorbed and is present as a soluble ion unbound to plasma proteins. Peak plasma concentrations are reached 2–4 hours after an oral dose. Approximately 95% of a single dose is eliminated in the urine, with a half-life of 20–24 hours; steady-state plasma concentrations are reached 5–6 days after initiation of treatment. Approximately 80% of filtered lithium is reabsorbed by the renal proximal tubules.

Lithium has a low therapeutic index; therapeutic levels are 0.6–1.4 mEq/L, and toxicity is manifest at 1.6–2.0 mEq/L. Thus the concentration of lithium in plasma must be monitored routinely to ensure adequate therapeutic levels without toxicity.

TABLE 16.2   Side Effect Profile of Representative Antipsychotic Drugs

Drug	Anticholinergic	Antiadrenergic (α_1)	Antihistaminergic (H_1)
Typical Antipsychotics			
Chlorpromazine	++	++++	+++
Fluphenazine	−	+++	++
Haloperidol	−	+++	−
Pimozide	−	−	−
Thioridazine	+++	++++	−
Thiothixene	−	+++	+++
Atypical Antipsychotics			
Aripiprazole	−	++	++
Asenapine	−	+++	+++
Clozapine	+++	+++	+++
Iloperidone	−	++++	++
Lurasidone	−	++	−
Olanzapine	+++	++	+++
Quetiapine	++	++	+++
Risperidone	−	+++	++
Ziprasidone	−	+++	++

The symbols represent the relative potency of each compound to produce anticholinergic (dry mouth, constipation, cycloplegia), antiadrenergic (sedation, postural hypotension) or antihistaminergic (sedation, weight gain) effects. The highest activity (++++) represents an inhibition constant (K_i) of <1 nM; +++, K_i from 1–10 nM; ++, K_i from 10–100 nM; +, K_i from 100–1000 nM; and −, K_i >1000 nM.

PHARMACOVIGILANCE: ADVERSE EFFECTS AND DRUG INTERACTIONS

Although most antipsychotics are relatively safe, they can elicit a variety of neurological, autonomic, neuroendocrine, and metabolic side effects. Many side effects are an extension of the general pharmacological actions of these drugs and result from blockade of several neurotransmitter receptors (Table 16.2), whereas other side effects are specific to particular compounds. In addition, because most of these agents are metabolized by cytochrome P450s, their plasma levels can be greatly influenced by the concurrent use of other compounds, both enzyme inducers and inhibitors, as well as by pharmacogenomics (Chapters 3 and 4). Both the typical and atypical antipsychotics have a boxed warning indicating an increased risk of mortality in elderly patients treated for dementia-related psychoses.

Typical Antipsychotics

All typical antipsychotics block muscarinic cholinergic receptors, leading to dry mouth, urinary retention, and memory impairment (Chapter 8). These effects are more common with the lower potency agents such as chlorpromazine and thioridazine. They also block α_1-adrenergic and histamine (H_1) receptors, leading to orthostatic hypotension and reflex tachycardia, and sedation, respectively. Blocking DA receptors in the pituitary gland results in elevated prolactin secretion, and this **hyperprolactinemia** may lead to menstrual irregularities in females and breast enlargement and galactorrhea in both sexes. In addition, **thioridazine** and **pimozide** have a propensity to prolong the cardiac QT interval, predisposing to a risk for ventricular arrhythmias. High-dose thioridazine therapy (>800 mg/day) has been associated with the development of retinitis pigmentosa and should be used with caution at all times, whether it is used as monotherapy or with other agents.

Blocking DA receptors in the basal ganglia leads to **acute extrapyramidal symptoms**. Acute **dystonic reactions**, characterized by spasms of the facial or neck muscles, may be evident, as well as a **parkinsonian syndrome** characterized by bradykinesia, rigidity, tremor, shuffling gait, and **akathisia** or motor restlessness. These symptoms occur early (1–60 days) after initiation of drug treatment, improve if the antipsychotic is terminated, and, if severe enough to cause noncompliance, may be treated with centrally active anticholinergic compounds such as those used for Parkinson disease (Chapter 15). In general, the high-potency butyrophenones, such as **haloperidol**, are associated with a greater incidence of extrapyramidal side effects, whereas the low-potency phenothiazines, such as **chlorpromazine**, are associated with a greater incidence of autonomic side effects and sedation.

After months to years of therapy, two late-onset effects may become apparent: **perioral tremor**, characterized by "rabbit-like" facial movements, and **tardive dyskinesia**, characterized by involuntary and excessive movements of the face and extremities, and more common in older women with a history of mood disorder. Severe tardive dyskinesia can be disfiguring and cause impaired feeding and breathing. There is no satisfactory treatment for tardive dyskinesia, and stopping drug treatment may unmask the symptoms, apparently exacerbating the condition. Tardive dyskinesia is thought to result from the hypersensitivity or up regulation of DA receptors that occurs after chronic DA receptor blockade induced by the antipsychotics. Together, clinician and patient must weigh the risks and benefits when considering whether to stop the antipsychotic medication or switch from one atypical to another once symptoms manifest themselves.

An idiosyncratic and potentially lethal effect of the typical antipsychotics is known as **neuroleptic malignant syndrome**, which occurs in 1%–2% of patients and is fatal in almost 10% of those affected. It is most commonly seen in young males recently treated with an intramuscular injection of a typical antipsychotic agent. This syndrome is observed early in treatment and is characterized by a near-complete collapse of the autonomic nervous system, causing fever, muscle rigidity, diaphoresis, and cardiovascular instability. As a consequence of the associated tissue damage, these individuals frequently have elevated blood levels of creatine phosphokinase (CPK). Immediate medical intervention with the DA receptor agonist bromocriptine (Chapter 15) and the skeletal muscle relaxant dantrolene (Chapter 22) is recommended to treat this condition.

Antipsychotics are not the only class of medications that can cause these types of side effects. In fact, any medication with significant

D_2-receptor blockade may induce extrapyramidal symptoms, akathisia, neuroleptic malignant syndrome, and other side effects normally associated with antipsychotics. The antidepressant amoxapine, which is a metabolite of the antipsychotic loxapine, has been associated with the development of extrapyramidal side effects, tardive dyskinesia, and neuroleptic malignant syndrome. In addition, prochlorperazine, metoclopramide, promethazine, and trimethobenzamide, agents used in gastroenterology, can have similar side effects.

Atypical Antipsychotics

The side effect profile of the atypical antipsychotics differs from that of typical antipsychotics. While the typical antipsychotics have a narrow therapeutic window in terms of acute extrapyramidal side effects, clozapine and the newer atypical compounds are associated with a low incidence of these problems, and most do not produce hyperprolactinemia. Risperidone has been associated with increased prolactin levels, which in some cases, especially in women, has been attributed to a drug-induced benign pituitary prolactinoma. Although the atypical compounds are not devoid totally of the ability to induce tardive dyskinesia or neuroleptic malignant syndrome, their incidence is lower than with the typical antipsychotics.

The most prominent side effects of the atypical compounds are metabolic and cardiovascular. Many of these compounds cause substantial weight gain (particularly olanzapine and clozapine) with the development of insulin resistance, leading to the onset of diabetes mellitus, which has been most commonly observed with olanzapine and clozapine. The atypical antipsychotics also increase plasma lipids, with as much as a 10% increase in cholesterol levels. Olanzapine, clozapine, and, to a lesser extent, quetiapine, are the atypical agents most likely to induce hyperlipidemia. Like the typical antipsychotics thioridazine and pimozide, the atypical compounds iloperidone and ziprasidone can increase the cardiac QT interval, predisposing to arrhythmias. Thus these drugs are contraindicated in individuals taking agents that have a similar effect, including some antiarrhythmics (Chapter 45), antimicrobials (Chapters 58 and 59), antidepressants (Chapter 17), and others. Quetiapine is very sedating and has been associated with significant hypotension, especially during the titration phase of treatment.

Clozapine is the only atypical compound that causes agranulocytosis, characterized by leukopenia. Because this condition can be fatal, weekly blood cell counts must be performed for the first 6 months of treatment. After that time, if counts are stable, blood counts are done every other week. The incidence of agranulocytosis with the other atypical antipsychotics is minimal and is no greater than that associated with the use of typical antipsychotics. Clozapine has also been associated with the development of seizures at doses greater than 60 mg daily and has been reported to cause myocarditis or cardiomyopathy that may be fatal. All of these effects are noted in the boxed warnings for clozapine. Clozapine use has also been linked to sialorrhea, which may be due to swallowing difficulties.

Lithium

Numerous side effects occur in patients treated with lithium, most of which involve the central nervous system, thyroid, kidneys, and heart. Subclinical hypothyroidism can develop in patients taking lithium. Although obvious hypothyroidism is rare, a benign, diffuse, nontender thyroid enlargement (goiter), indicative of compromised thyroid function, occurs in some patients. This results from the ability of lithium to interfere with the iodination of tyrosine and, consequently, the synthesis of thyroxine (Chapter 54).

Lithium blocks the responsiveness of the renal collecting tubule epithelium to vasopressin, leading to a nephrogenic diabetes insipidus.

In addition, polydipsia and polyuria are frequent problems, the latter resulting from uncoupling of vasopressin receptors from their G-proteins. It is important to monitor renal function in patients during treatment with lithium.

Lithium can cause substantial weight gain, which may be detrimental to health but also leads to patient noncompliance. Lithium may also cause nausea and diarrhea and daytime drowsiness. All these effects are quite common, even in patients with therapeutic plasma concentrations. Other side effects include allergic reactions, particularly an exacerbation of acne vulgaris or psoriasis. It may also cause a fine hand tremor in some patients.

Lithium is an important human teratogen, and there is evidence of human fetal risk. It has been noted to cause Ebstein anomaly, which is an endocardial cushion defect affecting the walls separating the chambers of the heart. It is also secreted in breast milk, so breastfeeding should be discouraged in mothers receiving lithium.

Potential changes in the plasma concentration of lithium resulting from changes in renal clearance can be dangerous because lithium exhibits a very narrow therapeutic index. The major drug class that poses a problem when administered with lithium is the class of thiazide diuretics, which block Na^+ reabsorption in renal distal tubules. The resulting Na^+ depletion promotes reabsorption of both Na^+ and lithium from proximal tubules, reducing lithium excretion and elevating its plasma concentrations. Similarly, nonsteroidal antiinflammatory agents can decrease lithium clearance and elevate plasma lithium concentrations, leading to lithium toxicity. Difficulties can arise if a patient on lithium becomes dehydrated, as that may also increase serum lithium levels to the toxic range.

Lithium toxicity is related to its absolute plasma concentration and its rate of rise. Symptoms of mild toxicity occur at the peak of lithium absorption and include nausea, vomiting, abdominal pain, diarrhea, sedation, and fine hand tremor. Because lithium is often administered concomitantly with antipsychotics, which may exhibit antinausea effects, it is critical to be aware of the potential of these compounds to mask the initial signs of lithium toxicity. More serious toxicity, which occurs at higher plasma concentrations, produces central effects, including confusion, hyperreflexia, gross tremor, cranial nerve and focal neurological signs, and even convulsions and coma. Cardiac dysrhythmias may also occur, and death can result from severe lithium toxicity.

The adverse effects of the anticonvulsants are discussed in Chapter 21. Those associated with the antipsychotics and lithium are listed in the Clinical Problems Box.

NEW DEVELOPMENTS

The development of new antipsychotic drugs has been a major focus, and numerous atypical compounds have been developed during the past decade. However, 20%–30% of diagnosed schizophrenics remain resistant to all currently available drugs, and currently available agents do not alleviate cognitive impairment, which is a core symptom of this disorder.

Although much attention has focused on the role of DA and 5-HT in schizophrenia, recent studies have begun to focus on glutamatergic neurotransmission. The glutamate NMDA receptor antagonist phencyclidine mimics schizophrenia better than any other compound. The behavioral effects of phencyclidine prompted investigators to postulate a glutamatergic deficiency in the etiology of schizophrenia, and recent studies have demonstrated that partial deletion of the gene encoding these receptors leads to the same behavioral abnormalities observed after phencyclidine. Thus attempts to enhance the activity of the NMDA receptor in schizophrenic patients with glycine or serine, both of which stimulate allosteric sites on the receptor, have resulted in some symptomatic improvement. Recent studies have suggested that muscarinic cholinergic receptors, specifically M_1 and M_4 subtypes, may be efficacious for treating all domains of schizophrenia. The utility of these agents as monotherapy for the disorder will be tested as selective agonists are being developed. The challenge remains to develop drugs that are effective in the schizophrenic population resistant to currently available antipsychotic agents and to improve side effect profiles to enhance patient compliance.

CLINICAL RELEVANCE FOR HEALTHCARE PROFESSIONALS

Treatments for psychoses and bipolar disorder have advanced over the past decade or more, with a significant increase in treatment options available. The second-generation ("atypical") antipsychotics have supplanted the first-generation ("conventional") compounds as the medications of choice for schizophrenia and related psychotic disorders because of some efficacy for the negative symptoms of schizophrenia and less troublesome side effects. Similarly, for bipolar disorder, a wider range of medications that can serve as mood stabilizers are now available, providing clinicians the opportunity to individualize treatments for each patient. As the use of these drugs becomes more widespread, all healthcare professionals in all settings will need to maintain awareness of the particular profiles of each agent.

CLINICAL PROBLEMS

Typical antipsychotics	Chlorpromazine: sedation, postural hypotension, severe sunburns, anticholinergic (constipation, dry mouth, urinary hesitancy)
	Thioridazine and pimozide: prolonged QT interval with risk of ventricular arrhythmias
	Haloperidol and fluphenazine: high propensity to produce extrapyramidal symptoms, tardive dyskinesia, and neuroleptic malignant syndrome
Atypical antipsychotics	Diabetes mellitus/weight gain (clozapine = olanzapine > quetiapine = risperidone), hypercholesterolemia, sedation, seizures and agranulocytosis (clozapine), hyperprolactinemia (risperidone, asenapine), prolonged QT interval, risk of ventricular arrhythmias (iloperidone, ziprasidone)
Lithium	Tremors, mental confusion, decreased seizure threshold, decreased thyroid function, polydipsia, polyuria, induced diabetes insipidus, cardiac dysrhythmias

TRADE NAMES

In addition to generic and fixed-combination preparations, the following trade-named materials are some of the important compounds available in the United States.

Typical (First-Generation) Antipsychotics
Chlorpromazine (Thorazine)
Fluphenazine (Permitil, Prolixin)
Haloperidol (Haldol)
Loxapine (Adasuve, Loxitane)
Perphenazine (Trilafon)
Pimozide (Orap)
Thioridazine (Mellaril)
Thiothixene (Navane)
Trifluoperazine (Stelazine)

Atypical (Second-Generation) Antipsychotics
Aripiprazole (Abilify)
Asenapine (Saphris)
Brexpiprazole (Rexulti)
Cariprazine (Vraylar)
Clozapine (Clozaril, Versacloz, FazaClo)
Iloperidone (Fanapt)
Lurasidone (Latuda)
Olanzapine (Zyprexa)
Paliperidone (Invega)
Pimavanserin (Nuplazid)
Quetiapine (Seroquel)
Risperidone (Risperdal)
Ziprasidone (Geodon)

Drugs for Bipolar Disorder
Carbamazepine (Tegretol, Carbatrol, Equetro)
Lithium (Eskalith, Lithobid)
Lamotrigine (Lamictal)
Olanzapine/fluoxetine (Symbyax)
Valproate/divalproex sodium (Depakene/Depakote)

SELF-ASSESSMENT QUESTIONS

1. A 30-year-old woman was newly diagnosed with bipolar disorder. Her physician reviewed her current medication list before initiating treatment with lithium to ensure that she was not taking any drugs that could alter lithium levels. Drugs that affect which of the following are most likely to increase plasma levels of lithium?
   A. Glomerular filtration.
   B. Bile formation.
   C. Muscarinic receptors.
   D. Tyrosine iodination.
   E. CYP2D6.

2. A 36-year-old man with schizophrenia was prescribed haloperidol 5 years ago and was responding very well. Recently, he developed involuntary facial movements that could only be alleviated by increasing his dose of the medication. This adverse reaction was likely due to which of the following mechanisms?
   A. 5-HT receptor sensitization.
   B. DA receptor sensitization.
   C. Decreased synthesis of 5-HT receptors.
   D. Decreased synthesis of DA receptors.
   E. Uncoupling DA receptors from their G-proteins.

3. A 32-year-old woman with schizophrenia responded very well to the typical antipsychotic medication prescribed to control her hallucinations and delusions, but she was very bothered by the dry mouth she was experiencing. This effect may be attributed to which action?
   A. Antiadrenergic.
   B. Anticholinergic.
   C. Antidopaminergic.
   D. Antihistaminergic.
   E. Antiserotonergic.

4. Blood cell counts are required for individuals prescribed clozapine because this agent can lead to:
   A. Parkinsonian symptoms.
   B. Hyperprolactinemia.
   C. Tardive dyskinesia.
   D. Agranulocytosis.
   E. Akathisia.

5. A 24-year-old woman with schizophrenia presents with negative symptoms of this disorder. Antagonism at which of the following receptors may have the greatest ability to temper her negative symptoms?
   A. Dopamine.
   B. Glutamate.
   C. Muscarinic.
   D. Nicotinic.
   E. Serotonin.

FURTHER READING

Amato D, Vernon AC, Papaleo F. Dopamine, the antipsychotic molecule: a perspective on mechanisms underlying antipsychotic response variability. *Neurosci Biobehav Rev.* 2018;85:146–159.

Jakobsson E, Arguello-Mirando O, Chiu S-W, et al. Towards a unified understanding of lithium action in basic biology and its significance for applied biology. *J Membr Biol.* 2017;50:587–604.

Javitt DC, Spencer KM, Thaker GK, et al. Neurophysiological biomarkers for drug development in schizophrenia. *Nature Rev Drug Disc.* 2008;7:68–83.

Ovenden ES, McGregor NW, Emsley RA, Warnich L. DNA methylation and antipsychotic treatment mechanisms in schizophrenia: progress and future directions. *Prog Neuropsychopharm Biol Psych.* 2017;81:38–49.

WEBSITES

https://www.psychiatry.org/patients-families/schizophrenia/what-is-schizophrenia
This is an excellent website maintained by the American Psychiatric Association and contains resources and links on psychotic disorders and treatment for patients, caregivers, and professionals.

https://www.nimh.nih.gov/index.shtml
This website is maintained by the National Institute of Mental Health and includes much information and links to numerous resources for both professionals and caregivers on signs and symptoms, risk factors, treatments, and therapies for all mental disorders.

Drug Therapy for Depression and Anxiety

Lynn Wecker, Deborah L. Sanchez, and Glenn W. Currier

MAJOR DRUG CLASSES

Antidepressants
  Tricyclic antidepressants
  Serotonin selective reuptake inhibitors
  Norepinephrine selective reuptake inhibitors
  Serotonin/norepinephrine reuptake inhibitors
  Multiaction agents
  Monoamine oxidase inhibitors
Anxiolytics
  Benzodiazepines
  Nonbenzodiazepine anxiolytics

ABBREVIATIONS

CNS	Central nervous system
DA	Dopamine
DAT	Plasma membrane dopamine transporter
5-HT	Serotonin
GABA	γ-Aminobutyric acid
IM	Intramuscular
IV	Intravenous
MAO	Monoamine oxidase
MAOI	Monoamine oxidase inhibitor
NE	Norepinephrine
NET	Plasma membrane norepinephrine transporter
NMDA	Glutamate *N*-methyl-D-aspartate receptor
NRI	Norepinephrine reuptake inhibitor
SERT	Plasma membrane serotonin transporter
SNRI	Serotonin/norepinephrine reuptake inhibitor
SSRI	Serotonin selective reuptake inhibitor
TCA	Tricyclic antidepressant

THERAPEUTIC OVERVIEW

Depression

Depression is a heterogeneous disorder that involves bodily functions, moods, and thoughts. It is characterized by feelings of sadness, anxiety, guilt, and worthlessness; disturbances in sleep and appetite; fatigue and loss of interest in daily activities; and difficulties in concentration. In addition, individuals with depression often experience suicidal thoughts. Symptoms of depression can last for weeks, months, or years, and depression is a major cause of morbidity and mortality. In any given year, nearly 10% of the population (almost 20 million adults in the United States) suffers from a depressive illness, and depression is a factor in more than 40,000 suicides per year in the United States, making it one of the most widespread of all life-threatening disorders. Although depression can affect any age, the current mean age of onset is 25 to 35 years. Of particular concern is the rate of depression and suicide among children, adolescents, and the aged, which is increasing at an alarming pace and often goes unrecognized. Depression is a symptom of many different illnesses and may arise as a result of substance abuse (alcohol, steroids, cocaine, etc.), a medical illness (pancreatic carcinoma, hypothyroidism, etc.), or a major life stress event. However, it may also arise from unknown causes.

Three of the most important psychiatric illnesses that present with depressive symptoms are major depressive disorder (also referred to as unipolar depression), persistent depressive disorder (formerly termed dysthymia), and bipolar disorder (Chapter 16). Major depressive disorder may be totally disabling (interfering with work, sleeping, and eating), and episodes may occur several times during a lifetime. Persistent depressive disorder is less severe and involves long-term chronic symptoms that do not disable totally but keep a person from functioning at his or her highest level. In addition, depression is often associated with comorbid anxiety disorders.

Although the molecular and cellular etiology of depression remains unknown, it is generally accepted that depression involves impaired monoaminergic neurotransmission, leading to alterations in the expression of specific genes. This is supported by studies demonstrating that antidepressants increase the expression of cyclic adenosine monophosphate response element-binding protein (CREB) and brain-derived neurotrophic factor (BNDF), both of which are critical for maintaining normal cell structure in limbic regions of the brain that are targets for monoaminergic projections. In addition, postmortem and imaging studies have demonstrated neuronal loss and shrinkage in the prefrontal cortex and hippocampus in depressed patients, alterations that could be tempered by antidepressants.

Within the past several years, as evidence of adult neurogenesis has become increasingly clear, the idea has emerged that depression may be caused by impaired neurogenesis in the adult hippocampus. Studies have demonstrated that new neurons can proliferate from progenitor cells in the hippocampus, a process impaired by stress and stress hormones such as the glucocorticoids and enhanced by antidepressants. Furthermore, it has been shown that neurogenesis is required for antidepressants to exert their behavioral effects in laboratory animals. Thus impaired monoaminergic transmission in specific brain regions may lead to a decreased expression of transcription or growth factors required for sustaining neurogenesis, dendritic branching, and synaptic connections, resulting in depression.

Major depressive disorder, persistent depressive disorder, and the depression associated with anxiety disorders are treated with compounds classified as antidepressants. These compounds fall into several categories:

- The amine reuptake inhibitors, which include the tricyclic antidepressants (TCAs), the serotonin selective reuptake inhibitors (SSRIs), the norepinephrine reuptake inhibitors (NRIs), and the serotonin/norepinephrine reuptake inhibitors (SNRIs)
- The multiaction agents, representing a heterogeneous group and including agents affecting serotonin (5-HT), norepinephrine (NE), dopamine (DA), and possibly glutamate neurotransmission
- The monoamine oxidase inhibitors (MAOIs)

Although the specific sites of action and neurotransmitter selectivity differ for agents in these categories, these drugs all increase monoaminergic neurotransmission in the brain.

Anxiety

Anxiety disorders affect 19 million adults in the United States. The term anxiety refers to a pervasive feeling of apprehension, characterized by diffuse symptoms such as feelings of helplessness, difficulties concentrating, irritability, and insomnia. Anxiety is also manifest by somatic symptoms including gastrointestinal disturbances, muscle tension, excessive perspiration, tachypnea, tachycardia, nausea, palpitations, and dry mouth.

Anxiety disorders are chronic and relentless, can progress if not treated, and include panic disorder, obsessive-compulsive disorder, social phobia, social anxiety disorder, generalized anxiety disorder, and specific phobias. Although posttraumatic stress disorder was classified as an anxiety disorder for many years, it has been reclassified as a "trauma and stressor-related disorder." Each disorder has its own distinct features, but they are all bound together by the common theme of excessive, irrational fear of impending doom, loss of control, nervousness, and dread. Depression often accompanies anxiety disorders, and when it does, it should be treated.

In many cases, anxiety symptoms may be mild and require little or no treatment. However, at other times, symptoms may be severe enough to cause considerable distress. When patients exhibit anxiety so debilitating that lifestyle, work, and interpersonal relationships are severely impaired, they may require drug treatment. Although these compounds may be of great benefit, concurrent psychological support and counseling are absolute necessities for the treatment of anxiety and cannot be overemphasized.

Both benzodiazepine and nonbenzodiazepine drugs are used to treat anxiety disorders, with the benzodiazepines the most commonly prescribed anxiolytics in the United States. Before the introduction of these compounds in the 1960s, the major drugs used to treat anxiety were primarily sedatives and hypnotics, including barbiturates, compounds with potent respiratory depressant effects that led to a high incidence of overdose and death. Although the benzodiazepines are not devoid of side effects, they have a wide margin of safety, with anxiolytic activity achieved at doses that do not induce clinically significant respiratory depression. The nonbenzodiazepine anxiolytics include buspirone and β-adrenergic receptor antagonists; many antidepressants are also approved for the treatment of anxiety.

The characteristics and treatment of depression and anxiety are summarized in the Therapeutic Overview Box.

MECHANISMS OF ACTION

Antidepressants

The antidepressants have been classified several different ways including structural, chronological, and mechanistic. Chemical structures of representative antidepressants are shown in Fig. 17.1.

THERAPEUTIC OVERVIEW

Depression
Characterized by feelings of sadness, guilt, and worthlessness; may exhibit suicidal ideation
Antidepressants increase aminergic neurotransmission by inhibiting 5-HT, NE, and/or DA reuptake, inhibiting 5-HT or NE catabolism, or other processes, leading to increased neurogenesis in the adult hippocampus, with increased dendritic branching and synaptic density

Anxiety Disorders
Characterized by feelings of apprehension and helplessness with an irrational fear of impending doom
Anxiolytics include the benzodiazepines that increase GABAergic inhibitory neurotransmission in the brain, the anxiolytic buspirone that decreases 5-HT and enhances DA and NE neuronal activity, and several 5-HT and NE reuptake inhibitors
β-Adrenergic receptor antagonists can also be used acutely for performance anxiety

---

Amine Reuptake Inhibitors

The amine reuptake inhibitors interact with and block plasma membrane transporters primarily for NE (NET) or 5-HT (SERT), thereby prolonging activation of postsynaptic NE or 5-HT receptors, respectively (Fig. 17.2). Based on the inhibitory constants of these agents to block the transporters, these compounds have been classified as SSRIs, NRIs, or SNRIs.

The TCAs were the first group of antidepressants developed in the 1950s, with the prototypical compound imipramine the first agent demonstrated to have antidepressant efficacy. The TCAs have a three-ring structure with a side chain containing a tertiary or secondary amine attached to the central ring (see Fig. 17.1), resembling the phenothiazine antipsychotics. This group of agents includes the primary amines amitriptyline, clomipramine, doxepin, and imipramine, and the secondary amines desipramine and nortriptyline. Most of these compounds have similar inhibitory activity at NET and SERT, whereas clomipramine is somewhat selective for SERT and desipramine for NET (Table 17.1); the TCAs do not affect DA reuptake.

Drugs developed as SSRIs include citalopram (a racemic mixture), escitalopram (the S-enantiomer of citalopram), fluoxetine, fluvoxamine, paroxetine, and sertraline. It is important to keep in mind, however, that specificity and selectivity are always dose related such that paroxetine and sertraline inhibit both 5-HT and NE reuptake at the upper end of their dose ranges. NET selective compounds (NRIs) include atomoxetine, maprotiline, and reboxetine, while agents with relatively high affinity for both NET and SERT (SNRIs) include amoxapine, duloxetine, and venlafaxine.

In addition to inhibiting NE and 5-HT reuptake, the reuptake inhibitors block muscarinic cholinergic receptors, α_1-adrenergic receptors, and histamine H_1 receptors to a variable extent (Table 17.2), actions that underlie many of the side effects of these compounds.

Multiaction Agents

The multiaction compounds, often referred to as atypical antidepressants, represent a very heterogeneous group and include bupropion, mirtazapine, nefazodone, trazodone, and vortioxetine.

Bupropion inhibits both NET and the DA transporter (DAT). It also increases the activity of the vesicular monoamine transporter-2 (VMAT2), which is responsible for transporting DA from the cytosol into the synaptic vesicle and is a noncompetitive antagonist at several

Tricyclic antidepressants (TCAs)

Serotonin selective reuptake inhibitors (SSRIs)

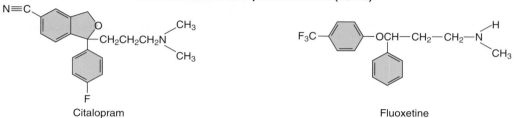

Norepinephrine selective reuptake inhibitors (NRIs)

Serotonin/norepinephrine reuptake inhibitors (SNRIs)

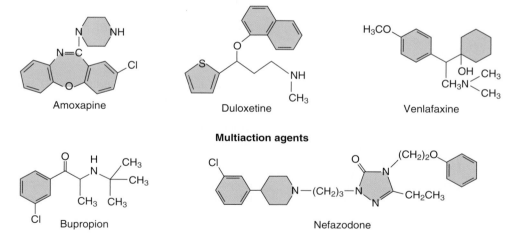

Multiaction agents

Monoamine oxidase inhibitors (MAOIs)

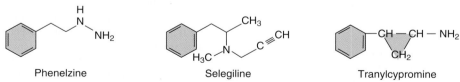

FIG. 17.1 Structures of Representative Antidepressants.

NE neuron

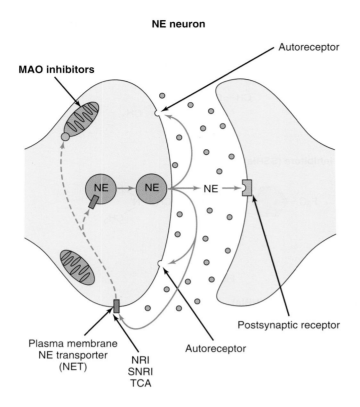

5-HT neuron

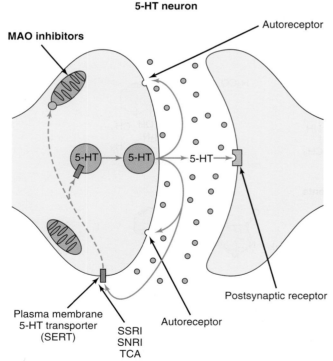

FIG. 17.2 A Noradrenergic and Serotonergic Synapse and Sites at Which Antidepressants May Exert Their Actions. TCAs, SSRIs, NRIs, SNRIs, and some multiaction antidepressants inhibit the reuptake transporters for NE (NET), 5-HT (SERT), or both. Monoamine oxidase (MAO), which is targeted by MAO inhibitors, is localized at the outer mitochondrial membrane. *NRIs,* Norepinephrine reuptake inhibitors; *SNRIs,* serotonin/norepinephrine reuptake inhibitors; *SSRIs,* serotonin selective reuptake inhibitors; *TCAs,* tricyclic antidepressants.

TABLE 17.1 **Relative Selectivity of Amine Reuptake Inhibitors**			
	NET	**SERT**	**DAT**
Tricyclic Antidepressants (TCAs)			
Amitriptyline	++	+++	−
Clomipramine	++	++++	−
Desipramine	++++	++	−
Doxepin	++	++	−
Imipramine	++	+++	−
Nortriptyline	+++	++	−
Serotonin Selective Reuptake Inhibitors (SSRIs)			
Citalopram	−	+++	−
Escitalopram	−	+++	−
Fluoxetine	+	++++	−
Fluvoxamine	−	+++	−
Paroxetine	++	++++	+
Sertraline	+	++++	++
Norepinephrine Selective Reuptake Inhibitors (NRIs)			
Atomoxetine	+++	++	−
Maprotiline	++	−	+
Reboxetine	+++	++	−
Serotonin/Norepinephrine Reuptake Inhibitors (SNRIs)			
Amoxapine	++	++	−
Duloxetine	++	+++	−
Venlafaxine	+	+++	−

The symbols represent the relative potency of each compound to inhibit the reuptake of the amines. The highest activity (++++) represents an inhibition constant (K_i) of <1 nM; +++, K_i from 1–10 nM; ++, K_i from 10–100 nM; +, K_i from 100–1000 nM; and −, K_i >1000 nM. *DAT,* Dopamine transporter; *NET,* norepinephrine transporter; *SERT,* serotonin transporter.

neuronal nicotinic receptors, including $\alpha 4\beta 2$-and $\alpha 3\beta 2$-receptors and, to a lesser extent, $\alpha 7$-receptors.

Mirtazapine blocks α_2-adrenergic receptors on noradrenergic and serotonergic nerve terminals and on noradrenergic dendrites (Fig. 17.3). Stimulation of α_2-autoreceptors on noradrenergic neurons decreases NE release, whereas stimulation of α_2-heteroreceptors on serotonergic neurons inhibits 5-HT release. In addition, stimulation of α_1-adrenergic receptors on serotonergic cell bodies and dendrites increases their firing rate. Thus mirtazapine, by inhibiting α_2-autoreceptors, enhances noradrenergic cell firing and the release of NE, which activates α_1-adrenergic receptors to increase 5-HT release while concurrently blocking α_2-heteroreceptors, further facilitating the release of 5-HT. Mirtazapine also blocks 5-HT_{2A} receptors with high potency.

Trazodone and **nefazodone** both inhibit amine reuptake, with trazodone more selective for SERT and nefazodone more selective for NET. In addition, these drugs block 5-HT_{2A} receptors with high potency and are at least fivefold more potent in vitro as 5-HT_{2A} receptor antagonists than SERT or NET inhibitors. These receptors are widely distributed throughout the brain in regions containing 5-HT nerve terminals, with stimulation leading to depolarization. Interestingly, chronic antagonism of these receptors leads to their paradoxical down regulation, although the role of this mechanism in mediating the antidepressant actions of these compounds remains to be elucidated.

Vortioxetine is a relatively new agent that blocks SERT but is also an agonist at presynaptic 5-HT_{1A} receptors; an antagonist at 5-HT_3,

TABLE 17.2 Activity of Representative Antidepressants at Muscarinic, Adrenergic, and Histaminergic Receptors

Compound	Anticholinergic	Antiadrenergic (α_1)	Antihistaminergic (H_1)
Tricyclic Antidepressants (TCAs)			
Amitriptyline	++	++	+++
Clomipramine	++	++	++
Desipramine	+	+	++
Doxepin	++	++	++++
Imipramine	+	++	+++
Nortriptyline	+	++	+++
Serotonin Selective Reuptake Inhibitors (SSRIs)			
Citalopram	−	−	+
Escitalopram	−	−	+
Fluoxetine	−	−	−
Fluvoxamine	−	−	−
Paroxetine	++	−	+
Sertraline	+	+	−
Norepinephrine Selective Reuptake Inhibitors (NRIs)			
Atomoxetine	−	−	−
Maprotiline	+	++	+++
Reboxetine	−	−	+
Serotonin/Norepinephrine Reuptake Inhibitors (SNRIs)			
Amoxapine	+	++	++
Duloxetine	−	−	−
Venlafaxine	−	−	−
Multiaction Agents			
Bupropion	−	−	−
Mirtazapine	+	+	++++
Nefazodone	−	++	++
Trazodone	−	++	+

The symbols represent the relative potency of each compound to produce anticholinergic (dry mouth, constipation, cycloplegia), antiadrenergic (postural hypotension), or antihistaminergic (sedation, weight gain) effects. The highest activity (++++) represents an inhibition constant (K_i) of <1 nM; +++, K_i from 1 to 10 nM; ++, K_i from 10 to 100 nM; +, K_i from 100 to 1000 nM; and −, K_i >1000 nM.

5-HT$_{1D}$, and 5-HT$_7$ receptors; and a partial agonist at 5-HT$_{1B}$ receptors. The contribution of these actions to the antidepressant efficacy of this compound is not yet understood.

Although ketamine and esketamine (the S-enantiomer of ketamine) are not approved for depression at the time of preparation of this chapter, it is expected that esketamine will obtain approval for the treatment of depression with suicidal ideation in 2018. Ketamine, which is used for anesthesia (Chapter 26), is an antagonist at glutamate N-methyl-D-aspartate (NMDA) receptors. It also has weak agonist activity at opioid μ and κ receptors (Chapter 28), is an antagonist at D$_2$-receptors, and blocks both Na$^+$ and Ca^{++} channels. Esketamine appears somewhat more selective as a noncompetitive and subtype-selective NMDA receptor antagonist.

Monoamine Oxidase Inhibitors

The MAOIs used for the treatment of depression include phenelzine, tranylcypromine, isocarboxazid, and the selegiline transdermal patch (see Fig. 17.1). Phenelzine, selegiline, and isocarboxazid are irreversible MAO inhibitors, and tranylcypromine is a long-lasting MAO inhibitor. At the doses used for depression, all these compounds are nonselective and inhibit both MAO-A and MAO-B. These enzymes are distinct gene products, with MAO-A present in human placenta, intestinal mucosa, liver, and brain, and MAO-B present in human platelets, liver, and brain. MAO-A catabolizes 5-HT, NE, and tyramine, whereas MAO-B catabolizes predominantly DA and tyramine. These enzymes are located in the outer membrane of mitochondria (see Fig. 17.2) and function to maintain low cytoplasmic concentrations of the monoamines, facilitating inward-directed transporter activity (i.e., monoamine reuptake). MAO inhibition causes an increase in monoamine concentrations in the cytosol of the nerve terminal. All the effects of the MAOIs have been attributed to enhanced aminergic activity resulting from enzyme inhibition.

Research with selective MAOIs has shown that inhibition of MAO-A is necessary for antidepressant activity. Thus although selegiline is a selective inhibitor of MAO-B at low doses and is used at these doses for the treatment of Parkinson disease (Chapter 15), selectivity is lost at the higher doses required for antidepressant activity, with selegiline inhibiting both MAO-A and MAO-B at these doses.

Anxiolytics

Anxiety may be treated with the benzodiazepines, buspirone, β-adrenergic antagonists such as propranolol, and several antidepressants. Structures of representative benzodiazepines, buspirone, and propranolol are shown in Fig. 17.4.

Benzodiazepines

The **benzodiazepines** are **positive allosteric modulators (PAMs)** of the γ-aminobutyric acid type A (GABA$_A$) receptor that increase the effect of GABA but have no effect in the absence of agonist. GABA$_A$ receptors are pentameric ligand-gated ion channels, and stimulation of these receptors by GABA leads to the influx of Cl$^-$ and a resultant hyperpolarization of the postsynaptic cell (Chapter 2). This hyperpolarization renders the cell less likely to fire in response to an incoming excitatory stimulus, thus mediating the inhibitory effects of GABA throughout the central nervous system (CNS).

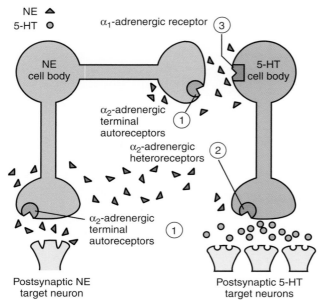

FIG. 17.3 Receptor Mechanisms Controlling Norepinephrine and 5-Serotonin Release. (1) Stimulation of α_2-adrenergic autoreceptors on NE nerve terminals decreases NE release by a negative feedback process. (2) Stimulation of α_2-adrenergic heteroreceptors on 5-HT nerve terminals decreases 5-HT release. (3) Stimulation of α_1-adrenergic receptors on 5-HT dendrites and perikarya increases the firing of 5-HT neurons. Thus a drug that blocks α_2- but not α_1-adrenergic receptors increases NE and 5-HT release. *5-HT,* Serotonin; *NE,* norepinephrine.

GABA$_A$ receptors contain orthosteric binding sites for GABA, allosteric sites that can be occupied to modify the interaction of GABA with the receptor, and additional sites that can be occupied by other compounds to activate or block the receptor, as depicted in Fig. 17.5 and listed in Table 17.3. Benzodiazepines bind to one of these modulatory sites, often referred to as the benzodiazepine binding site or benzodiazepine receptor. When benzodiazepines bind to the benzodiazepine binding site, they induce a conformational change in the receptor, resulting in an increased frequency of chloride ion channel opening upon stimulation of the receptor by GABA. **Barbiturates** bind to another allosteric site, while compounds such as the poison picrotoxin bind to other sites on the receptor.

The β-carbolines, such as harmine and harmaline, which occur widely throughout the plant and animal kingdoms, also interact with the benzodiazepine binding site. However, when these compounds bind, they allosterically reduce Cl$^-$ conductance by decreasing the affinity of GABA for its binding site. Because the β-carbolines increase CNS excitability and may produce anxiety and precipitate panic attacks, effects opposite to those of the benzodiazepines, they are called **inverse agonists** (Chapter 2). The inverse agonists block the effects of the benzodiazepines but have no therapeutic use. Rather, they are thought to be responsible for the psychedelic properties of some plant species.

Flumazenil is a **competitive antagonist** that binds to the benzodiazepine site on the GABA$_A$ receptor. As a competitive antagonist, flumazenil occupies the benzodiazepine site with high affinity but does not have the ability to activate it and does not affect GABA-mediated Cl$^-$ influx. Rather, flumazenil competitively antagonizes the actions of the benzodiazepines and is used therapeutically to treat benzodiazepine overdose. Flumazenil also competitively antagonizes the effects of the inverse agonists and the benzodiazepine receptor agonists because they also bind at the same allosteric site.

Nonbenzodiazepine Anxiolytics

Buspirone is unrelated chemically to the benzodiazepines or the barbiturates. It is as effective as the benzodiazepines as an anxiolytic but does not have anticonvulsant, muscle relaxant, or sedative effects. Buspirone is a partial agonist at serotonin 5-HT$_{1A}$ receptors on presynaptic neurons in the dorsal raphe nucleus and on postsynaptic neurons in the hippocampus, actions that decrease the firing rate of dorsal raphe neurons and may mediate the anxiolytic effects of this compound. Buspirone also increases the firing rate of NE neurons in the locus

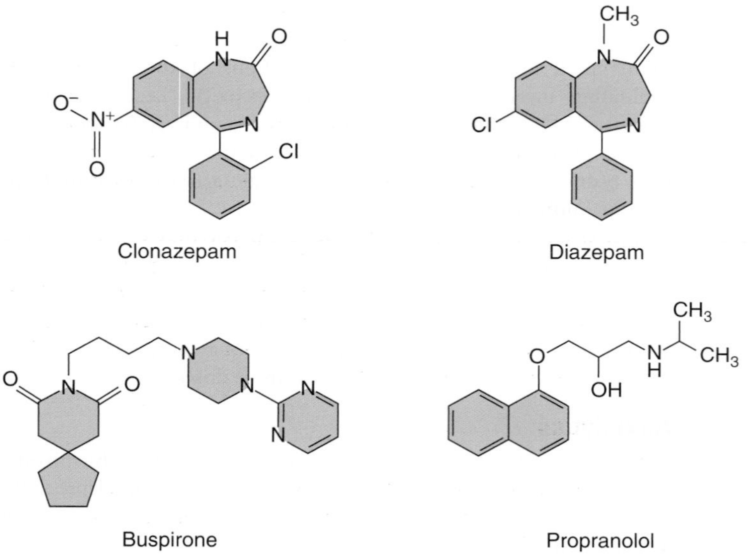

FIG. 17.4 Structures of Representative Benzodiazepines, Buspirone, and Propranolol.

Clonazepam

Diazepam

Buspirone

Propranolol

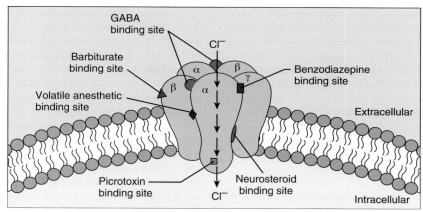

FIG. 17.5 The GABA_A Receptor. The GABA_A receptor is a membrane-associated protein composed of five subunits surrounding a Cl⁻ channel. Shown are the relative locations of binding sites for GABA, benzodiazepines, barbiturates, volatile anesthetics, neurosteroids, and picrotoxin.

TABLE 17.3 Agents Affecting the GABA_A Receptor

Site of Action	Compound	Mechanism	Action
GABA binding site	GABA, muscimol	Agonist	Promotes Cl⁻ influx, hyperpolarization
	Bicuculline	Competitive antagonist	Blocks effects of agonist
Benzodiazepine binding site	Benzodiazepines	Allosteric agonist	Potentiates effects of GABA
	β-Carboline	Allosteric inverse agonist	Inhibits effects of GABA and the benzodiazepines
	Flumazenil	Competitive antagonist	Blocks effects of the benzodiazepines
	Eszopiclone, zaleplon, zolpidem	Benzodiazepine receptor agonists	Potentiates effects of GABA at specific receptor subtypes
Barbiturate binding site	Barbiturate	Allosteric agonist	Potentiates effects of GABA
Cl⁻ channel	Picrotoxin	Noncompetitive antagonist	Blocks Cl⁻ influx

coeruleus and has moderate affinity for DA type 2 (D_2) receptors, but the relationship between anxiety and dopaminergic activity is unclear. Buspirone has no affinity for either GABA or benzodiazepine binding sites on GABA_A receptors.

The β-adrenergic receptor antagonists, such as **propranolol** (Chapter 12), are useful for the short-term relief of anxiety, such as for the treatment of performance anxiety. These agents are competitive antagonists at all β-adrenergic receptors and suppress the sympathetically mediated somatic and autonomic symptoms of anxiety.

RELATIONSHIP OF MECHANISMS OF ACTION TO CLINICAL RESPONSE

Depression

Currently available antidepressants significantly improve symptoms in 50%–65% of patients. The mood-elevating properties of antidepressants are associated with a blunting or amelioration of the depressive state, such that there is an improvement in all signs and symptoms of depression, although rates of improvement of individual symptoms may differ. A major problem, however, is that it takes several weeks for the maximal therapeutic benefit of these compounds to become apparent. This limitation is particularly disturbing given the potential for depressed patients to commit suicide, underscoring the clinical importance of esketamine for immediate treatment. Esketamine was granted a "breakthrough therapy designation" by the United States Food and Drug Administration in 2013 for treatment-resistant depression and in 2016 for depression with an imminent risk for suicide.

Although the antidepressants facilitate monoaminergic transmission immediately, their therapeutic efficacy may not be evident for several weeks. This apparent temporal discrepancy may be explained by the antidepressant-induced increase in neurogenesis and dendritic sprouting in the hippocampus, which is not immediate and which may underlie the therapeutic efficacy of these agents. Studies have suggested that depression may involve an impairment of these processes, which can be reversed by all classes of antidepressants. In addition, the repeated administration of many antidepressants produces several adaptive changes in the brain, particularly at serotonergic and noradrenergic receptors. For example, studies have shown that acute administration of the SSRIs stimulates both somatodendritic and terminal autoreceptors on serotonergic neurons to decrease firing and inhibit 5-HT release. However, chronic administration of the SSRIs down regulates or desensitizes these autoreceptors, producing a disinhibition, thereby promoting neuronal firing and 5-HT release. Similarly, several other agents reduce responses elicited by activation of central β-adrenergic receptors and decrease their density after chronic administration. Because these and other adaptive changes induced by antidepressants take weeks to develop, it is likely that antidepressant-induced neuroplasticity is crucial to the clinical efficacy of these drugs.

Because of the frequency of recurrences of depression, attention has focused on whether antidepressants can prevent recurrences, and if so, for how long these agents should be prescribed. Eighty percent of recurrently depressed patients maintained for 3 years on the same dose of imipramine used to treat their initial acute episode had no recurrence of a serious depressive episode. Prophylactic effects of other antidepressants have been described as well. Studies have reported that

50% of patients who have a depressive episode will have a recurrence. Of patients who have two depressive episodes, 70% will have a third episode. If a patient has three depressive episodes, there is a 90% chance there will be another. Therefore if a patient has three depressive episodes, he or she should remain on long-term antidepressant therapy. If the patient has two severe episodes (reaching psychotic proportions or the patient becomes suicidal), the clinician should consider maintaining the patient on long-term antidepressant therapy at that time. However, it is not yet clear when, if ever, patients can be taken off long-term maintenance treatment without the risk of recurrence of a depressive episode.

Anxiety

Anxiety is managed effectively with the benzodiazepines, particularly **alprazolam**, **lorazepam**, and **clonazepam**. Their intermittent use for acute attacks or limited long-term use (4–8 weeks) for recurring symptoms is often beneficial. However, all benzodiazepines should be used cautiously in patients with a history of addiction or more chronic and severe emotional disturbances. Panic attacks respond favorably to **alprazolam**, which has been shown to possess antidepressant activity similar to that of the TCAs, which are also used for the treatment of panic attacks. A debilitating anxiety caused by another illness can be controlled by short-term treatment with anxiolytic drugs while treatment for the primary condition is implemented.

Due to their ability to produce sedation and anterograde amnesia and reduce the anxiety, stress, and tension associated with surgical or diagnostic procedures, benzodiazepines are used both as **preanesthetic medications** and for **induction** and **maintenance of anesthesia** (Chapter 26). For procedures that do not require anesthesia, such as endoscopy, cardioversion, cardiac catheterization, specific radiodiagnostic procedures, and reduction of minor fractures, benzodiazepines may be administered orally, intramuscularly (IM), or intravenously (IV).

The benzodiazepines produce skeletal muscle relaxation by inhibiting polysynaptic reflexes. However, most evidence suggests that with the exception of diazepam, skeletal muscle relaxation occurs only with doses of the benzodiazepines that have significant CNS depressant effects. **Diazepam** has a direct depressant effect on monosynaptic reflex pathways in the spinal cord and thus produces skeletal muscle relaxation at doses that do not induce sedation. This effect renders diazepam of benefit for **relief of skeletal muscle spasms**, spasticity, and athetosis.

In addition to these major indications, the benzodiazepines are used for the treatment of **alcohol withdrawal**. Because the benzodiazepines exhibit cross-tolerance with alcohol, have anticonvulsant activity, and do not have major respiratory depressant effects, they have become drugs of choice for treatment of acute alcohol withdrawal symptoms (Chapter 23). In particular, **chlordiazepoxide**, **lorazepam**, and **diazepam** have now replaced other drugs for this purpose. Choosing between these medications for alcohol withdrawal is often based on metabolic considerations. If a patient has hepatic impairment, lorazepam is often preferred to treat the symptoms of alcohol withdrawal because it is metabolized in both liver and kidney. If hepatic dysfunction is not an issue, the use of drugs metabolized primarily by the liver (such as chlordiazepoxide and diazepam) would be appropriate.

Although all benzodiazepines act at benzodiazepine-binding sites on $GABA_A$ receptors, they differ in their pharmacological profiles. For example, some anxiolytic benzodiazepines are nonsedating, whereas other benzodiazepines are used selectively for their sedative properties. Similarly, the incidence of muscle relaxation differs among compounds, and not all benzodiazepines have anticonvulsant activity. Such differences may be attributed to two primary factors: the specific subunit composition of the $GABA_A$ receptor involved and the nature of the interaction of the benzodiazepine with its binding site.

Current evidence indicates that multiple $GABA_A$ receptors exist in the brain. These receptors have different subunit compositions and different anatomical distributions. Studies have shown that receptors containing α_2, α_3, and/or α_5 subunits may mediate anxiolytic and muscle relaxant effects of the benzodiazepines, whereas receptors containing α_1 subunits may mediate the sedative and motor effects, as well as contribute to the abuse potential of these agents. In addition to receptor subtype selectivity, the divergent pharmacological and behavioral profiles of the benzodiazepines may be explained on the basis of differences in intrinsic efficacy. The benzodiazepines exhibit a broad range of intrinsic efficacies, and studies have shown that partial agonists with anxiolytic and anticonvulsant activities are nonsedating and do not cause muscle relaxation. Thus as we learn more about benzodiazepine receptor subtypes and the nature of the interactions between these receptors and drugs, therapeutic compounds with selective and specific pharmacological and behavioral profiles may be developed.

As indicated, β-adrenergic receptor antagonists such as **propranolol** are useful for the treatment of performance anxiety, or "stage fright," and suppress the somatic and autonomic symptoms of anxiety but do not alter emotional symptoms. Interestingly, the α_2-adrenergic receptor agonist clonidine has also been reported to have anxiolytic properties.

PHARMACOKINETICS

Antidepressants

Pharmacokinetic parameters of representative antidepressants are presented in Table 17.4. In general, antidepressants are readily absorbed, primarily in the small intestine, and undergo significant first-pass hepatic metabolism. Peak plasma concentrations are achieved within hours after ingestion, with steady-state concentrations achieved after 4–7 days at a fixed dose.

Most agents are extensively bound to plasma proteins, are oxidized by hepatic microsomal enzymes to inactive metabolites, and are excreted in the urine as glucuronides or sulfates. A small amount may be excreted in the feces via the bile. Some antidepressants are metabolized to active compounds, which themselves have antidepressant efficacy. For example, **fluoxetine**, **nefazodone**, and **trazodone** are metabolized relatively rapidly into active compounds with varying half-lives. In addition, **desipramine** and **nortriptyline** are major metabolites of **imipramine** and **amitriptyline**, respectively. Some metabolites have properties similar to those of the parent compounds, which may contribute to their antidepressant activity.

Ketamine is readily absorbed following oral, IV, and IM administration. Following oral administration, peak plasma levels are achieved within 30 minutes. Ketamine is metabolized primarily by CYP3A4 to N-demethylketamine (norketamine), which is active and may contribute to the pharmacological activity of ketamine. The duration of action following oral administration is 4–6 hours, and both parent and metabolites are excreted in the urine. **Esketamine** is typically administered IV or IM, with current investigations on both inhaled and intranasal delivery.

The MAOIs **phenelzine**, **isocarboxazid**, and **tranylcypromine** are absorbed readily after oral administration, and maximal inhibition of MAO occurs in 5–10 days. The binding of these compounds to MAO leads to their cleavage to active products (hydrazines), which are inactivated primarily by acetylation. Because acetylation depends on genotype, **slow acetylators** may exhibit an exaggerated effect when given these compounds.

The transdermal administration of **selegiline** increases systemic delivery of drug because it does not undergo first-pass metabolism. After transdermal absorption, selegiline is metabolized by several hepatic CYP enzymes, and metabolites are excreted in the urine.

TABLE 17.4 Pharmacokinetic Parameters of Representative Antidepressant Drugs

Compound	Elimination t$_{1/2}$ (hrs)	Plasma Protein Binding (%)	Disposition/ Elimination
Tricyclic Antidepressants (TCAs)			
Amitriptyline	9–25	90–95	M, R
Clomipramine	19–37	97	M, R, B
Desipramine	14–24	90–95	M, R
Doxepin	6–24.5	80	M, R
Imipramine	6–18	90	M, R
Nortriptyline	18–38	90	M, R
Serotonin Selective Reuptake Inhibitors (SSRIs)			
Citalopram	35	80	M, R
Escitalopram	27–32	56	M, R
Fluoxetine	1–3 days (acute) 4–6 days (chronic)	95	M, R
Fluvoxamine	15–20	80	M, R
Paroxetine	20	95	M, R, B
Sertraline	26	98	M, R, B
Norepinephrine Selective Reuptake Inhibitors (NRIs)			
Atomoxetine	5	98	M, R
Maprotiline	51	88	M, R, B
Reboxetine	12.5	98	M, R
Serotonin/Norepinephrine Reuptake Inhibitors (SNRIs)			
Amoxapine	8	90	M, R
Duloxetine	12	>90	M, R, B
Venlafaxine	3–4	30	M, R
Multiaction Agents			
Bupropion	14	85	M, R, B
Mirtazapine	20–40	85	M, R, B
Nefazodone	3–4	>99	M, R
Trazodone	4–8	90–95	M, R

B, Biliary; *M*, metabolism; *R*, renal.

TABLE 17.5 Pharmacokinetic Parameters for Representative Benzodiazepines After Oral Administration

Drug	Onset of Action[a]	t$_{1/2}$[b]
Alprazolam	Intermediate	Intermediate
Chlordiazepoxide	Intermediate	Long
Clorazepate	Rapid	Long
Diazepam[c]	Rapid	Long
Flurazepam	Rapid	Long
Halazepam	Intermediate	Long
Lorazepam[c]	Intermediate	Intermediate
Oxazepam	Slow	Short
Prazepam	Slow	Long
Temazepam	Slow	Intermediate
Triazolam	Rapid	Short

[a]Rapid = 15–30 min; intermediate = 30–45 min; slow = 45–90 min.
[b]Short, <10 hours; intermediate, 10–36 hours; long >48 hours.
[c]Also administered by injection.

Because phenelzine, selegiline, and isocarboxazid inhibit MAO irreversibly and tranylcypromine inhibits it persistently but noncovalently, the biological effects of these compounds outlast their physical presence in the body; that is, a loss of enzyme activity persists after the drugs are metabolized and eliminated. New enzymes must be synthesized for MAO activity to return to normal, a process that takes several weeks.

Anxiolytics

In general, the benzodiazepines are well absorbed after oral administration and reach peak blood and brain concentrations within 1–2 hours. Clorazepate is an exception because it is the only benzodiazepine that is rapidly converted in the stomach to the active product N-desmethyldiazepam. The rate of conversion of clorazepate is inversely proportional to gastric pH.

Whereas the benzodiazepines are typically taken orally, diazepam, chlordiazepoxide, and lorazepam are available for IM and IV injection. Lorazepam is well absorbed after IM injection, but absorption of diazepam and chlordiazepoxide is poor and erratic after this route of administration and should be avoided. When administered IV as an anticonvulsant or for induction of anesthesia, diazepam enters the brain rapidly and is redistributed to peripheral tissues, providing CNS

depression for less than 2 hours. In contrast, lorazepam is less lipid soluble and depresses brain function for as long as 8 hours after IV injection.

The duration of action and plasma protein binding of the benzodiazepines varies considerably, with the formation of active metabolites playing a major role in the effects of these compounds (Table 17.5). The benzodiazepines and their active metabolites are highly bound to plasma proteins, with diazepam exhibiting the greatest binding (99%) and alprazolam the lowest (70%). The distribution of diazepam and other benzodiazepines is complicated somewhat by a considerable degree of biliary excretion, which occurs early in distribution. This enterohepatic recirculation occurs with both metabolites and parent compounds and may be important clinically for compounds with a long elimination half-life. The presence of food in the upper bowel delays reabsorption and contributes to the late resurgence of plasma drug levels and activity.

The benzodiazepines are metabolized extensively by hepatic microsomal enzymes, including CYP3A4 and CYP2C19 (Fig. 17.6). The major biotransformation reactions are N-dealkylation and aliphatic hydroxylation, followed by conjugation to inactive glucuronides that are excreted in the urine. The long-acting benzodiazepines clorazepate, diazepam, chlordiazepoxide, prazepam, and halazepam are dealkylated to the active compound N-desmethyldiazepam (nordiazepam). This compound has an elimination half-life of 30–200 hours and is responsible for the long duration of action of these compounds. N-desmethyldiazepam is hydroxylated to oxazepam, which is glucuronidated and excreted in the urine. Alprazolam undergoes hydroxylation by CYP3A4 followed by glucuronidation, and lorazepam is directly glucuronidated.

Flurazepam is a long-acting drug that is converted to desalkylflurazepam, a long-acting active metabolite. Relatively little flurazepam and desalkylflurazepam are excreted unchanged in urine because they are biotransformed in the liver. Hence, their elimination half-lives are long in young adults and even longer in older patients and those with hepatic disease.

The nonbenzodiazepine anxiolytic buspirone is rapidly absorbed and undergoes extensive first-pass metabolism. It is highly bound to plasma proteins (>90%) and oxidized by CYP3A4 to an active metabolite. The elimination half-life is approximately 2–3 hours, and less than 50% of the drug is excreted in the urine unchanged.

The pharmacokinetics of propranolol are discussed in Chapter 12.

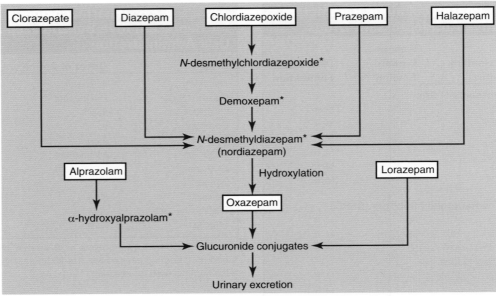

FIG. 17.6 Major Metabolic Interrelationships Among the Benzodiazepines. *Active metabolite.

PHARMACOVIGILANCE: ADVERSE EFFECTS AND DRUG INTERACTIONS

Antidepressants

Many of the most common side effects of the TCAs and multiaction antidepressants result from their antagonist actions at muscarinic cholinergic, α_1-adrenergic, and H_1 histaminergic receptors, leading to atropine-like effects including dry mouth, constipation, and cycloplegia, prazosin-like effects such as orthostatic hypotension, and marked sedative effects, respectively (Table 17.2). As a group, these drugs are more potent at blocking H_1 than either muscarinic or α_1-adrenergic receptors, but several agents have fairly marked anticholinergic activity at clinical doses. The antihistaminergic, antimuscarinic, and antiadrenergic side effects of the antidepressants are especially bothersome in aged patients, with postural hypotension a particularly severe problem because it can lead to falls and broken bones. Clinically, amitriptyline has the most pronounced orthostatic hypotensive effect.

Several of the amine reuptake inhibitors affect the heart through a combination of anticholinergic activity, inhibition of amine reuptake, and direct depressant effects. Although these effects may be manifested by mild tachycardia, conduction disturbances and electrocardiographic changes can occur. The quinidine-like depressant effects on the myocardium can precipitate slowing of atrioventricular conduction or bundle-branch block or premature ventricular contractions. These effects are much more common in patients with preexisting cardiac problems. Abnormalities of cardiac conduction occur in less than 5% of patients receiving therapeutic doses, with most being clinically insignificant. There have been several cases (some fatal) of citalopram-induced cardiac conduction delay in patients who have taken an overdose of this compound. One of citalopram's metabolites is cardiotoxic, and when patients take an overdose, this metabolite increases enough to cause changes in the electrocardiogram and clinical symptoms. Therefore citalopram and escitalopram should not be a first-line agent in patients with preexisting cardiac disease.

These agents can lower seizure thresholds and are potentially epileptogenic. This is a particularly pronounced problem with maprotiline and bupropion, especially in patients receiving high doses. In fact, bupropion is contraindicated for use in any patient with a history of seizures. By contrast, the incidence of seizures is very low in patients receiving mirtazapine, nefazodone, trazodone, the SSRIs, or other amine reuptake inhibitors.

Toxicity of the CNS can produce delirium, especially in the aged, which is easily recognizable. Such delirium is usually preceded by what appears to be a worsening of depression, which may lead to administration of increased drug doses, with further worsening of the delirium. Antimuscarinic activity correlates with the delirium, which can be reversed in hospitalized patients with the cholinesterase inhibitor physostigmine. The incidence of insomnia, nervousness, restlessness, and anxiety appears to be relatively high in patients taking fluoxetine. It has an activating effect that can be anxiogenic in some patients and should be started at a lower dose in those with an anxiety component to their illness.

Sexual dysfunction, including abnormal ejaculation, anorgasmia, impotence, and decreased libido, are receiving increasing attention in patients receiving antidepressants. These effects occur at least as frequently in patients treated with TCAs or MAOIs as in patients receiving SSRIs. There appears to be little impairment of sexual function in patients treated with bupropion or mirtazapine and perhaps nefazodone. However, care must be taken because nefazodone has been associated with the development of priapism, along with the structurally similar trazodone.

Several extensive retrospective analyses have indicated no association between amine reuptake inhibitor or multiaction agent exposure during pregnancy and the occurrence of fetal malformations or defects. Although most agents show little evidence of teratogenicity in humans, there have been a few isolated reports of possible birth defects in the offspring of mothers taking paroxetine, imipramine, nortriptyline, and amitriptyline during the first trimester. In newborns of mothers who take these agents late in pregnancy, signs and symptoms of withdrawal can occur, and fetal development and birth weight may be affected. Although these agents are not known to have teratogenic or embryocidal effects, further research is warranted, given the relatively short time these agents have been in use and their increasing use as maintenance therapies.

Nefazodone is associated with hepatic failure and has a boxed warning. Amoxapine produces many of the same side effects as antipsychotic agents, including dystonic reactions, tardive dyskinesia, and neuroleptic malignant syndrome (Chapter 16). Bupropion can cause nervousness and insomnia as well as tremors and palpitations and has more of a stimulant than a sedative effect; therefore, it should not be administered in the evening.

Many SSRIs are potent inhibitors of several cytochrome P450 enzymes and thus can lead to potentially dangerous drug interactions. Fluoxetine, paroxetine, and duloxetine inhibit CYP2D6, whereas fluvoxamine inhibits both CYP1A2 and CYP3A4. Sertraline, escitalopram, citalopram, and venlafaxine have little, if any, effect on cytochrome P450s.

Although there is limited information on the long-term adverse effects of ketamine, a recent systematic review has indicated that following acute dosing to patients with depression, tachycardia, hypertension, and tremor are relatively common. Confusion, delirium, and hallucinations may also occur.

The side effects of the MAOIs are an extension of their pharmacological effects, reflecting enhanced catecholaminergic activity. Primary side effects are CNS excitation (hallucinations, agitation, hyperreflexia, and convulsions), a large suppression of REM sleep that may lead to psychotic behavior, and drug interactions, the latter of which are potentially life-threatening. The MAOIs have not been associated with extensive human teratogenicity.

Because MAOIs lead to increased intracellular stores of NE within adrenergic nerve terminals, these compounds can enhance the action of indirect-acting sympathomimetics that stimulate the release of NE from these sites. Of major importance is the potential for the MAOIs to induce a hypertensive reaction after the ingestion of tyramine-containing compounds, an action known as the tyramine or cheese effect. Tyramine, which is an indirect-acting sympathomimetic, is normally metabolized by MAO within the gastrointestinal tract after ingestion. When MAO activity in the gastrointestinal tract is inhibited, such as occurs after the oral administration of MAOIs, tyramine is not metabolized and enters the circulation, where it can release stored NE from sympathetic nerve endings. Because the amount of NE in the adrenergic nerve ending is increased as a consequence of MAO inhibition, the result is a massive increase in NE released into the synapse, with a resultant hypertensive crisis (Chapter 11). Therefore, patients taking MAOIs are maintained on a tyramine-restricted diet. This may not be a problem with the use of the selegiline transdermal system, because sufficient MAO activity in the gastrointestinal tract remains intact after transdermal drug administration. Although hypertensive crises are associated with tyramine ingestion during MAOI treatment, in all actuality, hypotension is a much more common side effect of MAOI treatment.

The amine reuptake inhibitors, multiaction agents, and MAOIs all have the potential to lead to serious consequences if combined with other compounds that increase brain levels of 5-HT or stimulate 5-HT receptors. Among these are the MAOIs and other antidepressants, as well as meperidine and dextromethorphan, which are potent inhibitors of 5-HT reuptake, and tryptophan, which can enhance 5-HT synthesis. This interaction can lead to a condition known as serotonin syndrome. This syndrome is characterized by alterations in autonomic function (fever, chills, and diarrhea), cognition and behavior (agitation, excitement, hypomania), and motor systems (myoclonus, tremor, motor weakness, ataxia, hyperreflexia) and may often resemble neuroleptic malignant syndrome (Chapter 16). Currently it is believed that activation of 5-HT receptors in the brainstem and spinal cord may mediate these effects. The incidence of the disorder is not known, but as the use of SSRIs increases, it may become more prevalent. Thus a heightened awareness is required for prevention, recognition, and prompt treatment, which involves discontinuation of the suspected drugs, administration of 5-HT antagonists such as cyproheptadine or methysergide, administration of the skeletal muscle relaxant dantrolene, and other supportive measures. The syndrome usually resolves within 24 hours but can be fatal.

Another important side effect of many of the antidepressants, including the MAOIs, is weight gain, which reduces patient compliance. Most

SSRIs and SNRIs have an anorectic effect and do not cause any clinically significant weight gain. Venlafaxine can cause weight loss, although paroxetine has been reported to cause weight gain over time. Among the multiaction antidepressants, bupropion does not cause weight gain, but mirtazapine can cause significant weight gain, perhaps because of its potent antihistamine activity.

An important consideration for all of the antidepressants is induction of mania or hypomania in depressed patients with a bipolar disorder (Chapter 16). This manic overshoot requires urgent care because a patient can switch from deep depression to an agitated manic state overnight. Anecdotally, fluoxetine is believed to be the drug most likely to induce such an overshoot and bupropion the least likely to do so.

All antidepressants have a boxed warning indicating an increased risk of suicidal ideation in children, adolescents, and young adults less than 24 years of age. Poisoning accounts for approximately 20% of all suicides, and although the TCAs have been the most commonly used drugs in such cases, all antidepressants have been and continue to be used.

Anxiolytics

The adverse reactions most frequently encountered with benzodiazepine use are an extension of their CNS depressant effects and include sedation, lightheadedness, ataxia, and lethargy. Sedation is the most common effect of the benzodiazepines, and its intensity and duration depend on the dose and concentration of drug in plasma and brain. For example, lorazepam has a prolonged sedative action compared with the other benzodiazepines, even though it clears the body rapidly. Tolerance occurs to the sedative but not the anxiolytic effect of the benzodiazepines. Occasional reactions observed with hypnotic doses of the benzodiazepines include impaired mental and psychomotor function, confusion, euphoria, delayed reaction time, uncoordinated motor function, dysarthria, headache, and xerostomia. Rare reactions may include syncope, hypotension, blurred vision, altered libido, skin rashes, nausea, menstrual irregularities, agranulocytosis, lupus-like syndrome, edema, and constipation.

Anterograde memory disturbances have been observed in patients taking diazepam, chlordiazepoxide, and lorazepam. Thus patients cannot recall information acquired after drug administration. This effect has been attributed to interference with the memory consolidation process and may be beneficial when the benzodiazepines are administered parenterally for presurgical or diagnostic procedures such as endoscopy. In this situation, patients should be warned of this effect, especially if they are being treated on an outpatient basis. When administered orally, most benzodiazepines do not cause this effect.

Adverse reactions associated with the IV use of benzodiazepines include pain during injection, thrombophlebitis, hypothermia, restlessness, cardiac arrhythmias, coughing, apnea, vomiting, and a mild anticholinergic effect. Deaths from overdose rarely occur. Patients have taken as much as 50 times the therapeutic doses of benzodiazepines without causing mortality. This particular property of these drugs is another example of how they differ from the potent respiratory depressant sedatives and hypnotics. Unlike the barbiturates, the benzodiazepines have only a mild effect on respiration when given orally, even with toxic doses. However, when they are administered parenterally or are taken in conjunction with other depressants such as alcohol, all benzodiazepines have the potential of causing significant respiratory depression and death.

The benzodiazepines are well known to produce physical dependence, and withdrawal reactions ensue upon abrupt discontinuation. The dependence associated with the benzodiazepines is not the same as that observed with alcohol, opioids, or the barbiturates. Although physical dependence is more likely to occur with high drug doses and long-term treatment, it has also been reported after usual therapeutic regimens. The onset of withdrawal symptoms is related to the elimination half-life and is more rapid in onset and more severe after discontinuation of the shorter acting benzodiazepines such as oxazepam, lorazepam, and alprazolam. With the longer-acting benzodiazepines, the onset of withdrawal is much slower because of their longer half-lives and slower disappearance from the plasma. Therefore doses of the benzodiazepines with short half-lives should be decreased more gradually. In addition, alprazolam, estazolam, and triazolam, which have a chemical structure (triazolo ring) that differs from the other benzodiazepines and are referred to as triazolobenzodiazepines, cause more serious withdrawal reactions than the other compounds.

The withdrawal symptoms accompanying abrupt discontinuation from the benzodiazepines are generally autonomic and include tremor, sweating, insomnia, abdominal discomfort, tachycardia, systolic hypertension, muscle twitching, and sensitivity to light and sound. In rare instances, severe withdrawal reactions may develop, characterized by convulsions. These reactions are usually manifest in individuals maintained on high doses of the benzodiazepines for prolonged (more than 4 months) periods of time. In addition to these autonomic manifestations, abrupt withdrawal of benzodiazepines can often cause patients to "rebound," exhibiting symptoms of anxiety and insomnia sometimes worse than before drug treatment was initiated, with a rebound increased REM sleep, characterized by bizarre dreams.

The benzodiazepines have been reported to have a high abuse potential. However, evidence suggests that psychological dependence occurs mainly in people with a history of drug abuse; appropriate therapeutic use by persons not predisposed to drug abuse should not lead to abuse of the benzodiazepines.

The benzodiazepines are powerful CNS depressants, and additive effects are apparent when they are administered with other CNS depressants. These include ethanol, antihistamines, other sedative/hypnotic agents, antipsychotics, antidepressants, and opioid analgesics. Because ethanol is readily available and widely used, the CNS depressant interaction between the benzodiazepines and ethanol is common. Individuals may experience episodes of mild to severe ataxia and "drunkenness" that severely retards performance levels. No single compound is considered safer than another in combination with ethanol. This is especially important for patients not exposed previously to the benzodiazepines. Individuals who have been drinking alcohol and taking benzodiazepines for long periods of time experience this interaction but to a milder degree.

Another drug interaction is a consequence of the biotransformation of the benzodiazepines. Because many of the benzodiazepines are metabolized by hepatic microsomal enzymes, therapeutic agents that inhibit cytochrome P450s decrease the biotransformation of the long-acting compounds. The histamine H_2-receptor antagonist cimetidine and oral contraceptives prolong the elimination half-life of the benzodiazepines by inhibiting their metabolism. Cisapride is a potent inhibitor of CYP3A4 and can cause significant increases in blood levels of many medications, including alprazolam, midazolam, and triazolam. Conversely, compounds that induce this enzyme, such as the barbiturates and carbamazepine, increase their rate of metabolism. Of course, the biotransformation of benzodiazepines that proceed by a route other than hepatic oxidation is unaltered. Although the benzodiazepines are biotransformed via the hepatic microsomal enzymes, they do not significantly induce enzyme activity and do not accelerate the metabolism of other agents biotransformed via this system.

As with any drug or class of drugs, the benzodiazepines should be avoided in patients with a known hypersensitivity to these agents. Alprazolam, clorazepate, diazepam, halazepam, lorazepam, and prazepam are contraindicated in individuals with acute narrow-angle glaucoma because of their anticholinergic side effects. In addition, because of the considerable lipid solubility of most benzodiazepines, they cross the placenta and are secreted in breast milk. It should be noted that the benzodiazepines may be teratogenic and should be avoided in pregnant and nursing women.

Again, because of the hepatic biotransformation of these compounds, special care must be taken when prescribing benzodiazepines for individuals with hepatic dysfunction and for the aged and debilitated population. These patients generally have a diminished liver-detoxifying capacity and often show cumulative toxicity in response to the usual adult dosage, especially of agents metabolized to active metabolites with long half-lives (diazepam, chlordiazepoxide). The aged are also more prone to acute depression of attention, alertness, motor dexterity, and sensory acuity as well as memory disturbance and confusion. For this reason, doses in the aged should be started at 25% of the usual adult dose and administered less frequently.

As with other psychoactive medications, precautions should be given with respect to administration of the drug and the amount of the prescription for severely depressed patients or for those in whom there is reason to suspect concealed suicidal ideation or plans.

Adverse reactions of buspirone include dizziness, drowsiness, dry mouth, headaches, nervousness, fatigue, insomnia, weakness, lightheadedness, and muscle spasms. When administered chronically, buspirone causes less tolerance and potential for abuse than the benzodiazepines and does not produce a rebound effect after discontinuation.

The problems associated with the use of the antidepressants and anxiolytics are summarized in the Clinical Problems Box.

CLINICAL PROBLEMS

Antidepressants

Tricyclic antidepressants (TCAs)	Anticholinergic (urinary retention, constipation, dry mouth, memory impairment), antiadrenergic (orthostatic hypotension), antihistaminergic (sedation), sexual dysfunction
Serotonin selective reuptake inhibitors (SSRIs)	Restlessness, nervousness, agitation, sweating and fatigue; sleep disturbances, sexual dysfunction, weight gain
Serotonin/norepinephrine reuptake inhibitors (SNRIs)	Similar to the SSRIs with the addition of increased sweating, tachycardia and urinary retention; dose-dependent hypertension
Multiaction agents	Bupropion: agitation, anxiety, headache, insomnia with dose-related seizures, especially in patients with eating disorders
	Mirtazapine: sedation, dizziness, weight gain, dry mouth, constipation
Monoamine oxidase inhibitors (MAOIs)	Sleep disturbances, orthostatic hypotension, sexual dysfunction, weight gain, serotonin syndrome, hypertensive crisis

Anxiolytics

Benzodiazepines	Sedation, lethargy, ataxia, anterograde memory impairment, physical dependence, abuse potential
Buspirone	Dizziness, drowsiness, nervousness, fatigue

NEW DEVELOPMENTS

Although the introduction of the SSRIs, SNRIs, and multiaction antidepressants represent major advances in the treatment of depression, these compounds still have limitations related to efficacy, tolerability, and rapidity of action. Unfortunately, only approximately 50% of patients treated with standard doses of currently available antidepressants exhibit favorable responses after 6–8 weeks of treatment, whereas others exhibit suboptimal improvement, and some individuals do not respond at all. Some lack of response may be attributed to patient compliance because many individuals cannot tolerate the side effects of these compounds. Last, and most important, slow response time is a major issue because many depressed individuals are prone to suicidal ideation.

Clearly, new approaches to the pharmacological treatment of depression are needed, including developing compounds aimed at new targets such as drugs that promote neurogenesis and agents that normalize the hypothalamic-pituitary-adrenal axis, which is hyperactive in many depressed patients. The challenge remains to develop therapeutic agents that are effective in the population of depressive patients that are resistant to currently available antidepressant medications and to decrease side effects to enhance patient compliance.

Studies with both ketamine and esketamine, as well as rapastinel (GLYX-13), which also targets NMDA receptors, and the opioid-based compound ALKS5461 (a combination of buprenorphine and samidorphan), represent the most significant advances in antidepressant therapy in a long time. Only time will tell whether these agents represent safer or more efficacious alternatives to currently available compounds.

In addition to new developments for the treatment of depression, there is also a need for newer, better tolerated, and more efficacious treatments for anxiety, especially drugs without abuse potential. To this end, our understanding of the role of different GABA$_A$ receptor subtypes in the brain is of paramount importance. If each of the pharmacological actions of the benzodiazepines could be ascribed to a specific receptor subtype, then it may be possible to develop compounds with selective actions on these receptors.

Additional approaches to the development of newer compounds depend on our understanding the molecular and cellular events mediating the pathophysiology of stress and stress-related disorders. Studies have suggested that the ability to cope with stress involves corticotropin-releasing factor signaling pathways, involving several peptides and their receptors that may represent new targets for the development of anxiolytic compounds.

CLINICAL RELEVANCE FOR HEALTHCARE PROFESSIONALS

Because the antidepressants are among the most commonly prescribed, if not the most commonly prescribed group of drugs, it is quite likely that all healthcare professionals will encounter patients taking these medications. Further, unlike the antipsychotics, the antidepressants, as well as the anxiolytics, are prescribed by individuals in all medical specialties, not only psychiatrists. Thus it is critical for all healthcare professionals to be aware of the adverse effects of these agents, with particular attention given to the possible increased suicidal ideation in children, teenagers, and young adults prescribed antidepressants, and the physical dependence and abuse potential of the benzodiazepines prescribed for anxiety for individuals of any age. Last, because both the antidepressants and anxiolytics are CNS depressants, all healthcare professionals must caution their patients not to drink alcoholic beverages while taking any of these compounds.

TRADE NAMES

In addition to generic and fixed-combination preparations, the following trade-named materials are some of the important compounds available in the United States.

TCAs
Amitriptyline (Elavil)
Clomipramine (Anafranil)
Desipramine (Norpramin)
Doxepin (Adapin, Sinequan, Silenor, Zonalon, Prudoxin)
Imipramine (Tofranil)
Nortriptyline (Pamelor)

SSRIs
Citalopram (Celexa)
Escitalopram (Lexapro)
Fluoxetine (Prozac, Sarafem)
Fluvoxamine (Luvox)
Paroxetine (Paxil, Pexeva)
Sertraline (Zoloft)

NRIs
Atomoxetine (Strattera)
Maprotiline (Ludiomil)
Reboxetine (Edronax)

SNRIs
Amoxapine (Asendin)
Desvenlafaxine (Pristiq)
Duloxetine (Cymbalta)
Levomilnacipran (Fetzima)
Milnacipran (Savella)
Venlafaxine (Effexor)

Multiaction Agents
Bupropion (Wellbutrin, Zyban)
Mirtazapine (Remeron)
Nefazodone (Serzone)
Trazodone (Desyrel)
Vilazodone (Viibryd)
Vortioxetine (Brintellix)

MAOIs
Isocarboxazid (Marplan)
Phenelzine (Nardil)
Selegiline (Emsam)
Tranylcypromine (Parnate)

Anxiolytics
Alprazolam (Xanax)
Chlordiazepoxide (Librium)
Clonazepam (Klonopin)
Clorazepate (Tranxene)
Diazepam (Valium)
Halazepam (Paxipam)
Lorazepam (Ativan)
Oxazepam (Serax)
Prazepam (Centrax)

Nonbenzodiazepines
Buspirone (BuSpar)
Propranolol (Inderal)

SELF-ASSESSMENT QUESTIONS

1. A woman who just landed her first job in a big marketing firm started to deliver a major presentation in the boardroom. Suddenly her hands began to sweat, and she felt her heart beat so fast that she began to feel lightheaded. Prescribing which of the following medications would be the best choice to alleviate this patient's symptoms before she gives her presentations?
   A. A benzodiazepine.
   B. A β-adrenergic receptor blocker.
   C. A monoamine oxidase A inhibitor.
   D. A serotonin selective reuptake inhibitor.
   E. A serotonin/norepinephrine reuptake inhibitor.

2. A 34-year-old man was brought into the emergency department by the police, who rescued him from the ledge of a five-story building. The man was totally despondent and had no interest in continuing to live. He was administered a medication intravenously, and within 2 hours, the darkness seemed to lift, and he indicated an interest in reuniting with his family. Which of the following medications was administered?
   A. Fluoxetine.
   B. Selegiline.
   C. Imipramine.
   D. Ketamine.
   E. Mirtazapine.

3. A 42-year-old woman was prescribed an SSRI and has been taking her medication diligently for more than a year. During the winter, she developed a cough that kept her up at night. She decided to get some cough medicine to help her sleep, but she woke up in the middle of the night with tremors, chills, and diarrhea. It is likely that she was exhibiting:
   A. A tyramine reaction.
   B. Neuroleptic malignant syndrome.
   C. Serotonin syndrome.
   D. REM sleep deprivation.
   E. The flu.

4. A 43-year-old man is requesting medication for treatment of depression and anxiety. His psychiatric history is notable for previous substance abuse treatment, and his medical history is significant for seizure disorder. Which medication would be *least* appropriate?
   A. Sertraline.
   B. Venlafaxine.
   C. Bupropion.
   D. Mirtazapine.

5. A 38-year-old woman with alcohol use disorder in remission for 2 years is requesting medication for treatment of anxiety. Which of the following drugs would be the *least* appropriate choice to target anxiety symptoms in this patient?
   A. A benzodiazepine such as lorazepam.
   B. A serotonin selective reuptake inhibitor such as sertraline.
   C. A nonbenzodiazepine anxiolytic such as buspirone.
   D. A serotonin/norepinephrine reuptake inhibitor such as venlafaxine.

FURTHER READING

Berton O, Nestler EJ. New approaches to antidepressant drug discovery: beyond monoamines. *Nature Rev Neurosci.* 2006;7:137–151.

Lang E, Mallien AS, Vasilescu AN, et al. Molecular and cellular dissection of NMDA receptor subtypes as antidepressant targets. *Neurosci Biobehav Rev.* in press, 2017.

Short B, Fong J, Galvez V, et al. Side-effects associated with ketamine use in depression: a systematic review. *Lancet.* 2018;5:65–78.

WEBSITES

https://www.nimh.nih.gov/index.shtml
This website is maintained by the National Institute of Mental Health and includes much information on depression and anxiety, including signs and symptoms, risk factors, treatments and therapies, and links to numerous resources for both professionals and caregivers.

https://www.psychiatry.org/patients-families/depression/what-is-depression
This website is maintained by of the American Psychiatric Association and is a valuable resource with links for patients, caregivers, and professionals.

https://adaa.org/understanding-anxiety
This website is maintained by the Anxiety and Depression Association of America (ADAA) with information for the public and professionals.

Drug Therapy for the Management of Attention Deficit-Hyperactivity Disorder

D. Samba Reddy

MAJOR DRUG CLASSES

Stimulants
    Amphetamines
    Nonamphetamines
Nonstimulants
    Norepinephrine reuptake inhibitors
    α_2-Adrenergic receptor agonists

ABBREVIATIONS

ADHD	Attention deficit-hyperactivity disorder
CNS	Central nervous system
DA	Dopamine
DAT	Dopamine transporter
GI	Gastrointestinal
5-HT	Serotonin
MAO	Monoamine oxidase
NE	Norepinephrine
NET	Norepinephrine transporter
VMAT2	Vesicular monoamine transporter-2

THERAPEUTIC OVERVIEW

Attention deficit-hyperactivity disorder (ADHD) is one of the most common childhood neurobehavioral disorders; it affects 4%–12% of children. ADHD affects males more than females (3–9 : 1) and can persist into adulthood. The most common symptoms of ADHD in children are impulsiveness, inattention, and hyperactivity, with individuals manifesting one or all of these symptoms to varying degrees. As a consequence, three subtypes of ADHD have been defined: (1) predominantly hyperactive-impulsive, (2) predominantly inattentive, and (3) combined hyperactive-impulsive and inattentive.

THERAPEUTIC OVERVIEW

Symptoms of ADHD	Inattentiveness
	Hyperactivity
	Impulsivity
Drug treatment of ADHD	Stimulants (amphetamines and nonamphetamines)
	Non-stimulants (norepinephrine reuptake inhibitors and α_2-adrenergic receptor agonists)

Pathophysiology

The exact pathophysiology of ADHD is unclear but is believed to involve suboptimal norepinephrine (NE) and dopamine (DA) neurotransmission in the frontal lobe. Although studies do not show any definitive pathologic marker for ADHD, the prefrontal cortex, which regulates attention, and the basal ganglia, which regulate movements and impulsivity, are consistently reported as smaller than normal and/or deformed. There are, however, several factors that may contribute to ADHD, including genetics and environment.

ADHD often shows a familial pattern, and genetics is believed to play a role in about 75% of cases. Polymorphisms in several genes have been reported, including those coding for DA receptor subtypes (D1, D4, and D5), adrenergic α_{2A} receptors, the DA transporter (DAT), and several enzymes including DA β-hydroxylase, monoamine oxidase A

(MAO-A), and catechol-O-methyltransferase (COMT). In addition, twin studies have suggested that approximately 9%–20% of the variance in ADHD symptoms can be attributed to environmental or nongenetic factors including alcohol use and tobacco smoke exposure during pregnancy and lead exposure in very early life. Complications during pregnancy and birth, such as hypoxia, might also play a role. Thus multiple factors may contribute to weakened prefrontal cortical circuits regulating cognitive control and attention.

There is currently no cure for ADHD. The most effective treatment, which can dramatically improve the key behavioral symptoms and improve the quality of life for both patients and their families, is the combination of behavioral therapy and drug treatment. Two broad classes of drugs are used for the pharmacotherapy of ADHD, stimulants and nonstimulants (Fig. 18.1). These drugs have been shown to be safe and efficacious for many children when used appropriately. The symptoms of ADHD and drugs used to control these symptoms are presented in the Therapeutic Overview Box.

MECHANISMS OF ACTION

Stimulants

The stimulant drugs used to treat ADHD are sympathomimetic amines that act on the central nervous system (CNS) by enhancing DA and NE neurotransmission. The amphetamine drugs include dextroamphetamine and the prodrug lisdexamfetamine, and the non-amphetamine drugs include methylphenidate and dexmethylphenidate. The effects of the amphetamines arise primarily from enhanced DA and NE neurotransmission through increased release and possibly decreased reuptake. The amphetamines target both DAT and the vesicular monoamine transporter-2 (VMAT2). Similarly, the nonamphetamine stimulant methylphenidate and its derivatives enhance DA and NE neurotransmission by inhibiting both DAT and NE reuptake (NET) and directly increasing DA release by affecting presynaptic storage of the monoamine.

Nonstimulants: Norepinephrine Reuptake Inhibitors and α₂-Adrenergic Receptor Agonists

Atomoxetine is a selective norepinephrine reuptake inhibitor (SNRI) and the first nonstimulant approved for the treatment of ADHD. Because the prefrontal cortex has a relative lack of DA transporters, DA is taken back into nerve terminals by NET. Thus, atomoxetine increases synaptic levels of both NE and DA in the prefrontal cortex.

Guanfacine is a selective agonist of α_{2A}-adrenergic receptors, similar to clonidine. These postsynaptic receptors are widely distributed in the brain, including the prefrontal cortex, and their activation promotes optimal adrenergic transmission in these regions.

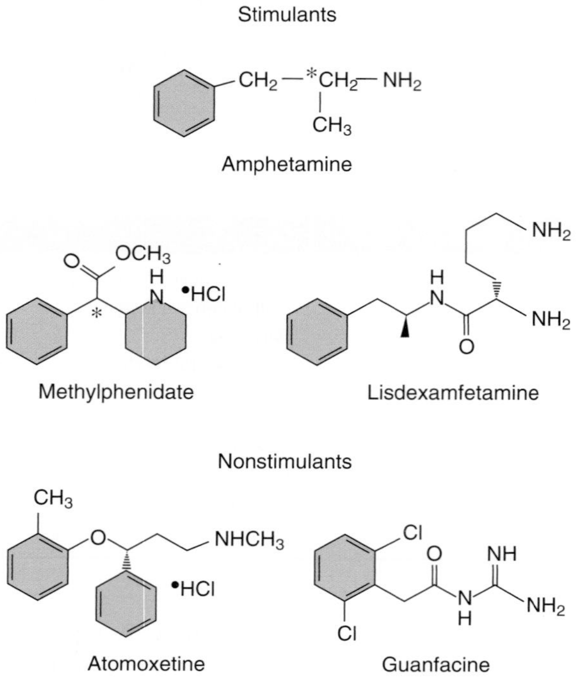

RELATIONSHIP OF MECHANISMS OF ACTION TO CLINICAL RESPONSE

Stimulants

Amphetamines are very effective for the treatment of ADHD. They increase DA and NE neurotransmission in the prefrontal cortex at doses lower than those required to affect DA transmission in subcortical structures such as the nucleus accumbens (Fig. 18.2). As a consequence, when used at doses appropriate for ADHD, they do not lead to addiction.

Methylphenidate is the most commonly prescribed stimulant for ADHD and is available in several formulations. Clinically used methylphenidate is a racemic mixture (50:50) comprised of the *d*- and *l*-enantiomers. The *d*-enantiomer is more pharmacologically active than the *l*-enantiomer. Methylphenidate has been shown to be safe and effective, with no tolerance to its therapeutic effects, for more than 1 year.

The amphetamines are comparable in efficacy with methylphenidate but are twice as potent. Dextroamphetamine is three to four times more potent than the *l*-isomer to produce CNS stimulation. There is no evidence that mixed amphetamine salts (salts of the two isomers) are superior to dextroamphetamine; however, some clinicians prefer the mixed formulations.

Although lisdexamfetamine was initially approved to treat children aged 6–12, it is now approved to treat children older than 12 as well as adults.

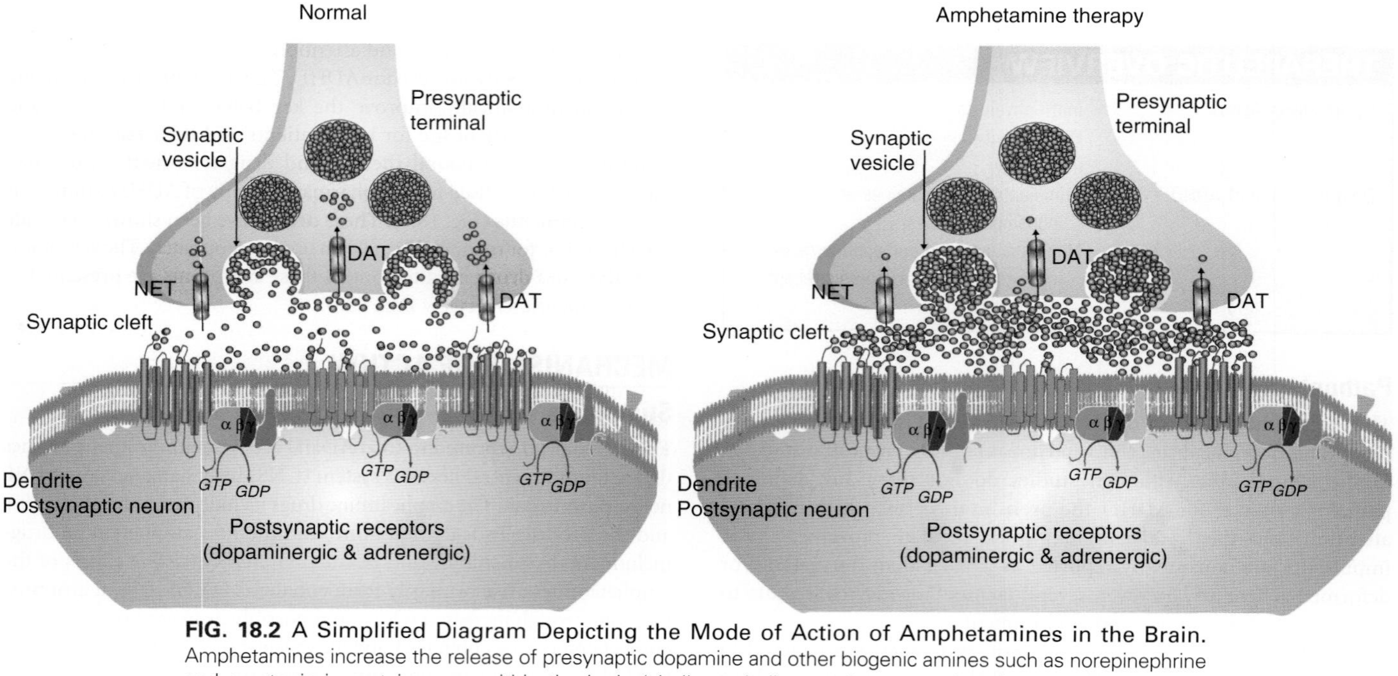

FIG. 18.1 Chemical Structures of Amphetamines and Related Agents Used to Treat ADHD. The asterisks denote an asymmetric (chiral) carbon.

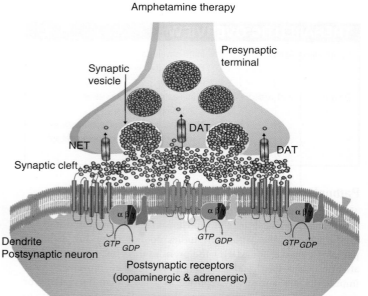

FIG. 18.2 A Simplified Diagram Depicting the Mode of Action of Amphetamines in the Brain. Amphetamines increase the release of presynaptic dopamine and other biogenic amines such as norepinephrine and serotonin in certain areas within the brain (similar to indirect-acting sympathomimetics). They modify the uptake of these neurotransmitters within the synaptic cleft by inhibiting the reuptake process or reuptake transporters, such as dopamine transporter (DAT) and norepinephrine transporter (NET). GTP, Guanosine triphosphate; GDP, guanosine diphosphate.

Nonstimulants

Several placebo-controlled clinical trials have demonstrated the effectiveness of atomoxetine for ADHD. However, it is less efficacious than either amphetamine or methylphenidate. Atomoxetine is typically prescribed for individuals who do not respond to the stimulants or who cannot tolerate the adverse effects of these agents, including children of low weight or stature.

Guanfacine is also used for individuals who cannot tolerate the adverse effects of the stimulants, particularly for those with tics. It may be used alone or added to an ADHD stimulant medicine as part of a total treatment plan, including behavioral therapy.

PHARMACOKINETICS

Stimulants

Amphetamine is available as a racemic mixture, the dextro isomer, and a mixture of the two, in both immediate and extended-release formulations. Amphetamine is readily absorbed after oral administration, enters the brain rapidly due to its high lipophilicity, and reaches peak plasma levels within 1–2 hours, with a duration of several hours. Dextroamphetamine is also absorbed orally, with a peak effect at 3 hours and a half-life of 6.8 hours. Mixed amphetamine salts are available in an extended-release capsule that provides 12 hours of symptom control. Amphetamines are eliminated via the kidneys, with approximately 30%–40% of the drug excreted unchanged at normal urinary pH. Because amphetamine is a weak base with a pKa of 9.9, urinary pH has a marked effect on excretion; alkalinization of the urine will lead to more amphetamine as the free base and will decrease excretion, while urinary acidification will increase excretion. Amphetamine is also metabolized by CYP2D6, DA β-hydroxylase, and other enzymes to several metabolites, some of which are active sympathomimetics, including 4-hydroxyamphetamine and norephedrine.

Lisdexamfetamine is a prodrug that is rapidly absorbed from the gastrointestinal (GI) tract and converted to dextroamphetamine and the amino acid L-lysine via enzymatic hydrolysis by red blood cells. It is the dextroamphetamine that is responsible for the drug's activity. Lisdexamfetamine was developed to create a longer lasting and more difficult to abuse version of dextroamphetamine to reduce abuse potential.

Methylphenidate is orally absorbed with a bioavailability of approximately 25%. Methylphenidate is available in short-acting, intermediate-acting, and long-acting once-daily preparations. The racemic mixture has an overall half-life of 4–6 hours, with elimination by metabolism via hepatic ester hydrolysis to ritalinic acid. Single-pulse, sustained-release methylphenidate products use a wax matrix to prolong release. These intermediate-acting agents are used infrequently because of their unpredictable absorption, variable duration of action, and availability of long-acting beaded double-pulse or osmotic-release preparations. The half-life of dexmethylphenidate is 2.2 hours.

Once-daily preparations, including modified-release methylphenidate, once-daily extended-release methylphenidate, and the osmotically released oral system (OROS) formulation, have gained popularity because they avoid frequent dosing and provide all-day symptom coverage. The OROS methylphenidate formulation has an advantage of lower abuse potential because it cannot be crushed and snorted. The tablet uses an osmotic delivery system to extend the duration of action of methylphenidate for up to 12 hours and is coated with immediate-release methylphenidate (22% of the dose) for immediate action within 1 hour. The remainder of the dose is delivered by an osmotic pump that gradually releases the drug over a 10-hour period. Therefore, the total methylphenidate dose is released over 6–10 hours. Beaded methylphenidate products use an extended-release formulation with a bimodal release mechanism containing 50% of the dose in immediate-release beads and 50% in enteric-coated, delayed-release beads. These delivery systems mimic the twice-daily administration release pattern of methylphenidate.

All extended-release once-daily preparations of methylphenidate have the potential for increased insomnia compared with conventional preparations, given that drug levels persist into the late afternoon and evening hours. It is unknown whether the cardiovascular adverse effects are more problematic with extended-release preparations due to persistent blood drug levels over 8–12 hours.

A methylphenidate transdermal patch is available that produces comparable drug levels to those of regular preparations given three times a day. The patch is a useful option for children who are unable to swallow pills; wearing the patch for 9 hours provides a full day of symptom coverage.

Nonstimulants

Atomoxetine is absorbed orally, with a bioavailability of 63%. It is metabolized by CYP2D6 to the 4-hydroxy metabolite, which is equal in potency to the parent compound. Atomoxetine is administered as a single daily dose in the morning or as evenly divided doses in the morning and late afternoon/early evening. It binds extensively (98%) to plasma proteins and can be discontinued without being tapered.

Guanfacine is also readily absorbed following oral administration and 70% bound to plasma proteins, irrespective of dose. Guanfacine is metabolized primarily by CYP3A4 followed by glucuronidation. Both parent and metabolites are excreted via the urine.

PHARMACOVIGILANCE: ADVERSE EFFECTS AND DRUG INTERACTIONS

All drug products approved for ADHD should be dispensed with a patient medication guide to alert patients or parents to boxed warnings, possible cardiovascular risks, and adverse psychiatric symptoms associated with the use of these drugs. Drugs for the treatment of ADHD can pose serious risks, particularly when they are misused; precautions must be taken.

Stimulants

Stimulant medications elicit a biphasic action: low doses reduce locomotor activity and distractibility, while high doses cause sleeplessness and other symptoms of excessive stimulation. In the CNS, the potency is methamphetamine > d-amphetamine > l-amphetamine. In the periphery, the potency is l-amphetamine > d-amphetamine; methamphetamine has few or no peripheral effects.

Amphetamines have potent CNS stimulant actions in addition to peripheral sympathomimetic effects common to indirect-acting adrenergic agents. All amphetamines stimulate medullary centers, leading to increased respiration and motor activity. Common adverse effects include headaches, insomnia, anorexia, tic exacerbation, dry mouth, GI upset, weight loss, and reduced growth velocity.

Amphetamines cause a dose-dependent acute and chronic toxicity. Acute toxic CNS effects include restlessness, dizziness, pupillary dilation, delusion, hallucinations, increased sexual activity, tremor, hypertensive reflexes, talkativeness, tenseness, irritability, weakness, fever, and euphoria. Cardiovascular effects include headache, chilliness, flushing, palpitation, cardiac arrhythmias, hypertension, and circulatory collapse. Excessive sweating is also evident following amphetamine administration.

Massive overdoses lead to loss of consciousness following seizures and a hypertensive crisis. The drug of choice for treating amphetamine toxicity is haloperidol, a D2 receptor antagonist and typical antipsychotic agent (Chapter 16). With chronic amphetamine use, a loss of biogenic amine neurons has been reported. Recommended monitoring parameters while taking these medications include cardiac evaluation in patients with risk factors including monitoring blood pressure and heart rate, height and weight in pediatrics, and complete blood count with differential annually, if prolonged treatment is required.

Drug interactions may occur with amphetamines and other agents that increase NE or DA levels including MAO inhibitors and other antidepressants. Amphetamines are contraindicated in patients with hardening of the arteries, heart disease, hypertension, hyperactive thyroid, and glaucoma. Patients should be monitored for signs of abuse and dependence while on amphetamine therapy.

Methylphenidate leads to many of the same adverse effects as the amphetamines, including nervousness, insomnia, headache, anorexia, GI upset, weight loss, slow growth, and psychiatric effects. Methylphenidate use can cause cardiovascular effects such as sudden death in susceptible patients, strokes and heart attacks, and hypertension. In addition, it can lead to psychiatric effects such as exacerbating psychotic symptoms in bipolar illness, manic symptoms, and aggression. Methylphenidate is contraindicated in patients with symptomatic cardiovascular disease, moderate to severe hypertension, hyperthyroidism or glaucoma, psychiatric conditions of anxiety, tension, and agitation. No methylphenidate product should be used during or within 14 days following MAO inhibitors.

The stimulants are all Schedule II controlled substances and have a high potential for abuse. Drug dependence on and addiction to these compounds are discussed in Chapter 24.

Nonstimulants

Common side effects of atomoxetine in children include upset stomach, decreased appetite, nausea or vomiting, dizziness, somnolence, and mood swings. In adults, insomnia, constipation, dry mouth (xerostomia), nausea, decreased appetite, dizziness, sexual side effects, urinary hesitancy/retention, problems urinating, and menstrual cramps are not uncommon. Atomoxetine is contraindicated in persons with narrow-angle glaucoma and MAO inhibitor usage within 14 days. Dose adjustment is needed for individuals with hepatic or renal impairment. The major potential risks and side effects of atomoxetine include suicidal thoughts or actions, hepatotoxicity, weight loss/slowed growth, and impaired motor skills. Recommended monitoring parameters while taking this drug include cardiac evaluation in patients with risk factors, height and weight in pediatrics, liver function, and suicidal evaluation in teens, especially during initial treatment or after dose changes. Atomoxetine carries boxed warnings and additional warnings regarding hepatotoxicity and suicidal ideation.

As a consequence of atomoxetine metabolism by CYP2D6, CYP2D6 phenotype will greatly affect circulating levels (Chapter 4).

Guanfacine had little effect in a study in healthy volunteers. Adverse reactions include hypotension, somnolence, bradycardia, and syncope.

Guanfacine should be discontinued carefully to avoid abrupt withdrawal effects.

Adverse effects associated with use of drugs for the treatment of ADHD are presented in the Clinical Problems Box.

NEW DEVELOPMENTS

Currently available treatments for ADHD focus on reducing symptoms and improving functioning at home, school, or work through both behavioral and drug therapy. Despite the fact that stimulant medications have been proven safe and effective for the treatment of ADHD, an estimated 30%–50% of children and adults with ADHD either do not respond to or cannot tolerate treatment with stimulants. Although the nonstimulant medications atomoxetine and guanfacine were developed for individuals who could not tolerate the stimulants, many patients fail to respond to these compounds.

Interest in the use of modafinil, which is approved for promoting wakefulness in individuals with narcolepsy, shift work sleep disorder, and sleep apnea, for patients with inattentive and combined ADHD was spurred by off-label clinical findings that it reduced the symptoms of ADHD. Although double-blind randomized trials supported the efficacy and tolerability of modafinil for pediatric patients with ADHD, enthusiasm was tempered because of the development of serious adverse skin reactions and Stevens-Johnson syndrome.

New information on the neurobiology of ADHD, including elucidating the role of genetics and environmental factors, will hopefully give rise to the development of newer and more selective medications.

CLINICAL RELEVANCE FOR HEALTHCARE PROFESSIONALS

Most children are treated with drugs for ADHD for a prolonged period of time. As a consequence, all healthcare professionals should reevaluate the efficacy and safety issues of pharmacotherapy in individual patients periodically. The substantial increase in the number of people prescribed stimulants for longer periods of time may increase reports of adverse psychiatric events and cardiovascular toxicity. All individuals involved in the treatment of children and young adults with ADHD must be vigilant on these issues. Furthermore, all healthcare professionals are urged to educate patients and their families about the potential dangers of misusing stimulants.

SELF-ASSESSMENT QUESTIONS

1. A 7-year-old boy is having major difficulty in school with inattentiveness and hyperactivity. Which neurotransmitter systems in the brain may be functioning suboptimally?
   A. Dopamine and serotonin.
   B. Dopamine and norepinephrine.
   C. Norepinephrine and serotonin.
   D. Dopamine and glutamate.

2. A 10-year-old girl was diagnosed with ADHD and prescribed a stimulant. One of the most common adverse effects associated with the use of the stimulants is:
   A. Sedation.
   B. Hypotension.
   C. Elevated liver function tests.
   D. Itching.
   E. Anorexia.

3. An 8-year-old boy in the 50th percentile of height and weight for his age was recently diagnosed with ADHD. Which of the following is the best drug to begin treatment with for this boy?
   A. Amphetamine.
   B. Methylphenidate.
   C. Dextroamphetamine.
   D. Lisdexamfetamine.
   E. Atomoxetine.

4. One of the most common adverse effects of guanfacine experienced by a 14-year-old boy prescribed the drug for ADHD is:
   A. Insomnia.
   B. Tachycardia.
   C. Nervousness.
   D. Hypotension.
   E. Arrhythmias.

5. Which of the following is a prodrug that must be hydrolyzed to be active for the treatment of ADHD?
   A. Methylphenidate.
   B. Atomoxetine.
   C. Dextroamphetamine.
   D. Lisdexamfetamine.
   E. Methamphetamine.

6. The primary mechanism of action of amphetamines that is beneficial in the treatment of ADHD in children is:
   A. Selective agonism of α_2-adrenergic receptors.
   B. Selective inhibition of NE reuptake.
   C. Release of DA and NE from presynaptic nerve terminals.
   D. Selective inhibition of vesicular DA transport.
   E. Selective inhibition of β-adrenergic receptors.

FURTHER READING

Minzenberg MJ. Pharmacotherapy for attention-deficit/hyperactivity disorder: from cells to circuits. *Neurother.* 2012;9:610–621.

Reddy DS. Current pharmacotherapy of attention deficit hyperactivity disorder. *Drugs Today.* 2013;49:647–665.

Dopheide JA. A calming influence: an analysis of ADHD treatments. *Pharm Times.* 2006, August;1–16.

WEBSITES

https://www.nimh.nih.gov/health/topics/attention-deficit-hyperactivity-disorder-adhd/index.shtml

The National Institute of Mental Health maintains an excellent website with links to resources for healthcare professionals, teachers, and parents on this topic, as well as clinical trial information.

https://www.cdc.gov/ncbddd/adhd/treatment.html

The Centers for Disease Control and Prevention also has an excellent website with links to numerous resources.

Drug Therapy for Insomnia and the Hypersomnias

Lynn Wecker

ABBREVIATIONS

CNS	Central nervous system
DORA	Dual orexin receptor antagonist
GABA	γ-Aminobutyric acid
GABA$_A$	γ-Aminobutyric acid type A receptor
REM	Rapid eye movement
SCN	Suprachiasmatic nucleus

THERAPEUTIC OVERVIEW

It has been estimated that 30% of all adults in the United States have insomnia, characterized by difficulty both initiating and maintaining sleep. Insomnia often accompanies anxiety, stress, and depression and may result from medical conditions, an underlying sleep disorder such as sleep apnea, the adverse effect of drugs, or an unhealthy lifestyle. Women are twice as likely as men to experience insomnia, with increased prevalence during hormonal changes, such as occur during menopause and the third trimester of pregnancy. Further, the incidence of insomnia increases with age and is particularly common in the aged; estimates indicate that 66% of the population older than 65 years of age experience insomnia.

The benzodiazepines were the mainstay treatment of insomnia for many years, followed by the development of the benzodiazepine receptor agonists, or "z-drugs": zopiclone, zaleplon, and zolpidem. However, these agents are not without their share of adverse effects, may lead to dependence, and most important, appear to promote nonrapid eye movement (NREM) sleep at the expense of REM sleep, failing to produce a physiological sleep state. Thus much research has been devoted to the development of drugs that reproduce normal sleep. To this end, both the melatonin receptor agonist ramelteon, and, most recently, the dual orexin receptor antagonist (DORA) suvorexant have been introduced. In addition, several antidepressants and over-the-counter antihistamine preparations may be useful for insomnia.

While many individuals suffer from insomnia, a limited number of persons exhibit hypersomnia. The central hypersomnias are characterized by excessive daytime sleepiness, despite a long sleep the night before and normal circadian rhythms, and include narcolepsy with and without cataplexy, idiopathic and recurrent hypersomnia, and others. These disorders are treated with conventional central nervous system (CNS) stimulants, including amphetamines and methylphenidate, as well as nonamphetamine stimulants, including modafinil (Chapter 18) and some antidepressants (Chapter 17).

Therapeutic issues related to insomnia and the hypersomnias and the goals of treatment are summarized in the Therapeutic Overview Box.

THERAPEUTIC OVERVIEW

Conditions That Manifest Insomnia
Age: increased incidence in individuals >65 years old
Gender and hormonal status: twice as prevalent in females relative to males and increased incidence after menopause and during the third trimester of pregnancy
Psychiatric disorders: depression, anxiety, substance use, posttraumatic stress disorder
Stress
Drug withdrawal

Goals of Pharmacological Treatment of Insomnia
Decrease sleep latency
Increase sleep maintenance
Mimic normal healthy physiological sleep: do not increase non-REM sleep at the expense of REM sleep

Conditions That Manifest Hypersomnia
Narcolepsy with and without cataplexy
Idiopathic insomnias

Goals of Pharmacological Treatment of Hypersomnias
Maintain arousal without sympathetic stimulation

MECHANISMS OF ACTION

Drugs for Insomnia

GABA-Enhancing Drugs

The benzodiazepines, which are used for several disorders, including anxiety and seizures, are positive allosteric modulators at γ-aminobutyric acid type A (GABA$_A$) receptors and enhance inhibitory neurotransmission in the CNS (Chapter 17). There are currently five benzodiazepines approved for the treatment of insomnia, including estazolam, flurazepam, quazepam, temazepam, and triazolam.

The benzodiazepine receptor agonists (z-drugs), including the racemic zopiclone and its active stereoisomer eszopiclone, zaleplon, and zolpidem

GABA-enhancing drugs

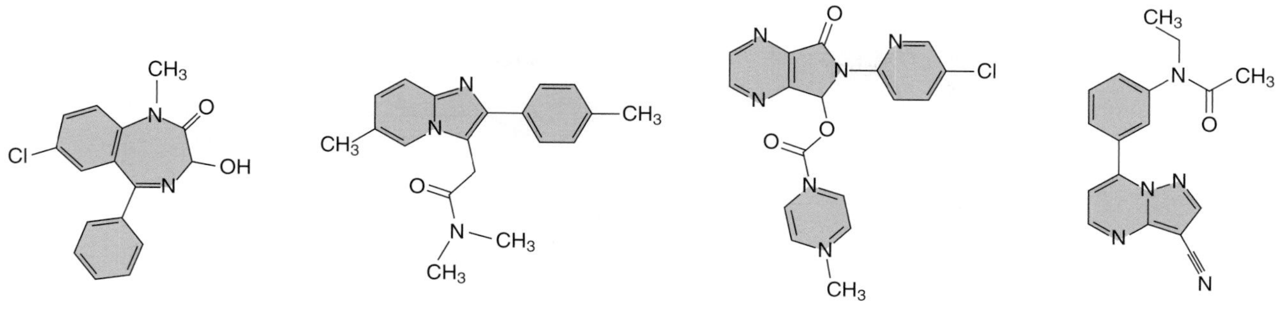

Temazepam   Zolpidem   Zopiclone   Zaleplon

Melatonin receptor agonists

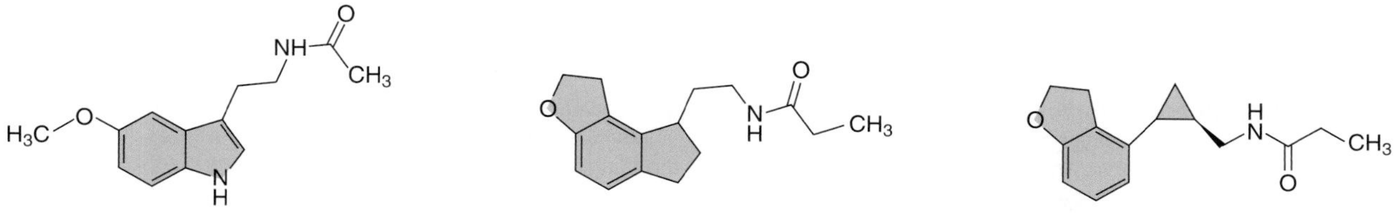

Melatonin   Ramelteon   Tasimelteon

FIG. 19.1 Structures of GABA-Enhancing Drugs and Melatonin Receptor Agonists. For the GABA-enhancing drugs, note the differences between the structure of the prototypical benzodiazepine temazepam and the other compounds, which are benzodiazepine receptor agonists. Also note the similarities in structure between melatonin and its analogues ramelteon and tasimelteon.

are also approved to treat insomnia. These agents are chemically unrelated to the benzodiazepines (Fig. 19.1) but bind to the same allosteric site on the $GABA_A$ receptor that binds the benzodiazepines. However, in contrast to the benzodiazepines, which bind to sites on all $GABA_A$ receptors irrespective of their subunit composition, the benzodiazepine agonists bind with high affinity only to receptors containing α_1 subunits and with lower affinity to α_2- or α_3-containing subunits. Thus these compounds have a different pharmacological profile than the benzodiazepines.

Melatonin Receptor Agonists

Melatonin is a neurohormone produced in the pineal gland whose expression is modulated in response to light and that plays a major role in the regulation of circadian rhythms. As shown in Fig. 19.2, when the retina is exposed to light, the optic nerve transmits the signal to GABA neurons in the suprachiasmatic nucleus (SCN) of the hypothalamus. The SCN is an area intimately involved in regulating circadian rhythms and sleep and is often referred to as the circadian pacemaker, or "master clock." Activation of the SCN inhibits the firing of paraventricular neurons, which synapse in the intermediolateral column with cholinergic neurons that modulate the activity of noradrenergic neurons in the superior cervical ganglion. These postganglionic neurons relay information to the pineal gland, regulating melatonin synthesis.

Melatonin is synthesized by a two-step process catalyzed by the enzymes serotonin-N-acetyltransferase (NAT) and hydroxyindole-O-methyltransferase, respectively, converting serotonin to melatonin. NAT is rate limiting, with low activity during the day and peaking in the dark. Thus light exposure of the retina decreases melatonin synthesis,

while dark promotes synthesis. Following synthesis, melatonin is released from the pineal gland and activates its receptors, MT_1 and MT_2, both of which are G-protein receptors coupled to $G_{i/o}$, whose activation leads to decreased adenylyl cyclase activity. MT_1 and MT_2 receptors are expressed throughout the brain and highly abundant in the SCN, anterior pituitary, and retina. In the SCN, activation of MT_1 receptors decreases neuronal firing, thereby promoting sleep, whereas activation of MT_2 receptors, which desensitize following exposure to melatonin, are involved in phase shifting circadian rhythms.

Ramelteon is the first and only selective melatonin receptor agonist approved for the treatment of insomnia, while tasimelteon is the first and only selective melatonin receptor agonist approved for non-24-hour sleep-wake disorder (N24HSWD) in which individuals are not entrained and have a free-running circadian rhythm. Both of these compounds are structural analogues of melatonin (see Fig. 19.1) and, like melatonin, have high affinity for both MT_1 and MT_2 receptors, with minimal affinity for other receptors. Both agents mimic the effects of the neurohormone on receptors in the SCN, with ramelteon promoting the induction of sleep and tasimelteon resynchronizing circadian rhythms.

Orexin Receptor Antagonists

The orexins, also referred to as hypocretins, are neuropeptides (Fig. 19.3) synthesized in the lateral hypothalamus by the posttranslational cleavage of prepro-orexin, yielding orexin-A, a 33–amino acid peptide, and orexin-B, a 28–amino acid peptide. Orexin-A is more lipid soluble and stable than orexin-B and, as a consequence, crosses the blood-brain barrier; orexin-B is rapidly degraded in the circulation. The orexins activate two receptors, OX_1, which is activated by orexin-A, and OX_2,

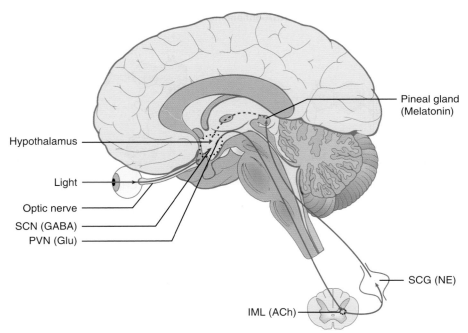

FIG. 19.2 Melatonin and Sleep. Shown are the pathways involved in the regulation of sleep by melatonin. The retina is activated by light, with the signal relayed to the suprachiasmatic nucleus (SCN) of the hypothalamus via the optic nerve. These GABAergic interneurons inhibit the firing of excitatory glutamatergic paraventricular nuclei (PVN) of the hypothalamus that ultimately control noradrenergic input from the superior cervical ganglion (SCG) to the pineal gland, the site of melatonin synthesis. Melatonin synthesized in and released from the pineal gland activates MT$_1$ receptors concentrated in the SCN, which decreases neuronal firing, disinhibiting noradrenergic input, increasing melatonin synthesis, and promoting sleep. *ACh*, Acetylcholine; *GABA*, γ-aminobutyric acid; *Glu*, glutamate; *IML*, intermediolateral nucleus of the spinal column; *NE*, norepinephrine.

which is activated by both orexins. Both receptors are G-protein–coupled to G$_{q/11}$, whose activation increases phospholipase C activity, leading to the hydrolysis of phosphatidylinositol to inositol triphosphate and diacylglycerol, increasing intracellular Ca^{++}.

Orexin neurons project to regions in the brainstem involved in promoting arousal, including the histaminergic tuberomammillary nucleus, the cholinergic laterodorsal and pedunculopontine tegmental nuclei, the serotonergic dorsal raphe nucleus, and the noradrenergic locus coeruleus (Fig. 19.4). Activation of these nuclei by orexin promotes arousal and vigilance, with orexin serving as a physiologically relevant modulator of sleep-wakefulness. Orexin neurons also project to brain regions involved in appetitive activity and reward, promoting eating and, possibly, addictive behavior.

Suvorexant is currently the only orexin receptor antagonist approved for the treatment of insomnia. The drug blocks orexin neuropeptides from binding to both receptors, hence the name dual orexin receptor antagonist (DORA). Thus the action of suvorexant differs from all other compounds for insomnia as it inhibits arousal signaling rather than promoting sleep signaling. Further, in contrast to other compounds approved for sleep-onset insomnia, suvorexant is approved for both sleep-onset and sleep-maintenance insomnia.

Others

Several antidepressants as well as over-the-counter histamine receptor antagonists have also been shown to be useful for insomnia. Doxepin, a tricyclic antidepressant, is currently the only antidepressant approved for the treatment of sleep-maintenance insomnia, although other antidepressants are often used, including trazadone, mirtazapine, and amitriptyline. The sedative effects of these agents have been attributed

to their antagonist effect at histamine H$_1$ receptors that occurs at doses lower than those required for an antidepressant effect. Similarly, antihistamines have been used for many years to help aid sleep. Diphenhydramine and doxylamine are approved for this indication, again, due to antagonism at histamine H$_1$ receptors.

Drugs for Hypersomnias

Agents currently available for hypersomnia include amphetamine compounds, methylphenidate, and modafinil, typically used to treat attention deficit-hyperactivity disorder (Chapter 18), and some antidepressants (Chapter 17), all of which increase norepinephrine in the CNS. Most recently, the first histamine H$_3$ receptor inverse agonist/antagonist (Chapter 2) pitolisant was approved for the treatment of narcolepsy. H$_3$ receptors are autoreceptors that negatively feed back to inhibit histamine release from the tuberomammillary nucleus, thereby promoting drowsiness. By acting as an inverse agonists/antagonist, pitolisant has the opposite effect, producing arousal.

RELATIONSHIP OF MECHANISMS OF ACTION TO CLINICAL RESPONSE

GABA-Enhancing Drugs

The effects of the benzodiazepines are discussed in depth in Chapter 17. For insomnia, these compounds decrease sleep latency and prolong the first two stages of sleep.

The benzodiazepine receptor agonists produce sedation without anxiolytic, anticonvulsant, or muscle relaxant effects. These compounds have been shown to be highly efficacious for the treatment of transient and chronic insomnia and are approved for use in patients with

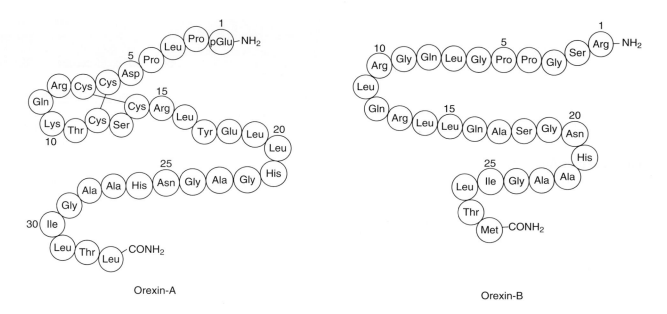

Orexin-A

Orexin-B

Suvorexant

FIG. 19.3 Amino Acid Sequence of Orexin-A and Orexin-B and the Structure of the Orexin Receptor Antagonist Suvorexant.

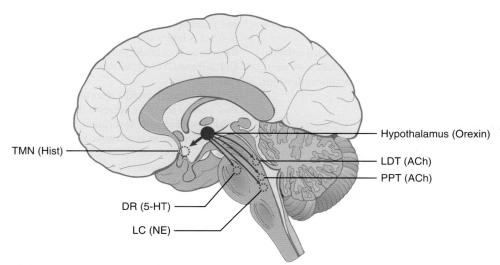

FIG. 19.4 Orexin Pathways Mediating Sleep. Orexin neurons in the hypothalamus project to many brain regions involved in sleep including the tuberomammillary nucleus (TMN), the dorsal raphe nucleus (DR), the locus coeruleus (LC), and the laterodorsal and pedunculopontine tegmental nuclei (LDT and PPT, respectively). Shown are these pathways and their associated neurotransmitters. *ACh,* Acetylcholine; *Hist,* histamine; *NE,* norepinephrine; *5-HT,* serotonin.

sleep-onset insomnia, with zolpidem the most widely prescribed sedating drug in the United States. These drugs are also used for circadian rhythm disorders and high-altitude insomnia. The major difference among these agents is duration of action, with zaleplon having the shortest duration of action, causing less daytime sedation. These compounds have been reported to be devoid of abuse potential because high doses induce nausea and vomiting. However, there is some evidence of addictive effects of zaleplon and zolpidem but not eszopiclone.

Melatonin Receptor Agonists

The sleep-promoting actions of ramelteon are related to its ability to mimic the endogenous hormone melatonin. Ramelteon is approved for sleep-onset insomnia and produces a significant decrease in sleep latency; it does not affect sleep maintenance. Ramelteon should be taken within 30 minutes of going to bed and should not be taken with or immediately after a high-fat meal because its absorption will be delayed. Studies have shown that ramelteon decreases sleep latency by 8–16 minutes, is devoid of residual effects the day after administration, and does not produce rebound insomnia. It is often used off-label for the treatment of circadian disorders.

Tasimelteon is indicated for the treatment of non-24-hour sleep-wake disorder (N24HSWD, which occurs commonly in blind individuals without light perception and is characterized by nighttime insomnia and daytime sleepiness. Further, the 24-hour circadian cycle is typically lengthened due to a lack of light stimulation, leading to progressively delayed sleep onset. Tasimelteon improves sleep by resynchronizing the circadian rhythm. It is currently the only drug available for the treatment of this disorder.

Orexin Receptor Antagonists

Suvorexant is unique because it is approved for both sleep-onset and sleep-maintenance insomnia. Studies indicate that patients fall asleep sooner and stay asleep longer than placebo.

Others

Doxepin exerts its sedative effects at doses lower than those required for the treatment of depression, as well as doses lower than those leading to anticholinergic actions. It increases total sleep time in both healthy volunteers and the aged with chronic insomnia.

The antihistamines are approved as sleep aids and are clearly sedating, but it is unclear that they improve the quality or duration of sleep. Further, tolerance to the sedative effects of the antihistamines develops rapidly.

PHARMACOKINETICS

Selected pharmacokinetic parameters for drugs used for the treatment of insomnia are shown in Table 19.1.

The pharmacokinetics of the benzodiazepines are discussed extensively in Chapter 17. The benzodiazepine receptor agonists are well absorbed following oral administration. Eszopiclone is weakly bound to plasma proteins (52%–59%), reaches peak plasma levels in 1 hour, and has an elimination half-life of 6 hours. It is metabolized extensively by CYP3A4 and CYP2E1 to mostly inactive metabolites that are excreted in the urine as glucuronides. Zolpidem is rapidly adsorbed and highly bound to plasma proteins (>90%). Peak plasma levels are reached in 1.6 hours, and the drug has an elimination half-life of 2.6 hours. It is inactivated primarily by CYP3A4, and glucuronidated metabolites are excreted in the urine. Zaleplon is nearly completely absorbed following administration, exhibits weak to moderate plasma protein binding (60%), reaches peak plasma levels in 1 hour, and has an elimination half-life

TABLE 19.1 Pharmacokinetic Parameters for Representative Drugs for the Treatment of Insomnia

Drug	Time to Peak Effect (hours)	Elimination $t_{1/2}$ (hours)	Elimination
Benzodiazepines			
Estazolam	2	10–25	M, R (87%), B
Flurazepam	1	50–100	M, R
Quazepam	2	25–85	M, R
Temazepam	1.5	3.5–20	M, R (80–90%)
Triazolam	2	1.5–5.5	M, R (80%)
Benzodiazepine Receptor Agonists			
Eszopiclone	1	6	M, R
Zaleplon	1	1	M, R
Zolpidem	1.6	2.6	M, R
Melatonin Receptor Agonists			
Ramelteon	0.5–1.5	2.5	M, R (84%), B (4%)
Tasimelteon	0.5–3	1.3–3.7	M, R (80%), B (4%)
Orexin Receptor Antagonist			
Suvorexant	2	12–15	M, R (23%), B (66%)
Other			
Doxepin	2	6–25	M, R

B, Biliary excretion; *M*, metabolized by liver; *R*, renal elimination.

of 1 hour. It is metabolized extensively by aldehyde oxidase, with CYP3A4 playing a secondary role. The inactive metabolites are glucuronidated and excreted in the urine.

Ramelteon is rapidly absorbed following oral administration, is moderately bound to plasma proteins (82%), and undergoes rapid and extensive first-pass metabolism. High-fat meals decrease adsorption and prolong the time to reach peak plasma levels, which are achieved in 0.5–1.5 hours after fasting. The elimination half-life is 2–5 hours. Ramelteon is oxidized primarily by CYP1A2, and to a lesser extent by CYP2C9 and CYP3A4, followed by glucuronidation and primarily urinary excretion.

Tasimelteon is rapidly absorbed and 90% bound to plasma proteins. Peak plasma levels are achieved 0.5–3 hours after fasting, and high-fat meals decrease both absorption and the time to reach peak plasma levels. Tasimelteon is extensively oxidized and dealkylated at multiple sites via CYP1A2 and CYP3A, and inactive glucuronidated metabolites are excreted in urine (80%) and feces (4%). The mean elimination half-life for tasimelteon ranges from 1.3–3.7 hours.

Suvorexant is well absorbed following oral administration, with peak plasma concentrations reached at 2 hours. It is extensively bound to plasma proteins (>99%) and metabolized to inactive products primarily by CYP3A4, with a minor contribution by CYP2C19. Elimination is through the feces (66%) and urine (23%).

Doxepin is rapidly absorbed following oral administration and exhibits 80% plasma protein binding, and appreciable first-pass metabolism. Peak plasma levels are achieved at 2 hours. Doxepin is metabolized mainly by CYP2D6 to *N*-desmethyldoxepin, which is an active metabolite; CYP1A2 and CYP3A4 also contribute to metabolism. The elimination half-life is 6–25 hours, with metabolites excreted mainly in the urine.

PHARMACOVIGILANCE: ADVERSE EFFECTS AND DRUG INTERACTIONS

GABA-Enhancing Drugs

The adverse effects of the benzodiazepines are discussed in Chapter 17 and include impaired next-day performance and anterograde amnesia, especially with triazolam. Most important, these compounds depress REM sleep and have a high risk of causing physical dependence, with rebound insomnia and increased anxiety manifest following cessation of drug treatment after as little as a few weeks of therapy. The aged may exhibit muscle weakness and impaired coordination, leading to an increased incidence of falls and hip fractures. Because these compounds are metabolized by CYP3A4, drug interactions are expected with inhibitors and inducers of this cytochrome P450. Further, the CNS depressant actions of the benzodiazepines are additive with other CNS depressants, such as the opioids or alcohol.

Although the benzodiazepine receptor agonists were developed to overcome some of the adverse effects associated with the benzodiazepines, these agents share many negative aspects with the benzodiazepines, particularly the inability to produce "physiological sleep." Further, these agents lead to dose-related anterograde amnesia, headache, and dizziness. They also lead to daytime sedation, as with the benzodiazepines, leading to impaired driving or falls in the aged. Although uncommon, complex sleep-related behaviors have been reported, including sleepwalking, sleep-eating, and sleep-driving without conscious awareness, particularly after high drug doses. These effects led the United States Food and Drug Administration to lower the recommended doses of these drugs.

Eszopiclone and zaleplon may cause chest pain and anticholinergic effects, while zolpidem may lead to confusion and ataxia. There have also been reports of zolpidem inducing delirium, psychotic reactions, and nightmares. The most common side effect of eszopiclone is an unpleasant taste; patients have also reported abnormal dreams and hallucinations.

The abuse liability of zaleplon and zolpidem is less than that of the benzodiazepines when used at the doses recommended. However, when used at higher doses, zolpidem may lead to some physical dependence, and abrupt discontinuation may lead to withdrawal, although less severe than that observed with the benzodiazepines. There is no evidence for abuse liability with eszopiclone.

Because these drugs, like the benzodiazepines, are metabolized by CYP3A4, interactions may occur with the concomitant use of enzyme inhibitors or inducers. Further, the CNS depression induced by these agents is additive with other CNS depressants.

Melatonin Receptor Agonists

Ramelteon, unlike the benzodiazepines and benzodiazepine receptor agonists, is not a controlled drug, and there are no reports of rebound insomnia, dependence, tolerance, or withdrawal. The most common side effects are dizziness, nausea, fatigue, and headache. Ramelteon has been reported to be associated with decreased testosterone and increased prolactin levels, although the clinical significance of these alterations is unclear. Because ramelteon is metabolized by several cytochrome P450s, drug interactions with inhibitors or inducers of these enzymes are expected.

Tasimelteon can lead to headache, nightmares, and upper respiratory or urinary tract infections, as well as increased alanine aminotransferase. It is unclear whether tasimelteon is teratogenic in humans because controlled studies have not been performed, but animal studies support adverse effects in the offspring when administered during pregnancy. Tasimelteon, like ramelteon, does not appear to have the potential for abuse.

CLINICAL PROBLEMS

Benzodiazepines (estazolam, flurazepam, quazepam, temazepam, triazolam)	Central nervous system and respiratory depression, abuse potential, REM sleep depression, impaired next-day performance, anterograde amnesia
Benzodiazepine receptor agonists (eszopiclone, zaleplon, zolpidem)	Central nervous system and respiratory depression; REM sleep depression; anterograde amnesia; headache; dizziness; daytime sedation; complex sleep-related behaviors including sleepwalking, sleep-eating, and sleep-driving without conscious awareness
Ramelteon	Dizziness, nausea, fatigue, headache
Tasimelteon	Headache, nightmares, upper respiratory or urinary tract infections
Suvorexant	Somnolence

Orexin Receptor Antagonists

The most serious adverse effect of suvorexant is daytime somnolence due to its long half-life, which can impair performance. Further, muscle weakness in the extremities has been reported. Because suvorexant is metabolized by CYP3A4, drug interactions may ensue in the presence of enzyme inducers or inhibitors. Like all other drugs used for insomnia, the CNS depressant effects of suvorexant are additive with other CNS depressants.

Others

Doxepin and the antihistamines may lead to daytime hangover, which may be particularly troublesome in the aged. Although the doses of doxepin for insomnia are less than those that produce anticholinergic activity, the antihistamines routinely lead to dry mouth and urinary retention, again troublesome for the aged.

The adverse effects associated with agents used for the treatment of insomnia are in the Clinical Problems Box.

NEW DEVELOPMENTS

There is a need for newer, better tolerated, and more efficacious treatments for insomnia. As more is learned about the cellular and molecular events regulating specific functional pathways in the brain, research should provide better agents to treat sleep disorders. Our knowledge of the role of orexin and its signaling system in regulating sleep has increased very rapidly and led to the development of the DORAs, which are more selective than the benzodiazepines and benzodiazepine receptor agonists and produce a natural sleep without disturbing the normal sleep cycle. As we learn more about the specific roles of OX_1 and OX_2 in sleep, even more compounds that target these receptors will be developed. In addition, other areas of special interest include sleep-promoting fatty acid amides, neurosteroids, prostaglandins, and peptides.

For the hypersomnias, recent studies have suggested that the benzodiazepine receptor antagonist flumazenil and orexin receptor agonists may be effective. Obviously, more research is needed in these areas.

CLINICAL RELEVANCE FOR HEALTHCARE PROFESSIONALS

Due to the prevalence of insomnia in the population, most, if not all, healthcare professionals will have patients who have taken or are taking these drugs. All healthcare professionals need to be aware of the side effects of these drugs, especially issues related to daytime sedation, which can be especially troublesome in the aged, leading to falls and hip fractures. All healthcare professionals should advise their patients not to use excessive amounts of ethanol or other CNS depressants because the effects of these compounds will be additive with those of the benzodiazepines and benzodiazepine receptor agonists. In addition, because of the potential of these compounds to cause physical dependence, all healthcare professionals should caution their patients on this matter.

TRADE NAMES

In addition to generic and fixed-combination preparations, the following trade-named materials are some of the important compounds available in the United States.

Benzodiazepines
Estazolam (Prosom)
Flurazepam (Dalmane)
Quazepam (Doral)
Temazepam (Restoril)
Triazolam (Halcion)

Benzodiazepine Receptor Agonists
Eszopiclone (Lunesta)
Zaleplon (Sonata)
Zolpidem (Ambien, Edluar, Intermezzo)

Melatonin Receptor Agonists
Ramelteon (Rozerem)
Tasimelteon (Hetlioz)

Orexin Receptor Antagonist
Suvorexant (Belsomra)

SELF-ASSESSMENT QUESTIONS

1. A 62-year-old man is having trouble both falling asleep and staying asleep. Which of the following medications should be prescribed?
   A. Alprazolam.
   B. Flumazenil.
   C. Fluoxetine.
   D. Ramelteon.
   E. Suvorexant.

2. A 55-year-old woman with insomnia took medication every night to help her sleep. After several weeks, she began exhibiting psychotic-like symptoms, including delusions. Which of the following medications was she most likely prescribed?
   A. Buspirone.
   B. Flumazenil.
   C. Ramelteon.
   D. Temazepam.
   E. Zaleplon.

3. Ramelteon, recently approved for the treatment of insomnia, has a mechanism of action very different from zaleplon, which is also used to treat insomnia. Ramelteon has its effects by interacting with which receptors in the hypothalamus?
   A. Melatonin receptors.
   B. GABA$_A$ receptors.
   C. 5-HT receptors.

   D. Glutamate receptors.
   E. Muscarinic receptors.

4. Although the benzodiazepines and the benzodiazepine receptor agonists improve sleep latency, these agents are not ideal for the treatment of chronic insomnia because they:
   A. Cause CNS depression.
   B. Cause anterograde amnesia.
   C. Have the potential for dependence.
   D. Lead to daytime sedation.
   E. All of the above.

5. The action of the orexin receptor antagonist suvorexant differs from all other agents used for the treatment of insomnia because it:
   A. Inhibits arousal rather than promotes sleep.
   B. Interacts with a naturally occurring protein in the brain.
   C. Does not lead to daytime somnolence.
   D. Is not metabolized by cytochrome P450s.
   E. Reaches peak plasma levels in less than 3 hours.

FURTHER READING

Jacobson LH, Chen S, Mir S, Hoyer D. Orexin OX$_2$ receptor antagonists as sleep aids. *Curr Topics BehaV Neurosci.* 2017;33:105–136.

Kuriyama A, Honda M, Hayashino Y. Ramelteon for the treatment of insomnia in adults: a systematic review. *Sleep Med.* 2014;15:385–392.

Kuriyama A, Tabata H. Suvorexant or the treatment of primary insomnia: a systematic review and meta-analysis. *Sleep Med.* 2017;35:1–7.

Sonka K, Susta M. Diagnosis and management of central hypersomnias. *Ther Adv Neurol Disord.* 2012;5:297–305.

WEBSITES

https://www.ncbi.nlm.nih.gov/pubmedhealth/PMHT0023679/
This website is maintained by the United States National Library of Medicine and is an excellent resource on sleep disorders, with links for both medical professionals and patients.

https://www.nhlbi.nih.gov/health/health-topics/topics/inso
This is an excellent website maintained by the National Heart, Lung, and Blood Institute of the National Institutes of Health, and has numerous links to all aspects of insomnia, including causes, signs and symptoms, treatments, and clinical trials.

https://aasm.org/
The American Academy of Sleep Medicine provides excellent resources on sleep disorders, including guidelines for their diagnosis and treatment.

Drug Therapy for Managing Obesity and Eating Disorders

Charles Rudick

MAJOR DRUG CLASSES

Antiobesity agents
  Sympathomimetics
  Serotonin receptor 2C agonist
  Glucagon-like peptide-1 receptor agonist
  Lipase inhibitor
Drugs for anorexia, bulimia, and binge-eating disorder
  Antidepressants
  Lisdexamfetamine dimesylate
Drugs for cachexia
  Progestational agents
  Corticosteroids
  Anabolic steroids
  Cannabinoid receptor agonist

ABBREVIATIONS

CNS	Central nervous system
DA	Dopamine
GI	Gastrointestinal
GLP-1	Glucagon-like peptide-1
5-HT	Serotonin
MAO	Monoamine oxidase
NE	Norepinephrine

THERAPEUTIC OVERVIEW

Obesity

Obesity, defined as a body mass index (BMI) of greater than 30 kg/m^2, is approaching epidemic proportions in the United States and throughout the world. The most recent studies suggest that 69% of adults in the United States are either overweight (a BMI of 25–29.9 kg/m^2) or obese, with the latter accounting for 36% and affecting both women and men equally. Additionally, studies estimate that 18% of all adolescents between the ages 12 and19 years old are obese.

Obesity is a significant risk factor for many common conditions, including type 2 diabetes mellitus, hypertension, dyslipidemia, coronary artery disease, congestive heart failure, stroke, hepatic steatosis, sleep apnea, osteoarthritis, endometrial, breast, prostate, and colon cancers, and reduced cognitive function. In addition, mortality rates from all causes increase with obesity.

The cause of obesity is still unknown, but research suggests that it results from several genetic, metabolic, physiological, behavioral, and social factors. Weight reduction lowers the risk of morbidity and mortality, and obesity is currently accepted as one of the most preventable health risk factors. Drugs available currently for the short-term treatment of obesity include the sympathomimetics benzphetamine, diethylpropion, phentermine, phendimetrazine and phentermine/topiramate, the serotonin (5-HT) 2C receptor agonist lorcaserin, the glucagon-like peptide 1 (GLP-1) receptor agonist liraglutide, and the peripherally active gastrointestinal (GI) lipase inhibitor orlistat.

Anorexia Nervosa, Bulimia Nervosa, and Binge-Eating Disorder

In contrast to obesity, anorexia nervosa and bulimia nervosa are commonly recognized eating disorders in which there is an exaggerated concern about body weight and shape. Traditionally, these disorders have been more prevalent in young women; however, increasing numbers of older women, men, and boys are developing these illnesses. Anorexia is the more disabling and lethal, characterized by the obsessive pursuit of thinness that results in serious, even life-threatening, weight loss. Bulimia differs from anorexia because many individuals are of normal body weight. Bulimic patients indulge in binge-eating, followed by excessive inappropriate behavior to lose weight such as vomiting, the use of laxatives, or compulsive exercising. Anorexic and bulimic patients have common characteristics, and although the physiological disturbances resulting from bulimia are less severe than from anorexia, both disorders are associated with serious medical complications. Treatment involves the management of these complications and restoring and maintaining normal body weight through psychotherapy and pharmacotherapy with antidepressants. Currently, fluoxetine is the only medication approved by the United States Food and Drug Administration (FDA) for bulimia (with or without depression), with no medication currently approved for anorexia.

Binge-eating disorder is characterized by frequently consuming unusually large amounts of food and the compulsion to continue eating even when full or not hungry. This disorder can occur at any age, but most commonly begins in the late teens or early 20s, with men and women affected equally. Many people with binge-eating disorder have a history of dieting, and they include approximately one-third of obese patients enrolled in weight-loss clinics; a relationship between binge-eating disorder and obesity is beginning to be recognized. The only drug approved by the FDA for binge-eating disorder is lisdexamfetamine dimesylate, originally approved for attention deficit-hyperactivity disorder (Chapter 18).

169

Cachexia

Cachexia is not a primary eating disorder but is a loss of appetite and weight as a consequence of cancer, infectious diseases such as AIDS, and other major chronic disorders. Cachexia is often very debilitating and is associated with weakness, a loss of fat and muscle, fatigue, decreased survival, and diminished responses to cytotoxic therapeutic compounds. The orexigenic agents may be naturally occurring or synthetic and include progestational agents, corticosteroids and anabolic steroids, and the orally active synthetic cannabinoid dronabinol. All of these compounds stimulate appetite and cause weight gain in these patients.

The etiology of eating disorders and the involvement of developmental, social, and biological factors are beyond the scope of this chapter. The pharmacological treatment of eating disorders is presented in the Therapeutic Overview Box.

THERAPEUTIC OVERVIEW

Obesity
Significant risk factors should be present before initiating drug therapy.
Patients with concurrent diseases such as diabetes and hypertension require close monitoring.
Exercise and a supervised dietary plan are essential.
Sympathomimetics, 5-HT$_{2C}$ agonists, GLP-1 agonists, or lipase inhibitors may be of benefit.

Anorexia, Bulimia, and Binge-Eating Disorder
Baseline medical and psychological assessment with psychotherapy.
Antidepressants may be of benefit for bulimia and lisdexamfetamine for binge-eating.

Cachexia
Associated with advanced cancers and AIDS.
Corticosteroids, progestational agents, anabolic steroids, and stimulation of cannabinoid type 1 receptors stimulate appetite and weight gain.

MECHANISMS OF ACTION

Antiobesity Agents

Four sympathomimetics are available to treat obesity including benzphetamine, diethylpropion, phentermine, and phendimetrazine. These drugs are β-phenethylamine derivatives structurally related to the biogenic amines norepinephrine (NE) and dopamine (DA) and to the stimulant amphetamine (Fig. 20.1). As a consequence of the latter, these agents have been deemed to have the potential for abuse and are classified by the United States Drug Enforcement Administration (DEA) as Schedule III (benzphetamine and phendimetrazine) and Schedule IV (diethylpropion and phentermine) drugs, with diethylpropion and phentermine producing less central nervous system (CNS) stimulation than benzphetamine and phendimetrazine. Phentermine has also been combined with the antiseizure drug topiramate, which leads to anorexia and weight loss, for the treatment of obesity. Although the exact mechanism mediating these well-known side effects of topiramate is not readily apparent, the two-drug combination decreases the excitatory side effects of phentermine, perhaps reflecting the inhibitory effects of topiramate (Chapter 21). Nevertheless, all of these agents increase the release of NE or DA and suppress appetite through effects on the satiety center in the hypothalamus rather than effects on metabolism.

Lorcaserin is a unique agent that is an agonist at 5-HT$_{2C}$ receptors. These receptors are distributed in the hypothalamus, amygdala, hippocampus, and cortex, and receptor activation in the hypothalamus has been shown to increase the synthesis of proopiomelanocortin (POMC), increasing satiety. Thus evidence to date suggests that lorcaserin may directly activate anorexigenic neurons or may modify the emotional, cognitive, or decision-making components of appetite. Lorcaserin is a Schedule IV drug with hallucinogenic properties.

The combination of the antidepressant bupropion and the opioid receptor antagonist naltrexone has been approved recently to treat obesity in adults. The precise mechanism of action of this preparation is unknown but likely reflects the ability of bupropion to inhibit both NE and DA reuptake. Evidence has shown that the combination of

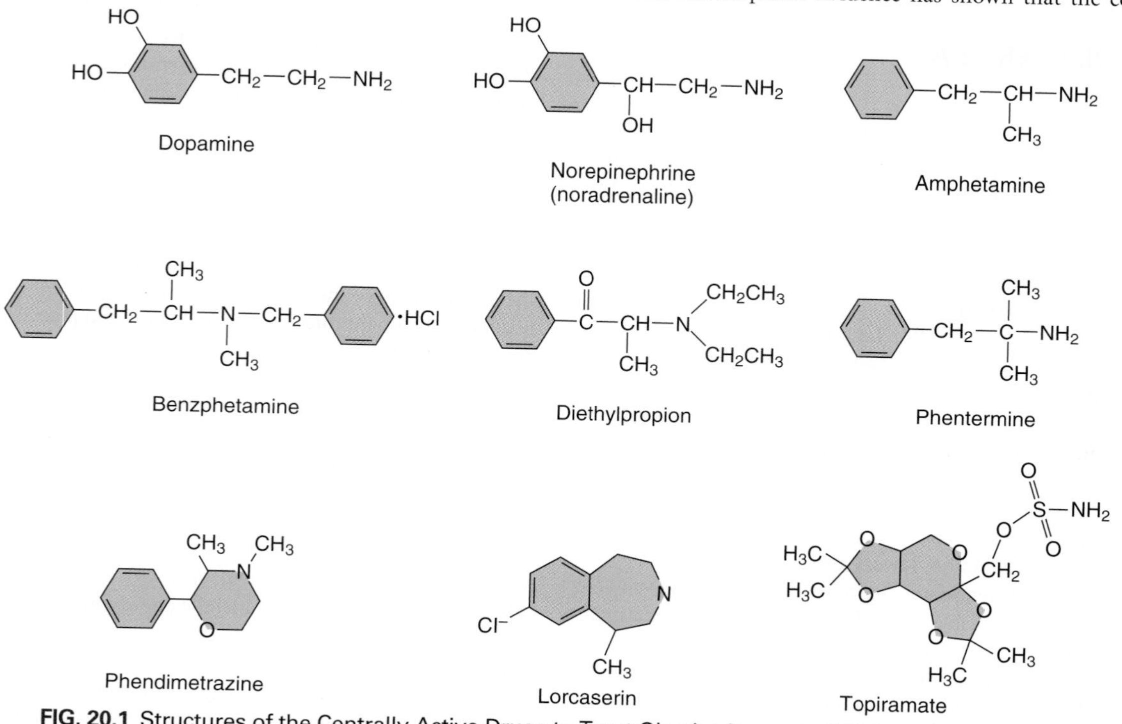

FIG. 20.1 Structures of the Centrally Active Drugs to Treat Obesity Compared With the Endogenous Neurotransmitters NE and DA, and Amphetamine.

these drugs is synergistic and leads to greater weight loss than with either drug alone.

Liraglutide is a long-acting GLP-1 receptor agonist approved for type 2 diabetes and for the treatment of obese adults or overweight adults with a BMI of 27 and at least one weight-related condition. Liraglutide represents one of the first in a new class of drugs that mimics the actions of the naturally occurring peptide GLP-1. Although the specific mechanisms mediating the ability of liraglutide to suppress appetite and lead to weight loss remain unknown, they may be related to the incretin mimetic effects of this compound to increase glucose-dependent insulin release from pancreatic β cells and decrease glucagon secretion from pancreatic α cells, as well as extra-pancreatic effects to slow gastric emptying and increase satiety.

Orlistat is the only weight-loss drug that does not suppress appetite. Rather, orlistat binds to and inhibits the enzyme lipase in the lumen of the stomach and small intestine, thereby decreasing the production of absorbable monoglycerides and free fatty acids from triglycerides. Orlistat is a synthetic derivative of lipstatin, a naturally occurring lipase inhibitor produced by *Streptomyces toxytricini*. Normal GI lipases are essential for the dietary absorption of long-chain triglycerides and facilitate gastric emptying and secretion of pancreatic and biliary substances. Because the body has limited ability to synthesize fat from carbohydrates and proteins, most accumulated body fat in humans comes from dietary intake. Orlistat reduces fat absorption up to 30% in individuals whose diets contain a significant fat component. Reduced fat absorption translates into significant calorie reduction and weight loss in obese individuals. In addition, the lower luminal free fatty acid concentrations also reduce cholesterol absorption, thereby improving lipid profiles. Orlistat is not a controlled substance, is approved for the long-term treatment of obesity, and is now available over the counter.

Drugs for Anorexia, Bulimia, and Binge-Eating

Based on evidence that individuals with anorexia and bulimia are prone to mood disturbances, the pharmacological treatment of these disorders has focused on use of antidepressants, and evidence supports the efficacy of these compounds for the treatment of bulimia. Antidepressants in all classes have been shown to be equally efficacious, but because of side effects associated with the use of the tricyclic antidepressants and monoamine oxidase inhibitors (Chapter 17), selective serotonin reuptake inhibitors may be considered first-line agents. Antidepressants reduce vomiting and depression and improve eating habits in bulimia but do not affect poor body image and are ineffective for binge-eating disorder. It is unclear whether the actions of these compounds are due primarily to their antidepressant effects or whether they are directly orexigenic. Currently, fluoxetine is the only antidepressant approved for the treatment of bulimia. The mechanisms of action of the antidepressants are discussed in Chapter 17.

Lisdexamfetamine dimesylate is a stimulant prodrug used primarily for the treatment of attention deficit-hyperactivity disorder (Chapter 18) and was recently approved for the treatment of binge-eating disorder. Lisdexamfetamine is metabolized to amphetamine and thus acts as a sympathomimetic. It is classified as a Schedule II drug.

Orexigenics

Similar to the goal for therapy with anorectic and bulimic patients is the need to stimulate appetite in individuals with cachexia. In concert with nutritional counseling, progestational agents such as megestrol acetate, corticosteroids such as dexamethasone, and anabolic steroids such as oxandrolone have been shown to stimulate appetite and cause weight gain in these patients. The mechanisms of action of these compounds are discussed in Chapters 50, 51, and 52.

In addition to steroids, the orally active synthetic cannabinoid dronabinol is approved for promoting appetite in individuals with cachexia. Dronabinol, which is also used to prevent the nausea and vomiting associated with cancer chemotherapy in individuals who fail to respond to other antiemetics, produces a dose-related stimulation of appetite through activation of cannabinoid type 1 (CB_1) receptors in the hypothalamus and has sympathomimetic activity, and is a Schedule III agent.

RELATIONSHIP OF MECHANISMS OF ACTION TO CLINICAL RESPONSE

Antiobesity Agents

The sympathomimetic antiobesity drugs increase synaptic concentrations of biogenic amines in the CNS, leading to their anorectic effect. In addition, increases in peripheral amine levels may promote thermogenesis, contributing to weight loss. Although clinical studies have demonstrated that the use of these drugs produces more weight loss than placebo when used as an adjunct to a supervised diet and exercise routine, their effects were maximal during initial use, and continued treatment did not lead to further weight loss; as a matter of fact, weight regain usually occurs within 6 months after discontinuation. Unfortunately, it is unclear whether chronic use of these drugs continues to decrease mechanisms controlling appetite or whether tolerance develops. Further studies are needed to understand the loss of effectiveness after chronic use.

Liraglutide, by mimicking the actions of the naturally occurring peptide GLP-1, is effective as an adjunct to diet and exercise for weight loss. Studies have shown that liraglutide leads to weight loss that is maintained for at least 1 year and that it may prevent the development of obesity-activated diabetes.

Orlistat has no effect on appetite-regulating pathways in the CNS, and, as such, there is no potential for CNS tolerance or abuse. Continued treatment with orlistat increases the intake of low-fat foods and decreases high-fat intake by patients, perhaps reflecting the desire to decrease the GI side effects that accompany its use. In addition to decreasing fat absorption, orlistat decreases cholesterol absorption and reduces plasma low-density lipoprotein cholesterol beyond that produced by weight loss alone in obese individuals, an added benefit of this drug.

Drugs for Anorexia, Bulimia, and Binge-Eating Disorder

Anorexia nervosa, bulimia nervosa, and binge-eating disorder have multifactorial etiologies, and, as such, drug therapy alone is likely to be ineffective. Studies indicate that antidepressants do not lead to the remission of bulimia, although a single course of drug is better than placebo. In addition, with continued treatment, patients have a high rate of relapse. Thus, although antidepressants have been shown to be efficacious for bulimia, their long-term utility remains to be determined.

Orexigenics

Weight gain in patients with cachexia may be achieved by increasing the appetite and caloric intake of these individuals. Megestrol has been found to be effective in increasing body weight, primarily reflecting increased fat weight rather than lean body mass. In contrast, the anabolic agent oxandrolone promotes appetite and physical activity and increases muscle anabolism and protein synthesis, decreases catabolism, and stimulates growth hormone and insulin-like growth factors. Thus the anabolic steroids increase lean body mass in men; the effectiveness of anabolic steroids has not been thoroughly evaluated in women.

Dronabinol produces a modest increase in weight gain relative to both megestrol and the anabolic steroids and may be additive with these other agents.

It is important to keep in mind that none of the orexigenic compounds has been shown to affect the course of either cancer or AIDS, but they do enhance the quality of life for patients with these diseases.

PHARMACOKINETICS

All centrally acting anorectic drugs are well absorbed from the GI tract and reach peak plasma levels within 2 hours. However, they differ somewhat in their pharmacokinetic profiles (Table 20.1).

Most of the sympathomimetics undergo extensive first-pass metabolism. Benzphetamine is metabolized to two para-hydroxylated derivatives that are excreted in urine within 24 hours, whereas diethylpropion is metabolized via N-dealkylation and reduction, producing active metabolites with half-lives of approximately 4 to 6 hours that are excreted mainly by the kidneys.

Phentermine and phendimetrazine are available in both immediate- and sustained-release formulations. Phentermine is not metabolized, and 70% to 80% of an administered dose is excreted unchanged by the kidneys. Phendimetrazine is metabolized by the liver and excreted by the kidneys with an apparent $t_{1/2}$ of 1.9 and 9.8 hours for the immediate- and slow-release preparations, respectively.

Lisdexamfetamine dimesylate is a prodrug that is enzymatically hydrolyzed by red blood cells to dextroamphetamine. The pharmacokinetics of lisdexamfetamine are discussed in Chapter 18.

Lorcaserin is extensively metabolized in the liver by multiple CYP450 enzymes (CYP1A1, 1A2, 1A6, 2B2, 2C19, 2D6, 2E1, and 3A4) as well human flavin-containing mono-oxygenase 1. The apparent $t_{1/2}$ is 11 hours, and both parent drug and metabolites are excreted in the urine (~93%) and feces (~3%).

Liraglutide is handled by the body in a manner similar to that of endogenous GLP-1. It is completely metabolized by two peptidases, and metabolic products are excreted equally in the urine and feces. Liraglutide has a $t_{1/2}$ of 13 hours.

Orlistat is not absorbed to any appreciable extent, is metabolized in the GI tract to two inactive metabolites, and is excreted primarily in the feces.

Dronabinol is nearly completely absorbed after oral administration and undergoes extensive first-pass hepatic metabolism. It has a high lipid solubility with a large (10 L/kg) apparent volume of distribution, and is 97% bound to plasma proteins. Hepatic metabolism yields both active and inactive metabolites, with 11-OH-Δ-9-THC representing the primary active metabolite, which reaches plasma levels equal to that of the parent compound. Dronabinol and its metabolites are excreted in both urine and feces, with biliary excretion representing the primary route. Dronabinol has a terminal half-life of 25–36 hours.

The pharmacokinetics of the antidepressants are discussed in Chapter 17; those of the corticosteroids are discussed in Chapter 50, those of the progestational agents in Chapter 51, and those of the anabolic steroids in Chapter 52.

PHARMACOVIGILANCE: ADVERSE EFFECTS AND DRUG INTERACTIONS

Antiobesity Agents

The centrally active anorexigenics and lisdexamfetamine dimesylate have similar side effect profiles, related to their ability to increase central and peripheral aminergic activity. Use is contraindicated in patients with a history of stroke, coronary artery disease, congestive heart failure, arrhythmias, and drug abuse.

These drugs should be used as monotherapy and are contraindicated in patients receiving sympathomimetic amines, tricyclic antidepressants, serotonin or serotonin/norepinephrine reuptake inhibitors, or monoamine oxidase (MAO) inhibitors because of the possibility of hypertensive crises. In addition, for compounds such as lorcaserin that affect 5-HT activity, a 5-HT syndrome can be precipitated (Chapter 17). A minimum drug-free period of 14 days is required for anyone using MAO inhibitors before therapy is initiated with these agents.

Glaucoma can be exacerbated as a result of the mydriasis produced by these agents and is also a contraindication to their use.

Increased insulin sensitivity has been reported in type 2 diabetics receiving diethylpropion, and thus careful monitoring of serum glucose, insulin, and oral hypoglycemic agents is required in these patients.

These drugs also cause insomnia and tremors and induce anxiety through their CNS actions. Because of their CNS stimulation, these drugs carry a potential for abuse. Although they have less abuse potential than amphetamine, they are contraindicated in abusers of cocaine, phencyclidine, and methamphetamine.

As a consequence of significant hepatic metabolism of these agents, a potential for drug interactions exists.

Liraglutide has well-documented adverse effects that include nausea, vomiting, and the potential for development of an allergic reaction including a rash, itching, and difficulty breathing. It may also lead to acute pancreatitis and kidney failure. Liraglutide can lead to the formation of antibodies and has a boxed warning from the FDA indicating the possible development of thyroid tumors, including cancer.

Orlistat is unique for the treatment of obesity, as it does not carry a risk of cardiovascular side effects. Because its actions involve the GI system, its adverse effects are limited to this area. The most commonly reported GI complaints, which occur in as many as 80% of individuals, are most pronounced in the first 1 to 2 months and decline with continued use. Malabsorption of fat-soluble vitamins (A, D, E, and K) and β-carotene occur, but no notable changes in the pharmacokinetic profiles of other drugs have been reported. Long-term use of orlistat has not resulted in any documented cases of serious reactions.

Side effects associated with use of the antiobesity drugs are listed in the Clinical Problems Box.

Orexigenics

The adverse effects of the corticosteroids, progestational agents, and anabolic steroids are presented in Chapters 50, 51, and 52, respectively.

Dronabinol produces dose-related CNS effects including a "high" characterized by laughing, elation, altered time perception, and a heightened sensory awareness at low doses; memory impairment and depersonalization at moderate doses; and motor incoordination at high

TABLE 20.1	Selected Pharmacokinetic Parameters	
Drug	**T$_{1/2}$ (Hrs)**	**Metabolism and Elimination**
Benzphetamine	Unknown	M, R
Diethylpropion	4–6 for metabolites	M, R
Phendimetrazine	1.9 for immediate-release preparation	M, R
	10 for sustained-released preparation	
Phentermine	19–24	R
Phentermine/ Topiramate	19–24/21	M, R
Lorcaserin	11	M, R
Liraglutide	13	R, F

T$_{1/2}$, Half-life; *F*, fecal; *M*, metabolized; *R*, renal.

CLINICAL PROBLEMS

Benzphetamine, Diethylpropion, Phentermine, Phendimetrazine
Headaches, nervousness, insomnia, tachycardia

Lorcaserin
Headache, depression, anxiety, and suicidal ideation

Liraglutide
Antibody development with allergic manifestations, thyroid cancer, acute pancreatitis

Orlistat
Malabsorption of fat-soluble vitamins; steatorrhea (soft and oily stools) and fecal incontinence; cramping, diarrhea, and flatulence; liver and pancreatic disease

TRADE NAMES

In addition to generic and fixed-combination preparations, the following trade-named materials are some of the important compounds available in the United States.

Antiobesity Drugs
Benzphetamine (Didrex)
Bupropion/naltrexone (Contrave)
Diethylpropion (Tenuate, Tepanil)
Liraglutide (Saxenda)
Lorcaserin (Belviq)
Orlistat (Xenical, Alli)
Phendimetrazine (Bontril, Plegine, Prelu-2, X-Trozine)
Phentermine (Adipex-P, Anoxine, Fastin, Ionamin, Obenix, Obephen, Oby-Cap, Oby-Trim, Phentercot, Phentride, Pro-Fast, Teramine, Zantryl)
Phentermine/Topiramate (Qsymia)

Drugs for Anorexia, Bulimia, and Binge-Eating Disorder
Antidepressants
Lisdexamfetamine dimesylate (Vyvanse)

Orexigenics
Dronabinol (Marinol)
Megestrol (Megace)
Oxandrolone (Anavar, Oxandrin)

doses. Dronabinol may decrease seizure threshold and has variable effects on the cardiovascular system. Thus it should be used with caution in patients with a history of either seizure or cardiac disorders.

NEW DEVELOPMENTS

Novel drugs and therapies will emerge as the basic understanding of the pathways and neurotransmitters involved in eating disorders expands. To date, most research is focused on treatment of obesity, which has provided few new drugs despite a better understanding of the pathways and mechanisms. Anorexia and bulimia are still not well understood, and psychotherapy remains the cornerstone of therapy. However, as the role of specific neurotransmitters becomes more clearly defined, new treatment options may become available.

Orexigenic signals appear to be redundant in the body and involve numerous peptides, hormones, and neurotransmitters. When body fat stores decrease, serum concentrations of leptin secreted by adipocytes and insulin secreted by the pancreas also decrease while endocrine cells within the GI tract secrete ghrelin. Ghrelin readily crosses the blood-brain barrier to exert its effects in the arcuate nucleus of the hypothalamus and stimulates production of orexigenic signals that regulate appetite and energy use. As we continue to learn about these systems, new targets for drug development will emerge.

CLINICAL RELEVANCE FOR HEALTHCARE PROFESSIONALS

Because obesity is associated with the development of numerous disorders and increased mortality, it is imperative for all healthcare professionals to discuss this issue with their patients and educate them and their families. Both psychosocial and economic factors come into play, and all efforts should be taken to provide obese and overweight individuals with information on resources available to them.

SELF-ASSESSMENT QUESTIONS

1. A 47-year-old obese man with a history of hypertension and angina requires pharmacological intervention for weight loss. Which of the following drugs would be *best* for this patient?
   A. Diethylpropion.
   B. Fluoxetine.
   C. Orlistat.
   D. Phentermine.
   E. Phentermine/topiramate.

2. A 22-year-old woman with binge-eating disorder is seeking help for her condition. Which of the following drugs might be prescribed by her family physician?
   A. Lisdexamfetamine.
   B. Fluoxetine.
   C. Phentermine.
   D. Liraglutide.
   E. Diethylpropion.

3. Which of the following agents is not absorbed into the systemic circulation and has its actions locally in the gastrointestinal tract?
   A. Amitriptyline.
   B. Dronabinol.
   C. Phentermine.
   D. Orlistat.
   E. Phentermine/topiramate.

4. Which of the following is an agonist at cannabinoid type 1 receptors in both the brain and gastrointestinal tract?
   A. Benzphetamine.
   B. Lorcaserin.
   C. Dronabinol.
   D. Phentermine/topiramate.
   E. Phentermine.

5. A 42-year-old obese man with hyperglycemia seeks his physician for help. A drug that is approved for both diabetes and obesity that may prove to be useful for this patient is:
   A. Amphetamine.
   B. Lorcaserin.
   C. Liraglutide.
   D. Phentermine/topiramate.

FURTHER READING

Khera R, Murad MH, Chandar AK, et al. Association of Pharmacological Treatments for Obesity With Weight Loss and Adverse Events: A Systematic Review and Meta-analysis. *JAMA.* 2016;315(22):2424–2434.

WEBSITES

https://www.cdc.gov/obesity/
The Centers for Disease Control and Prevention has an excellent website with links to numerous resources on obesity.

https://www.niddk.nih.gov/health-information/health-statistics/Pages/overweight-obesity-statistics.aspx
The National Institute of Diabetes and Digestive and Kidney Diseases has an excellent website on obesity, statistics, and associated disorders with links to numerous resources.

https://www.cancer.gov/about-cancer/treatment/research/cachexia
The National Cancer Institute maintains a website on "Tackling the Conundrum of Cachexia in Cancer" with information on mechanisms involved and treatments.

Treatment of Seizure Disorders

Michael A. Rogawski

MAJOR DRUG CLASSES

Voltage-gated ion channel modulators
  Voltage-gated sodium channel blockers
  T-type voltage-gated calcium channel blockers
  Gabapentinoids ($\alpha 2\delta$ ligands)
  K_v7 voltage-gated potassium channel openers
GABA enhancers
  $GABA_A$ receptor modulators
  GABA transporter inhibitors
  GABA transaminase inhibitors
AMPA receptor antagonists
SV2A ligands
Mixed-acting compounds

ABBREVIATIONS

ACTH	Adrenocorticotropin
ARS	Acute repetitive seizures
EEG	Electroencephalogram
GABA	γ-Aminobutyric acid
GAT-1	GABA transporter

THERAPEUTIC OVERVIEW

Epilepsy is a chronic episodic disorder of brain function characterized by the unpredictable occurrence of seizures. Epileptic seizures are transitory alterations in behavior, sensation, or consciousness caused by abnormal, excessive, or synchronous neuronal activity in the brain that can be detected with the electroencephalogram (EEG). Approximately 0.8% of the population suffers from epilepsy. Epilepsy can occur at any age, but onset is more frequent in children younger than about age 10 and in adults over age 50. Recurrent seizures, if frequent, interfere with a patient's ability to carry out day-to-day activities. However, daily oral use of antiseizure medications allows approximately 70% of patients to remain seizure free.

Seizures are classified into two major types: focal onset (formerly partial onset) seizures and generalized onset seizures. Focal seizures arise in a localized region in one cerebral hemisphere and are accompanied by EEG abnormalities that are restricted to the epileptic focus. In contrast, generalized seizures are associated with EEG features indicating simultaneous hemispheric activation.

Focal seizures are further classified as aware, impaired awareness, or focal to bilateral tonic-clonic. The seizures are termed aware (formerly simple) if consciousness is preserved and impaired awareness (formerly complex) if consciousness is impaired or lost. In impaired awareness seizures, motor activity often appears as a complicated and seemingly purposeful movement referred to as an automatism. If a focal seizure spreads to encompass both hemispheres, the focal seizure can transition to a bilateral tonic-clonic seizure (formerly secondarily generalized) resulting in tonic-clonic manifestations, which involve rigid extension of the trunk and limbs (tonic phase) followed by rhythmic contractions of the arms and legs (clonic phase).

In generalized seizures, both hemispheres are involved at the onset. There are various types of generalized seizures, including generalized tonic-clonic seizures, which are similar to focal to bilateral tonic-clonic seizures except that they do not begin focally; absence seizures, characterized by impaired consciousness and minimal motor manifestations; and other types of seizures, including myoclonic, clonic, tonic, or atonic (astatic), depending on the specific clinical manifestations. The classification of seizures and their characteristics are presented in the Therapeutic Overview Box.

Status epilepticus, clinically defined as abnormally prolonged or repetitive seizures, presents in several forms, including (1) tonic-clonic (convulsive) status epilepticus, (2) nonconvulsive status epilepticus, (3) focal status epilepticus, and (4) absence status epilepticus. Convulsive status epilepticus is a life-threatening medical emergency that requires immediate treatment. Traditionally, convulsive status epilepticus was defined as more than 30 minutes of either (1) continuous seizure activity or (2) two or more sequential seizures without full recovery of consciousness between seizures. Because persistent seizure activity is believed to cause permanent neuronal injury and the majority of seizures terminates in 2 to 3 minutes, it is now generally accepted that treatment should begin when the seizure duration reaches 5 minutes for generalized tonic-clonic seizures and 10 minutes for focal seizures with or without impairment of awareness.

Convulsive status epilepticus can lead to systemic hypoxia, acidemia, hyperpyrexia, cardiovascular collapse, and renal shutdown. Nonconvulsive status epilepticus, a persistent change in behavior or mental processes with continuous epileptiform EEG but without major motor signs, also requires urgent treatment.

All people are capable of experiencing seizures. Brain insults such as fever, hypoglycemia, hypocalcemia, hyponatremia, and extreme lactic acidosis, or exposure to certain drugs or toxins, can trigger a seizure, but if the condition is corrected, seizures do not recur, and the condition is not considered epilepsy. Epilepsy is a disease (also variously described as a disorder) characterized by an enduring predisposition to epileptic seizures and by the neurobiological, cognitive, psychological, and social consequences of this condition. The diverse causes of seizures and epilepsy are listed in Box 21.1.

The goal of antiseizure drug therapy is to prevent seizures while minimizing adverse effects. If seizures continue after drug therapy is initiated, the dose may be increased until unacceptable adverse effects

---

prevent further dosage increases, at which point another drug can be substituted or a second drug added. Children who are seizure free for periods longer than 2–4 years while on antiseizure medications will remain so when medications are withdrawn in 70% of cases so that a trial of discontinuation may be warranted. Resolution of seizures is common for certain syndromes, such as childhood absence epilepsy and benign epilepsy of childhood with centrotemporal spikes (BECTS), but infrequent for others, such as juvenile myoclonic epilepsy. Resolution is unlikely in adults with an abnormal neurologic examination or an abnormal EEG so that drug treatment will likely be required for the life of the patient.

Pathophysiology

Many cases of epilepsy are the result of damage to the brain, as occurs in traumatic brain injury, stroke, or infections, whereas in other cases, the epilepsy is caused by a brain tumor or developmental lesion such as a cortical or vascular malformation; these epilepsies are referred to as symptomatic. Mesial temporal lobe epilepsy associated with hippocampal sclerosis is a symptomatic epilepsy that is a common cause of medication refractory seizures.

In 40% of all epilepsies, genetic factors are believed to be the root cause. In some cases, the epilepsy is a component of a genetic syndrome, such as tuberous sclerosis, that has other associated structural or metabolic brain abnormalities. In other cases, the genetic epilepsy has seizures as its only clinical manifestation, and there is no apparent structural or metabolic disorder of the brain. Such idiopathic epilepsies include benign epilepsy of childhood with centrotemporal spikes (BECTS), benign familial neonatal convulsions, childhood absence epilepsy, and juvenile myoclonic epilepsy. In most genetic epilepsies, the inheritance is complex (polygenic); rarely, a single gene defect can be identified. Some monogenic epilepsies and associated gene mutations are listed in Box 21.2. In some cases, these genetic epilepsies are benign, and in other cases, they are severe and termed epileptic encephalopathies.

It is noteworthy that many of the genes in the monogenic epilepsies encode subunits of ion channels, which are the fundamental mediators of neuronal excitability. These types of epilepsies can be considered channelopathies. However, some monogenic epilepsies are caused by mutations in non–ion channel genes, including neural adhesion molecules, such as PCDH19 (protocadherin 19), and proteins involved in synapse development, such as LGI1 (leucine-rich glioma inactivated 1).

The cellular and molecular events leading to the development of focal epilepsies in cases of cortical injury are poorly understood. There is better understanding of the physiology of the seizures. Focal seizures are thought to occur as a consequence of the loss of surround inhibition, a process that normally prevents the activation of neurons adjacent to a focus (Fig. 21.1). This loss of surround inhibition may result from impaired γ-aminobutyric acid (GABA) transmission, loss of GABA interneurons, changes in GABA type A (GABA$_A$) receptors, or alterations in intracellular chloride or bicarbonate ion concentrations. Excessive glutamate-mediated excitation may also lead to focal seizures. Impaired GABA-mediated inhibition or excessive glutamate-mediated excitation predisposes to abnormal hypersynchronous activity manifest as epileptiform discharges, which, if they encompass a large enough area of cortex, are associated with the motor, sensory, psychic, or autonomic symptoms of a focal seizure.

Generalized seizures involve both hemispheres and thalamic synchronizing mechanisms. In tonic-clonic convulsions, the tonic phase of muscle contraction is thought to reflect prolonged neuronal depolarization as a consequence of the loss of GABA-mediated inhibition and the dominance of excitatory glutamate neurotransmission. As the seizure evolves, neurons repolarize and afterhyperpolarizations are apparent, which reflect the reappearance of GABA-mediated inhibition and diminished glutamate excitation, producing the clonic phase. Drugs that increase surround inhibition and prevent the spread of synchronous activity are effective in the treatment of focal seizures.

Our understanding of the onset of generalized tonic-clonic seizures is limited. However, there are some clues concerning the cellular mechanisms underlying absence seizures, which are characterized by the sudden appearance of spike-wave discharges synchronized throughout the brain. The EEGs recorded during an absence seizure compared with a generalized tonic-clonic seizure are shown in Fig. 21.2. Studies support a major role of thalamocortical circuits in the pathogenesis of absence seizures with abnormal oscillations generated by excitatory glutamatergic cortical pyramidal and thalamic relay neurons and inhibitory GABAergic thalamic reticular neurons (Fig. 21.3). Thalamic relay neurons project to the cortex, and cortical pyramidal neurons project back to the thalamus

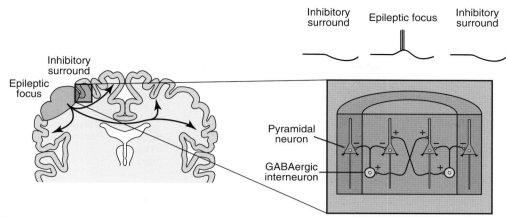

FIG. 21.1 Seizure Generation and Spread in a Focal Seizure. Epileptiform activity begins in a localized area (epileptic focus) and spreads to adjacent and contralateral cortical regions. Epileptic activity reflects the synchronized activity of excitatory (+) glutamate cortical pyramidal neurons. Spread is restrained by inhibitory (−) γ-aminobutyric acid (GABA) interneurons. Seizure spread is believed to reflect the loss of surround inhibition. Antiseizure drugs that enhance GABA inhibition restrain seizure spread. Spread can also be prevented by sodium-channel blocking drugs (Fig. 21.4) and AMPA receptor antagonists.

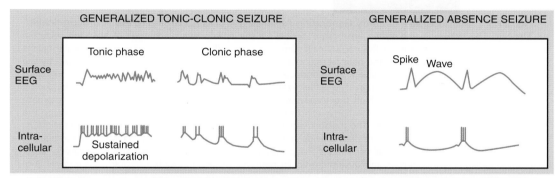

FIG. 21.2 Comparison of the Electrical Behavior of the Surface Electroencephalogram (EEG) and Single-Neuron Recording During Generalized Tonic-Clonic and Absence Seizures on a Time Scale of Hundreds of Milliseconds. Surface EEG signals are field responses detected with flat metal electrodes on the scalp. Intracellular recordings represent the membrane potential changes of individual cortical neurons. A generalized tonic-clonic seizure begins with a tonic phase consisting of rhythmic high-frequency discharges recorded in the surface EEG; cortical neurons undergo sustained depolarization, which generates high-frequency action potential firing. Subsequently, the seizure converts to a clonic phase, characterized by groups of spikes on the EEG; cortical neurons exhibit periodic depolarizations with clusters of action potentials on the crests. In an absence seizure, 3-Hz spike-and-wave discharges are recorded in the surface EEG. During the spike phase, cortical neurons generate short-duration depolarizations, which trigger a brief burst of action potentials. During the wave phase, cortical neurons are hyperpolarized. Recognizing the differences between the single neuron electrical events in tonic-clonic and absence seizures helps in understanding why antiseizure drugs that inhibit sustained repetitive firing of action potentials (see Fig. 21.4) are effective in the treatment of tonic-clonic, but not absence, seizures.

in a recurrent excitatory loop. Thalamic relay neurons exhibit spike-wave discharges that generate normal cortical rhythms and participate in the generation of sleep spindles. The normal bursting pattern of these neurons results from the activation of low voltage-gated T-type calcium channels during depolarization, followed by GABA release from thalamic reticular neurons and hyperpolarization. The circuit transitions to abnormal rhythmicity at the onset of an absence seizure. T-type calcium channels in relay neurons and thalamic reticular neurons play a critical role in the pathological behavior of absence seizures, as blockade of these channels, most notably by ethosuximide, is effective for the treatment of such seizures.

MECHANISMS OF ACTION

Selection of the correct antiseizure drug depends on accurate diagnosis of the patient's seizure type and epilepsy syndrome. Focal onset seizures must be distinguished from generalized onset seizures because some drugs effective for focal seizures do not prevent and may exacerbate some generalized seizure types. Certain epilepsy syndromes, such as infantile spasms, require treatment with special agents.

Epileptic activity may occur as a consequence of either decreased inhibition or increased excitation of neurons. Agents used for the treatment of epilepsy depress aberrant neuronal firing primarily by

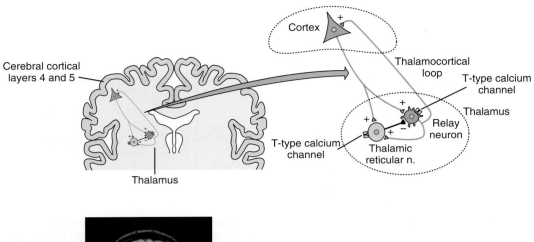

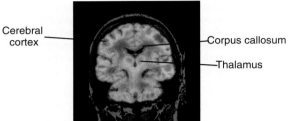

FIG. 21.3 Thalamocortical Circuitry Generating Absence Seizures According to the "Corticoreticular" Theory. The thalamus and cortex are both essential for the spike-wave discharges of absence seizures; bilateral synchrony depends on the corpus callosum connecting the two hemispheres. Spike-wave bursts are likely initiated in the cortex (the perioral region of the somatosensory cortex has been implicated) by the discharge of a network of massively interconnected excitatory neurons in the presence of insufficient γ-aminobutyric acid (GABA) inhibition. This initial event is followed by entrainment of the thalamus leading to synchronized oscillations in which the thalamus and cortex drive each other. Excitatory (+) glutamate thalamic relay neurons project to the cortex, and excitatory glutamate cortical neurons project back to the thalamus, forming a recurrent loop. The thalamic reticular nucleus, a shell-like structure covering the thalamus, is composed of GABA interneurons that provide massive inhibitory (−) input to thalamic relay neurons and may contribute to the pathological oscillations. T-type voltage-gated calcium channels are necessary for burst firing in thalamic relay neurons and thalamic reticular neurons. Shown below the diagram is a coronal fluorodeoxyglucose positron emission tomography image of a human brain superimposed on T1 magnetic resonance image, illustrating the location of the relevant structures. (Courtesy of Johnson KA, Becker JA. *Whole Brain Atlas.* http://www.med.harvard.edu/aanlib/cprt.html)

THERAPEUTIC OVERVIEW

Focal Onset (Partial Onset) Seizures

Focal aware seizure (formerly simple partial seizure)

Sensory, motor, autonomic, or psychic symptoms, without altered awareness

Focal impaired awareness seizure (formerly complex partial seizure)

Dreamy disaffective state with or without automatisms, with altered awareness

Focal to bilateral tonic-clonic seizure (formerly secondarily generalized tonic-clonic seizure or grand mal seizure)

Evolution of focal aware or focal impaired awareness seizure to convulsion with rigid extension of trunk and limbs (tonic phase) and rhythmic contractions of arms and legs (clonic phase)

Generalized Onset Seizures

Generalized tonic-clonic seizure (formerly primary generalized tonic-clonic seizure or grand mal seizure)

Similar to focal to bilateral tonic-clonic seizure except that onset is in both hemispheres; occurs in patients with genetic (idiopathic) generalized epilepsies

Generalized absence seizures

Abrupt loss of consciousness with staring and cessation of ongoing activity with or without eye blinks; occurs in patients with genetic (idiopathic) generalized epilepsies, including childhood absence epilepsy

Other types of generalized onset seizures

Myoclonic seizure: rapid shock-like (jerking) muscle contraction

Atonic seizure (drop seizure or astatic seizure): loss of muscle tone

Epileptic spasm: sudden flexion, extension or flexion-extension of neck, trunk, arms, and legs

BOX 21.3   Mechanisms of Action of Antiseizure Drugs

Voltage-Gated Ion-Channel Modulators
Voltage-Gated Sodium-Channel Blockers
Phenytoin
Carbamazepine
Oxcarbazepine
Eslicarbazepine acetate (prodrug)
Lamotrigine
Lacosamide

T-Type Calcium-Channel Blocker
Ethosuximide

α2δ Ligands
Gabapentin
Pregabalin

Voltage-Gated Potassium-Channel Opener
Retigabine (ezogabine)

GABA Enhancers
GABA$_A$ Receptor Positive Modulators
Phenobarbital
Primidone
Benzodiazepines including diazepam, lorazepam, and clonazepam

GABA Transporter (GAT-1) Inhibitor
Tiagabine

GABA Transaminase Inhibitor
Vigabatrin

Glutamate AMPA Receptor Antagonist
Perampanel

SV2A Ligand
Levetiracetam
Brivaracetam

Mixed/Unknown
Valproate
Topiramate
Zonisamide
Felbamate
Rufinamide
Adrenocorticotropin

GABA, γ-Aminobutyric acid.

altering ion channel activity, enhancing GABA-mediated inhibitory neurotransmission, or dampening glutamate-mediated excitatory neurotransmission. Although some drugs have a single mechanism of action, several of these agents have more than one mechanism. Antiseizure drugs classified according to mechanisms of action are listed in Box 21.3.

Voltage-Gated Ion-Channel Modulators

The voltage-gated sodium-channel blockers are widely used antiseizure drugs with demonstrated effectiveness for focal seizures. These drugs include phenytoin, carbamazepine, oxcarbazepine, eslicarbazepine acetate (a prodrug), lamotrigine, and lacosamide. These agents reduce the repetitive firing of neurons by producing a use-dependent and voltage-dependent blockade of sodium channels (Fig. 21.4). By prolonging the inactivated state of the sodium channel and thus the relative refractory period, these drugs do not alter the first action potential in a train but rather reduce the likelihood of repetitive action potentials. Neurons retain their ability to generate action potentials at the lower frequencies common during normal brain function. The discrimination between normal firing from usual membrane potential levels and high-frequency firing under the abnormally depolarized conditions of the epileptic discharge allows these drugs to inhibit seizures without affecting normal brain function at therapeutic concentrations.

T-type calcium channels provide for rhythmic firing of thalamic neurons and are thought to be involved in generating spike-wave discharges in absence seizures. Ethosuximide inhibits T-type calcium channels, thus suppressing absence seizures.

The α2δ auxiliary subunit of voltage-gated calcium channels modulates the trafficking and biophysical properties of these membrane channels but can also be non–channel associated and interact with proteins in the extracellular matrix and alter synaptogenesis. Although the specific role of α2δ in seizure disorders is unclear, this protein is the primary target of the gabapentinoid drugs gabapentin and pregabalin. These compounds have a close structural resemblance to GABA but do not affect GABA receptors or any other mechanism related to GABA-mediated neurotransmission. Rather, the gabapentinoids appear to exert their antiseizure and analgesic activity by interacting with α2δ, although how this action protects against seizures is unknown.

Ezogabine opens K$_v$7 voltage-gated potassium channels (K$_v$7.2–K$_v$7.5) but does not affect the cardiac channel (K$_v$7.1). Potassium channels are inhibitory and cause neuronal hyperpolarization when activated. Both K$_v$7.2 and K$_v$7.3 contribute to the M-current, a potassium-channel current that increases as the membrane potential in neurons approaches action potential threshold and serves as a "brake" on epileptic burst firing.

GABA Enhancers

GABA, the major inhibitory neurotransmitter in the brain, causes fast inhibition through its action on GABA$_A$ receptors (Chapter 17) to reduce circuit hyperexcitability. Barbiturates including phenobarbital exert antiseizure activity in part by acting as positive allosteric modulators (PAMs) of GABA$_A$ receptors to prolong the duration of channel openings upon receptor activation by GABA. The benzodiazepines, such as diazepam, lorazepam, and clonazepam, are also PAMs of GABA$_A$ receptors, acting at a site distinct from that of the barbiturates to increase the frequency of channel openings upon receptor activation by GABA.

Several drugs increase GABAergic inhibition by either decreasing the reuptake of GABA or by inhibiting its catabolism. Tiagabine blocks GABA reuptake into presynaptic neurons and glia by inhibiting the GABA transporter (GAT-1), while vigabatrin is an irreversible inhibitor of GABA transaminase, the enzyme that inactivates GABA.

AMPA Receptor Antagonist

AMPA receptors mediate glutamate excitation in the brain and are critical for both the local generation of seizure activity in epileptic foci and for the spread of excitation to distant sites. Activation of these tetrameric ion channels by glutamate leads to sodium (and in some receptors, calcium) influx, contributing to the excitatory postsynaptic potential (EPSP). Perampanel is a potent noncompetitive antagonist of AMPA receptors that binds to an allosteric site on the extracellular side of the channel, acting as a wedge to prevent channel opening.

SV2A Ligands

Levetiracetam and brivaracetam exert their antiseizure activity by binding to SV2A, a ubiquitous synaptic vesicle membrane glycoprotein

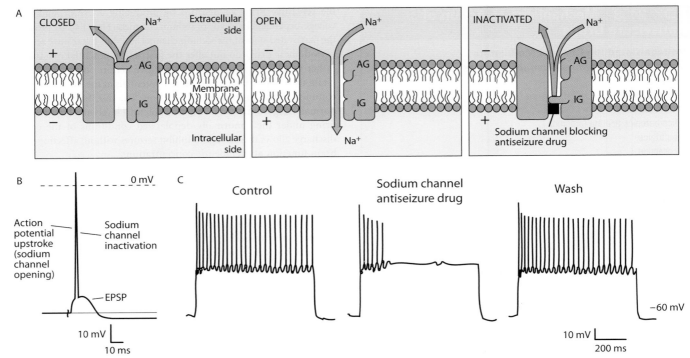

FIG. 21.4 Action of Sodium-Channel Blocking Antiseizure Drugs on Voltage-Gated Sodium Channels. (A) At hyperpolarized membrane potentials, the sodium-channel activation gate (AG) is closed, blocking sodium influx. Depolarization of the neuron causes AG to open, allowing sodium flux. Within less than 1 ms, the inactivation gate (IG) closes, terminating sodium flux. When the membrane potential is repolarized, the AG closes (not shown), and after 1–2 ms, the IG opens, and the channel reverts to its closed (resting) state, where it can be opened again by depolarization. Sodium-channel blocking drugs selectively bind to and stabilize the inactivated state of the channel. (B) Membrane potential changes in a neuron activated by an excitatory postsynaptic potential (EPSP) generated by stimulation of excitatory (glutamate) afferents. When the depolarization of the EPSP reaches threshold, an action potential is generated. The upstroke of the action potential results from sodium influx through voltage-gated channels opened by the EPSP depolarization. The downstroke is largely due to sodium-channel inactivation. (C) Depolarization of a neuron in vitro causes a high-frequency train of action potentials. In the presence of a sodium-channel blocking drug, the train terminates because sodium channels are progressively inhibited in a use-dependent fashion as the sodium channels cycle into the inactivated state where drug binding occurs. Wash out of the drug restores the ability of the neuron to discharge long trains.

involved in exocytosis. The precise role of SV2A in the exocytotic process is not well understood, but evidence suggests that it interacts with synaptotagmin, a trigger for calcium-mediated exocytosis. It is possible that the binding of levetiracetam and brivaracetam to SV2A reduces the release of glutamate during trains of high-frequency activity as occurs during epileptic activity.

Mixed-Acting Compounds

The mechanisms of action of many antiseizure drugs involve mixed effects or are poorly understood. These compounds include valproate, felbamate, topiramate, zonisamide, rufinamide, and adrenocorticotropin (ACTH).

The antiseizure effects of valproate have been attributed to increases in the turnover of GABA in a regionally selective manner, which might be associated with enhanced synaptic or extrasynaptic inhibition, but this mechanism is not well established and there is no consensus on the drug's antiseizure mechanism. Felbamate acts as a PAM at $GABA_A$ receptors and blocks glutamate NMDA receptors, although the relationship between this latter action and the antiseizure activity of felbamate is questionable. Topiramate may modulate voltage-gated sodium channels and glutamate receptors and may potentiate GABA activity, but again, the relationship between these actions and antiseizure activity is not

well understood. Zonisamide blocks voltage-gated sodium and T-type calcium channels, while rufinamide also modulates voltage-gated sodium-channel activity but may also have other actions.

ACTH, which is used for the treatment of infantile spasms, stimulates glucocorticoid (cortisol) synthesis and release from the adrenal cortex. The cortisol could influence infantile spasms through an antiinflammatory action or in some other fashion. Synthetic glucocorticoids such as prednisone and prednisolone also have therapeutic activity in the treatment of infantile spasms.

RELATIONSHIP OF MECHANISMS OF ACTION TO CLINICAL RESPONSE

Drugs Used in the Treatment of Focal Seizures

The sodium-channel blockers (except lamotrigine), gabapentinoids, and tiagabine are used exclusively for the treatment of focal seizures and focal to bilateral tonic-clonic seizures (Box 21.4). Some of these drugs have also shown efficacy in generalized onset tonic-clonic seizures, including oxcarbazepine and phenytoin. These drugs may exacerbate certain types of generalized onset seizures, including absence and myoclonic seizures, and seizures in Dravet syndrome.

BOX 21.4   Drugs Effective for Specific Seizure Types

Focal Seizures Exclusively
Carbamazepine
Oxcarbazepine
Eslicarbazepine acetate
Lacosamide
Phenytoin
Gabapentin
Pregabalin
Tiagabine
Vigabatrin (also infantile spasms)
Ezogabine

Focal Seizures and Certain Generalized Seizure Types
Lamotrigine
Levetiracetam
Brivaracetam (evidence only available in focal seizures)
Perampanel
Phenobarbital
Primidone
Felbamate

Broad Spectrum (Generalized Seizures and Focal Seizures)
Valproate (divalproex sodium)
Topiramate
Zonisamide

Absence Seizures
Ethosuximide
Divalproex sodium
Lamotrigine

Myoclonic Seizures
Divalproex sodium
Levetiracetam

Zonisamide
Topiramate
Lamotrigine

Atonic Seizures
Valproate (divalproex sodium)
Clobazam
Rufinamide
Topiramate
Felbamate
Lamotrigine

Dravet Syndrome
Clobazam
Valproate (divalproex sodium)
Topiramate
Stiripentol

West Syndrome
Adrenocorticotropic hormone
Vigabatrin

Status Epilepticus
Intravenous lorazepam or diazepam, intramuscular midazolam
Intravenous fosphenytoin or phenytoin
Intravenous phenobarbital, valproic acid, lacosamide, levetiracetam
For refractory status epilepticus, anesthesia with intravenous pentobarbital, propofol, midazolam, thiopental, ketamine

Acute Repetitive Seizures (Seizure Clusters)
Diazepam rectal gel
Rectal paraldehyde
Buccal (oromucosal) midazolam
Intranasal midazolam, diazepam, lorazepam

Drugs Used in the Treatment of Focal Seizures With Efficacy in Certain Generalized Seizure Types

Some antiseizure drugs are effective for the treatment of both focal seizures and certain generalized seizures. For example, lamotrigine is first choice for focal seizures and is also useful in treating absence seizures, although it is not as effective as ethosuximide or valproate. Levetiracetam is also first choice for focal seizures and is probably useful for myoclonic seizures. Brivaracetam, a drug related to levetiracetam, likely has the same spectrum of activity as levetiracetam but has not been studied in the treatment of other seizure types. Perampanel is useful in the treatment of focal and focal to bilateral tonic-clonic seizures and in the treatment of generalized onset tonic-clonic seizures. Phenobarbital is effective in the treatment of focal seizures, focal to bilateral tonic-clonic seizures, generalized onset tonic-clinic seizures, and other seizure types, but it is not effective in absence seizures and is not commonly used because it is sedating and has many drug-drug interactions. Primidone is not commonly used, as it is metabolized to phenobarbital and has many of the same issues. Felbamate is effective for the treatment of focal seizures, focal to bilateral tonic-clonic seizures, generalized onset tonic-clinic seizures, and seizures associated with Lennox-Gastaut syndrome in children but is rarely used because of the risk of aplastic anemia and hepatic failure.

Valproate, topiramate, and zonisamide have the broadest spectrum among antiseizure drugs and are useful in the treatment of focal seizures and diverse generalized seizure types. Valproate is especially effective and considered the first choice for patients who exhibit multiple generalized seizure types. It is widely used for myoclonic, atonic, and generalized tonic-clonic seizures. Valproate is also effective in focal seizures, but it may not be as effective as carbamazepine or phenytoin.

Drugs Used in the Treatment of Absence Seizures

Ethosuximide and valproate are the drugs of choice for absence seizures. Although less effective than these two drugs, lamotrigine also has activity in the treatment of absence seizures and may be prescribed because of its greater tolerability or fewer fetal risks than valproate.

Drugs Used in the Treatment of Lennox-Gastaut Syndrome

Lennox-Gastaut syndrome is a severe type of childhood epilepsy with multiple seizure types, including atonic (drop) seizures. Seizures in Lennox-Gastaut syndrome are difficult to treat and usually require drug combinations. Valproate, in combination with lamotrigine and a benzodiazepine such as clonazepam, is the most widely used combination. Topiramate, clobazam, rufinamide, felbamate, and lamotrigine are also used. Sodium-channel blocking antiseizure drugs other than lamotrigine are not used, as they may worsen atonic seizures.

Drugs Used in the Treatment of Status Epilepticus and Acute Seizures

The initial treatment of choice for status epilepticus is a benzodiazepine administered intravenously; lorazepam or diazepam are most commonly used. Recent evidence indicates that intramuscular midazolam delivered with an autoinjector system is equally effective and may be easier and more rapid to administer in an out-of-hospital setting. If seizures continue, or if there is a concern that seizures may recur, a second therapy is administered. Intravenous fosphenytoin or phenytoin is most common in the United States, although there is no evidence that these choices are superior to intravenous valproate or levetiracetam. Phenobarbital is also an acceptable second therapy, but it causes persistent sedation and may have serious cardiorespiratory adverse effects, including respiratory depression and hypotension. Lacosamide is available in an intravenous formulation, but there is little published experience to assess its efficacy. If the second therapy fails to stop the seizures, an additional second therapy agent is often tried.

Refractory status epilepticus occurs when seizures continue or recur at least 30 minutes following treatment with first and second therapy agents. Refractory status epilepticus is treated with anesthetic doses of pentobarbital, propofol, midazolam, thiopental, or ketamine, usually in combination. If status epilepticus continues or recurs 24 hours or more after the onset of anesthesia, the condition is considered superrefractory. Often superrefractory status epilepticus is recognized when anesthetics are withdrawn and seizures recur. There are no established therapies for superrefractory status epilepticus other than to reinstitute general anesthesia.

Acute repetitive seizures (ARS), or seizure clusters, are groups of seizures that occur more frequently than usual, typically three or more seizures within 24 hours. There is complete recovery between seizures so that patients do not meet the definition of status epilepticus. However, ARS can progress to status epilepticus and may be associated with other medical complications, including injury. Optimal management of ARS begins at home, before the need for emergency room care arises. In the United States, diazepam rectal gel is the only approved treatment for ARS. Although it has been demonstrated to be effective, administering the rectal gel can be a cumbersome, time-consuming, and embarrassing experience for the patient and caregivers. Rectal gel is most commonly used in children and rarely in adults because of stigma and difficulty positioning the patient. Buccal (oromucosal) midazolam, in which the treatment solution is administered to the buccal mucosa using an oral syringe, is commonly used in Europe and elsewhere in the world. Intranasal midazolam, diazepam, and lorazepam have also been shown to be efficacious; these drugs are not approved for this route of administration in the United States, but some clinicians use intranasal midazolam or oral benzodiazepines on an off-label basis.

PHARMACOKINETICS

Antiseizure drugs used in the chronic therapy of epilepsy must be orally bioavailable. Even fosphenytoin and benzodiazepines, including midazolam, which are primarily administered parenterally, have excellent oral bioavailability and can be administered orally if necessary.

Seizures are a disorder of brain circuits; consequently, antiseizure agents must cross the blood-brain barrier to be active. Many antiseizure drugs are metabolized by the hepatic cytochrome P450 (CYP) system, and several have active metabolites, including primidone and diazepam. Some of these agents are prodrugs that require activation, including

oxcarbazepine, which is activated to S-licarbazepine, and fosphenytoin, which is converted to phenytoin. Some antiseizure drugs, including gabapentin, pregabalin, vigabatrin, and levetiracetam, are not metabolized and are excreted unchanged in the urine. These drugs have a low propensity for drug-drug interactions.

Some antiseizure drugs, including phenytoin, tiagabine, valproate, diazepam, and perampanel, are highly (>90%) bound to plasma proteins and can be displaced by other protein-bound drugs, resulting in a transitory rise in the active free fraction that may be associated with adverse effects until metabolism or renal excretion reduces the free levels. The usual clinical laboratory determination of blood concentrations represents the total drug exposure (bound plus free) in plasma and may fail to reveal the cause of such toxicity. In states of hypoalbuminemia, free levels may be increased, leading either to toxicity, more rapid hepatic metabolism, or both. The half-life ($t_{1/2}$) of antiseizure drugs varies with the age of the patient and exposure to other drugs. The pharmacokinetic parameters of antiseizure agents are summarized in Table 21.1. The pharmacokinetics of the benzodiazepines are presented in Chapter 17.

Carbamazepine is nearly completely metabolized by CYP3A4 (although CYP2C8 and CYP3A5 may contribute) in the liver to produce carbamazepine-10,11-epoxide, which is relatively stable, accumulates in the blood, and has antiseizure activity. Carbamazepine also induces its own metabolism, with the rate of metabolism increasing during the first 4 to 6 weeks. After this time, larger doses become necessary to maintain constant plasma concentrations.

Oxcarbazepine is a prodrug and completely absorbed and extensively metabolized by hepatic cytosolic enzymes to its active 10-hydroxy metabolite licarbazepine, which is responsible for its clinical effects; both enantiomeric forms of licarbazepine [$R(+)$ and $S(-)$] have antiseizure activity. Oxcarbazepine is administered twice daily. Eslicarbazepine acetate is a prodrug for $S(-)$-licarbazepine and is available as a marketed antiseizure drug recommended for once-daily administration.

Ethosuximide has a long half-life, which allows for once-a-day dosing. However, it has significant gastrointestinal side effects that are frequently intolerable with once-a-day dosing and may be mitigated with divided dosing, which reduces the peak plasma concentration and thereby reduces the incidence of side effects.

Lamotrigine is well absorbed and has negligible first-pass metabolism so that its bioavailability is >95%. However, it has a variable half-life, dependent on concomitant medications. Lamotrigine with valproate is considered to be a particularly effective combination, but valproate inhibits the metabolism of lamotrigine, decreasing its clearance by 60% so that plasma lamotrigine levels are increased. The interaction is a consequence of the effect of valproate on the UGT1A4 glucuronidation of lamotrigine. The addition of lamotrigine to a patient already taking valproate must be done especially slowly to avoid a skin rash (potentially Stevens-Johnson syndrome or toxic epidermal necrolysis) caused by lamotrigine levels rising too rapidly. In contrast, the addition of valproate to a patient already on a stable lamotrigine regimen does not increase the risk, as the patient is desensitized to the immunotoxic effect that causes Stevens-Johnson syndrome.

Phenytoin metabolism is characterized by saturation (zero order) kinetics (Chapter 3). At low doses, there is a linear relationship between the dose and the plasma concentration of the drug. At higher doses, however, there is a much greater rise in plasma concentration for a given increase in dose (nonlinear) because when plasma concentrations rise above a certain value, the liver enzymes that catalyze phenytoin metabolism become saturated. The dose at which this transition occurs varies from patient to patient but is usually between 400 and 600 mg/day (Fig. 21.5). Because of the unusual pharmacokinetic properties of phenytoin, dosing must be individualized.

TABLE 21.1   Pharmacokinetic Parameters

Drug	$t_{1/2}$ (Hours)[a]	Bound to Plasma Proteins (%)	Disposition	Therapeutic Concentration Range (μg/mL)
Brivaracetam	7–8	17	M, R	Not available
Carbamazepine	3–55	75	M	4–12
Clobazam	10–30; 36–46 (N-desmethylclobazam)	70–90	M	0.03–0.30; 0.3–3.0 (N-desmethylclobazam)
Eslicarbazepine acetate	<2 h conversion to eslicarbazepine	30	M	3–35 (based on licarbazepine value for oxcarbazepine)
Ethosuximide	30–60	<10	M, R	40–100
Felbamate	16–22	25	M, R	30–60
Gabapentin	5–9	<3	R	2–20
Lacosamide	13	<15	M, R	10–20
Lamotrigine	7–70	55	M, R	3–15
Leviracetam	6–8	0	M, R	12–46
Oxcarbazepine	7–15 (licarbazepine)	60 (parent), 40 (licarbazepine)	M	3–35 (licarbazepine)
Perampanel	51–129; with inducing comedications, 25	95	M	0.1–1
Phenobarbital	53–118	55	M, R	10–40
Phenytoin	12–36	90	M, R	10–20
Pregabalin	5–7	0	R	0.9–14.2
Primidone	6–8	10	M, R	5–10 (primidone), 10–40 (phenobarbital)
Rufinamide	6–10	35	M	30–40
Tiagabine	7–9	96	M	20–200
Topiramate	10–30	15	R	5–20
Valproate	8–17	90	M	50–100
Vigabatrin	5–8	0	R	0.8–36
Zonisamide	60–65	40	M, R	10–40

[a]Age dependent.

M, Metabolized by liver; R, renal elimination (>3%); $t_{1/2}$, half-life.

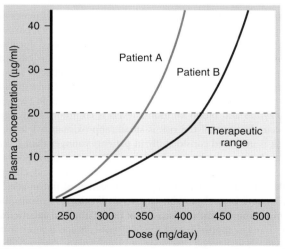

FIG. 21.5 Relationship between the dose and steady-state plasma concentration of phenytoin is illustrated for two patients. In both patients, there is a linear relationship between the dose and plasma concentration at low doses. As the dose increases, there is saturation of metabolism and a shift from first-order to zero-order kinetics, in which a small increase in dose results in a large increase in concentration. This transition occurs at different doses in the two patients so that Patient A would not tolerate an increase in dose from 300 mg/day to 400 mg/day, whereas Patient B would require the higher dose to obtain a therapeutic plasma concentration.

Valproate has a relatively short half-life and is metabolized by both the hepatic microsomal cytochrome P450 system and mitochondria to approximately the same extent. In excess of 25 metabolites have been identified, but valproic acid glucuronide and 3-oxo-valproic acid are the most abundant.

Gabapentin is absorbed in the proximal small intestine by the L-amino acid transport system. Bioavailability is dose limited because of transporter saturation (<60%). Gabapentin blood levels increase linearly with dose, up to about 1.8 g per day. Plasma levels continue to increase at higher doses, but less than expected. Once absorbed, gabapentin is not bound to plasma proteins and is not metabolized. It has a relatively short half-life in the circulation and is excreted unchanged by the kidneys. **Pregabalin** is absorbed throughout the small intestine and by the ascending colon; it is not subject to saturation. Pregabalin is absorbed more rapidly and has higher bioavailability than gabapentin (>90%). Gabapentin can be administered as a gastroretentive formulation, which swells in gastric fluid and remains in the upper gastrointestinal tract, gradually releasing gabapentin over approximately 10 hours. The prodrug **gabapentin enacarbil** is absorbed through the small intestine by the proton-linked monocarboxylate transporter MCT-1, increasing the bioavailability somewhat (about 75%), and eliminating saturation kinetics inasmuch as MCT-1 is expressed at high levels in the intestine.

Levetiracetam is nearly completely absorbed and is not bound to plasma proteins. It is partially metabolized by hydrolysis of the acetamide group to the acid metabolite ucb L057 (24% of the dose), and approximately two-thirds of an administered dose is excreted unchanged by the kidneys.

Perampanel is completely absorbed following oral administration and exhibits linear dose-proportional kinetics. Plasma protein binding is 95%–96%. Perampanel is extensively metabolized, primarily by CYP3A4 followed by glucuronidation. Clearance is increased with inducing drugs such as carbamazepine, oxcarbazepine, and phenytoin, and the concomitant use of these drugs reduces perampanel exposure, necessitating higher doses of perampanel. Because of the long half-life and the propensity for adverse effects, the dose should be up titrated slowly, generally no more rapidly than 2 mg in a 2-week interval.

Phenobarbital is a weak acid that is absorbed with a bioavailability of >90% and rapidly distributed to all tissues. The drug is metabolized by hepatic CYP (CYP2C9 with minor contributions from CYP2C19 and CYP2E1) and by N-glucosidation. Phenobarbital is a major inducer of CYP, accelerating its own metabolism and that of other drugs taken concurrently. Phenobarbital dosing may need upward adjustment as a result of autoinduction. Approximately 20%–40% of an administered dose is excreted unchanged, while the metabolites are excreted as glucuronide conjugates in the urine. Phenobarbital has a long half-life and is usually administered on a once-daily schedule.

Primidone is an analogue of phenobarbital with antiseizure activity but is metabolized slowly to phenobarbital, which gradually accumulates to plasma concentrations comparable to those in patients receiving therapeutic doses of phenobarbital itself. Another active metabolite is phenylethylmalonamide (PEMA). Because of its metabolism to phenobarbital, primidone leads to cytochrome P450 induction. Approximately 65% of the administered dose of primidone is excreted unchanged in the urine.

Tiagabine is well absorbed (bioavailability >90%), but its rate of absorption is decreased by the presence of food. Tiagabine is oxidized primarily by CYP3A4 to inactive metabolites excreted in both the urine and feces. Drug-drug interactions with tiagabine are minimal. However, CYP3A4 induction by the concurrent administration of drugs such as phenobarbital, carbamazepine, or phenytoin increases the clearance of tiagabine by approximately 60%, resulting in approximately a 50% decreased half-life.

Topiramate is well absorbed (bioavailability >80%), and it is not extensively metabolized; typically 40%–50% is excreted unchanged by the kidneys. Elimination is accelerated in the presence of enzyme-inducing antiseizure drugs.

Zonisamide is well absorbed (bioavailability >90%) and undergoes moderate metabolism in the liver, primarily by acetylation (20%) and reduction by CYP3A4 (50%). Zonisamide binds extensively to erythrocytes, resulting in an approximate eightfold higher concentration in erythrocytes than the plasma.

PHARMACOVIGILANCE: ADVERSE EFFECTS AND DRUG INTERACTIONS

Antiseizure drugs have dose-limiting adverse effects that can be avoided by reducing the dose. In addition, there are diverse serious idiosyncratic reactions, including allergic reactions, that are rare but can be life-threatening. These usually occur within several weeks or months of starting a new drug and tend to be dose-independent. Most antiseizure drugs should be introduced slowly to minimize adverse effects.

The adverse effects associated with the use of the benzodiazepines are presented in Chapter 17.

Carbamazepine often causes nausea and visual disturbances during initiation of therapy, but these effects can be minimized by slow titration. With high initial doses or rapid dose escalation, carbamazepine has been associated with rash. In some cases, the dermatological reactions are serious (Stevens-Johnson syndrome and toxic epidermal necrolysis); these reactions are more common in patients of Chinese ancestry, and there is a strong association with the inherited HLA-B*1502 variant. Testing for this variant is recommended in patients of Chinese ancestry. HLA-B*3101 has also been associated with increased risk of the serious skin reactions and is present in a broader ethnic population. It may be worthwhile to test for this allele prior to initiating carbamazepine therapy in all ethnic groups. Carbamazepine causes leukopenia in 12% of children and 7% of adults, which may be transient or persistent and does not usually require discontinuation of treatment. The most problematic hematological effect is aplastic anemia (pancytopenia), which is a rare (less than 1 in 50,000), idiosyncratic (non–dose related) complication that usually occurs early in treatment. Oxcarbazepine is associated with similar adverse effects as carbamazepine. Both drugs may cause hyponatremia, which is usually asymptomatic, but the risk is greater with oxcarbazepine. Multiorgan hypersensitivity reactions have been reported with oxcarbazepine, and cross-reactivity with carbamazepine is not uncommon.

Ethosuximide causes a variety of dose-related side effects including nausea, vomiting, sleep disturbance, drowsiness, and hyperactivity. Psychotic behaviors can be precipitated, and blood dyscrasias and bone marrow suppression have been reported, but rarely.

Lamotrigine produces dose-related side effects that include dizziness, headache, diplopia, nausea, and sleepiness. A rash can occur as either a dose-related or idiosyncratic reaction. The rash may progress to Stevens-Johnson syndrome, toxic epidermal necrolysis, or angioedema, which can be life-threatening. Slow dose titration is essential to reduce the risk of developing a rash.

Phenytoin has many dose-related adverse effects, including ataxia and nystagmus, commonly detected when total plasma concentrations exceed 20 μg/mL. Other adverse effects of long-term therapy are hirsutism, coarsening of facial features, gingival hyperplasia, and osteomalacia. Less common reactions are hepatitis, a lupus-like connective tissue disease, lymphadenopathy, and pseudolymphoma. Because of the propensity for adverse effects and the availability of safer agents with fewer drug-drug interactions, phenytoin is rarely prescribed except for patients who initiated therapy prior to the availability of newer agents.

Valproate may cause nausea, vomiting, and lethargy, particularly early in therapy. The availability of an enteric-coated formulation containing valproate in the form of divalproex sodium has led to a decrease in the incidence of gastrointestinal side effects. Today, the divalproex form is almost always used for oral dosing. Common adverse effects of valproate are weight gain, alopecia, and tremor. Elevation of liver enzymes and blood ammonia levels is common. Fatal hepatitis may occur, but overall the risk is small (approximately 1 in 40,000). The risk is increased considerably in patients younger than 2 years of age treated with multiple antiseizure drugs. Two uncommon dose-related adverse effects of valproate are thrombocytopenia and changes in coagulation parameters resulting from depletion of fibrinogen.

Felbamate is used only in patients with seizures uncontrolled by other medications because of the risk of potentially fatal aplastic anemia, which occurs in approximately 1 in 5000 patients and is more common in individuals with blood dyscrasias and autoimmune disease. Felbamate use has also been associated with hepatic failure, but the risk may not be greater than that of valproate. Felbamate treatment is also associated with typical antiseizure drug adverse effects of anorexia, headache, nausea, dizziness, and gait disturbance. The drug is not sedative and often causes insomnia.

The gabapentinoids gabapentin and pregabalin are relatively safe drugs that are well tolerated and devoid of pharmacokinetic interactions with other agents. They can produce transient fatigue, dizziness, somnolence, and ataxia, which are dose related and usually transitory, as well as edema and weight gain. Gabapentinoids can exacerbate myoclonic seizures.

Levetiracetam is generally well tolerated, but the drug can cause sedation and behavioral adverse effects, including irritability. In some patients, agitation and aggression have been a problem, particularly for those who are intellectually disabled and have a history of behavioral disturbances. Psychotic-like reactions can occur, especially in individuals with a previous psychiatric illness.

Perampanel is generally well tolerated but can cause dizziness, somnolence, headaches, and falls. Because of the tendency to produce sedation, administration at bedtime is advised. Some patients receiving perampanel experience troubling adverse behavioral effects, including irritability, aggression, hostility, anger, and homicidal ideation and threats. The incidence of these symptoms increases with dose, and younger patients are at greater risk.

Phenobarbital is highly sedative, although the sedation may resolve with chronic therapy. Cognitive disturbances are not uncommon, particularly in children. Additional adverse effects in children include hyperactivity, irritability, decreased attention, and mental slowing.

Tiagabine produces abdominal pain and nausea and should be taken with food to minimize these effects. Additional major side effects include dizziness, lack of energy, somnolence, nervousness, tremor, and difficulty concentrating. Tiagabine can also impair cognition and produce confusion and in some circumstances may have proconvulsant actions causing nonconvulsive status epilepticus.

Topiramate often leads to cognitive disturbances characterized by impairment in working memory, cognitive processing speed, motor speed, and verbal fluency and naming. It may also produce nervousness, weight loss, and diplopia. Renal stones have been reported, likely as a consequence of the ability of topiramate to cause a metabolic acidosis resulting from carbonic anhydrase inhibition.

Vigabatrin is only used in exceptional cases where other treatments have failed, or in catastrophic infantile spasms, as it can cause permanent bilateral concentric visual field constriction that is often asymptomatic but can be disabling. In addition, vigabatrin can damage the central retina. Other adverse effects are somnolence, headache, dizziness, and weight gain. Vigabatrin can worsen myoclonic seizures and cause nonconvulsive status epilepticus.

Zonisamide adverse effects include lethargy, dizziness, ataxia, anorexia, and weight loss. Zonisamide is a carbonic anhydrase inhibitor and, like topiramate, is rarely associated with renal stones. In children, oligohydrosis may lead to hyperthermia and heat stroke.

Common adverse effects of the antiseizure drugs are listed in the Clinical Problems Box.

Antiepileptic Drugs During Pregnancy

Seizures during pregnancy present risks to the mother and fetus. Therefore most women with epilepsy who become pregnant require antiseizure drug therapy. If at all possible, valproate, phenobarbital, and topiramate should be avoided, most importantly at the time of conception and early in the pregnancy. Valproate exposure during pregnancy is associated with neural tube defects and other malformations including cardiac, orofacial/craniofacial, and skeletal and limb malformations. In addition, there is evidence of reduced cognitive ability in the offspring, and there may be an increased risk of autism spectrum disorders. The risk with valproate increases with dose. Phenobarbital use during pregnancy is associated with a risk of major congenital malformations, including cardiac defects. Topiramate increases the risk of oral clefts. Other antiseizure drugs may also present a risk of congenital malformations, but the risk may be lower than that of valproate, phenobarbital, and topiramate. Lamotrigine is often considered for use in pregnancy, as pregnancy registries have failed to find evidence of a substantial increase in the risk of major birth defects. The prevalence of malformations following levetiracetam exposure is not significantly different from lamotrigine and the rate in controls. Based on current evidence, lamotrigine and levetiracetam present the lowest level of risk to the fetus, whereas the risk with valproate is clear. Despite the risks, most pregnant patients exposed to antiseizure drugs deliver normal infants. Children of mothers who have epilepsy are at increased risk for malformations even if antiseizure drugs are not used during pregnancy. Whenever possible, women with epilepsy should be counseled before they become pregnant. It is recommended that the lowest possible doses of antiseizure drug be used during pregnancy.

Newborn infants of mothers who have received enzyme-inducing antiseizure drugs during pregnancy may develop a deficiency of vitamin K–dependent clotting factors, which can result in serious hemorrhage during the first 24 hours of life. This situation can be prevented by administering vitamin K to the newborn by intramuscular injection shortly after birth.

NEW DEVELOPMENTS

Several potential new drug treatments for seizures and epilepsy are in clinical development. Many of the treatments are being studied for rare childhood epilepsy syndromes. For example, **cannabidiol**, a nonpsychoactive component of the cannabis plant, is being studied for the treatment of Dravet syndrome and Lennox-Gastaut syndrome. **Fenfluramine** is also being studied for these two syndromes. **Stiripentol**, which is available in Europe, Canada, and Japan as a treatment for Dravet syndrome, is being evaluated for marketing in the United States. The neurosteroid **allopregnanolone** and related compounds, which act as positive modulators of synaptic and extrasynaptic $GABA_A$ receptors, are being studied for various clinical indications. Allopregnanolone is being evaluated for refractory status epilepticus and its 3β-methyl analogue **ganaxolone** for status epilepticus and rare epilepsy syndromes. Various treatments for ARS are under investigation, including thermal aerosol (inhaled) **alprazolam** and intranasal **midazolam** and **diazepam**. Finally, the carbamate **cenobamate** (YKP3089) is being studied for focal seizures.

CLINICAL RELEVANCE FOR HEALTHCARE PROFESSIONALS

Individuals with seizure disorders often require long-term medication. Because many of these antiseizure drugs induce CYPs, it is incumbent on all healthcare professionals to ensure that their patients present a complete drug history. It is also incumbent on healthcare professionals to be aware of the primary adverse reactions associated with the antiseizure drugs so that they can recognize issues readily when they arise.

CLINICAL PROBLEMS

Carbamazepine

Induction of its own metabolism; nausea, dizziness, blurred vision, ataxia (dose-related); rash and rarely Stevens-Johnson syndrome; hyponatremia; leukopenia; aplastic anemia; hepatic failure

Divalproex (Valproate)

Nausea, vomiting, and other gastrointestinal complaints; fine tremor; hair loss; weight gain; thrombocytopenia; teratogenicity; hepatic failure, pancreatitis, hyperammonemia, aplastic anemia; many drug interactions

Ethosuximide

Abdominal pain and vomiting; valproate increases ethosuximide levels; abrupt discontinuation may precipitate absence status epilepticus

Felbamate

Anorexia; aplastic anemia; hepatic failure

Gabapentin and Pregabalin

At initiation of therapy: sedation, fatigue, dizziness, ataxia

Lacosamide

Dizziness, headache, nausea, vomiting, diplopia; prolonged PR interval

Lamotrigine

Dizziness, blurred vision, headache, insomnia; rash, Stevens-Johnson syndrome, toxic epidermal necrolysis; hepatic failure

Levetiracetam

Irritability, aggression

Oxcarbazepine

Nausea and vomiting, dizziness, blurred vision, ataxia (dose-related); rash and rarely Stevens-Johnson syndrome; hyponatremia; leukopenia; aplastic anemia

Perampanel

Behavioral adverse effects: irritability, aggression, hostility, anger; dizziness, somnolence, headache, falls; increases clearance of carbamazepine, oxcarbazepine, phenytoin

Phenobarbital

Fatigue, dizziness, ataxia, confusion; in children: hyperactivity; hepatic failure, rash, Stevens-Johnson syndrome; many drug interactions; rebound seizures on abrupt discontinuation

Phenytoin

Nystagmus (benign sign); diplopia and ataxia (dose-related); cognitive impairment; hirsutism, coarsening of facial features, gingival hyperplasia; saturation metabolism kinetics

Tiagabine

Fatigue, dizziness, somnolence, irritability; spike-wave status epilepticus

Topiramate

Impaired expressive language function, impaired verbal memory, slowing of cognition; paresthesias at initiation of therapy; anorexia and weight loss; kidney stones; heat stroke (children); metabolic acidosis; acute close-angle glaucoma; teratogenicity (oral clefts)

Vigabatrin

Fatigue, somnolence; irreversible visual loss

Zonisamide

Anorexia and weight loss; kidney stones; heat stroke (children)

TRADE NAMES

Many antiseizure drugs are available in generic form, but some are proprietary. Trade names for some branded products available in the United States are shown in this table.

Acetazolamide (Diamox)

Carbamazepine (Tegretol, Carbatrol,[a] Equetro,[a] Carnexiv[b])

Clobazam (Onfi)

Clonazepam (Klonopin)

Diazepam (Valium, Diastat Acudial[c])

Divalproex (Depakote)

Eslicarbazepine acetate (Aptiom)

Ethosuximide (Zarontin)

Ezogabine (Potiga)

Felbamate (Felbatol)

Fosphenytoin (Cerebyx)

Gabapentin (Neurontin, Gralise[a,e])

Gabapentin enacarbil (Horizant[a])

Lacosamide (Vimpat)

Lamotrigine (Lamictal)

Levetiracetam (Keppra, Keppra XR,[a] Spritam)

Lorazepam (Ativan)

Methsuximide (Celontin)

Oxcarbazepine (Trileptal, Oxtellar XR[a])

Perampanel (Fycompa)

Phenobarbital (Luminal)

Phenytoin (Dilantin)

Pregabalin (Lyrica)

Primidone (Mysoline)

Rufinamide (Banzel)

Stiripentol (Diacomit)[d]

Tiagabine (Gabitril)

Topiramate (Topamax, Trokendi XR,[a] Qudexy XR[a])

Valproic acid (Depakene)

Valproate sodium injection (Depacon[b])

Zonisamide (Zonegran)

[a]Extended release.
[b]Intravenous.
[c]Rectal.
[d]Not yet available in United States.
[e]Gastroretentive.

SELF-ASSESSMENT QUESTIONS

1. A 6-year-old girl and her mother come to see you because the girl's teacher observed episodes of staring and inability to communicate. These episodes last 3–5 seconds and occur 10–20 times during the school day. An EEG shows synchronized three-per-second spike-wave discharges generalized over the entire cortex. Which antiepileptic medication would you try first in this young girl?
   A. Phenytoin
   B. Clonazepam
   C. Primidone
   D. Carbamazepine
   E. Ethosuximide

2. A young patient's seizures have been well controlled with phenytoin for many years, but he recently had two seizures. You determine that the phenytoin concentration in his blood is low because of his recent growth, and increase the phenytoin dose, calculating it based on his weight gain (same mg/kg as before). Several weeks later, the patient calls and tells you that he has not had any seizures, but he is having trouble walking and is dizzy. Which of the following statements best describes what has happened?
   A. The patient did not follow your instructions and has been taking too many pills.
   B. After the dose increase, phenytoin was eliminated by zero-order kinetics, and plasma concentrations were in the toxic range.
   C. His metabolism of phenytoin has increased as a result of induction of liver microsomal enzymes.
   D. His phenytoin concentrations are too low.
   E. An inner ear infection has developed.

3. What is the best initial treatment for a 3-year-old girl experiencing generalized tonic-clonic seizures daily?
   A. Brain surgery to remove the focus of her seizures
   B. Monotherapy with primidone
   C. Treatment with carbamazepine
   D. Treatment with phenytoin
   E. No drug therapy at this time

4. Generalized tonic-clonic seizures are characterized by a sustained depolarization of cortical neurons with high-frequency repetitive action potential firing. An antiseizure drug that acts by which of the following mechanisms is best suited to treat such seizures?
   A. A voltage-gated sodium-channel blocker
   B. A T-type calcium-channel blocker
   C. A GABA$_A$ receptor positive modulator
   D. A GABA transporter inhibitor
   E. A GABA transaminase inhibitor

5. A 45-year-old woman with newly diagnosed epilepsy is started on an antiseizure drug. She initially does well, but she has two seizures approximately 4 weeks after the start of treatment. She has taken the same number of pills each day, but during therapeutic drug monitoring, it is noticed that the plasma level of her drug has decreased. Which antiseizure drug is she taking?
   A. Ethosuximide
   B. Primidone
   C. Phenytoin
   D. Carbamazepine
   E. Valproic acid

FURTHER READING

Brodie MJ. Pharmacological treatment of drug-resistant epilepsy in adults: a practical guide. *Curr Neurol Neurosci Rep*. 2016;16:82.

Burakgazi E, French JA. Treatment of epilepsy in adults. *Epileptic Disord*. 2016;18:228–239.

Patsalos PN. *Antiepileptic Drug Interactions: A Clinical Guide*. 2nd ed. Springer Verlag, Switzerland; 2013.

Pellock JM, Nordli DR Jr, Sankar R, Wheless JW. *Pediatric Epilepsy: Diagnosis and Therapy*. 4th ed. Demos Medical; 2016.

Rao VR, Lowenstein DH. Epilepsy. *Curr Biol*. 2015;25:R742–R746.

Rogawski MA, Löscher W, Rho JM. Mechanisms of action of antiseizure drugs and the ketogenic diet. *Cold Spring Harb Perspect Med*. 2016;6:pii: a022780.

Wyllie E, Gidal BE, Goodkin HP, et al. *Wyllie's Treatment of Epilepsy: Principles and Practice*. Wolters Kluwer; 2015.

WEBSITES

http://www.epilepsy.com/learn/treating-seizures-and-epilepsy
This site is maintained by the Epilepsy Foundation and is an excellent resource for both healthcare professionals and patients, as it has links to many resources.

https://www.aesnet.org/clinical_resources/guidelines
The American Epilepsy Society website presents current evidence-based guidelines for the treatment of seizure disorders.

https://www.aan.com/Guidelines/Home/ByTopic?topicId=23
The American Academy of Neurology also maintains evidence-based guidelines for the treatment of seizure disorders.

22

Drug Therapy for Spasticity Disorders

Michael Saulino

MAJOR DRUG CLASSES
GABA-enhancing drugs
Adrenergic α_2-receptor agonists
Direct-acting skeletal muscle relaxant
Motor neuron blocker

ABBREVIATIONS	
BTX	Botulinum toxin
CNS	Central nervous system
GABA	γ-Aminobutyric acid
ITB	Intrathecal baclofen

THERAPEUTIC OVERVIEW

Spasticity, which presents as intermittent or sustained involuntary skeletal muscle activation, represents a disordered control of sensorimotor function resulting from a central or upper motor neuron lesion. Spasticity is present in many commonly encountered disorders, including spinal cord injury, multiple sclerosis, amyotrophic lateral sclerosis, cerebral palsy, stroke, and brain injury. The management of spasticity involves a complex and diverse array of approaches involving neuromodulation, physical therapy, and pharmacological therapy. Pharmacological approaches include the use of agents that have distinct actions at different sites, ranging from generalized central nervous system (CNS) depression to specific blockade of motor neuron activity and muscle contraction.

Disorders that manifest spasticity and goals of the pharmacological treatment of spasticity are shown in the Therapeutic Overview Box.

THERAPEUTIC OVERVIEW

Conditions That Manifest Spasticity

- Cerebral palsy
- Multiple sclerosis
- Traumatic brain injury
- Spinal cord injury
- Brain damage due to oxygen deprivation
- Stroke
- Encephalitis
- Meningitis
- Adrenoleukodystrophy
- Amyotrophic lateral sclerosis
- Phenylketonuria

Goals of Pharmacological Treatment

- Improve passive range of motion
- Decrease hyperreflexia
- Decrease spasm frequency and severity
- Improve clonus
- Decrease muscle tone
- Increase muscle strength

MECHANISMS OF ACTION

The structures of drugs commonly used for spasticity are shown in Fig. 22.1.

GABA-Enhancing Drugs

Historically, **diazepam** has been used clinically to treat spasticity for almost half a century. This agent, which is a benzodiazepine (Chapter 17), is a positive allosteric modulator at γ-aminobutyric acid (GABA) type A (**GABA-A**) receptors located primarily in the brain stem and spinal cord. GABA-A receptors are ligand-gated ion channels, whose activation results in Cl^- influx and hyperpolarization, leading to neuronal inhibition. Both pre- and postsynaptic GABA-A receptors in the dorsal and ventral horns of the spinal cord are activated by diazepam, leading to decreased glutamate release, increased GABA activity, and inhibition of motor neuron activity (Fig. 22.2). In addition, diazepam, like all of the benzodiazepines, has depressant effects on the central nervous system (CNS). Several other CNS depressants used to treat spasticity, including **methocarbamol**, **metaxalone**, and **meprobamate**, share many actions of the benzodiazepines and may enhance GABA activity via modulation of GABA-A receptors, leading to skeletal muscle relaxation.

The most commonly used oral medication to treat spasticity that also enhances GABA activity is **baclofen**. Baclofen is structurally similar to GABA (see Fig. 22.1) and is an agonist at **GABA-B receptors** within the brainstem, the dorsal horn of the spinal cord, and other pre- and postsynaptic sites (see Fig. 22.2). GABA-B receptors are G-protein–coupled receptors (GPCRs) belonging to the $G_{i/o}$ family whose activation leads to inhibition of adenylyl cyclase, inhibition of voltage-gated Ca^{2+} channels that decrease glutamate release, and activation of inwardly rectifying K^+ channels, all of which contribute to inhibition of motor neuron activity and skeletal muscle relaxation.

Adrenergic α_2-Receptor Agonists

Another commonly used oral medication is **tizanidine**, an imidazoline that is a selective adrenergic α_2-receptor agonist structurally similar to **clonidine**, which may also be used for its antispastic effect (Chapters 11 and 37). Tizanidine is active at both spinal and supraspinal levels (see Fig. 22.2). At the spinal level, it activates presynaptic α_2 receptors, inhibiting the release of glutamate and substance P. In the brain, tizanidine inhibits neuronal firing within the locus coeruleus, an action that dampens the facilitatory influence of the descending cerebrospinal tract on motor neuron activity. In addition to tizanidine and clonidine, cyclobenzaprine is a centrally acting skeletal muscle relaxant and CNS depressant whose action is also mediated by inhibition of the firing of locus coeruleus neurons, perhaps via α_2 receptor activation. Cyclobenzaprine also antagonizes serotonin (5-HT) type 2 (5-HT$_2$) receptors, thereby decreasing the activity of descending serotonergic neurons. All of these actions contribute to inhibition of motor neuron activity and thus skeletal muscle relaxation.

Direct-Acting Skeletal Muscle Relaxant

Dantrolene, a hydantoin derivative, is a direct-acting skeletal muscle relaxant. Dantrolene binds to the ryanodine receptor 1 (RyR1) located in the sarcoplasmic reticulum of skeletal muscle and inhibits the ability of RyR1 to release Ca^{2+}, essential for muscle contraction (Fig. 22.3).

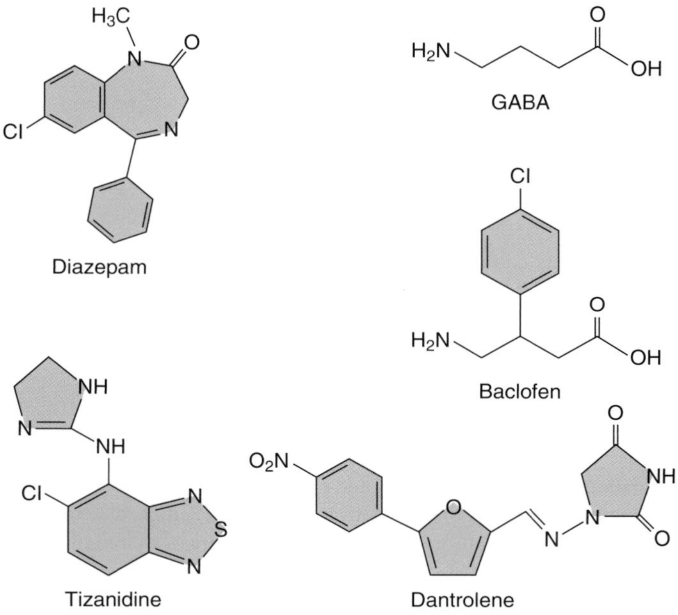

H$_3$C

GABA

Diazepam

Baclofen

Tizanidine   Dantrolene

FIG. 22.1 Structures of Drugs Used For the Treatment of Spasticity.

Motor Neuron Blocker

Seven antigenically and serologically distinct but structurally similar neurotoxins are produced by the anaerobic bacterium *Clostridium botulinum*. These botulinum toxins (BTXs) are termed A, B, C1, C2, D, E, F, and G, with only type A (BTX-A) and B (BTX-B) toxins utilized currently for medical purposes. BTX-A and BTX-B interfere with the release of acetylcholine (ACh) from motor neurons, thereby preventing the activation of skeletal muscle nicotinic receptors required for muscle contraction. The exocytotic release of ACh involves docking and fusion of the synaptic vesicle with the plasma membrane, processes facilitated by protein-protein interactions between the vesicular membrane protein synaptobrevin (also known as vesicle-associated membrane protein or VAMP) and the plasma membrane proteins SNAP-25 and syntaxin (see Fig. 22.3). BTX-A cleaves nine amino acids from the C-terminus of SNAP-25, while BTX-B cleaves a site on the extravesicular loop of synaptobrevin. As a consequence, the interactions required between these proteins for proper docking and fusion of the vesicle with the plasma membrane are perturbed, resulting in inhibition of ACh release and neurotransmission at the skeletal neuromuscular junction.

RELATIONSHIP OF MECHANISMS OF ACTION TO CLINICAL RESPONSE

Spasticity is frequently managed by the administration of oral medications. The use of these agents is relatively easy without the need for specialized technical expertise. They are often considered "first-line" agents and are generic, inexpensive, and, with the exceptions of the benzodiazepines, not scheduled medications. Other advantages of oral spasticity medications include their utility as a breakthrough strategy, as well as for secondary indications such as pain, insomnia, epilepsy, and mood disorders. Oral medications are best suited for global or multisite muscle overactivity.

Diazepam has shown clinical efficacy in patients with multiple sclerosis and spinal cord injury. Pediatric use has also been described. However, because all of the benzodiazepines are CNS depressants, the usefulness of these compounds is limited by their sedative effects.

Baclofen has been demonstrated to be most effective in patients with spasticity of spinal origin, including spinal cord injury, multiple sclerosis, and amyotrophic lateral sclerosis. Intrathecal baclofen (ITB) therapy is a powerful technique for the management of spastic hypertonia.

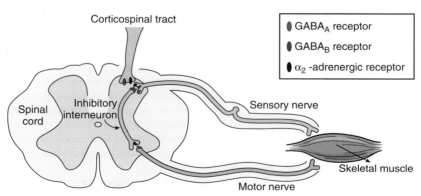

FIG. 22.2 Sites of Drug Action at the Spinal Level. Shown are presynaptic GABA-A receptors on glutamatergic nerve terminals that are activated by diazepam to decrease glutamate release, and postsynaptic GABA-A receptors on motor neurons whose activation by diazepam decreases nerve activity. Also shown are GABA-B receptors on both corticospinal and sensory nerve terminals whose activation by baclofen decreases glutamate and substance P release. Tizanidine and clonidine stimulate presynaptic α_2 receptors to decrease glutamate release from corticospinal and sensory nerve terminals.

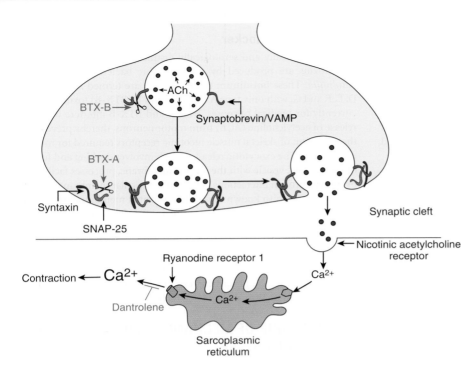

FIG. 22.3 Mechanisms of Action of Botulinum Toxins and Dantrolene at the Skeletal Neuromuscular Junction. Botulinum toxin type A (BTX-A) cleaves amino acids from the C-terminus of the plasma membrane protein SNAP-25, while BTX-B cleaves amino acids from the extravesicular loop of the vesicular protein synaptobrevin. These effects prevent the protein-protein interactions necessary for the docking of vesicles and the exocytotic release of acetylcholine (ACh). Also shown is the site of action of dantrolene, which binds to and inhibits the ryanodine receptor 1 in the sarcoplasmic reticulum in skeletal muscle to prevent the release of Ca^{2+} required for muscle contraction.

ITB infusion delivers baclofen directly into the cerebrospinal fluid (CSF) using an implanted pump and catheter. This system affords enhanced distribution to target neurons in the spinal cord and is considered to be several hundred times more potent than oral baclofen. In general, patients can be considered candidates for ITB therapy when:

- Spasticity is poorly controlled, despite maximal therapy with other modalities
- Spasticity is poorly controlled because of limited patient tolerance of other modalities
- Adjustable spasticity reduction afforded by a programmable variable flow pump would be advantageous

Prior to implanting the system, patients are temporarily exposed to ITB via a test or trial dose by injecting a bolus of liquid baclofen after a lumbar puncture. If a positive response is present during the test dose, the patient can undergo pump implantation. Dose adjustments can commence immediately. During the titration phase of ITB therapy, patients are usually weaned from oral antispasticity medications. The amount of each intrathecal adjustment varies depending on patient tolerability. If ITB is anticipated to affect the patient's active functional status, a rehabilitation program after implantation is appropriate. Following the titration phase of ITB therapy, the patient enters the chronic maintenance phase of therapy. Aspects of this treatment phase include refilling the pump reservoir with new medication, troubleshooting any infusion system malfunction, and replacing the pump for battery replenishment.

Tizanidine is used primarily for the treatment of multiple sclerosis, spasticity following a stroke, and amyotrophic lateral sclerosis. It has also been used for myofascial pain disorders, for which it decreases spasms in the neck and shoulder, and may be efficacious for spasms associated with cerebral palsy. **Clonidine** has also been shown to have efficacy for alleviating spasticity in patients with spinal cord injury but is not used as a single agent because of its cardiovascular and CNS depressant effects. Tizanidine has less of an effect on heart rate and blood pressure than clonidine.

Dantrolene has demonstrated efficacy for spasticity in a number of disorders, including spinal cord injury, cerebral palsy, and multiple

sclerosis. This compound is particularly useful for the treatment of spasticity after brain injury. Pediatric use has also been described.

Dantrolene is also the drug of choice for the prevention and treatment of **malignant hyperthermia**, a life-threatening genetic disorder triggered by volatile anesthetics and the depolarizing neuromuscular blocking agent succinylcholine (Chapter 10). Susceptible individuals have a mutation in the ryanodine receptor, which leads to an abnormal release of Ca^{2+} in skeletal muscle, resulting in numerous metabolic alterations, including respiratory and metabolic acidosis, heat production, sympathetic nervous system activation, hyperkalemia, disseminated intravascular coagulation (DIC), and multiple organ dysfunction and failure.

No technique has affected the management of spasticity more than the introduction of focal neurolysis with **BTX**. BTX must be injected directly into the overactive muscle with a variety of techniques available for localization. Some clinicians use visual inspection and palpation to guide toxin injection, while others use electromyographic, electrical stimulation, or ultrasound techniques for guidance. The choice of localization technique should be based on local expertise and resources. While BTX therapy is an effective treatment for muscle overactivity, the duration of effect can be limited. At the human neuromuscular junction, the effect typically lasts from 2 to 4 months, with repeat injections often necessary. BTX is the first-line treatment for both hemifacial spasm and blepharospasm, the former characterized by tonic or clonic contractions of muscle innervated by the facial nerve, typically unilaterally, while the latter is characterized by bilateral, symmetrical, and synchronous contractions of the orbicularis oculi muscles. It is also used for the treatment of migraine headaches (Chapter 31).

PHARMACOKINETICS

In general, oral medications have relatively short half-lives, which necessitates multiple administrations per day. The pharmacokinetics of the benzodiazepines are discussed in Chapter 17.

When administered orally, **baclofen** is absorbed through a relatively small section of the upper portion of the small intestine. The drug has a mean half-life of 3.5 hours, with limited (<15%) hepatic metabolism. It is excreted primarily unchanged by the kidneys.

Tizanidine is nearly completely absorbed following oral administration, with absorption increased by food. The drug is 30% bound to plasma proteins and undergoes extensive first-pass metabolism. The half-life of tizanidine is 2.5 hours, and 95% of the drug is metabolized to inactive products in the liver by CYP1A2. The metabolites are excreted in the urine (60%) and feces (20%). Thus the drug must be used with caution in patients with either hepatic or renal impairment. The effects of the drug peak at 1–2 hours and last approximately 3–6 hours. Tizanidine has a shorter duration of action than clonidine. The pharmacokinetics of clonidine are presented in Chapter 11.

Dantrolene may be administered orally or by intravenous injection. The half-life following oral administration is 8–9 hours, where that following intravenous administration is 4–8 hours. Dantrolene is metabolized by the liver primarily to a 5-hydroxy and an acetylamino derivative. It may also be hydrolyzed and oxidized to 5-(p-nitrophenyl)-2-furoic acid. Dantrolene is excreted as both the unchanged drug and as metabolites in both the feces (45%–50%) and urine (25%).

The pharmacokinetics of BTX have not been studied in humans. The toxin is injected directly into skeletal muscle, and thus bioavailability is not of clinical relevance. The elimination half-life for native (non-metabolized) toxin in serum is approximately 4 hours.

PHARMACOVIGILANCE: ADVERSE EFFECTS AND DRUG INTERACTIONS

There are many limitations to the use of oral spasticity medications. Tolerability of these agents, especially in patients with acquired cerebral injury, is often significant. Concerns with sedation, drowsiness, lethargy, and impairment in cognitive processing can be seen with many oral preparations.

As noted, the CNS depressant effects often limit the utility of benzodiazepines. At higher doses, somnolence can progress to respiratory depression, coma, or death. The use of benzodiazepines can also lead to physiologic dependence, with the potential for a withdrawal syndrome if the medication is abruptly discontinued or tapered too rapidly. The adverse effects of the benzodiazepines are discussed in Chapter 17.

Baclofen leads to sedation, confusion, dizziness, and nausea, with respiratory suppression, hypotension, and bradycardia at high doses. The abrupt withdrawal of baclofen may lead to mental health alterations and seizures, which, if untreated, may lead to death. Significant adverse effects have been demonstrated in both the elderly stroke population and a mixed population with acquired brain injury. Baclofen lowers seizure threshold, regardless of whether the dose is increased or decreased.

Both overdose and withdrawal from ITB are potentially serious entities and may result from pump programming mishaps, erroneous drug formulations, and mechanical problems involving the pump or catheter (e.g., kinks, holes, occlusions, etc.).

The most frequent side effects reported with tizanidine are dry mouth, drowsiness, dizziness, and fatigue. Comparative studies have indicated that tizanidine has a similar clinical efficacy to baclofen and diazepam, with less subject withdrawal due to adverse events. Approximately 5% of patients treated with chronic tizanidine exhibit elevated hepatic enzymes, which typically resolve with either drug discontinuation or dose reductions. Because tizanidine is nearly totally metabolized by CYP1A2, potential drug interactions exist with other agents metabolized by this enzyme, such as the fluoroquinolones, amiodarone, verapamil, and others. The concomitant use of tizanidine with fluvoxamine may lead to hypotension and increased psychomotor performance and is contraindicated.

Frequent adverse effects of dantrolene include drowsiness, dizziness, and diarrhea, all of which are short lasting, occur early in treatment, and can be obviated by titrating the dose gradually until an optimal dose is obtained. The most significant limitation of dantrolene is hepatotoxicity. Approximately 1% of patients treated with this agent develop significant liver abnormalities, and the risk is elevated at daily doses greater than the 400 mg/day maximum.

Adverse effects of BTX can be grouped into three broad categories. First, diffusion of the toxin away from the intended sites of action can lead to unwanted inhibition of neurotransmission at neighboring nerve endings. While localized diffusion is undesirable, it is rarely a serious problem. More worrisome is distal diffusion to muscles controlling respiration and swallowing. In 2008, the United States Food and Drug Administration reported that BTX has "… been linked in some cases to adverse reactions, including respiratory failure and death, following treatment of a variety of conditions using a wide range of doses." Several of these cases involved pediatric use for which weight-based dosing strategies must be considered. Administration of BTX with other agents that affect neuromuscular function, such as the aminoglycosides, may increase the effect of BTX. The second issue is that sustained blockade of transmission can produce effects similar to anatomic denervation, including muscle atrophy. The third undesirable effect is immunoresistance to BTX resulting from the development of circulating antibodies that bind to the heavy chain of the toxin and prevent its association with nerve membranes, thus preventing internalization of the functionally active light chain. Auxiliary proteins in the toxin complex could theoretically promote an immune response to the toxin. Further, it is important to note that bruising or bleeding at the site of injection is not a side effect of the toxin but rather a consequence of the injection procedure. Clinicians should be sensitive to this consequence in patients who are using antiplatelet or anticoagulant therapy. Other adverse events of BTX include flu-like syndromes, blurred vision, dry mouth, and fatigue.

A summary of the adverse effects of agents used to treat spasticity is presented in the Clinical Problems Box.

NEW DEVELOPMENTS

Because of the limited gastrointestinal absorption and short plasma half-life of baclofen requiring dosing throughout the day, the R isomer of racemic baclofen, which is pharmacologically more active, has been formulated with a carrier molecule that affords enhanced absorption. A small clinical trial with this preparation demonstrated spasticity reduction in individuals with spinal cord injury with only twice-daily dosing. However, a subsequent trial with multiple sclerosis was reportedly negative, although the results have never been published. Further studies are being conducted to ascertain whether this preparation is advantageous relative to the currently available formulation.

There is considerable interest in the modulation of spasticity via the endocannabinoid system (Chapter 30). Agonists at CB_1 receptors have an antispastic effect in experimental animals, likely reflecting decreased excitatory amino acid release. Muscle spasms are a very common qualifying condition for medicinal marijuana therapy use, and the nabiximols have received approval in many countries for the treatment of spasticity in multiple sclerosis when conventional antispastic therapy is not adequately effective. Clinical trials in the United States are ongoing.

Last, there is a growing interest in the antispastic effects of both gabapentin and pregabalin, agents developed for the treatment of seizures, whose mechanism of action involves decreased glutamate release. These drugs are currently the treatment of choice for managing neuropathic pain in patients with spinal cord injury. Further studies are needed

CLINICAL PROBLEMS

Benzodiazepines (diazepam, clonazepam)	Central nervous system and respiratory depression, abuse potential
Baclofen (oral)	Sedation, confusion, dizziness, hypotension, bradycardia, seizures
Baclofen (intrathecal)	Seizures
Adrenergic α_2-receptor agonists (tizanidine, clonidine)	Dry mouth, drowsiness, fatigue, elevated hepatic enzymes
Dantrolene	Hepatotoxicity
Botulinum toxin	Unwanted neuromuscular blockage, muscle atrophy, immunoresistance

TRADE NAMES

In addition to generic and fixed-combination preparations, the following trade-named materials are some of the important compounds available in the United States.

Diazepam (Valium)
Clonazepam (Klonopin)
Baclofen (Lioresal)
Tizanidine (Zanaflex)
Clonidine (Catapres, Kapvay)
Dantrolene (Dantrium)
Onabotulinum toxin A (Botox)
Incobotulinum toxin A (Xeomin)
Abobotulinum toxin A (Dysport)
Rimabotulinum toxin B (Myobloc)
Cyclobenzaprine (Flexeril)
Metaxalone (Skelaxin)
Methocarbamol (Robaxin)

to ascertain the efficacy of these compounds for the treatment of spasticity.

CLINICAL RELEVANCE FOR HEALTHCARE PROFESSIONALS

Patients with spasticity disorders will typically be undergoing physical therapy, with pharmacological treatment serving as adjunctive therapy. It is imperative that healthcare providers be aware of the side effects and limitations associated with these treatments and distinguish them from the primary disease process. Clinicians are encouraged to develop their own treatment approach based on familiarly with these medications. As medical science continues to explore the fundamental underpinnings of spasticity, and as new treatments become available, the breadth and depth of this management will continue to expand.

SELF-ASSESSMENT QUESTIONS

1. The ability of baclofen to alleviate spasticity is due to:
   A. Activation of GABA-B receptors on spinal interneurons.
   B. Excitation of α motor neuron activity.
   C. Sequestration of calcium at muscle spindles.
   D. All of the above.
   E. None of the above.
2. Dantrolene is an antispasticity drug often used for the treatment of spasticity associated with cerebral palsy or multiple sclerosis. Dantrolene relaxes skeletal muscle by:
   A. Stimulating GABA receptors on spinal motor neurons.
   B. Inhibiting excitatory amino acid release.
   C. Inhibiting calcium release from the sarcoplasmic reticulum.
   D. Blocking glutamate NMDA receptors.
   E. Inhibiting the exocytotic release of ACh.
3. Which of the following represents the primary reason limiting the use of many orally available antispasticity agents?
   A. Hepatotoxicity.
   B. Seizures.
   C. Immunoresistance.
   D. Muscle atrophy.
   E. Sedation.

FURTHER READING

Watanabe TK. Role of oral medications in spasticity management. *PM R.* 2009;1(9):839–841.

Phadke CP, Balasubramanian CK, Holz A, et al. Adverse clinical effects of botulinum toxin intramuscular injections for spasticity. *Can J Neurol Sci.* 2016;43:298–310.

Simon O, Yelnik AP. Managing spasticity with drugs. *Eur J Phys Rehabil Med.* 2010;46:401–410.

Taricco M, Pagliacci MC, Telaro E, Adone R. Pharmacological interventions for spasticity following spinal cord injury: results of a Cochrane systematic review. *Eura Medicophys.* 2006;42:5–15.

Boster AL, Bennett SE, Bilsky GS, et al. Best practices for intrathecal baclofen therapy: screening test. *Neuromodulation.* 2016;19:616–622.

Boster AL, Adair RL, Gooch JL, et al. Best practices for intrathecal baclofen therapy: dosing and long-term management. *Neuromodulation.* 2016;19:623–631.

WEBSITES

http://www.aans.org/Patients/Neurosurgical-Conditions-and-Treatments/Spasticity

This website is maintained by the American Association of Neurological Surgeons and presents an overview of spasticity and its treatment in several neurological disorders.

https://www.ninds.nih.gov/Disorders/All-Disorders/Spasticity-Information-Page

This page is maintained by the National Institute of Neurological Disorders and Stroke and has links to many resources on spasticity including current treatment approaches, research, and clinical trials.

Ethanol, Other Alcohols, and Drugs for Alcohol Use Disorder

Charles A. Whitmore and Christian J. Hopfer

MAJOR DRUG CLASSES

Alcohols
Drugs for alcohol use disorder
    Aldehyde dehydrogenase inhibitor
    Glutamate receptor antagonist
    Opioid receptor antagonist
    Anticonvulsant

ABBREVIATIONS

ADH	Alcohol dehydrogenase
ALDH	Aldehyde dehydrogenase
AUD	Alcohol use disorder
BAC	Blood alcohol concentration
CNS	Central nervous system
DA	Dopamine
FDA	United States Food and Drug Administration
GABA	γ-Aminobutyric acid
GI	Gastrointestinal
5-HT	Serotonin
NA	Nucleus accumbens
NAD$^+$	Nicotinamide adenine dinucleotide
NADH	Nicotinamide adenine dinucleotide, reduced
NADP$^+$	Nicotinamide adenine dinucleotide phosphate
NADPH	Nicotinamide adenine dinucleotide phosphate, reduced
NMDA	*N*-methyl-D-aspartate
VTA	Ventral tegmental area

THERAPEUTIC OVERVIEW

Ethanol belongs to a class of compounds known as the central nervous system (CNS) depressants that includes the barbiturate and nonbarbiturate sedative/hypnotics and the benzodiazepines. Although these latter compounds are used for their sedative and anxiolytic properties, ethanol is not prescribed for these purposes. Rather, ethanol is used primarily as a social drug, with only limited applications as a therapeutic agent administered by injection to produce irreversible nerve block or tumor destruction. Ethanol is effective for the treatment of methanol and ethylene glycol poisonings because it inhibits the metabolism of these alcohols to toxic intermediates, but fomepizole is now preferred.

In cultures in which ethanol use is accepted, the substance is misused and abused by a fraction of the population and is associated with social, medical, and economic problems, including life-threatening damage to most major organ systems and psychological and physical dependence in people who use it excessively. It is estimated that in the United States, roughly 70% of the population use ethanol, and more than 16 million adults have an alcohol use disorder (AUD). An additional 10 million people are subject to negative consequences of alcohol abuse such as arrests, automobile accidents, violence, occupational injuries, and deleterious effects on job performance and health. Approximately 30% of all traffic fatalities are estimated to involve alcohol, and the annual cost of alcohol-related problems in the United States is more than $180 billion. Alcohol use is the fourth leading preventable cause of death in the United States, and alcohol dependence is the third leading preventable cause of morbidity and mortality, resulting in roughly 88,000 alcohol-related deaths per year.

This chapter covers the pharmacology of ethanol, including the behavioral and toxicological problems associated with its use, reviews the deleterious effects of other alcohols, and presents the pharmacology of three medications approved by the United States Food and Drug Administration (FDA) for the treatment of AUD, and two medications commonly used, yet not approved, for treating AUD. Approved medications include the aldehyde dehydrogenase inhibitor disulfiram, the glutamate receptor antagonist acamprosate, and the opioid receptor antagonist naltrexone. Commonly used medications include the anticonvulsants topiramate and gabapentin.

The uses of ethanol and treatment of ethanol dependence are summarized in the Therapeutic Overview Box.

THERAPEUTIC OVERVIEW

Ethanol can be used:
    Topically to reduce body temperature and as an antiseptic
    By injection to produce irreversible nerve block by protein denaturation
    By inhalation to reduce foaming in pulmonary edema
    For the treatment of methanol and ethylene glycol poisoning
Ethanol dependence may be treated with psychosocial/behavioral therapy and an:
    Aldehyde dehydrogenase inhibitor (Disulfiram)
    Glutamate receptor antagonist (Acamprosate)
    Opioid receptor antagonist (Naltrexone)
    Anticonvulsant (Topiramate and Gabapentin)

MECHANISMS OF ACTION

Ethanol

Before the advent of ether, ethanol was used as an "anesthetic" agent for surgical procedures, and, for many years, ethanol and the general anesthetic agents were assumed to share a common mechanism of action to "fluidize" or "disorder" the physical structure of cell membranes, particularly those low in cholesterol. Although ethanol may interfere with the packing of molecules in the phospholipid bilayer of the cell membrane, increasing membrane fluidity, this bulk fluidizing effect is small and not primarily responsible for the depressant effects of ethanol on the CNS. This action, however, may play a role in disrupting membranes surrounding neurotransmitter receptors or ion channels, proteins thought to mediate the actions of ethanol.

Studies suggest that the effects of ethanol may be attributed to its direct binding to lipophilic areas in or near ion channels and multiple receptors. The ion channels influenced by ethanol are listed in Table 23.1. Ethanol may have either inhibitory or facilitatory effects, depending on the channel, but its resultant action is CNS depression. Because the barbiturates and benzodiazepines exhibit cross-tolerance to ethanol, and their CNS depressant effects are additive with those of ethanol, they may share a common mechanism, perhaps through the γ-aminobutyric acid (GABA) type A (GABA$_A$) receptor (Chapter 17). Ethanol may also exert some of its effects by actions at glutamate N-methyl-D-aspartate (NMDA) or serotonin (5-HT) receptors.

The reinforcing actions of ethanol are complex but are mediated in part through its ability to stimulate the dopamine (DA) reward pathway in the brain (Chapter 24, Fig. 24.2). Evidence has indicated that ethanol increases the synthesis and release of the endogenous opioid β-endorphin in both the ventral tegmental area (VTA) and the nucleus accumbens (NA). Increased β-endorphin release in the VTA dampens the inhibitory influence of GABA on the tonic firing of VTA DA neurons, whereas increased β-endorphin release in the NA stimulates DA nerve terminals to release neurotransmitter. Both of these actions to increase DA release may be involved in the rewarding effects of ethanol.

Other Alcohols

Methanol, ethylene glycol, and isopropanol are commonly encountered alcohols. Methanol and ethylene glycol have applications in industry and are fairly toxic to humans, whereas isopropyl alcohol, like ethanol, is bactericidal and used as a disinfectant. Industrial ethanol contains small amounts of methanol, making it unsafe for consumption, and is used to create products such as cosmetics, solvents, and detergents.

Drugs for Alcohol Dependence

Disulfiram, used for the treatment of alcoholism since the 1940s, is an inhibitor of the enzyme aldehyde dehydrogenase (ALDH), a major enzyme involved in the metabolism of ethanol (Fig. 23.1). Inhibiting the catabolism of acetaldehyde produced by the oxidation of ethanol leads to the accumulation of acetaldehyde in the plasma, resulting in aversive effects.

Acamprosate is a synthetic taurine derivative resembling GABA and was the first glutamate receptor antagonist approved by the FDA in 2004 for the treatment of alcoholism. Acamprosate affects glutamate NMDA receptors in a state-dependent manner, such that it functions as an antagonist when glutamatergic activity is high, as following chronic alcohol administration. It also modulates the ability of glutamate to activate the metabotropic type 5 glutamate receptor. Both of these effects decrease the excitatory actions of glutamate in the CNS. Based on studies indicating that ethanol disrupts the balance between excitatory and inhibitory neurotransmission in the CNS, acamprosate is thought to restore this balance by inhibiting the excitatory component. Imaging studies in human volunteers have supported the ability of acamprosate to inhibit glutamatergic activity within the brain.

TABLE 23.1	**Ion Channels Affected by Ethanol**	
Channel	**Effects**	**Ethanol Concentration (mM)**
Na$^+$ (voltage-gated)	Inhibition	100 and higher*
K$^+$ (voltage-gated)	Facilitation	50–100
Ca^{2+} (voltage-gated)	Inhibition	50 and higher
Ca^{2+} (glutamate receptor–activated)	Inhibition	20–50
Cl$^-$ (GABA$_A$ receptor–gated)	Facilitation	10–50
Cl$^-$ (glycine receptor–gated)	Facilitation	10–50
Na$^+$/K$^+$ (5HT$_3$ receptor–gated)	Facilitation	10–50

*100 mM ethanol is 460 mg/dL.

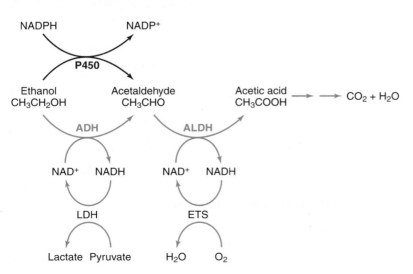

FIG. 23.1 Metabolism of Ethanol by ADH, ALDH, and Cytochrome P450. *ETS,* Electron transport system; *LDH,* lactate dehydrogenase.

Naltrexone is an opioid receptor antagonist at both κ and μ opioid receptors. Its ability to inhibit alcohol consumption has been attributed to blockade of μ receptors in both the VTA and NA, thereby decreasing the ethanol-induced activation of the DA reward pathway. The pharmacology of the opioids and opioid antagonists is discussed in Chapter 28.

Topiramate is a broad-spectrum anticonvulsant with multiple actions that inhibit seizure activity. Its ability to inhibit alcohol consumption has been attributed to enhancing GABAergic and decreasing glutamatergic activity within the NA.

Gabapentin belongs to a class of anticonvulsants known as gabapentinoids. Although gabapentin is an analogue of GABA, its anticonvulsant activity appears unrelated to GABA activity in the brain, Rather, gabapentin interacts with a subunit of voltage-gated Ca^{2+} channels and may decrease glutamate activity at excitatory synapses in the CNS. The pharmacology of the anticonvulsants is discussed in detail in Chapter 21.

RELATIONSHIP OF MECHANISMS OF ACTION TO CLINICAL RESPONSE

Ethanol

Like general anesthetics and most CNS depressants, ethanol decreases the function of inhibitory centers in the brain, releasing normal mechanisms controlling social functioning and behavior, leading to an initial excitation. Thus ethanol is described as a **disinhibitor** or **euphoriant**. The higher integrative areas are affected first, with thought processes, fine discrimination, judgment, and motor function impaired sequentially. These effects may be observed with **blood alcohol concentrations (BACs)** of 0.05% or lower. Specific behavioral changes are difficult to predict and depend to a large extent on the environment and the personality of the individual. As BACs increase to 100 mg/dL, errors in judgment are frequent, motor systems are impaired, and responses to complex auditory and visual stimuli are altered. Patterns of involuntary motor action are also affected. Ataxia is noticeable, with walking becoming difficult and staggering common as the BAC approaches 0.155%–0.2%. Reaction times are increased, and the person may become extremely loud, incoherent, and emotionally unstable. Violent behavior may occur. These effects are the result of depression of excitatory areas of the brain. At BACs of 0.2%–0.3%, intoxicated people may experience periods of amnesia, or "blackout," and fail to recall events occurring at that time.

Anesthesia occurs when BAC increases to 0.25%–0.30%. Ethanol shares many properties with general anesthetics but is less safe because of its low therapeutic index (Chapter 26). It is also a poor analgesic. Coma in humans occurs with a BAC above 0.3%, and the lethal range for ethanol, in the absence of other CNS depressants, is 0.4%–0.5%, though people with much higher concentrations have survived. Death from acute ethanol overdose is relatively rare compared with the frequency of death resulting from combinations of alcohol with other CNS depressants, such as barbiturates and benzodiazepines. Death is due to a depressant effect on the medulla, resulting in respiratory failure. Physiological and behavioral changes as a function of BAC are summarized in Table 23.2.

Measures of BAC are important for providing adequate medical care to intoxicated individuals. BAC is calculated based on the amount of ethanol ingested, the percentage of alcohol in the beverage (usually volume/volume, with 100 proof equivalent to 50% ethanol by volume), and the density of 0.8 g/mL of ethanol. BACs are expressed in a variety of ways. The legal limit for operating a motor vehicle in most states is 80 mg/dL, or 0.08%. An example of a typical calculation for a 70-kg

TABLE 23.2	**Physiological and Behavioral States as a Function of Blood Ethanol Concentrations**	
BLOOD ETHANOL CONCENTRATIONS		
(mg/dL)	**%**	**Reactions**
0–50	0–0.05	Loss of inhibitions, excitement, incoordination, impaired judgment, slurred speech, body sway
50–100	0.05–0.1	Impaired reaction time, further impaired judgment, impaired driving ability, ataxia
100–200	0.1–0.2	Staggering gait, inability to operate a motor vehicle
200–300	0.2–0.3	Respiratory depression, danger of death in presence of other CNS depressants, blackouts
>300	>0.3	Unconsciousness, severe respiratory and cardiovascular depression, death
>1200	>1.2	Highest known blood concentration with survival in a chronic alcoholic

person ingesting 1 oz, or 30 mL, of 80-proof (80 proof/2 = 40%) distilled spirits is as follows:

$$(40\%)(30\,mL) = 12\,mL\,100\%\,ethanol\,(by\,volume)$$

$$(12\,mL)(0.8\,g/mL) = 9.6\,g\,ethanol\,(by\,weight)$$

If absorbed immediately and distributed in total body H_2O (assuming blood is 80% H_2O and body H_2O content averages 68% of body weight in men and 55% in women):

$$BAC\,(male) = \frac{9.6\,g}{(70\,kg)(0.68)} \times 0.8$$

$$= 0.16\,g/L\,or\,16\,mg/dL, which\,is\,0.016\%$$

$$BAC\,(female) = \frac{9.6\,g}{(70\,kg)(0.55)} \times 0.8$$

$$= 0.199\,g/L\,or\,20\,mg/dL, which\,is\,0.02\%$$

The average rate at which ethanol is metabolized in nontolerant individuals is 100 mg/kg body weight/hr or 7 g/hr in a 70-kg person. Chronic alcoholics metabolize ethanol faster because of hepatic enzyme induction. In the calculation above, a male with a body burden of 9.6 g of ethanol would metabolize the alcohol totally in less than 2 hours.

Fig. 23.2 shows approximate maximum BACs in men of various body weights ingesting one to five drinks in 1 hour. Rapid absorption is assumed. This figure emphasizes how little consumption is required to impair motor skills and render a person unable to drive safely.

The BAC varies with hematocrit; that is, people living at higher altitudes have a higher hematocrit and a lower H_2O content in blood. It is therefore essential to know whether the BAC was determined by using whole blood, serum, or plasma. Urine, cerebrospinal fluid, and vitreous concentrations of ethanol have also been used in estimating BAC.

Because expired air contains ethanol in proportion to its vapor pressure at body temperature, the ratio of ethanol concentrations between exhaled air and blood alcohol (1/2100) forms the basis for the **breathalyzer test**, in which BAC is extrapolated from the alcohol content of the expired air.

BACs can also be calculated from the weight and sex of the person if the amount of ethanol consumed orally is known. However, this

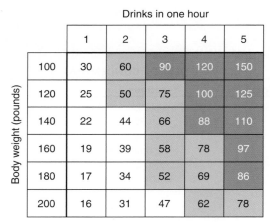

Drinks in one hour

Body weight (pounds)	1	2	3	4	5
100	30	60	90	120	150
120	25	50	75	100	125
140	22	44	66	88	110
160	19	39	58	78	97
180	17	34	52	69	86
200	16	31	47	62	78

Blood alcohol concentration (BAC) mg/dL

FIG. 23.2 Approximate Percentages of Ethanol in Blood *(BAC)* in Male Subjects of Different Body Weights, Calculated as Percentage, Weight/Volume (W/V), After Indicated Number of Drinks. One drink is 12 oz of beer, 5 oz of wine, or 1 oz of 80%-proof distilled spirits. People with BACs of 0.08% (80 mg/dL) or higher are considered intoxicated in most states; those with BACs of 0.05% to 0.079% (50 to 79 mg/dL) are considered impaired. *Light rust–colored area*, impaired; *dark rust–colored area*, legally intoxicated. BAC can be 20% to 30% higher in female subjects. Notice the small number of drinks that can result in a state of intoxication.

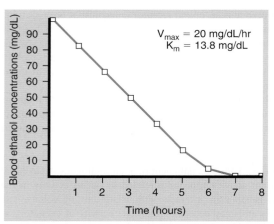

V_{max} = 20 mg/dL/hr
K_m = 13.8 mg/dL

FIG. 23.3 Disappearance of Ethanol After Oral Ingestion Follows Zero-Order Kinetics.

estimate is somewhat higher than actual concentrations because of rapid first-pass metabolism after oral administration (see Pharmacokinetics).

Drugs for Alcohol Dependence

The inhibitory effects of disulfiram are attributed to its adverse effects that directly result from ethanol ingestion. Although disulfiram does not have any effect on alcohol craving, it may help prevent relapse in compliant individuals. For disulfiram to be effective, individuals must be highly motivated to abstain from alcohol and remain treatment compliant. Furthermore, like other medications used to treat AUD, treatment appears to be most effective when combined with effective psychotherapy and social support.

Acamprosate is modestly effective in maintaining abstinence after alcohol withdrawal. The approval of acamprosate for the treatment of alcoholism in the United States was based largely on results from clinical trials conducted in Europe. Acamprosate appears to have a small therapeutic effect but may be of greater benefit in alcoholics who exhibit increased anxiety rather than the entire population of alcohol-dependent individuals.

Short-term, double-blind, placebo-controlled trials have shown that naltrexone decreased the craving for alcohol, the number of drinking days, the number of drinks per occasion, and the relapse rate. Naltrexone appears to have the greatest benefits in individuals with a family history of alcohol dependence and high craving, decreasing the rewarding efficacy of ethanol. The long-acting injectable formulation of naltrexone has the potential to maintain sobriety through greater compliance.

In randomized placebo-controlled trials involving patients with AUD, topiramate has been shown to reduce the number drinks per day and the frequency of heavy drinking and to increase the number of days when patients abstain from alcohol. Similarly, gabapentin has been shown to increase rates of abstinence and reduce the risk of heavy drinking in a dose-related relationship.

PHARMACOKINETICS

Ethanol

Alcohol taken orally is absorbed throughout the gastrointestinal (GI) tract. Absorption depends on passive diffusion and is governed by the concentration gradient and the mucosal surface area. Food in the stomach will dilute the alcohol and delay gastric emptying time, thereby retarding absorption from the small intestine (where absorption is favored because of the large surface area). High ethanol concentrations in the GI tract cause a greater concentration gradient and therefore hasten absorption. Absorption continues until the alcohol concentration in the blood and GI tract are at equilibrium. Because ethanol is rapidly metabolized and subsequently removed from the blood, all the alcohol is eventually absorbed from the GI tract.

Once ethanol reaches the systemic circulation, it is distributed to all body compartments at a rate proportional to blood flow to that area; its distribution approximates that of total body H_2O. Because the brain receives a high blood flow, high concentrations of ethanol occur rapidly in the brain.

Ethanol absorbed through the GI tract undergoes significant first-pass metabolism. Most (>90%) of the ethanol ingested is metabolized in the liver, with the remainder excreted through the lungs and in urine. Alcohol dehydrogenase (ADH) catalyzes the oxidation of ethanol to acetaldehyde, which is oxidized further by ALDH to acetate (see Fig. 23.1). Acetate is oxidized primarily in peripheral tissues to CO_2 and H_2O. Both ADH and ALDH require the reduction of nicotinamide adenine dinucleotide (NAD+), with 1 mole of ethanol producing 2 moles of reduced NAD+ (NADH). The NADH is reoxidized to NAD+ by conversion of pyruvate to lactate by lactate dehydrogenase (LDH) and the mitochondrial electron transport system (ETS). During ethanol oxidation, the concentration of NADH can rise substantially, and NADH product inhibition can become rate-limiting. Similarly, with large amounts of ethanol, NAD+ may become depleted, limiting further oxidation through this pathway. At typical BACs, the metabolism of ethanol exhibits zero-order kinetics, that is, it is independent of concentration and occurs at a relatively constant rate (Fig. 23.3). Fasting decreases liver ADH activity, decreasing ethanol metabolism.

Ethanol may also be metabolized to acetaldehyde in the liver by cytochrome P450 (CYP2E1), a reaction that requires 1 mole of reduced nicotinamide adenine dinucleotide phosphate (NADPH) for every ethanol molecule (see Fig. 23.1). Although the P450-mediated oxidation does not normally play a significant role, it is important with high concentrations of ethanol ($\geq$100 mg/dL), which saturate ADH and deplete NAD^+. Because CYP2E1 also metabolizes other compounds, ethanol may alter the metabolism of many other drugs. In addition, this system may be inhibited or induced (Chapter 3), and induction by ethanol may contribute to the oxidative stress of chronic alcohol consumption by releasing reactive O_2 species during metabolism.

A third system capable of metabolizing ethanol is a peroxidative reaction mediated by catalase, a system limited by the amount of hydrogen peroxide available, which is normally low. Small amounts of ethanol are also metabolized by formation of phosphatidylethanol and ethyl esters of fatty acids. The significance of these pathways is unknown.

The metabolism of ethanol differs significantly between men and women. Women have a smaller volume of distribution than men as a consequence of a greater percentage of adipose tissue that does not contain as much H_2O as do other tissues. In addition, the first-pass metabolism of ethanol, which occurs primarily in gastric tissue, is less in women than men because ADH activity in the female gastric mucosa is less than that in the male. Thus with low doses of ethanol, first-pass metabolism is lower in women, leading to higher BACs than in men after consumption of comparable amounts of ethanol, even after correcting for differences in body weight; at higher doses, the percentage of ethanol that undergoes first-pass metabolism is relatively small. Women are also more susceptible to alcoholic liver disease for this reason as well as a consequence of interactions with estrogen. This applies to both nonalcoholic and alcoholic women and partially explains the increased vulnerability of women to the deleterious effects of acute and chronic alcoholism. It was once assumed that higher BACs in women were entirely the result of differences in apparent volumes of distribution between men and women; however, this does not account entirely for this difference.

Significant genetic differences exist for both ADH and ALDH that affect the rate of ethanol metabolism. Several forms of ADH exist in human liver, with differing affinities for ethanol. Whites, Asians, and African-Americans express different relative percentages of the genes and their respective alleles that encode subunits of ADH, contributing to ethnic differences in the rate of ethanol metabolism. Similarly, there are genetic differences in ALDH. Approximately 30%–50% of Asians have an inactive ALDH, caused by a single base change in the gene that renders them incapable of oxidizing acetaldehyde efficiently, especially if they are homozygous. When these individuals consume ethanol, high concentrations of acetaldehyde are achieved, leading to flushing and other unpleasant effects. People with this condition rarely become alcoholic. As discussed, the unpleasant effects of acetaldehyde accumulation form the basis for the aversive treatment of chronic alcoholism with disulfiram. The pharmacokinetics of ethanol are summarized in Table 23.3.

Other Alcohols

Methanol, which may be accidentally or intentionally ingested, is metabolized by ADH and ALDH in a manner similar to ethanol, but at a much slower rate, forming formaldehyde and formic acid. Because ethanol can compete with methanol for ADH and saturate the enzyme, ethanol can be used successfully for methanol intoxication.

Ethylene glycol and isopropyl alcohol are also metabolized by ADH; thus ethanol can be used as a competitive antagonist for these compounds. Because of high rates of ethanol abuse and developments in the treatment of methanol and ethylene glycol poisoning, fomepizole was developed as a competitive inhibitor of ADH. Both ethanol and fomepizole appear equally effective, but the latter is now preferred, as

TABLE 23.3 **Pharmacokinetic Considerations of Ethanol**	
Pharmacokinetic Parameter	**Considerations**
Route of administration	Topically, orally, inhalation, by injection into nerve trunks, or intravenously for poison management
Absorption	Slight topically
	Complete from stomach and intestine by passive diffusion
	Rapid via lungs
Distribution	Total body H_2O; volume of distribution is 68% of body weight in men and 55% in women; varies widely
Metabolism	>90% to CO_2 and H_2O by liver and other tissues
	Follows zero-order kinetics
	Rate is approximately 100 mg/kg/hr of total body burden; higher or lower with hepatic enzyme induction or disease
Elimination	Excreted in expired air, urine, milk, sweat

the use of ethanol is associated with a higher incidence of complications and mortality.

Drugs for Alcohol Dependence

Disulfiram is administered orally and absorbed from the GI tract. It is highly lipid soluble, accumulates in fat stores, and is slowly eliminated. Disulfiram is metabolized primarily by the liver. Acutely, it is a mechanism-based inhibitor of CYP2E1, and chronically it inhibits CYP1A2, thereby preventing the metabolism of several drugs, including phenytoin and oral anticoagulants.

Acamprosate is administered orally with a bioavailability of approximately 11%. It exhibits negligible plasma protein binding, is not metabolized, is excreted unchanged by the kidneys, and has an elimination half-life of 20–33 hours.

Naltrexone is available both orally and as depot injections for the treatment of alcohol dependence. The pharmacokinetics of naltrexone are discussed in Chapter 28. The depot microsphere preparations are administered intramuscularly once per month and release naltrexone steadily to maintain constant plasma levels.

Topiramate is administered orally and rapidly absorbed within the GI tract. Its bioavailability is not affected by food, and it is slowly excreted unchanged by the kidneys, with a half-life of 10–30 hours. Gabapentin is administered orally and absorbed within the small intestine. Its bioavailability is not affected by food, and it is excreted unchanged by the kidneys with a half-life of 5–9 hours. The pharmacokinetics of topiramate and gabapentin are discussed in depth in Chapter 21.

PHARMACOVIGILANCE: ADVERSE EFFECTS AND DRUG INTERACTIONS

Ethanol

Ethanol has detrimental effects on many organs and tissues, and knowledge of these actions is important for understanding its hazards. Deleterious effects of ethanol on the liver and other organs resulting from chronic alcoholism are listed in the Clinical Problems Box.

Gastrointestinal Tract

The oral mucosa, esophagus, stomach, and small intestine are exposed to higher concentrations of ethanol than other tissues of the body and are susceptible to direct toxic effects. Acute gastritis resulting in nausea and vomiting results from ethanol abuse; bleeding ulcers and cancer of the upper GI tract are possible consequences.

Liver

Ethanol metabolism by the liver causes a large increase in the NADH/NAD$^+$ ratio, which disrupts liver metabolism. The cell attempts to maintain NAD$^+$ concentrations in the cytosol by reducing pyruvate to lactate, leading to increased lactic acid in liver and blood. Lactate is excreted by the kidney and competes with urate for elimination, which can increase blood urate concentrations. Excretion of lactate also apparently leads to a deficiency of zinc and Mg^{2+}. A more direct effect of increased NADH concentrations in the liver is increased fatty acid synthesis because NADH is a necessary cofactor. Because NADH participates in the citric acid cycle, the oxidation of lipids is depressed, further contributing to fat accumulation in liver cells.

The increase in NADH/NAD$^+$ ratio and the inability to regenerate NAD$^+$ may cause hypoglycemia and ketoacidosis. The former occurs in the fasting user of alcohol when hepatic glycogen stores are exhausted (72 hours), and gluconeogenesis is inhibited as a result of the increased NADH/NAD$^+$ ratio. The metabolic acidosis observed in nondiabetic alcoholics is an anion gap acidosis, with an increase in the plasma concentration of β-hydroxybutyrate and lactate.

Acetaldehyde may also play a prominent role in liver damage. If there is an initial insult to the liver, the concentration of ALDH decreases, and acetaldehyde is not removed efficiently and can react with many cell constituents. For example, acetaldehyde blocks transcriptional activation by **peroxisome proliferator-activated receptor-α (PPAR-α)**. Normally, fatty acids activate this receptor, and this action of acetaldehyde may contribute to fatty acid accumulation in liver. Acetaldehyde also increases collagen in the liver.

During ethanol ingestion, the intestine releases increased amounts of lipopolysaccharide (endotoxin), which are taken up from the portal blood by the Kupffer cells of the liver. In response to this, these cells release **tumor necrosis factor-α (TNF-α)** and a host of other proinflammatory cytokines. In the face of depleted glutathione and *S*-adenosylmethionine, liver cells die. This process of secondary liver injury occurs over and above the primary liver injury caused directly by ethanol. In spite of this, there are many heavy drinkers who never develop severe liver damage, indicating a significant genetic effect in producing alcoholic hepatic damage.

The use of acetaminophen by alcoholics may result in hepatic necrosis. This reaction can occur with acetaminophen doses that are less than the maximum recommended (4 g/24 hours). Ethanol has this effect because it induces the cytochrome P450s (primarily CYP3A4) responsible for formation of a hepatotoxic acetaminophen metabolite, which cannot be detoxified when glutathione stores are depleted by ethanol or starvation. This condition is characterized by greatly elevated serum aminotransferase concentrations. *N*-acetylcysteine is given orally to provide the required glutathione substrate in such patients.

Pancreas

Ethanol use is a known cause of acute pancreatitis, and repeated use can lead to chronic pancreatitis, with decreased enzyme secretion and diabetes mellitus as possible consequences.

Endocrine System

Large amounts of ethanol decrease testosterone concentrations in males and cause a loss of secondary sex characteristics and feminization. Ovarian function may be disrupted in premenopausal females who abuse alcohol, and this may be manifest as oligomenorrhea, hypomenorrhea, or amenorrhea. Ethanol also stimulates release of adrenocortical hormones by increasing secretion of adrenocorticotropic hormone.

Cardiovascular System

Alcoholic cardiomyopathy is a consequence of chronic ethanol consumption. Other cardiovascular effects include mild increases in blood pressure and heart rate and cardiac dysrhythmias. Cardiovascular complications also result from hepatic cirrhosis and accompanying changes in the venous circulation that predispose to upper GI bleeding. Coagulopathy, caused by hepatic dysfunction and bone marrow depression, increases the risk of bleeding.

Epidemiological studies have demonstrated an association between alcohol use and a reduced risk of cardiovascular disease, including nonfatal myocardial infarction and fatal coronary heart disease. Alcohol increases the levels of high-density lipoprotein cholesterol. However, the biological foundations of the observed cardioprotective effects of alcohol have not been established. Ethanol relaxes blood vessels, and, in severe intoxication, hypothermia resulting from heat loss as a consequence of vasodilatation may occur.

Kidney

Ethanol has a diuretic effect unrelated to fluid intake that results from inhibition of antidiuretic hormone secretion, which decreases the renal reabsorption of H$_2$O.

Immune System

Alcoholics are frequently immunologically compromised and are subject to infectious diseases. The mortality resulting from cancers of the upper GI tract and liver is also excessively high in alcoholics, and alcohol consumption is a known risk factor for cancer.

Nervous System

There are several well-documented neurological conditions resulting from excessive ethanol intake and concomitant nutritional deficiencies. These include Wernicke-Korsakoff syndrome, cerebellar atrophy, central pontine myelinolysis, demyelination of the corpus callosum, and mammillary body destruction.

Fetal Alcohol Spectrum Disorders

Fetal alcohol spectrum disorders include a range of abnormalities resulting from the prenatal effects of alcohol on the fetus. Consequences of the maternal ingestion of alcohol can include miscarriage, stillbirth, low birth weight, slow postnatal growth, microcephaly, dysmorphic facial features, mental retardation, and many other organic and structural abnormalities. Despite the general public being well aware of the deleterious effects of prenatal exposure to alcohol, fetal alcohol syndrome remains the most frequent preventable cause of birth defects. The prevalence of fetal alcohol syndrome in the United States is estimated to be 0.3–1.5 per 1000 live births.

Tolerance

Both acute and chronic tolerance occur in response to ethanol use. Acute tolerance can occur in a matter of minutes and rapidly dissipates when ethanol is applied directly to nerve cells. Chronic tolerance occurs in people who ingest alcohol daily for weeks to months, with very high tolerance developing in some individuals. As a person develops tolerance to the effects of alcohol, they must consume greater amounts of alcohol to produce similar effects to people who have not developed a tolerance. The development of tolerance to alcohol has greater implications than that to other agents because organ systems are exposed to much higher concentrations of ethanol with deleterious consequences, particularly to the liver. Because the liver becomes injured as a function of the dose and duration of ethanol exposure, metabolism of ethanol may be impaired in late-stage alcoholism with serious liver damage.

Dependence

It can be difficult to diagnose alcohol dependence based upon a brief history and physical examination. An accurate diagnosis depends on obtaining a reliable history from the patient or sufficient collateral information from a member of the patient's family. Even if a diagnosis can be made, it is frequently difficult to manage the problem because treatment is often initiated when the disorder is already well advanced.

Over the past 10–15 years, the role of genetic factors in the development of chronic alcoholism has been identified with the hope that early intervention may be more successful. Results of studies involving family members of alcoholics and twins support a predisposition and an increased risk among close relatives. This conclusion that primary alcoholism is genetically influenced is based on several interesting findings.

Studies indicate that children of alcoholic parents have a higher risk of developing an AUD. Comparisons in identical twins versus fraternal twins should reveal whether alcoholism is related to childhood environment. Because both types of twins have similar backgrounds, if alcoholism is related to childhood environment, its incidence should be the same in identical and fraternal twins. Most studies show that there is a twofold higher concordance for alcoholism in identical twins than in fraternal twins. In another study, alcoholic risk was assessed in male children of alcoholics raised by adoptive parents who were nonalcoholic. A threefold to fourfold higher risk of alcoholism was found in these males. Being raised by alcoholic adoptive parents did not increase the risk for alcoholism but may instead confer a protective effect.

Other studies have categorized alcoholics into several subgroups. One is the alcoholism most frequently seen in males and is associated with criminality; the second is a subtype observed in both sexes and influenced by the environment. Genetic predisposition, however, is merely one of several factors leading to alcoholism. Studies are attempting to reveal biological markers with which to identify potential alcoholics (e.g., differences in blood proteins, enzymes involved in ethanol degradation, and enzymes concerned with brain neurotransmitters and signaling components, including G proteins) to encourage such people to seek assistance sooner.

Effective management of chronic alcoholism includes social, environmental, and medical approaches and involves the family of the person undergoing treatment. Several types of treatments are available, including group psychotherapy (e.g., Alcoholics Anonymous) that may be rendered in private and public clinics outside of a hospital setting. Hypnotherapy and psychoanalysis have been used. Studies have shown that pharmacological therapy is of benefit when added to psychosocial/behavioral therapy.

Both psychological and physical dependence are characteristic of chronic alcohol use. The clinical manifestations of ethanol withdrawal are divided into early and late stages. Early symptoms occur between a few hours and up to 48 hours after relative or absolute abstinence. Peak effects occur around 24–36 hours. Tremor, agitation, anxiety, anorexia, confusion, and signs of autonomic hyperactivity occur individually or in combinations. Seizures occurring in the early phase of withdrawal may reflect decreased neurotransmission at GABA$_A$ receptors and increased neurotransmission at NMDA receptors. Late withdrawal symptoms (delirium tremens) occur 1–5 days after abstinence, and while relatively rare, can be life-threatening if untreated. Signs of sympathetic hyperactivity, agitation, and tremulousness characterize the onset of the syndrome. There are sensory disturbances, including auditory or visual hallucinations, confusion, and delirium. Death may occur, even in treated patients. Complicating factors in alcohol withdrawal include trauma from falls or accidents, bacterial infections, and concomitant medical problems such as heart and liver failure. The alcohol withdrawal syndrome is more likely to be life-threatening than that associated with opioids.

Management of withdrawal is directed toward protecting and calming the person while identifying and treating underlying medical problems. Clinical data have demonstrated that the longer-acting benzodiazepines (chlordiazepoxide, diazepam, or lorazepam) have a favorable effect on clinically important outcomes, including the severity of the withdrawal syndrome, risk of delirium and seizures, and incidence of adverse responses to the drugs used. The benzodiazepines are the treatment of choice. The phenothiazine antipsychotics and haloperidol are less effective in preventing seizures or delirium. Phenobarbital is problematic because its long half-life makes dose adjustment difficult, and, in high doses, it may cause respiratory depression. β-Adrenergic receptor blockers and centrally acting α_2-adrenergic receptor agonists are useful as adjuvants to limit autonomic manifestations. Neither class of drugs reduces the risk of seizures or delirium tremens.

Treatment of Intoxication

Emergency treatment of acute alcohol intoxication includes maintenance of an adequate airway and support of ventilation and blood pressure. In addition to depressant actions on the CNS, other organs, including the heart, may be affected. It is also important to assess the level of consciousness relative to the BAC because other drugs may influence the apparent degree of intoxication. An acetaminophen concentration, complex metabolic panel, complete blood count, thyroid-stimulating hormone level, and urine toxicology screen should also be performed as part of an adequate workup in patients presenting with CNS depression. A short-acting opioid receptor antagonist (naloxone) is generally administered in patients presenting with altered consciousness as a precaution against opioid overdose. Glucose may need to be administered in the event of hypoglycemia, ketoacidosis, or dehydration. Loss of body fluids may necessitate intravenous infusion of fluids containing potassium, magnesium, and phosphate. Thiamine and other vitamins, such as folate and pyridoxine, are usually administered with intravenous glucose to prevent neurological deficits. Extreme caution is needed when modifying sodium concentrations in such patients, however, because correcting sodium concentrations too quickly has been associated with central pontine myelinolysis.

Other Alcohols

Methanol has a toxicological profile quite different from that of ethanol. The metabolic products of methanol are formaldehyde and formic acid, which can cause optic nerve damage and lead to blindness and severe acidosis. Maintenance of the airways and ventilation are required with methanol intoxication. Management also includes attempts to remove residual methanol, treatment of the metabolic acidosis, electrolyte monitoring and replacement, and administration of intravenous fomepizole or intravenous ethanol to reduce the formation of toxic metabolic products while awaiting the initiation of hemodialysis. Intravenous fomepizole has been shown to be as effective as intravenous ethanol for the treatment of methanol poisoning, and fomepizole can be used alone or in conjunction with hemodialysis.

Ingestion of ethylene glycol may cause severe CNS depression and renal damage. In addition, the glycolic acid produced from metabolism by ADH can cause metabolic acidosis, whereas the oxalate formed is responsible for renal toxicity. Management of intoxication in this context is similar to that for methanol.

Isopropanol is a CNS depressant that is more toxic to the CNS than ethanol. Signs and symptoms of intoxication are similar to those of ethanol intoxication, but toxicity is limited because isopropanol produces severe gastritis with accompanying pain, nausea, and vomiting. In severe intoxication, hemodialysis is used to remove isopropanol from the body.

Drugs for Alcohol Dependence

Disulfiram causes a rise in blood acetaldehyde concentrations, producing flushing, headache, nausea and vomiting, sweating, and hypotension. Disulfiram also inhibits DA β-hydroxylase, the enzyme that converts DA to norepinephrine (NE) in sympathetic neurons (Chapter 6). Thus there is an altered ability to synthesize NE in a person with an AUD taking disulfiram, possibly contributing to the hypotension when alcohol is taken in conjunction with disulfiram. Disulfiram carries a Category C warning.

The most common adverse effects associated with acamprosate are diarrhea and asthenia. Other reported effects include nervousness, nausea, depression, and anxiety. Acamprosate has been shown to be teratogenic in animals and carries a Category C warning. It is contraindicated in patients with a sulfite allergy.

The most common adverse effects noted by alcohol-dependent individuals taking naltrexone included nausea, headache, dizziness, nervousness, and fatigue. A small percentage of individuals experience withdrawal-like symptoms consisting of abdominal cramps, bone or joint pain, and myalgia. A long-acting injection form of naltrexone approved for the treatment of AUD can lead to injection site reactions and eosinophilia. At high doses, naltrexone can produce hepatic injury, and a boxed warning noting this effect is included in its labeling. Baseline liver enzyme testing should be performed prior to initiating treatment and subsequently monitored throughout its use. Naltrexone carries a Category C warning.

The most common adverse effects associated with topiramate are fatigue, poor concentration, nausea, diarrhea, anxiety, and depression. Similar to other anticonvulsant drugs, the use of topiramate has been associated with more frequent thoughts of suicide and suicidal behavior. Topiramate is associated with an increased risk of cleft palate and cleft lip deformities and carries a Category D warning, discussed in Chapter 21.

The most common adverse effects associated with gabapentin are sedation, dizziness, and restlessness. Sudden discontinuation carries the risk of withdrawal seizures, especially among patients with a seizure history. Similar to other anticonvulsant drugs, the use of gabapentin has been associated with more frequent thoughts of suicide and suicidal behavior. Gabapentin has been shown to be developmentally toxic in animal studies and carries a Category C warning, discussed in Chapter 21.

NEW DEVELOPMENTS

Alcohol dependence is accepted as a medical problem, much like other chronic illnesses such as asthma, type 2 diabetes, and hypertension. To this end, drugs are being investigated for both the treatment of alcohol craving and the prevention of relapse. Several nonapproved medications being studied include other NMDA receptor antagonists, such as memantine (Chapter 14), the GABA$_B$ receptor agonist baclofen (Chapter 22), and the DA receptor antagonists such as aripiprazole and quetiapine (Chapter 16). In addition, based on data from animal studies and limited clinical trials, agents affecting 5-HT transmission are being studied, including 5-HT reuptake inhibitors, 5-HT$_1$ receptor partial agonists, and 5-HT$_{2/3}$ receptor antagonists.

Much effort is also being expended in identifying genes associated with both a risk for alcohol dependence and prediction of the success of drug therapy. In particular, studies have postulated that the ability of naltrexone to alter alcohol craving and consumption may be related to variants in the μ opioid receptor gene *OPRM1*. Data from both human and animal studies are revealing new avenues for development of tools for early detection of risk.

CLINICAL RELEVANCE FOR HEALTHCARE PROFESSIONALS

It is critical for all healthcare professionals to understand the frequency of "at-risk" alcohol consumption and its associated terms. Binge drinking is used to describe consuming five or more alcoholic beverages in a single setting within the past month. Heavy drinking involves consuming five or more alcoholic beverages in a single setting during 5 or more days in the past month. In 2014, approximately 25% of American adults reported binge drinking in the past month, while roughly 7% of American adults reported heavy drinking in the past month. Therefore a medical history designed to elicit information on a person's frequency and duration of alcohol use is an essential feature of a thorough medical interview that should be conducted by all healthcare professionals.

AUD is a chronic and relapsing condition much like diabetes and hypertension and can be treated with pharmacological agents to enhance the efficacy of psychological and behavioral therapy.

SELF-ASSESSMENT QUESTIONS

1. An adequate medical history from a patient should include information concerning alcohol usage because alcohol may be implicated in:
   A. Cardiovascular disease.
   B. Liver malfunction.
   C. Cancer of the larynx and pharynx.
   D. Mental retardation of children.
   E. All of the above.

2. A 53-year-old man with chronic excessive alcohol intake exhibits ascites that is most likely caused by:
   A. Obstructed hepatic venous return.
   B. Increased osmolality of the blood.
   C. Increased blood uric acid concentrations.
   D. Increased Mg^{++} excretion.
   E. Increased blood lactate concentrations.

3. Which organ in a 45-year-old woman is at a greater risk for alcohol-induced disorders than a similarly aged man?
   A. Pancreas.
   B. Stomach.
   C. Larynx.
   D. Liver.
   E. Heart.

4. Flushing reactions in response to ethanol in Asians resemble the response to ethanol in people who have taken:
   A. Benzodiazepines.
   B. Barbiturates.
   C. Antihistamines.
   D. Disulfiram.
   E. Chloral hydrate.

5. Which of the following may occur as a consequence of ethanol metabolism by the cytochrome P450 system and the induction of this system by ethanol?
   A. Increased rate of metabolism of other drugs.
   B. When ethanol is present, a decreased rate of metabolism of some drugs.
   C. Increased production of carcinogenic compounds from procarcinogens.
   D. Increased clearance of ethanol.
   E. All of the above.

FURTHER READING

Johnson BA. Update on neuropharmacological treatments for alcoholism: Scientific basis and clinical findings. *Biochem Pharmacol.* 2008;75(1):34–56.

Jonas DE, Amick HR, Feltner C, et al. Pharmacotherapy for adults with alcohol use disorders in outpatient settings: a systematic review and meta-analysis. *JAMA.* 2014;311:1889.

Mason BJ, Quello S, Goodell V, et al. Gabapentin treatment for alcohol dependence: a randomized clinical trial. *JAMA Intern Med.* 2014;174(1):70–77.

McLellan AT, Lewis DC, O'Brien CP, Kleber HD. Drug dependence, a chronic medical illness. *JAMA.* 2000;284(13):1689–1695.

Mukamal KJ, Conigrave KM, Mittleman MA, et al. Roles of drinking pattern and type of alcohol consumed in coronary heart disease in men. *N Engl J Med.* 2003;348(2):109–118.

Spanagel R, Kiefer F. Drugs for relapse prevention of alcoholism: Ten years of progress. *Trends Pharmacol Sci.* 2008;29(3):109–115.

WEBSITES

https://www.niaaa.nih.gov/
The National Institute on Alcohol Abuse and Alcoholism maintains an excellent website that contains information and links to a multitude of resources for all healthcare professionals that pertain to ethanol use by both children and adults.

Illicit Psychoactive Compounds and Substance Use Disorder

Rex M. Philpot and Peter W. Kalivas

MAJOR DRUG CLASSES

Cannabinoids
Depressants
Opioids
Stimulants
Dissociative compounds
Hallucinogens
Inhalants

ABBREVIATIONS

CNS	Central nervous system
CBD	Cannabidiol
DA	Dopamine
GABA	γ-Aminobutyric acid
GHB	γ-Hydroxybutyrate
5-HT	Serotonin
IV	Intravenous
LSD	D-Lysergic acid diethylamide
MDMA	Methylenedioxymethamphetamine
NAcc	Nucleus accumbens
NE	Norepinephrine
PCP	Phencyclidine
SAMHSA	Substance Abuse and Mental Health Services Administration
SUD	Substance use disorder
THC	Tetrahydrocannabinol
VTA	Ventral tegmental area

THERAPEUTIC OVERVIEW

The nonmedical use of drugs and other substances affecting the central nervous system (CNS) represents a significant health, social, and economic issue. Many compounds used historically to alter mood and behavior are still commonly used today. In addition, many drugs intended for medical use, such as stimulants, antianxiety agents, and drugs to alleviate pain, are obtained illicitly and used for their mood-altering actions. Although the short-term effects of these drugs may be exciting or pleasurable, recreational use or misuse can promote substance abuse and lead to addiction and dependence. In the United States alone, drugs of abuse are estimated to cost nearly $700 billion annually for healthcare expenses, lost productivity, crime, incarceration, and drug enforcement.

Drug Use Trends

According to the 2015 United States Substance Abuse and Mental Health Services Administration (SAMHSA) survey, 27.1 million Americans aged 12 and older had used illicit substances in the prior month, representing approximately 10.1% of the population. (Note: the terms drug and substance are used interchangeably and refer to all agents that interact with the body.) The most commonly used substance was marijuana, followed by prescription pain relievers, prescription tranquilizers and cocaine, prescription stimulants, hallucinogens, methamphetamine, inhalants, prescription sedatives, and heroin (Table 24.1). In addition to illicit drug use, more than 50% of Americans are current users of alcohol, and 25% are current users of tobacco products. The major drugs and substances abused, grouped by pharmacological class, are presented in the Therapeutic Overview Box.

Misuse, Abuse, and Addiction

Substance use, substance misuse, and substance abuse are terms that are often wrongly used interchangeably and misunderstood.

- **Recreational substance use** is the use of a substance for its psychoactive effects.
- **Substance misuse** is the use of a prescription drug for a purpose other than medically intended, such as using higher doses or a frequency other than prescribed or using someone else's medication.
- **Substance abuse** is a pattern of licit or illicit drug use that results in significant social, occupational, and/or medical impairment. This pattern of use often progresses to **addiction**, the compulsive use of a substance despite adverse consequences, and **dependence**, the manifestation of aversive physical and/or psychological symptoms as a consequence of drug withdrawal that can motivate further drug use.

Tolerance and Dependence

Many individuals often misuse the terms tolerance and dependence. **Tolerance** is a reduced drug effect with repeated use and a need for higher doses of drug to produce the same effect. Tolerance does not occur to the same extent for all the effects of a single drug, and individuals who take increasing amounts of drug risk an increase in those effects to which less tolerance develops. For example, chronic heroin abusers increase the dose of drug necessary to achieve a euphoric high to which tolerance develops but may die from respiratory depression at this dose.

Dependence is characterized by psychological or physiological changes after discontinuation of drug use, effects that are reversible on resumption of drug administration. Psychological dependence is characterized by intense drug craving and compulsive drug-seeking behavior. Abused substances often produce intense euphoria and feelings of well-being that motivate use and produce reinforcing effects that promote habitual, stimulus-driven drug use. The development of habitual use patterns can make it very difficult to stop using a drug of abuse and can also precipitate relapse in abstinent individuals.

Physical dependence is associated with characteristic withdrawal signs upon cessation of drug administration. Physical dependence occurs when substances are used for days, weeks, or months and becomes increasingly severe with repeated use. Occasional drug use does not typically result in clinically significant dependence. Spontaneous withdrawal occurs upon cessation of drug administration, with a similar withdrawal syndrome for drugs within a pharmacological class. The time course and severity of withdrawal vary according to the rate of elimination of the drugs or their active metabolites. Withdrawal from long-acting drugs has a delayed onset, is relatively mild, and occurs over many days or weeks (Fig. 24.1), whereas withdrawal from more rapidly inactivated or eliminated drugs is more intense but of shorter duration (see Fig. 24.1). Precipitated withdrawal occurs when an antagonist is administered to displace the drug from its receptors, causing more rapid and severe effects, such as occurs following the administration of the opioid antagonist naltrexone to heroin-dependent individuals (see Fig. 24.1).

Different drugs in the same class can maintain physical dependence produced by other drugs in the same class, termed cross-dependence. Thus heroin withdrawal can be prevented by administration of other opioids, part of the rationale for the use of methadone for the treatment of opioid abuse. Alcohol, barbiturates, and benzodiazepines exhibit cross-dependence with each other but not with opioids; thus benzodiazepines are effective in suppressing symptoms of alcohol, but not opioid, withdrawal. Cross-tolerance is similar to cross-dependence and indicates that people tolerant to a drug in one class will usually be tolerant to other drugs in the same class but not to drugs in other classes.

Substance Use Disorder and Treatment

According to SAMHSA, more than 20 million Americans were classified with a substance use disorder (SUD) in 2015. SUDs occur when the use of a drug leads to significant adverse consequences, such as health problems, disability, and failure to meet major responsibilities at work, school, or home. Among those diagnosed with SUDs, 7.9 million individuals exhibited a comorbid mental disorder. Thus individuals with SUDs often require treatment for acute overdose and withdrawal, as well as for associated mental health and medical conditions. Although primary caregivers provide diagnoses, referral, and short-term treatment, long-term treatment of substance abuse is the province of specialized, multidisciplinary programs that use several strategies. Detoxification is used to treat physical dependence and consists of abruptly or gradually reducing drug doses, whereas maintenance therapy involves using drugs such as methadone to manage drug cravings and symptoms of dependence, with psychological, social, and vocational therapies used to reduce the adverse consequences of chronic drug use.

TABLE 24.1 **Prevalence of Illicit Drug Use in the United States in 2015**[a]	
Marijuana	22.2
Prescription pain relievers	3.8
Prescription tranquilizers	1.9
Cocaine	1.9
Prescription stimulants	1.7
Hallucinogens	1.2
Methamphetamine	0.9
Inhalants	0.53
Prescription sedatives	0.45
Heroin	0.33

[a]Data from the SAMHSA; numbers represent millions of persons.

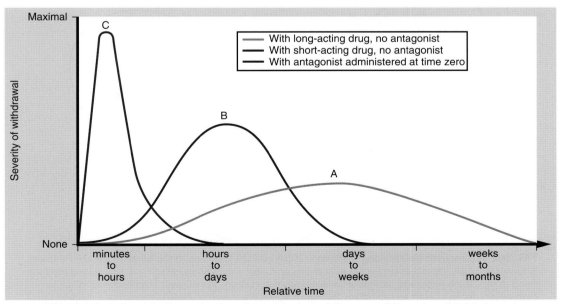

FIG. 24.1 Relationship Between Duration of Action of Drugs and Severity of Withdrawal.

MECHANISMS OF ACTION

Several pharmacological classes of abused drugs, including the cannabinoids, depressants, opioids, and stimulants, share the ability to activate the mesolimbic dopamine (DA) reward pathway in the brain (Chapter 13). Activation of this pathway is associated with satisfaction of basic needs and contributes energy and direction (i.e., motivation) to behavior. Drugs of abuse either directly activate these DA neurons or alter the activity of other neurotransmitters affecting the activity of these neurons, such as acetylcholine, γ-aminobutyric acid (GABA), glutamate, serotonin (5-HT), and norepinephrine (NE). The effects of GABA on the activity of ventral tegmental area (VTA)-nucleus accumbens (NAcc) DA neurons is shown in Fig. 24.2.

Cannabinoids

Marijuana (cannabis) is the dried leaf material, buds, and flowering tops from the *Cannabis sativa* and *Cannabis indica* plants. Hashish is the dried resinous material exuded by mature plants. Among illicit substances (as per the United States Drug Enforcement Administration), cannabis is the most commonly used drug in the United States (Table 24.1). It is important to note that as of 2016, cannabis has been legalized for recreational or medical use or decriminalized in 26 states, including the District of Columbia.

The major active chemicals in marijuana are Δ^9-tetrahydrocannabinol (Δ^9-THC) and cannabidiol (CBD); structures are shown in Fig. 24.3. CBD, Δ^9-THC, and related molecules are termed cannabinoids and exert their effects by binding to specific cannabinoid receptors, CB_1 and CB_2, which are G-protein–coupled receptors (Chapter 30). Synthetic cannabinoids are ingredients in popular products named K2 and Spice, and typically marketed as "incense." These synthetic compounds include: CP-47, 497, HU-210, JWH-018, JWH-073, JWH-250, JWH-398, and oleamide. Synthetic cannabinoids bind to CB_1 and CB_2 with an affinity 100–800 times that of Δ^9-THC, exhibit full receptor agonism, and have several active metabolites.

Depressants

CNS depressants such as barbiturates, nonbarbiturate sedatives, and benzodiazepines enhance the action of endogenous GABA at $GABA_A$ receptors, which are ligand-gated ion channels (Chapter 17). GABA interneurons in the VTA express $GABA_A$ receptors containing α_1 subunits

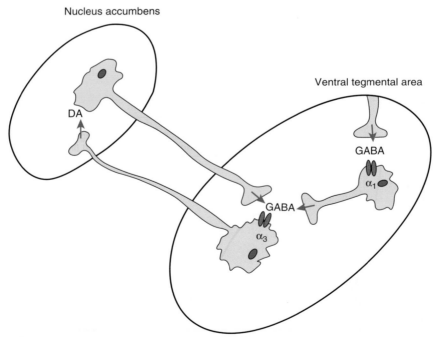

FIG. 24.2 A Simplistic Relationship Between GABA and DA Neurons in the Mesolimbic DA Pathway. Shown are $GABA_A$ receptors containing α_1 subunits on GABA interneurons, which normally control the tonic firing of the DA neurons, and receptors containing α_3 subunits on DA neurons. The benzodiazepines have a high affinity for α_1-containing receptors, leading to hyperpolarization of GABA interneurons, leading to DA release.

Cannabinoids

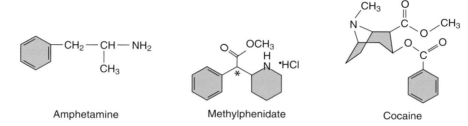

Δ⁹–Tetrahydrocannabinol (THC)   Cannabidiol (CBD)

Stimulants

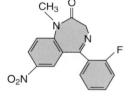

Amphetamine   Methylphenidate   Cocaine

Depressants   **Dissociative compounds**

Flunitrazepam   γ-Hydroxybutyrate (GHB)   Phencyclidine (PCP)   Ketamine

Opioids

Morphine

Heroin

Hallucinogens

Mescaline   *D*–Lysergic acid diethylamide (LSD)

FIG. 24.3 Structures of Some Commonly Abused Drugs.

on their perikarya, while DA neurons in the VTA express GABA$_A$ receptors containing α_3 subunits (see Fig. 24.2). Under normal conditions, the tonic firing of these DA neurons is controlled by GABA interneurons. The benzodiazepines, which have a higher affinity for α_1-containing receptors, hyperpolarize GABA interneurons, thereby releasing DA neurons from tonic inhibition and increasing DA release.

A related CNS depressant is γ-hydroxybutyrate (GHB). The structure of GHB is shown in Fig. 24.3. GHB is synthesized in trace amounts in the brain and functions as a precursor for and a metabolite of GABA. GHB modulates GABA activity in brain; it is a low-affinity full agonist at GABA$_B$ receptors, a full or partial agonist at specific subtypes of GABA$_A$ receptors, and a high-affinity full agonist at GHB-specific receptors.

Ethanol is also a CNS depressant that activates the mesolimbic DA pathway; its mechanism of action is discussed in Chapter 23.

Opioids

Heroin (diacetylmorphine) is the most commonly abused illicit opioid and is approximately three times more potent than morphine, but the two have very similar effects. The structures of these compounds are shown in Fig. 24.3. The mechanism of action of the opioids is discussed in Chapter 28 and involves activation of μ, κ, and δ opioid receptors, which are G-protein–coupled receptors. The action of heroin is attributed to its metabolites 6-acetylmorphine and morphine, which are both potent μ opioid receptor agonists. Similarly, codeine (methylmorphine) is a μ opioid receptor agonist with weaker affinity than morphine.

Other synthetic opioids are widely available and abused, often as diverted prescription medications. Desomorphine is a synthetic derivative of morphine that acts as a μ opioid receptor agonist, producing effects that are more potent than heroin. In recent years, desomorphine has been derived from "cooking" codeine using organic solvents and other compounds. When these solvents are present in the injected drug preparation, they produce greenish-black, scalelike skin, lending to the street name "krokodil."

Kratom is a tropical tree (Mitragyna speciosa) found in southeast Asia, where it is used in traditional medicine. At least 40 alkaloids are present in kratom that interact with opioid and monoaminergic receptors. The indole alkaloid mitragynine is likely responsible for the opioid-like effects of kratom and is an agonist at opioid receptors. Mitragynine is also an agonist at the A$_{2A}$ adenosine receptor, α$_2$-adrenergic receptor, D2 receptor, and 5-HT receptors, all of which may contribute to the subjective properties of this drug.

Stimulants

The stimulant drugs are sympathomimetic amines that act on the CNS by enhancing NE and DA neurotransmission (Chapter 18). Amphetamines are structurally related to the catecholamine neurotransmitters and ephedrine and include amphetamine, N-methylamphetamine, and others such as methylphenidate; these structures are shown in Fig. 24.3. Many stimulants are naturally occurring, including cocaine, the active ingredient of the South American coca bush, and cathinone, the main psychoactive compound in the shrub Catha edulis (khat), a plant chewed by the indigenous people of eastern Africa. Synthetic cathinones, or bath salts, are analogues of naturally occurring cathinones, which are monoamine alkaloids chemically similar to ephedrine, cathine, methcathinone, and other amphetamines.

The reinforcing effects of stimulants arise from enhanced neurotransmission at DA synapses in the mesolimbic pathway (see Fig. 24.2). Cocaine binds to DA transporters and blocks reuptake, increasing synaptic concentrations of DA. Amphetamines also affect DA transporters to enhance DA release and may increase DA concentrations by inhibiting monoamine oxidase. Amphetamines may also directly activate postsynaptic receptors. The cathinones act on monoamine transporters, increasing synaptic concentrations of 5-HT, DA, and NE.

Dissociative Compounds

Phencyclidine (PCP) and ketamine were originally developed as anesthetics; their structures are shown in Fig. 24.3. Ketamine is still used for changing burn dressings, for anesthesia in children, for short-duration anesthesia in veterinary medicine, and, most recently, as a rapid-acting antidepressant. PCP is not used therapeutically because of the severity of emergence delirium in patients. The over-the-counter cough suppressant dextromethorphan produces effects similar to those of PCP and ketamine when taken in high doses. All of these compounds produce their effects through a use-dependent noncompetitive antagonism at excitatory glutamate N-methyl-D-aspartate (NMDA) receptors throughout the CNS.

Salvia is a dissociative hallucinogen derived from Salvia divornorum (Lamiaceae), a plant native to Mexico. Unlike other dissociative drugs, salvia is a κ opioid receptor agonist and produces its dissociative effect via activation of this receptor. Although activation of κ opioid receptors is frequently associated with aversive experiences, low doses of salvia (0.1–40.0 μg/kg) have rewarding properties and increase DA release in the NAcc. However, higher doses have been shown to reduce DA release in this region.

Hallucinogens

Abused hallucinogens fall into two chemical classes, the substituted phenethylamines, of which mescaline is the prototype, and the indoleamines, of which D-lysergic acid diethylamide (LSD) is the prototype (see Fig. 24.3). Other common hallucinogens include psilocybin (from mushrooms) and dimethyltryptamine. The unique effects of hallucinogens result from modulation of 5-HT neurotransmission, in particular, activation of 5-HT$_{2A}$ receptors in the cerebral cortex, a region involved in mood, cognition, and perception, and in the locus coeruleus, an area concerned with response to external stimuli.

Methylenedioxymethamphetamine (MDMA) is a substituted amphetamine with both hallucinogenic and stimulant activity attributed to its ability to increase the release of both DA and 5-HT.

Inhalants

The inhalants are comprised of solvents, aerosol sprays, gases, and nitrites. The volatile solvents include toluene-containing materials (paint thinners and sprays, correction fluids, and plastic adhesives), alkylbenzene-containing cleaners, and chlorinated hydrocarbon cleaners/degreasers. Aerosol propellants include ethyl chloride and chlorofluorocarbon-containing compounds. Although the specific mechanisms mediating the intoxicating effects of these compounds are not well understood, they produce CNS actions similar to those of alcohol, producing initial excitation, disinhibition, lightheadedness, and agitation. In sufficient amounts, they can produce anesthesia. They also limit the delivery of oxygen to the brain.

The inhalants also include nitrous oxide (N$_2$O) and aliphatic nitrites such as amyl nitrite. The nitrites are abused for their vasodilating properties (Chapter 41) and produce dizziness and euphoria as a consequence of hypotension and cerebral hypoxia.

RELATIONSHIP OF MECHANISMS OF ACTION TO CLINICAL RESPONSE

Cannabinoids

The effects of the cannabinoids are discussed in Chapter 30. Marijuana, hashish, and the synthetic cannabinoids are abused for their psychotropic effects, producing a euphoric state and leading to alterations in mood and sensory experiences that are generally perceived as pleasant. The psychoactive effects of marijuana and hashish are attributed to the actions of Δ^9-THC, while the calming, hypnotic effects are attributed to the actions of CBD. Because the synthetic cannabinoids are full agonists and have higher affinity than Δ^9-THC and CBD for CB_1 and CB_2 receptors, the effects of the synthetic cannabinoids can be more intense than those with marijuana or hashish.

Depressants

The benzodiazepines are prescribed to treat anxiety, acute stress reactions, panic attacks, and the short-term treatment of insomnia. The barbiturates can also be used to reduce anxiety or help with sleep difficulties but are not used frequently due to a higher risk of overdose. CNS depressants have a high abuse potential, and physical dependence can develop rapidly.

Flunitrazepam is a highly efficacious, high-potency, particularly abused benzodiazepine that is tasteless and odorless and has achieved notoriety as a "date-rape" drug. GHB is used for its ability to cause euphoria, relaxation, and lack of inhibition. Like flunitrazepam, GHB has been used as a date-rape drug because of its short-lived hypnotic effects. It is also abused by bodybuilders for its purported anabolic properties and is used by alcoholics to reduce alcohol cravings.

The effects of alcohol are discussed in Chapter 23.

Opioids

Opioids are widely abused for their intense euphoric effects and numbing psychological calm, occasionally characterized as a feeling of postorgasm bliss. The intravenous (IV) administration of heroin causes a surge of intense euphoria, a "rush" accompanied by a warming of the skin, dry mouth, and heavy feelings in arms and legs. The rush subsides after a few minutes, and the user feels relaxed, carefree, and somewhat dreamy but able to carry on many normal activities. The prescription opioids are abused and often misused for their pain-relieving properties, leading to serious consequences for the users, their families, and the community.

Chewing kratom leaves produces both opiate- and stimulant-like effects, alleviating pain and increasing energy and sexual desire. The stimulant effects occur with lower doses (1–5 g of leaves), while the depressant and opiate-like euphoric effects occur when higher doses (>5 g of leaves) are used.

Stimulants

Stimulants produce increased alertness, feelings of elation and well-being, increased energy, feelings of competence, increased sexuality, and suppression of appetite, reflecting activation of both the CNS and autonomic nervous system. Athletic performance has been reported to be enhanced in those who use stimulants, particularly in sports requiring sustained attention and endurance. Although these effects are small, they provide a significant advantage. Thus all sympathomimetic drugs, including over-the-counter medications such as pseudoephedrine, are banned by most athletic associations. Several of these agents are used for the treatment of attention deficit-hyperactivity disorder (Chapter 18) but are also misused and abused. The cathinones are similar to other stimulants and increase alertness and energy, act as an appetite suppressant, increase sociability and sex drive, and can produce hallucinations.

Dissociative Compounds

Ketamine and PCP produce a "dissociative" anesthesia, i.e., amnesia and profound analgesia, although the patient is not asleep, and respiration and blood pressure are unaltered. This is different from anesthesia produced by the general anesthetics (Chapter 26). PCP produces a unique profile of effects and combines aspects of the actions of stimulants, depressants, and hallucinogens. The subjective experience of PCP intoxication is unlike that of other hallucinogens; perceptual effects are not as profound and relate more to somesthesia. Distortions of body image are common, and one of the motivations for PCP abuse is to enhance sexual experience. Ketamine is a less potent version of PCP. These compounds are abused for their visual and auditory distortions, as well as the altered sense of self and sensation of floating that accompanies dissociative effects.

High-dose dextromethorphan produces dissociative effects similar to PCP and ketamine and is often taken in cough medications containing stimulant decongestants increasing the risks of adverse effects. Dextromethorphan is particularly abused by teenagers and young adults. Similarly, salvia has dissociative properties that result in an altered sense of self and causes hallucinations. It has been used in Mexico to produce "visionary" experiences for centuries. To date, there is no evidence to suggest that salvia is an addictive compound.

Hallucinogens

The unique psychological effects of hallucinogens include enjoyment of perceptual alterations, stress reduction, and a feeling of enlightenment. Hallucinogens produce changes in mood, thought, and sensory perceptions such that colors, sounds, and smells are intensified. Because of the latter actions, these compounds are referred to as psychedelic or psychotomimetic agents. The hallucinogens have no recognized medical uses.

Inhalants

Most inhalants produce a brief high similar to alcohol, followed by a period of drowsiness and disinhibition. Additional effects can vary considerably, depending on the chemicals present in the product being abused. Inhalants are abused by young children who obtain these compounds readily at low to no cost. Abuse of inhalants peaks at eighth grade and represents a cheap entry into drug abuse.

PHARMACOKINETICS

Abused substances include many compounds whose pharmacokinetic profiles depend highly on their mode of administration. A rapid effect is sought by opioid and stimulant abusers, and methods such as smoking or IV injection are preferred. Smoking allows the drug to pass rapidly from the lungs into the blood and brain. This is not true for slower-acting depressants such as alcohol or GHB or longer-lasting compounds such as LSD. The difference in degree of euphoria and the length of stimulant action for cocaine administered by different routes is shown in Fig. 24.4.

Cannabinoids

Marijuana and hashish are usually smoked in cigarettes ("joints" or "reefers") or in pipes or "bongs" (water pipes) but are also taken orally. Effects following inhalation begin almost immediately, peak in 15–30 minutes, and last for 1–3 hours. When taken orally, effects begin in 1 hour and last up to 4 hours. Because of their high lipophilicity, cannabinoids remain in the body for weeks and accumulate with repeated use. The pharmacokinetics of the cannabinoids are discussed in detail in Chapter 30.

Synthetic cannabinoids may be smoked, ingested, or injected. The onset and duration of effects are generally similar to that of marijuana; however, there is considerable variability depending on the specific compound. For example, smoking JWH-018 leads to detectable serum levels within 5 minutes and produces subjective effects for 6–12 hours, considerably longer than the effects of marijuana.

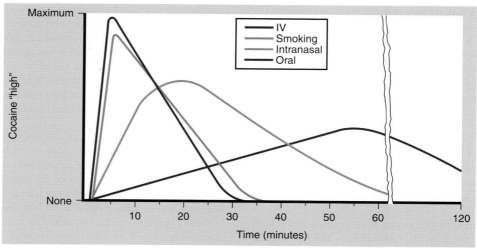

FIG. 24.4 The Intensity and Time Course (in Minutes) of Cocaine Intoxication at Equivalent Doses By Different Routes of Administration.

Depressants

CNS depressants are taken orally, with rapid-acting barbiturates, such as secobarbital and pentobarbital, more widely abused than those with a slower onset, such as phenobarbital or the benzodiazepines. Fluni-trazepam shows effects after 30 minutes and lasts up to 8 hours. GHB is rapidly absorbed and readily penetrates the CNS, producing effects within 15–30 minutes and lasting 2–3 hours. The pharmacokinetics of the benzodiazepines are discussed in Chapter 17.

Opioids

Heroin, like morphine, has poor oral bioavailability and is usually snorted, smoked ("chasing the dragon"), or injected, providing a feeling of euphoria in 10–15 minutes when snorted or smoked, or in 7–8 seconds when injected, the latter leading to very rapid euphoria that contributes to powerful addictive actions. The effects of heroin last approximately 4–6 hours, depending on dose. Heroin is metabolized to 6-acetylmorphine and morphine, while codeine is demethylated to morphine by CYP2D6.

Desomorphine is typically injected and has an onset of action within 2 minutes and a duration of action of 1–2 hours. Its rapid onset and shorter duration of action make it more likely to be abused than morphine.

Kratom is usually sold as leaves, powder, capsules, pellets, or gum and can be smoked, chewed, or consumed as a tea. When kratom is ingested, the onset of action occurs within 5–10 minutes, with a duration of 2–5 hours.

Stimulants

Pure cocaine is used as a water-soluble salt or as a free base. Cocaine salt is a bitter-tasting, white crystalline material that is generally snorted or injected. Crack (free-base cocaine), sold as small hard pieces, or "rocks," is volatilized and inhaled. It is rapidly absorbed and provides an almost instantaneous action. When administered by IV injection, cocaine takes effect in a few seconds, whereas when it is snorted, onset is 5–10 minutes, but the duration of effects is increased. The IV administration or inhalation of cocaine produces a rapid-onset rush with intense positive-reinforcing effects. Oral cocaine is slowly absorbed (see Fig. 24.4) and produces a less intense effect. The effect of IV or inhaled cocaine generally lasts only 30 minutes, and repeated administration is common in an attempt to maintain intoxication. Cocaine is

rapidly metabolized by blood and liver esterases, with urinary metabolites present for up to a week after use. Some N-demethylation occurs in the liver, with metabolites excreted in urine.

Amphetamines and similar stimulants, such as methylphenidate, are usually taken orally but may be snorted. Oral methamphetamine produces effects within 15–20 minutes, but when snorted, effects are apparent within 3–5 minutes, lasting for several hours. A smoked form of methamphetamine is used in a manner similar to crack cocaine.

Synthetic cathinones are typically available as a powder, pills, or capsules and are usually snorted or ingested but can be smoked or injected as well. Onset of psychoactive effects occurs between 10–45 minutes following administration and persist for 2–4 hours, depending on the specific compound taken and the route of administration.

Dissociative Compounds

For a rapid onset of action, PCP is generally mixed with plants (dried parsley, tobacco, or marijuana) and smoked, but it may also be snorted. The effects of oral PCP occur within minutes and last for several hours. Ketamine has a shorter duration of action (30–60 minutes). For illicit use, injectable ketamine (often diverted from veterinarians' offices) is dried, powdered, and snorted or converted into pills.

Salvia can be absorbed through the buccal membranes by chewing, or an extract of the leaves can be ingested or smoked. The preferred route of administration is smoking or vaporization, as the effects of the drug following oral administration are extremely limited due to first-pass metabolism. Onset of action after ingestion typically occurs within 30 minutes, while the onset of effects when inhaled is within 30 seconds. The typical duration of action is very short, lasting about 15 minutes.

Hallucinogens

LSD is usually taken orally as capsules, tablets, or on small paper squares but can also be injected or smoked. Effects begin in 30–90 minutes and last up to 12 hours. MDMA is usually taken orally. Effects last up to 6 hours, but more drug is often taken when effects start to fade.

Inhalants

Inhalants are sniffed or snorted from containers or bags into which aerosols have been sprayed, are sprayed directly into the nose or mouth, or are inhaled from balloons as gases. They are quickly absorbed, producing intoxication within minutes. However, effects last only a few minutes, and repeated administration is needed for a prolonged high.

Amyl nitrite ampules are diverted from medical supplies, while other organic nitrites are available in specialty stores as room "odorizers." The industrial solvents γ-butyrolactone and 1,4-butanedione are abused because they are metabolized to GHB. N₂O produces a short-lived intoxication similar to early stages of anesthesia.

PHARMACOVIGILANCE: ADVERSE EFFECTS AND DRUG INTERACTIONS

Cannabinoids

Marijuana produces alterations in thought processes, judgment, and time estimation. Users have a reduced ability to form memories, although recall of previously learned facts is unaltered. Marijuana has little effect on psychomotor coordination, although altered perception and judgment can impair performance, including driving. Because of the prevalence of its use, accidents and injury are important concerns. High doses can induce personality changes, while physiological effects include tachycardia and reddening of conjunctival vessels. Death from acute overdose is extremely rare. Heavy smokers of marijuana will experience respiratory problems, including bronchitis and emphysema. Tolerance to marijuana develops after heavy use, and withdrawal causes irritability and restlessness. Addiction can develop with long-term use, referred to as cannabis use disorder (CUD).

The adverse effects associated with the use of synthetic cannabinoids include anxiety, paranoia, psychosis, sedation, seizures, and hallucinations. Additionally, these compounds have been reported to produce tachycardia, hypertension, nausea, vomiting, acute kidney injury, and heart attacks. Long-term use may be associated with an increased risk of psychosis. Withdrawal symptoms include headaches, anxiety, irritability, and depression.

Depressants

Dose-response curves for the effects of the barbiturates, nonbarbiturate sedatives, and GHB are essentially the same as those for ethanol, whereas curves for the benzodiazepines are much shallower (Fig. 24.5). Thus, for ethanol, the dose causing intoxication is only one-quarter to one-third of the lethal dose (Chapter 23), whereas for a benzodiazepine, the doses that induce the depressant effects are much less than those leading to death. Flunitrazepam and GHB cause sedation and anterograde amnesia.

Increased doses of GHB can produce a state of anesthesia, coma, respiratory and cardiac depression, seizures, and death.

After an overdose with depressant drugs, patients are unresponsive, pupils are sluggish and miotic, respiration is shallow and slow, and deep tendon reflexes are absent or attenuated. There are no known antagonists for barbiturates, nonbarbiturate sedatives, or GHB, whereas the competitive benzodiazepine antagonist flumazenil can completely reverse benzodiazepine intoxication. Although benzodiazepines are rarely lethal when taken alone, they enhance the effects of other depressants taken concurrently, including alcohol.

Repeated use of depressants produces physical dependence, and cross-dependence occurs among barbiturates, nonbarbiturate sedatives, benzodiazepines, and alcohol. Signs and symptoms of withdrawal are often opposite to their acute effects. Occasional convulsions and delirium make depressant withdrawal a medical emergency. Long-acting benzodiazepines or phenobarbital can be used as substitution therapy to treat alcohol and barbiturate withdrawal. The withdrawal symptoms after abrupt discontinuation of depressants and a comparison with those associated with opioid withdrawal are summarized in Table 24.2.

TABLE 24.2 **Comparison of Opioid and Depressant Withdrawal**	
Opioid Withdrawal	**Depressant Withdrawal**[a]
Anxiety and dysphoria	Anxiety and dysphoria
Craving and drug-seeking behavior	Craving and drug-seeking behavior
Sleep disturbance	Sleep disturbance
Nausea and vomiting	Nausea and vomiting
Lacrimation	Tremors
Rhinorrhea	Hyperreflexia
Yawning	Hyperpyrexia
Piloerection and gooseflesh	Confusion and delirium
Sweating	Convulsions
Diarrhea	Life-threatening convulsions
Mydriasis	
Abdominal cramping	
Hyperpyrexia	
Tachycardia and hypertension	

[a]Alcohol, barbiturates, or benzodiazepines.

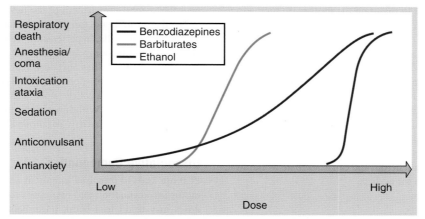

FIG. 24.5 Comparison of Dose-Response Relationships For the Acute Effects of Ethanol, Barbiturates, and Benzodiazepines.

Opioids

Opioid overdose leads to unconsciousness, respiratory depression, and extreme miosis, although the latter is not always apparent because asphyxia can result in pupillary dilation. Death is due to respiratory failure. The IV injection of an opioid antagonist, such as naloxone or nalmefene, can reverse all effects immediately and produce rapid recovery. However, it is important not to administer too large a dose because severe withdrawal could be precipitated in a physically dependent patient. Patients should be observed to ensure severe intoxication does not reemerge.

Heroin users often begin by smoking, but many eventually progress to IV injection because of the increased rapidity of effect, leading to many medical problems. Particularly dangerous is sharing of needles and other injection paraphernalia, which dramatically increases blood-borne infections. Street heroin is not pure but is "cut" with several compounds, including sugar, starch, powdered milk, quinine, and strychnine, the latter leading to convulsions. These substances are also dangerous because they can block small arteries to vital organs. Long-term effects of the IV administration of heroin include collapsed veins, infection of heart linings and valves, abscesses, and pulmonary complications.

Because desomorphine has a very rapid onset, is extremely potent, and has a short half-life, it promotes binge patterns of use, making addiction and dependence highly likely. The most common complication associated with use and abuse is serious damage to veins, soft tissue infection, necrosis, and gangrene.

The adverse effects of kratom are similar to those of heroin or morphine. High doses can produce a state of stupor and/or sedation that can be life-threatening. Long-term use can lead to weight loss, insomnia, dry mouth, frequent urination, and constipation.

Most opioid abusers become physically dependent over time. Initial users are generally confident that they can control their use and are only dimly aware of their gradual dependence. Taking multiple daily doses of heroin or other opioids usually results in significant dependence within a few weeks. The unavoidable withdrawal syndrome begins approximately 6 hours after the last heroin injection. Many dependent abusers are tolerant to the positive reinforcing effects of the opioids, and continued drug use only provides relief from withdrawal. If a person is not treated, withdrawal reaches peak severity in approximately 24 hours and ceases in 7–10 days. This rarely constitutes a medical emergency and is considerably less dangerous than withdrawal from alcohol or barbiturates.

Opioids cross the placental barrier, and a newborn of an opioid-dependent mother will undergo withdrawal within 6–12 hours of birth. The long-term consequences of prenatal opioid dependence are poorly understood, but it may be best to maintain the mother on methadone and treat the infant with opioids rather than withdraw the mother before parturition.

Cross-dependence occurs among all full opioid agonists. Hydromorphone, meperidine, oxycodone, and others can reverse withdrawal and, at appropriate doses, can produce a heroin-like intoxication in addicts. Less efficacious agonists, such as codeine and dextropropoxyphene, also show cross-dependence. Mixed opioid agonist-antagonists and partial agonists such as pentazocine, butorphanol, nalbuphine, and buprenorphine are less abused than full agonists, although each has a slightly different profile. Except for buprenorphine, these compounds show little cross-dependence with heroin and can exacerbate withdrawal; thus they offer little attraction for addicts.

Stimulants

Stimulant overdose results in excessive activation of the sympathetic nervous system. The resulting tachycardia and hypertension may result in myocardial infarction and stroke. Cocaine can cause coronary vasospasm and cardiac dysrhythmias. Cocaine salts are often cut with inert substances, with other local anesthetics similar in appearance and taste, or with other stimulants. The IV administration of stimulants is associated with the same problems as IV heroin. Abuse of cocaine by snorting may lead to irritation of the nasal mucosa, sinusitis, and a perforated septum.

CNS symptoms in cocaine users include anxiety, feelings of paranoia and impending doom, and restlessness. Users exhibit unpredictable behavior and sometimes become violent. Adrenergic receptor antagonists alleviate some of these symptoms, although they are often ineffective.

A dangerous pattern of stimulant abuse is the extended, uninterrupted sequences referred to as "runs" or "binging." Runs result from attempts to maintain a continuous state of intoxication, to extend the pleasurable feeling, and to postpone the postintoxication crash. Acute tolerance can occur, particularly in those injecting the substance, resulting in a need for increasingly larger doses. This spiral of tolerance and increased dose is often continued until drug supplies are depleted or the person collapses from exhaustion. During runs, drug-taking and drug-seeking behavior take on a compulsive character, making treatment intervention difficult.

Another typical abuse pattern begins with self-medication. Some individuals, such as long-distance truck drivers or students, use stimulants to achieve sustained attention, while others use these drugs to make tasks (e.g., housework) appear easier and to complete them faster. These patterns lead to increased doses and frequency of use, producing tolerance and further dose increases. Alcohol or depressant drugs are frequently used to counteract the resultant anxiety and insomnia, establishing a cycle of "uppers and downers."

Dependence on stimulants is characterized principally by uncontrolled compulsive episodes of use. An important component of stimulant intoxication is the "crash" that occurs as drug effects subside or upon cessation of use. Dysphoria, tiredness, irritability, and mild depression often occur within hours after stimulant ingestion, resulting in drug craving and relapse. Sleep disturbances, hyperphagia, and brain abnormalities have also been noted. These psychological sequelae are important in fostering continued abuse and are important treatment targets.

Personality changes often occur in stimulant abusers and include delusions, preoccupation with self, hostility, and paranoia. A toxic psychosis can develop. Often difficult to distinguish from paranoid schizophrenia, severe amphetamine and cocaine psychoses require psychiatric management.

Cocaine use during pregnancy may be associated with complications including abruptio placentae, premature birth, lower birth weight, and neurobehavioral impairment of the newborn.

Synthetic cathinones can produce agitation, confusion, hallucinations, paranoia, tachycardia, hypertension, tremor, and fever. They have also been linked to rhabdomyolysis, renal failure, seizures, and death. Aggressive violent behavior has also been reported. The synthetic cathinone α-pyrrolidinopentiophenone (α-PVP) is believed to be responsible for the 2016 incident of a college student killing and attempting to eat the faces of two victims. Withdrawal symptoms from the use of synthetic cathinones include anxiety, paranoia, sleep difficulties, tremors, and depression.

Dissociative Compounds

PCP use leads to impaired judgment and bizarre behaviors, including motor incoordination and catalepsy accompanied by nystagmus; high doses may result in a blank stare. Behavior may be more disrupted when PCP is taken with depressant drugs, including alcohol. Major dangers are risk-taking behavior and the progressive development of personality changes, culminating in a toxic psychosis. PCP overdose is rarely lethal but may require careful management because of severe incapacitation. No PCP antagonist is available. High doses of PCP or ketamine can produce a state of almost complete sensory detachment, resembling catatonic schizophrenia; this state is referred to as the "K-hole."

The adverse effects of salvia are not well established. The most frequent side effects reported are confusion/disorientation, dizziness, flushed sensation, and tachycardia. There do not appear to be any significant risks to cardiac tissue or other internal organs, although salvia use may precipitate acute psychotic episodes. There are no established withdrawal symptoms, perhaps because salvia is not used with great frequency.

Hallucinogens

The hallucinogens can lead to mood swings ranging from profound euphoria to anxiety and terror. Panic states ("bad trips") are more common with larger doses and result from the propensity of the drug experience to be rapidly transformed because it is highly dependent on environmental context. Bad trips often lead abusers to seek assistance, and they usually respond to calm reassurance and removal from a threatening environment until the drug wears off. Medication is rarely needed, although antipsychotic treatment may be useful. Nearly all hallucinogens produce varying degrees of sympathomimetic effects, and psychomotor stimulation may be evident. These effects are more common in people who use substituted amphetamines such as MDMA, particularly at higher doses.

Although acute overdose is not a common problem with hallucinogens, there is the risk of injury stemming from impaired judgment. In addition, even occasional use of hallucinogens may precipitate a psychiatric illness in predisposed subjects that is exacerbated by repeated use. A poorly understood aspect is the "flashback" in which previous users reexperience aspects of intoxication while drug-free. Flashbacks may also occur in those who have used marijuana or PCP and may be no more than déjà vu experiences triggered by drug-associated environments or cues, or episodes that reflect an emerging psychopathological condition. LSD does not produce withdrawal symptoms or the intense cravings caused by other drugs of abuse. However, strong tolerance (tachyphylaxis) occurs, with cross-tolerance to other hallucinogens, and increasingly higher doses may be used, leading to unpredictable consequences.

Inhalants

Abused solvents and gases lead to motor performance deficits similar to those produced by alcohol and depressant drugs. Prolonged use can lead to arrhythmias, heart failure, and death, especially with butane, propane, and aerosols. Death may also occur as a consequence of suffocation, asphyxiation, choking, and accidents while intoxicated. Inhalants are highly toxic, and chronic use can cause damage to the central and peripheral nervous systems, including well-defined axonopathies. In addition, chlorofluorocarbons are cardiotoxic. Treatment of acute toxicity is supportive to stabilize vital signs. There is no antidote or treatment for chronic exposure.

The nitrites are vasodilators, and dizziness and euphoria result from the hypotension and cerebral hypoxia caused by peripheral venous pooling. Nitrites are often abused in conjunction with sexual activity and are popular among homosexual men for their ability to enhance orgasms, probably as a result of penile vasodilation. Nitrite use can result in accidents related to syncope.

Pharmacotherapies for Substance Abuse

In considering treatment, it is important to remember that SUDs are chronic, relapsing diseases. Treatment can be very effective, especially if one accepts reduction in drug use and its resultant harm as an important goal. Complete cessation of drug use can also be achieved but may require multiple attempts. Thus repeated treatment of SUDs should be considered in a similar light as treatment of other chronic diseases. It is important to distinguish physically dependent from nondependent abusers because treatment strategies differ considerably. Unfortunately, most treatment programs are for dependent abusers. Strategies for preventing escalation from occasional use would be desirable but are rare. Although there are several pharmacological interventions for the treatment of opioid use disorders (Chapter 28) and alcohol use disorders (Chapter 23), there are no approved medications to treat SUDs involving cannabinoids, dissociative compounds, hallucinogens, or inhalants.

Physical and psychological symptoms associated with drug abuse are summarized in the Clinical Problems Box.

NEW DEVELOPMENTS

Increasing knowledge of the mechanisms of action of abused drugs could lead to medications that stabilize the user in the same way as methadone and buprenorphine for opioid addicts, or even allow for abstinence. The development of substitute agonists of the DA transporter may provide similar benefits across several drug classes by substituting for the effects of the drug on the mesolimbic DA pathway. This approach has had some success in preventing the self-administration of cocaine in nonhuman primates. Researchers are also exploring pharmacotherapies that act on D_3 receptors, which are expressed in the mesolimbic system and in brain regions mediating emotion.

Other neurotransmitter systems may also be targets for novel pharmacotherapies. The use of N-acetylcysteine to stabilize glutamate activity and improve impulse control has been investigated as a treatment intervention for SUDs, with promising preclinical and clinical results. Similarly, alteration of 5-HT receptor activity may reduce compulsive drug taking by improving behavioral regulation. Because cognitive functions are frequently impaired by chronic drug abuse, approaches that improve cognitive function, particularly the ability of the drug user to self-regulate, may prove to be very useful when combined with established cognitive behavioral therapies.

CLINICAL RELEVANCE FOR HEALTHCARE PROFESSIONALS

Approximately 15% of the population over the age of 12 years suffer from some form of SUD each year. Therefore most healthcare professionals will frequently encounter individuals with addiction and dependence issues. It is unlikely that patients with an SUD will readily disclose their ongoing struggles; thus it is important for all healthcare professionals to identify signs and symptoms and address substance use concerns.

Detoxification from most abused substances does not require medical assistance. However, individuals who have become dependent on depressants typically require medically managed detoxification to control withdrawal symptoms that could otherwise be fatal. Additionally, although the withdrawal symptoms associated with opiate withdrawal are not fatal, physician-prescribed substitution drug treatment can greatly reduce discomfort during detoxification and increase the likelihood of recovery. For all SUDs, the use of cognitive-behavioral therapeutic approaches and recovery support groups (i.e., Alcoholics Anonymous, Narcotics Anonymous) following detoxification greatly reduces the likelihood of relapse and should be encouraged.

CLINICAL PROBLEMS

Cannabinoids
- Dry mouth, high blood pressure, rapid heart rate, poor coordination, red eyes, slow reaction times
- Decreased sociability, difficulty concentrating, increased appetite, memory problems

Depressants
- Dizziness, drowsiness, low blood pressure, nystagmus, poor coordination, slow respiration, slurred speech
- Depression, difficulty concentrating, lack of inhibition, memory problems

Opioids
- Constipation, constricted pupils, poor hygiene, sweaty/clammy skin
- Blackouts, complaints of pain, irritability, lack of external awareness or attention, memory problems, mood swings

Stimulants
- Dilated pupils, high blood pressure, irregular heart rate, nasal congestion (when snorted), weight loss
- Acute psychosis, anxiety, insomnia, irritability, paranoia, rapid speech, restlessness, sudden mood changes

Dissociative Compounds
- High blood pressure, nystagmus, pain insensitivity, poor coordination, rapid heart rate
- Aggression, difficulty concentrating, hallucinations, increased sensitivity to noise, memory problems

Hallucinogens
- High blood pressure, rapid heart rate, tremors
- Distorted and possible permanent changes in perception, hallucinations, lack of inhibition, rapid mood swings

Inhalants
- Irregular heartbeat, nystagmus, poor coordination, rashes around the nose and mouth, slow movements, slurred speech, tremors
- Difficulty concentrating, lack of inhibition, memory problems

DRUG NAMES

The following are common "street" or "slang" names for abused drugs in the United States.

Class	Substance	Street Names
Cannabis	Hashish	Charas, Hash, Kiff, Nup, Shish
	Marijuana	420, Bud, Cheeba, Chronic, Dope: Ganja, Grass, Herb, Hippie lettuce, Hay, Hydro, Kiff, Maryjane, Pot, Sticky icky, Wacky tobaccy, Weed
	Synthetic Cannabinoids	Black mamba, Bliss, Bombay blue, Flakka, Genie, K2, Spice, Zohai
Depressants	Benzodiazepines	Candy, Dead flower powers, Downers, Goofballs, Heavenly blues, Moggies, Qual, Sleepers, Stupefy, Tranx, Valley girl, Z bars
	Flunitrazepam	Circles, Mexican valium, Rib, Roofies, Rope, Rophies, Ruffies
	GHB	Liquid ecstasy, G, Georgia home boy, Grievous bodily harm
Opiates	Codeine	Doors, Fours, Lean, Loads, Purple drank, Schoolboy, syrup
	Desomorphine	Crocodile, Krokodil, Russian magic
	Fentanyl	Apache, China girl, China town, Friends, Great bear, He-Man, Jackpot, King ivory
	Heroin	Black stuff, Brown sugar, China white, Dope, Golden girls, H, Smack, Tar, White horse
	Kratom	Blak, Kakuam, Ketum, Thang, Thom
	Morphine	Aunti Em, Dance fever, Drone, Goodfellas, M, Monkey, Morph, Murder 8, Roxanol, Tango and cash, TNT, White stuff
Stimulants	Amphetamines	Bennies, Copilots, Uppers, Scooby snacks, Speed, Truck drivers
	Cathinones	Bath salts, Bloom, Chat, Cloud 9, Ivory wave, Khat, Miraa, Quaadka, Red dove, Snow day, Vanilla sky, White lightning
	Cocaine	Base, Blow, Coke, Cola, Crack, Powder, Snow
	Methamphetamine	Crank, Dunk, Ice, Meth, Tweek
	Methylphenidate	Diet coke, Kiddy coke, R-ball, R pop, Rids, Rittles, Skippy, Skittles, Smart drug, Smarties, Study buddies, Vitamin R, West coast
Dissociative Compounds	Dextromethorphan	Dex, Drex, DMX, Orange crush, Poor man's PCP, Red devils, Robo
	Ketamine	Cat valium, K, Kit kat, Jet, Purple, Special K, Super K, Vitamin K
	Phencyclidine	Angel dust, Embalming fluid, Hog, PCP, Super dust, Tic tac
	Salvia	Diviner's sage, Purple sticky, Magic mint, Sage of the seers, Sally-D, Ska pastora
Hallucinogens	Dimethyltryptamine	Businessman's lunch, Businessman's special
	LSD	Acid, Blotter, Dots, Fry, Gel, Hawk, L, Lucy, Purple haze, Smilies, Tab, Trips, Window
	MDMA	Adam, Beans, Ecstasy, Hug drug, Molly, XTC
	Mescaline	Buttons, Cactus, Peyote
	Psilocybin	Boomers, Little smoke, Magic mushrooms, Shrooms
Inhalants	Amyl Nitrate; N_2O	Boppers, Poppers, Laughing gas, Whippets
	Volatile Solvents	Quicksilver, Snotballs, Whiteout
	Nitrites	Bullet, Snappers, Thrust

SELF-ASSESSMENT QUESTIONS

1. A person who has been taking one drug chronically and experiences a withdrawal syndrome upon discontinuation finds relief from these symptoms by taking a different drug. This is an example of:
    A. Craving.
    B. Psychological dependence.
    C. Cross-dependence.
    D. Tolerance.
    E. Drug addiction.

2. The reinforcing effects of drugs of abuse are thought to reflect:
    A. Increased raphe serotonergic transmission.
    B. Increased mesolimbic dopaminergic transmission.
    C. Increased glutamatergic activity.
    D. increased cardiovascular and psychomotor effects.

3. A 32-year-old known drug abuser ran out of drugs and had no way to purchase more to support his habit. As a consequence, he began exhibiting symptoms of withdrawal. Which of the following drugs results in a life-threatening withdrawal?
    A. Cocaine.
    B. Pentobarbital.
    C. Heroin.
    D. LSD.
    E. Methamphetamine.

4. The withdrawal symptoms following barbiturate cessation are similar to the withdrawal symptoms from:
    A. Heroin.
    B. Alcohol.
    C. Phenothiazines.
    D. Morphine.

5. An 18-year-old college student took a pill she bought from a friend and began hallucinating. Which neurotransmitter system is thought to underlie the manifestation of hallucinations?
    A. Dopamine.
    B. GABA.
    C. Norepinephrine.
    D. Serotonin.

FURTHER READING

Everitt BJ, Robbins TW. From the ventral to the dorsal striatum: devolving views of their roles in drug addiction. *Neurosci Biobehav Rev*. 2013;37(9): 1946–1954.

Jasinska AJ, Zorick T, Brody AL, Stein EA. Dual role of nicotine in addiction and cognition: a review of neuroimaging studies in humans. *Neuropharmacology*. 2014;84:111–122.

Nutt DJ, Lingford-Hughes A, Erritzoe D, Stokes PRA. The dopamine theory of addiction: 40 years of highs and lows. *Nat Rev Neurosci*. 2015;16: 305–312.

Rech MA, Donahey E, Cappiello Diedic JM, et al. New drugs of abuse. *Pharmacotherapy*. 2015;35(2):189–197.

WEBSITES

https://www.drugabuse.gov/

The National Institute on Drug Abuse maintains an excellent website with information and many resource links for healthcare professionals, caregivers, and others seeking information on drug abuse.

https://www.samhsa.gov/

The United States Substance Abuse and Mental Health Services Administration, which was established in 1992 by an act of Congress, provides links to numerous resources on substance use and mental health disorders.

Drug Therapy for Pain Management

25

Introduction

Susan L. Ingram

Pain (or nociception) is an important sensory experience that protects organisms from tissue damage and potentially harmful environments. In some situations, acute pain transitions to chronic pain that persists long after the initial insult. In other cases, chronic pain exists in the absence of any observed tissue or nerve damage. This pathological pain is not protective but reflects changes in the central nervous system that increase the "perception of pain." In these cases, the normal processing of nociceptive inputs in the spinal cord by descending projections from cortical and subcortical brain circuits is sensitized so that patients perceive pain in the absence of painful stimuli. The plasticity involved in the neural control of pain highlights the fact that the "perception" of tissue damage is rarely explained by the sensory inputs from the periphery, but rather includes the cognitive and emotional states of the patient, i.e., pain is highly subjective. Chronic pain typically lasts greater than 3 months and impacts quality of life and social interactions because it is associated with negative emotional and behavioral symptoms. This critical distinction acknowledges that the brain is a key player in the perception of pain and is particularly relevant when considering the etiology of chronic pain.

Many years of research have delineated the different processes and circuits that mediate acute and chronic pain, and many pain clinics recognize the need to treat pain using multiple modalities (Table 25.1). Unfortunately, the cellular and molecular mechanisms underlying the transition from acute pain to chronic pain states are not well understood and represent an active area of research.

NEUROPHYSIOLOGY OF PAIN

Peripheral Transmission of Pain

Noxious or nociceptive stimuli activate highly developed endings on primary afferent neurons, termed nociceptors (pain receptors). Primary afferents innervate the skin, viscera, deep muscle, and joints and have their soma in the dorsal root or trigeminal ganglia with axons extending bidirectionally into the periphery and centrally into the spinal cord. Specialized receptors transduce mechanical and thermal nociceptive signals via different primary afferent fibers. Activation of these specialized receptors and ligand-activated ion channels produces depolarization (or a generator potential) in afferent nerve endings. Summation of multiple events produces a generator potential of sufficient amplitude in the nerve endings to activate voltage-gated Na^+ and K^+ channels, and initiate action potentials that are transmitted to the dorsal horn of the spinal cord.

Primary afferents include both touch (nonnociceptive) and nociceptive fibers (Chapter 27, Fig. 27.5). Nonnociceptive afferents include myelinated Aβ fibers that innervate pacinian corpuscles and Merkel cells that detect vibration and light pressure and respond to low-intensity touch stimulation. These afferents do not play a role in acute pain processing. Nociceptive primary afferents include both myelinated Aδ and unmyelinated C fibers, both of which respond to high-intensity nociceptive stimulation and express many chemoreceptors that detect tissue damage. Aδ fibers are small, rapidly conducting, afferent neurons that terminate in lamina I of the spinal cord. They have a relatively high threshold for activation by mechanical and thermal stimuli and mediate sharp and localized pain, often termed somatic pain. C fibers are even smaller unmyelinated afferent neurons that conduct action potentials more slowly. They are polymodal and are activated by mechanical, thermal, or chemical stimuli. They terminate in lamina II of the spinal cord (substantia gelatinosa) and mediate dull, diffuse, aching, or burning pain, sometimes called visceral pain. The receptors for nociceptive fibers are channels and receptors expressed on free nerve endings that extend into the skin and respond to high-intensity mechanical stimulation and specific chemical mediators released in the periphery. The intensity of a painful stimulus is encoded by action potential frequency.

Upon tissue damage, damaged cells release large quantities of adenosine triphosphate (ATP) and glutamate that activate free nerve endings of nociceptive Aδ and C fibers in the skin. This damage sets off a cascade of events involved in the inflammatory response. The activation of free nerve endings elicits the release of pronociceptive neurotransmitters, including the neuropeptides substance P, calcitonin gene–related peptide (CGRP), and neuropeptide Y that trigger inflammatory responses. Immune cells are recruited to the site of injury and release many inflammatory mediators known collectively as "the inflammatory soup," including prostaglandins, bradykinin, cytokines, serotonin (5-HT), and histamine. There are many receptors and channels expressed on free nerve endings that are either activated by these inflammatory mediators or are sensitized by these chemicals. For example, the family of transient receptor potential (TRP) channels includes several proteins involved in nociceptive transduction. TRPV1 is gated by multiple chemical

ABBREVIATIONS	
CGRP	Calcitonin gene–related peptide
GABA	γ-Aminobutyric acid
5-HT	Serotonin (5-hydroxytryptophan)
NE	Norepinephrine
NSAID	Nonsteroidal antiinflammatory agent
TRP	Transient receptor potential
WDR	Wide dynamic range

TABLE 25.1   Multiple Approaches to Pain Therapies

Nonpharmacological	
Psychosocial	Use cognitive behavioral therapies to learn to cope with negative beliefs and fears and decrease catastrophizing
Behavioral approaches	Decrease stress through meditation, mindfulness, yoga, and biofeedback
Exercise/activity	Focus on returning to functional activity
Spinal manipulation, acupuncture	Efficacy demonstrated for pain
Group support	Increase social interaction
Education	Promote patient and caregiver knowledge of pain processing
Spiritual support	Promote meaning and purpose in life
Sleep hygiene	Use strategies to improve sleep and decrease stress
Pharmacological	
Opioids	Gold standard for acute pain; little evidence for effectiveness for chronic pain
NSAIDs (aspirin, ibuprofen)	Equally or more effective (especially when used with acetaminophen) for mild to moderate pain with less risk for harm than opioids
Acetaminophen	See above
Sleep medications	Melatonin and antidepressants can increase sleep
Antidepressants (TCAs/SSRIs)	Effective in several clinical trials for chronic pain conditions
Anticonvulsants (gabapentin and pregabalin)	Effective for diabetic peripheral neuropathy, other neuropathies, and fibromyalgia
Muscle relaxants and antispasticity drugs	Some evidence effective for pain, but are sedating

Adapted/created from Interagency Guideline on Prescribing Opioids for Pain, Developed by the Washington State Agency Medical Directors' Group [AMDG] in collaboration with an Expert Advisory Panel, Actively Practicing Providers, Public Stakeholders, and Senior State Officials [2015]. http://www.agencymeddirectors.wa.gov/Files/2015AMDGOpioidGuideline.pdf

stimuli, including capsaicin, the active ingredient in hot peppers, but it is also gated by increases in temperature in the noxious range (>43°C for humans). In addition, lipid neuromodulators, kinases, and protons also sensitize TRPV1 channels. This type of complex regulation holds for several of the receptors and channels that respond to nociceptive stimuli that have been cloned and studied in detail.

Central Transmission of Pain

Action potentials that are generated in peripheral axons of Aδ and C primary afferents travel centrally to release excitatory amino acids and neuropeptides in the dorsal horn of the spinal cord. The primary afferent axons enter the spinal cord at multiple levels via the dorsal roots, and release glutamate and other neuropeptides onto second-order projection neurons to the brain and interneurons that can contain γ-aminobutyric acid (GABA), glycine, or glutamate. Secondary neurons that form the ascending spinothalamic pathway project to supraspinal

nuclei in the thalamus, and then to the limbic system and cerebral cortex (Fig. 25.1A).

Considerable processing of nociceptive information occurs in the dorsal horn. Some second-order dorsal horn neurons respond selectively to nociceptive stimuli, termed "nociceptive-specific," and have small receptive fields that give information as to the location of the stimulus. Other neurons respond to multiple inputs and are polymodal nociceptive neurons. Another population of cells in the deeper lamina V are known as **wide-dynamic-range (WDR) neurons** because they respond to both innocuous and nociceptive stimuli and have large, complex receptive fields. Second-order projection neurons that respond to nociceptive stimuli send axons across the midline at the level that they enter the spinal cord and ascend to the contralateral side of the brain.

The brain also has an endogenous descending circuit that can regulate pain in both directions: facilitation and inhibition. Descending pain control systems originate in the periaqueductal gray region of the midbrain and from several nuclei of the rostroventral medulla oblongata and project downward to the dorsal horn. These descending systems release norepinephrine (NE), 5-HT, and other neurotransmitters that modulate the activity of the ascending pain pathways, either through direct synaptic contacts or indirectly by activating inhibitory interneurons. These pathways are illustrated in Fig. 25.1B.

Sensitization of nociceptive inputs can occur in the spinal cord, as well as higher brain structures, and is known as **central sensitization**. Synaptic plasticity is initiated by intense stimulation or inflammation and can result in increased neurotransmitter release from primary afferent terminals and/or enhanced postsynaptic responses of dorsal horn neurons. In some cases, this plasticity recruits changes in typically nonnoxious myelinated Aβ touch fibers that result in **paresthesias** and **diathesis**. Plasticity also occurs in the descending pain control pathways so that the normal pain inhibition function of the system shifts to pain facilitation. It is clear that the balance between inhibitory and facilitatory control of pain by the descending pathways is shifted in states of neuropathic or chronic pain.

DRUGS TO ALLEVIATE PAIN

Numerous pharmacological agents, both prescription and nonprescription compounds, are available to alleviate pain. Studies have indicated that more than 100 million adult Americans experience chronic pain and use pain-relieving medications on a daily basis. The chronic use of medications for alleviating pain may do more harm than good and can lead to numerous adverse effects ranging from gastrointestinal, hepatic, or cardiovascular issues following the use of the nonsteroidal antiinflammatory agents (NSAIDs) for mild pain (Chapter 29) to depression and addiction following the long-term use of opioids for severe pain (Chapter 28).

The general anesthetics produce a controlled state of unconsciousness and analgesia, and their pharmacology is discussed in Chapter 26, while the use and pharmacology of the local anesthetics are presented in Chapter 27. Although evidence suggests that the cannabinoids and endocannabinoid system may not be effective for the treatment of acute pain, they may modulate neuropathic pain and the pain associated with fibromyalgia (Chapter 30).

SPECIFIC PAIN SYNDROMES
Neuropathic Pain

Neuropathic pain is the result of injury to peripheral sensory nerves and involves different cellular mechanisms than those involved in inflammatory pain. There are many causes of nerve injury including physical trauma, alcoholism, metabolic and autoimmune disorders, viral

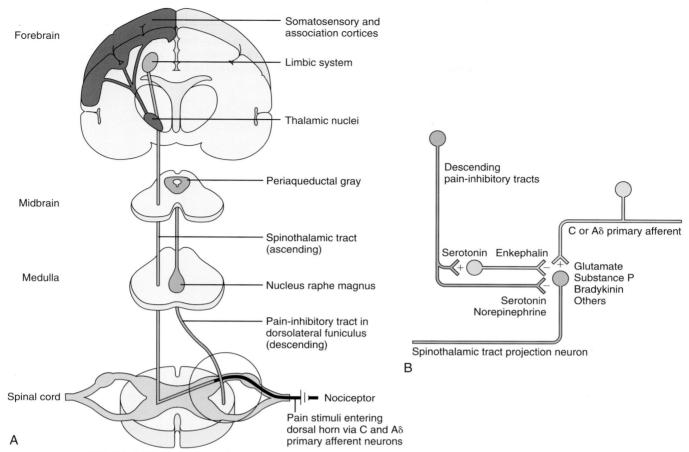

FIG. 25.1 (A) Ascending spinothalamic tract pain-transmitting pathway and descending pain-modulatory pathway originating in the midbrain. (B) Possible synaptic connections in the dorsal horn and mediators that may influence the transmission of pain stimuli.

infection, chemotoxicity, and chronic inflammation. Nearly half of all diabetic patients eventually experience peripheral neuropathies. Neuropathic pain states often are associated with hyperalgesia (increased sensitivity to normally painful stimuli) and allodynia (pain caused by stimuli that are not normally painful; e.g., touch). These manifest as either shooting and burning pain or tingling and numbness.

In neuropathic pain, primary afferent neurons are hyperactive, discharging spontaneously (in the absence of an identifiable noxious stimulus), and there is a cascade of changes to neurons in dorsal root ganglia and in the dorsal horn of the spinal cord indicating sensitization of central pain pathways. These changes present multiple targets for pharmacological intervention, among which are increases in the expression and activity of Na^+ and Ca^{2+} channels and decreases in the expression of K^+ channels. Several drugs introduced to treat seizure disorders have been shown to be effective in the treatment of neuropathic pain, including carbamazepine and lamotrigine, which inhibit voltage-dependent Na^+ channels, and pregabalin and gabapentin, which bind to an auxiliary subunit of voltage-gated Ca^{2+} channels to decrease the release of several neurotransmitters (Chapter 21). The tricyclic antidepressants (Chapter 17) have also been shown to be effective for this condition, and several studies support the use of the cannabinoids (Chapter 30).

Fibromyalgia

Fibromyalgia is a disorder characterized by widespread musculoskeletal pain accompanied by fatigue and sleep, memory, and mood issues. The causes of fibromyalgia are not known, but it is believed to result from central sensitization of pain pathways that decrease pain thresholds. The anticonvulsant pregabalin was the first drug approved by the United States Food and Drug Administration in 2007 specifically for the management of fibromyalgia. Other drugs shown to be effective for some fibromyalgia patients include the antidepressants such as amitriptyline, muscle relaxants such as cyclobenzaprine, and the cannabinoids.

Others

In addition to neuropathic pain and fibromyalgia, pain is a primary characteristic of several debilitating disorders including migraines, arthritis, and gout. The pharmacology of drugs to alleviate the pain associated with migraine and other headaches is presented in Chapter 31. Chapter 35 presents the pharmacology of agents used to alleviate the pain associated with rheumatoid arthritis, while Chapter 32 deals with drugs used to alleviate the pain and inflammation associated with gout and the hyperuricemias.

FURTHER READING

Fillingim RB, Loeser JD, Baron R, Edwards RR. Assessment of chronic pain: domains, methods, and mechanisms. *J Pain*. 2016;17(suppl 9):T10–T20.

Kuner R. Central mechanisms of pathological pain. *Nat Med*. 2010;16(11): 1258–1266.

Sluka KA, Clauw DJ. Neurobiology of fibromyalgia and chronic widespread pain. *Neuroscience*. 2016.

WEBSITES

http://www.painmed.org/patientcenter/facts_on_pain.aspx
This is the American Academy of Pain Medicine website and contains very useful facts related to the incidence of pain and the use of pain medications.

26

General Anesthetics

David R. Wetzel and Jeffrey J. Pasternak

MAJOR DRUG CLASSES

Inhalational anesthetics
Intravenous anesthetics

ABBREVIATIONS

CNS	Central nervous system
ED$_{50}$	Median effective dose
GABA	γ-Aminobutyric acid
MAC	Minimum alveolar concentration
N$_2$O	Nitrous oxide
NMDA	*N*-methyl-D-aspartate
PCO$_2$	Partial pressure of carbon dioxide

THERAPEUTIC OVERVIEW

General anesthesia is a controlled state of loss of sensation, loss of consciousness, and analgesia combined with relaxation of skeletal muscles and suppression of somatic, autonomic, and endocrine reflexes. An ideal anesthetic drug would provide all of these properties along with easy reversibility and limited side effects. However, in current practice, no single drug can reliably produce all of these effects, often requiring the use of multiple drugs, a technique known as "balanced anesthesia."

Sedative/hypnotic drugs, often referred to as "general anesthetics," are a class of compounds that produce a state of sedation or loss of consciousness (i.e., hypnosis) and have been used to facilitate surgery and various medical procedures for over 170 years. Some of the original anesthetics, such as nitrous oxide (N$_2$O), are still in use today, while others, like ether and chloroform, are no longer in contemporary practice. Modern anesthetic drugs are most commonly administered via two routes, through inhalation and intravenously, although some drugs may be given intramuscularly. The safe and effective use of general anesthetics is a dynamic process that must be individualized for each patient and surgical situation. Further, the needs of both the surgical team and the patient may change during a procedure, altering anesthetic requirements and drug choices.

Anesthesiologists play a critical role in the facilitation of surgical, medical, and diagnostic procedures for patient management. Although some medical and surgical procedures can be performed with the use of local anesthetics, many procedures often require either sedation or general anesthesia. Generally, the spectrum of sedation and general anesthesia can be stratified into four primary states (sedation, excitation, general anesthesia, and deep general anesthesia) that can be facilitated by the addition of other medications, such as the benzodiazepines (Chapter 17), neuromuscular blocking agents (Chapter 10), and the opioids (Chapter 28).

1. Sedation is generally achieved with lower doses of medications. When patients are sedated, they may be responsive to verbal or sensory stimuli and often continue breathing with minimal support. Although they report a sense of relaxation, they still will respond to moderately or severely painful stimuli and may not have amnesia for the events.

2. As drug doses increase, many inhaled and injectable sedative/hypnotic drugs induce a state of excitation during which increases in high-frequency activity are observed on the electroencephalogram. Clinically, this is manifest as heart-rate irregularities, abnormal breathing patterns, involuntary movements, and enhanced reflexes such as airway reflexes and increased risk for vomiting. As such, it is prudent to minimize the time that the patient spends in this stage.

3. As further sedative/hypnotic medications are administered, vital signs stabilize, and patients no longer respond to verbal or sensory stimuli, representing general anesthesia. During this stage, patients are unconscious and amnestic for events. Respiration may be regular but significantly depressed, and airway reflexes are reduced, requiring mechanical airway support, often by endotracheal intubation. Patients are often pharmacologically placed into this stage during most procedures that require complete unconsciousness.

4. If excessive doses of anesthetic drugs are administered, patients may transition to deep general anesthesia, during which time they become hemodynamically unstable and may exhibit significant suppression of electrical activity in the brain. Rarely, surgical procedures may require a patient to be pharmacologically placed into deep general anesthesia, but it is often avoided if possible.

The administration and facilitation of the state of general anesthesia can be divided into three distinct phases, induction, maintenance, and emergence.

1. During the induction phase, an awake patient is placed into a state of general anesthesia through the administration of a sedative/hypnotic drug. An intravenous drug is usually administered in adults who have an intravenous catheter in place, whereas induction of anesthesia with inhalation drugs is usually reserved for children or other patients who are unable to tolerate intravenous catheter placement while awake. Other drugs, such as opioids or neuromuscular blocking agents, may also be administered during this time. One of the primary goals of induction is to minimize the duration of time that the patient spends in the excitation phase of anesthesia. Therefore patients often receive a large dose of injectable drugs or high concentrations of inhaled drugs.

2. The maintenance phase involves assuring hypnosis (i.e., anesthesia), attenuation of noxious stimuli and pain control (i.e., analgesia),

prevention of awareness and memory consolidation (i.e., amnesia), and prevention of patient movement by relaxation of skeletal muscles. Continued administration of inhaled and intravenous sedative/hypnotics provides anesthesia with varying degrees of analgesia, amnesia, and muscle relaxation, thereby requiring the addition of other medications to provide a "balanced anesthesia."

3. Following the surgical procedure, the administration of sedative/hypnotic drugs is discontinued, enabling emergence, during which time the patient regains consciousness.

The primary therapeutic considerations are summarized in the Therapeutic Overview Box.

THERAPEUTIC OVERVIEW

Requirements of Anesthetic Drugs
Inhalational
Chemical stability
Minimal irritation upon inhalation
Speed of onset (time to loss of consciousness)
Ability to produce analgesia, amnesia, and skeletal muscle relaxation
Minimal side effects, especially cardiovascular and respiratory depression and hepatic toxicity
Speed and safety of emergence
Minimal metabolism

Intravenous
Chemical stability
No pain at injection site
Rapid onset
Minimal side effects
Ability to produce analgesia, amnesia, and skeletal muscle relaxation
Speed and safety of emergence
Rapid metabolism or redistribution

MECHANISMS OF ACTION

Inhalational Anesthetics

The molecular basis for the anesthetic action of inhalational drugs is poorly understood. The inhalational anesthetics (Fig. 26.1) include diethyl ether, halogenated compounds containing an ether (-O-) link and a halogen such as desflurane, enflurane, or halothane, and the inorganic drug N_2O. No obvious structure-activity relationships have been defined for this group of agents, and several theories have been posited to explain the mechanism of action of inhaled anesthetics.

Desflurane	CHF_2—O—CF_3
Diethyl ether	CH_3—CH_2—O—CH_2—CH_3
Enflurane	$CHFCl$—CF_2—O—CHF_2
Halothane	CF_3—$CHBrCl$
Isoflurane	CF_3—$CHCl$—O—CHF_2
Methoxyflurane	$CHCl_2$—CF_2—O—CH_3
Nitrous oxide	N_2O
Sevoflurane	CH_2F—O—$CH(CF_3)_2$

FIG. 26.1 Chemical Structure of Inhalational Anesthetic Drugs.

According to the volume expansion theory, molecules of an anesthetic dissolve in the phospholipid bilayer of the neuronal membrane, causing it to expand and impede opening of ion channels necessary for generation and propagation of action potentials. Another hypothesis suggests that anesthetic molecules bind to specific hydrophobic regions of lipoproteins in the neuronal membrane that are part of, or close to, an ion channel. The resulting conformational change in the protein prevents effective operation of the channel. Anesthetics also have been considered to alter the fluidity of membrane lipids, which could prevent or limit increases in ion conductance. Alternatively, evidence suggests that anesthetics may affect specific cell-surface receptors for neurotransmitters or neuromodulators. For example, clinically relevant concentrations of halogenated inhalational anesthetics increase Cl^- conductance induced by γ-aminobutyric acid (GABA) in in vitro neuronal preparations. Because GABA is the principal inhibitory neurotransmitter in the brain, activation or enhancement of GABA-mediated Cl^- conductance would inhibit neuronal activity in the central nervous system (CNS). Similarly, N_2O decreases cation conductance in the ion channel controlled by the N-methyl-D-aspartate (NMDA) glutamate receptor, thereby blocking the actions of the principal excitatory neurotransmitter in the brain. Thus, through mechanisms as yet undefined, inhalational anesthetics disrupt the function of ligand-gated ion channels, increasing inhibitory and decreasing excitatory synaptic transmission.

The potency of an inhalational anesthetic is expressed in terms of the minimum alveolar concentration (MAC), which is the end-expired concentration that prevents 50% of subjects from responding to a painful stimulus. MAC is analogous to the median effective dose (ED_{50}) and is used to express the relative potency of inhaled drugs. Meyer and Overton observed that the potencies of anesthetic drugs correlate highly with their lipid solubilities, as measured by the oil:gas partition coefficient (Table 26.1; Fig. 26.2). Indeed, this relationship holds not only for drugs in current clinical use but also for inert gases that are not used clinically, such as xenon and argon.

Intravenous Anesthetics

Most anesthetic drugs administered intravenously contain substituted benzene rings (Fig. 26.3), have well-documented effects at specific cell-surface receptors, and include the barbiturates and benzodiazepines, propofol, ketamine, etomidate, and dexmedetomidine.

The barbiturate anesthetics include thiopental, phenobarbital, and methohexital, while the benzodiazepine anesthetics include diazepam and midazolam. These drugs act at two distinct allosteric sites on the

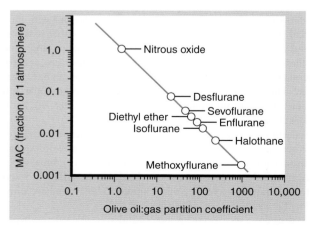

FIG. 26.2 The potency of an inhalational anesthetic drug is determined by its lipid solubility, as measured by its oil:gas partition coefficient.

TABLE 26.1 Characteristics of Modern Inhalational Anesthetic Drugs

Anesthetic Drug	Blood:Gas Partition Coefficient	Brain:Blood Partition Coefficient	Fat:Blood Partition Coefficient	Oil:Gas Partition Coefficient	MAC (% of 1 Atmosphere Pressure)	Approximate Percentage of Drug Metabolized	Airway Irritancy
Desflurane	0.42	1.3	27	19	6.0	0.5%	Significant
Halothane	2.3	2.9	60	225	0.75	15%	Minimal
Isoflurane	1.4	2.6	45	98	1.2	0.5%	Some
Nitrous oxide	0.47	1.1	2.3	1.4	105	<0.1%	None
Sevoflurane	0.63	1.7	48	53	2.0	3%	Minimal

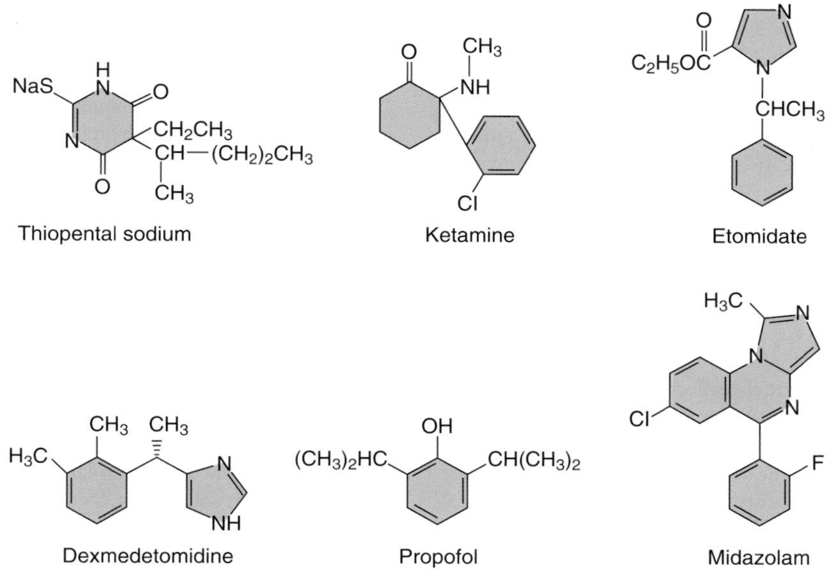

FIG. 26.3 Structures of Representative Intravenous General Anesthetic Drugs.

GABA$_A$ receptor Cl$^-$ channel complex to potentiate GABA-mediated Cl$^-$ conductance and neuronal inhibition (Chapter 17).

Propofol, the most widely used anesthetic in the United States, appears to facilitate GABA$_A$ receptor–mediated inhibition, inhibits high affinity GABA reuptake without affecting release, and inhibits glutamate NMDA receptor–mediated excitation. Similarly, etomidate also facilitates GABA$_A$ receptor–mediated neuronal inhibition and at clinically relevant concentrations in vitro also blocks the specific high-affinity neuronal uptake of GABA without affecting release. Ketamine appears to act by blocking neuronal excitation; it binds to the phencyclidine site within the NMDA glutamate receptor cation channel and inhibits cation conductance through the channel.

The action of dexmedetomidine is unlike the other intravenous anesthetics, as it induces sedation via agonism at α$_2$-adrenergic receptors in locus coeruleus neurons. The locus coeruleus, which is the major noradrenergic nucleus in the brain (Chapter 13), has efferents projecting to the reticular activating system including the midbrain reticular formation, thalamus, and hypothalamus; efferents also project to the spinal cord and peripheral nervous system. Locus coeruleus neurons contain the highest density of α$_2$ autoreceptors in the CNS that function to reduce neuronal firing. Thus an α$_2$ receptor agonist such as dexmedetomidine leads to sedation and inhibition of the sympathetic nervous system.

RELATIONSHIP OF MECHANISMS OF ACTION TO CLINICAL RESPONSE

Inhalational Anesthetics

As indicated, MAC is used to express the concentration of anesthetic vapor that prevents 50% of patients from responding to a painful stimulus. The MAC needed to blunt awareness and induce sleep is much lower than that needed to prevent movement. A MAC of 1.3 correlates with the ED$_{99}$, where 99% of the patients will not move to painful stimuli. If neuromuscular blockade is used as part of the anesthetic, a lower MAC of inhaled anesthetic can be used to maintain amnesia and blunting of surgical responses without the side effects of a high MAC anesthetic. MAC equivalents of a mixture of drugs are additive. For example, 0.6 MAC of N$_2$O is 63% (479 mm Hg at 1.0 atmosphere of pressure), and 0.4 MAC of isoflurane is 0.48% (3.6 mm Hg). Therefore an inspired gas mixture containing 63% N$_2$O and 0.48% isoflurane has a MAC of 1.0.

The MAC of an inhalational anesthetic also relates to the lipid solubility of the drug and is quantified by the oil:gas partition coefficient (see Table 26.1). Specifically, greater lipid solubility (i.e., a higher oil:gas partition coefficient) is associated with increased drug potency and a lower concentration necessary to produce a specific effect (i.e., lower

MAC value). For example, desflurane has a lower lipid solubility than isoflurane as indicated by the lower oil:gas partition coefficient of the former. Thus desflurane is less potent than isoflurane, and a higher concentration, or partial pressure, is required to achieve 1 MAC.

Except for N_2O (MAC of 104), all inhalational anesthetics in clinical use are sufficiently potent to produce surgical anesthesia when administered in a mixture containing at least 25% O_2. Although MAC is not a prime factor in determining the inhalational anesthetic selected, it does provide a convenient point of reference for comparing their properties. For example, it can be useful to compare the extent of hypotension or relaxation of skeletal muscle produced by two different anesthetic drugs administered at a MAC of 1.0.

The MAC is independent of the duration of the surgical procedure, remaining unchanged with time, and is unaffected by the sex of the patient. It also is relatively independent of the type of noxious stimulus applied (e.g., pressure versus heat). Indeed, increasing the intensity of the noxious stimulus, within limits, has little effect on MAC, although higher anesthetic concentrations are required for some extremely noxious surgical events. MAC is also independent of the patient's body mass. However, at a fixed alveolar concentration, it takes longer to anesthetize a larger patient because of differences in the apparent volume of distribution. Although the MAC of an anesthetic is relatively independent of many patient and surgical variables, it is affected by age. MAC is maximum in young children and lower in neonates and geriatric patients. N_2O, which cannot be used safely by itself to produce surgical levels of anesthesia, is a common component of anesthetic-gas mixtures and can serve to allow for a decrease in the requirements for other anesthetic drugs.

The general health of the patient also affects the anesthetic requirements, as critically ill patients or those with significant systemic disease often have lower anesthetic requirements. Another consideration is the presence of other drugs. In general, the MAC of an inhalational anesthetic is reduced in patients receiving other CNS depressants. In surgical patients, these drugs are commonly opioid analgesics, antianxiety drugs, or other sedative/hypnotic drugs. Indeed, CNS depressants are frequently administered preoperatively or intraoperatively to lower the MAC for an inhalational anesthetic. Alcoholic patients who have acquired a tolerance to the CNS depressant effects of ethanol often have an increased anesthetic requirement, as do patients who are tolerant to barbiturates and benzodiazepines. CNS stimulants also cause the anesthetic requirement to be increased. Although a stimulant is unlikely to be administered to a hospitalized patient, the widespread abuse of stimulants increases the probability of encountering patients undergoing emergency surgery with appreciable tissue concentrations of cocaine or amphetamine.

Intravenous Anesthetics

The onset of hypnosis following administration of an intravenous drug is determined by administering a single dose and monitoring for a loss of responsiveness to either verbal or sensory stimuli, such as loss of eyelash reflex. Factors that alter the apparent volume of distribution, including protein binding, alter the amount of drug required to obtund body reflexes. An insufficient dose of a single intravenous hypnotic drug may lead to transient excitation, which varies for different drugs. Excitation may be manifest by nonpurposeful movements. For example, thiopental may cause laryngeal spasm in an asthmatic patient, especially if the dose is insufficient.

Most intravenous anesthetics do not have muscle relaxant effects and, with the exception of ketamine and dexmedetomidine, have no analgesic properties. Because ketamine has sympathomimetic properties, it does not reduce cardiac output or blood pressure, making it a useful induction drug for patients in shock. Care should be taken, however, because if the patient's sympathetic tone is depleted, as can be the case

in prolonged shock, ketamine is a myocardial depressant, and without the sympathetic stimulation, this side effect can be unmasked. In addition, ketamine can cause bronchodilation, making it useful for induction in patients with status asthmaticus. Ketamine can cause significant dysphoria, even at small doses, which can be alleviated with a small dose of a benzodiazepine.

Due to its slower onset of action and inability to induce reliable unconsciousness at recommended doses, dexmedetomidine can be used for sedation, but not for the induction of general anesthesia. Dexmedetomidine can be used as an adjunct during maintenance of general anesthesia in addition to other medications. In this role, dexmedetomidine can be useful because it will supplement analgesia without causing respiratory depression and will allow a decrease in the dosing of other sedative/hypnotics and opioids.

PHARMACOKINETICS

Inhalational Anesthetics

The depth of anesthesia is determined by the partial pressure of the inhaled anesthetic drug in the brain. Therefore to produce concentrations adequate for surgery, it is necessary to deliver an appropriate amount of drug to the brain. Unlike most drugs, inhalational anesthetics are administered as gases or vapors. Therefore a specific set of physical principles applies to the delivery of these drugs.

In a mixture of gases, the **partial pressure** of an anesthetic drug is directly proportional to its fractional concentration in the mixture (Dalton's Law). Thus, as depicted in Fig. 26.4, in a mixture of 70% N_2O, 25% O_2, and 5% halothane, the partial pressures of the component gases are 532, 190, and 38 mm Hg, respectively, at 1 atmosphere (760 mm hg) of pressure.

When a gas is dissolved in the blood or other body tissues, its partial pressure is directly proportional to its concentration but inversely proportional to its solubility in that tissue. The concept of partial pressure is of central importance because the difference in the partial pressure of a gas at various locations is the driving force that moves the gas from

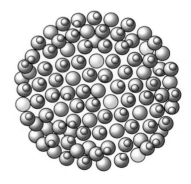

	Concentration %		Partial pressure (mm Hg)
Nitrous oxide	70	(x 760 =)	532
Oxygen	25	(x 760 =)	190
Halothane	5	(x 760 =)	38
	100%	(=)	760 mm Hg (1 atmosphere)

FIG. 26.4 The partial pressure of a gas in a mixture of gases is directly proportional to its concentration.

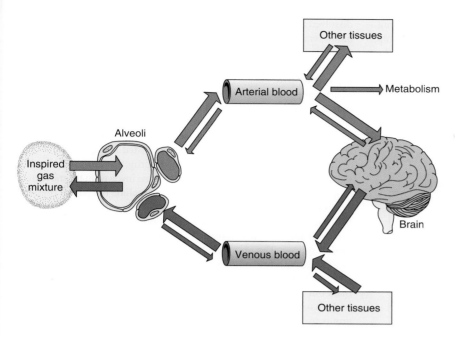

FIG. 26.5 The pathway of an inhalational anesthetic drug is indicated during induction of *(red arrows)* and emergence from *(blue arrows)* anesthesia. The *large arrows* indicate the direction of net movement.

the anesthetic machine to the lungs, from the lungs to the blood, and from the blood to the brain. Because solubility varies from tissue to tissue as a consequence of differences in tissue lipophilicity, the concentration of anesthetic must also vary from tissue to tissue if partial pressures are equal throughout the body. The partial pressure (or concentration) of the anesthetic in the inspired gas mixture is the factor controlled most easily by the anesthesiologist by adjusting the concentration of the anesthetic in the gas mixture from the anesthesia machine. The path followed by an inhalational anesthetic during induction of, and emergence from, anesthesia is diagrammed in Fig. 26.5. As the partial pressure of the anesthetic vapor increases in the alveoli, it drives the gas to the blood and is then delivered to the site of anesthetic action in the brain. The rate of this process depends on multiple factors. Induction of the state of general anesthesia is facilitated by rapidly increasing the partial pressure of the anesthetic in the alveoli. Increased alveolar ventilation [respiratory rate multiplied by (tidal volume minus dead space)] and gas flow allow for an increase in the delivery of the anesthetic vapor to the alveolar space. When delivery of the anesthetic gas is started, and the concentration is high with high gas flow, the partial pressure of the anesthetic gas increases in the alveoli, driving down its partial pressure gradient into the blood. The alveolar membrane poses no barrier to anesthetic gases, permitting unhindered diffusion in both directions. Therefore once the anesthetic gas reaches the alveolar space, it obeys the law of mass action and moves down its partial pressure gradient into the blood. The solubility of the anesthetic gas in the blood plays a role as well, as the less soluble the vapor is in blood, the faster the partial pressure will increase in the alveolar space, allowing the blood and alveolar partial pressures to equilibrate more quickly. In addition to these factors, pulmonary blood flow plays a role in the rate of induction of anesthesia. With lower cardiac output and therefore lower pulmonary blood flow, the blood has more time to equilibrate with the anesthetic partial pressure within the alveoli, leading to a faster induction because a greater quantity of anesthetic drug can be delivered to the blood. With higher cardiac output, the blood does not have as much time to become saturated with anesthetic gas; therefore the partial pressure cannot increase as quickly, and induction of general anesthesia is slowed (Table 26.2). As the partial pressure of the anesthetic drug in blood increases, the gradient between the alveolar space and blood

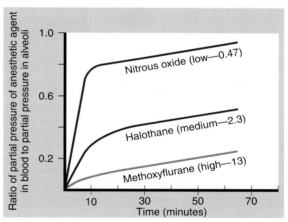

FIG. 26.6 Rate of rise of partial pressure of an inhalational anesthetic drug in arterial blood is determined by its solubility in blood (blood:gas partition coefficient).

TABLE 26.2 Factors Affecting the Rate of Induction With an Inhalational Anesthetic

Condition	Rate of Induction
Increased concentration of anesthetic in inspired gas mixture	Increased
Increased alveolar ventilation	Increased
Increased solubility of anesthetic in blood (blood:gas partition coefficient)	Decreased
Increased cardiac output	Decreased

decreases, and uptake slows (Fig. 26.6). Eventually, equilibrium is approached between the alveolar partial pressure, the arterial partial pressure, and the cerebral partial pressure of the anesthetic gas, and anesthesia can be maintained with stable gas flow and continued anesthetic administration.

As mentioned, the solubility of the anesthetic gas plays an important role in the rate of uptake and induction of anesthesia. This relationship is expressed as the **blood:gas partition coefficient**. The higher the solubility of an anesthetic gas in blood, the more must be dissolved to produce a change in partial pressure (because partial pressure is inversely proportional to solubility) and the slower the increase in the partial pressure of the gas, leading to a slower induction of anesthesia. This relationship is illustrated for N_2O and halothane in Fig. 26.7. N_2O has a blood:gas partition coefficient of 0.47, so relatively little must be

dissolved in blood for its partial pressure in blood to rise. In contrast, blood serves as a large reservoir for halothane, retaining at equilibrium 2.3 parts for every 1 part in the alveolar space. Induction depends not on dissolving the anesthetic in blood but on raising arterial partial pressure to drive the gas from blood to brain. Therefore the rate of rise of arterial partial pressure and speed of induction are fastest for gases that are least soluble in blood, such as N_2O or desflurane. The rate of rise of blood concentration is slowest for gases with greater blood solubility, such as isoflurane or halothane (see Fig. 26.6). The blood:gas partition coefficients of inhalational anesthetics are listed in Table 26.1.

The transfer of an inhaled anesthetic drug from arterial blood to the brain depends on factors analogous to those involved in the movement of gas from alveoli to arterial blood. These include the partial pressure gradient between blood and brain, the solubility of the anesthetic in the brain, and cerebral blood flow. The brain is part of the **vessel-rich group** of tissues that compose 9% of body mass but receive 75% of cardiac output. The anesthetic uptake curve rapidly reaches a plateau (see Fig. 26.6), reflecting early approach of equilibrium by the vessel-rich group of tissues. In contrast, the muscle group constitutes 50% of body mass but receives only 18% of cardiac output. Fat represents 19% of body mass and receives 5% of cardiac output, whereas the vessel-poor group, including bone and tendon, accounts for 22% of body mass, yet receives less than 2% of cardiac output. Thus approximately 41% of total body mass receives a mere 7% of cardiac output. As a consequence, in most surgical procedures, poorly perfused tissues do not contribute meaningfully to the apparent volume of distribution of the inhalational anesthetic. The importance of tissue perfusion as a factor determining the uptake of an anesthetic is illustrated for halothane in Fig. 26.8.

When the anesthetic gas concentration is decreased or administration is halted, alveolar partial pressure decreases. The sequence leading to uptake and induction of anesthesia is reversed, and the net movement of inhaled anesthetic drug will involve leaving the brain to enter the blood and then the alveolar space, again guided by partial pressure gradients. Like induction of anesthesia, the rate of removal of the anesthesia gas depends on minute ventilation, fresh gas flow, pulmonary blood flow, and solubility. Also, inhaled drugs with low solubility in blood, which lead to rapid uptake and induction of anesthesia, will be cleared more rapidly, allowing for a more rapid emergence from

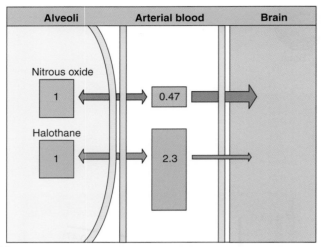

FIG. 26.7 The solubility of an inhalational anesthetic in blood determines how rapidly its partial pressure rises in blood and brain with a change in partial pressure in the inspired gas mixture. If the alveolar space and blood were a closed system and N_2O and halothane were allowed to equilibrate between the two, there would be 0.47 parts of N_2O in blood for every 1 part in alveoli, and 2.3 parts of halothane in blood for every 1 part in alveoli. An increase in the partial pressure of N_2O in the inspired gas mixture would result in an almost fivefold larger increase in its partial pressure in blood compared to a similar increase in the partial pressure of halothane in the inspired gas mixture, thus driving N_2O into the brain more rapidly.

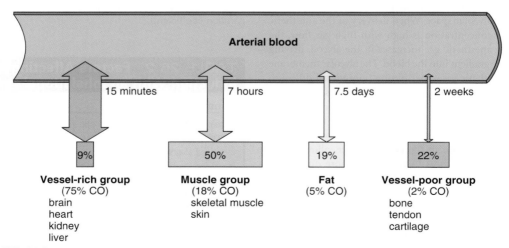

FIG. 26.8 The rate at which an inhalational anesthetic drug is taken up by a tissue depends on the fraction of the cardiac output *(CO)* that the tissue receives. The approximate time for halothane to equilibrate between blood and tissues is indicated next to the *arrows*; the percentage of body mass that the tissue represents is shown in the boxes. The numbers in parentheses represent the relative percentage of CO received by each tissue group.

anesthesia. However, the rate of elimination of inhaled anesthetic drugs also depends on their solubility in brain parenchyma and fat. The solubility of each drug in brain can be quantified by the brain:blood partition coefficient (see Table 26.1), where greater values indicate greater brain solubility. Drugs with higher solubility in the brain can be stored to a greater extent, taking longer to decrease in concentration and thereby delaying offset of drug action. Body fat can also serve as a depot for inhaled anesthetic drugs. After a decrease or cessation of delivery, drug that was stored in fat also enters the blood and serves to decrease the partial pressure gradient between the brain and blood by attenuating the decrease in the partial pressure of drug in the blood. Drugs with a higher fat:blood partition coefficient (see Table 26.1), indicating greater fat solubility, can be stored to a larger extent in fat and can serve to prolong the attenuation of the decrease in partial pressure of drug in the blood and delaying emergence from anesthesia to a larger extent than inhaled drugs with lower fat solubility. For example, sevoflurane has a lower blood:gas partition coefficient than isoflurane leading to a more rapid induction of general anesthesia due to relatively lower solubility in the blood by the former. However, both drugs have similar solubilities in fat as indicated by their similar fat:blood partition coefficients. Therefore following a period of general anesthesia during which time both drugs are allowed to accumulate in fat, all else being equal, rates of emergence will be relatively similar.

Although inhaled anesthetics are cleared from the body largely via the lung, most undergo some degree of metabolism, and several metabolites have been implicated in organ toxicity. The extent of biotransformation of inhalational anesthetics ranges from approximately 15% for halothane to negligible amounts for N_2O (see Table 26.1). Halothane and, to a much lesser extent, isoflurane and desflurane are metabolized by cytochrome P4502E1 (CYP2E1) in the liver, producing a trifluoroacetyl metabolite, which can bind to hepatic proteins, leading to an immune-mediated liver injury. Some of the liver injury may also be related to the reduction in liver blood flow. Inhalational anesthetics that are not appreciably metabolized generally exhibit less toxic sequelae, and while hepatic injury is still reported with current inhalational anesthetics, it is quite rare.

Intravenous Anesthetics

Box 26.1 describes the characteristics of the ideal intravenous anesthetic drug. This drug would be a fast-acting medication with short duration of action and no active or toxic metabolites. Additionally, this medication should have a wide margin of safety, limited side effect profile, and consistent effects across all patients. Further, it should have physiochemical stability and be soluble in blood at physiologic pH. No current medications meet all of these criteria.

The onset of action of intravenous drugs is determined by the time it takes the drug to reach the brain, as well as how quickly it crosses the blood-brain barrier. Because blood flow to the brain is also important, the onset of action may be delayed in a patient with low cardiac output and therefore a relatively low blood flow to the brain. The duration of effect of a single dose of an intravenous anesthetic is determined predominantly by its rate of redistribution from the brain and vessel-rich group into less well-perfused tissues (i.e., abdominal viscera, skeletal muscle). Redistribution can occur within minutes of induction of anesthesia with a single dose of anesthetic, resulting in recovery of reflex activity and consciousness. Once the anesthetic drug has redistributed out of the brain, it can then be metabolized and removed from the body. Following a large dose or repeated doses, drug concentration in less perfused organs increases and attenuates the rate of redistribution. In this circumstance, drug duration of action depends increasingly on the rate of metabolism, thus prolonging duration of action. The intravenous anesthetic drugs have varying speeds of onset, durations of action, and rates of redistribution.

BOX 26.1 Characteristics of an Ideal Intravenous Anesthetic Drug

Physicochemical
- H_2O soluble
- Stable on shelf and to light exposure
- Lipophilic
- Small injection volume

Pharmacokinetic
- Rapid onset of action
- Short duration of action
- Nontoxic metabolites

Pharmacodynamic
- Wide margin of safety
- No interpatient variability in effects
- Nonallergenic
- Nontoxic to tissues

Propofol is the most commonly used intravenous induction drug. It is twice as potent as thiopental, with loss of consciousness within 30 seconds. Induction doses of propofol are highest in young children and decrease with age. A single induction dose lasts for 5–10 minutes due to redistribution, but it has a long terminal elimination half-life and high lipid solubility, leading to accumulation in fat. As a result, the context-sensitive half-time increases as an infusion continues. Propofol is metabolized by the liver via conjugation to water-soluble metabolites and eliminated through the kidneys.

Etomidate is another commonly used anesthetic drug. Like propofol, etomidate has a rapid onset of action, but the recovery is more prolonged as compared to propofol. It has the advantage of causing less hemodynamic changes than propofol and has little respiratory depression. Etomidate undergoes ester hydrolysis in plasma and hepatic metabolism, forming water-soluble, inactive metabolites.

Ketamine has been used for induction of anesthesia and is unique because it tends to increase sympathetic nervous system outflow, thus minimizing hypotension. It causes a dissociative state during which patients maintain breathing, and the eyes often stay open despite a deep level of anesthesia. Onset is fairly rapid, although patients may take quite some time, 10–20 minutes, to emerge after bolus dosing. Initial recovery is due to redistribution, followed by metabolism in the liver. Ketamine is metabolized by the P450 system to water soluble compounds and then excreted renally. Ketamine, unlike other intravenous sedative/hypnotics, can also be administered intramuscularly if needed.

Thiopental was used widely for intravenous induction of anesthesia prior to the development of propofol because of its rapid and smooth onset and its short duration of action. It is highly lipid soluble, rapidly crosses the blood-brain barrier, and is rapidly redistributed from brain to other body tissues. However, because of its long terminal elimination half-life (Table 26.3), thiopental accumulates in the body, and its repeated administration increases its duration of action, causing some patients to have residual sedation after surgery is completed. Thiopental is metabolized primarily in the liver to water soluble metabolites that are excreted in the urine. The pharmacokinetic properties of other barbiturates used as intravenous anesthetics, such as methohexital and phenobarbital, are generally similar to those of thiopental. Due to these issues, the barbiturates have primarily been replaced by newer induction drugs.

Induction of anesthesia with the benzodiazepine diazepam is relatively slow, often taking several minutes. It has a long redistribution half-life

TABLE 26.3   Comparison of Intravenous Anesthetics in Healthy Adults

Drug	H$_2$O Soluble	Solution Characteristics	Dose (mg/kg)	Elimination t$_{1/2}$ (hrs)	Active Metabolites
Dexmedetomidine	Yes	Clear	Loading dose: 1 μg/kg over 10 min Maintenance: 0.2–0.7 μg/kg/h	2–3	No
Etomidate	No	Clear	Induction: 0.2–0.5 mg/kg	1–1.5	No
Ketamine	Yes	Clear	Induction: 1–2 mg/kg IV or 3–5 mg/kg IM	2–3	Yes
Methohexital	Yes	Clear	Induction: 1–2 mg/kg	3–6	No
Midazolam	Yes	Clear	Sedation: 0.01–0.1 mg/kg Induction: 0.1–0.4 mg/kg*	2–6	Yes
Propofol	No	Milky white	Induction: 1–2.5 mg/kg Maintenance of GA: 50–200 μg/kg/min Maintenance of sedation: 25–100 μg/kg/min	3–12	No
Thiopental	Yes	Clear, light yellow	Induction: 3–6 mg/kg	3–8	Yes

*Rarely used as sole induction agent for general anesthesia.

(30 to 60 minutes), a long duration of action, and a long terminal elimination half-life (see Table 26.3). It is metabolized by the microsomal enzyme system in liver, and most of its metabolites are pharmacologically active and have long half-lives (Chapter 17). **Midazolam** is a water-soluble benzodiazepine twice as potent as diazepam. It takes midazolam 2 to 3 minutes to induce anesthesia, which is faster than diazepam, but slower than thiopental. **Lorazepam** is a long-acting benzodiazepine with a long onset time, limiting its use as an induction drug, but the duration of action can be useful in some circumstances, such as for the acute treatment of seizures.

Dexmedetomidine is often administered as an intravenous infusion with or without a preceding loading dose. Approximately 94% of the serum content of drug is protein bound, mostly to albumin with a volume of distribution of approximately 1.33 L/kg. In healthy patients, the half-lives for redistribution and elimination are approximately 6 minutes and 2–3 hours, respectively. Metabolism is primarily in the liver by cytochrome P4502A6 (CYP2A6) to inactive metabolites that are excreted by the kidney.

The physicochemical properties of some intravenous anesthetic drugs render them insoluble in water at physiological pH, necessitating use of solvents or adjusting the pH of the injectate (see Table 26.3), either of which can lead to problems. The propofol emulsion can cause a burning pain on injection. Commonly, lidocaine is injected prior to administration, or mixed with the propofol to help with the injection site pain. Acidic etomidate solutions can cause pain and thrombophlebitis after intravascular injection. All alcohol-based solvents and buffers are venous irritants, causing pain when injected intravenously. The alkaline pH of a 2.5% solution of thiopental makes it unsuitable for mixing with acidic drugs, especially opioids and neuromuscular blocking agents. Thiopental solutions also cause tissue damage if injected intraarterially or extravascularly.

PHARMACOVIGILANCE: ADVERSE EFFECTS AND DRUG INTERACTIONS

Clinical problems associated with the use of both the inhalational and intravenous anesthetics are summarized in the Clinical Problems Box.

Inhalational Anesthetics
Respiratory and Cardiovascular Effects

With the exception of N$_2$O, all inhalational anesthetics reduce spontaneous respiration in a concentration-dependent manner by depressing medullary centers in the brainstem. They decrease the responsiveness

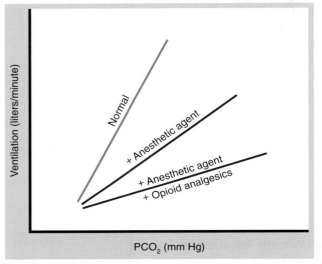

FIG. 26.9 Anesthetic drugs reduce the ventilatory response to increases in the arterial carbon dioxide tension (PCO$_2$) in blood and cerebrospinal fluid. This effect is exacerbated by opioid analgesics.

of chemoreceptors in respiratory centers to elevations in carbon dioxide tension (PCO$_2$) in blood and cerebrospinal fluid, which normally serve as a potent stimulus for increasing minute ventilation. The result is a shift to the right and flattening of the PCO$_2$ ventilation-response curve (Fig. 26.9). Thus the ventilatory response to hypercapnia is attenuated. Opioids also reduce the responsiveness of brainstem chemoreceptors to elevations in PCO$_2$ and shift the PCO$_2$ ventilation-response curve in a similar manner. When an opioid is given concurrently with an inhalational anesthetic, the effects of the two on respiration are additive and often synergistic, as shown in Fig. 26.9. CO$_2$ exerts a local effect on the cerebral vasculature by dilating small vessels. The resultant increase in intracranial pressure is a cause for concern in patients with preexisting intracranial hypertension. Inhalational drugs can induce varying degrees of airway irritation, as shown in Table 26.1, making desflurane and isoflurane unsuitable for inhalational induction of general anesthesia.

All inhalational anesthetics depress the force of myocardial contraction in a concentration-dependent manner in isolated heart preparations. In patients, the effect on myocardial function varies depending on the drug, the concentration needed for surgical anesthesia, and the drug's effects on the sympathetic nervous system. Isoflurane and sevoflurane have minimal direct effects on myocardial contractility but cause peripheral vasodilation resulting in hypotension. Desflurane increases sympathetic outflow and can result in hypertension and tachycardia, especially when the dose is increased rapidly. Halothane has the most direct myocardial depression, resulting in a reduced cardiac output. Additionally, it reduces the central outflow of the sympathetic nervous system, depresses the baroreceptor reflex, and relaxes peripheral vascular smooth muscle. The overall effect is hypotension and decreased organ perfusion. N_2O causes vasoconstriction of the pulmonary artery and should be used with caution in patients with preexisting pulmonary hypertension. Halothane also sensitizes the myocardium to dysrhythmias induced by catecholamines, an action shared to a lesser extent with enflurane. Therefore caution must be exercised when pressor drugs are administered to counteract the hypotension induced by these anesthetics. As a result, halothane and enflurane have fallen out of common use in favor of the newer volatile anesthetics (i.e., desflurane, isoflurane, and sevoflurane).

Hepatic and Renal Effects

The liver and kidney are the most prominent targets of undesirable effects of anesthetics. Generally, metabolites of the anesthetics are implicated in organ toxicity, but it is often difficult to determine which toxic effects are attributable to the anesthetic itself or to its metabolites. Some adverse effects are caused by the anesthetic-induced decreases in cardiac output and blood flow to the liver. Halothane hepatitis occurs in 1 in 10,000 to 1 in 20,000 patients, with fatal hepatic necrosis occurring in approximately half. Of patients who develop halothane hepatitis, a metabolite of halothane, trifluoroacetyl, combines with hepatic microsomal proteins, triggering an immune response that can lead to hepatitis and possibly severe liver injury. Isoflurane and desflurane are also metabolized in the same manner but to a much lesser extent. Sevoflurane has been implicated, rarely, in fulminant hepatic failure, although through different mechanisms than trifluoroacetyl metabolites. Although halothane has been administered safely in most patients, it is now used less frequently, particularly in the United States, in favor of newer halogenated drugs because of the specter of hepatic toxicity.

Renal blood flow and glomerular filtration rate are decreased during general anesthesia, resulting in decreased urine formation. Enflurane and sevoflurane undergo some metabolism in the liver and release free fluoride ions, which can be nephrotoxic in sufficiently high concentrations during lengthy surgical procedures. It is best not to use either drug in patients with impaired renal function. Additionally, sevoflurane can produce Compound A when degraded by CO_2 absorbents, which, in supratherapeutic doses, can cause renal injury. Halothane, though metabolized to an appreciable extent (see Table 26.1), does not release significant amounts of free fluoride.

Malignant Hyperthermia

Halogenated inhalational anesthetics, and halothane in particular, can precipitate malignant hyperthermia in genetically susceptible patients. Depolarizing neuromuscular blocking drugs (i.e., succinylcholine, Chapter 10) can also trigger this reaction, which is manifest as a sustained contraction of the musculature with a dramatic increase in O_2 consumption and an increased body temperature. The syndrome results from a failure of the sarcoplasmic reticulum to resequester Ca^{++}, preventing the dissociation of actin and myosin filaments of muscle. The resultant hyperthermia is an emergency requiring prompt treatment, including rapid cooling and administration of the skeletal muscle relaxant dantrolene (Chapter 22). Overall, malignant hyperthermia occurs in 1 in 15,000 to 1 in 50,000 cases. The combined use of halothane and

succinylcholine is associated with the highest incidence, and the combined use of a halogenated anesthetic other than halothane and a nondepolarizing muscle relaxant significantly decreases the risk for malignant hyperthermia. Risk is eliminated by avoiding succinylcholine and all halogenated inhaled anesthetic drugs, and would be the technique of choice in patients at high risk for malignant hyperthermia, such as those with a personal or family history of prior episodes.

Central Nervous System Effects

As indicated, N_2O lacks sufficient potency to produce surgical levels of anesthesia safely by itself. It can produce analgesia and can induce a state of behavioral disinhibition. It is this latter action of N_2O that has given it the name "laughing gas." N_2O can reduce memory consolidation but, by itself, does not produce reliable amnesia, likely due in part to its low potency. Most often, N_2O is administered in combination with a halogenated anesthetic to lower the anesthetic requirement for the latter and to promote rapid induction and emergence from anesthesia.

Concentrations of enflurane and sevoflurane above MAC can cause characteristic seizure activity on an electroencephalogram. This excitatory effect has minimal or no adverse consequences to the patient. Nevertheless, it may be a consideration in patients with known seizure disorders. Isoflurane, a structural isomer of enflurane, does not evoke seizures. In fact, it suppresses electrical activity of the brain and, like propofol and barbiturates, can be used to treat seizure activity.

Other Effects

N_2O diffuses into enclosed air-filled cavities in the body, where it exchanges with nitrogen. N_2O diffuses out of the blood and into air-filled cavities approximately 35 times faster than nitrogen leaves those cavities and enters the blood. This results in an increase in pressure and distention of enclosed air-filled, nitrogen-containing spaces. This situation might be encountered in patients with an occlusion of the middle ear, pneumothorax, obstructed intestine, air emboli in the bloodstream, or in a patient with pneumocephalus. These conditions, if not absolute contraindications to the use of N_2O, are at least signals for caution.

N_2O also oxidizes moieties of vitamin B_{12}, which decreases the availability of this vitamin and inhibits the activity of methionine synthetase, a vitamin B_{12}-dependent enzyme. This results in a decrease in protein and nucleic acid synthesis, megaloblastic anemia, and other signs of vitamin B_{12} deficiency. Inhalation of N_2O for as little as 2 hours can result in a detectable decrease in methionine synthetase activity, and megaloblastic anemia has been observed in severely ill patients several days after exposure. Generally, clinical problems do not occur unless exposure is lengthened from hours to days. However, long-term exposure to low concentrations of N_2O has been linked to neuropathies stemming from vitamin B_{12} deficiency. Prolonged exposure to all inhalational anesthetics, but N_2O in particular, has been associated with an increased risk of spontaneous abortion.

Intravenous Anesthetics

General side effects, clinical problems, and toxicities associated with the use of the benzodiazepines and opioids are presented in Chapters 17 and 28, respectively.

Respiratory and Cardiovascular Effects

The barbiturates and propofol are well-known respiratory and cardiovascular depressants and should be used only in a setting in which instrumentation is available to provide assisted ventilation. Barbiturates and propofol decrease myocardial contractile force and dilate peripheral vessels and should be used with caution in patients with cardiovascular instability, such as shock.

Etomidate is useful for its minimal effect on the cardiovascular system and can be used to maintain hemodynamic stability on induction of anesthesia in patients with limited hemodynamic reserves. Ketamine has sympathomimetic effects and can cause tachycardia. The increase in sympathetic outflow can be helpful in induction of patients with status asthmaticus, as it can cause bronchodilation. However, caution should be used because ketamine also has myocardial depressant effects, and in patients with depleted catecholamine reserves, such as patients in shock, this depressant effect can be unmasked and result in hypotension.

Dexmedetomidine induces sympatholysis, leading to hypotension and bradycardia. However, hypertension can also occur with dexmedetomidine. This latter effect is often observed during or immediately following a loading dose and is attributed to stimulation of peripheral α_{2B}-adrenergic receptors, leading to vasoconstriction. One of the major advantages of dexmedetomidine is its lack of respiratory depression, making it an attractive drug for intravenous sedation or as a component of a balanced general anesthetic, where it can provide analgesia and allow for a decrease in the dose requirements of other sedative/hypnotic drugs.

Central Nervous System Effects

Ketamine is related structurally to phencyclidine, and both drugs have many pharmacological actions in common. At appropriate doses, the patient may appear to be awake but is unresponsive to or dissociated from the environment (hence the term "dissociative anesthesia"). The usefulness of ketamine for maintenance of anesthesia is limited by the high incidence of unpleasant dreams and other dysphoric episodes occurring in patients during emergence from anesthesia. This is one reason why ketamine is used primarily as an induction drug in patients for brief painful procedures, such as changing burn dressings, where its analgesic and amnestic effects are advantageous. A benzodiazepine is often coadministered with ketamine to minimize postoperative psychotomimetic reactions. Etomidate can disinhibit the CNS as well and lead to myoclonic movements during induction.

Other Effects

The barbiturates are contraindicated in patients who may be allergic or have a familial history of acute intermittent porphyria. Etomidate is not suitable for intravenous infusion for maintenance of anesthesia because it causes pain on injection, myoclonus, and thrombophlebitis at the injection site. Its propensity to cause nausea and vomiting postoperatively limits its use in an outpatient setting. Etomidate suppresses 11β-hydroxylase, which is involved in the synthesis of corticosteroids. The clinical relevance of this adrenal suppression remains to be determined but is the major factor that limited its use for long-term infusion, such as for sedation in critically ill patients.

NEW DEVELOPMENTS

Efforts to reduce the rising cost of healthcare in the United States may result in 70%–75% of all surgical procedures being performed in ambulatory surgical facilities. Surgery in hospitals will be reserved for patients requiring the most intensive medical care. This trend has important implications in terms of drug development. Because most surgical patients are discharged within hours of their surgery, the effects of anesthetic drugs have to be dissipated rapidly and completely, enabling the patient to have a clear sensorium and no residual postoperative nausea or impairment of motor function, judgment, or memory. This requires intravenous anesthetic drugs that have a fast onset and offset of action, like propofol. Therefore intravenous drugs that are inactivated rapidly by simple mechanisms (such as plasma esterase activity or rapid redistribution) will be relied on more heavily for general anesthesia because their effects disappear within moments of terminating drug administration. Newer drugs should possess increasing numbers of the characteristics of the ideal drug, listed in Box 26.1.

Inhalational drugs will still be used widely. They should have good potency and low solubility in blood for rapid onset and offset of effects, and they should undergo minimal biotransformation because the metabolites of inhalational anesthetics are responsible for some undesirable side effects.

CLINICAL RELEVANCE FOR HEALTHCARE PROFESSIONALS

General anesthetics represent a unique group of compounds that are typically administered only by anesthesiologists. In some states within the United States, general anesthetics may also be administered by certified registered nurse anesthetists (CRNAs) or a certified anesthesiology assistant (CAA) directly supervised by an anesthesiologist. Because these compounds may be used for lengthy procedures and carry risk with their benefits, all individuals using these compounds must understand the principles governing the use of these compounds and possible adverse effects that may ensue.

SELF-ASSESSMENT QUESTIONS

1. Which of the following agents would be expected to lead to the greatest decrease in cardiac output and blood pressure in a patient during surgery?
   A. Nitrous oxide (N_2O).
   B. Halothane.
   C. Ketamine.
   D. Isoflurane.
   E. Etomidate.

2. A young man preparing for surgery read all about the effects of general anesthetics on ventilation and learned that the ventilatory response to CO_2 is blunted during anesthesia with which agent(s)?
   A. Halothane.
   B. Propofol.
   C. Morphine.
   D. Isoflurane.
   E. All of the above.

3. The MAC of an inhalational anesthetic is higher:
   A. In an obese patient than in a patient of average body weight.
   B. During a long surgical procedure than during a short surgical procedure.
   C. In a young child than in an elderly patient.
   D. In a patient pretreated with morphine than in an otherwise drug-free patient.
   E. In males than in females.

4. Which of the following drugs should be avoided in a patient with intracranial air due to concern for expansion of intracranial gas volume?
   A. Propofol.
   B. Isoflurane.
   C. Thiopental.
   D. Nitrous oxide (N_2O).
   E. Halothane.

5. Which of the following properties is most closely correlated with the rate of induction of general anesthesia with inhalational drugs?
   A. Blood:gas partition coefficient.
   B. Oil:gas partition coefficient.
   C. Brain:blood partition coefficient.
   D. Fat:blood partition coefficient.
   E. Muscle:blood partition coefficient.

FURTHER READING

Bovill JG. Inhalation anaesthesia: From diethyl ether to xenon. *Handb Exp Pharmacol.* 2008;182:121–142.

Campagna JA, Miller KW, Forman A. Mechanisms of actions of inhaled anesthetics. *N Engl J Med.* 2003;348:2110–2124.

Farag E, Argalious M, Abd-Elsayed A, et al. The use of dexmedetomidine in anesthesia and intensive care. *Curr Pharm Des.* 2012;18:6257–6265.

Hendrickx JF, DeWolf A. Special aspects of pharmacokinetics of inhalation anesthesia. *Handb Exp Pharmacol.* 2008;182:159–186.

Henthorn TK. The effects of altered physiological states on intravenous anesthetics. *Handb Exp Pharmacol.* 2008;182:363–377.

Vanlersberghe C, Camu F. Propofol. *Handb Exp Pharmacol.* 2008;182:227–252.

WEBSITES

https://www.asahq.org/resources/clinical-information
This website is maintained by the American Society of Anesthesiologists (ASA) and contains standards, guidelines, and practice parameters for all aspects of the profession for both anesthesiologists and nonanesthesiologists.

Local Anesthetics

Joshua R. Edwards

THERAPEUTIC OVERVIEW

Local anesthetics have been used as therapeutic agents for well over 100 years to alleviate pain. The primary effects of these agents are to inhibit the propagation of action potentials in sensory neurons at the site of administration. In medical practice today, local anesthetics have a wide range of uses, from numbing tissue for dental procedures to surgical site–specific peripheral regional anesthesia. The first known local anesthetic was the natural product cocaine, but its abuse potential (Chapter 24) limits its clinical use. All local anesthetics available today are synthetic derivatives of cocaine (they have similar chemical structures) that lack the high abuse potential and have fewer side effects or toxicities, but share the same mechanism of action. Local anesthetics are considered safer than intravenous (IV) or inhalational general anesthetics (Chapter 26), especially for patients who may have a genetic predisposition for adverse reactions to general anesthetics (e.g., malignant hyperthermia). However, severe side effects and death may occur if local anesthetics are administered improperly or given to patients with heart disease or a history of seizures who could be at higher risk of developing adverse effects. The specific local anesthetic selected and the location and type of administration (e.g., topical, subcutaneous injection, epidural injection, etc.) determine, in large part, the duration and depth of anesthesia. Factors in drug selection and side effects are summarized in the Therapeutic Overview Box.

THERAPEUTIC OVERVIEW
Factors in drug selection
Speed of onset
Duration of effect
Side effects
Seizures
Cardiovascular depression
Methemoglobinemia
Prolonged numbness or paresthesia

MECHANISMS OF ACTION

All local anesthetics eliminate sensations of pain by blocking action potential propagation in pain-receiving (nociceptive) neurons. Local anesthetics affect sensory, motor, and autonomic neurons to varying degrees. In this respect, the local anesthetic ropivacaine is notable because this relatively newer drug has selective inhibitory effects on sensory neurons as compared to motor neurons, making it ideal for use during natural childbirth by providing the expectant mother beneficial analgesic effects while retaining motor and autonomic function, enabling her to help push during childbirth.

The molecular targets for local anesthetics are the **voltage-gated sodium channels (VGSCs)**, which exist in all neurons and are responsible for propagation of action potentials. VGSCs are usually closed at normal resting membrane potentials, which prevents the high concentration of Na^+ in the extracellular fluid from entering the cell. When membranes are depolarized, these channels sense the change in intracellular charge or polarity and open to allow Na^+ to flow into the cell down its concentration gradient. This influx of positively charged ions leads to further depolarization, causing more channels to open and leading to a self-regenerating action potential. Sustained depolarization causes:
- spontaneous inactivation of VGSCs, which terminates Na^+ influx; and
- concurrent opening of voltage-gated K^+ channels.

The resultant K^+ efflux through these and non–voltage gated K^+ channels returns the membrane potential to its normal resting value. This mechanism is depicted in Fig. 27.1.

Local anesthetics bind selectively to VGSCs at the intracellular surface of the channel pore near the pore's vestibule, preventing the channels from opening and inhibiting Na^+ influx, resulting in blocking the propagation of action potentials (Fig. 27.2). A critical concentration of local anesthetic is needed at the axon because the drugs dissociate from VGSCs very rapidly. Diffusion of the local anesthetic away from the site of administration and absorption into the circulatory system is the most significant factor determining the duration of effects.

The ability of local anesthetics to block VGSCs is highly dependent on the activity (or state) of individual channels. Na^+ channels exist in

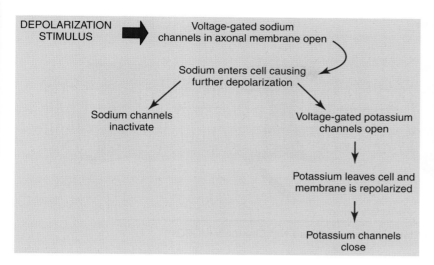

FIG. 27.1 Sequence of Events Occurring During an Action Potential.

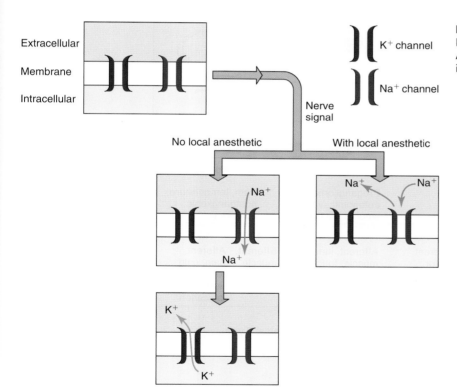

FIG. 27.2 Movement of Na⁺ and K⁺ Through Their Membrane Channels During Propagation of an Action Potential and Blockade of the Na⁺ Channel in the Presence of Local Anesthetics.

three main conformational states—namely, the resting, open, and inactivated states, with a minor intermediate resting state, depending on the voltage (Fig. 27.3). In the resting state, the channels do not allow Na⁺ influx and are highly sensitive to depolarization-induced opening. In the open state, the channels allow Na⁺ influx. However, as mentioned, these channels exhibit spontaneous inactivation after sustained depolarization, and when the channels are in the inactivated state, they do not allow Na⁺ influx and are not opened by depolarization. Local anesthetics are much more likely to bind when the channels are open or inactivated and are less likely to bind to VGSCs in the resting state. This modulation of affinity is called activity (or state) dependence and has practical importance. Because local anesthetics preferentially block

nerves in which VGSCs are open or inactivated (activity dependent), they are more potent in rapidly firing nerves than in nerves in which action potentials occur less frequently. Because sensory neurons fire at greater frequencies in response to more intense noxious stimuli, impulse blockade by local anesthetics is greater under this condition.

RELATIONSHIP OF MECHANISMS OF ACTION TO CLINICAL RESPONSE

Neurons differ substantially in terms of their axonal diameter, degree of myelination, conduction velocity, and frequency of firing, all of which influence the ability of local anesthetics to inhibit action potential

| | Resting | Intermediate | Open | Inactivated |

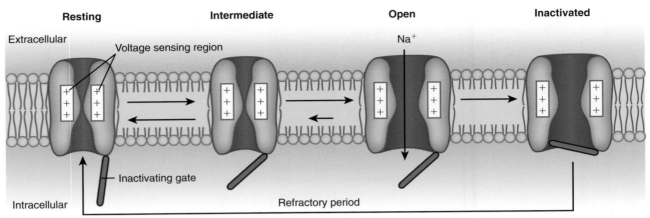

FIG. 27.3 Conformational States of Voltage-Gated Na$^+$ Channels (VGSCs).

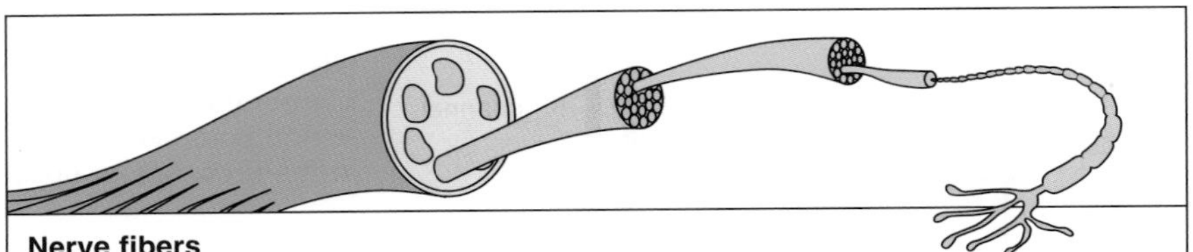

Nerve fibers

Fiber type	A	B	C*
Diameter μm	2–20	<3	<1.5
Conduction velocity (m/sec)	5–100	3–15	0.1–2.5
Myelinated	Yes	Yes	No
		Preganglionic, autonomic, vascular smooth muscle	Pain, temperature, postganglionic, autonomic

Subtypes of A fibers	Aα	Aβ	Aγ	Aδ*
	Efferent, motor, somatic, reflex activity	Afferent, innervate muscle, touch sensation, pressure sensation	Efferent, muscle spindle tone	Afferent, pain, cold, temperature, tissue damage indication*

*Pain transmission fibers.

FIG. 27.4 Nerve Fibers According to Anatomical Type.

propagation. The three major types of nerve fibers are classified as A, B, or C, and A fibers have several subtypes: Aα, Aβ, Aγ, and Aδ (Fig. 27.4). A fibers are myelinated and have the fastest conduction velocity, B fibers are myelinated with a slower conduction velocity, and C fibers are unmyelinated and have the slowest conduction velocity. Most pain impulses in humans are carried by the Aδ and C fibers. The Aδ fibers, which are distributed primarily in skin and mucous membranes, are the smallest subtype of A fibers (2 to 5 μm diameter) and are associated with a sharp, pricking pain termed "fast pain." C fibers, which are more widely distributed, are smaller than Aδ fibers (<1.5 μm diameter) and are associated with a duller, long-lasting, burning pain termed "slow pain."

Local anesthetics are not equally potent or effective in all cells that express VGSCs and exhibit selectivity for different neuronal cell types. Local anesthetics preferentially block neurons with smaller-diameter axons as compared to neurons with larger-diameter axons due to the spatial relationship between axon diameter and the number of VGSCs present per length of axon. Consider that an axon with a diameter over 20 times larger than a smaller axon will contain a greater number of VGSCs within the same length of axon. Therefore the larger the axon diameter, the greater amount or dose of local anesthetic needed to inhibit a greater number of VGSCs for any given length of axon; with smaller-diameter axons, a smaller dose of local anesthetic is needed to achieve the same effect. The degree of myelination of the axon also affects sensitivity to the local anesthetics. VGSCs are present only at the nodes of Ranvier in myelinated axons, thus limiting the number of VGSCs present per length of axon; nonmyelinated axons do not have such a limitation. In general, the presence of local anesthetics at three consecutive nodes is required to prevent further depolarization and inhibit propagation of action potentials. Myelination also leads to faster action potential firing frequency, and rapidly firing neurons are generally blocked at lower local anesthetic concentrations than more slowly firing neurons because these agents exhibit activity dependence, as discussed. Therefore small axonal diameter/myelinated Aδ fibers are blocked before blockade of small axonal diameter/unmyelinated C fibers. Blockade of impulses in Aγ fibers produces a flaccid paralysis and probably accounts for the early signs of motor weakness. In summary, fast pain fibers that have small axonal diameters and are myelinated (Aδ) are inhibited before a loss of touch or pressure sensations (from larger axonal diameter/myelinated Aβ fibers), slow pain (from small-axonal-diameter/unmyelinated C fibers), or motor function (from large-axonal-diameter/myelinated Aα fibers).

The anatomical location of different nerve types also influences the ability of local anesthetics to produce nerve block. For example, peripheral nerves are never affected uniformly by a local anesthetic because a concentration gradient of the drug from the mantle (peripheral neurons) to the core (centrally located neurons) of the nerve bundle is established during the onset of the block; a steady-state distribution of drug in the nerve is rarely achieved. Axons in the mantle are generally exposed to higher local anesthetic concentrations than are axons in the core, where drug diffusion is more restricted. Although these principles help explain the differential sensitivity of nerve fibers to local anesthetics, it is difficult to predict what will happen in every given situation. Sensory modalities are lost in the following general order: cold > warmth > pain > touch > deep pressure. As indicated, motor functions appear to be more resistant to blockade by local anesthetics, but this may result from the relatively complex motor tasks that are tested in the clinical setting, wherein the patient can recruit several different groups of muscles to accomplish a similar movement. Indeed, when simple muscle movements, e.g., extensor postural thrust, are isolated in experimental animals during peripheral nerve block, their deficiencies are greater and longer in duration than the loss of pain sensitivity.

Local anesthetics are used to simultaneously provide analgesia and muscle relaxation through spinal or epidural administration, and this route is also used to administer dilute solutions of local anesthetics mixed with opioids for postoperative pain relief. These combinations provide effective analgesia and have the advantage of using a lower total dose of the opioid than would be required alone. Local anesthetics are used as both diagnostic and therapeutic tools in the management of more complicated acute and chronic pain states.

PHARMACOKINETICS

Certain practical pharmacokinetic properties make local anesthetics particularly useful in temporarily blocking the sensory transmission of pain impulses. The greatest advantage of local anesthetics is their reversibility, i.e., once local anesthetic concentrations decrease at the site of administration by diffusion, the nerve resumes normal function. Of note is the local anesthetic articaine that tends to cause prolonged numbness or paresthesia (tingling sensation) hours or days after administration.

The structures of local anesthetics have a direct bearing on their therapeutic actions (Fig. 27.5). All local anesthetics contain a hydrophobic group linked by either an ester or an amide bond to a relatively hydrophilic group (usually a tertiary or quaternary amine). This hydrophilic group makes the drug water soluble, enabling the agent to diffuse from the site of administration to the nerve. The hydrophobic group makes the agent lipid soluble and enables the drug to penetrate the lipid membranes (sheath, perineural tissue, and nerve membrane) to reach its binding site on the inner surface of VGSCs.

Local anesthetics must cross the neuronal cell membrane to reach their sites of action. Therefore sufficient amounts of the drug must be in the unionized form to gain entry to the axon. However, only the

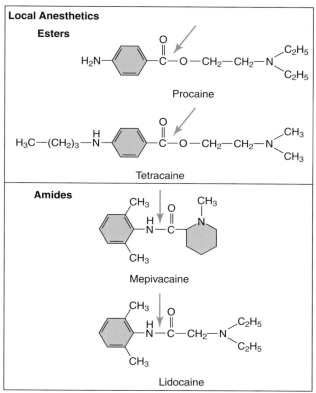

FIG. 27.5 Structures of the Two Types of Local Anesthetics Depicting Sites of Hydrolysis (Shown with Arrows).

charged form of the local anesthetic binds to VGSCs to cause effects. Thus an important chemical property of local anesthetics is that most are weak bases, with pK_a values of 8 to 9; one exception is benzocaine with a pK_a of 2.5. At physiological pH (~7.4), most (80% to 90%) of the drug is in the ionized (charged) form (Chapter 3). At an acidic pH, the portion of drug in the nonionized form is reduced markedly, resulting in reduced penetration of cell membranes and reducing the amount of drug reaching its site of action (Chapter 3). The consequence is that local anesthetics are less effective in inflamed or infected tissues that tend to have lower pH than in normal noninflamed tissues. The one exception is benzocaine. Although the pK_a of benzocaine is 2.5, it is very lipophilic, so tissue pH is not a factor, as the drug will gain access to the intracellular space of the axon to block VGSCs at any pH range.

The rate of onset of clinical local anesthesia is determined by drug concentration and potency, binding to local tissues, the rate of metabolism (for ester-type agents), and the degree of vascularity, especially if the drug is administered by injection. The last factor is of primary importance because any diffusion of the agent into blood reduces drug concentration at the nerve fibers, resulting in diminished potency. This is especially problematic because, with the exception of cocaine, all local anesthetics cause mild vasodilation. Therefore vasoconstrictors (adrenergic agonists) such as epinephrine are frequently combined with local anesthetics to reduce systemic absorption by reducing local blood flow. These vasoconstrictors double the duration of anesthesia, decrease rate of absorption into the circulatory system, and reduce the amount of local anesthetic needed by one-third to reach the desired effect. While commercially available formulations of local anesthetics that contain vasoconstrictors are very common, certain anatomical sites, such as

TABLE 27.1 Pharmacokinetic Parameters

Drug	Route of Administration	Elimination $t_{1/2}$ (hrs)	Disposition	Plasma Protein Bound (%)[a]	Onset Time (min)
Articaine	PN	1.8	M, R	54	1–6
Bupivacaine	PN	2.7 (adults)	M	95	10–20
		8.1 (neonates)	R, M		
Etidocaine	PN	2.5	M, R	95	3–5
Lidocaine	PN, IV[b]	1.5–2.0	M[c] (95%), R	70	3–15
Mepivacaine	PN	1.9–3.2 (adults)	R, M (main)	75	3–20
		2.7–9.0 (neonates)			
Procaine	PN, IV[b]	<3 min	M	10	5–20
Ropivacaine	PN	4.2	M	94	15–30

[a]Binding of local anesthetics to plasma proteins is rapidly reversible, such that a substantial fraction of the drug bound at equilibrium becomes free during hepatic extraction, making it a substrate for biotransformation.
[b]Intravenous (IV) lidocaine and procaine used at very low concentrations to relieve neuropathic pain may have effects lasting weeks to months.
[c]Large first-pass effect; significant pulmonary biotransformation.
M, Metabolism; *PN*, perineural; *R*, renal.

digits, penis, and scrotum cannot receive coinjections of vasoconstrictors because these compounds would cause severe and prolonged vasoconstriction such that the appendage (e.g., digit) would become necrotic and gangrenous. Thus topical application is considered safer at these anatomical sites.

Local anesthetics vary considerably in the rates at which they are metabolized. Because all of these compounds diffuse into the systemic circulation to some extent, metabolism is a prominent factor in the potential ability of these agents to produce adverse side effects and toxicity. In addition to metabolism, the binding to plasma proteins (α_1-acid glycoprotein and serum albumin) also causes the concentration of free drug in the circulation to be reduced.

The ester local anesthetics, including procaine and tetracaine (see Fig. 27.5), are rapidly hydrolyzed to inactive products by plasma cholinesterase (butyrylcholinesterase) and liver esterases. Therefore compounds such as procaine have a very short $t_{1/2}$ in the body (Table 27.1). Certain anatomical sites lack esterase activity, notably the spinal fluid, which extends the duration of action with "spinal" (intrathecal) anesthesia. The amide local anesthetics, by contrast, are metabolized in the liver by cytochrome P450s (CYPs) through *N*-dealkylation, followed by hydrolysis. Articaine is the exception because it is metabolized by both plasma cholinesterase and hepatic P450 drug-metabolizing enzymes (see Table 27.1).

Bupivacaine and etidocaine are bound to plasma proteins extensively, and nonspecific tissue binding also occurs near the injection site. These agents are more likely to cause toxicity in patients with preexisting liver disease as a result of the reduced drug biotransformation and lower plasma protein concentrations in these patients because plasma proteins are synthesized in the liver.

PHARMACOVIGILANCE: ADVERSE EFFECTS AND DRUG INTERACTIONS

Many of the local anesthetics used today, including lidocaine, which is one of the most widely-used compounds, were introduced and used before drug safety testing was required or common practice. As a consequence, there are few wide-scale or large population studies to identify toxicities or dangerous side effects.

Because local anesthetics ultimately redistribute from the site of administration into the systemic circulation, side effects and toxicity can result from both properly conducted nerve blocks and from accidental IV injection. Local anesthetics, especially the amides, are lipophilic and redistribute to many sites in the body, including the central nervous system (CNS). If blood concentrations are high enough, initial excitatory CNS effects are apparent and may include muscle twitching, visual disturbances, extreme patient anxiety, and tonic-clonic convulsions, followed by inhibitory effects including coma and respiratory arrest (Clinical Problems Box). However, a variety of signs and symptoms, including general depression and drowsiness, or euphoria with lidocaine, are common clinical consequences. Seizures can be treated rapidly or prevented by the IV administration of anticonvulsants, such as lorazepam or levetiracetam, along with oxygen administration to protect against hypoxemia in the convulsing patient. An overdose of a local anesthetic can result in the reduced transmission of impulses at the neuromuscular junction, producing weakness or muscle paralysis. Support of respiration is an important component of treatment. Smooth muscle is only minimally affected by local anesthetics.

The local anesthetics benzocaine, prilocaine, and lidocaine have been reported to cause the formation of methemoglobin, an altered form of hemoglobin. Methemoglobin does not carry oxygen like hemoglobin, resulting in methemoglobinemia, a rare but potentially life-threatening condition primarily reported in young children. The signs and symptoms include cyanosis, headache, fatigue, respiratory depression, and seizures. As little as 5 mL of a 20% solution of benzocaine may result in severe methemoglobinemia in children weighing under 40 kilograms. The potential adverse health effects are so severe that the United States Food and Drug Administration requires boxed warnings indicating the possibility of methemoglobinemia on over-the-counter medications that contain benzocaine or lidocaine. Parents of young children who are teething may apply too much topical local anesthetic, resulting in this potentially life-threatening condition.

Local anesthetics have potentially deleterious effects on cardiac pacemaker activity, electrical excitability, conduction times, and contractile force. Dysrhythmias are possible when high blood concentrations of local anesthetics are attained. Bupivacaine is considered the most cardiotoxic due to its ability to inhibit both VGSCs and voltage-gated Ca^{++} channels in cardiac myocytes. Local hypersensitivity reactions can result from the use of some ester-type local anesthetics, particularly procaine and related compounds, which cause the formation of para-aminobenzoic acid, which may cause severe allergic reactions, including dermatitis. In addition, some sulfite-based preservatives used in formulations of local anesthetics containing vasoconstrictors can lead to an

CNS—anxiety, visual disturbances, seizures
PNS—neuromuscular blockade leading to respiratory arrest
Cardiovascular—arrhythmias due to blockade of cardiac Na^+ and Ca^{++} channels
Hypersensitivity reactions—dermatitis

TRADE NAMES

In addition to generic and fixed-combination preparations, the following trade-named materials are some of the important compounds available in the United States.

Articaine (Septocaine)
Bupivacaine (Marcaine, Sensorcaine)
Chloroprocaine (Nesacaine)
Etidocaine (Duranest)
Levobupivacaine (Chirocaine)
Lidocaine[a] (Dilocaine, Lidoject, Octocaine, Xylocaine)
Mepivacaine (Carbocaine, Isocaine, Polocaine)
Procaine (Novocain)
Ropivacaine (Naropin)
Tetracaine[b] (Pontocaine)

[a]In the United Kingdom, the drug name is lignocaine.
[b]In the United Kingdom, the drug name is amethocaine.

allergic reaction. These can be ameliorated by the systemic administration of antihistamines (H_1 antagonists).

NEW DEVELOPMENTS

Although the local anesthetics are important therapeutic compounds for pain management, their usefulness is somewhat limited by their potential side effects. The therapeutic profile of these agents would be improved significantly if one were able to:

- control and predict the duration of block;
- enhance selectivity for pain suppression relative to motor and autonomic blockade; and
- improve safety, especially cardiotoxicity.

Recent advances in MRI have allowed for the precise localization and verification of local anesthetic injection in deep tissue to ensure the accurate site of administration of the drug. Although this practice is limited, use of imaging techniques to confirm needle placement in the administration of local anesthetics may become more commonplace in the future.

The recent finding that local anesthetics, at doses below those that block nerve impulse propagation, have systemic antiinflammatory actions by acting on specific G-protein–coupled receptors on circulating neutrophils and platelets, may lead to local anesthetics having a greater role in postsurgical pain management where inflammation may be problematic.

Several advances in drug development have been made to mitigate the harmful side effects associated with local anesthetics. Ropivacaine is a newer drug that is very similar in chemical structure to bupivacaine. However, unlike all other local anesthetics, ropivacaine is not a racemic mixture (both levorotatory and dextrorotatory molecules are present) but rather a pure levorotatory stereoisomer. This is thought to be responsible for the decreased cardiotoxicity of ropivacaine compared to bupivacaine. Future formulations of local anesthetics that are pure levorotatory stereoisomers may become available as the use of these compounds increases and becomes more widespread. In addition, there are multiple isoforms of the VGSCs α-subunit, and some are implicated in neuropathic and inflammatory pain. Because specific isoforms are expressed by somatosensory primary afferent neurons and not by skeletal or cardiac muscle, the possibility exists that future isoform-specific local anesthetics may have diminished cardiotoxicity and neurotoxicity.

The use of local anesthetics to control pain may increase in the future as the long-term abuse of opioids is increasing dramatically and being recognized as deleterious for pain management. New longer-acting (72 hour) formulations of liposomal bupivacaine are being used to control postoperative surgical site pain following procedures such as bunion and hemorrhoid removal, and further developments will likely lead to additional compounds with fewer adverse effects.

CLINICAL RELEVANCE FOR HEALTHCARE PROFESSIONALS

Local anesthetics are the most used group of drugs in modern dental practice. The short onset, reversibility, and localized effects render these agents ideally suited for treating patients in the dental office setting. Further, the advent of longer-acting formulations may allow these drugs to be used for single drug therapy for postsurgical pain management instead of prescription opioids. This is especially likely considering the addictive and dangerous nature of opioids and the added systemic antiinflammatory effects of local anesthetics at low blood levels.

Currently, only highly trained anesthesiologists and other healthcare providers (e.g., dentists or dermatologists) administer local anesthetics by injection. The ability to avoid both damaging deep nerve tissue and injecting these drugs into large blood vessels requires a high level of education and experience. With the advent of new imaging technology such as MRI, the administration of local anesthetics in deep tissue may become safer and more commonplace, performed by more physician assistants or nurse practitioners. In addition, advances in the safety profile of newer local anesthetics such as ropivacaine may allow for more widespread use of these drugs in the office setting administered by general healthcare providers. In addition, advances in patient screening may result in fewer complications and deaths due to local anesthetics. Specifically, the ability to identify patients with preexisting conditions such as arrhythmias or seizure disorders as being potentially at risk for toxicities may lead to the more widespread use of local anesthetics by family doctors or general healthcare providers.

SELF-ASSESSMENT QUESTIONS

1. A 64-year-old woman had a mole on her back that required dermatological removal using a local anesthetic. These drugs exert their therapeutic effects primarily by:
   A. Stimulating activity–dependent Na^+ channels.
   B. Blocking activity–dependent Na^+ channels.
   C. Stimulating activity–independent Na^+ channels.
   D. Blocking activity–independent Na^+ channels.
   E. Blocking activity–dependent K^+ channels.

2. A 24-year-old motorcyclist had an accident a week ago that resulted in an open wound on his knee that became infected. When he decided to seek medical help, the physician told him that he could not use lidocaine as a local anesthetic prior to suturing the wound because:
   A. The wound was too old.
   B. Lidocaine is a strong acid.
   C. Lidocaine would be destroyed by plasma esterases.
   D. Lidocaine would be in a charged form in the infected area and would not readily penetrate the cell membrane.
   E. Could easily gain entry to the brain.

3. Local anesthetics exert their therapeutic effects by selectively blocking which one of the following nerve fibers?
   A. Type Aα.
   B. Type Aβ.
   C. Type Aγ.
   D. Type Aδ.
   E. Type B.

4. Termination of the action of local anesthetics:
   A. Depends on the type of local anesthetic, i.e., ester or amide.
   B. Involves hydrolysis by plasma cholinesterases.
   C. Involves plasma-protein binding.
   D. Involves primarily vascular redistribution.
   E. Is enhanced in the presence of vasoconstrictors such as epinephrine.

5. A 6-month-old baby begins the teething process, which can be painful at times. In an effort to reduce pain and suffering, the parents of the baby give an over-the-counter oral analgesic that contains benzocaine. What is the specific risk to the baby if too much of the analgesic is given?
   A. Thromboembolism
   B. Botulism
   C. Methemoglobinemia
   D. Diarrhea
   E. Sudden infant death syndrome

FURTHER READING

Beiranvand S, Eatemadi A, Karimi A. New updates pertaining to drug delivery of local anesthetics in particular bupivacaine using lipid nanoparticles. *Nanoscale Res Lett.* 2016;11:307–317. PMID: 27342601.

Boyce RA, Kirpalani T, Mohan N. Updates of topical and local anesthesia agents. *Dent Clin North Am.* 2016;60(2):445–471. PMID: 27040295.

Curatolo M. Regional anesthesia in pain management. *Curr Opin Anaesthesiol.* 2016;29(5):614–619. PMID: 27137511.

Verlinde M, Hollmann MW, Stevens MF, et al. Local anesthetic-induced neurotoxicity. *Int J Mol Sci.* 2016;17:339. PMID: 26959012.

WEBSITES

https://www.asra.com/advisory-guidelines/article/3/checklist-for-treatment-of-local-anesthetic-systemic-toxicity

This website is from the American Society of Regional Anesthesia and Pain Medicine and contains valuable information on the treatment of local anesthetic toxicity.

https://www.guideline.gov/summaries/summary/48871/guideline-for-care-of-the-patient-receiving-local-anesthesia

This website is maintained by the Agency for Healthcare Research and Quality of the United States Department of Health and Human Services and contains major guidelines for care of patients receiving local anesthesia for perioperative nurses.

Opioid Analgesics

Susan L. Ingram and Elena E. Bagley

MAJOR DRUG CLASSES

Morphine-like compounds
Partial agonists and mixed-acting compounds
Antagonists

THERAPEUTIC OVERVIEW

Opioid analgesics are compounds that relieve moderate to severe visceral or somatic pain by binding to and activating a specific family of G-protein–coupled receptors (GPCRs) known as opioid receptors. Opioids are synthetic or natural compounds of any structural type that interact with opioid receptors and include peptides, as well as small organic molecules. In contrast, opiates are compounds isolated from the milky exudate of the poppy plant *(Papaver somniferum)* and include morphine, the first alkaloid isolated in 1806 by Sertürner and named after the Greek god of dreams, *Morpheus*, and codeine (3-methoxymorphine). The terms *opioid* and *opiate* are erroneously often used interchangeably.

Reference to the use of poppy plant extracts dates back centuries when preparations were used therapeutically as antidepressants to alleviate grief. In modern medicine, the opioids are used for a diverse array of effects, ranging from alleviation of pain to inhibiting the cough reflex. Despite the beneficial effects of these compounds, their use is accompanied by serious side effects, including respiratory depression, which is a major cause of death.

There is currently an opioid epidemic in the United States, with a major increase in the number of prescriptions written during the past 25 years. Increases in the availability of opioids have led to increases in the number of individuals using and abusing these drugs recreationally for their euphoric effects. Further, the increased use of these compounds has been accompanied by an escalation in the number of overdoses (Chapter 24). Unfortunately, this is now a critical health issue that has not been remedied. The primary uses and adverse effects of the opioids are shown in the Therapeutic Overview Box.

MECHANISMS OF ACTION

Endogenous Opioid Peptides

Opium derivatives and other opioid drugs mimic the actions of our own endogenous opioid peptides. Three major families of opioid peptides have been identified: enkephalins, endorphins, and dynorphins. These peptides are processed from precursor molecules encoded by three separate genes: proenkephalin, proopiomelanocortin, and prodynorphin, respectively (Fig. 28.1). The opioid peptides are found throughout the body and regulate many different peripheral and central processes (Table 28.1). The enkephalins (met-enkephalin and leu-enkephalin) are

ABBREVIATIONS

CNS	Central nervous system
ERK	Extracellular signal–related kinase
GABA	γ-Aminobutyric acid
GPCRs	G-protein–coupled receptors
MAPK	Mitogen-activated protein kinase
PAG	Periaqueductal gray
RVM	Rostral ventromedial medulla

THERAPEUTIC OVERVIEW

Primary Uses

Analgesia—gold standard for strong pain relief
Anesthesia—adjunct with general anesthetics
Antitussive—impairs cough reflex
Antidiarrheal—leads to constipation
Euphoria—the "rush" or feeling of well-being (dependence liability)

Adverse Effects

Dependence—withdrawal syndrome, intense craving
Respiratory depression—major cause of death
Miosis—pupillary constriction; may be indicator of opioid use
Nausea and vomiting—usually early; may need antiemetics
Pruritis—itching, particularly following intravenous or intrathecal administration

pentapeptides that are widely distributed in many regions of the central nervous system (CNS), including those involved in pain, such as the periaqueductal gray and spinal cord. The endorphins, primarily β-endorphin, are larger peptides with a distribution in the CNS more restricted to the hypothalamus and nucleus solitarius but are also expressed in other regions; the release of endorphins from the anterior lobe of the pituitary is a critical component of the stress response. The dynorphin family contains several peptides, of which dynorphin A (1-17) has been most studied and found to be expressed in the magnocellular cells of the hypothalamus and posterior lobe of the pituitary gland, where it colocalizes with vasopressin (antidiuretic hormone). Other dynorphin peptides are widely distributed in the CNS and have been shown to have roles in pain and dysphoria.

Opioid Receptors

The opioid receptor family consists of three receptors named μ, κ, and δ, also known as MOP, KOP, and DOP, respectively, all of which bind

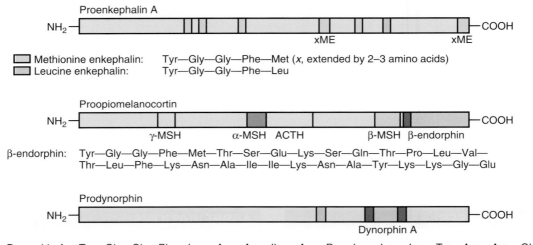

FIG. 28.1 The major families of opioid peptides, the enkephalins, endorphins, and dynorphins, are derived from distinct precursor molecules, proenkephalin A, proopiomelanocortin, and prodynorphin, respectively, and are encoded by three distinct genes.

TABLE 28.1 Principal Endogenous Opioid Peptides

Opioid Family	Precursor	Distribution
Enkephalins	Proenkephalin	Widely throughout the CNS, especially in interneurons, including those associated with pain pathways and emotional behavior; also found in some peripheral tissues
Endorphins	Proopiomelanocortin	β-Endorphin in hypothalamus, nucleus tractus solitarius, and anterior lobe of the pituitary, where it is coreleased with adrenocorticotropin in response to stress
Dynorphins	Prodynorphin	Dynorphin A (1-17) in the magnocellular cells of the hypothalamus and posterior lobe of the pituitary gland, where it colocalizes with vasopressin; shorter-chain dynorphins distributed widely in the CNS, some associated with pain pathways, especially in the spinal cord

TABLE 28.2 Opioid Receptors and Their Ligands

IUPHAR[a] nomenclature	Prior Nomenclature	Endogenous Ligand	Exogenous Ligand
μ Receptor (MOP)	OP$_3$	Enkephalins β-Endorphin Endomorphins	Morphine Buprenorphine[b] Codeine Fentanyl Meperidine Methadone Oxycodone
κ Receptor (KOP)	OP$_2$	Dynorphins	Butorphanol[b] Pentazocine
δ Receptor (DOP)	OP$_1$	Enkephalins β-Endorphin	None to date

[a]International Union of Basic and Clinical Pharmacology.
[b]Partial agonist.

endogenous and exogenous compounds with varying affinities (Table 28.2); the Greek nomenclature is now recommended. These receptors are GPCRs (Chapter 2) and are expressed to varying degrees throughout peripheral tissues and the CNS. All three opioid receptors couple to Gα$_{i/o}$ to inhibit neuronal activity through inhibition of adenylyl cyclase and calcium conductance and activation of potassium conductance. The receptors mediate long-term signaling through activation of the extracellular signal–related kinase (ERK)/mitogen-activated protein kinase (MAPK) pathway and regulation of transcription. Through these signaling cascades, opioid receptors located postsynaptially on neuronal cell bodies and dendrites inhibit neuronal activity and regulate signaling to the nucleus; receptors localized presynaptically on nerve terminals inhibit the release of neurotransmitter, as shown for the μ receptor in Fig. 28.2. Given the similarity of signaling of the three opioid receptors, the differing effects observed when these receptors are activated by endogenous opioid peptides or opioid drugs are dependent on receptor locations in different cell compartments in single neurons and location of the neurons within the CNS.

Opioid Agonists

Morphine, whose structure is shown in Fig. 28.3, is the prototypical agonist at the μ-opioid receptor, and compounds like morphine represent the strongest analgesics but also produce constipation, nausea, respiratory depression, euphoria, reduction in the cough reflex, tolerance, and

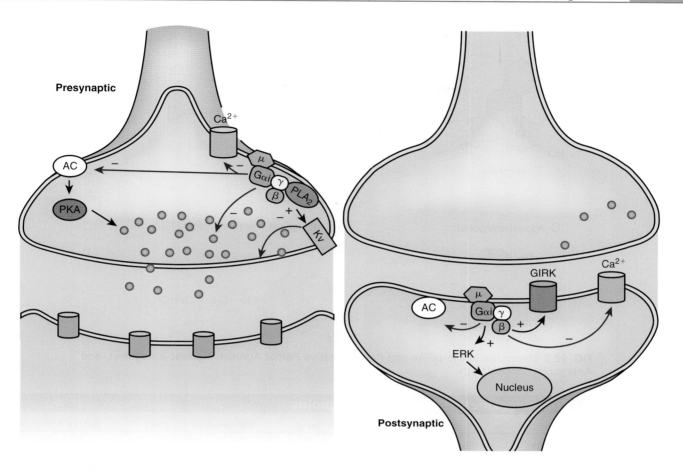

FIG. 28.2 μ-Opioid Receptors Couple to Different Effectors Depending on Location. Receptors localized to presynaptic terminals decrease neurotransmitter release through multiple mechanisms including activation of voltage-gated K⁺ channels; inhibition of adenylyl cyclase; inhibition of voltage-activated Ca^{2+} channels; and through interactions with proteins involved with exocytosis. Receptors in postsynaptic perikarya and dendritic locations are coupled to GIRK and calcium channels, as well as adenylyl cyclase and ERK. The overall effect of μ-opioid receptor actions at these effectors is to inhibit neuronal activity. *AC,* Adenylyl cyclase; *ERK,* extracellular signal–regulated kinase; *Gαβγ,* subunits of G proteins; *GIRK,* G-protein–activated inwardly rectifying potassium channel; *Kv,* voltage-activated potassium channel; *PKA,* protein kinase A; *PLA₂,* phospholipase A2.

dependence. These multiple actions are due to the widespread localization of μ-opioid receptors and limit the clinical usefulness of these compounds for pain, especially long-term chronic pain. Opioid analgesics are most effective in the management of dull, diffuse, and continuous pain. A standard dose produces satisfactory relief in approximately 90% of patients with mild to moderate postoperative pain and in 65%–70% of patients with moderate to severe postoperative pain. The degree of relief may decline after several days or more of frequent administration as tolerance develops. Within limits, increasing the dose can restore the analgesic response. Long-term use has also been shown to produce opioid-induced hyperalgesia, or a worsening of pain in some patients. Opioid-induced pain relief is often accompanied by drowsiness, mental clouding, and an elevated mood (i.e., euphoria). Although the euphoria is associated with a potential for abuse, in patients with pain, it is more likely to be a secondary consequence of pain relief.

In general, all morphine-like drugs are equally efficacious in alleviating pain except for codeine and tramadol, which are less effective. Codeine by itself is not suitable for treating severe pain and is often administered in combination with a nonopioid antipyretic analgesic, especially aspirin or acetaminophen. Synergistic effects of these drug combinations have been shown to occur because opioids and cyclooxygenase inhibitors target different molecules in the arachidonic acid signaling cascade. A related compound, propoxyphene, and its relative, dextropropoxyphene, also target cardiac sodium channels and have been withdrawn from the market. Since most opioid drugs are effective for analgesia, a particular opioid is often chosen based on its speed of onset, duration of action, ability to cross the blood-brain barrier, and oral bioavailability (Table 28.3).

Virtually all opioids exert their analgesic effects through μ-opioid receptors in the brain and spinal cord. Tramadol is an exception, being a racemic mixture with the "d or +" isomer binding to μ-opioid receptors and inhibiting neuronal serotonin (5-HT) reuptake, and the "l or –" isomer inhibiting norepinephrine (NE) reuptake and stimulating α₂-adrenergic receptors. The analgesic effects of tramadol are only partially

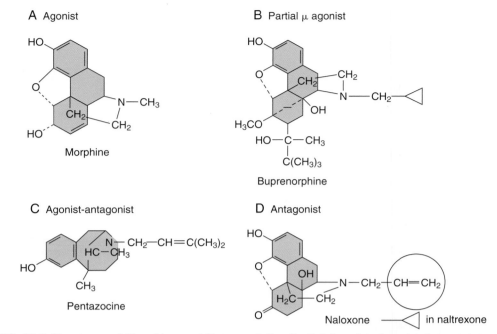

FIG. 28.3 Structures of Morphine and Representative Partial Agonist, Agonist-Antagonist, and Antagonist Opioid Drugs.

TABLE 28.3 Pharmacokinetic Parameters of Opioids

Drug	Route	Duration of Action (hrs)	Elimination $t_{1/2}$ (hrs)	Active Metabolites
Morphine-like Compounds				
Alfentanil	Parenteral[a]	0.5	1.5	No
Codeine	Oral, parenteral	4–6	3	Yes
Fentanyl	Parenteral, transdermal	0.5–1	3.7	No
Hydrocodone	Oral	4–5	3.8	Yes
Hydromorphone	Parenteral, oral	4–5	2.6	No
Levorphanol	Parenteral, oral	4–5	11	No
Meperidine[b]	Parenteral, oral	3–4	3	Yes
Methadone	Oral, parenteral	4–5	23	No
Morphine	Parenteral, oral	4–5	2.3	Yes
Oxycodone	Oral	3–5	3	Yes
Oxymorphone	Parenteral, rectal	4–5	1.5	No
Propoxyphene	Oral	4–5	9	Yes
Remifentanil	Parenteral	0.25	0.2	No
Sufentanil	Parenteral	0.5	2.7	No
Tramadol	Parenteral, oral	3–5	6	Yes
Partial Agonists and Mixed-acting Compounds				
Buprenorphine	Parenteral, sublingual	4–6	5	No
Butorphanol	Parenteral, intranasal	3–4	3	No
Dezocine	Parenteral	3–4	2.5	No
Nalbuphine	Parenteral	4–5	5	No
Pentazocine	Parenteral, oral	3–5	4	No
Antagonists				
Naloxone	Parenteral	1–2[c]	1	No
Nalmefene	Parenteral	9–11[c]	10	No
Naltrexone	Oral, depot injection[d]	24[c]	4	Yes

[a]Parenteral refers to administration by injection.
[b]Pethidine in many countries.
[c]Duration of antagonist activity.
[d]For treatment of alcoholism.
$t_{1/2}$, Half-life.

blocked by the opioid receptor antagonist naloxone, indicating that these other targets play a role in tramadol-mediated analgesia.

Activation of the κ-opioid receptor can also produce analgesia, and several compounds such as butorphanol and pentazocine, known as mixed-acting opioids, have partial agonist activity at both κ and μ receptors; the structures of these compounds are shown in Fig. 28.3. Although the contribution of κ-receptor activity to the analgesia produced by these agents is not well understood, evidence suggests that κ agonists are better analgesics in females than males, possibly due to differential expression patterns in the sexes. The κ agonists produce many of the same side effects as μ agonists but also lead to dysphoria, hallucinations, and diuresis.

Selective agonists for the δ receptor produce some analgesia, although these compounds are not as efficacious as agonists at the μ receptor. The δ-receptor agonists are not currently used clinically, although there is evidence that these receptors may be induced in chronic pain states and that selective δ-receptor agonists may be analgesic in chronic pain. There are some early-phase clinical trials testing δ-receptor–selective compounds. However, activation of δ receptors can produce seizures.

Opioid Antagonists

Most clinically used opioid-receptor antagonists are relatively nonselective at opioid receptors. However, given that almost all clinically used opioids produce their effects through the μ receptor, these antagonists produce their response primarily through competitive inhibition at this receptor. These drugs are used for reversal of opioid overdose and are components in some opioid formulations to discourage nonprescribed use and addiction.

Naloxone, whose structure is shown in Fig. 28.3, and naltrexone are competitive antagonists at opioid receptors. Naloxone is often used in conjunction with an opioid agonist taken orally to reduce constipation (naloxone + oxycodone [Targin]). When taken orally, naloxone reduces opioid actions in the gastrointestinal system but is metabolized before reaching the brain and therefore doesn't block CNS-mediated oxycodone analgesia. This combination may also reduce drug diversion if administered intravenously because intravenous delivery bypasses the first-pass metabolism of naloxone, leading to increased blood levels and entry into the CNS, thereby blocking the CNS actions of oxycodone. Naltrexone has been used successfully to reduce craving in alcohol dependence but has had little success in treating opioid dependence partly due to compliance issues in some patients. Nalmefene is a competitive opioid antagonist that is structurally similar to naltrexone and is also effective for the treatment of alcohol dependence. Recently, the United States Food and Drug Administration approved long-lasting naltrexone implants that reduce compliance issues and may be useful for some individuals.

Methylnaltrexone is a newer μ-receptor antagonist with a quaternary nitrogen, limiting its ability to cross the blood-brain barrier. As a peripherally acting antagonist, methylnaltrexone reduces opioid-induced constipation, but this drug may also reduce opioid analgesia through its antagonist effects at peripheral opioid receptors located on primary afferents that are involved in analgesia.

Partial Agonists and Mixed-Acting Compounds

In addition to the pure agonists and antagonists, compounds with partial agonist activity or mixed-acting compounds are also used to treat opioid addiction, including both buprenorphine and pentazocine, whose structures are shown in Fig. 28.3. Buprenorphine has partial agonist activity at μ-opioid receptors, as well as antagonist activity at κ and possibly δ receptors, rendering it useful for both the treatment of addiction and for the relief of acute and moderate chronic pain. Pentazocine is another mixed-acting compound with agonist activity

at κ receptors and weak antagonist effects at μ receptors, resulting in analgesic activity, but capable of weakly antagonizing the analgesic effects of morphine and related compounds.

RELATIONSHIP OF MECHANISMS OF ACTION TO CLINICAL RESPONSE

Pain is a subjective experience that includes emotional processing of sensory stimuli and is quite dependent on the overall emotional and cognitive state of the patient. Opioids, through their widespread expression, modulate all aspects of pain, including transduction, transmission, and cortical processing. Opioids in the periphery reduce activation of nociceptive primary afferents, as well as the second-order ascending neurons in lamina I and II of the spinal cord. The receptors are localized on both central terminals of the primary afferents and on postsynaptic perikarya of spinal cord neurons to reduce excitatory neurotransmitter release and decrease ascending transmission, respectively. The receptors are also a key component of the descending pain modulatory pathway from the periaqueductal gray (PAG) to the rostral ventromedial medulla (RVM) to the spinal cord, which, when activated by opioids acting in the PAG, inhibit ascending pain transmission at the level of the spinal cord. The PAG serves as an integration center for the emotional processing of pain and fear through activation of the limbic system and the amygdala. The overall effect of activating this system is an increase in pain thresholds.

Although opioids activate inhibitory GPCRs in many brain areas, they have excitatory effects on neural circuits because μ-opioid receptors are expressed by inhibitory γ-aminobutyric acid (GABA) neurons. Opioid activation of these receptors disinhibits circuits by inhibiting the activity of GABA neurons and decreasing release of GABA. Neuronal excitation via this mechanism occurs in the PAG, where opioids inhibit the release of GABA onto the PAG to RVM output neurons, thereby activating the descending pain inhibition circuit. The disinhibition of circuits by opioids is also apparent in the mesolimbic system, where activation of μ-opioid receptors on GABA terminals impinging on dopamine neurons in the ventral tegmental area (VTA) ultimately results in the increased release of dopamine. This increased dopamine release is associated with opioid-induced euphoria. In contrast, κ-opioid receptors expressed on dopamine neurons in the VTA directly inhibit the release of dopamine, and thus their activation contributes to the dysphoria elicited by κ-receptor agonists.

Opioids are well known for their antitussive effects, and dextromethorphan is present in many over-the-counter preparations for its ability to suppress cough. The specific mechanisms mediating this effect are not well understood and have been attributed to agonist activity at μ-, κ-, and δ-opioid receptors, as well as to nonopioid-receptor–mediated activity. Similarly, the specific anatomical site of action mediating the ability of the opioids to suppress cough have been attributed to the nucleus tractus solitarius in the medulla, to the autonomic nervous system, and to a direct action on airway smooth muscle.

PHARMACOKINETICS

Opioid Agonists

The pharmacokinetic profile of an opioid is a major determinant of its therapeutic use. Opioids have been studied extensively for the past 50 years, and many agonists and antagonists have been designed that have different physiochemical properties. Most opioids are well absorbed from the gastrointestinal tract, but some have greatly reduced bioavailability due to extensive first-pass metabolism in the liver. Thus parenteral administration is much more effective for opioid drugs, especially morphine. Drugs with greater lipophilicity, including fentanyl and buprenorphine, are well absorbed through the nasal and buccal mucosa. The most lipophilic of opioids, including fentanyl, are absorbed transdermally as well. Serum protein binding ranges from approximately 30% for morphine to 80%–90% for fentanyl and its derivatives.

Various physicochemical properties of the opioid drugs make it difficult to correlate the speed of onset and duration of action of opioids with their plasma concentrations or elimination half-lives. For example, the rise in plasma concentrations of morphine long precedes the onset of analgesia because this hydrophilic drug penetrates the blood-brain barrier very slowly. In contrast, plasma concentrations of fentanyl closely parallel therapeutic effects. The rapid redistribution of lipophilic fentanyl from brain to lean body mass results in a short duration of action that is not predictable from its elimination half-life, which exceeds that of the longer acting morphine. Remifentanil, a fentanyl analogue ester, is so rapidly metabolized by plasma esterases that its plasma half-life is only 10–20 minutes, and it does not accumulate upon repeated or slow continuous administration. Opioids with relatively long elimination half-lives can accumulate in the body upon repeated dosing, thereby prolonging their duration of action. Methadone and buprenorphine have long-lasting effects and are currently used as treatments for opioid addiction in medication-assisted therapy (MAT) centers.

Opioids are metabolized mainly by the liver, usually to more polar and less active or inactive compounds. The mechanisms involved include N-dealkylation, conjugation of hydroxyl groups, and hydrolysis. However, metabolites account for much of the opioid activity of codeine, which is O-demethylated to morphine, heroin (diacetylmorphine), which is deacetylated to morphine, and tramadol, whose O-desmethyl metabolite has a 200 times greater affinity for the μ receptor than tramadol. There is considerable variability in the hepatic metabolism of the largely inactive codeine to morphine due to genetic factors influencing the activity of the CYP2D6 enzyme. About 5%–10% of the Caucasian population will experience weak analgesia from codeine as they are poor metabolizers, while up to 7% may experience greater effects because they are fast metabolizers (Chapter 4).

The two hydroxyl groups of morphine (Fig. 28.3) are conjugated with glucuronic acid to produce two metabolites. Morphine-3-glucuronide is inactive, but morphine-6-glucuronide has a higher affinity for the μ opioid receptor and is a more potent analgesic than morphine. Morphine-6-glucuronide accumulates during long-term morphine treatment, and measurable amounts are found in cerebrospinal fluid. However, morphine-6-glucuronide is relatively polar and penetrates the blood-brain barrier poorly. Thus the extent to which it contributes to the analgesic effect of morphine administered acutely is unknown.

Meperidine is N-demethylated, resulting in the production of normeperidine, which can lead to convulsions at moderately high levels. Significant amounts of normeperidine accumulate in patients receiving multiple large doses of meperidine over a relatively short time, in patients with renal insufficiency, and in people taking drugs that interfere with its metabolism, including monoamine oxidase (MAO) inhibitors. The pharmacokinetic parameters of opioid drugs are summarized in Table 28.3.

Several newer delivery systems for opioids are now available. A fentanyl transdermal patch is used to treat patients with chronic pain, and fentanyl administered intranasally is used to relieve acute pain. Morphine and other morphine-like opioids, especially fentanyl, are administered intrathecally and epidurally to control pain during and after surgery and to treat otherwise intractable pain. Patient-controlled analgesia allows patients to deliver opioids on demand within preset limits by activating a microprocessor-controlled pump that delivers a bolus dose through an intravenous or epidural catheter. With this method of administration, patients can self-medicate whenever the need arises, and the quality of pain control is usually better than that provided by doses administered at predetermined intervals. When high drug concentrations need to be maintained over long periods, as in certain chronic pain syndromes and in pain associated with cancer and other terminal illnesses, there are sustained-release oral formulations of morphine and oxycodone.

Opioid Antagonists

Naloxone is a short-acting antagonist with low oral bioavailability due to marked first-pass metabolism. Its short half-life may require multiple doses to reverse overdose of longer acting agonists. Nalmefene has an intermediate duration of action and is metabolized by the liver via N-dealkylation and glucuronidation, resulting in metabolites that are minimally or entirely inactive. Naltrexone is long acting with high oral bioavailability and is also available as a depot injection, used for the treatment of alcoholism. Interestingly, studies have shown that alcoholics who express a variant of the μ-opioid receptor (carrying the Asp40 allele) are more likely to achieve success following naloxone administration than alcoholics who do not express this variant. This finding underscores the importance of pharmacogenetics as a prime determinant of the efficacy of opioid antagonist treatment for alcoholism (Chapter 4).

PHARMACOVIGILANCE: ADVERSE EFFECTS AND DRUG INTERACTIONS

Common Adverse Effects

The most common cause of death from opioid overdose is respiratory depression. The μ-opioid agonists act on respiratory centers in the medulla, including the pre-Bötzinger complex, and decrease the sensitivity of neurons in these centers to the partial pressure of CO_2 in the blood. If these centers cannot detect CO_2, then the usual response to breathe is inhibited. Insufficient O_2 leads to cardiac arrest and hypoxia (reduced O_2 in the brain and possible brain damage). The intravenous administration of the opioid antagonist naloxone competes with the opioid agonist at μ-receptors in the medulla, thus reducing agonist receptor occupancy and reducing opioid inhibition of these respiratory centers.

The opioids are also well known to cause emesis. This effect is thought to be mediated by activation of opioid receptors in the area postrema, also known as the chemotrigger zone, located on the dorsal surface of the medulla. The area postrema is not protected by the blood-brain barrier and has evolved to react to environmental chemicals in the cerebrospinal fluid. Opioid receptors in the area postrema regulate the activity of this brain region and therefore can cause nausea and vomiting. Nausea and vomiting usually affect about 40% of people receiving morphine, but tolerance develops to this side effect with repeated administration. Often antiemetic medications are required on treatment initiation.

Opioids stimulate the Edinger-Westphal nucleus, the parasympathetic preganglionic fiber that innervates the sphincter of the iris and ciliary muscle, leading to miosis (Chapters 6 and 7). Tolerance does not develop to this effect.

Another major side effect of chronic opioid use is constipation. Activation of μ-opioid receptors in the enteric nervous system of the gastrointestinal tract blocks propulsive peristalsis, inhibiting the secretion of intestinal fluids and increasing fluid absorption. Unlike some of the other side effects, constipation is not reduced following the chronic use of the opioids. This adverse effect can be so painful that people will choose to stop analgesic therapy. Combining an opioid agonist with a peripherally restricted opioid antagonist or oral

CLINICAL PROBLEMS

Respiratory depression
Drowsiness
Nausea and vomiting
Constipation[a]
Endocrine disturbances
Tolerance to analgesic effect
Physical dependence
Abuse potential
Interactions with other CNS-depressant drugs

[a]Can also be a therapeutic effect.

TRADE NAMES

In addition to generic and fixed-combination preparations, the following trade-named materials are some of the important compounds available in the United States.

Agonists
Alfentanil (Alfenta)
Fentanyl (Actiq, Duragesic, Fentora, Ionsys, Sublimaze)
Hydrocodone (Hycodan)
Hydromorphone (Dilaudid)
Levorphanol (Levo-Dromoran)
Loperamide (Imodium)
Meperidine (Demerol)
Methadone (Dolophine)
Morphine (MS Contin, Oramorph, Astramorph PF)
Oxycodone (OxyContin, Roxicodone)
Oxymorphone (Numorphan)

Partial Agonists and Agonist-Antagonists
Buprenorphine (Buprenex, Subutex)
Butorphanol (Stadol)
Dezocine (Dalgan)
Nalbuphine (Nubain)
Pentazocine (Talwin)

Antagonists
Nalmefene (Revex)
Naloxone (Narcan)
Naltrexone (Revia, Depade)

naloxone that has high first-pass metabolism can reduce opioid-induced constipation (OIC).

Chronic Use

Chronic morphine treatment produces long-term changes (i.e., tolerance and dependence) in the opioid system, indicating that opioid-sensitive signaling in the brain is very plastic. Opioid tolerance is characterized by a diminished responsiveness to the inhibitory actions of opioids and is thought to involve a functional uncoupling between the opioid receptors and their effectors. In contrast, opioid dependence is characterized by withdrawal behaviors or rebound responses after administration of an antagonist and cannot be explained by opioid receptor/effector uncoupling. Withdrawal by dependent individuals results in increased neuronal excitability in several brain areas and an increase in adenylyl cyclase activity. Functional and biochemical studies have suggested a role for the PAG in the expression of many signs of withdrawal.

Adaptations in opioid signaling following chronic administration have been studied at the cellular level and involve a series of events that occur after agonist binding to the receptor (Fig. 28.4). Following activation by agonist, opioid receptors are phosphorylated by a G-protein–coupled receptor kinase (GRK) that enables the binding of β-arrestin to the phosphorylated receptor, leading to receptor internalization and terminating signaling from the plasma membrane. Internalized receptors have several possible fates, similar to those described for the β-adrenergic receptor (Figs. 2.15 and 2.16, Chapter 2). These processes occur at different rates and contribute to the tolerance observed in patients following the repeated use of the opioids.

Opioid-induced hyperalgesia is another potential consequence of repeated opioid administration, particularly high doses. There is evidence that some patients exhibit worsening of their pain symptoms with chronic opioid treatment. The cellular mechanisms are not completely understood but may involve adaptations in the descending pain control system (Chapter 25).

NEW DEVELOPMENTS

The increase in prescription opioid use and overdose deaths has led to a public health crisis and several shifts in policy and education initiatives at the national level. Although these initiatives may be leading to a leveling off of escalating opioid use, they do not address the underlying issue: the lack of effective long-term treatments for chronic pain. Several different avenues are currently being explored for new therapies, including antibodies to nerve growth factor (NGF), specific inhibitors or small molecule inhibitors of ion channels differentially expressed in primary afferents, allosteric modulators for GPCRs involved in pain pathways, and biased ligands for opioid receptors. Combined formulations of opioids and opioid inhibitors may have enhanced efficacy as therapies for opioid dependence, addiction, and overdose.

CLINICAL RELEVANCE FOR HEALTHCARE PROFESSIONALS

All healthcare professionals must be aware that opioid dependence and addiction are serious consequences associated with the long-term use of the opioids. Opioid prescriptions have risen substantially in the past 10 years, and in 2014, more than 240 million prescriptions were written for opioids in the United States. The number of overdose incidents related to opioid pain medication and heroin use also escalated 200% from 2000 to 2014. Heroin use appears to be escalating because heroin is cheaper on the black market than prescription opioids. One reason for the escalation is the increase in chronic pain rates and the lack of effective treatments for chronic pain, leaving physicians with few options for treating their patients. There is particular concern because there is little evidence to support the long-term efficacy of chronic opioid analgesic therapy for improving function or alleviating overall pain, and the likelihood of developing opioid overuse disorder ranges from 3-fold for acute low doses to 120-fold for chronic high doses. The Centers for Disease Control and Prevention (CDC) recently prepared guidelines for prescribing opioids for chronic pain to help physicians and other healthcare professionals make difficult decisions regarding the use of opioids for their patients with chronic pain (www.cdc.gov/media/modules/dpk/2016/dpk-pod/rr6501e1er-ebook .pdf).

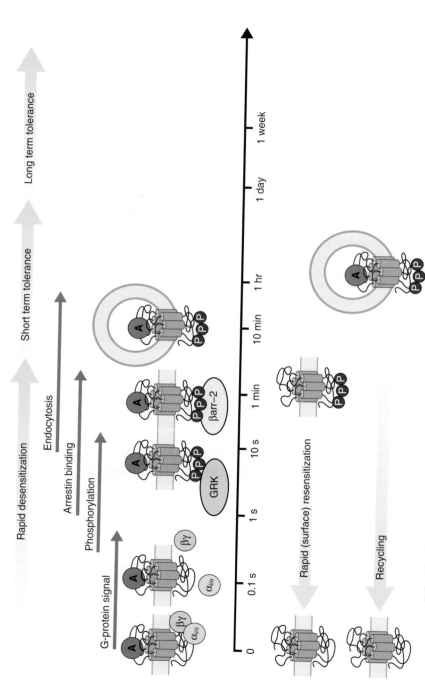

FIG. 28.4 Timescale for μ-Opioid Receptor Regulation. The time (log scale) following binding of an efficacious agonist such as [Met⁵] enkephalin is depicted. Phosphorylation by G-protein–coupled receptor kinase (GRK) is very rapid, saturating in less than 20 seconds. β-arrestin binding saturates in several minutes, and desensitization reaches steady state in approximately 5 minutes. The steady state of rapid desensitization represents the equilibrium between the forward desensitizing process, presumably phosphorylation and β-arrestin binding and dephosphorylation at the cell surface. Endocytosis reaches steady state in approximately 30 minutes, and recycling occurs over approximately 60 minutes, although this varies for different splice variants. Desensitization is defined as a rapid process preceding significant endocytosis (approximately 2–5 minutes), short-term tolerance includes endocytosis and other mechanisms (up to 1 day), and long-term tolerance (greater than 1 day) presumably involves multiple regulatory processes. *βarr-2,* β-arrestin 2. (From Williams JT, Ingram SL, Henderson G, et al. Regulation of μ-opioid receptors: desensitization, phosphorylation, internalization, and tolerance. *Pharmacol Rev.* 2013 Jan 15;65(1):223-54. https://www-ncbi-nlm-nih-gov.liboff.ohsu.edu/pubmed/23321159.)

SELF-ASSESSMENT QUESTIONS

1. J.D. received severe burns while escaping from a burning building and was rushed to the emergency department, where he was given the intravenous opioids morphine and oxycodone. These drugs relieved his pain by activating opioid receptors that:
   A. Increased calcium channel activity.
   B. Increased sodium channel activity.
   C. Inhibited potassium channels.
   D. Hyperpolarized neurons.
   E. Depolarized neurons.

2. P.K. is a well-known drug addict around town with many neuromuscular problems. When he came to your office for his last visit, you noted that he had "pinpoint" pupils and decreased respiration and heart rate. These effects are likely the result of:
   A. Morphine-activating μ receptors.
   B. Oxycodone-activating κ receptors.
   C. Methadone-activating κ receptors.
   D. Naloxone-activating μ receptors.
   E. Buprenorphine-activating δ receptors.

3. Which of the following correctly matches the prototype compound with its clinical use?
   A. Naloxone for opioid overdose.
   B. Oxycodone for diarrhea.
   C. Morphine for mild pain.
   D. Naloxone for cough.
   E. Methadone for opioid toxicity.

4. A 72-year-old cancer patient was prescribed morphine for her pain. After taking the drug daily for more than a month, she noted that her pain worsened. This is referred to as opioid-induced:
   A. Hyperalgesia.
   B. Tolerance.
   C. Dependence.
   D. Neuroplasticity.
   E. Phosphorylation.

5. A 32-year-old homeless woman was found unresponsive with a needle in her arm. The response team quickly administered a dose of naloxone to:
   A. Desensitize opioid receptors.
   B. Antagonize the ability of opioids to cross the blood-brain barrier.
   C. Competitively inhibit opioid-induced respiratory depression.
   D. Stimulate the hepatic metabolism of the opioids.
   E. Counteract opioid-induced constipation.

FURTHER READING

Dowell D, Haegerich TM, Chou R. CDC Guideline for Prescribing Opioids for Chronic Pain - United States, 2016. *MMWR Recomm Rep*. 2016;65(1):1–49.

Edlund MJ, Martin BC, Russo JE, et al. The role of opioid prescription in incident opioid abuse and dependence among individuals with chronic noncancer pain: the role of opioid prescription. *Clin J Pain*. 2014;30(7):557–564.

Kolodny A, Courtwright DT, Hwang CS, et al. The prescription opioid and heroin crisis: a public health approach to an epidemic of addiction. *Annu Rev Public Health*. 2015;36:559–574.

Rudd RA, Aleshire N, Zibbell JE, Gladden RM. Increases in Drug and Opioid Overdose Deaths–United States, 2000-2014. *MMWR Morb Mortal Wkly Rep*. 2016;64(50–51):1378–1382.

Williams JT, Ingram SL, Henderson G, et al. Regulation of mu-opioid receptors: desensitization, phosphorylation, internalization, and tolerance. *Pharmacol Rev*. 2013;65(1):223–254.

WEBSITES

https://www.hhs.gov/opioids/about-the-epidemic/
This website is maintained by the United States Government Department of Health and Human Services and documents information about the opioid epidemic in the United States.

https://www.cdc.gov/mmwr/volumes/65/rr/rr6501e1.htm
This is the Centers for Disease Control and Prevention (CDC) website that contains the CDC Guideline for Prescribing Opioids for Chronic Pain—United States, 2016.

Nonsteroidal Antiinflammatory Agents and Acetaminophen

Jennelle Durnett Richardson and Jill Fehrenbacher

THERAPEUTIC OVERVIEW

Nonsteroidal antiinflammatory drugs (NSAIDs) and acetaminophen are among the most commonly used drugs in the United States. They are available over-the-counter and by prescription, as well as in combination with other medications. Both NSAIDs and acetaminophen are used as analgesics and antipyretics. NSAIDs, but not acetaminophen, have antiinflammatory actions and also are used in the treatment of several inflammatory disorders including gout, osteoarthritis, and rheumatoid arthritis. It is important to note that NSAIDs treat the symptoms associated with these inflammatory diseases, but they do not affect disease progression.

The therapeutic action of the NSAIDs is mediated by their ability to inhibit the synthesis of prostaglandins (PGs). Prostaglandins are members of the eicosanoid class, a family of endogenous compounds containing oxygenated unsaturated 20-carbon fatty acids. Other members of the eicosanoid class include thromboxanes (TX), which are involved in platelet aggregation, and leukotrienes, which mediate vasodilation and chemotaxis associated with allergy and asthma. Eicosanoids are considered nonclassical signaling molecules because they are not stored in vesicles but are synthesized on demand and released via facilitated transport to act as local hormones (autacoids) in the cell, tissue, or structure where they are synthesized. The eicosanoids are derived from arachidonic acid (AA), which can be liberated from cell membrane phospholipids by the action of phospholipase A_2. The enzyme cyclo-oxygenase (COX) catalyzes the formation of the PGs and TX from AA, as shown in Fig. 29.1. AA is converted to PGG_2, which is immediately converted to PGH_2, followed by the enzymatic formation of other PGs or TXs, mediated by specific PG or TX synthases. Once transported out of the cell, eicosanoids interact with a diverse array of G-protein–coupled receptors (GPCRs) to produce biological effects. PGs are involved in many processes in the body, and PG analogues and inhibitors of PG synthesis are used therapeutically to mimic or inhibit many of these actions. Indications for the use of the NSAIDs and acetaminophen are in the Therapeutic Overview Box.

THERAPEUTIC OVERVIEW

NSAIDs and Acetaminophen
Relief of mild to moderate somatic pain, including headache, toothache, myalgia, and arthralgia
Relief of moderate to severe postoperative pain as combination therapy with opioids and/or as part of a multimodal analgesia regimen
Reduction of fever

NSAIDs Only
Relief of pain due to inflammatory disorders such as rheumatoid arthritis, osteoarthritis, gout, and ankylosing spondylitis
Prevention of trauma-induced local inflammation

Low-Dose Aspirin Only
Prophylaxis of thrombosis (myocardial infarction, stroke, pulmonary embolism, venous thromboembolism)

MECHANISMS OF ACTION

COX is the enzyme involved in the synthesis of PGG_2 and PGH_2, the precursors for the prostanoids. The prostanoid class consists of PGs, prostacyclin (PGI_2), and TXs (see Fig. 29.1). Different cell types express specific prostanoid synthases, thus determining which prostanoid will be synthesized and released from which cells. There are two isoforms of the COX enzyme: COX-1 and COX-2. COX-1 is constitutively active in many cell types and plays a role in many homeostatic functions, such as PG-mediated suppression of gastric acid secretion, whereas, in

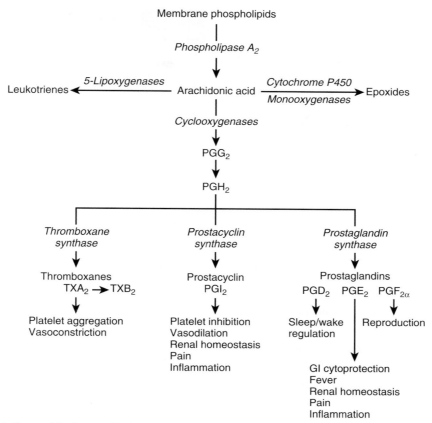

FIG. 29.1 General Pathways Mediating the Synthesis of the Eicosanoids. The first step in prostanoid synthesis is the release of arachidonic acid from membrane phospholipids, a reaction catalyzed by phospholipase A_2. Arachidonic acid is oxidized by cyclooxygenases, and the PGH_2 produced is further metabolized by specific synthases, leading to the on-demand production of various prostanoids, which elicit diverse physiological effects.

general, COX-2 is induced in response to inflammatory mediators and plays a role in the inflammatory process. However, in specific instances, COX-1 may be induced, and COX-2 constitutively expressed, perhaps mediating some of the adverse effects associated with inhibition of these enzymes.

NSAIDs inhibit the COX enzymes and thus decrease the synthesis of PGs, PGI_2, and TXs. This action accounts for both the therapeutic and adverse effects associated with the use of NSAIDs. Most NSAIDs inhibit both COX-1 and COX-2 in a reversible manner—that is, the COX enzyme is able to resume its function once the concentration of the NSAID decreases to a certain level. However, acetylsalicylic acid, also known as aspirin, inhibits both COX-1 and COX-2 in an irreversible manner via acetylation of the enzyme, which permanently inhibits the function of the enzyme, such that new COX must by synthesized to regain functional activity. This has long-term implications in platelets, which have no nuclei; to regain COX function in platelets new platelets must be synthesized, which takes 8–10 days. In nucleated cells, regeneration of COX can occur in 6–12 hours.

The selective COX-2 inhibitors were developed to target the pro-inflammatory functions of PGs while avoiding inhibition of their homeostatic functions, such as cytoprotection of the gastric epithelium. While these compounds are effective antiinflammatory agents, they also block the production of PGI_2 in endothelial cells. PGI_2 serves a cardioprotective role and balances the effects of COX-1–mediated TXA_2 synthesis on vasoconstriction and platelet aggregation. Thus the selective

COX-2 inhibitors increase the risk of certain cardiovascular events and do so with a higher incidence than with nonselective COX inhibitors (Fig. 29.2).

The mechanism of action of acetaminophen is not well understood, as it is only a weak inhibitor of COX enzymes. It has been suggested that acetaminophen may preferentially inhibit a COX splice variant expressed in the brain, which could explain its weak antiinflammatory effects in peripheral tissues. More research is needed in this area to better understand the mechanism underlying the analgesic and antipyretic effects of acetaminophen.

It is important to note that in addition to inhibiting the COX enzymes, the synthesis of the prostanoids may be inhibited by limiting the availability of AA. The corticosteroids manifest their antiinflammatory effects by inhibiting phospholipase A_2, thereby decreasing the release of AA from membrane phospholipids; these compounds also reduce the expression of enzymes that mediate PG synthesis (Chapter 50).

RELATIONSHIP OF MECHANISMS OF ACTION TO CLINICAL RESPONSE

Fever

The current approach to fever is to treat it only if it is debilitating and if lowering the elevated temperature will make the patient feel better. The NSAIDs and acetaminophen are antipyretic at doses that produce analgesia. By lowering the hypothalamic thermoregulatory set

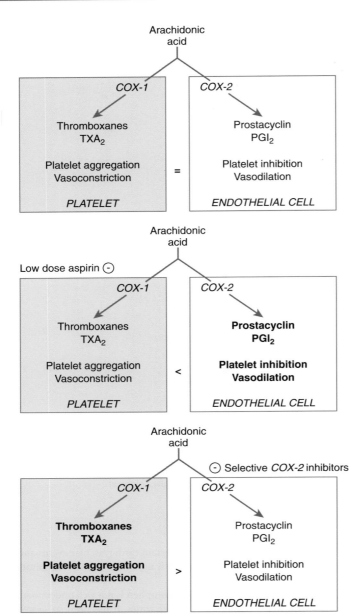

FIG. 29.2 The Effects of Low Doses of Aspirin Versus Selective COX-2 Inhibitors on Cardiovascular Risk. There is a dynamic interplay between platelet-derived thromboxane A_2 (TXA$_2$) and endothelium-derived prostacyclin (PGI$_2$) to maintain vascular homeostasis. Low-dose aspirin shifts the balance between TXA$_2$ and PGI$_2$, favoring the antiaggregation and vasodilation effects of endothelial cell–derived PGI$_2$. In contrast, selective COX-2 inhibitors shift the balance in the opposite direction to favor platelet-derived TXA$_2$, with aggregation and vasoconstriction dominating.

TABLE 29.1	Comparison of the Analgesic Effects of Morphine and Aspirin	
Parameter	**Morphine**	**Aspirin**
Type of pain relieved	Visceral, somatic	Somatic
Intensity of pain relieved	Moderate to severe	Mild to moderate
Tolerance development	Yes	No
Physical dependence development	Yes	No
Abuse potential	High	None

including bradykinin, cytokines, and certain amino acids and neuropeptides. Aspirin, the prototype NSAID, remains one of the most commonly used and effective agents for treating headache and mild to moderate pain arising from muscles, tendons, and joints. A dose of 650–1000 mg produces acceptable relief in 60%–80% of patients. Aspirin is far less effective in providing relief of severe pain and pain from visceral organs, which usually require an opioid (Chapter 28). However, unlike the opioids, aspirin and other NSAIDs do not cause analgesic tolerance or physical dependence and are not abused. Some of the major differences between aspirin and morphine, the prototype opioid analgesic, are listed in Table 29.1.

Other NSAIDs have analgesic effects similar to those of aspirin. Ibuprofen and naproxen, which are available over-the-counter, have become popular alternatives to aspirin. Ketorolac is most often used to treat postoperative pain because it can be administered parenterally. Celecoxib, a selective COX-2 inhibitor, is approved for the treatment of acute pain in adults and primary dysmenorrhea in women; however, its greatest value appears to be in relieving pain caused by chronic inflammatory conditions such as osteoarthritis and rheumatoid arthritis (Chapter 35).

Acetaminophen is also a popular alternative to aspirin for treating pain, especially by patients who are discomforted by the side effects of aspirin. Acetaminophen has analgesic potency and efficacy similar to aspirin. However, because it is devoid of antiinflammatory activity, it may be less effective in treating pain caused by inflammation. The mechanism of the analgesic effect of acetaminophen has been something of a quandary. It shares analgesic and antipyretic activity with the NSAIDs but lacks other actions associated with COX inhibition. It is possible that its analgesic effect, like its antipyretic effect, is mediated via an action on the central nervous system (CNS). Alternatively, acetaminophen could act through another, as-yet-unknown variant or isoform of COX.

NSAIDs and acetaminophen are commonly administered with other analgesics for perioperative pain management. The combination of NSAIDs or acetaminophen with an opioid analgesic can increase analgesic efficacy compared to either drug alone and also has an opioid-sparing effect.

Inflammatory Conditions

PGs and PGI$_2$ promote blood flow to injured tissues, resulting in leukocyte infiltration. These effects, together with leukotriene-induced increases in vascular permeability and attraction of polymorphonuclear leukocytes, lead to edema and inflammation. Peripheral inflammation is also associated with an increased expression of COX-2 in the dorsal horn of the spinal cord. Thus treatment with NSAIDs could reverse both peripheral and central sensitization to attenuate inflammatory pain. Indeed, the NSAIDs are used to alleviate pain associated with inflammatory disorders affecting the CNS, such as headache (Chapter 31), as

point, they promote autonomic reflexes that cause the loss of body heat, notably peripheral vasodilation and sweating. However, they are effective only in instances where elevated body temperature is caused by the increased synthesis of PGs, such as in infectious disease and autoimmune disorders.

Pain

PGs are released at the site of injury and act to sensitize nociceptors—that is, lower the threshold for sensory neuron firing in response to mechanical and thermal stimuli, as well as to many chemical mediators of pain,

TABLE 29.2 Pharmacokinetic Parameters of NSAIDs and Acetaminophen

Drug	Hours to Peak Plasma Level[a]	Elimination $t_{1/2}$ (hrs)	Plasma Protein Binding (%)	COX-2:COX-1 Ratio[b]
Acetaminophen[c]	0.5–1	2–4	25	3.7[d]
Aspirin	–[e]	0.25	60–80	0.3
Celecoxib	3	10–12	97	7.6
Diclofenac	1	1–2	99	2.8
Diflunisal	2–3	8–12	99	4.5
Etodolac	1.5–2	6–7	99	10
Fenoprofen	2	2–3	99	–
Flurbiprofen	1–2	2–3	99	–
Ibuprofen	2	2–4	90–99	0.1
Indomethacin	2	4–5	99	0.1
Ketoprofen	1.2	2–2.5	99	0.3
Ketorolac	1	2–9	99	1.8
Meclofenamic acid	0.5–2	0.8–2	99	-
Mefenamic acid	2–4	2	>90	–
Meloxicam	4–5	15–20	99	11.2
Nabumetone	–[e]	22–30	99	1.5
Naproxen	2–4	12–16	99	0.1
Oxaprozin	1.5–3.5	≥40	99	0.4
Piroxicam	3–5	50	99	0.1
Sodium salicylate	1–2	2–12	60–80	–
Sulindac	–[e]	8	93–98	0.1
Tolmetin	0.5–1	1–5	99	0.4
Valdecoxib	3	8–11	98	28

[a]For regular-release tablet or capsule taken orally without food in the stomach.
[b]Determined in whole blood.
[c]Paracetamol in many countries.
[d]Low affinity for both isoforms of COX.
[e]Converted rapidly to an active metabolite.

well as the periphery, including arthritis (Chapter 35) and gout (Chapter 32).

One mechanism by which the perioperative administration of NSAIDs reduces postoperative pain is by minimizing procedure-induced tissue inflammation. For example, NSAIDs are administered prior to surgical removal of mandibular third molars to limit the development of peripheral and central sensitization and ultimately reduce postoperative pain. Topical administration of NSAIDs is used during ophthalmic surgeries to maintain pupil dilation, reduce postoperative inflammation, and minimize pain and discomfort.

The adequacy of the therapeutic effect (and adverse effects) of the NSAIDs varies, and one NSAID may be preferred over another based upon the selectivity margin of the drug for COX-2 versus COX-1 (Table 29.2).

Platelet Aggregation

The dynamic interplay at the platelet-endothelium interface between mediators of proaggregation/vasoconstriction and antiaggregation/vasodilation influences the outcome of arterial insufficiency, thrombosis, and ischemia (Chapter 46). COX-1 produces TXA_2 in platelets, which has a proaggregation effect and produces vasoconstriction. COX-2 produces PGI_2 in endothelial cells, which has an antiaggregation effect and produces vasodilation. Therapeutic strategies with aspirin to reduce thrombosis strive to maximize its effects on platelet COX-1 while sparing endothelial cell COX-2. As mentioned, aspirin irreversibly inhibits COX by covalent acetylation, and because platelets lack nuclei and cannot synthesize new COX-1, the aspirin-induced deficient production of

TXA_2 by platelets continues for the life of the platelet, which can exceed 10 days. In contrast, vascular COX-2 can be replaced within a few hours by resynthesis in endothelial cells, and thus a low dose of aspirin can be used to reduce the risk of recurrent myocardial infarction, stroke, and vascular death.

The selective COX-2 inhibitors reduce the production of PGI_2, which has an antiaggregation effect, but does not affect the production of TXA_2, which has a proaggregation effect. Thus these compounds are associated with an increased risk of adverse cardiovascular events. These effects are illustrated in Fig. 29.2.

The nonselective, reversible NSAIDs are also associated with an increased risk of adverse cardiovascular events, particularly in patients with known cardiovascular disease. The absolute risk of adverse cardiovascular events in patients who have not been diagnosed with cardiovascular disease is small when treating with standard doses of nonselective NSAIDs.

Ductus Arteriosus

The ductus arteriosus, which is the blood vessel connecting the pulmonary artery to the proximal descending aorta in the developing fetus, generally closes spontaneously at birth. In some cases, especially in infants born prematurely, it remains patent (open) so that 90% of the cardiac output is shunted away from the lungs. The patency of the vessel seems to be maintained as a result of the high production of PGs after delivery. Neonates with certain congenital heart defects depend on an open ductus arteriosus for survival until corrective surgery can be performed. These defects include interruption of the aortic arch, transposition of the great vessels, and pulmonary atresia or stenosis. In this situation, PGE₁ (alprostadil) can be administered by continuous intravenous infusion or by catheter through the umbilical vein to maintain dilation of the ductus until surgery. When surgical ligation is not indicated, the NSAIDs indomethacin and ibuprofen can be administered intravenously to inhibit PG production and close the ductus arteriosus.

PHARMACOKINETICS

All of the antipyretic analgesics have good oral bioavailability, ranging from 80%–100%, and are distributed throughout the body. Some are formulated as rectal suppositories or topical preparations and have good bioavailability by those routes as well. Ketorolac is often administered parenterally; bioavailability via intravenous administration is essentially 100%. The pharmacokinetic parameters for the NSAIDs and acetaminophen are shown in Table 29.2.

Aspirin (acetylsalicylic acid) has a low pK_a and is well absorbed from the acidic environment of the stomach and duodenum, the part of the gastrointestinal (GI) tract largely responsible for absorption of orally administered NSAIDs. Aspirin has a plasma half-life of only 15 minutes because it undergoes rapid hydrolysis to salicylic acid, which has therapeutic effects similar to those of the parent drug. The half-life of salicylic acid ranges from 2–3 hours at doses used to treat pain and fever, to as high as 12 hours at doses sometimes used to treat inflammatory disorders. Approximately 75% is conjugated with glycine in the liver to form the inactive salicyluric acid, which is excreted by the kidneys, along with glucuronide conjugates and 10% free salicylic acid. The limited hepatic pool of glycine and glucuronide available for conjugation results in elimination of salicylate by first-order kinetics at low doses and by zero-order kinetics at higher doses. This accounts for the increasing half-life with increasing dose. At alkaline pH, up to 30% of a dose may be excreted as free salicylic acid, which is why sodium bicarbonate is administered to alkalinize the urine for the treatment of aspirin overdose. The effects of pH on the excretion of salicylic acid are shown in Fig. 29.3.

Other NSAIDs are metabolized to inactive compounds in the liver by cytochrome P450 enzymes and other pathways. Some drugs, such as naproxen and indomethacin, are demethylated before being conjugated and excreted. Piroxicam and fenoprofen are hydroxylated, whereas ibuprofen and meclofenamate are hydroxylated and carboxylated before they are conjugated with glucuronic acid and excreted. Sulindac is somewhat unique because it is metabolized to an active sulfide and undergoes extensive enterohepatic cycling, accounting for its relatively long elimination half-life. Nabumetone, like sulindac, is a prodrug; approximately 35% undergoes rapid hepatic metabolism to the active compound 6-methoxy-2-naphthylacetic acid.

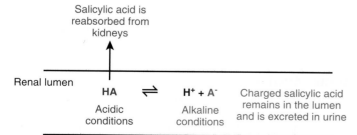

FIG. 29.3 Effect of pH on Salicylic Acid Excretion. In acidic conditions, salicylic acid is protonated and uncharged, which enables diffusion across the renal lumen and reabsorption into the body. In alkaline conditions, more of the salicylic acid is in the unprotonated, charged form favoring its urinary excretion.

Approximately half of the NSAIDs now in clinical use are cleared from the body rapidly and have an elimination half-life <6 hours, whereas others have a longer duration of action, with half-lives in excess of 8 hours. Because the liver plays a key role in inactivating (or activating) and excreting NSAIDs, drug doses should be adjusted and some drugs avoided entirely in patients with impaired hepatic function. Most NSAIDs are highly bound to plasma proteins, especially albumin, creating the potential for interactions with other drugs that also bind extensively to plasma proteins. The binding of some NSAIDs is saturable, and free drug concentration rises at higher doses.

Acetaminophen (paracetamol in many countries), like the NSAIDs, is a weak acid that is almost completely absorbed from the GI tract and the rectum. Peak plasma concentration is achieved within 1 hour, and distribution is relatively uniform throughout the body. Acetaminophen is converted almost completely to inactive metabolites in the liver. A small proportion is oxidatively metabolized via cytochrome P450 enzymes to N-acetyl-p-benzoquinone imine (NAPQI), which is conjugated with sulfhydryl groups in glutathione and excreted.

PHARMACOVIGILANCE: ADVERSE EFFECTS AND DRUG INTERACTIONS

GI Effects

Epigastric distress is the most common side effect produced by the NSAIDs and the one most likely to cause a patient to stop taking an NSAID. Symptoms include nausea, dyspepsia, heartburn, and abdominal discomfort. While a single dose of aspirin will rarely cause clinically significant GI irritation, repeated dosing of low-dose aspirin causes gastroesophageal reflux and dyspepsia in 15%–20% of patients. The incidence and severity of GI effects are increased by the dose and duration of NSAID administration. Antiinflammatory doses of aspirin taken chronically result in peptic ulcers in 15%–25% of patients and major upper GI events such as ulceration, bleeding, and perforation in 2%–5% of patients.

The adverse GI effects are due to two distinct actions. The first is a physical interaction between the drug and the gastric mucosa and can be reduced by taking the medication with meals and with adequate amounts of fluids to facilitate complete dissolution of tablets. The second is due to COX-1 inhibition and the resultant loss of the cytoprotective effects of PGE₁ and PGE₂ in the gastric mucosa. Because the selective COX-2 inhibitors largely spare COX-1, they produce a lower incidence of significant upper GI complications than do nonselective NSAIDs.

Acetaminophen produces minimal GI side effects, even with prolonged administration, and is a good alternative for patients who require an analgesic but cannot tolerate the GI effects of NSAIDs.

Renal Effects

The eicosanoids have only a modest role in renal homeostasis under normal physiological conditions—that is, PGE₂ inhibits Na⁺ and K⁺ reabsorption. The NSAIDs have little effect on renal function in healthy individuals, with the most common side effects being transient fluid retention and edema. However, in patients who have either actual or effective circulatory volume depletion (e.g., congestive heart failure or renal insufficiency), renal perfusion is maintained largely by PGI₂. Thus these patients are at greater risk to develop edema and other NSAID-induced renal side effects such as hyperkalemia, hypertension, interstitial nephritis, and rarely, renal failure. For the most part, side effects are dose dependent and reversible. The kidney is one of several tissues in which COX-2 is expressed constitutively; thus renal side effects also occur with COX-2–selective NSAIDs.

Cardiovascular Effects

Aspirin and other nonselective NSAIDs prolong bleeding time by inhibiting COX-1 in platelets, preventing the synthesis of TXA_2. Clinical manifestations of this effect are usually negligible because TXA_2 is only one of several mediators of platelet aggregation. Upper GI bleeding is the most common spontaneous bleeding event associated with the use of nonselective NSAIDs. Inhibition of clotting can also be a concern during surgical procedures, particularly in patients with impaired hemostasis or taking other drugs that inhibit clotting. Selective COX-2 inhibitors do not inhibit platelet aggregation or prolong bleeding time because COX-2 is not expressed in platelets. On the other hand, selective COX-2 inhibitors can increase the incidence of major cardiovascular events (e.g., myocardial infarction) in high-risk patients because they prevent the production of PGI_2 in vascular epithelial cells, which inhibits platelet aggregation without the benefit of blocking TXA_2 production in platelets.

CNS Effects

Aspirin can cause salicylism, a syndrome characterized by tinnitus, hearing loss, dizziness, confusion, and even headache. Salicylism is dose dependent and reversible. It is usually associated with high doses, but sensitive individuals may experience these effects after a single analgesic dose.

Hypersensitivity

Hypersensitivity to aspirin occurs in a small percentage of the population and is manifest by an anaphylactic reaction that can include rhinitis, urticaria, flushing, hypotension, and bronchial asthma. Middle-aged patients with asthma, nasal polyps, or urticaria are at a higher risk for aspirin hypersensitivity than the general population. The mechanisms are unknown but may be due to increased levels of lipoxygenase products formed by diversion of AA metabolism. Patients with aspirin hypersensitivity also are hypersensitive to other nonselective NSAIDs. Although there is no current evidence for hypersensitivity to selective COX-2 inhibitors, these drugs are not recommended for use in patients with known NSAID hypersensitivity.

Reye Syndrome

Although a causal relationship has yet to be established, there is a significant epidemiological relationship between the use of aspirin in children with certain viral infections (e.g., influenza or chickenpox) and the occurrence of Reye syndrome, which can result in brain swelling and liver dysfunction. It is not known if similar relationships exist for other NSAIDs. Because of these uncertainties, acetaminophen has become the drug of choice for treating fever in children.

Acute Overdose

Acute overdose with aspirin results in effects not manifest at therapeutic doses and includes ventilatory changes, metabolic acidosis, nausea, vomiting, hyperthermia, and stupor, as shown in Table 29.3. Treatment, which is largely supportive, depends upon the severity of intoxication determined by measuring plasma salicylate levels and includes gastric lavage, alkalinizing the urine, cooling the body, and intravenous fluids containing bicarbonate and glucose. Acute aspirin overdose is a leading cause of accidental poisoning in children.

Acute overdose or chronic daily administration of acetaminophen may result in liver toxicity as a consequence of the cytochrome P450–mediated production of hepatotoxic amounts of NAPQI (Fig. 29.4). Although NAPQI is normally inactivated through its binding to glutathione sulfhydryl groups, if the glutathione content of the liver is

decreased by disease, fasting, or acute acetaminophen overdose, then NAPQI can interact with sulfhydryl-containing hepatocellular proteins, leading to hepatic necrosis. Hepatotoxicity can occur in adults after a single ingestion of 7.5 g of acetaminophen or after lower doses (4–7.4 g/day) under conditions that enhance the oxidative metabolism of acetaminophen. Symptoms that occur within the first 24 hours are relatively nonspecific and include lethargy, nausea, and anorexia. Indicators of abnormal liver function appear gradually over the next few days, followed by jaundice, coagulation defects, other signs of hepatic necrosis, and finally hepatic failure. Overdose is treated with N-acetylcysteine, which restores hepatic glutathione. Early treatment is essential to prevent or minimize hepatic damage.

The adverse events associated with the use of the NSAIDs and acetaminophen are summarized in the Clinical Problems Box.

NEW DEVELOPMENTS

Epidemiological data suggest that inhibitors of COX-1 and COX-2 might prevent the initiation and progression of several cancers. The strongest association between NSAID use and a decreased development of cancer has been demonstrated for colorectal cancer. Additional studies are emerging, which suggest that multiple cancers, for which inflammation plays a large role in the expansion and metastasis of tumor growth, are also inhibited by NSAIDs. Research is ongoing to elucidate how modulation of PG synthesis and metabolism could alter local inflammation and the immune response, platelet activity, or the activation of the WNT/β-catenin pathway to decrease the initiation and maintenance of tumorigenesis.

CLINICAL RELEVANCE FOR HEALTHCARE PROFESSIONALS

Because the NSAIDs and acetaminophen are commonly used over-the-counter medications, many individuals use these drugs on a chronic basis and may not be aware of their potential toxicities. It is imperative for all healthcare professionals to educate their patients to avoid potential adverse effects.

TABLE 29.3 Relationship Between Blood Salicylate Levels and Therapeutic and Toxic Effects

Increasing Salicylate Blood Levels	Effect	Consequence
↓	Analgesia, antipyresis Antiinflammatory	
	Salicylism	Tinnitus, dizziness, nausea
	Hyperventilation	Respiratory alkalosis
	Disrupted carbohydrate metabolism, sweating, vomiting, uncoupled oxidative phosphorylation, depressed respiration, increasing acidosis and body temperature	Metabolic acidosis, dehydration, hyperthermia, respiratory acidosis, delirium, convulsions, coma

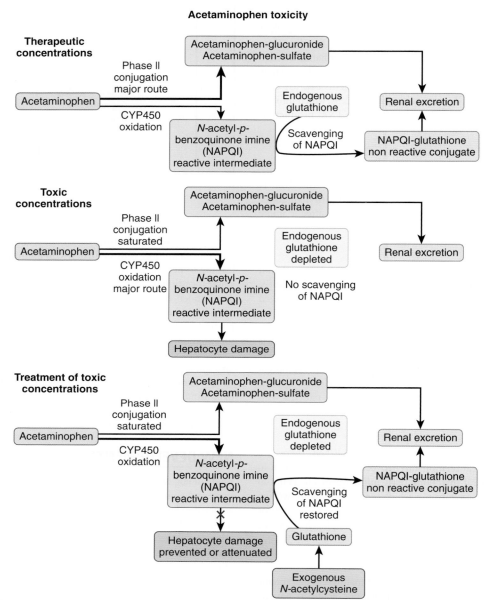

FIG. 29.4 Acetaminophen Toxicity. At therapeutic concentrations, acetaminophen is primarily glucuronidated and excreted by the kidneys. Oxidative metabolism is a minor pathway and results in the formation of the toxic metabolite NAPQI, which is normally scavenged by glutathione. At high concentrations of acetaminophen, NAPQI accumulates and can lead to hepatotoxicity; N-acetylcysteine is administered to replenish glutathione. (Courtesy Bardal SK, Waechter JE, Martin DS. *Toxicology*. In: *Applied Pharmacology*. St. Louis: Saunders; 2011.)

CLINICAL PROBLEMS

NSAIDs
GI tract disturbances
Renal dysfunction
Prolonged bleeding time (Chapter 46)
Hypersensitivity reactions
Salicylism
Interactions with highly plasma protein–bound drugs

Acetaminophen
Hepatic toxicity

TRADE NAMES

In addition to generic and fixed-combination preparations, the following trade-named materials are some of the important compounds available in the United States.
NSAIDs
Celecoxib (Celebrex)
Diclofenac (Cataflam, Voltaren)
Diflunisal (Dolobid)
Etodolac (Lodine)
Fenoprofen (Nalfon)
Flurbiprofen (Ansaid)
Ibuprofen (Advil, Motrin, Nuprin)
Indomethacin (Indocin)
Ketoprofen (Orudis)
Ketorolac (Toradol)
Meclofenamic acid (Meclomen)
Mefenamic acid (Ponstel)
Meloxicam (Mobic)
Nabumetone (Relafen)
Naproxen (Aleve, Anaprox, Naprosyn)
Oxaprozin (Daypro)
Piroxicam (Feldene)
Sodium salicylate (Uracel)
Sulindac (Clinoril)
Tolmetin (Tolectin)
Acetaminophen (Tylenol)

SELF-ASSESSMENT QUESTIONS

1. A 10-year-old girl recovering from leg surgery comes into the clinic hyperventilating and sweating and begins to vomit. You talk to her mother and find out that her daughter had a high fever last night, and she gave her "something" to alleviate it. Which of the following drugs is likely the cause?
   A. Aspirin.
   B. Ibuprofen.
   C. Acetaminophen.
   D. Morphine.
   E. Lidocaine.

2. Sally overslept and was in a rush to get dressed so that she would not be late for work. As a consequence, she slipped on the shower floor and sprained her ankle. Which of the following would not be helpful in this situation?
   A. Aspirin
   B. Ibuprofen
   C. Naproxen
   D. Celecoxib
   E. Acetaminophen

3. The FDA recommends that individuals taking the COX-2 inhibitor celecoxib should take a drug holiday to decrease the risk associated with this drug. The increased risk associated with the chronic use of COX-2 inhibitors may be attributed to:
   A. Gastrointestinal bleeding.
   B. Renal insufficiency.
   C. Respiratory depression.
   D. Increased platelet aggregation.
   E. A hypersensitivity reaction.

4. How does naproxen control the pain of an inflamed temporomandibular joint?
   A. It inhibits the activation of sodium channels and prevents abnormal signal transmission.
   B. It inhibits COX and prevents the formation of prostaglandins.
   C. It stimulates μ receptors and inhibits the release of neurotransmitters in the spinal cord.
   D. It is an agonist at spinal cord prostanoid receptors.
   E. It has both monoaminergic and opioid effects in the CNS.

5. The NSAIDs are used on a chronic basis by many who suffer headache and inflammation. Many individuals do not realize that the chronic use of these compounds can lead to major adverse effects on which organ system(s)?
   A. Cardiovascular.
   B. Hepatic.
   C. Renal.
   D. Gastrointestinal.
   E. None of the above.

FURTHER READING

Gupta A, Bah M. NSAIDs in the treatment of postoperative pain. *Curr Pain Headache Rep*. 2016;0:62.

Liao Z, Mason KA, Milas L. Cyclooxygenase-2 and its inhibition in cancer: Is there a role? *Drugs*. 2007;67:821–845.

Patrono C. Cardiovascular effects of cyclooxygenase-2 inhibitors: a mechanistic and clinical perspective. *Br J Clin Pharmacol*. 2016;82(4):957–964.

WEBSITES

http://www.mayoclinic.org/diseases-conditions/reyes-syndrome/basics/definition/con-20020083
This website is maintained by the Mayo Clinic and is a resource on Reye syndrome.

https://livertox.nih.gov/Acetaminophen.htm
This website is maintained by the American College of Emergency Physicians and presents information on acetaminophen toxicity and treatment.

Cannabinoids as Analgesics

Rex M. Philpot and Lynn Wecker

MAJOR DRUG CLASSES

Phytocannabinoids
Synthetic cannabinoids

ABBREVIATIONS

2-AG	2-Arachidonoylglycerol
AEA	Arachidonoylethanolamide; anandamide
CBD	Cannabidiol
CNS	Central nervous system
FAAH	Fatty acid amide hydrolase
GPCR	G-protein–coupled receptor
PPAR	Peroxisome proliferator-activated receptor
THC	Δ^9-Tetrahydrocannabinol
TRPV1	Transient receptor potential vanilloid receptor 1

THERAPEUTIC OVERVIEW

The cannabis plant has been used as a source of medicine since antiquity, evidenced in some of the earliest written documents, and prominent in the United States pharmacopeia in the early 20th century. Popular lore, anecdotal evidence, and historical indications for cannabis use across various cultures support the therapeutic potential of this plant for several disorders. Unfortunately, investigations into the scientific basis for the use of cannabis and the cannabinoids, the unique active compounds in cannabis, have been limited by regulatory barriers, such as schedule I classification of the plant. Additionally, the development of cannabinoids as therapeutic agents has been tempered by the perceived risk of medicinal use progressing to substance use disorders. Although cannabinoids from plants, the phytocannabinoids, have not been approved for medical use in the United States, two synthetic compounds were approved more than 30 years ago for medical use: namely, dronabinol and nabilone.

The use of botanical cannabis, or marijuana, is on the rise in the United States, supported by a patchwork of state laws that allow for medicinal use of at least some forms of cannabis across a majority of states. Since 1996, 28 states, plus the District of Columbia, have approved the use of cannabis or cannabis-derived products for medicinal purposes, and at the time of writing, another 16 states allow the use of specific cannabinoids for medicinal use.

Although the evidence is incomplete for most medical applications of cannabis, owing to a limited number of evidence-based clinical studies and case reports, the cannabinoids may have therapeutic value for a diverse array of clinical conditions. Scientific support for the use of the cannabinoids is conclusive/substantial for pain control and as an antiemetic, and most recently, evidence has supported use for severe forms of childhood epilepsy. The strength or lack of scientific support for the use of cannabinoids for other medical disorders ranges from insufficient to moderate and is summarized in the Therapeutic Overview Box.

MECHANISMS OF ACTION

The Endocannabinoid System

Studies have shown that the cannabinoids exert widespread effects on numerous systems throughout the body, mediated primarily through

THERAPEUTIC OVERVIEW

Strength of evidence	Indications
Conclusive/Substantial	Chronic pain in adults
	Chemotherapy-induced nausea/vomiting
Moderate	Severe forms of epilepsy in children including Dravet syndrome and Lennox-Gastaut syndrome
	AIDS-associated cachexia
	Patient-reported spasticity associated with multiple sclerosis
	Sleep disturbances associated with obstructive sleep apnea, fibromyalgia, chronic pain, and multiple sclerosis
Limited to insufficient	Posttraumatic stress disorder, social anxiety disorder, Tourette syndrome, traumatic brain injury, addiction, amyotrophic lateral sclerosis, cancer, dystonia, Huntington disease, irritable bowel syndrome, Parkinson disease, schizophrenia, spasticity related to spinal cord injury

actions on cannabinoid receptors. These receptors are part of the endogenous cannabinoid system, which is comprised of the cannabinoid receptors, the endogenous cannabinoids (endocannabinoids), and the enzymes involved in the synthesis and degradation of the endocannabinoids. This system is thought to play a pivotal role in diverse functions including, but not limited to, pain modulation, inflammation, nervous system development, and gastrointestinal and hepatic function.

Cannabinoid Receptors

Two cannabinoid receptors have been identified to date, CB_1 and CB_2. These are $G_{i/o}$-protein–coupled receptors, with activation leading to inhibition of adenylyl cyclase and activation of mitogen-activated protein kinases (MAPKs). In addition, CB_1 receptors inhibit N-type and P/Q-type calcium channels and activate inwardly rectifying potassium channels. Both CB_1 and CB_2 receptors have allosteric binding sites and are phosphorylated by G-protein–coupled receptor (GPCR) kinases and associate with arrestins.

CB_1 receptors are prevalent at nerve terminals in both the central (CNS) and peripheral (PNS) nervous systems, where they function to attenuate the release of several neurotransmitters, including acetylcholine, dopamine, γ-aminobutyric acid, glutamate, histamine, norepinephrine, and serotonin. Very high levels of CB_1 receptors are expressed by both neurons and astrocytes in the cerebral cortex, hippocampus, basal ganglia, basolateral amygdala, thalamus, and cerebellum, all of which are involved in the perception of nociceptive stimuli. They are also expressed in the periaqueductal gray (PAG) matter of the midbrain and in the substantia gelatinosa and dorsal horn of the spinal cord, supporting the role of CB_1 receptors in the processing of nociceptive information and pain. CB_1 receptors are also expressed by immune and nonneuronal cells, and these receptors have been detected in numerous organs including, but not limited to, the adrenal gland, gastrointestinal tract, liver, skeletal muscle, heart, and lung, albeit at lower levels than CB_2 receptors. CB_1 receptors on primary afferent neurons, primarily on myelinated A-fibers, as well as those on mast cells, are believed to modulate the pain associated with inflammation. Thus evidence supports a pain-modulating role for CB_1 receptors at both peripheral and central levels.

CB_2 receptors are expressed primarily by immune cells, including lymphocytes, monocytes, and macrophages, and are present in the tonsils, spleen, and thymus. These receptors are also expressed by microglia, astrocytes, and some neurons and have been identified on transient receptor potential vanilloid receptor 1 (TRPV1)-positive nociceptive neurons in dorsal root ganglia (Chapter 25). Interestingly, the expression of CB_2 receptors is induced markedly following peripheral nerve damage and inflammation, and activation modulates the migration of immune cells in both the CNS and PNS and inhibits the release of proinflammatory cytokines by nonneuronal cells in areas near the nerve terminals of nociceptive neurons. Thus activation of CB_2 receptors, especially following an inflammatory response, also contributes to the pain-modulating effects of the cannabinoids.

Endocannabinoids

The endocannabinoids are eicosanoids derived from arachidonic acid (Chapter 29) and include arachidonoylethanolamide (anandamide; AEA), 2-arachidonoylglycerol (2-AG), 2-arachidonyl glyceryl (noladin) ether, and O-arachidonoyl ethanolamine (virodhamine), with anandamide and 2-AG the best characterized. Like other eicosanoids and unlike classical neurotransmitters, the endocannabinoids are synthesized and released on demand rather than stored. Further, they are engaged in retrograde signaling, activating presynaptic receptors. The synthesis and degradation of anandamide and 2-AG are shown in Fig. 30.1.

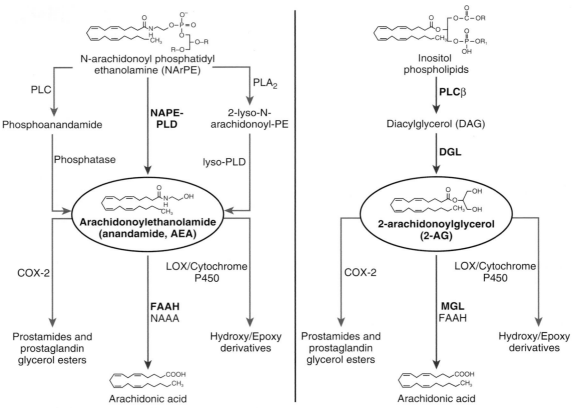

FIG. 30.1 Synthetic and Degradative Pathways for the Endocannabinoids. Arachidonoylethanolamide (anandamide, AEA) and 2-arachidonoylglycerol (2-AG) are synthesized from membrane lipids and catabolized as shown with the major pathways in red. Abbreviations: *COX-2*, Cyclooxygenase-2; *DAG*, diacylglycerol; *DGL*, diacylglycerol lipase; *FAAH*, fatty acid amide hydrolase; *LOX*, lipoxygenase; *lyso-PLD*, lysophospholipase D; *MGL*, monoacylglycerol lipase; *NAAA*, N-acyl-ethanolamine-hydrolyzing acid amidase; *NAPE-PLD*, N-acyl-phosphatidylethanolamine-specific phospholipase D; *PLA₂*, phospholipase A₂; *PLC*, phospholipase C.

Anandamide is synthesized primarily via the phospholipase D–mediated enzymatic hydrolysis of the membrane lipid precursor N-arachidonoyl phosphatidyl ethanolamine (NArPE), the latter derived from phosphatidylethanolamine. It can also be synthesized via two parallel pathways, the first catalyzed by phospholipase C with phosphoanandamide produced as an intermediate, followed by dephosphorylation, and the second mediated by phospholipase A$_2$, followed by lysophospholipase D cleavage. Following release and receptor activation, anandamide is actively taken back into cells and catabolized primarily to arachidonic acid by the hydrolytic action of fatty acid amide hydrolase (FAAH). It can also be metabolized by enzymes involved in the arachidonic acid cascade, cyclooxygenase-2 (COX-2), and lipoxygenases (LOXs), as well as by cytochrome P450s.

The synthesis of 2-AG is mediated by the hydrolysis of membrane phospholipids by the action of phospholipase C to yield the intracellular second messenger diacylglycerol (DAG), followed by cleavage by diacylglycerol lipase (DGL), the latter reaction process activated by calcium. Released 2-AG is subsequently taken into cells and hydrolyzed to arachidonic acid by monoacylglycerol lipase (MGL). 2-AG can also be catabolized by enzymes of the arachidonic acid cascade and cytochrome P450s.

Both anandamide and 2-AG are synthesized in postsynaptic neurons from which they are released and bind to presynaptic CB$_1$ and CB$_2$ receptors with high affinity to inhibit neurotransmitter release; anandamide has greater affinity for these receptors than 2-AG. However, the levels of anandamide in brain are 100 times lower than those of 2-AG. In addition to the activation of CB$_1$ and CB$_2$ receptors, the endocannabinoids activate several other receptors, including TRPV1 channels and peroxisome proliferator–activated receptors (PPARs). TRPV1 channels are located primarily on nociceptive neurons and in the hippocampus, cerebral cortex, and substantia nigra. These channels are gated by chemical stimuli and temperature (Chapter 25) and are sensitized by lipid neuromodulators, such as the endocannabinoids. Indeed, high concentrations of anandamide have been shown to increase postsynaptic currents via activation of these channels; 2-AG has no effect at TRPV1 channels. Several PPARs are activated by the endocannabinoids. Both anandamide and 2-AG activate PPARα, which is involved in feeding and the regulation of fat metabolism and body weight, as well as neuroprotection, and PPARγ, mediating the antiinflammatory effects of these endocannabinoids.

Phytocannabinoids

Over 100 different phytocannabinoids have been identified in cannabis. Phytocannabinoids exist in the plant as carboxylic acid precursors (i.e., Δ^9-tetrahydrocannabinolic acid and cannabidiolic acid) that are decarboxylated by light or heat (Fig. 30.2). Of the numerous phytocannabinoids, only Δ^9-tetrahydrocannbinol (THC) and cannabidiol (CBD) are known to activate cannabinoid receptors. THC is a high-affinity

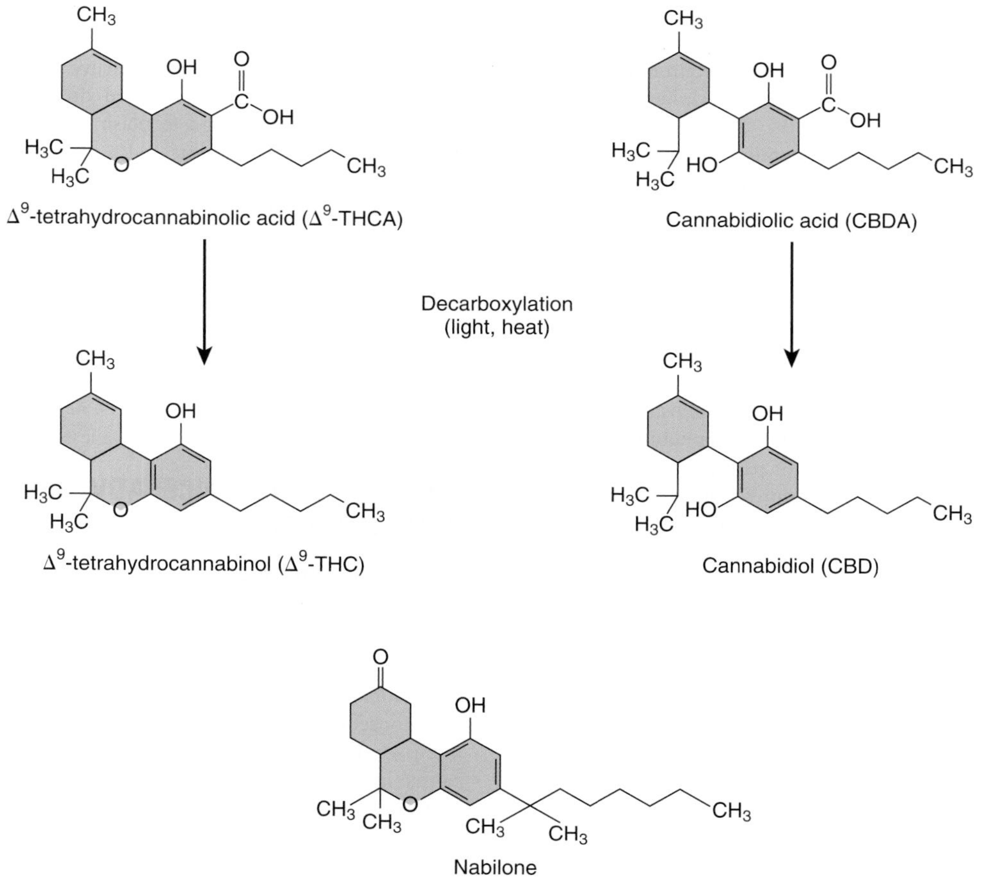

FIG. 30.2 Structures of the Phytocannabinoids. These compounds exist as carboxylic acid precursors in plants that are decarboxylated by light and heat to the active compounds Δ^9-THC and CBD. Also shown is the structure of nabilone.

partial agonist at CB_1 and CB_2 receptors, while CBD has a low affinity for these receptors. THC and CBD also activate TRPV1 channels, with CBD more potent than THC. Both THC and CBD activate PPARγ but not PPARα.

In addition to actions at these receptors, the phytocannabinoids have been shown to affect several orphan GPCRs, including GRP55 and GPR18. Of these, GPR55 is highly expressed in dorsal root ganglia neurons and is activated by THC but not CBD. Similarly, GRP18 is expressed in microglia and appears to modulate microglial-neuronal interactions. THC is an agonist, while CBD appears to act as an antagonist at this receptor. The functional implications of these interactions are equivocal.

Synthetic Cannabinoids

Several synthetic cannabinoids have been developed over the years. Dronabinol is the (−)-*trans*-isomer of THC, which is 6–100 times more potent than the (+)-*trans*-isomer. Nabilone is a THC analogue whose structure is shown in Fig. 30.2. Both compounds act at CB_1 and CB_2 receptors. Nabilone is more efficacious than THC.

RELATIONSHIP OF MECHANISMS OF ACTION TO CLINICAL RESPONSE

THC and CBD have antinociceptive and antiinflammatory activity mediated by central and peripheral CB_1 and CB_2 receptors, as well as TRPV1 channels, PPARγ, and possibly orphan GPCRs. THC, which has higher psychoactive potency than CBD, also appears to have the greater analgesic activity, with a potency comparable to that of the opioids. Further, low doses of THC devoid of psychoactive effects have been shown to decrease neuropathic pain. In addition, several analogues of CBD that do not cross the blood-brain barrier retain antinociceptive and antiinflammatory activity, supporting a peripherally mediated action.

The cannabinoids modulate the perception of pain at the central level, as well as the peripheral activation of pain receptors. Multiple randomized and controlled clinical studies have demonstrated that the cannabinoids are effective for alleviating both acute and chronic pain. Indeed, studies have demonstrated that smoking marijuana significantly decreased HIV-associated neuropathic pain and significantly attenuated capsaicin-induced pain responses in healthy volunteers. Further, several studies have shown dose-dependent effects for several pain conditions.

In addition to structured clinical trials, several published case reports and anecdotal evidence have demonstrated that cannabinoids decrease the doses of opioid analgesics required for pain control. Interestingly, the annual opioid mortality rates and use of prescription pain medications in states with medical cannabis laws are lower than in states without such laws.

The synthetic THC analogue nabilone is approved for the treatment of chemotherapy-related nausea and vomiting, while dronabinol is approved for the treatment of chemotherapy-related nausea and vomiting and for the stimulation of appetite and weight gain in AIDS patients (Chapter 20). Although these agents are not currently approved as analgesics, patients with fibromyalgia have reported a significant reduction in pain with nabilone compared to placebo.

PHARMACOKINETICS

Phytocannabinoids

The pharmacokinetics of THC and CBD are highly dependent on the method of intake. When cannabis is smoked, approximately 30% of the THC is lost due to pyrolysis, with the remaining 70% delivered to the lungs and bloodstream. Because THC is highly lipid soluble, it distributes rapidly and quickly diffuses across the blood-brain barrier, leading to a rapid onset. Blood levels of THC peak about 30 minutes following inhalation and subside within 1–3.5 hours. When cannabis is consumed, bioavailability is low and variable (6%–20%), the onset of effects is between 0.5 and 2 hours after ingestion, and the effects are prolonged relative to inhaled THC, subsiding within 5–8 hours.

THC is metabolized in the liver to more than 20 compounds, the majority of which are inactive. The major metabolite, 11-OH-THC, formed by the action of CYP2C9, is the most important active psychotropic metabolite, while the further oxidation of 11-OH-THC yields THC-COOH, which is the most important nonpsychotropic metabolite, with antiinflammatory and analgesic properties. Plasma concentrations of 11-OH-THC following ingestion of cannabis increase to approximately 10% of the initial concentration of THC, with the presence of this long-lasting metabolite likely contributing to the prolonged effects of ingested cannabis. Approximately 70% of THC is excreted within 72 hours of intake.

Similar to THC, CBD is rapidly absorbed following inhalation, with peak plasma levels in 10–12 minutes and a duration of effect of 2–3 hours. Following ingestion, only about 6% of CBD reaches the systemic circulation due to extensive first-pass metabolism. The onset of effects of ingested CBD is about 30 minutes, and the duration of effects may last for as many as 12 hours. CBD is excreted intact or as glucuronidated metabolites, with excretion of the parent in the feces twice that as in the urine.

Synthetic Cannabinoids

Dronabinol is almost completely absorbed (90%–95%) following oral administration and undergoes extensive first-pass metabolism, with only 10%–20% of the administered dose reaching the circulation. Dronabinol is highly bound to plasma proteins (>95%) and has an onset of action of 0.5–1 hour and a peak psychoactive effect in 4–6 hours. Dronabinol is metabolized predominantly by hepatic CYP2C9 to the active compound 11-OH-THC; metabolism via CYP3A4 yields inactive metabolites. Dronabinol and its metabolites are excreted in both urine and feces, with biliary excretion representing the major (>50%) route.

Orally administered nabilone is completely absorbed from the gastrointestinal tract, with plasma concentrations peaking within 2 hours and a plasma half-life of approximately 2 hours. It is metabolized extensively by several cytochrome P450 enzymes and is eliminated primarily (>50%) in the feces and to a lesser extent (25%) in the urine.

PHARMACOVIGILANCE: ADVERSE EFFECTS AND DRUG INTERACTIONS

Phytocannabinoids

The adverse effects of the cannabinoids depend on both the route and frequency of administration and involve both psychological and physiological actions. Acute administration can alter perception, lead to confusion, and disrupt attention, as well as cause anxiety and agitation. As a consequence of these perceptual and cognitive effects, cannabis increases the risk of motor vehicle accidents. When used chronically, cannabinoids alter short-term explicit memory.

Cannabinoids also increase symptoms of mania in individuals with bipolar disorder, increase the risk for depression, increase the incidence of suicidal ideation and suicide completion, and increase the incidence of social anxiety disorder. Additionally, statistical evidence supports an association between the chronic use of cannabis and an increased risk

CLINICAL PROBLEMS

Acute cannabinoid exposure	Agitation, anxiety, altered perception, confusion, disrupted attention, conjunctiva redness, diarrhea, dizziness, dry mouth, fatigue, hypotension, nausea, postural imbalance, sedation, tachycardia
Chronic cannabinoid exposure	Hyperemesis syndrome, short-term memory deficits
Smoke-related	Bronchitis, increased pregnancy complications, obstructive pulmonary disease, poor neonatal health
	Heart attack, hemorrhage, and stroke in vulnerable individuals
Dronabinol	Anxiety, altered perception, confusion, fatigue, seizures, delirium, tachycardia, orthostatic hypotension
Nabilone	Anxiety, altered perception, confusion, fatigue, seizures, delirium, tachycardia, orthostatic hypotension

TRADE NAMES

In addition to generic and fixed-combination preparations, the following trade-named materials are some of the important compounds available in the United States.

Dronabinol (Marinol, Syndros)

Nabilone (Cesamet)

Cannabidiol (Epidiolex; currently awaiting FDA approval)

for the development of schizophrenia and other psychoses. However, these outcomes may reflect a relationship between predisposing factors and the tendency to use cannabis rather than a consequence of cannabinoid effects. Further research is warranted.

There have not been any substantiated cases of cannabinoid-induced fatalities in humans, indicating that the cannabinoids are relatively safe. However, there is some evidence that the acute use of these agents can precipitate heart attack, ischemic stroke, and/or subarachnoid hemorrhage in vulnerable individuals. Additional adverse effects include conjunctiva redness, fatigue, sedation, hypotension, dry mouth, nausea, diarrhea, dizziness, poor balance, and tachycardia among older adults. The chronic use of cannabinoids can also lead to hyperemesis syndrome, a rare form of cannabinoid toxicity characterized by cyclical episodes of nausea, vomiting, and abdominal pain, symptoms that can be alleviated temporarily by a hot shower or bath and that can be reversed by cessation of cannabis use.

There is substantial evidence that smoking cannabis leads to frequent chronic bronchitis episodes and respiratory symptoms and limited evidence that chronic smoking of cannabis increases the risk of developing chronic obstructive pulmonary disease, not unlike that associated with smoking cigarettes. Cannabis smoking is also associated with increased complications during pregnancy, lower birth weights in offspring, and more frequent admissions to neonatal intensive care units.

Synthetic Cannabinoids

The adverse effects of dronabinol are discussed in Chapter 20 and include dose-related CNS effects similar to the phytocannabinoids. Dronabinol may decrease seizure threshold and has variable effects on the cardiovascular system, including tachycardia and orthostatic hypotension. Dronabinol is additive with other CNS depressants, and CYP2C9 inhibitors or individuals with genetic variants associated with diminished CYP2C9 function exhibit increased plasma levels of dronabinol, while inducers decrease plasma levels.

The adverse effects associated with the use of nabilone include CNS and cardiovascular effects similar to those of dronabinol.

The adverse effects of the cannabinoids are summarized in the Clinical Problems Box.

NEW DEVELOPMENTS

The preclinical literature on cannabinoid pharmacology is rapidly expanding and supports the development of compounds that target several elements of the endocannabinoid system, including direct-acting receptor agonists and degradative enzyme inhibitors. Agents that activate the endocannabinoid system may be particularly useful for alleviating pain, refractory to currently available medications. Drug development in this area is not without issues, particularly developing medications that have a therapeutic effect with lower psychoactivity than THC. To this end, the FAAH inhibitors have been investigated actively. In general, results from clinical trials indicate that these compounds are well tolerated with few side effects. Although a 2016 trial in France of the FAAH inhibitor BIA-10-2474 was terminated when one participant died and five were hospitalized with serious neurological damage, this particular compound has been determined to have numerous off-target effects responsible for the unfortunate outcomes. Although there are no clinical trials scheduled in the United States with other FAAH inhibitors as of the writing of this chapter, the United States Food and Drug Administration has completed a safety review of this class of agents and pledges to work with sponsors for future studies.

CLINICAL RELEVANCE FOR HEALTHCARE PROFESSIONALS

Because the use of cannabinoids continues to increase in concert with major developments in cannabinoid-based therapeutics, all healthcare professionals need to be aware of the effects of the cannabinoids. Professionals also need to be aware of the fact that the types and qualities of cannabinoid preparations in use vary widely, and strains can differ considerably in the content of THC, CBD, and the THC/CBD ratio. Although evidence from controlled scientific studies continues to support the medicinal properties of cannabis, individuals should be discouraged from attempting to self-medicate using unregulated products.

A common concern for medical professionals considering the use of cannabinoids for the treatment of a health-related condition is the risk for misuse or progression to a substance use disorder. However, evidence to date indicates that transitioning from medical to problematic use of a cannabinoid is rare. The most common risk factors for transitioning to problematic use are the presence of depression or sleep disturbances. An additional concern is that the medical use of cannabinoids will act as a "gateway" to the abuse of other substances; however, there is little scientific evidence to support the idea that the use of cannabinoids leads to other substance use disorders.

SELF-ASSESSMENT QUESTIONS

1. There is conclusive evidence-based support for the use of cannabinoids for the treatment of which condition?
   A. Parkinson disease.
   B. Traumatic brain injury.
   C. Cancer.
   D. Chronic pain in adults.
   E. Social anxiety disorder.

2. The ability of the cannabinoids to alleviate pain and inflammation may be attributed to activation of:
   A. CB_1 and CB_2 receptors.
   B. G-protein–coupled receptors.
   C. Transient receptor potential channels.
   D. Peroxisome proliferator-activated receptors.
   E. All of the above.

3. A 35-year-old man experienced chronic pain following removal of a facial tumor that was initially controlled by opioids, but tolerance developed, and he could not increase his drug dose further without toxic effects. The addition of which of the following agents may help alleviate his pain and allow him to decrease his dose of opioids?
   A. Nabilone.
   B. Dronabinol.
   C. CBD.
   D. Anandamide.
   E. None of the above.

4. Which of the following represents a logical target for the development drugs to alleviate pain?
   A. FAAH.
   B. MGL.
   C. PPARs.
   D. TRPV1 channels.
   E. All of the above.

FURTHER READING

Devinsky O, Cross JH, Laux L, et al. Trial of cannabidiol for drug-resistant seizures in the Dravet syndrome. *N Eng J Med.* 2017;376:2011–2020.

Ligresti A, De Petrocellis L, Di Marzo V. From phytocannabinoids to cannabinoid receptors and endocannabinoids: pleiotropic physiological and pathological roles through complex pharmacology. *Physiol Rev.* 2016;96:1593–1659.

Manzanares J, Julian MD, Carrascosa A. Role of the cannabinoid system in pain control and therapeutic implications for the management of acute and chronic pain episodes. *Curr Neuropharmacol.* 2006;4:239–257.

National Academies of Sciences, Engineering, and Medicine. *The Health Effects of Cannabis and Cannabinoids: The Current State of Evidence and Recommendations for Research.* Washington, DC: The National Academies Press; 2017.

Yuill MB, Hale DE, Guindon J, Morgan DJ. Anti-nociceptive interactions between opioids and a cannabinoid receptor 2 agonist in inflammatory pain. *Mol Pain.* 2017;13:1–15.

WEBSITE

https://nccih.nih.gov/health/marijuana

This website is maintained by the National Institute of Complementary and Integrative Health of the National Institutes of Health and is an excellent resource on medical marijuana.

Treatment of Inflammatory, Allergic, and Immunological Disorders

Drug Therapy for Migraine Headache

D. Samba Reddy

THERAPEUTIC OVERVIEW

Migraine headaches are a common neurological condition with a prevalence of 10%–20% within the adult population. The typical manifestations of migraine headaches are a debilitating throbbing pain around the eyes and temples lasting for hours, nausea, heightened sensitivity to light and sound, and other neurological disturbances. Migraines may be classified into two primary categories, viz., migraine with aura (also referred to as classic migraine) and migraine without aura (common migraine), with several rarer subtypes. Approximately 20%–30% of migraine patients manifest migraine with aura, characterized by flashes of light, blind spots, or tingling in the extremities within 60 minutes prior to headache onset.

According to the American Migraine Study, migraines affect approximately 30 million people in the United States, and migraines affect many adults during their productive years (25–50 years of age), with a threefold greater incidence in women than men. Approximately 80% of patients report a family history of migraines, suggesting a genetic link, with a highly variable frequency and duration. Thus migraine headaches have a significant impact on the quality of life. It is estimated that $13 billion are lost in productivity each year due to the burden of migraines in the United States. Migraines are ranked by the World Health Organization as number 19 among all diseases worldwide causing disability.

The characteristics of migraine are shown in the Therapeutic Overview Box.

Pathophysiology

Both neural and vascular theories of migraine have been posited for more than 50 years, with much debate and controversy. While it is beyond the scope of this chapter to present evidence for or against either theory, studies to date suggest that migraine may represent a neurovascular disorder involving genetic alterations in both neuronal and vascular pathways. It has been suggested that the pathophysiology of migraine may represent an imbalance between excitatory and inhibitory nerve impulse activity, resulting in a hyperexcitable cerebral cortex. Studies suggest that an intense wave of depolarization and increased blood flow over the cerebral cortex, perhaps initiated in the visual or somatosensory areas, leads to a cortical spreading depression (CSD), which is a long-lasting inhibition of neuronal and glial activity, and concomitant decreased cerebral blood flow. The CSD is believed to be responsible for causing the migraine aura and activating trigeminal nerve afferents.

Although the specific contributions of vascular and neural factors are debatable, it is clear that both neuronal activity and blood vessel dilation lead to activation of the trigeminal nerve and that serotonin (5-HT) plays a central role. The 5-HT receptor family is composed of seven distinct subfamilies and, with the exception of the 5-HT$_3$ receptor, are G-protein–coupled receptors distributed throughout the body. The 5-HT$_1$ subfamily is coupled to G$_{i/o}$, and activation leads to inhibition of adenylyl cyclase (Chapter 2). These receptors are located throughout the central nervous system, and presynaptic 5-HT$_{1D}$ and 5-HT$_{1F}$ receptors negatively regulate the release of norepinephrine (NE) and several nociceptive and inflammatory mediators. Specifically, activation of these receptors inhibits the release of calcitonin gene–related peptide (CGRP) and substance P, endogenous compounds that produce inflammation of the pain-sensitive meninges and potently vasodilate affected cranial blood vessels. These mediators also activate and up regulate matrix metalloproteinases, increasing the permeability of the blood-brain barrier. In addition, 5-HT$_{1B}$ receptors are located pre- and postsynaptically and inhibit dopamine (DA), 5-HT, and glutamate release, as well as on cranial arteries (middle meningeal, pial, and temporal) and peripheral

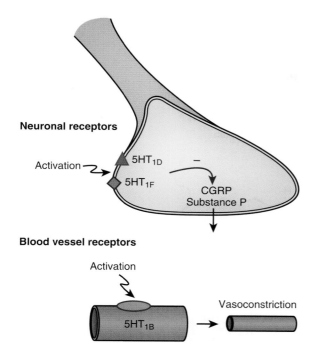

FIG. 31.1 Effects of Serotonin 1 (5-HT₁) Receptor Activation on Neurons and Blood Vessels. The 5-HT$_{1D}$ and 5-HT$_{1F}$ receptors are located presynaptically where they function to inhibit the release of calcitonin gene–related peptide (CGRP) and substance P. 5-HT$_{1B}$ receptors are located on blood vessels where activation leads to vasoconstriction.

(uterine artery and saphenous vein) blood vessels, where they promote vasoconstriction (Fig. 31.1).

THERAPEUTIC OVERVIEW

Migraine Without Aura
Recurrent attacks of moderate to severe intensity lasting 4–72 hours with a pulsating quality and unilateral location. Typically associated with nausea/vomiting or photophobia/phonophobia.

Migraine With Aura
Recurrent attacks lasting minutes that typically develop (from 5–20 minutes) and last for less than 60 minutes with unilateral visual (most common), sensory, speech and/or language, motor, brainstem, or retinal symptoms.

Chronic Migraine
Frequent attacks (more than 15/month) for more than 3 months with more than half having characteristic migraine features.

MECHANISMS OF ACTION

Migraine treatment may be classified as symptomatic (abortive; drugs used only during an attack) or prophylactic (chronic continuous treatment or treatment when a migraine is expected, i.e., menstruation). Symptomatic therapy is the mainstay of migraine management, with the goal of alleviation of symptoms. Further, for treatment considerations, migraine attacks can be classified as: (1) severe (more than three migraines in a month, significant functional impairment, and marked nausea and vomiting); (2) moderate (moderate to severe headache, some impairment of functioning, and nausea); or (3) mild (occasional throbbing headache with no major functional impairment).

Symptomatic Treatment
Triptans and Ergot Alkaloids
Moderate to severe migraine attacks are generally treated with the "triptans," or ergot alkaloids. Triptans are the mainstay of therapy and the most effective drugs for acute migraines. Triptans are indole derivatives, with substituents on the 3 and 5 positions (Fig. 31.2). Sumatriptan was the first triptan marketed in the United States (1992), followed by the development and approval of other triptans, which are similar in efficacy to sumatriptan but differ in pharmacokinetic properties.

The triptans are potent 5-HT$_{1B}$/5-HT$_{1D}$/5-HT$_{1F}$ agonists with little or no affinity for other receptor types or subtypes. Through activation of presynaptic 5-HT$_{1D}$ and 5-HT$_{1F}$ receptors, the triptans inhibit the release of CGRP and other peptides implicated in the dilation of intracranial blood vessels, thereby preventing this effect and contributing to vasoconstriction. Further, triptans also activate 5-HT$_{1B}$ receptors on blood vessels, leading to a direct vasoconstriction. Clinically effective doses of the triptans correlate well with their affinities for 5-HT$_{1B}$/5-HT$_{1D}$/5-HT$_{1F}$ receptors, supporting the hypothesis that these receptors are most likely involved in the mechanism of action of these drugs.

In addition to relieving the pain associated with migraine, triptans also decrease associated nausea and vomiting, which may reflect the 5-HT$_{1B}$ receptor–mediated decreased DA release, similar to the antiemetic effects of the DA-receptor antagonists chlorpromazine or prochlorperazine.

The ergot alkaloids (ergotamine and dihydroergotamine [DHE]) produced by the rye fungus were the first antimigraine drugs available. DHE is an ergotamine analogue wherein the ergotamine molecule is hydrogenated in the 9, 10 position (see Fig. 31.2). The ergot alkaloids are agonists at several 5-HT$_1$ receptors, including 5-HT$_{1A}$, 5-HT$_{1B}$, 5-HT$_{1D}$, and 5-HT$_{1F}$. They also affect 5-HT$_2$, adrenergic, and DA receptors. As a consequence, the ergot alkaloids decrease the release of inflammatory neuropeptides and produce both arterial and venous vasoconstriction, similar to the triptans. These compounds, however, do not alleviate the nausea and vomiting associated with migraines, and thus an antiemetic is often used in conjunction.

Analgesics

Mild to moderate migraines often respond to nonsteroidal antiinflammatory agents (NSAIDs) and acetaminophen, or combinations of these agents with a vasoconstrictor such as caffeine. The mechanism of action of the NSAIDs and acetaminophen are discussed in Chapter 29. In addition, the oral and injected opioids (butorphanol nasal spray) are often prescribed, but should not be considered first-line because they lead to dependence and abuse (Chapters 24 and 28) and may produce a heightened sensitivity to pain.

Prophylactic Treatment

Several groups of drugs are available for the prophylaxis of migraine and are indicated to reduce the frequency, duration, and severity of attacks. This approach is typically used for individuals who experience two or more migraines per week or two or more migraines per month lasting 3 or more days, or those who do not respond to acute treatment. These drugs are also indicated for individuals who cannot tolerate vasoconstrictors.

Several classes of antihypertensives reduce the prevalence of migraines. These agents include: the β-adrenergic receptor blockers propranolol, timolol, and metoprolol, discussed in Chapter 12; the Ca²⁺-channel blockers discussed in Chapter 40; the angiotensin-converting enzyme (ACE) inhibitors and angiotensin-receptor blockers (ARBs) discussed in Chapter 39; the anticonvulsants (topiramate, valproate, and gabapentin) discussed in Chapter 39; several antidepressants (amitriptyline

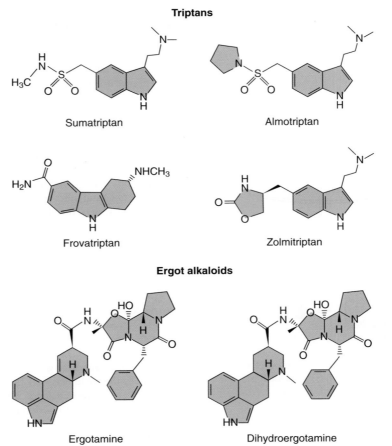

FIG. 31.2 Chemical Structures of Some Triptans and the Ergotamine Alkaloids.

and possibly venlafaxine) discussed in Chapter 17; and the motor-neuron blocker botulinum toxin (discussed in Chapter 22).

RELATIONSHIP OF MECHANISMS OF ACTION TO CLINICAL RESPONSE

The choice of migraine drug or drug combinations for a given patient remains largely empirical. A patient with migraine may be started on monotherapy with an NSAID or a combination regimen chosen to relieve the headache by reducing inflammation. The ergot alkaloids provided a foundation for migraine therapeutics, and the discovery and development of the triptans revolutionized the treatment of acute migraine attacks.

Triptans are highly effective for short-term treatment of acute migraine attacks, and various triptans have comparable efficacy in providing relief. If a specific triptan is ineffective, a different one should be tried before switching to a different class of drugs. The triptans are effective for migraine with or without aura but are not intended for use in prophylaxis of migraine, except frovatriptan, which is used in short-term prophylaxis for menstrual-associated migraine. As indicated, triptans also decrease symptoms of nausea and vomiting, a highly desirable feature. These drugs are considered safe when used appropriately but are contraindicated for patients with cardiovascular disease because they are direct coronary vasoconstrictors.

Ergotamine and dihydroergotamine are used to alleviate migraine headaches with or without aura, but clinical studies have shown that oral ergotamine plus caffeine is less effective than the triptans for acute migraine. The use of these compounds should be restricted for patients

having frequent moderate migraines or infrequent severe migraine attacks.

Route of administration is an important consideration for effective pain relief. Abortive drugs can be given by self-injection, by oral route, or by nasal spray. Although oral preparations have the slowest onset, they are the first choice. Suppositories are useful when the patient has nausea but are not preferred by patients; therefore recent efforts are focused on intranasal formulations.

Recent data suggest that a combination of a triptan and an NSAID has increased efficacy. Rational polytherapy is emerging with drugs that enhance migraine control when given together (sumatriptan + naproxen sodium). Such a combination is suggested to produce faster and better control of acute migraine. NSAID combinations have been reported to be effective in the abortive therapy of mild to moderate migraine. Rational polytherapy presupposes that two drugs with different mechanisms of action may provide better disease control than two drugs with a similar mechanism. However, the adverse effects or toxicity of a drug combination can be additive or synergistic, creating serious or fatal toxicity, as ergot alkaloids and triptans are both powerful vasoconstrictors.

The Pediatric Population

Migraine with and without aura is common among adolescents, with a prevalence in the pediatric population of 7.7%. Among pediatric patients, migraine headaches occur frequently, but pharmacologic therapies for the management of migraine in children and adolescents are limited. Among over-the-counter treatments, ibuprofen is considered first line for pediatric patients, with acetaminophen effective in individuals who cannot tolerate NSAIDs. Zolmitriptan nasal spray and topiramate have been approved in the United States for prophylaxis in patients aged 12 to 17 years of age. Aspirin should not be used in pediatric patients due to Reye's syndrome (Chapter 29).

PHARMACOKINETICS

Triptans are available in oral (disintegrating lingual tablet) and injectable formulations, as well as a nasal spray. Pharmacokinetic features vary with individual triptans and as per route of administration. In general, the triptans have an onset of action ranging from 10 minutes to 2 hours with an elimination half-life of 2–6 hours or longer.

Sumatriptan is administered orally, subcutaneously, or intranasally. Sumatriptan injections should not be given intravenously because of its potential to cause coronary vasospasm. Oral bioavailability is 15%, and peak plasma concentrations are reached in 1.5–2 hours. In contrast, subcutaneous administration results in 97% bioavailability, with peak plasma concentrations reached in 10–20 minutes. Protein binding is low, and the elimination half-life is 2–2.5 hours. Sumatriptan is metabolized in the liver by monoamine oxidase type A (MAO-A). After subcutaneous administration, approximately 60% of a dose is excreted renally (20% unchanged) and the rest by the biliary-fecal route.

Some of the triptans have better oral bioavailability than sumatriptan, ranging from 40% for zolmitriptan to 60%–75% for almotriptan and naratriptan. In addition, many of these compounds, with the exception of zolmitriptan, including almotriptan, eletriptan, frovatriptan, and naratriptan, are available in tablet form only; zolmitriptan is available as a nasal spray. Most of these compounds are metabolized 25%–50% in the liver by MAO-A, and both metabolites and unchanged drug are excreted in the urine and bile. Eletriptan and almotriptan are metabolized by CYP3A4 and therefore must be used with caution with known CYP3A4 inhibitors (ketoconazole, clarithromycin). Among the available drugs, only zolmitriptan has an important active metabolite that is more potent than the parent compound and likely contributes to its therapeutic effect. Elimination half-lives for the triptans range from 2–6 hours with the exception of frovatriptan, which has an elimination half-life of about 26 hours.

Ergot Alkaloids

Ergotamine is available as lingual tablets and as rectal suppositories, while DHE is available as a nasal spray or by injection only because it has very poor bioavailability following tablet administration. DHE bioavailability is comparable following subcutaneous and intramuscular injections but is only 32% relative to the injections following administration by nasal spray. Ergotamine and DHE are absorbed erratically and undergo significant first-pass metabolism. Both alkaloids are metabolized in the liver and excreted in the bile.

Ergotamine is less widely used than the triptans due to limited availability and its adverse side effect profile. In addition, the injected, oral, and nasal spray forms are all inferior to the triptans; only the rectal form of ergotamine is superior. Ergotamine may still be helpful for patients with status migrainous or those with frequent recurring headaches. DHE is a weaker vasoconstrictor with fewer adverse effects than ergotamine and may be effective in patients who do not respond to a triptan.

PHARMACOVIGILANCE: ADVERSE EFFECTS AND DRUG INTERACTIONS

Triptans

The triptans cause few side effects when used for acute treatment of migraine. Triptans can cause tingling; asthenia; fatigue; flushing; feeling of pressure, tightness, or pain in the chest, neck, and jaw; drowsiness; dizziness; and sweating. The rapid onset of action of subcutaneously injected sumatriptan may lead to heaviness in the chest and throat and paresthesias of the head, neck, and extremities. A burning sensation at the injection site is common following the subcutaneous administration of sumatriptan.

Serious but rare cardiac events, including coronary artery vasospasm, transient myocardial ischemia, atrial and ventricular arrhythmias, and myocardial infarction, have been reported with triptans. Triptans alter vascular tone, which can cause arterial vasospasms and hypertension, and are contraindicated in patients with ischemic, cardiac, cerebrovascular or peripheral vascular disease, or uncontrolled hypertension. In addition, patients with other significant underlying cardiovascular diseases should not receive a triptan.

Triptans should not be taken within 24 hours of another triptan or an ergot alkaloid due to additive vasoconstrictor effects. Further, many compounds have been shown to increase serum levels of the triptans with MAO inhibitors increasing levels of rizatriptan, sumatriptan, and zolmitriptan, and propranolol increasing serum levels of eletriptan, frovatriptan, rizatriptan, and zolmitriptan. In addition, serum levels of eletriptan and almotriptan are increased in patients taking inhibitors of CYP3A4. The triptans are classified as category C (risk cannot be ruled out) for use in pregnancy.

Triptans should not be used concomitantly with any other drug that increases serotonergic activity, as it could precipitate serotonin syndrome, which could be life threatening. Such drugs include the serotonin selective reuptake inhibitors (SSRIS) or serotonin/norepinephrine reuptake inhibitors (SNRIs). These commonly used antidepressants and the signs and symptoms of serotonin syndrome are discussed in Chapter 17.

Ergot Alkaloids

The side effects of the ergot alkaloids include nausea and vomiting in 10% of patients. Adverse effects and vasoconstrictive complications of a serious nature may occur at times. As for the triptans, the argot alkaloids are also contraindicated in patients with cardiovascular disease. The compounds also have the potential to cause teratogenic effects and are contraindicated during pregnancy (pregnancy category X) because they cause uterine contractions, fetal distress, gastrointestinal atresia, and miscarriage.

Ergot alkaloids contain a boxed warning indicating that serious or life-threatening peripheral ischemia has been associated with the coadministration of ergotamine and potent CYP3A4 inhibitors, including protease inhibitors and macrolide antibiotics. Because CYP3A4 inhibition elevates serum levels of ergotamine, the risk for vasospasm leading to cerebral ischemia and/or ischemia of the extremities is increased. Hence, concomitant use of these medications is contraindicated.

Recent clinical studies have shown that excessive use of symptomatic medications on a daily basis may result in chronic migraines; thus prophylactic and symptomatic medications become ineffective. Medication overuse headache is a major issue in headache medicine. It is a secondary chronic headache that is an evolution from episodic headaches as a consequence of overuse of symptomatic medications.

Common adverse effects are summarized in the Clinical Problems Box.

NEW DEVELOPMENTS

Several new drugs are being developed for migraine with an overall goal of higher efficacy and an improved side effect profile. CGRP has long been hypothesized to play a key role in migraine pathophysiology, and much effort has been expended on the development of CGRP-receptor antagonists. While these agents have demonstrated clinical

CLINICAL PROBLEMS

Triptans
Chest heaviness, paresthesias, arterial vasospasms, cardiac events, fatigue
Vasoconstriction additive with the ergot alkaloids

Ergot Alkaloids
Nausea and vomiting, vasoconstriction, teratogenic, oxytocic

TRADE NAMES

In addition to generic and fixed-combination preparations, the following trade-named materials are some of the important compounds available in the United States:

Ergot Alkaloids
Dihydroergotamine (Migranal)
Ergotamine (Ergomar)
Ergotamine/caffeine (Cafergot)

Triptans
Almotriptan (Axert)
Eletriptan (Relpax)
Frovatriptan (Frova)
Naratriptan (Amerge)
Rizatriptan (Maxalt)
Sumatriptan (Imitrex)
Zolmitriptan (Zomig)

Specific NSAID Preparations
Aspirin + caffeine (Anacin)
Acetaminophen + aspirin + caffeine (Excedrin migraine)
Acetaminophen + isometheptene + dichloralphenazone (Midrin)
Ibuprofen (Advil migraine, Motrin migraine)

efficacy, their hepatic toxicities have proven to be a major concern. More recently, monoclonal antibodies to the CGRP receptor have been developed, have shown to be efficacious for migraine and devoid of major toxicity, and are now in phase III clinical trials.

Nevertheless, the field of migraine therapeutics is still in its infancy. Despite intense efforts in migraine research, the molecular pathophysiology of migraine attacks is poorly understood and remains controversial. Therefore migraine therapeutics lack the target-based, rational therapy to provide migraine control or prevent migraine attacks.

CLINICAL RELEVANCE FOR HEALTHCARE PROFESSIONALS

The Commission on Clinical Policies and Research of the American Academy of Family Physicians, and the Clinical Efficacy Assessment Subcommittee of the American College of Physicians (ACP) and American Society of Internal Medicine (ASIM) made several management guidelines in 2012 that are listed below:
- For most migraine sufferers, NSAIDs are first-line therapy.
- In patients whose migraine attacks have not responded to NSAIDs, use migraine-specific agents (triptans, ergot products).
- Select a nonoral route of administration for patients whose migraines present early with nausea or vomiting as a significant component of the symptom complex. Treat nausea and vomiting with an antiemetic.

- Migraine sufferers should be evaluated for use of preventive therapy.
- Recommended first-line agents for the prevention of migraine are propranolol, timolol, amitriptyline, divalproex sodium, and sodium valproate.
- Educate migraine sufferers about the control of acute attacks and preventive therapy, and engage them in the formulation of a management plan. Therapy should be reevaluated on a regular basis.

SELF-ASSESSMENT QUESTIONS

1. A 32-year-old women presented with a severe unilateral headache. The patient indicated that she experienced nausea, could not handle moderately loud noises and bright lights, and was confused several hours prior to onset of the pain. She was not able to go to work, as throbbing pain around the eyes and temples impaired her for several hours. The drug of choice for treatment of this type of migraine attack is:
   A. Acetaminophen.
   B. Sumatriptan.
   C. Topiramate.
   D. Losartan.
   E. Amitriptyline.

2. The triptans such as sumatriptan, naratriptan, and zolmitriptan can cause serious adverse reactions, and are contraindicated in patients with:
   A. Epilepsy.
   B. Cardiovascular disorders.
   C. Anxiety.
   D. Attention deficit-hyperactivity disorder.
   E. Asthma.

3. The ability of drugs to relieve the pain associated with migraine headaches is attributed to the ability of these compounds to:
   A. Activate 5-HT receptors.
   B. Enhance GABA inhibition.
   C. Inhibit glutamate excitotoxicity.
   D. Block calcium channels.
   E. Increase endorphin release.

4. The release of calcitonin gene-related peptide (CGRP) from the trigeminal nerve may be decreased by:
   A. Beta blockers.
   B. Anticonvulsants.
   C. Calcium channel blockers.
   D. Serotonin agonists.
   E. None of the above.

5. Joe began to develop migraine headaches when he was 62 years old, a year after he was diagnosed with coronary artery disease. His doctor was hesitant to prescribe a triptan to alleviate his headache pain because these compounds:
   A. Constrict blood vessels in the heart.
   B. Activate noradrenergic alpha receptors.
   C. Activate cardiac calcium channels.
   D. Cause vasodilation leading to reflex tachycardia.
   E. Inhibit several P450s.

6. Mary was prone to developing migraines and wanted to take a drug to prevent their occurrence. A drug used for the prevention of severe migraines whose mechanism of action involves inhibition of vesicular ACh release is:
   A. Verapamil.
   B. Valproate.
   C. Amitriptyline.
   D. Botulinum toxin.
   E. Naproxen.

FURTHER READING

Anonymous. Drugs for migraine. *Treat Guidel Med Lett.* 2008;6:17–22.

Diener HC, et al. Chronic migraine-classification, characteristics and treatment. *Nat Rev Neurol.* 2012;8:162–171.

Olesen J, Ashina M. Emerging migraine treatments and drug targets. *Trends Pharmacol Sci.* 2011;32:352–359.

Reddy DS. The pathophysiological and pharmacological basis of current drug treatment of migraine headache. *Expert Rev Clin Pharmacol.* 2013;6:271–288.

Schürks M, et al. Update on the prophylaxis of migraine. *Curr Treat Options Neurol.* 2008;10:20–29.

Vecchia D, Pietrobon D. Migraine: a disorder of brain excitatory-inhibitory balance? *Trends Neurosci.* 2012;35:507–520.

WEBSITES

https://www.ichd-3.org/

This website is maintained by the International Headache Society and has the third edition of the International Classification of Headache Disorders.

https://americanheadachesociety.org/guidelines/

This website is maintained by the American Headache Society and contains guidelines for both professionals and patients on several topics, including drug use.

Drug Therapy for Gout and Hyperuricemia

Keith S. Elmslie

MAJOR DRUG CLASSES

Prophylactic treatment
  Xanthine oxidase inhibitors
  Uricosuric drugs
  Uricases
Symptomatic treatment
  Colchicine
  Corticosteroids
  Nonsteroidal antiinflammatory agents

ABBREVIATIONS

GI	Gastrointestinal
GLUT9	Glucose transporter 9
IL-1β	Interleukin-1β
NSAIDs	Nonsteroidal antiinflammatory drugs
URAT1	Renal urate transporter 1

THERAPEUTIC OVERVIEW

Hyperuricemia refers to abnormally high levels of circulating uric acid (urate), which are >6.8–7.0 mg/dL. For many years, hyperuricemia was thought to be synonymous with **gout**, but high levels of uric acid can be associated with several metabolic and hemodynamic abnormalities, as well as lifestyle. Factors that may increase levels of uric acid include alcohol consumption, a high body mass index (being overweight), recent surgery, uncontrolled hypertension, diabetes, metabolic syndrome, and cardiovascular and renal disease. In addition, adults receiving chemotherapy for some cancers exhibit elevated uric acid levels due to accelerated purine degradation accompanying tumor lysis. Uric acid may also be overproduced in individuals with enzymatic defects such as those with Lesch-Nyhan syndrome (often referred to as juvenile gout) or a related disorder, Kelley-Seegmiller syndrome. In addition, several drugs can increase uric acid, including thiazide diuretics (Chapter 38).

Gout, often called gouty arthritis, is a common disease, with 6 million adults experiencing symptoms at some time in their lives. Gout occurs more often in men 40–50 years of age because their uric acid levels are typically higher than those in women. However, uric acid levels increase in women after menopause, leading to symptoms.

The characteristics of gout are presented in the Therapeutic Overview Box.

THERAPEUTIC OVERVIEW

Gout is a form of inflammatory arthritis characterized by:
  increased blood urate levels
  deposition of urate crystals in the joints, often in the big toe
  release of inflammatory mediators
  hot, swollen, and tender joints
  sudden pain onset, typically at night

Pathophysiology

Approximately one-third of the uric acid in the body comes from dietary sources (red meat, seafood, organ meats), while the other two-thirds are produced endogenously from the breakdown of purines within cells. Normally, the circulation carries dissolved uric acid from cells to the kidneys, where it is excreted into the urine. When the body produces too much uric acid, does not excrete enough, or increases the renal reabsorption of uric acid, **hyperuricemia** results. When circulating uric acid levels are high (>6–7 mg/dL), the uric acid can form crystals in joint synovial fluid, which initiate an inflammatory reaction that yields the pain and swelling associated with gout. The inflammatory reaction is mediated by the migration of leukocytes into the synovial fluid, where they phagocytose the crystals and release inflammatory cytokines, particularly **interleukin-1β** (**IL-1β**).

Two approaches are used to treat gout: a prophylactic approach and a treatment approach. Drugs that lower plasma uric acid levels can prevent the development of crystals within the joints; this is accomplished by decreasing uric acid production, increasing uric acid secretion, or catabolizing circulating uric acid. If crystals have already developed, leading to disease, lowering uric acid levels will enhance the reabsorption of the crystals so that the affected joints can heal. Treatment approaches focus on alleviating the pain during a gout attack, whereas prophylactic approaches focus on preventing further attacks.

MECHANISMS OF ACTION

Prophylactic Treatment

First-line treatment for gout involves using drugs that decrease the synthesis of uric acid. Uric acid is synthesized from hypoxanthine in a two-step process, both of which are catalyzed by the enzyme **xanthine oxidase**, as shown in Fig. 32.1. Xanthine oxidase can be inhibited by **allopurinol** or **febuxostat**. Allopurinol is a purine substrate for xanthine oxidase, leading to the production of alloxanthine (also known as oxypurinol); both allopurinol and alloxanthine inhibit xanthine oxidase, with allopurinol a reversible inhibitor and alloxanthine an irreversible inhibitor. Febuxostat is a nonpurine drug that reversibly inhibits xanthine oxidase.

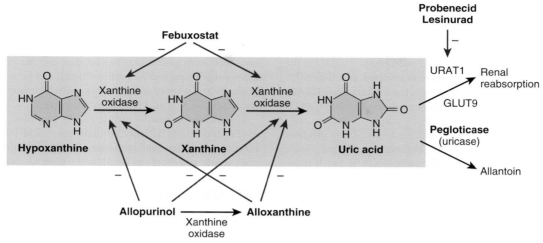

FIG. 32.1 Uric Acid Synthesis and Metabolism and the Sites of Action of Drugs Used for the Prophylactic Treatment of Gout. URAT1 and GLUT9 are the primary transporters in the renal proximal tubule.

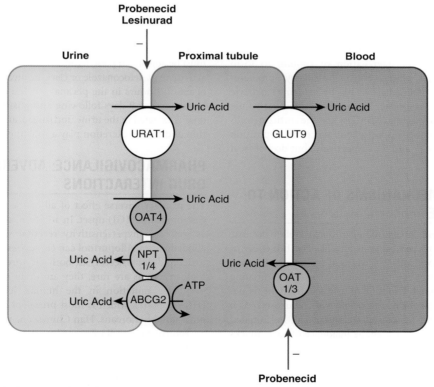

FIG. 32.2 Transport Proteins Involved in Uric Acid Reabsorption and Secretion. Several transporters in the renal proximal tubule have been proposed to be involved with uric acid homeostasis. Both URAT1 and GLUT9 are thought to play a primary role, with URAT1 responsible for the reabsorption of uric acid into the tubular lumen, followed by GLUT9 transport into the circulation. Other proteins capable of transporting uric acid have been identified, including the organic anion transporters OAT3 and OAT4, which function in opposite directions; the NPT1 and NPT4 transporters mediating secretion; and the ABCG2 transporter, representing an active secretory transporter. Although several other transporters have also been identified, the preponderance of evidence strongly favors the primary roles of URAT1 and GLUT9.

Second-line treatment for gout involves increasing uric acid excretion. Uric acid undergoes glomerular filtration and is 90% reabsorbed within the renal proximal tubule. Several transporter proteins have been proposed to participate in uric acid reabsorption (Fig. 32.2), with the urate transporter 1 (URAT1) and glucose transporter 9 (GLUT9) the best characterized as the main transporters involved and targets for drug action. The uricosuric agent probenecid inhibits both URAT1 and OAT1/3, while the recently approved drug lesinurad inhibits URAT1, thereby increasing the renal secretion of uric acid.

The third approach to decrease circulating uric acid is to promote its oxidation. Most mammals express the enzyme uricase (urate oxidase) that oxidizes uric acid to allantoin, which is much more soluble than uric acid and does not form crystals (Fig. 32.1). Humans, however, do not express a functional enzyme. To overcome this issue, recombinant enzymes have been created to reduce uric acid levels in the same manner that the human enzyme would, if it were functional. The first recombinant enzyme created was rasburicase, produced by a genetically modified strain of yeast. Although rasburicase is effective in decreasing uric acid levels, its toxicity has limited its use for adults with elevated uric acid levels as a consequence of tumor lysis, and not for the treatment of gout. The second enzyme created was pegloticase, a porcine-baboon recombinant uricase covalently attached to polyethylene glycol (pegylated) to increase its elimination half-life and decrease immunogenicity.

Symptomatic Treatment

Drugs from several pharmacological classes are used for the symptomatic treatment of gout. Colchicine does not affect uric acid levels but decreases the intensity of the inflammatory response to urate crystals. Colchicine disrupts the aggregation of tubulin to form microtubules within leukocytes, which is critical for leukocyte proliferation and migration into the inflamed area. Thus by reducing leukocyte activity, the inflammatory response is controlled. Similarly, the nonsteroidal antiinflammatory agents (NSAIDs) and the corticosteroids can also reduce the inflammatory response to urate crystal deposition and alleviate pain (Chapters 29 and 50, respectively) but do not treat the underlying problem.

RELATIONSHIP OF MECHANISMS OF ACTION TO CLINICAL RESPONSE

Allopurinol is the first-line drug for controlling uric acid levels to decrease the frequency and severity of painful gout attacks. The full effect of allopurinol is typically observed after 2–3 weeks of treatment. However, gout attacks can increase over the first month or so after initiating allopurinol treatment due to redistribution of uric acid from the tissues into the plasma. The same problem can occur with febuxostat. As a consequence, allopurinol and febuxostat treatment can be initiated concomitantly with colchicine to reduce the incidence of such attacks until the uric acid stored in tissues has been depleted. The colchicine treatment can then be stopped.

Probenecid and lesinurad are uricosuric drugs and are effective at lowering plasma uric acid levels, particularly in patients with low urinary uric acid. Because these compounds increase urinary uric acid levels, patients should be encouraged to drink plenty of fluids to reduce the risk of renal stones. Neither probenecid nor lesinurad should be used in individuals with compromised renal function. Interestingly, the angiotensin II receptor blocker (ARB) losartan (Chapter 39) and the diuretic furosemide (Chapter 38) both inhibit URAT1. Although the antagonist effects of these drugs are modest relative to probenecid and lesinurad, for gout patients who are also hypertensive and have not reached target uric acid levels (<6–7 mg/dL) following treatment with allopurinol or febuxostat alone, the addition of these antihypertensives to their treatment regimen may be beneficial.

Pegloticase is prescribed typically for individuals who fail to respond or are intolerant to other medications. As with the xanthine oxidase inhibitors, acute gout attacks can increase over the first few months of treatment with pegloticase, and colchicine can be used to reduce the frequency and severity of these attacks with treatment terminated once tissue stores of uric acid have been dissipated.

Colchicine is primarily used to rapidly terminate flare-ups but can also be used prophylactically. For flare-ups, colchicine can shorten the duration of pain and inflammation if taken within the first 36 hours of an attack, and relief can be realized within 12–24 hours.

PHARMACOKINETICS

The drugs used for the treatment of gout have good bioavailability following oral dosing. Allopurinol has a half-life of 1–2 hours, but its clinical effect is much longer due to its metabolism to alloxanthine and irreversible inhibition of xanthine oxidase. Allopurinol and its primary metabolite are eliminated via the kidneys. Febuxostat is metabolized extensively by hepatic glucuronidation, with metabolites excreted via the kidney. Probenecid has a half-life of 5–8 hours and is metabolized by glucuronidation and oxidation of it alkyl side chains. The metabolites are excreted by the kidneys.

Pegloticase is a protein administered by intravenous infusion. Serum concentrations increase proportionately with dose administered and, following removal of the polyethylene glycol moieties, cells take up the free protein and degrade it to the component amino acids.

Colchicine is demethylated in the liver via CYP3A4; thus dosing must be adjusted if patients are also taking drugs that modulate CYP3A4 activity (e.g., ketoconazole or clarithromycin). The half-life of colchicine is about 9 hours in the plasma, but the drug can be detected within leukocytes for 9 days following administration. About half of an oral dose is excreted in the urine unchanged, and both enterohepatic circulation and biliary excretion play a role in elimination.

PHARMACOVIGILANCE: ADVERSE EFFECTS AND DRUG INTERACTIONS

The primary adverse effect of all of the orally administered drugs is gastrointestinal (GI) upset. In addition, allopurinol can lead to a rash, as well as a hypersensitivity reaction with hepatic and blood cell abnormalities. Allopurinol can cause Stevens-Johnson syndrome and toxic epidermal necrolysis, both life-threatening disorders. Although these reactions are rare, they are quite severe and associated with a particular mutation in the human leukocyte antigen B protein (HLA-B*5801), which is most prevalent in patients of Asian descent, most notably Koreans, Han Chinese, or people of Thai descent.

Febuxostat is well tolerated by patients with allopurinol intolerance. Primary adverse effects include liver abnormalities, nausea, diarrhea, GI intolerance, and headache.

Drug interactions with allopurinol and febuxostat are not uncommon because the metabolism of several drugs is mediated by xanthine oxidase. Mercaptopurine, used to treat acute lymphatic leukemia (Chapter 68), and azathioprine, used primarily to prevent rejection in renal homotransplantations (Chapter 34), but also approved for the treatment of rheumatoid arthritis (Chapter 35), are metabolized by xanthine oxidase. Thus the coadministration of a xanthine oxidase inhibitor with mercaptopurine or azathioprine will interfere with the metabolism of these drugs.

In general, probenecid is well tolerated with a low incidence of side effects. Rare hypersensitivity reactions have been reported, and glucose-6-phosphate dehydrogenase (G6PD) deficiency increases the risk of probenecid-induced hemolytic anemia. Probenecid was developed originally to inhibit the renal transporter responsible for the excretion of some antibiotics such as penicillin, thereby maintaining plasma levels of these drugs. This inhibition extends to other drugs that are also weak acids, such as some NSAIDs, cephalosporins, and β-lactam antibiotics. Thus the concomitant use of probenecid with these agents will impair their renal clearance and increase serum levels.

Similarly, uric acid is not the only organic compound transported by URAT1. Some drugs are also substrates for this transporter, including allopurinol and its metabolite alloxanthine. Combination therapy with allopurinol and probenecid can increase allopurinol secretion, which requires increasing the dose. Aspirin has the opposite effect on URAT1 and increases uric acid reuptake. Thus even at low doses, aspirin is contraindicated for patients with gout and may reduce the effectiveness of probenecid.

As a recombinant foreign protein, pegloticase can lead to several adverse events, including anaphylaxis, as well as delayed-type hypersensitivity reactions. Infusion reactions may ensue, and premedication with antihistamines (Chapter 33) and corticosteroids (Chapter 50) is suggested. Similar to probenecid, patients with a high risk for glucose-6-phosphate dehydrogenase deficiency (individuals of African and Mediterranean descent) are at a greater risk of pegloticase-induced hemolysis and methemoglobinemia.

The primary adverse effects of colchicine are nausea and vomiting, abdominal pain, and diarrhea. These GI problems can occur in a large percentage of patients receiving colchicine but have been reduced by the administration of divided doses. Additionally, serious adverse hypersensitivity reactions are rare but have been reported and include a rash and difficulty breathing. Further, colchicine has been reported to lead to leukopenia, granulocytopenia, thrombopenia, and rhabdomyolysis, all of which are generally reversed by decreasing drug dose or stopping drug administration.

NEW DEVELOPMENTS

Several agents are being investigated for both the prophylactic and symptomatic treatment of gout and other hyperuricemic disorders. For prophylaxis, new inhibitors of xanthine oxidase and renal transport inhibitors are being tested alone and in combination with each other. A new approach involves inhibition of purine nucleoside phosphorylase, the enzyme that metabolizes inosine to hypoxanthine—that is, the step prior to the xanthine oxidase–catalyzed reactions. Ulodesine is the first agent in this class and is actively being developed. In addition to drugs targeting uric acid, based on the central role of IL-1β in mediating gouty inflammation, this proinflammatory cytokine is also being investigated as a drug target.

CLINICAL RELEVANCE FOR HEALTHCARE PROFESSIONALS

All healthcare providers, particularly those involved in point-of-care service, such as physical therapists, occupational therapists, nurses, and physician assistants, must always keep in mind that gout is a chronic disorder and that patients will be using both prophylactic and pain-relieving medications on a long-term basis. Thus it is critical for all to be aware of the potential adverse effects that may ensue following the chronic use of these compounds. Sensitivity reactions that may develop are rare, but are potentially life-threatening, requiring all healthcare providers to recognize the signs and symptoms of serious adverse effects.

■ SELF-ASSESSMENT QUESTIONS

1. A 62-year-old man with gout experienced a flare-up. Which drug did he take to alleviate the acute pain and swelling he experienced?
   A. Allopurinol.
   B. Febuxostat.
   C. Colchicine.
   D. Pegloticase.
   E. Probenecid.

2. A 75-year-old woman taking allopurinol had her blood uric acid levels measured, and they were above 7 mg/dL. Current guidelines recommend that she add which drug to her regimen to decrease serum uric acid?
   A. NSAIDs.
   B. Febuxostat.
   C. Colchicine.
   D. Pegloticase.
   E. Probenecid.

3. A 56-year-old female presents to her primary care physician complaining of an increased urgency to urinate. Her history is significant for gout, for which she takes probenecid. The physician diagnoses the patient with an infection of her urinary tract and prescribes cephalexin. Because of potential drug-drug interactions, what does the physician do?
   A. Decrease the dose of probenecid.
   B. Increase the dose of probenecid.
   C. Increase the dose of cephalexin.
   D. Decrease the dose of cephalexin.
   E. Discontinue the probenecid while the patient is taking cephalexin.

4. A 61-year-old male continues to experience acute gout attacks even though he has been taking the maximum doses of allopurinol and probenecid. His plasma urate level is 7.9 mg/dL. What additional approach can be used to decrease serum uric acid levels?
   A. Use a uricase to oxidize circulating uric acid.
   B. Use a uricosuric agent to inhibit xanthine oxidase.
   C. Use colchicine to promote uric acid excretion.
   D. Use an IL-1β activator.
   E. Have the patient increase his exercise regimen.

FURTHER READING

Khanna D, Fitzgerald JD, Khanna PP, et al. 2012 American College of Rheumatology guidelines for management of gout. Part 1: systematic nonpharmacologic and pharmacologic therapeutic approaches to hyperuricemia. *Arthritis Care Res.* 2012;64:1431–1446.

Khanna D, Khanna PP, Fitzgerald JD, et al. 2012 American College of Rheumatology guidelines for management of gout. Part 2: therapy and antiinflammatory prophylaxis of acute gouty arthritis. *Arthritis Care Res.* 2012;64:1447–1461.

Sattui S, Gaffo AL. Treatment of hyperuricemia in gout: current therapeutic options, latest developments and clinical implications. *Ther Adv Musculoskelet Dis.* 2016;8(4):145–159.

WEBSITES

http://www.rheumatology.org/Practice-Quality/Clinical-Support/Clinical-Practice-Guidelines/Gout

This website is maintained by the American College of Rheumatology and contains information on gout and its treatment for both healthcare professionals and patients.

https://www.guideline.gov/summaries/summary/47897

This website is maintained by the United States Department of Health and Human Services Agency for Healthcare Research and Quality and contains clinical practice guidelines for the management of gout.

Drug Treatment for Allergic Reactions

Kirk E. Dineley and Latha Malaiyandi

MAJOR DRUG CLASSES
Antihistamines (H$_1$ receptor antagonists)
Mast cell stabilizers
Corticosteroids

ABBREVIATIONS	
CNS	Central nervous system
GI	Gastrointestinal
IgE	Immunoglobulin E

THERAPEUTIC OVERVIEW

Allergic reactions are commonplace in society and represent the fifth leading group of chronic diseases, affecting 40% of the world population. Estimates have indicated that more than 50 million Americans suffer from some type of allergic disorder, which represents a heterogeneous group ranging from seasonal allergies to reactions to specific foods (e.g., peanuts), insect venom, cosmetics, animal dander, latex, and medications. In addition, the manifestations of allergic reactions are very diverse and can range from mild **urticaria** (hives), **pruritus** (itching), or **rhinorrhea** (runny noses) to **anaphylaxis**, a severe, life-threatening allergic reaction requiring immediate treatment.

Pathophysiology

Allergic reactions represent an immune response involving **mast cells** that produce an array of biologically active mediators. Mast cells are present in mucosal and epithelial tissues close to small blood vessels, as well as in connective tissue, and contain secretory granules containing **histamine** and other **inflammatory mediators** (leukotrienes, prostaglandins, and cytokines). These cells express the high-affinity Fcε receptor I constitutively on their surface that binds to IgE. When antigens cross-link IgE bound to these receptors, **degranulation** of mast cells ensues within seconds to release the granular contents, leading to the early phase response (Fig. 33.1). The histamine released causes **vasodilation**, increased **gastrointestinal** (GI) and **mucous secretions**, **peristalsis**, and **bronchoconstriction**. Histamine also increases **vascular permeability**, enabling the extravasation of plasma, proteins, and immune mediators from the vasculature to the surrounding tissues. Depending on the allergen and the amount of exposure, a severe reaction may ensue, leading to **anaphylaxis**, which is treated with epinephrine (Chapter 11).

The **H$_1$-antihistamines**, or H$_1$ receptor antagonists, play an important role in the treatment of allergic reactions. These drugs are also used frequently to treat the common cold. Although some H$_1$-antihistamines are available by prescription only, others are over-the-counter, contributing to their widespread use.

Histamine signaling can also be impeded by the **mast cell stabilizers** that inhibit degranulation, potentially mitigating the effects of both the early- and late-phase responses, the latter involving the de novo synthesis of chemokines and cytokines. The first-generation mast cell stabilizers, the **chromone** drugs, are second-line or adjunctive therapy in allergy and histamine disorders, whereas the newly developed, often termed *second-generation* group, represents dual-action agents with both mast cell–stabilizing activity and antihistamine activity.

Although the H$_1$-antihistamines are efficacious for relieving the symptoms of allergies, the corticosteroids are commonly used for several allergic conditions including allergic rhinitis, dermatitis, and reactions to foods, drugs, and insect bites. The pharmacology of these compounds is discussed in Chapter 50.

Common allergic manifestations are shown in the Therapeutic Overview Box.

THERAPEUTIC OVERVIEW	
Allergic Manifestations	
Mild	Urticaria (hives), pruritus (itching), rhinitis (nasal congestion), rash, scratchy throat, watery or itchy eyes
Severe	Abdominal cramping or pain, pain or tightness in the chest, diarrhea, difficulty swallowing, dizziness (vertigo), anxiety, flushing and swelling of the face, nausea and vomiting, heart palpitations, weakness, wheezing and difficulty breathing, unconsciousness

MECHANISMS OF ACTION

Histamine signaling via H$_1$ receptors plays a primary role in allergic responses. These receptors are G-protein–coupled receptors (GPCRs) linked to G$_q$, and activate phospholipase C to produce inositol triphosphate (IP$_3$) and diacylglycerol (DAG), and increase intracellular Ca^{2+}. H$_2$ receptors are also present in mast cells, the heart, and the GI system, where they regulate the activity of gastric parietal cells with histamine, a most important stimulus of acid secretion into the stomach. The role of histamine and H$_2$ receptors in the GI system is discussed in Chapter 71. Histamine and histamine receptors are also present in the central nervous system (CNS) in which histamine signaling is involved in sleep, coupling neuronal activity with glucose utilization, and other critical processes (Chapters 13 and 19).

The H$_1$-antihistamines demonstrate excellent selectivity for H$_1$ receptors and have no meaningful effects at other histamine receptors. However, many of these compounds also inhibit muscarinic receptors, contributing to their physiological effects. These compounds, whose structures are shown in Fig. 33.2, are competitive at low concentrations

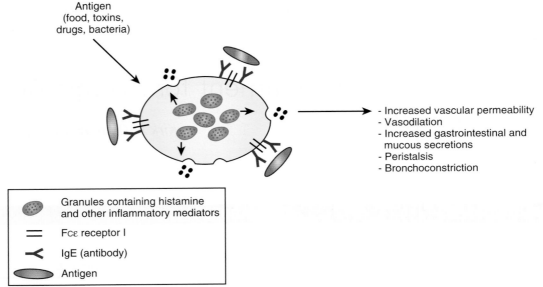

FIG. 33.1 Processes Involved in Degranulation of Mast Cells. Antigens, such as food, toxins, drugs, etc., cross-link IgE, which is bound to the Fcε receptor I constitutively expressed by mast cells, leading to Ca^{2+} influx and the release of histamine and other inflammatory mediators, which cause allergic and systemic effects.

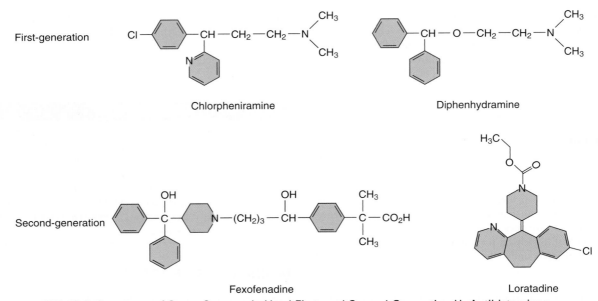

FIG. 33.2 Structures of Some Commonly Used First- and Second-Generation H_1-Antihistamines.

and noncompetitive at higher concentrations and are classified mainly on their ability to penetrate the CNS. The first-generation, or "classic" H_1-antihistamines, typified by chlorpheniramine and diphenhydramine, represent a large and diverse group of lipophilic compounds that readily cross the blood-brain barrier. The second-generation H_1-antihistamines, typified by fexofenadine and loratadine, represent a smaller group of compounds that have a low tendency to cross the blood-brain barrier at therapeutic doses and are largely devoid of CNS effects.

The first-generation mast cell stabilizers, typified by disodium cromoglycate and nedocromil, prevent degranulation by blocking Ca^{2+} channels in the mast cell membrane, preventing Ca^{2+}-mediated granule exocytosis and the release of histamine and other inflammatory mediators. Several newer drugs, such as azelastine, ketotifen, and olopatadine, actually represent dual-acting compounds with both classical mast cell–stabilizing activity and noncompetitive antihistamine activity; azelastine also has antiinflammatory activity.

RELATIONSHIP OF MECHANISMS OF ACTION TO CLINICAL RESPONSE

Effects for Allergies

Antihistamines have been the mainstay for the treatment of seasonal allergic disorders and allergic rhinitis for many years. With the advent of the second-generation compounds lacking in sedative effects, these agents have become suitable for daily use. Indeed, the H_1-antihistamines work well for mild to moderate symptoms. Recent studies, however, have shown that nasal steroids relieve symptoms of seasonal allergies more effectively than the antihistamines and that the daily use of an intranasal steroid may be superior to the use of H_1-antihistamines daily for patients with perennial rhinitis.

The H_1-antihistamines are the preferred drugs for allergic conjunctivitis, and several are formulated as eye drops, including the dual-acting agents azelastine, ketotifen, and olopatadine. Some ophthalmic over-the-counter versions combine an antihistamine with a topical α-adrenergic receptor agonist to produce vasoconstriction and fast relief of redness. Use of these preparations should be limited to a few days because extended use of α-adrenergic receptor agonists may lead to a loss of efficacy.

The H_1-antihistamines are also first-line agents for acute and chronic urticarial disorders. Second-generation agents are preferred, but first-generation drugs may help some patients who do not respond to initial therapy. Weak evidence suggests that H_1- and H_2-antihistamine combination therapy can be more effective than H_1-antihistamines alone. In chronic forms of urticaria, patients may require doses greater than those for other indications.

Despite dubious efficacy and frequent side effects, the first-generation H_1-antihistamines are pervasive in the treatment of the common cold. Some experts hold that drying mucous membranes, which may be more attributable to muscarinic antagonism, is actually harmful. Weak evidence suggests that the combination of an antihistamine and decongestant is more effective than either agent alone, but marginal in any case, as these therapies do not alter the course of the illness. Perception of improvement may be due to the somnolence associated with the long-lasting effects of some of these compounds that are included in many popular selling formulations. Nondrowsy cough and cold formulations do not include any antihistamines in their preparations.

Systemic Effects

The release of histamine from mast cells leads to effects on the GI system, the airways, and blood vessels. Within the GI tract, increased fluid secretion and peristalsis ensue, with expulsion of the GI contents (diarrhea and emesis). Thus as would be expected, the H_1-antihistamines are efficacious at decreasing GI tone, motility, and secretions and are also antiemetic agents. Whether these effects are attributed to histamine or muscarinic receptor blockade is debatable.

Histamine leads to bronchoconstriction and increased mucous secretion, leading to congestion and airway blockage (wheezing and coughing), with swelling of the nasal passages. Again, as would be expected, the antihistamines are effective in relieving these symptoms by blocking either histamine or muscarinic receptors.

In terms of the vasculature, histamine is a fairly potent vasodilator and increases blood flow and vascular permeability, often with a profound drop in blood pressure, a key component of the anaphylactic reaction. Most antihistamines do not affect blood pressure in normotensive individuals.

Antiemetic Effects

The sedative antihistamines with marked antimuscarinic activity were one of the first groups of drugs used as antiemetics and are still used for this purpose today in several contexts. However, other agents, including the serotonin receptor ($5\text{-}HT_3$) antagonist ondansetron, the dopamine receptor (D_2) agonist metoclopramide, the neurokinin receptor (NK1) antagonist aprepitant, and other more recently developed agents, may be preferred.

Other Indications

The antihistamines or mast cell–stabilizing agents are used to control symptoms in mastocytosis, a rare disorder involving the proliferation of mast cells in some tissues and organs. The antihistamines can also be used for gastric carcinoids or tumors of the GI tract that secrete abundant amounts of histamine, but surgery is usually preferred.

TABLE 33.1   Pharmacokinetic Parameters of Selected Antihistamines

Drug	Elimination $t_{1/2}$ (hrs)	Disposition
Azelastine	22	M, A, N
Cetirizine	7–9	R, N
Chlorpheniramine	~20	M
Desloratadine	~27	M, N
Diphenhydramine	~8	M
Doxylamine	10–13	M
Fexofenadine	14	R, N
Ketotifen	7–27	M
Loratadine	2–15	M, A, N
Olopatadine	8–12	R
Promethazine	7–15	M

M, Metabolism; *A*, active metabolite that contributes to therapeutic effect; *N*, nonsedating; *R*, renal elimination; $t_{1/2}$, half-life.

PHARMACOKINETICS

Most of the commonly used antihistamines are well absorbed after oral administration, have good bioavailability, and have onsets of action of approximately 30 to 60 minutes; they vary in duration of action due to varying half-lives, and most are metabolized extensively by the liver (Table 33.1). The first-generation compounds distribute throughout the body and readily penetrate the CNS. Because second-generation antihistamines are more hydrophilic and are substrates for the P-glycoprotein transporter, they do not easily enter the CNS. However, not all nonsedating antihistamines have the same low tendency to cross the blood-brain barrier at therapeutic doses and have led to sedation; cetirizine causes sedation in about 10% of individuals.

The antihistamines often induce hepatic cytochrome P450 enzymes and may facilitate their own metabolism or that of other drugs, leading to drug-drug interactions. Their actions and toxicities can be enhanced in patients with hepatic failure. Cetirizine and fexofenadine are not metabolized appreciably by the liver.

Absorption of cromolyn from the GI tract is negligible. For most applications, cromolyn is formulated in topical applications—that is, nasal spray, ophthalmic drops, and inhalable solutions. In the rare instances where oral administration is warranted—for example, in mastocytosis—its benefits are apparently derived from effects on the luminal surface of the GI epithelium.

PHARMACOVIGILANCE: ADVERSE EFFECTS AND DRUG INTERACTIONS

The most important adverse effects associated with the first-generation H_1-antihistamines result from CNS penetration and muscarinic antagonism. As a consequence of the sedative side effects of these drugs, they should not be taken by individuals operating heavy equipment and mass transportation vehicles, and in fact, the United States Federal Aviation Administration forbids pilots from using first-generation antihistamine as well as cetirizine. It is also important to note that the CNS depression resulting from the antihistamines is additive with other CNS depressants such as alcohol, benzodiazepines, and opioid analgesics.

Other anticholinergic effects of these agents include xerostomia, visual disturbances, constipation, and urinary retention. In severe poisoning, antihistamines can cause paradoxical excitement, hallucinations, ataxia, and seizures. The clinical presentation of antihistamine toxicity resembles atropine poisoning (Chapter 8), and the agitation and delirium are treated with benzodiazepines.

CLINICAL PROBLEMS

First generation	Sedation, dizziness, blurred vision, tinnitus, CNS depression, cognitive impairment, paradoxical excitation in children
Second generation	Headache, nausea
	May be sedating at recommended doses (cetirizine)
	May be sedating at higher-than-recommended doses (loratadine but not fexofenadine)

TRADE NAMES

In addition to generic and fixed-combination preparations, the following trade-named materials are some of the important compounds available in the United States.

First-Generation Antihistamines

Brompheniramine (Atrohist, Bromarest, Bromfed, Dimetane)
Chlorpheniramine (Chlor-Trimeton, Teldrin)
Clemastine (Tavist)
Cyclizine (Marezine)
Dexchlorpheniramine (Dexchlor, Polaramine)
Dimenhydrinate (Dimetabs, Dramamine, Marmine)
Diphenhydramine (Benadryl)
Doxylamine (NyQuil, Unisom SleepTabs; with pyridoxine, Diclegis)
Meclizine (Antivert, Bonikraft, Medivert)
Phenindamine (Nolahist)
Promethazine (Phenameth, Phenergan)
Tripelennamine (PBZ, Vaginex)
Triprolidine (Zymine)

Second-Generation Antihistamines

Azelastine (Astelin, Optivar)
Cetirizine (Zyrtec)
Desloratadine (Clarinex)
Fexofenadine (Allegra)
Ketotifen (Zaditor)
Loratadine (Claritin)
Olopatadine (Patanol, Pataday, Pazeo)

Mast Cell Stabilizers

Cromolyn (Gastrocrom, Opticrom)
Nedocromil (Tilade, Alocril)

The first-generation antihistamines should be avoided in children under 12 because they impair learning and memory, and there are rare instances of fatal excitement and seizures. The labeling of cough and cold formulations explicitly warns against the use of over-the-counter remedies in children under 4 years old, and many authorities suggest that they should not be used in children under 12.

Two second-generation H_1-antihistamines, terfenadine and astemizole, were withdrawn from the market due to cardiac arrhythmias as a consequence of prolongation of the Q-T interval. The problem with terfenadine, which is a prodrug, was obviated with the introduction of its active metabolite, fexofenadine. Other second-generation agents including cetirizine, loratadine, and desloratadine are not associated with cardiotoxicity and are rarely associated with serious adverse effects.

Because antihistamines are secreted into breast milk, first-generation agents should be avoided in nursing mothers. The Clinical Problems Box presents an overview of the adverse effects of the antihistamines.

NEW DEVELOPMENTS

During the past several years, efforts have focused on dual-acting compounds (antihistamine and mast cell–stabilizing activity) such as ketotifen and olopatadine, or even triple-acting compounds such as azelastine that has antihistamine, mast cell–stabilizing, and antiinflammatory activity. Further, some compounds, like fexofenadine, have been erroneously referred to as "third-generation" antihistamines but do not represent a class with a new mechanism of action.

Advances are being made, however, in the discovery and development of the next generation of mast cell stabilizers. Many natural products have been isolated with such activity, and synthetic compounds are being developed that inhibit signal transduction within the mast cell, including agents directed toward tyrosine kinases and phosphodiesterases, inhibiting Ca^{2+} influx and the release of histamine and other inflammatory mediators.

CLINICAL RELEVANCE FOR HEALTHCARE PROFESSIONALS

Antihistamines are conveniently available as over-the-counter preparations and are used for the relief of allergic rhinitis as well as other purposes, such as sleep aids (Chapter 19), and many individuals do not consider these compounds as drugs. Thus they are not aware of potential adverse reactions or drug-drug interactions, particularly the additive effects of the antihistamines with other CNS depressants, such as benzodiazepines and ethanol. All healthcare professionals should be aware of the potential adverse effects of these agents and educate their patients on potential issues.

SELF-ASSESSMENT QUESTIONS

1. The mother of a 5-year-old child with allergic rhinitis is seeking an approved treatment to make her child feel better. Which of the following is recommended?
   A. Diphenhydramine.
   B. Cetirizine.
   C. Meclizine.
   D. Promethazine.
   E. Doxylamine.

2. A 25-year-old man comes to your office complaining of sneezing, coughing, runny nose, and itchy eyes, all symptoms of allergic rhinitis. He also notes that he has been tired lately and has been self-medicating with an over-the-counter antihistamine. Which agent is most likely the cause of his fatigue?
   A. Loratadine.
   B. Diphenhydramine.
   C. Ketotifen.
   D. Fexofenadine.
   E. Olopatadine.

3. A 35-year-old woman with seasonal allergies decides to use an over-the-counter antihistamine. About an hour later, she felt dizzy and confused and was very thirsty. It is likely that these effects are a consequence of:
    A. Activation of H_2 receptors.
    B. Blockade of serotonin receptors.
    C. Blockade of cholinergic muscarinic receptors.
    D. Blockade of cholinergic nicotinic receptors.
    E. Activation of H_1 receptors.

4. The primary difference between the first- and second-generation H_1-antihistamines is their:
    A. Ability to enter the CNS.
    B. Efficacy at H_1 receptors.
    C. Metabolism by cytochrome P450s.
    D. Efficacy at H_2 receptors.
    E. Ability to cause vasoconstriction.

5. The antigen-mediated degranulation of mast cells leads to histamine-induced:
    A. Vasoconstriction.
    B. Decreased vascular permeability.
    C. Bronchodilation.
    D. Increased gastrointestinal motility.
    E. Decreased mucous secretions.

FURTHER READING

Finn DF, Walsh JJ. Twenty-first century mast cell stabilizers. *Br J Pharmacol.* 2013;170:23–37.

Juel-Berg N, Darling P, Bolvig J, et al. Intranasal corticosteroids compared with oral antihistamines in allergic rhinitis: a systematic review and meta-analysis. *Am J Rhinol Allergy.* 2017;31(1):19–28.

Pali-Schöll I, Namazy J, Jensen-Jarolim E. Allergic diseases and asthma in pregnancy, a secondary publication. *World Allergy Organ J.* 2017;10(1):10.

WEBSITES

https://www.fda.gov/ForConsumers/ConsumerUpdates/ucm273617.htm
This is a website maintained by the United States Food and Drug Administration and contains numerous resources on allergies and their treatment in children.

https://www.aaaai.org/conditions-and-treatments/library/at-a-glance/allergic-reactions
This website is maintained by the American Academy of Allergy, Asthma and Immunology and is an excellent resource for all things pertaining to allergies.

34

Immunosuppressants for Autoimmune Disorders and Organ Transplantation

Kymberly Gowdy

MAJOR DRUG CLASSES

Antiproliferative/Antimetabolic agents
Glucocorticoids
Immunophilin-binding agents (calcineurin and mTOR inhibitors)
Biopharmaceuticals (antibodies and fusion proteins)

ABBREVIATIONS

Ag	Antigen
APC	Antigen presenting cell
CTL	Cytolytic T lymphocyte
Ig	Immunoglobulin
IFN	Interferon
IL	Interleukin
mAb	Monoclonal antibody
MHC	Major histocompatibility complex
mTOR	Mechanistic target of rapamycin
NF-κB	Nuclear factor κ–light-chain-enhancer of activated B cells
Th	T-helper (cells)
TGF	Transforming growth factor
TNF	Tumor necrosis factor
Treg	Regulatory T cells

THERAPEUTIC OVERVIEW

Autoimmune disorders, including rheumatoid arthritis, inflammatory bowel disease, psoriasis, and others are characterized by dysregulation of various aspects of normal immunity and inflammation. The National Institutes of Health estimates up to 23.5 million people in the United States currently suffer from autoimmune diseases and that the prevalence of these potentially chronic and life-threatening diseases is rising. Current medications that suppress and/or polarize the immune system are utilized to treat these diseases and have dramatically improved patient outcomes. A vast majority of these drugs can also be used to suppress the immune system to prevent transplant rejection.

Alterations of the highly regulated immune system, which protects the host from invading organisms and growing neoplastic cells while sparing host cells, can change the delicate balance of host defenses toward immune reactions against "self" proteins and generate auto-immune diseases. Many agents with different mechanisms of action and side-effect profiles have been developed with increased specificity and minimal toxicity and nonspecific immunosuppression. The drugs used currently to treat autoimmunity and/or prevent transplantation rejection can be classified as antiproliferative/antimetabolic agents, glucocorticoids, immunophilin-binding agents, and biopharmaceuticals, each class with unique mechanisms to suppress the immune response and inhibit inflammatory processes. The common autoimmune diseases and classes of drugs used for treatment are in the Therapeutic Overview Box.

THERAPEUTIC OVERVIEW

Common autoimmune diseases
 Crohn disease, dermatomyositis, diabetes (type 1), glomerulonephritis, Graves' disease, myasthenia gravis, multiple sclerosis, polymyositis, psoriatic arthritis, rheumatoid arthritis, systemic lupus erythematosus, ulcerative colitis, vasculitis
Classification of immunosuppressant drugs
 Antiproliferative/Antimetabolic agents
 Glucocorticoids
 Immunophilin-binding agents (calcineurin and mTOR inhibitors)
Biopharmaceuticals (antibodies and fusion proteins)

The Immune Response

The role of the immune system is to recognize and remove invading organisms and tumor cells, while ignoring host cells, through innate and acquired immune responses. Innate immunity, which is nonspecific, represents the first line of immediate defense against detecting foreign antigens (Ags), whereas acquired (adaptive) immunity is an Ag-specific response and requires reexposure to invading organisms; key differences in response types are listed in Table 34.1.

Acquired immunity is commonly divided into cell-mediated and humoral responses. Initiation of acquired immunity involves antigen-presenting cells (APCs) processing antigens into peptide fragments that interact with major histocompatibility complexes (MHCs). This coupling produces signals to fully activate the response, schematically shown in Fig. 34.1. Activation of naïve T-helper (Th) cells by different interleukins (ILs) or transforming growth factors (TGFs) leads to the formation of four types of Th cells, each subserving different functions. Cell-mediated immune responses involve Th1 cells, which secrete cytokines (IFN-γ, IL-2, tumor necrosis factor [TNF]-α/β), leading to the recruitment and activation of macrophages (type IV hypersensitivity) and generation of CD8$^+$ cytotoxic T-lymphocytes (CTLs). Humoral responses involve Th2 cells, which produce cytokines (IL-4, IL-5, and IL-13) that drive the formation of antibodies (i.e., immunoglobulin, Ig). Activation of naïve Th cells can also lead to the formation of regulatory T cells (Tregs), which produce antiinflammatory cytokines (IL-10 and TGF-β) that control inflammation and promote wound healing responses, and Th17 cells that produce cytokines (IL-17, IL-21, and IL-22), which promote the activation of neutrophils to clear bacterial pathogens.

Th1 cell–mediated macrophage activation can kill intracellular bacteria and produce a localized inflammatory response, whereas

TABLE 34.1	**Differences Between Innate and Acquired Immune Responses**	
Characteristic	**Innate Immune Response**	**Acquired Immune Response**
Onset	Immediate	Days to weeks
Mechanism of antigen recognition	Pattern recognition receptors recognize common molecules on microbes and viruses	Antigen-specific receptors (T-cell receptor, B-cell receptor)
Cell types involved	Macrophages, neutrophils, mast cells, natural killer cells, NK T cells, innate lymphoid cells	Dendritic cells, T cells, B cells
Soluble factors	Complement, type I interferon, select cytokines and chemokines	Select cytokines and chemokines

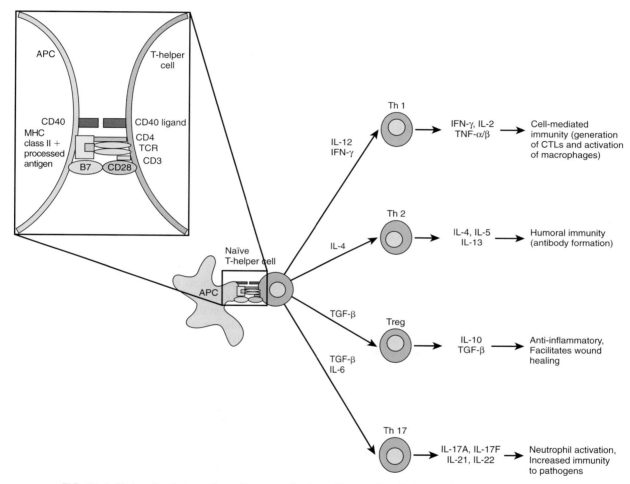

FIG. 34.1 Molecular Interactions Between Antigen-Presenting Cells (APCs) and Naïve T-Helper (Th) Cells. The T-cell receptor (TCR) and CD4 complex on Th cells act as coreceptors for the immunogenic peptide associated with the MHC Class II molecule with MHC Class II antigens located on dendritic cells, macrophages, B cells, and other specialized APCs. (Not shown are CD8⁺ molecules on cytotoxic T lymphocytes (CTLs) that act as coreceptors for the immunogenic peptide associated with the MHC Class I molecule; MHC Class I antigens are present on all somatic cells.) T cells require two signals to become activated. The first involves the binding of the TCR and CD4 or CD8⁺ with the antigen-MHC complex, resulting in the transduction of a signal via the CD3 molecule. The second signal is mediated by the costimulatory molecules CD28 and B7. The stimulated T cell activates the APC via CD40 ligand-CD40 interactions, resulting in activation and proliferation of effector T cells. IFN-γ and IL-12 stimulate the formation of Th1 cells, IL-4 drives the formation of Th2 cells, whereas TGF-β stimulates the formation of Treg cells and TGF-β and IL-6 induce Th17 cell formation.

generation of CTLs mediates the Ag-specific lysis of tumor cells, virally infected cells, and graft/transplant cells. The generation of CTLs for these functions involves activation of naïve precursor CTLs (pCTLs) in a manner similar to that for activation of naïve Th cells and can occur in the presence or absence of Th1 cells (Fig. 34.2). For the former, two signals are required; the first involves binding of peptide antigens associated with MHC Class I molecules on APCs to the T-cell receptor on CD8⁺ pCTLs, and the second is receptor-ligand interaction of costimulatory molecules. APCs with high levels of costimulatory molecules activate CD8⁺ CTLs without the presence of Th1 cells. Antigen recognition and binding of activated CTLs to antigen on tumor cells, virally infected cells, or graft/transplant cells result in cell lysis.

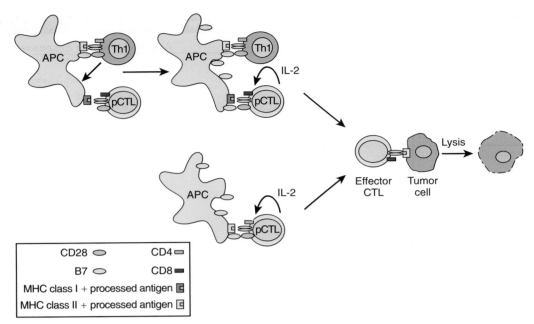

FIG. 34.2 Activation of Cytolytic T-Lymphocytes (CTLs). CTLs may be generated with or without support from Th1 cells. Antigens taken up by antigen-presenting cells (APCs) are processed and presented with MHC class II molecules to CD4⁺ Th cells, leading to the generation of effector Th1 cells. Activated Th1 cells stimulate the up regulation of costimulatory molecules (B7) on APCs and provide the second signal to antigen-activated precursor CTLs (pCTL). Activated CTLs secrete IL-2 and stimulate their own proliferation and differentiation to effector CTLs. Infected or foreign cells are recognized and lysed by effector CTLs.

The Th2 cell–mediated humoral immune response involves the secretion of cytokines that stimulate the proliferation and differentiation of B cells to antibody-secreting plasma cells or long-lived memory cells (Fig. 34.3). This process involves the internalization of Ag either by phagocytosis for APCs or by antibody-mediated endocytosis for B cells. Following Ag processing, the T-cell receptor couples with the Ag-bound MHC class II molecule, and with the costimulatory molecules B7 and CD28, activates the T cells. These activated T cells produce IL-2, which up regulates both CD25 and CD40L, the former a component of the IL-2 receptor. In lymphoid organs such as the spleen, the activated T cells interact with B cells specific for the Ag, and through the interaction of CD40L and CD40, this leads to the production of cytokines (IL-4) that promote the proliferation of B cells, which can differentiate into memory cells or antibody-producing plasma cells. The antibodies produced by plasma cells bind to and neutralize foreign Ags. Ag-antibody complexes can also activate the complement cascade to elicit local inflammation that furthers Ag removal. Once antibodies are bound to foreign proteins or bacteria, the Fc region can bind to receptors on phagocytic cells, as well as cause agglutination of pathogens, leading to internalization of the invading pathogens.

MECHANISMS OF ACTION

Pharmacological approaches to immunosuppressive therapy involve selective eradication of immunocompetent cells or down regulation of the immune response without deleting the target cell. In either case, the goal is to balance the activity and selectivity of the drug to optimize clinical efficacy while preventing adverse effects. The principal approaches used currently are highly effective in inhibiting the immune response and include antiproliferative/antimetabolite agents, glucocorticoids, immunophilin-binding agents, and biopharmaceuticals. The usefulness of these compounds is limited by their severe toxicities. Therefore synergistic combinations of drugs are used at lower doses to help minimize adverse effects. In autoimmune diseases, these agents are used primarily to prevent the immune system from recognizing self Ags as foreign and inducing inflammation and tissue damage. The primary use for transplantation is to maintain graft acceptance.

Antiproliferative/Antimetabolite Agents

The antiproliferative/antimetabolic drugs are cytotoxic and inhibit cell division and the proliferation of both T and B cells. The alkylating agents include cyclophosphamide, nitrogen mustards, and nitrosoureas that covalently complex to DNA. Cyclophosphamide is a prodrug that is metabolized to several active products, phosphoramide mustard and acrolein, that alkylate DNA. This mechanism mediates the antiproliferative and immunosuppressive effects of these compounds but is also responsible for their toxicity.

The antimetabolites are compounds that resemble normal metabolic compounds, including folic acid, pyrimidines, or purines, and block the proliferation of B and T cells by inhibiting the synthesis of building blocks necessary for cell replication. Methotrexate is a competitive inhibitor of dihydrofolate reductase, which coverts dihydrofolic acid to tetrahydrofolic acid, thereby preventing the regeneration of folic acid required for purine and pyrimidine synthesis. Azathioprine is a purine analogue prodrug metabolized to 6-mercaptopurine, which is further metabolized to the cytotoxic agents 6-thioguanine and 6-methylmercaptopurine that inhibit the de novo pathway for purine synthesis. Mycophenolate mofetil is another prodrug metabolized to mycophenolate that reversibly inhibits inosine monophosphate dehydrogenase, the enzyme catalyzing the synthesis of guanine monophosphate in the de novo pathway for purine synthesis required for proliferation by B and T cells.

All of these compounds are highly cytotoxic and decrease lymphocyte proliferation and function, thereby decreasing antibody formation. These

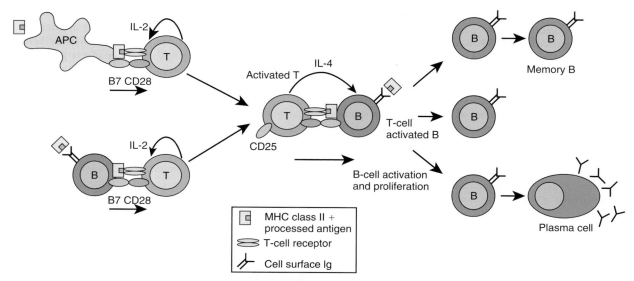

FIG. 34.3 Generation of the Humoral Response. Antigen-presenting cells (APCs) internalize Ag through phagocytosis, whereas B cells internalize Ag through antibody-mediated endocytosis. Following Ag processing, the resulting peptides are presented on the surface to naïve T cells in the setting of MHC class II molecules. The interactions between the processed Ag with the T-cell receptor and the costimulatory molecules B7 and CD28 are necessary for full activation. The activated T cell produces IL-2, leading to cell proliferation, and the up regulation of both CD25, a component of the IL-2 receptor, and CD40L. In the lymphoid organs such as the lymph nodes or the spleen, the activated T cell interacts with a B cell that is specific for the same Ag and provides help to the B cell through interaction of CD40L and CD40 and by producing cytokines such as IL-4 that lead to B-cell activation and proliferation. The activated B cells can differentiate into antibody-producing plasma cells or into memory cells.

drugs are used for their immunosuppressive effects; many are also used for the treatment of neoplastic diseases. The pharmacology of these compounds is discussed extensively in Chapter 68.

Glucocorticoids

The glucocorticoids are highly effective drugs for autoimmune and inflammatory diseases and for preventing graft rejection. **Prednisone** is the prototypical glucocorticoid and exerts its effects both directly and indirectly by binding to glucocorticoid receptors. Acutely, the glucocorticoids inhibit the vasodilation and increased vascular permeability that ensue upon inflammatory insult, as well as prevent leukocyte migration. They also decrease T-cell activation and the expression of IL-2, IL-1, IL-6, and nuclear factor κ–light-chain-enhancer of activated B cells (NF-κB). The glucocorticoids also bind to glucocorticoid-responsive elements on DNA to decrease the expression of proinflammatory and activate the expression of antiinflammatory genes. The glucocorticoids are among the most widely used immunosuppressive agents; their pharmacology is discussed extensively in Chapter 50.

Immunophilin-Binding Agents (Calcineurin and mTOR Inhibitors)

The immunophilins are proteins with both chaperone and enzymatic activity and have diverse functions ranging from neurotrophic actions to the regulation of cell proliferation. Of importance for immunosuppression are the immunophilins **cyclophilin** and **FKBP-12** (also known as FK-506 binding protein), both of which are targets for drug action (Fig. 34.4). In lymphocytes, **cyclosporine** binds to **cyclophilin A**. The complex formed binds to calcineurin and inhibits the phosphatase activity necessary for the expression of inflammatory cytokines such as IL-2 and TNF-α. Cyclosporin also binds to **cyclophilin D** in the mitochondrial matrix, preventing opening of the mitochondrial

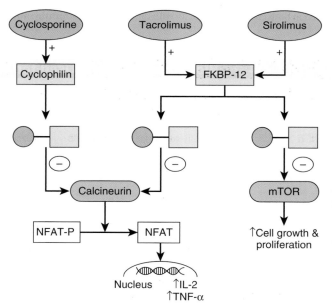

FIG. 34.4 Mechanism of Action of Calcineurin and mTOR Inhibitors. Calcineurin normally functions to dephosphorylate phosphorylated nuclear factor for activated T cells (NFAT-P) through its phosphatase activity, leading to translocation of NFAT into the nucleus, where it can bind to DNA and increase the expression of several proinflammatory cytokines, including IL-2 and TNF-α. Cyclosporine and tacrolimus are calcineurin inhibitors that bind to the immunophilins cyclophilin and FKBP-12, respectively, to form a complex that inhibits calcineurin. mTOR is a serine/threonine kinase involved in cell cycle progression. Sirolimus binds to the immunophilin FKBP-12, and the resulting complex inhibits mTOR, leading to the cell cycle arrest of B and T cells.

permeability transition pore, leading to inhibition of cytochrome c, an action thought to be important for apoptosis but not inflammation.

Tacrolimus, also referred to as FK-506, is another calcineurin inhibitor whose mechanism of action is similar to that of cyclosporine. Tacrolimus binds to the immunophilin FKBP-12 to form a complex that also binds calcineurin and inhibits its phosphatase activity. Thus the calcineurin inhibitors down regulate immune responses by inhibiting the production of IL-2 by activated T cells, a key driver of many immune responses and especially important in mediating organ transplant rejection.

Sirolimus, also known as **rapamycin**, is a macrolide that binds to FKBP-12 as does tacrolimus, but the complex formed inhibits the enzyme **mechanistic target of rapamycin (mTOR)**. mTOR is a serine/threonine kinase involved in cell growth and proliferation through the cell cycle, as well as a component of mTORC2, a tyrosine kinase involved in the activation of insulin receptors and the cytoskeleton. Thus sirolimus inhibits cell cycle progression of B and T cells by acting downstream of IL-2 and other T-cell growth factor receptors. It arrests cells in the G_1 phase, preventing them from progressing to the S phase of the cell cycle. **Everolimus** is an analogue of rapamycin.

Biopharmaceuticals

Biopharmaceuticals, or biologicals, represent a highly diverse group of compounds that include polyclonal and monoclonal antibodies, fusion proteins, and other products, most of which have been developed using recent advances in biotechnology.

Antibodies designed to bind to soluble proteins and surface receptors that mediate inflammatory processes and drive the immune response have demonstrated clinical efficacy in a variety of immune and neoplastic disorders. Both polyclonal and monoclonal antibodies have been generated against T-cell surface Ags. **Polyclonal antibodies** represented initial attempts to induce immunosuppression. However, these preparations varied in both efficacy and toxicity with different batches. **Antithymocyte**

globulin (ATG) was successful in decreasing circulating lymphocytes and their function, but major side effects were apparent, as might be expected from a polyclonal antibody. **Monoclonal antibodies (mAbs)** exert their effects by blocking the function of a target protein, altering the function of a target cell, directly inducing cytotoxicity, or removing target cells through immune-mediated complement-dependent cytotoxicity, antibody-dependent cellular cytotoxicity, or phagocytosis. The first-generation mAbs were derived from mice (murine), whereas newer mAbs are either humanized or fully human antibodies, thereby lacking antigenicity.

In addition to antibodies, **fusion proteins** have been developed to target specific sites in the immune system. Fusion proteins are created by combining two or more genes coding for two or more proteins, resulting in polypeptides with a combination of functional properties. Fusion proteins may also naturally occur in cancer cells, the best known example of which is BCR-ABL associated with the Philadelphia chromosome. Some of the most common currently available mAbs and fusion proteins with their targets, effects, and indications are shown in Table 34.2.

Agents Targeting Cytokines

Cytokine antagonists designed to bind to soluble proteins and surface receptors that mediate inflammatory processes and drive the immune response have demonstrated clinical efficacy in a variety of neoplastic and immune disorders. TNF-α and IL-1β are proinflammatory cytokines implicated in the pathogenesis of inflammatory disorders such as rheumatoid arthritis and Crohn disease. These cytokines are involved in activation and proliferation of synovial cells that produce endogenous substances involved in inflammation and bone resorption.

Both mAbs and fusion proteins have been developed that target TNF-α. **Adalimumab** is a recombinant humanized mAb that binds to soluble TNF-α, thereby preventing its interaction with its receptor. Similarly, **infliximab** is a murine/human chimeric mAb formed from

---

TABLE 34.2 Biopharmaceuticals Used for Immunosuppression

Target/Factor	Type of Molecule	Generic Name	Action/Indications
Multiple human T-cell Ags	Polyclonal	Anti-thymocyte globulin (ATG)	Depletes lymphocytes/transplantation
TNF-α	Recombinant humanized mAb	Adalimumab	Binds to TNF-α/autoimmune disorders: Crohn disease, ulcerative colitis, psoriasis, RA
	Chimeric mAb	Infliximab	Inhibits TNF-α binding to its receptor/autoimmune disorders: Crohn disease, ulcerative colitis, psoriasis, RA
	Recombinant fusion protein	Etanercept	Binds to TNF-α; functions as a decoy receptor/autoimmune disorders: psoriasis, RA
IL-1	Recombinant IL-1 receptor antagonist (IL-1RA)	Anakinra	Blocks IL-1 from binding to its receptor/RA
IL-1β	Human mAb	Canakinumab	Binds IL-1β, preventing it from interacting with its receptor/rare autoimmune disorders[a]
IL-2 receptor α chain on activated T cells (CD25)	Chimeric mAb	Basiliximab	Prevents T-cell replication and activation of B cells/transplantation
	Humanized mAb	Daclizumab	
IL-17A	Human mAb	Secukinumab	Binds IL-17A, preventing it from interacting with its receptor/psoriasis, multiple sclerosis
CD3 ε chain	Murine mAb	Muromonab-CD3	Depletes T cells/transplantation
CD2	Human fusion protein	Alefacept	Binds CD2 on T cells, interfering with T-cell activation/psoriasis
CD80	Human fusion protein	Abatacept	Binds CD80 on APCs, preventing its interaction with its receptor (CD28) on naïve T cells/RA
		Belatacept	
CD52 glycoprotein	Humanized mAb	Alemtuzumab	Prolonged T- and B-cell depletion/chronic lymphocytic leukemia

[a]For the treatment of cryopyrin-associated periodic syndromes (CAPS), including familial cold autoinflammatory syndrome, Muckle-Wells syndrome, and neonatal-onset multisystem inflammatory disease.
mAb, Monoclonal antibody; *RA*, rheumatoid arthritis.

the human constant region and the murine variable region of the antibody that also binds to soluble TNF-α and thereby prevents TNF-α–mediated immune responses. Etanercept is a dimeric fusion protein combining the p75 TNF receptor with the Fc portion of human IgG1. Like the mAbs, etanercept binds to TNF-α, but because it contains a portion of the receptor, it acts as a "decoy" receptor, preventing the cytokine from activating its receptor.

Agents that target ILs are also effective immunosuppressants. Anakinra is a recombinant IL-1 receptor antagonist (IL-1RA) that inhibits the binding of both IL-1α and IL-1β to the receptor, whereas canakinumab is a human mAb that binds specifically to IL-1β. Basiliximab, a chimeric mAb, and daclizumab, a humanized mAb, both bind to the α chain/subunit of the IL-2 receptor (CD25) on activated T cells and prevent IL-2 from binding to activated T-lymphocytes. Thus these antibodies target actively dividing cells that transiently express this receptor. Secukinumab is an IgG1κ mAb that binds to IL-17A, which has been implicated in the inflammatory response for several autoimmune diseases such as psoriasis and psoriatic arthritis, as well as the fibrosis associated with chronic graft rejection. Aldesleukin is an analogue of human IL-2 produced by recombinant technology and mimics the endogenous cytokine.

Several other fusion proteins and mAbs target other CD molecules, affecting T-cell activation (alefacept), the interaction of APCs with naïve T cells (abatacept and belatacept), T-cell–antigen interactions (muromonab-CD3), or mature lymphocytes targeting them for destruction (alemtuzumab).

In addition to the molecules that suppress the immune system, the interferons (IFNs) are known to stimulate the immune response and mediate antiinflammatory actions. These proteins activate natural killer cells and macrophages, and increase the expression of MHC antigens. Further, type II IFN (IFN-γ) is produced primarily by Th1 cells and blocks the proliferation of Th2 cells, thereby decreasing humoral immunity. Similarly, the immunomodulator glatiramer acetate is a synthetic copolymer composed of four amino acids, with a structure similar to myelin basic protein. This agent appears to activate a specific population of Th2 cells that depress immune responses to myelin basic protein, a unique Ag-specific mechanism of action.

RELATIONSHIP OF MECHANISMS OF ACTION TO CLINICAL RESPONSE

Immunosuppressive agents have dramatically improved patient outcomes in autoimmunity and transplantation rejection and transformed treatment paradigms for these diseases. The antiproliferative/antimetabolite agents are cytotoxic, which serves their function well for the treatment of neoplastic diseases (Chapter 68). Among these compounds, azathioprine is used as adjunctive treatment for the prevention of organ transplant rejection and for the treatment of severe rheumatoid arthritis (Chapter 35). It is also used to treat Crohn disease and ulcerative colitis. Mycophenolate is used in combination with calcineurin inhibitors and glucocorticoids for prevention of transplant rejection. It is also often used off-label for the treatment of systemic lupus erythematosus, while cyclophosphamide is approved for the treatment of systemic lupus erythematosus and is often used off-label as an immunosuppressant.

The glucocorticoids combined with other immunosuppressive agents are used to prevent and treat transplant rejections, particularly for graft-versus-host reactions in bone marrow transplants. They are also used for the treatment of several autoimmune disorders, including rheumatoid arthritis, systemic lupus erythematosus, psoriasis, inflammatory bowel disease, and multiple sclerosis.

The calcineurin inhibitor cyclosporine primarily affects T-cell–mediated responses. A lack of CTL precursor cell response to cyclosporine

indicates no effect on the proliferative response of activated CTLs to IL-2 or the lytic activity of CTLs, consistent with cyclosporine's effect only in very early stages of Ag activation of Th cells. There is also evidence for inhibition of macrophage Ag presentation and IL-1 production by macrophages. Both cyclosporine and tacrolimus are used for the prophylaxis of solid organ allograft rejection for kidney, heart, liver, and other organ transplants. Cyclosporine is also typically combined with other agents for the treatment of rheumatoid arthritis and psoriasis.

The mTOR inhibitor sirolimus is used prophylactically for preventing organ transplant rejection, usually in combination with a calcineurin inhibitor and glucocorticoid. Sirolimus and cyclosporine appear to act synergistically to inhibit lymphocyte proliferation, and aldesleukin is used for the treatment of malignant melanoma and renal cell cancer. The indications for the use of the biopharmaceuticals are presented in Table 34.2.

PHARMACOKINETICS

The immunosuppressants may be administered orally, as well as by injection, with variable pharmacokinetics because most of these drugs involve individual dosing with large intersubject variability. Several of these agents are active as administered, others are prodrugs that require metabolism to active forms, yet others are active and have active metabolites.

The antiproliferative/antimetabolic agent azathioprine is well absorbed after oral administration, with a half-life of 10 minutes for the parent drug and 1–5 hours for the active metabolites. Mycophenolate mofetil is a prodrug that is completely metabolized to mycophenolic acid after administration. The mycophenolic acid has a half-life of approximately 16 hours and is renally excreted as a phenolic glucuronide. The pharmacokinetics of the antiproliferative/antimetabolic compounds are discussed in detail in Chapter 68, methotrexate pharmacokinetics are discussed in Chapter 35, while the pharmacokinetics of the glucocorticoids are presented in Chapter 50.

The calcineurin inhibitors are administered both orally and via injection. Both cyclosporine and tacrolimus exhibit erratic and incomplete absorption from the gastrointestinal tract with much patient variability. Cyclosporine exhibits biphasic elimination with a half-life of 5–18 hours and is distributed extensively outside of the vascular compartment. Both cyclosporine and tacrolimus are metabolized in the liver by CYP3A4 and excreted primarily through the bile into the feces; some metabolites of tacrolimus are active. The mTOR inhibitor sirolimus is administered orally with rapid absorption and peak blood levels in 1–2 hours. It is also extensively metabolized by CYP3A4 with several active metabolites and mostly excreted in the feces. Everolimus is handled similarly to sirolimus, but it has a shorter half-life.

Antibodies are administered intravenously, except for adalimumab, which is administered subcutaneously, while fusion proteins are administered either intravenously or subcutaneously. Most compounds exhibit a fairly fast distribution after administration and a slower elimination phase with nonlinear pharmacokinetics at low doses but linear once the targets are saturated. Distribution is usually confined to the vascular compartment and the interstitial spaces because of molecular size and hydrophilicity. Proteolysis degrades antibodies and fusion proteins to amino acids, which can be reused in protein synthesis, with no renal clearance of the parent antibody or fusion protein.

PHARMACOVIGILANCE: ADVERSE EFFECTS AND DRUG INTERACTIONS

Despite the excellent efficacy of the immunosuppressives, these compounds affect normal immune responsiveness and can be associated

CLINICAL PROBLEMS

Myelosuppression
Predisposition to infection
Cytokine release syndrome
Vascular leak syndrome
Hypersensitivity and anaphylaxis
Dyslipidemias
Hypertension
Suppressed wound healing
Dysregulated glucose tolerance

TRADE NAMES

The following trade-named materials are some of the important compounds available in the United States.

Antiproliferative/Antimetabolite Agents

Azathioprine (Imuran, generic)
Cyclophosphamide (Cytoxan, Neosar)
Mycophenolate mofetil (CellCept, Myfortic)

Calcineurin Inhibitors

Cyclosporine (Sandimmune, Neoral, SangCya)
Tacrolimus/FK506 (Prograf)

mTOR Inhibitor

Rapamycin/Sirolimus (Rapamune)
Biopharmaceuticals
Abatacept (Orencia)
Adalimumab (Humira)
Aldesleukin (IL-2, Proleukin)
Alefacept (Amevive)
Anakinra (Kineret)
Anti-thymocyte globulin (ATG, Thymoglobulin)
Basiliximab (Simulect)
Belimumab (Benlysta, LymphoStat-B)
Certolizumab (Cimzia)
Daclizumab (Zenapax)
Etanercept (Enbrel)
Glatiramer acetate (Copaxone)
Golimumab (Simponi)
IFN-α2a (Roferon-A)
IFN-α2b (Intron A)
IFN-αn3 (Alferon N)
IFN-αcon-1 (Infergen)
IFN-α1a (Avonex, Rebif)
IFN-β1b (Betaseron)
Infliximab (Remicade)
Muromonab-CD3 (anti-CD3, Orthoclone OKT3)
Omalizumab (Xolair)
Oprelvekin (IL-11, Neumega)
Pegfilgrastim (G-CSF, Neulasta)
Rituximab (Rituxan)
Sargramostim (GM-CSF, Leukine)
Secukinumab (Cosentyx)
Tocilizumab (Actemra, RoActemra)
Ustekinumab (Stelara, Centocor)

with a variety of adverse and cytotoxic effects, including myelosuppression, that may predispose a patient to opportunistic infections. Thus antibacterial, antifungal, and/or antiviral agents should be considered prophylactically to guard against the potential development of an infection, activation of latent tuberculosis, or development of a lymphoproliferative disease, such as non-Hodgkin lymphoma. Additionally, specific for different immunosuppressant drug classes and their mechanisms of action, these drugs can elicit a variety of adverse effects, including insomnia, anxiety, increased appetite, osteoporosis, gastrointestinal issues, dysregulated glucose tolerance, dyslipidemias, hypersensitivity, hypertension, and poor wound healing.

Azathioprine is well known to suppress the bone marrow, leading to anemia and increasing susceptibility to infections. It also has hepatotoxic effects and causes alopecia and gastrointestinal disturbances. Mycophenolate mofetil has a similar adverse effect profile. A complete presentation of the adverse effects and drugs interactions of these cytotoxic agents is presented in Chapter 68.

The glucocorticoids are well known to retard growth in children, produce osteopenia and avascular necrosis of bone, and inhibit wound healing. The glucocorticoids decrease the number of circulating lymphocytes, basophils, and eosinophils over a 24-hour period, whereas the number of neutrophils increases. Lymphopenia is attributed to migration of cells into extravascular spaces, with more T cells than B cells or monocytes migrating. Most cells migrate to bone marrow. High-dose glucocorticoid therapy is also known to reduce the size of lymphoid organs. The adverse effects of these compounds are discussed extensively in Chapter 50.

Cyclosporine can lead to nephrotoxicity and hypertension, tremor, hirsutism, hyperlipidemia, gingival hyperplasia, and hyperuricemia. Because cyclosporine is metabolized by CYP3A4, drug interactions may ensue with the use of compounds that are metabolized by cytochrome P450 or inhibit this enzyme, including erythromycin, ketoconazole, Ca^{2+}-channel blockers, and grapefruit juice. Cyclosporine should not be administered with sirolimus or nonsteroidal antiinflammatory compounds that affect renal function. Adverse effects from tacrolimus are similar to those for cyclosporine with the addition of hyperkalemia and hyperglycemia. The direct effect of this drug on pancreatic β cells mediates the induced glucose intolerance.

Sirolimus increases serum cholesterol and triglycerides; leads to anemia, leukopenia, and thrombocytopenia; decreases serum potassium; and decreases wound healing. The adverse effect profile for everolimus is similar to that for sirolimus.

The use of antibody infusions, particularly following the administration of rituximab, muromonab, and other mAbs that activate T cells before they are destroyed can lead to a massive release of cytokines. Cytokine release syndrome includes a wide spectrum of symptoms such as fever, chills, dyspnea, nausea, and vomiting. It can lead to pulmonary edema and cardiovascular collapse. Somewhat similar to manifestations of anaphylactic reactions, it differs in onset, with anaphylactic reactions occurring within seconds to minutes, whereas cytokine release syndrome occurs 30 to 60 minutes after infusion.

A major effect of immunosuppressants that target IL-2 is vascular leak syndrome characterized by increased vascular permeability and extravasation of fluids and proteins that can result in interstitial edema and organ failure. This is one of the most serious adverse effects following the administration of aldesleukin, which has a very narrow therapeutic window.

Hypersensitivity and anaphylactic reactions are issues with all biopharmaceutical agents because there is a potential to induce an immune response. The relative immunogenicity of these compounds varies significantly among drugs and subjects and may have no clinical impact. However, rare cases in which specific IgE antibodies are generated may lead to type 1 hypersensitivity reactions that range from urticaria and angioedema to severe anaphylaxis.

Adverse effects associated with the use of immunosuppressants are presented in the Clinical Problems Box.

NEW DEVELOPMENTS

Our knowledge of the immune system is a growing field, with new cytokines and cell-signaling pathways being defined and investigated each day. Greater understanding of these soluble factors and pathways has and will reveal novel therapeutic targets. Currently, there are two new calcineurin inhibitors undergoing studies: CP-690550 (tasocitinib), an inhibitor of the downstream signaling molecule JAK 3, and AEB-071 (sotrastaurin), a protein kinase C inhibitor. Multiple biological agents are also undergoing development. Belatacept, a humanized antibody that blocks the T-cell costimulation pathway, and alefacept, a humanized antibody that inhibits T-cell adhesion, are currently undergoing investigation. New classes of T (Th17, follicular helper T cells, etc.) and B (innate B cells, regulatory B cells) cells are being defined that open up possibilities for developing drugs to target these classes. Discovery of single-nucleotide polymorphisms (SNPs) relevant to the immune system and other genotype discoveries may change the course of treatment, with personalized medicine leading to more effective and perhaps more selective immunosuppressants.

CLINICAL RELEVANCE FOR HEALTHCARE PROFESSIONALS

All healthcare providers should be vigilant in checking patients taking immunosuppressant agents for potential development of infections and/or cancers. Care should be taken to assure minimal exposure to potential infectious risks or adverse effects of procedures. This is particularly relevant during procedures that could be considered invasive, such as dentistry, or certain procedures performed by physician assistants or nurse practitioners. Additionally, all healthcare providers should be aware of the manifestations of immunosuppression complications, specifically in their particular profession. For example, oral complications associated with immunosuppressive drugs may present as gingival hypertrophy/enlargement, gingival bleeding, mouth ulcers, oral infections (bacterial, viral, and fungal), salivary gland enlargement, as well as abnormal taste and mouth odor, very apparent in dentistry. Physician assistants and nurse practitioners are crucial medical professionals in monitoring patients on immunosuppressant agents for any abnormal organ function, growth or change in tissue presentation, or drug responses indicative of drug interactions. Changes in bone density or muscle function may alter interventions by physical or occupational therapists. All healthcare providers should be familiar with changes that may occur with immunosuppressive agents, especially symptoms and signs that may foreshadow adverse effects that would be manifest through any procedures relevant to their profession. The frequency of these effects ranges from fairly common to rare, but knowledge of their potential can forewarn providers to be alert for manifestations.

SELF ASSESSMENT QUESTIONS

1. Corticosteroids are utilized extensively in the treatment of autoimmune disease and in the prevention of graft rejection because they:
   A. Alkylate DNA and inhibit the proliferation of B cells.
   B. Are also effective antiinflammatory agents.
   C. Stimulate cytokine production.
   D. Inhibit purine biosynthesis.
   E. B and C.
2. Cyclosporine is considered one of the more selective immunosuppressive agents because it:
   A. Alkylates DNA and inhibits B-cell proliferation.
   B. Specifically inactivates lymphocytes by binding to CD3 surface antigens on T cells.
   C. Specifically inhibits hypoxanthine-guanine phosphoribosyltransferase activity in T cells.
   D. Specifically inhibits production of cytokines by T lymphocytes.
   E. Specifically inhibits production of IL-1.

3. Which of the following immunosuppressive drugs is *not* correctly matched to its toxicity?
   A. Anti-CD3 monoclonal antibodies: flulike symptoms.
   B. Cyclosporine: bone marrow depression.
   C. Azathioprine: predisposition to opportunistic infections.
   D. Cyclophosphamide: myelosuppression.
4. After a liver transplant, your patient develops an infection with cytomegalovirus. Which of the following drugs could be responsible for the immunosuppression rendering your patient susceptible to an opportunistic infection?
   A. Muromonab-CD3.
   B. Azathioprine.
   C. Cyclophosphamide.
   D. A, B, and C.

FURTHER READING

Dessain SK, Adekar SP, Berry JD. Exploring the native human antibody repertoire to create antiviral therapeutics. *Curr Top Microbiol Immunol.* 2008;317:155–183.

Her M, Kavanaugh A. Alterations in immune function with biologic therapies for autoimmune disease. *J Allergy Clin Immunol.* 2016;137:19–27.

Liu PM, Handl H, Zou L, Kim B. Immunobiological aspects of therapeutic antibodies and related characterization approaches. *Curr Opin Drug Discov Devel.* 2007;10:515–522.

Loertscher R. The utility of monoclonal antibody therapy in renal transplantation. *Transplant Proc.* 2002;34:797–800.

Stucker F, Marti HP, Hunger RE. Immunosuppressive drugs in organ transplant recipients–rationale for critical selection. *Curr Probl Dermatol.* 2012;43:36–48.

WEBSITES

https://www.kidney.org/atoz/content/immuno
This website is maintained by the National Kidney Foundation and is a good resource on immunosuppressants for kidney transplants.

https://www.hopkinslupus.org/lupus-treatment/lupus-medications/immunosuppressive-medications/
This website is from the Johns Hopkins Lupus Center and has much information on using immunosuppressants for the treatment of lupus.

https://www.niams.nih.gov/health_info/autoimmune/
This website is maintained by the National Institute of Arthritis and Musculoskeletal and Skin Diseases and is an excellent resource on autoimmune disease.

35

Drug Therapy for Rheumatoid Arthritis

Keith S. Elmslie

THERAPEUTIC OVERVIEW

Rheumatoid arthritis (RA) is an autoimmune disorder that affects the lining of the joints and eventually leads to bone erosion and joint deformities. The etiology of RA involves the production of **autoantibodies** by an unknown mechanism that initiates and maintains a hyperactive inflammatory response in the affected joints. Therefore treatments rely on suppressing the immune system to minimize joint destruction. The nonsteroidal antiinflammatory drugs (NSAIDs) were used for years to alleviate the pain associated with RA, but these compounds do not affect the progression of the disease. The **disease-modifying antirheumatic drugs** (DMARDs) have a twofold action to decrease inflammation and significantly slow disease progression; in some cases, these compounds induce complete remission of RA. The characteristics of RA are shown in the Therapeutic Overview Box.

THERAPEUTIC OVERVIEW

Characteristics of Rheumatoid Arthritis

Articular	Joints are inflamed, swollen, tender, and stiff
	Smaller joints (fingers and toes) affected before larger joints (wrists, knees)
Extra-articular	Rheumatoid nodules, vasculitis, pericarditis, keratoconjunctivitis, uveitis, rheumatoid lung
Systemic	Acute phase protein production, anemia, cardiovascular disease, osteoporosis, fatigue, depression

Pathophysiology

Although the specific mechanisms involved in joint inflammation and bone destruction in RA are equivocal and still being investigated, the initial event involves the presentation of autologous arthritis-associated antigens to antigen presenting cells (APCs) and B cells, resulting in the activation of both T and B cells, leading to T-helper (Th)1 cell–mediated macrophage activation and an increased expression of Th17 cells. The cytokines produced by these cells, particularly tumor necrosis factor-α (TNF-α), interleukin-6 (IL-6), IL-1, and IL-17 all affect osteoclastogenesis and play a significant role in both the local and systemic pathophysiology of RA as shown in Fig. 35.1.

TNF-α and IL-6 are thought to play a major dominant role in the pathogenesis of RA, while IL-1, IL-17, and other cytokines and growth factors are implicated to play a lesser, but still important, role. The effects of these cytokines on bone integrity are shown in Fig. 35.1. TNF-α released from activated macrophages increases osteoclast survival and to a lesser extent decreases the proliferation of synovial fibroblasts (also referred to as fibroblast-like synoviocytes), resulting in bone resorption. IL-6, produced by both activated macrophages and synovial fibroblasts, increases the expression of receptor activator of NF-κB ligand (RANKL) on osteoblasts, leading to increased interaction with osteoclast precursor cells containing the receptor RANK, promoting osteoclast differentiation and survival, leading to bone resorption. IL-1 released from macrophages also promotes osteoclast differentiation and survival, while IL-17 released from Th17 cells (and mast cells) activates macrophages and synovial fibroblasts and directly induces the expression of RANKL. Thus all of these cytokines, as well as other factors, promote osteoclastogenesis, leading to bone resorption.

MECHANISMS OF ACTION

The DMARDs may be classified as conventional, biological, or targeted, representing chronological developments in the field and listed in Table 35.1. Irrespective of mechanisms, all of these agents reduce the inflammatory pathways involved in RA. The sites of action of these agents are shown in Fig. 35.2.

The **conventional DMARDs** include methotrexate, leflunomide, sulfasalazine, and hydroxychloroquine, with methotrexate and leflunomide more efficacious in slowing disease progression. These agents decrease the proliferation and function of T cells, macrophages, and B cells. **Methotrexate** is an antimetabolite that inhibits the synthesis of folic acid (Chapter 34) but also inhibits adenosine metabolism

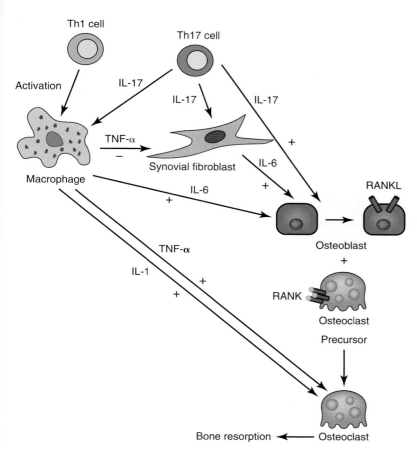

FIG. 35.1 Pathways Involved in Bone Reabsorption in RA. Following presentation of autologous arthritis-associated antigens to antigen-presenting cells (APCs) and B cells, naïve T cells are activated, promoting the formation of T-helper (Th)1 cells that activate macrophages to release tumor necrosis factor–α (TNF-α), interleukin-1 (IL-1), and IL-6, all of which promote osteoclastogenesis, with IL-6 increasing the expression of receptor activator of NF-κB ligand (RANKL). The proliferation of Th17 cells leads to the increased expression of IL-17, which stimulates macrophages and synovial fibroblasts, as well as directly increases the expression of RANKL, again promoting osteoclastogenesis, leading to increased bone resorption.

TABLE 35.1	Disease-Modifying Antirheumatic Drugs (DMARDs)		
Classification	**Mechanism/Target**	**Generic Name**	**Consequences**
Conventional	Antimetabolite	Methotrexate	Depletes T and B cells and macrophages
		Leflunomide	
	APC directed	Sulfasalazine	Prevents APC maturation; inhibits proliferation of T and B cells
		Hydroxychloroquine	Inhibits APC function; inhibits proliferation of T and B cells
		Chloroquine	
Biological	TNF-α	Infliximab	Binds TNF-α, preventing it from activating its receptor; protects bone
		Adalimumab	from destruction
		Golimumab	
		Certolizumab pegol	
		Etanercept	
	APC directed	Abatacept	Binds CD80 on APC; prevents activation of T cells; antiinflammatory
	B cells	Rituximab	Binds to CD20 on B cells, preventing their proliferation and differentiation
	IL-6 receptor (IL-6R)	Tocilizumab	Binds IL-6R, preventing activation of macrophages and osteoclasts
	IL-1 (IL-1R)	Anakinra	Antagonist at IL-1R, preventing immune activation
Targeted synthetic	Janus kinase (JAK)	Tofacitinib	Inhibits JAK blocking JAK-mediated intracellular signaling

and increases levels of extracellular adenosine, both of which lead to an antiinflammatory action. **Leflunomide**, a prodrug metabolized to teriflunomide, blocks pyrimidine synthesis and limits pyrimidine availability for the proliferation of immune cells. **Sulfasalazine** is both a drug and a prodrug largely hydrolyzed to sulfapyridine and mesalazine (5-aminosalicylic acid). Sulfapyridine and sulfasalazine are thought to be active, preventing the maturation of APCs to inhibit the activation

and proliferation of both T cells and B cells. **Hydroxychloroquine** and **chloroquine** are also thought to inhibit APC function by disrupting lysozyme activity. Other drugs previously considered to be conventional DMARDs, including azathioprine, cyclosporine, gold salts, and minocycline, are no longer recommended in treatment guidelines in the United States and Europe due to lack of efficacy and unfavorable adverse effects.

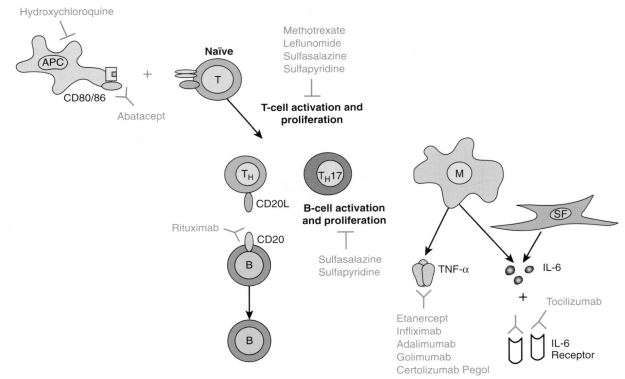

FIG. 35.2 Disruption of the Inflammatory Pathway by DMARDs. The nonspecific conventional DMARDs (methotrexate, leflunomide, sulfasalazine, and sulfapyridine) inhibit the proliferation and activation of T and B cells, whereas hydroxychloroquine affects the activation of antigen-presenting cells (APCs). The biological and targeted DMARDs interact with specific cytokines such as tumor necrosis factor-α (TNF-α), cytokine targets such as the interleukin-6 (IL-6) receptor, or cell surface proteins such as CD20 expressed by B-lymphocytes to potently inhibit inflammation.

The biological DMARDs are either **monoclonal antibodies** or **fusion proteins** representing receptors combined with the constant portion of human antibodies (Fc). The structures of these drugs are shown in Fig. 35.3. Some of these agents target **tumor necrosis factor-α** (TNF-α) to prevent this cytokine from activating its receptor, which prevents the signaling events that lead to the destruction of bone (see Fig. 35.1), and include **infliximab, adalimumab** and **golimumab, certolizumab pegol**, and **etanercept**. **Etanercept** is a fusion protein that combines two extracellular TNF-α binding domains of human p75 (TNF-α receptor) with the Fc portion of human IgG. In addition to binding TNF-α, etanercept is the only agent in this group that can also bind lymphotoxin-α. **Infliximab**, a chimeric murine-human antibody, and **adalimumab** and **golimumab**, fully humanized monoclonal antibodies, bind two TNF-α molecules, while **certolizumab pegol** is a pegylated Fab fragment of an anti–TNF-α monoclonal antibody.

Other biological DMARDs shown in Fig. 35.3 and listed in Table 35.1 target different components of the immune pathway. **Abatacept** is a human fusion protein that combines cytotoxic T-lymphocyte antigen-4 (CTLA-4), a CD80 receptor, with the human Fc IgG targeting CD80 on the APCs, effectively inhibiting T-cell activation and drive of the inflammatory process in RA. **Rituximab** is a mouse/human chimeric monoclonal antibody that targets CD20 expressed by B lymphocytes, effectively preventing proliferation and differentiation of these cells. The number of B lymphocytes is also decreased via complement-dependent cytotoxicity and apoptosis. **Tocilizumab** is a humanized monoclonal antibody that binds to IL-6 receptors to prevent IL-6 signaling and the subsequent activation of macrophages and osteoclasts.

Anakinra is a **decoy** receptor functioning as an IL-1 receptor antagonist that binds IL-1 to prevent activation of the immune system. It is now rarely used due to the existence of more effective drugs.

In addition to the conventional and biological DMARDs, a recently developed synthetic drug, **tofacitinib**, is a targeted DMARD. Tofacitinib is an orally available drug that inhibits Janus kinases (JAK), a family of protein kinases that couple activated type I/II cytokine receptors (e.g., IL-6 receptor) to intracellular signaling. Tofacitinib inhibits JAK to block the intracellular signaling of IL-6 and other type I/II cytokine receptors.

RELATIONSHIP OF MECHANISMS OF ACTION TO CLINICAL RESPONSE

The DMARDs inhibit the proliferation and activation of immune cells by multiple and nonoverlapping mechanisms of action to reduce inflammation in affected joints. The conventional DMARDs are weak immunosuppressives and can be combined to more effectively treat RA in patients who fail monotherapy. The biological and targeted DMARDs are potent inhibitors that cannot be prescribed together because of the high risk of infections. However, these agents can be used in combination with a conventional DMARD to improve treatment outcomes. The biological DMARDs are typically administered with methotrexate to increase effectiveness and decrease some adverse effects. The conventional DMARDs are also prescribed for rheumatic diseases, such as juvenile idiopathic arthritis, psoriatic arthritis, and systemic lupus erythematosus.

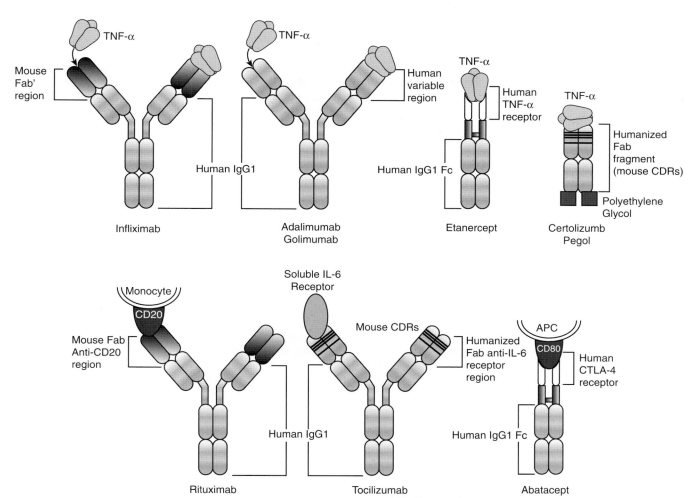

FIG. 35.3 Structures of the Biological and Targeted DMARDs. The light striped gray denotes the Fab and Fc portions of human antibodies (IgG1), while the darker striped gray indicates mouse Fab regions. The black stripes within the human Fab regions indicate mouse amino acids that form the complementary determining regions (CDR) in the humanized antibodies. The dark gray squares indicate polyethylene glycol moieties. *TNF-α,* Tumor necrosis factor-α; *APC,* antigen-presenting cell; *IL-6,* interleukin-6.

PHARMACOKINETICS

The onset of action of the conventional agents is slow so that patients may not realize a benefit for the initial 2–12 weeks of treatment. For this reason, a glucocorticoid such as prednisone is typically added to provide symptomatic relief until the DMARD treatment reaches full effect.

Methotrexate is administered orally or parenterally and has a bioavailability of 70% with oral administration. Dosing is typically a single dose once weekly. Methotrexate is transported into cells, where it is polyglutamated and protected from elimination. It is thought that polyglutamated methotrexate is the clinically relevant isoform because this form blocks the enzymes involved in adenosine metabolism with the highest efficacy. Methotrexate that is not polyglutamated is primarily eliminated via the kidneys, with a half-life of 6–9 hours. Weekly dosing results in a long delay in the drug reaching steady-state, with the full benefit of treatment in 3–6 months.

Leflunomide is a prodrug metabolized 100% in the intestines following oral administration to the active form, teriflunomide. The half-life of teriflunomide is 16 days, with steady state reached in 7–9 weeks following daily leflunomide dosing. Clinical effects are not observed for several weeks, with maximal effects after 12 weeks. Elimination is equally distributed via the liver and kidneys, with teriflunomide undergoing enterohepatic circulation, enhancing its duration of action.

Orally administered sulfasalazine is approximately 30% absorbed in the small intestines. The remaining 70% is converted by bacterial action into sulfapyridine and mesalazine in the large intestines. Sulfapyridine is well absorbed from the large intestines, but mesalazine remains in the large intestines and is excreted in the feces, where it mediates sulfasalazine treatment of ulcerative colitis. The half-life ranges from 4–14 hours for sulfasalazine and from 5–18 hours for sulfapyridine. Sulfasalazine is primarily eliminated unchanged via the kidney, while sulfapyridine is primarily metabolized in the liver by *N*-acetylation and excreted in the urine. Some individuals have a variant in the *N*-acetyltransferase gene that results in slow acetylation, which could result in sulfasalazine intolerance.

Hydroxychloroquine and chloroquine are orally administered with a high percent of absorption from the gastrointestinal (GI) tract (89% for chloroquine and 74% for hydroxychloroquine). These drugs are taken up by cells and protected from elimination, with a half-life of approximately 40–50 days. Steady-state concentrations are achieved after 3–4 months, and clinical effects are maximal after 36 months of administration. Both compounds are metabolized in the liver by CYP2C8 and CYP3A4, with metabolites excreted in the urine. Approximately 38% of chloroquine and 23% of hydrochloroquine are excreted unchanged by the kidneys, with about 25% of the drugs and metabolites excreted in the feces.

The biological DMARDs are proteins and administered parenterally to avoid degradation in the GI tract, with absorption following subcutaneous injection slower than intravenous administration because of diffusion for the former. The antibodies are metabolized like endogenous antibodies, with metabolism differing for antibodies bound to antigen versus those that are unbound. The unbound drugs are taken up by cells and processed, with component amino acids used by the cell. Certain cells will recycle antibodies following uptake, dependent on the Fc portion of the antibody, and may account for the long half-life of the unbound biological DMARDs. Any antigen-bound antibody is taken up and completely degraded by specific antibody-antigen elimination processes with no recycling, resulting in a shorter half-life of bound drug than unbound drug. The implication is that patients with severe inflammation will clear the biological agents faster than those patients with less inflammation (low disease state) or for whom the disease is under control (effective treatment). The addition of a conventional DMARD, such as methotrexate, can increase the half-life of the biological agents by decreasing inflammation. The half-life of certolizumab pegol is 12 days, which is shorter than most biological DMARDs. The shorter half-life could result from the polyethylene glycol moieties preventing recognition of the Fc portion of the molecule by the neonatal Fc-receptor (FcRn) recycling system. The half-life of tofacitinib is 3–3.5 hours, and the drug is about 70% metabolized in the liver by CYP3A4 and CYP2C19 into inactive metabolites, while the remaining 30% is excreted via the kidney unchanged.

PHARMACOVIGILANCE: ADVERSE EFFECTS AND DRUG INTERACTIONS

The major adverse effects of the conventional DMARDs are GI problems. Methotrexate can lead to dyspepsia, nausea, and anorexia. However, these problems can be reduced or eliminated if patients also take folic acid or folinic acid. Folinic acid should be taken 24 hours after methotrexate because it interferes with the GI uptake of methotrexate. Increased dosing frequency is associated with an increased risk of hepatotoxicity. Methotrexate is contraindicated for pregnant women and for both women and men actively trying to have children.

Leflunomide causes dyspepsia and nausea, diarrhea, abdominal pain, and hypertension. The most serious adverse effect is hepatotoxicity, and leflunomide is contraindicated in individuals with active liver disease or transaminase levels higher than twice normal, noted by a boxed warning issued by the United States Food and Drug Administration (FDA). Leflunomide is also contraindicated in pregnancy (FDA Category X). The active metabolite teriflunomide can remain in the body for several years after a patient has stopped taking leflunomide as a consequence of enterohepatic circulation. Women treated with leflunomide must be tested for teriflunomide if they become or plan to become pregnant. The elimination of teriflunomide can be increased by oral cholestyramine. The treatment is repeated until teriflunomide blood levels are <0.02 μg/mL for at least 14 days.

The most common adverse effects of sulfasalazine involve the GI system, including nausea, vomiting, and dyspepsia. Headache, rash, and dizziness are also common. The majority of these effects are experienced upon treatment initiation, and they generally subside with time. For this reason, it is common to begin with a low dose and increase weekly.

Sulfasalazine is perhaps the safest for pregnant women, classified as Category B. Sulfasalazine is also considered safe for women wishing to breastfeed.

Hydroxychloroquine and chloroquine commonly lead to GI problems and rashes. Retinal toxicity is a serious adverse effect, but the problem is minimal if dosing does not exceed guideline levels (>400 mg/day hydroxychloroquine or >250 mg/day chloroquine). Hydroxychloroquine can be prescribed for women during pregnancy (Category C).

The adverse effects common to the biological and targeted DMARDs are primarily a consequence of the major antiinflammatory actions of these agents. These drugs can lead to the acquisition of infections or the emergence of latent tuberculosis after treatment initiation, prompting the necessity for testing of all patients for tuberculosis prior to the initiation of treatment. These drugs have an FDA boxed warning of the risk of activating latent tuberculosis in patients and an increased risk of infections or cancer such as lymphoma. Although the overall cancer risk appears small, guidelines do recommend that patients be immunized against other relevant infections, such as pneumonia or influenza prior to beginning treatment. The combination of multiple biological DMARDs or a biological with a targeted DMARD results in a much higher risk for serious infection without a significant improvement in disease outcomes. Injection site or infusion reactions are common but typically mild. The injection site reaction is generally a rash, while infusion reactions include hypertension, fever, chills, headache, and rash.

Tocilizumab and tofacitinib can increase cholesterol levels, but this increase has not been associated with increased atherosclerosis or cardiovascular risk. As foreign proteins, all of the biologicals have the potential to generate antidrug antibodies, which have been associated with lower drug efficacy. To reduce this risk, the majority of these drugs are either human-derived proteins or humanized proteins from mouse. However, infliximab is comprised of a mouse Fab antibody portion and a human Fc portion and can generate antidrug antibodies in up to 40% of patients. The cotreatment with methotrexate can reduce the development of antidrug antibodies.

NEW DEVELOPMENTS

The inflammatory pathway in RA is complex, and there are many cytokines involved for which no drugs have yet been approved, including granulocyte-macrophage colony-stimulating factor (GM-CSF), IL-6, IL-17, IL-17 receptor, IL-20, and IL-12/23. Monoclonal antibodies against IL-6, IL-17, and IL-20 have shown efficacy against RA in phase II trials, but a monoclonal antibody against the IL-17 receptor was ineffective against RA, and the trial was terminated. Ustekinumab is a monoclonal antibody that targets IL-12/23 and is approved in the United States for psoriasis and psoriatic arthritis. Phase II trials testing the effectiveness of ustekinumab in treating RA showed some promise. In addition, there are a number of JAK inhibitors currently under investigation. Some of these are more specific than tofacitinib as they only target JAK1 or JAK3, instead of JAK1-3 like tofacitinib.

CLINICAL RELEVANCE FOR HEALTHCARE PROFESSIONALS

When dealing with patients with RA and patients being treated with DMARDs, healthcare professionals must be aware of the potential for compromising this treatment with exposure to potential infectious agents, particularly where invasive or semiinvasive procedures are used (e.g., dentistry or acupuncture), or the potential for inducing change in pain that may alter effectiveness of the RA treatment or treatment being applied, such as physical therapy.

CLINICAL PROBLEMS

Conventional DMARDs
   Gastrointestinal upset—dyspepsia and nausea and vomiting
   Hepatotoxicity
Biological DMARDs
   Increased risk of infection
   Increased risk of emergence of latent infections

TRADE NAMES

In addition to generic and fixed-combination preparations, the following trade-named materials are some of the important compounds available in the United States.
Conventional
   Hydroxychloroquine (Plaquenil)
   Chloroquine (Aralen)
   Leflunomide (Arava)
   Methotrexate (Trexall)
   Sulfasalazine (Azulfidine EN)
Biological
   Abatacept (Orencia)
   Adalimumab (Humira)
   Certolizumab pegol (Cimzia)
   Etanercept (Enbrel)
   Golimumab (Simponi)
   Infliximab (Remicade)
   Rituximab (Rituxan)
   Tocilizumab (Actemra)
Targeted
   Tofacitinib (Xeljanz)

SELF-ASSESSMENT QUESTIONS

1. A major side effect of methotrexate treatment can be mitigated if the patient also takes:
   A. Leflunomide.
   B. Prednisone.
   C. Sulfasalazine.
   D. Hydroxychloroquine.
   E. Folic acid.

2. Which of the following drug combinations has improved benefit with less risk of infection?
   A. Tofacitinib-tocilizumab.
   B. Etanercept-rituximab.
   C. Abatacept-infliximab.
   D. Adalimumab-methotrexate.
   E. Anakinra-tofacitinib.

3. Prior to treatment of rheumatoid arthritis with biological DMARDs, patients should be tested for:
   A. High levels of TNF-α.
   B. Latent tuberculosis.
   C. NSAID-induced gastrointestinal problems.
   D. Atherosclerosis.
   E. Liver disease.

4. A 59-year-old female being treated for rheumatoid arthritis with a biologic DMARD has developed autoantibodies toward the drug. Which DMARD was she most likely taking?
   A. Abatacept.
   B. Infliximab.
   C. Etanercept.
   D. Adalimumab.
   E. Tofacitinib.

FURTHER READING

Nurmohamed MT, Dijkmans BA. Efficacy, tolerability and cost effectiveness of disease-modifying antirheumatic drugs and biologic agents in rheumatoid arthritis. *Drugs.* 2005;65(5):661–694.

Schwartz DM, Bonelli M, Gadina M, O'Shea JJ. Type I/II cytokines, JAKs, and new strategies for treating autoimmune diseases. *Nat Rev Rheumatol.* 2016;12(1):25–36.

Scott DL. Biologics-based therapy for the treatment of rheumatoid arthritis. *Clin Pharmacol Ther.* 2012;91(1):30–43.

Singh JA, Saag KG, Bridges SL, et al. 2015 American College of Rheumatology Guideline for the Treatment of Rheumatoid Arthritis. *Arthritis Rheumatol.* 2016;68(1):1–26.

Smolen JS, Aletaha D. Rheumatoid arthritis therapy reappraisal: strategies, opportunities and challenges. *Nat Rev Rheumatol.* 2015;11(5):276–289.

Smolen JS, Steiner G. Therapeutic strategies for rheumatoid arthritis. *Nat Rev Drug Discov.* 2003;2(6):473–488.

WEBSITES

https://www.rheumatology.org/I-Am-A/Patient-Caregiver/Diseases-Conditions/Rheumatoid-Arthritis
This website is maintained by the American College of Rheumatology and contains information for patients, students and healthcare providers.

https://www.hopkinsarthritis.org/arthritis-info/rheumatoid-arthritis/ra-treatment/
This website is maintained by the John Hopkins Arthritis Center and contains information on treatments for rheumatoid arthritis.

SECTION 6

Drug Treatment for Cardiovascular Diseases

Introduction to the Regulation of Cardiovascular Function

David A. Taylor and Abdel A. Abdel-Rahman

Cardiovascular disease is the primary cause of death throughout the world, accounting for more than 17 million deaths per year, with an estimated increase to more than 23 million by 2030. Cardiovascular disease consists of a constellation of disorders that includes diseases of the heart (e.g., heart failure) and/or the blood vessels (e.g., hypertension). Recent statistics from the American Heart Association (2017) indicate that in the United States, approximately 92.1 million people suffer from cardiovascular disease or the aftereffects of stroke. Cardiovascular diseases are responsible for more deaths each year than cancer or lower respiratory diseases combined. Cardiovascular diseases appear more frequently in African-American adults, where estimates suggest that nearly one-half of this population exhibits some form of cardiovascular disease.

Hypertension is the most prominent risk factor contributing to the prevalence of cardiovascular disease. The importance of hypertension as a public health problem will increase as the population ages, and preventing hypertension will be a major public health challenge for this century. More than 85 million adults in the United States, which represents nearly 34% of the population, have hypertension. Of these individuals, approximately 76% are receiving antihypertensive therapy, but only 54% are adequately controlled. In addition, hypertension appears to be a prelude to stroke because 77% of individuals who experience a first stroke have blood pressures that exceed 140/90 mm Hg. Among cardiovascular diseases, stroke was the second leading cause of death behind coronary heart disease both globally and in the United States (Table 36.1) and was the fifth most common cause of overall mortality in the United States. The most recent report of the Joint National Committee on Prevention, Detection, Evaluation, and Treatment of High Blood Pressure (JNC-8) classifies hypertension based on both systolic and diastolic blood pressures. Most candidates for antihypertensive drug therapy have a systolic blood pressure above 140 mm Hg, a diastolic pressure above 90 mm Hg, or both. The presence of other risk factors (e.g., smoking, diabetes, hyperlipidemia, target organ damage) is also an important determinant in the decision to treat patients with drugs. To best understand pharmacological approaches to the management of these disorders, an overview of the processes by which cardiovascular function is regulated will provide insight regarding the target selections.

The function of the cardiovascular system is regulated by several components, including the autonomic nervous system (ANS); the kidneys; heart; vasculature, including the endothelium; and the blood. The ANS innervates the heart, blood vessels, kidney, and adrenal medulla and has the potential to modify cardiovascular function at several different levels (Chapter 6). Because these organ systems represent an integrated network, cardiovascular function can be affected by any single alteration. The heart, including the rhythmic nature of its electrical signals, force

ABBREVIATIONS	
ACh	Acetylcholine
ANS	Autonomic nervous system
CNS	Central nervous system
Epi	Epinephrine
NE	Norepinephrine

of contraction, and magnitude of the discharge pressure, is responsible for pumping the blood through the pulmonary system for oxygenation and delivering it through the vasculature to organs/tissues throughout the body. The circulation (both blood volume and composition), including H_2O, electrolyte and iron balances, cholesterol, lipid composition, and capabilities for clot formation and lysis, delivers O_2 and nutrients to, and carries CO_2 and waste away from, all tissues. The kidneys adjust the excretion of Na^+, K^+, and other electrolytes and H_2O to maintain extracellular fluid and volume; fluid retention by the kidney is a modifiable physiological parameter that can result in changes in blood pressure and cardiac function.

Cardiac performance and vascular caliber are controlled by several intrinsic regulatory mechanisms. The firing of pacemaker cells in the sinoatrial node determines heart rate, and several homeostatic mechanisms modulate cardiac pumping efficiency. Local regulation of the caliber of most resistance-producing blood vessels (i.e., capillaries) is influenced by the intrinsic contractile state of vascular smooth muscle, balanced by the production of vasodilator and vasoconstrictor substances originating from the endothelial cell monolayer lining the vessel lumen.

Superimposed on these intrinsic control processes to the heart and blood vessels are extrinsic factors that affect total cardiovascular function. These include the metabolic status of the tissues in which blood vessels are embedded and locally produced, and blood-borne vasoactive chemicals (autocrine/paracrine/endocrine regulators). It is essential to remember that arterial blood pressure is the product of cardiac output and total peripheral resistance. Blood flows through the vascular system, with cardiac output determined by the rate and efficiency of the pumping of the heart. Vascular resistance increases as the viscosity of the blood and the tone and length of blood vessels increases, particularly in precapillary arterioles, which represent the major structural determinant of vascular resistance. Thus understanding the physiological factors that regulate these three components (heart rate, stroke volume, and total peripheral resistance) will enable an individual to predict the activity of any given agent on cardiovascular function as it relates to blood pressure.

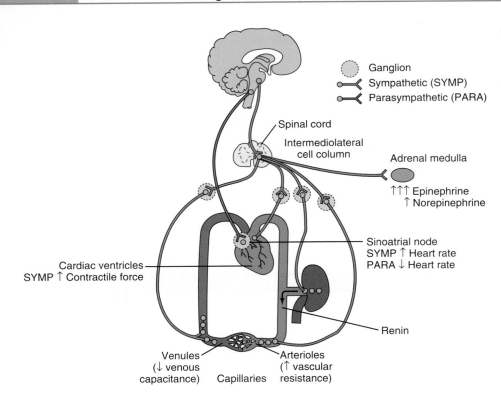

FIG. 36.1 Effects of the Autonomic Nervous System on Blood Pressure Control. Vascular resistance is affected almost exclusively by the sympathetic nervous system, whereas cardiac output is regulated by both sympathetic and parasympathetic influences.

TABLE 36.1	Deaths Due to Cardiovascular Disease in the United States[a]
Coronary heart disease	45.1
Stroke	16.5
Hypertension	9.1
Heart failure	8.5

[a]Data from the American Heart Association Statistics 2017; numbers represent percentages of the populations.

The overall coordination and integration of cardiovascular function is accomplished primarily by the ANS. Through its sympathetic and parasympathetic limbs, the ANS has powerful effects on both cardiac performance and blood vessel caliber. It is important to note that the sympathetic and parasympathetic innervations of cardiovascular end organs are tonically active, which means that activity can be modulated by either increasing or decreasing the firing rate of these nerves. Effects of autonomic nerve activity on the mechanisms that control blood pressure are summarized in Fig. 36.1. Parasympathetic effects are mediated by acetylcholine (ACh) released from postganglionic parasympathetic nerve endings, whereas sympathetic effects are mediated by norepinephrine (NE) released from postganglionic sympathetic nerve endings. Although there is little circulating ACh because of high cholinesterase activity in both tissue and blood, NE released from postganglionic sympathetic nerve endings escapes into the circulation because its degradation or uptake (by nerve endings) is incomplete. This source of NE, in concert with the epinephrine (Epi) and NE released into the blood from the adrenal medulla, influence cardiovascular function as circulating neurohormones. Chapter 6 has in-depth discussion of the ANS.

Overall cardiac performance is influenced by both parasympathetic and sympathetic actions at different sites within the heart. Heart rate is decreased by parasympathetic activity and increased by sympathetic activity at the sinoatrial node, but the parasympathetic effect is usually dominant. The heart rate is never stable, even during rest. The interaction between the parasympathetic and sympathetic innervation of the heart determines the heart rate measured at any particular time, as well as the heart rate variability. The latter is recognized as an important determinant of heart physiology, and its suppression is a predictor of myocardial pathology and mortality.

Ventricular contractile force is only modestly, if at all, directly influenced by parasympathetic activity but is greatly increased by sympathetic activity, including the actions of circulating Epi and NE. Increased sympathetic activity reduces vascular caliber by contracting vascular smooth muscle. Although there are parasympathetic influences on a few vascular beds, their contribution to overall vascular resistance is insignificant. Constriction of veins in response to sympathetic activity reduces venous capacitance, thereby increasing venous return to the heart, which augments right atrial and ventricular filling; under healthy conditions, these cardiovascular responses increase cardiac output. However, it must also be remembered that sympathetically mediated constriction of arterioles can reduce cardiac output by increasing the vascular resistance (afterload) against which the heart must pump blood. In addition, elevated sympathetic activity to the kidney increases renin release and subsequent angiotensin II and aldosterone formation, leading to Na^+ and H_2O retention (Chapter 39). All of these effects act in concert to elevate arterial blood pressure. Conversely, a reduction of sympathetic activity reduces blood pressure by diminishing the sympathetic stimulus and reduces the workload of the heart (O_2 consumption).

CENTRAL CONTROL OF AUTONOMIC NERVE ACTIVITY

The organization of autonomic cardiovascular control systems within the central nervous system (CNS) is summarized in Fig. 36.2. The final common (preganglionic) output neurons for cardiovascular control by

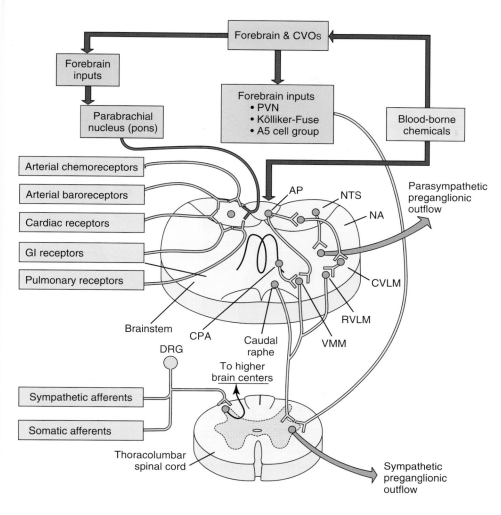

FIG. 36.2 Organization of Autonomic Cardiovascular Control Systems. Major inputs are in boxes. Many reciprocal connections are not illustrated. *AP*, Area postrema; *CPA*, caudal pressor area; *CVLM*, caudal ventrolateral medulla; *CVO*, circumventricular organs; *DRG*, dorsal root ganglia; *NA*, nucleus ambiguus; *NTS*, nucleus tractus solitarius; *PVN*, paraventricular nucleus; *RVLM*, rostral ventrolateral medulla; *VMM*, ventromedial medulla.

the parasympathetic nervous system are located principally in the nucleus ambiguus and the dorsal motor nucleus of the vagus in the brainstem. The preganglionic neurons of the sympathetic nervous system are located in the intermediolateral columns of the thoracolumbar region of the spinal cord. Antecedent to these final output neurons, much of the integration of neural signals contributing to autonomic regulation of cardiovascular function occurs at other sites in the brainstem, most notably the rostral ventrolateral medulla. These neurons, in turn, receive input from all levels of the CNS.

Origin and Regulation of Autonomic Activity

One of the primary functions of the ANS is to provide adaptive regulation and coordination of blood pressure and cardiac output to ensure adequate blood flow to various organs of the body in the face of an ever-changing internal environment. This is accomplished by neural circuits intrinsic to the CNS and as a response to mechanical and humoral signals originating in the periphery. Integration of these signals by the CNS produces patterns of autonomic activity that ensure adequate organ perfusion appropriate to such diverse demands as changes in posture, hemorrhage, digestion, stress, and exercise.

Parasympathetic preganglionic neurons that project to the heart via the vagus nerves have low levels of spontaneous firing, and their discharge rate is driven mostly by inputs from various afferents, particularly arterial baroreceptors. Inputs to spinal sympathetic preganglionic neurons originate in the brainstem, pons, and hypothalamus and are mostly excitatory, primarily by activating neurons located in the rostral

ventrolateral medulla, which is an important site in the central regulation of cardiovascular function and for many centrally active agents used to treat hypertension.

Under physiological and pathophysiological conditions, the activity of autonomic nerves is regulated by neural signals arising from the periphery. Activation of visceral sensory nerves projecting to the brain via the vagus afferent nerves generally reduces sympathetic activity and increases parasympathetic activity. These afferents include stretch receptors located in the cardiovascular system, which provide information about arterial pressure (arterial baroreceptors) and cardiac filling (cardiac stretch receptors), as well as stretch receptors and chemosensory receptors in the lungs, which provide information about respiratory mechanics and lung irritants, respectively. Afferents with chemosensory terminals located in the carotid body encode blood gas O_2 concentration, send projections to the brain via the glossopharyngeal nerve, and when activated by hypoxia, hypercapnia, or acidic pH, increase efferent sympathetic nerve activity. All of these afferents make their first central synapse within the nucleus of the tractus solitarius located in the dorsomedial brainstem. Aortic afferents (originating in the aortic arch) and sinus nerve afferents (originating in the carotid sinus) produce sympathoinhibition via activation of the caudal portion of the solitary tract nucleus, whereas glossopharyngeal afferents that produce sympathoexcitation project to more medial/rostral aspects of this nucleus.

Other visceral mechanosensitive and chemosensitive nerve terminals are located throughout the body. Some of these neurons, with cell bodies in the dorsal root ganglia, may initially commingle their axons within various sympathetic nerve trunks (sympathetic afferents) before synapsing on cells located in the dorsal horns of the spinal cord. Other sensory afferents do not travel with the sympathetic nerves and instead associate with various sensory-motor nerve trunks (somatic afferents) before synapsing in the spinal dorsal horns. All of these afferents typically encode noxious or painful chemical or mechanical stimuli, such as those associated with cardiac or visceral ischemia, visceral organ distention, or injury, and detect the metabolic products produced by exercising skeletal muscle. Activation of these afferents typically produces sympathoexcitation.

In addition to neural signals from the periphery, the brain also detects chemical signals (including drugs such as digitalis) that circulate in the blood. A wide variety of circulating humoral substances, including catecholamines, indoleamines, and peptides, directly contact neurons within the CNS by diffusing through the fenestrated capillaries of circumventricular organs that lack a blood-brain barrier. Activation of circumventricular organ neurons produces integrated autonomic, endocrine, and behavioral responses that can regulate a variety of physiological components, including salt and H_2O balance and nutrient homeostasis, as well as cardiovascular function. The most important of the circumventricular organs for central autonomic control are the area postrema, subfornical organ, and organum vasculosum of the lamina terminalis.

Baroreceptor Reflex

The baroreceptor reflex is the most rapidly acting ANS control system for regulating blood pressure. The principal role of this reflex is to ensure adequate organ perfusion, particularly to the brain, heart, and kidney, and to promote return of blood to the heart to counterbalance conditions that lower arterial blood pressure. Such conditions might include gravitational pooling of blood when assuming an upright posture and instances where blood volume is lost, such as during severe dehydration or hemorrhage. The baroreceptor reflex is also activated when drugs are used to lower blood pressure in hypertensive individuals, and this reflex may profoundly affect both the therapeutic outcomes and potential cardiac side effects caused by antihypertensive drug therapy.

Minute-to-minute control of arterial blood pressure is achieved when small blood pressure changes are linked to reflex alterations in ANS activity. Sensory nerve endings embedded in the wall of the carotid sinus and aortic arch (baroreceptors) are activated by wall stretch that occurs when arterial pressure increases or decreases from a recognized set point. An increase in blood pressure triggers within a few seconds a simultaneous increase in vagal (parasympathetic) and a reduction in sympathetic activity. Parasympathetic activation slows the heart rate, and sympathetic inhibition results in passive vasodilation, thus tending to return arterial pressure toward normal. Conversely, a decrease in arterial pressure is rapidly countered by increased sympathetic and decreased parasympathetic activity. This change in ANS activity results in vasoconstriction (increased vascular resistance) and an elevated cardiac rate and force of cardiac contraction (increased cardiac output). Organization of the baroreceptor reflex is illustrated in Fig. 36.3.

The baroreceptor reflex is important primarily in the short-term control of blood pressure. When changes in blood pressure persist beyond a few minutes, there is adaptation that involves both peripheral and CNS components. This change occurs to varying degrees with normal aging and in patients with heart failure or hypertension and is manifest by the failure of the baroreceptor reflex to respond when blood pressure is elevated for a prolonged period of time, referred to as baroreflex adaptation. Thus this impairment may help explain why some antihypertensive drugs are more effective in hypertensive than in normotensive patients, because lowering of blood pressure by

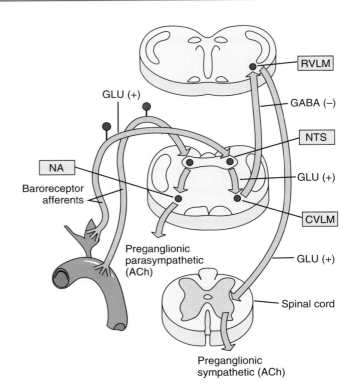

Blood pressure	NORMAL	INCREASED	DECREASED
Baroreceptor afferent activity	NORMAL	↑	↓
Sympathetic activity	NORMAL	↓	↑
Parasympathetic activity	NORMAL	↑	↓

FIG. 36.3 Brainstem Organization of the Baroreceptor Reflex and Associated Neurotransmitters. Primary pathways only are shown. Other afferents and interneurons are omitted. *CVLM,* Caudal ventrolateral medulla; *GABA,* γ-aminobutyric acid; *GLU,* 1-glutamate; *NA,* nucleus ambiguus; *NTS,* nucleus tractus solitarius; *RVLM,* rostral ventrolateral medulla; +, excitatory pathway; −, inhibitory pathway.

antihypertensive drugs may be less effectively counteracted by baroreflex-mediated sympathetic vasoconstriction in these individuals.

The influence of baroreceptors on sympathetic nerve activity can vary greatly in different vascular beds. Some beds, such as the cutaneous vasculature, are largely independent of arterial baroreceptor influence and contribute little to total peripheral vascular resistance. In contrast, the baroreceptor reflex predominates in controlling sympathetic regulation of vascular diameter in many organs that receive a significant fraction of the cardiac output, such as skeletal muscle and the kidneys. For this reason, baroreflex regulation of sympathetic vasoconstriction plays an important role in determining total peripheral resistance. In fact, except under some special circumstances (exercise, sleep, and certain behavioral states), baroreceptors are able to override all other inputs affecting autonomic regulation of arterial blood pressure. This may reflect the importance of maintaining a stable systemic blood pressure to ensure adequate organ perfusion under diverse environmental conditions. It is also imperative to note that some antihypertensive medications render the baroreceptor reflex dysfunctional by interrupting ganglionic transmission of sympathetic nerves, the release of NE from sympathetic nerve terminals, or blockade of vascular α_1-adrenergic receptors. Such drug-induced impairment compromises baroreceptor responsiveness and can result in orthostatic hypotension when the individual assumes the upright from the sitting position. On the other hand, some antihypertensive medications improve baroreceptor reflex function.

REGULATION OF SYMPATHETIC ACTIVITY

One potential cause of hypertension has been suggested to be sympathetic hyperactivity leading to an increase in vascular resistance, and a shift in the sympathetic to parasympathetic balance of the heart toward sympathetic dominance. Increased sympathetic effects can be produced by increased neural firing rate, increased catecholamine concentrations at the neuroeffector junction, and alterations at postjunctional receptors and signal transduction pathways. Although there is support for each of these mechanisms, the first two are most important, and drugs that inhibit sympathetic activity centrally and/or peripherally are useful for treating hypertension.

Under physiological conditions, the amount of NE released from sympathetic nerve terminals is influenced by various chemicals, some of which are coreleased substances, such as neuropeptide Y and adenosine triphosphate, whereas others are released from postjunctional tissues, including angiotensin II, or are present in the circulation, such as Epi (Table 36.2). Endogenous compounds that alter Ca^{++}, Na^+, or K^+ channel activity lead to alterations in vesicular NE release. In addition, the released transmitter itself, acting at prejunctional (presynaptic) **autoreceptors**, and other transmitters or hormones acting at prejunctional **heteroreceptors**, can affect NE release. Activation of prejunctional receptors modulates the probability that individual vesicles will discharge their contents by exocytosis congruent with depolarization; it does not affect the amount of transmitter released by individual vesicles. Activation of inhibitory presynaptic receptors by NE may function as a physiological brake on neurotransmitter secretion during periods of high-frequency nerve discharge, thus limiting postjunctional responses (negative feedback control). On the other hand, other circulating substances such as angiotensin II can activate their own presynaptic receptors at sympathetic nerve endings, leading to increased release of NE. In contrast, activation of inhibitory heteroreceptors, such as occurs with adenosine, reduces the probability of vesicular exocytosis and transmitter release. Some of these mechanisms are illustrated in Fig. 36.4. It is important to remember that because local mechanisms regulating NE release differ in different tissues, similar rates of sympathetic nerve firing may produce different effects in different tissues.

In addition to prejunctional regulation of release, the concentration of neurotransmitter at neuroeffector junctions can be influenced by alterations in transmitter synthesis, storage within the nerve terminal, and removal from the neuroeffector junction by diffusion, metabolism, and reuptake. These latter mechanisms are important targets for therapeutically active drugs. It must be remembered that the level of sympathetic activity, and ultimately blood pressure, is also modulated by central mechanisms. For example, activation of α_2-adrenergic receptors in the CNS, such as by the antihypertensive agent clonidine, decreases sympathetic activity. Other neuromodulators of sympathetic activity include locally synthesized neuropeptides such as angiotensin II, which activates the angiotensin receptors in the rostral ventrolateral medulla to increase sympathetic activity and elevate blood pressure, a mechanism implicated to play a role in human high renin hypertension.

Some of the factors proposed to play a causative role in hypertension as a consequence of increasing sympathetic activity are listed in Box 36.1. These central and peripheral factors constitute well-characterized molecular targets for therapeutically prescribed antihypertensive medications.

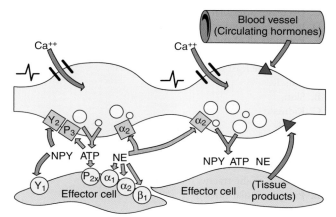

FIG. 36.4 Prejunctional Regulation at the Sympathetic Neuroeffector Junction. The left varicosity illustrates autoinhibition of neurotransmitter release, including possible "lateral" inhibition (i.e., transmitter from one varicosity inhibiting release from an adjacent varicosity). The right varicosity illustrates prejunctional regulation of transmitter release by tissue and blood-borne chemicals. See Table 36.2 for a list of involved substances. Postjunctional receptors are shown as yellow circles with the type of receptor noted, ○; prejunctional inhibitory autoreceptors are shown as squares, □; prejunctional heteroreceptors are shown as dark triangles, ▲. For abbreviations, see Table 36.2.

TABLE 36.2 Prejunctional Modulators of Sympathetic Neurotransmitter Release

Chemical	Source	Receptor	Mechanism	Effect
Norepinephrine (NE)	SNT	α_2	$\downarrow Ca^{++}$	$\downarrow$
Neuropeptide Y (NPY)	SNT	Y_2	$\downarrow Ca^{++}$	$\downarrow$
ATP	SNT	P_3, P_{2x}	$\downarrow Ca^{++}$	$\downarrow$
Epinephrine	Blood	β_2	$\uparrow cAMP$	$\uparrow$
Angiotensin II	Blood/PJT	AT_1	$\uparrow PLC$	$\uparrow$
Prostanoids	PJT	EP3	$\downarrow Ca^{++}$	$\downarrow$
Adenosine	PJT	P_1	$\downarrow Ca^{++}$	$\downarrow$
Opioids	Blood	μ, κ, δ	$\downarrow Ca^{++}$	$\downarrow$
Acetylcholine	Nerve	M_2	$\uparrow cGMP$	$\downarrow$
Dopamine	SNT	D_2	$\uparrow K^+$	$\downarrow$
Nitric oxide (NO)	EC	Guanylate cyclase	$\uparrow cGMP$	$\downarrow$

cAMP, Cyclic adenosine monophosphate; *cGMP,* cyclic guanosine monophosphate; *EC,* endothelial cell; *PJT,* postjunctional tissue; *PLC,* phospholipase C; *SNT,* sympathetic nerve terminal.

BOX 36.1   Factors Increasing Sympathetic Nervous System Activity That Lead to Hypertension

Elevated Sympathetic Discharge
Physiological Dysfunction
Sleep apnea
Stress
Obesity
Increased central sympathetic outflow
Impaired baroreceptor reflexes

Humoral
Increased plasma insulin
Increased plasma leptin

Increased plasma or tissue angiotensin II
Increased extracellular Na^+

Enhanced NE Release
Increased angiotensin II facilitation
Increased β_2-adrenergic receptor facilitation
Decreased neuropeptide Y inhibition

SELF-ASSESSMENT QUESTIONS

1. Increased activity of the sympathetic nervous system:
   A. Increases heart rate.
   B. Increases the force of cardiac contraction.
   C. Decreases arteriolar caliber.
   D. Increases venous return to the heart.
   E. Produces all of the above effects.

2. Sympathetic activity to which of the following vascular beds is influenced the least by arterial baroreflexes?
   A. Muscle.
   B. Skin.
   C. Kidney.
   D. Heart.
   E. Splanchnic viscera.

3. Peripheral information from the lungs and heart are transmitted via sensory afferents to which nucleus in the brain?
   A. Nucleus of the tractus solitarius.
   B. Paraventricular nucleus.
   C. Nucleus ambiguus.
   D. Caudal raphe nucleus.

4. A decrease in arterial pressure:
   A. Increases baroreceptor afferent activity.
   B. Decreases sympathetic nerve discharge.
   C. Decreases heart rate.
   D. Decreases vagal discharge.
   E. Decreases the release of NE from postganglionic sympathetic nerves.

5. Which of the following statements is correct with regard to autonomic control of blood vessels?
   A. Blood vessels are innervated by both divisions of the autonomic nervous system.
   B. Blood vessels are almost exclusively innervated by sympathetic nerves.
   C. Blood vessels are innervated exclusively by parasympathetic nerves.
   D. Blood vessels are not controlled by the autonomic nervous system.

FURTHER READING

Dampney RA. Central neural control of the cardiovascular system: current perspectives. *Adv Physiol Educ.* 2016;40(3):283–296.

Gordan R, Gwathmey JK, Xie L-H. Autonomic and endocrine control of cardiovascular function. *World J Cardiol.* 2015;7:204–214.

Mancia G, Grassi G. The autonomic nervous system and hypertension. *Circ Res.* 2014;114:1804–1814.

Robertson D, Biaggioni I, Burnstock G, Low PA. *Primer on the Autonomic Nervous System.* New York: Elsevier; 2004.

Sved AF, Ito S, Sved JC. Brainstem mechanisms of hypertension: role of the rostral ventrolateral medulla. *Curr Hypertens Rep.* 2003;5:262–268.

WEBSITES

http://www.heart.org/HEARTORG/
This site is maintained by the American Heart Association and is an excellent resource for all aspects of cardiovascular health, including links to a multitude of resources.

https://www.cdc.gov/heartdisease/facts.htm
This site is maintained by the United States Centers for Disease Control and Prevention and is another excellent resource on cardiovascular disorders, including statistical data on morbidity and mortality, as well as links to resources and educational materials.

Overview of Hypertension Management and Drugs That Decrease Sympathetic Tone

David A. Taylor and Abdel A. Abdel-Rahman

MAJOR DRUG CLASSES

Centrally acting sympatholytics
  α_2-Adrenergic receptor agonists
  Imidazoline receptor agonists
Peripherally acting sympatholytics

ABBREVIATIONS

ACE	Angiotensin-converting enzyme
ARB	Angiotensin receptor blocker
CCB	Calcium-channel blocker
CNS	Central nervous system
CO	Cardiac output
DBP	Diastolic blood pressure
Epi	Epinephrine
I_1-IR	Selective I_1-imidazoline receptor
JNC-8	Joint National Committee on Detection, Evaluation, and Treatment of High Blood Pressure
NE	Norepinephrine
RAAS	Renin-angiotensin-aldosterone system
TPR	Total peripheral resistance

THERAPEUTIC OVERVIEW

Hypertension is defined as an elevation of arterial blood pressure above an arbitrarily defined normal value. Although a small number (<10%) of people have hypertension traceable to specific causes such as renal disease or endocrine tumors, which are designated as **secondary hypertension**, the most common form of hypertension, which is present in over 90% of patients, has no readily identifiable cause and is termed **essential** or **primary hypertension**. Unless its onset is rapid and severe, hypertension does not produce noticeable symptoms. The purpose of treating hypertension is to circumvent end-organ injury and to prevent or reduce the severity of diseases such as atherosclerosis, coronary artery disease, aortic aneurysm, congestive heart failure, stroke, diabetes, and renal and retinal disease. The disorders for which hypertension represents a major risk factor and the treatments for hypertension designated by the Joint National Committee on Detection, Evaluation, and Treatment of High Blood Pressure (JNC-8) are presented in the Therapeutic Overview Box.

Therapy of hypertension involves both **pharmacological** and **nonpharmacological** interventions. The therapeutic goal is to reduce blood pressure to below 150/90 mm Hg in patients 60 years of age or older and below 140/90 mm Hg in patients between the ages of 18–59 or 60 years of age or older with other underlying conditions such as diabetes, chronic kidney disease, or both. The most recent recommendations from JNC-8 focus on achieving diastolic blood pressure (DBP) of <90 mm Hg, as a number of clinical trials provided compelling evidence that achieving a DBP <90 mm Hg significantly reduced the ri k of cerebrovascular events, heart failure, and overall mortality. Adoption of healthy lifestyles may lower blood pressure as much as some drugs and may also prevent the onset or progression of hypertension, although patients differ in their sensitivity to these lifestyle changes. For example, maintenance of normal body weight and increased physical activity lowers blood pressure in most sedentary and overweight hypertensive individuals, whereas Na^+ restriction lowers blood pressure mainly in hypertensive people categorized as "salt sensitive." The major advantage of nonpharmacological therapies is relative safety compared to drug therapy. While the lack of compliance by most people is a principal limitation of therapeutic lifestyle modification, lifestyle changes remain an important aspect of the management plan and should be recommended even when pharmacological therapy is initiated. Because drug therapy for hypertension must usually be continued for the lifetime of the patient, it is important to implement nonpharmacological interventions to enhance therapeutic outcome.

Systemic blood pressure is regulated redundantly by several physiological control systems to ensure optimal tissue perfusion throughout the body (Chapter 36). When blood pressure decreases by any means, including antihypertensive drug therapy, one or more of these regulatory mechanisms are activated to compensate for decreases in arterial blood pressure (Fig. 37.1). The compensatory systems involved include the sympathetic nervous system and the renin-angiotensin-aldosterone system (RAAS); these two systems regulate the function of the end organs responsible for maintaining blood pressure, which include the kidneys, heart, blood vessels, and brain. Therefore it should not be surprising that agents employed in the therapeutic management of hypertension influence molecular targets in these systems.

Although the goal of antihypertensive therapy is to reduce end-organ damage associated with chronically elevated blood pressure, the effects of therapy on other cardiovascular risk factors must also be considered. End-organ damage is not related exclusively to blood pressure. If an antihypertensive drug effectively lowers blood pressure but increases the influence of other risk factors for cardiovascular disease, the benefit of therapy may be reduced. In some studies, thiazide diuretics did not decrease the incidence of coronary artery disease, despite their ability to significantly reduce blood pressure. This may be related to the modest

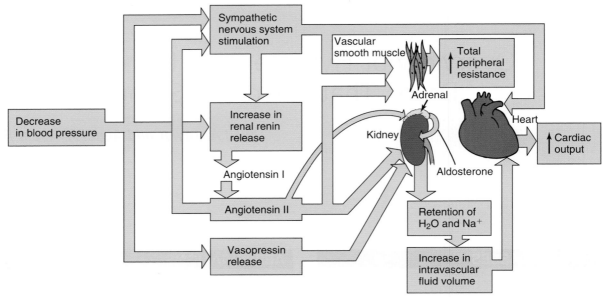

FIG. 37.1 Physiological Compensatory Mechanisms That Counteract Decreased Blood Pressure.

elevation of low-density lipoprotein and total triglycerides produced by K⁺-depleting diuretics, although the causative link or potential clinical significance of this finding has not been established. Other risk factors that can be affected by antihypertensive drugs include alterations in plasma levels of glucose and uric acid. In particular, insulin resistance is now recognized to be prevalent in patients with hypertension. Elevated insulin along with insulin resistance is a risk factor for coronary artery disease. Thus it is noteworthy that thiazide diuretics and β-adrenergic receptor blockers increase insulin resistance, angiotensin-converting enzyme (ACE) inhibitors and prazosin decrease insulin resistance, while Ca⁺⁺ channel blockers (CCBs) have no effect. Because of wide interpatient variability for risk factors and disease, therapeutic generalizations are difficult, and antihypertensive drug therapy must be tailored to each patient.

The classes of antihypertensive agents have their primary effects on different organs (Fig. 37.2) and produce different physiological responses (Table 37.1). These drugs have proven to be of clinical benefit, either alone or in combination, for several indications. The choice of therapy for a patient with essential hypertension depends on the initial blood pressure of the individual, as well as age, race, sex, family history of cardiovascular disease, and other risk factors, such as smoking, obesity, and sedentary lifestyle. Most important is the presence of other conditions such as kidney disease, ischemic heart disease, heart failure, previous myocardial infarction or stroke, or diabetes. Each of these must be given due consideration to determine an appropriate treatment plan as provided by the most recent recommendations of JNC-8.

MECHANISMS OF ACTION

Diuretics, which are discussed in Chapter 38, cause Na⁺ excretion and reduce fluid volume by inhibiting electrolyte transport in the renal tubules, which contributes to their antihypertensive action. **Drugs that affect the RAAS**, discussed in Chapter 39, are widely used in the treatment of several disorders of cardiovascular function, including hypertension, while the **CCBs** (Chapter 40) are now considered one of the first-line treatments for hypertension. The **direct vasodilators** are among the most powerful drugs used to lower blood pressure, and their use is usually reserved for the treatment of hypertension that is severe

or refractory to other drugs, as presented in Chapter 41. The **β-adrenergic receptor blockers** used for the treatment of hypertension share the common characteristic of competitively antagonizing the effects of norepinephrine (NE) and epinephrine (Epi) on β₁-adrenergic receptors in the heart and renin-secreting cells of the kidney, while clinically useful **α₁-adrenergic receptor antagonists** lower blood pressure

TABLE 37.1 Physiological Responses to Antihypertensive Drugs

Drug Class	Plasma Volume	CO	Heart Rate	TPR	Plasma Renin Activity	Sympathetic Nerve Activity
Diuretics	↓	↓	↔↑	↓	↑	↔↑
Angiotensin inhibitors	↔	↑↓↔	↔	↓	↑	↔
β-adrenergic receptor blockers	↔	↓	↓	↔↑	↓	↔↓
Centrally acting sympatholytics	↔↑	↓	↓	↓	↔↓	↓
Peripherally acting sympatholytics	↔↑	↔↓	↔↓	↓	↔	↑
Ca++ channel blockers	↔	↔	↔↑	↓	↔↑	↔↑
Orally active vasodilators	↑	↔↑	↑	↓	↑	↑

↑, Increase; ↓, decrease; ↔, no change.

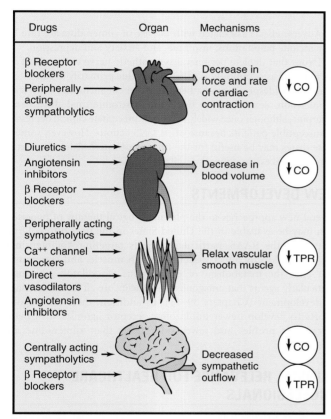

FIG. 37.2 Summary of the Sites and Mechanisms by Which Antihypertensive Drugs Reduce Blood Pressure. *CO,* Cardiac output; *TPR,* total peripheral resistance.

by blocking α_1 receptors on vascular smooth muscle (Chapters 11 and 12).

The agents that reduce sympathetic tone are generally reserved for the treatment of resistant forms of hypertension that are often clinically challenging. These agents include those that have an action in the central nervous system (CNS) or the peripheral nervous system or have mixed actions in the CNS and periphery. A common denominator for these drugs is their ability to elicit a direct or indirect sympatholytic effect.

Centrally acting sympatholytics lower blood pressure by reducing the firing rate of sympathetic nerves, principally by activation of α_2-adrenergic receptors. Drugs in this class include α-methyldopa, clonidine, guanfacine, and guanabenz and are referred to as the first-generation centrally acting sympatholytics. The antihypertensive

effects of α-methyldopa, which is the oldest centrally acting sympatholytic and is considered a pure α_2-receptor agonist, are attributed to its conversion in the brain to α-methyl-NE through reactions catalyzed by l-aromatic amino acid decarboxylase and dopamine-β-hydroxylase; thus α-methyl-NE is a prodrug. Clonidine, guanfacine, and guanabenz, which readily enter the brain after systemic administration, are also agonists at central α_2 receptors. The central site(s) where α_2-receptor agonists act to lower blood pressure have not been completely identified and characterized but may include the nucleus of the solitary tract and the C1 neurons of the rostral ventrolateral medulla (Chapter 36). It must also be remembered that clonidine and similar drugs also inhibit NE release from adrenergic nerves via activation of the presynaptic α_2-adrenergic receptors, which triggers the negative feedback inhibition of NE release.

The newer second-generation centrally acting drugs, or the selective I_1-imidazoline receptor (I_1-IR) agonists, include rilmenidine and moxonidine. It is important to note that these agents also retain α_2-adrenergic receptor agonist activity, albeit at a much weaker level than clonidine, which also has agonist activity at the I_1-IR. Although the exact molecular mechanisms implicated in the sympatholytic actions of these compounds remain to be fully elucidated, activation of both α_2-adrenergic receptors and I_1-IRs inhibit central sympathetic tone. The effect of the first-generation α_2-adrenergic receptor drugs is mediated via a reduction in intracellular cAMP resulting from activating the Gi-coupled α_2-adrenergic receptor, while that of the second-generation I_1-IR drugs involves the I_1-IR–mediated activation of phospholipase C, resulting in the generation of intracellular diacylglycerol. In addition, both drug subclasses increased the release of the inhibitory amino acid GABA within the rostral ventrolateral medulla, perhaps contributing to their sympatholytic effects.

Sympatholytics with a peripheral action include guanethidine, guanadrel, and reserpine. Guanethidine and guanadrel are no longer available in the United States, and reserpine is considered second line for some hypertensive situations. All of these agents act at sympathetic nerve endings to decrease NE release. Reserpine, which is a plant alkaloid, was the first drug to be used widely for the treatment of mild to moderate hypertension. It is highly lipophilic and binds almost irreversibly to the vesicular monoamine transporter in both peripheral and CNS catecholaminergic nerves, preventing the accumulation of monoamines. As a consequence, circulating NE levels are depleted, leading to reductions in vascular resistance and blood pressure.

RELATIONSHIP OF MECHANISMS OF ACTION TO CLINICAL RESPONSE

In general, more than 50% of patients require more than one drug to control their hypertension. If two or more drugs are used, each should target a different physiological mechanism (see Fig. 37.2). For example, it would be more beneficial to combine a diuretic with a vasodilator than to use two drugs that both reduce smooth muscle contraction. In most instances, a diuretic should be included in any regimen using two or more antihypertensive drugs. The recent recommendations from JNC-8 provide such a framework of drug combinations.

The centrally acting sympatholytics reduce sympathetic nerve discharge and lower blood pressure mainly by reducing total peripheral resistance (TPR) with an additional contribution from reduced cardiac output (CO). While centrally acting sympatholytics inhibit sympathetic activity, they do not inhibit (they actually enhance) the baroreceptor reflex. This favorable outcome should be distinguished from peripherally acting sympatholytics, which dramatically suppress the baroreceptor reflex. In addition, clonidine possesses a unique activity that is directly related to its central action. In patients with severe chronic pain (e.g., terminally ill patients receiving maximum doses of opioids) who are inadequately controlled, clonidine has become a useful adjunctive treatment to produce additional analgesia.

Centrally acting sympatholytics do not impair renal function and thus are suitable for patients with renal insufficiency. However, a mild fluid retention that might accompany therapy with α-methyldopa might be treated by the addition of a diuretic. The preferred drug for the treatment of hypertension during pregnancy is α-methyldopa (Chapter 11).

Sympatholytic drugs with actions primarily on peripheral sympathetic nerve terminals reduce TPR and CO, consistent with their effects on sympathetic nerves. Further, they produce more marked fluid retention and impairment of baroreceptor reflexes than do the centrally acting drugs. The use of reserpine declined dramatically as newer, more efficacious, and better tolerated agents became available. It is only used as a last resort for the management of extremely difficult cases of hypertension.

PHARMACOKINETICS

α-Methyldopa is available for oral administration and as a solution for intravenous administration to manage hypertensive emergencies or urgencies, but it is rarely used for this purpose.

Clonidine is available in oral and extended-release formulations and is well absorbed after systemic administration. It is also available as a transdermal formulation (patch) and for epidural administration to manage neuropathic pain in cancer patients for whom pain is inadequately controlled by opioids.

Guanabenz and guanfacine are available only for oral administration and are well absorbed following systemic administration.

PHARMACOVIGILANCE: ADVERSE EFFECTS AND DRUG INTERACTIONS

Centrally acting sympatholytics are notable for causing less orthostatic hypotension than many other antihypertensive agents, but they do lead to sedation and tiredness, dry mouth, and constipation. α-Methyldopa can also lead to weight gain and a swollen tongue. A unique problem associated with the use of these compounds, particularly drugs with short half-lives, is that a clinically serious rebound phenomenon characterized by a dramatic hypertensive response can occur after abrupt withdrawal. For this reason, these drugs should be terminated gradually, and clonidine-like drugs should be used cautiously, or not at all, in potentially noncompliant patients. If a hypertensive crisis does occur as a consequence of abrupt withdrawal, it may require the intravenous administration of sodium nitroprusside to bring blood pressure back toward normal levels.

TRADE NAMES

In addition to generic and fixed-combination preparations, the following trade-named materials are some of the important compounds available in the United States.

Clonidine (Catapres, Catapres-TTS, Duraclon, Kapvay, Nexiclon-XR)
Guanabenz (Wytensin)
Guanfacine (Tenex)
Methyldopa (Methyldopate HCl)
Reserpine

Adverse effects associated with the use of rilmenidine are rare but may include palpitations, insomnia, and anxiety and depression.

Drugs that deplete peripheral sympathetic nerve terminals of NE are not used as commonly as other classes due primarily to side effects related to widespread sympathetic impairment including orthostatic hypotension, sexual dysfunction, and gastrointestinal disturbance. Reserpine, although once widely used, may precipitate clinical depression in susceptible patients because of its CNS actions. However, some of these drugs may be useful for the therapy of catecholamine-secreting tumors or excessive sympathoexcitation.

NEW DEVELOPMENTS

Several new approaches to the pharmacological therapy of hypertension may be available in the United States in the near future. Drugs that affect the RAAS, particularly agents targeting Angiotensin II [1-7], that directly affect vascular smooth muscle, and compounds that alter the metabolism of endogenous vasodilator substances, particularly agents that antagonize endothelin, are all in various stages of development (Chapters 39–41). In addition, there are ongoing efforts to develop newer imidazoline receptor agonists with better therapeutic profiles and fewer side effects than rilmenidine and moxonidine.

CLINICAL RELEVANCE FOR HEALTHCARE PROFESSIONALS

Because hypertension is so prevalent, it is likely that all healthcare professionals will manage patients with hypertension. Physicians, physician assistants, and nurse practitioners will frequently need to initiate antihypertensive therapy in diverse populations of patients. These healthcare professionals must be aware of the recent recommendations of JNC-8 and consider comorbidities that may exist in a patient in order to select the appropriate regimen. Consideration of all of the adverse effects that these agents can produce will be a deciding factor to selection the most appropriate drug regimen. Physical therapists, occupational therapists, and other healthcare professionals need to be particularly aware of the ability of these agents to produce orthostatic hypotension. Cardiac output may be reduced in patients receiving one or more of several of the agents used, and drug-induced alterations of electrolytes could lead to reduced skeletal muscle function and an increased risk of cardiac dysfunction. Of particular importance, dentists should recognize that some of these agents possess significant antimuscarinic activity, drying mucous membranes in the oral cavity, rendering patients more sensitive during procedures and requiring more frequent hydrating of the oral cavity.

SELF-ASSESSMENT QUESTIONS

1. A 30-year-old hypertensive patient whose blood pressure has been adequately controlled with an angiotensin-receptor–blocking (ARB) agent just found out that she was pregnant. As a consequence, which of the following agents would be the best choice for an antihypertensive agent for a woman in this situation?
   A. β-Adrenergic receptor blockers.
   B. α-Methyldopa.
   C. Monoxidine.
   D. Clonidine.
   E. Guanfacine.

2. Which of the following adverse effects is commonly associated with the use of centrally acting sympatholytic agents?
   A. Orthostatic hypotension.
   B. Sedation.
   C. Diarrhea.
   D. Urticaria.
   E. Cycloplegia.

3. Which one of the following agents causes depletion of NE from sympathetic nerves?
   A. Rilmenidine.
   B. Clonidine.
   C. Reserpine.
   D. Guanfacine.
   E. α-Methyldopa

4. A 66-year-old woman with terminal cancer is receiving high doses of opioids to manage her neuropathic pain but requires an additional medication to alleviate the burning, shooting pain. Which of the following agents that are also used in the treatment of hypertension could be prescribed as an adjunct to opioid analgesics?
   A. Rilmenidine.
   B. Clonidine.
   C. Guanfacine.
   D. Reserpine.
   E. α-Methyldopa.

5. Which class of agents is recommended by the JNC-8 as first-line therapy for uncomplicated essential hypertension?
   A. α_1 Adrenergic receptor blocking agents
   B. Angiotensin converting enzyme inhibitors
   C. Angiotensin receptor blockers
   D. Loop diuretics
   E. Thiazide diuretics

FURTHER READING

Alves TB, Totola LT, Takakura AC, et al. GABA mechanisms of the nucleus of the solitary tract regulates the cardiovascular and sympathetic effects of moxonidine. *Auton Neurosci.* 2016;194:1–7.

Dampney RA. Central neural control of the cardiovascular system: current perspectives. *Adv Physiol Educ.* 2016;40(3):283–296.

James P, Oparil S, Carter B, et al. Eighth Joint National Committee: 2014 Evidence-Based Guideline for the Management of High Blood Pressure in Adults: Report From the Panel Members Appointed to the Eighth Joint National Committee. *JAMA.* 2014;507–520.

Sved AF, Ito S, Sved JC. Brainstem mechanisms of hypertension: role of the rostral ventrolateral medulla. *Curr Hypertens Rep.* 2003;5:262–268.

Taggart P, Critchley H, van Duijvendoden S, Lambiase PD. Significance of neuro-cardiac control mechanisms governed by higher regions of the brain. *Auton Neurosci.* 2016;pii:S1566-0702.

Whelton PK, Carey RM, Aronow WS. 2017 ACC/AHA/AAPA/ABC/ACPM/AGS/APhA/ASH/ASPC/NMA/PCNA Guideline for the Prevention, Detection, Evaluation, and Management of High Blood Pressure in Adults: A Report of the American College of Cardiology/American Heart Association Task Force on Clinical Practice Guidelines. *J Am Coll Cardiol.* 2017;S0735-1097(17):41519–1. doi:10.1016/j.jacc.2017.11.006.

WEBSITES

https://www.ncbi.nlm.nih.gov/pubmedhealth/PMHT0024199/

This website is maintained by the National Library of Medicine and contains links to numerous resources for both clinicians and researchers.

https://www.heart.org/HEARTORG/Conditions/HighBloodPressure/High-Blood-Pressure_UCM_002020_SubHomePage.jsp

This is the American Heart Association website with information for both healthcare professionals and patients and their families.

http://www.onlinejacc.org/content/accj/early/2017/11/04/j.jacc.2017.11.006.full.pdf

This link connects to the American College of Cardiology website that provides access to the manuscript by Whelton et al.

Diuretics and Drugs That Affect Volume and Electrolyte Content

Abdel A. Abdel-Rahman

MAJOR DRUG CLASSES

Osmotic diuretics
Carbonic anhydrase inhibitors
Thiazide diuretics
Loop diuretics
K⁺-sparing diuretics

ABBREVIATIONS

ATP	Adenosine triphosphate
cAMP	Adenosine 3′,5′ cyclic monophosphate
ECF	Extracellular fluid
ENaC	Epithelial Na^+ channel
GFR	Glomerular filtration rate
GI	Gastrointestinal
IV	Intravenous
NCC	Na^+/Cl^- cotransporter protein
NHE3	Na^+/H^+ exchange (antiport) protein
NKCC2	$Na^+/K^+/2Cl^-$ cotransporter protein
OA⁻	Organic anions
OC⁺	Organic cations
SIADH	Syndrome of inappropriate antidiuretic hormone

THERAPEUTIC OVERVIEW

The term **diuretic** defines an agent that increases the rate of urine flow via inhibition of electrolyte reabsorption in the kidney. Based on this definition, therefore, water ingestion (increases urine production without a substantial increase in the excretion of electrolytes) and digoxin (increases urine production via a cardiotonic effect) are not considered diuretics. The primary effect of diuretics is an increase in solute excretion, mainly Na^+ salts. The increase in urine flow is secondary and is a response to the osmotic force of the additional solute within the renal tubule lumen. Drugs that increase the net urinary excretion of Na^+ salts are called **natriuretics**.

Despite variations in dietary salt intake, the kidneys adjust the excretion of Na^+ and water to maintain the extracellular fluid (ECF) volume within narrow limits. In pathophysiological states such as chronic heart failure, cirrhosis of the liver, nephrotic syndrome, and renal failure, a deleterious expansion of the ECF leads to edema. Dietary Na^+ restriction is the mainstay of treatment, but frequently, ECF expansion persists, and diuretic drugs are needed. The prevalence of edema-forming states in clinical medicine has led to the widespread use of diuretics to enhance excretion of salts (mainly NaCl) and water.

Diuretics are used for the treatment of edema to normalize the volume of the ECF compartment without distorting electrolyte concentrations. The size of the ECF compartment is largely determined by the total body content of Na^+, which, in turn, is determined by the balance between dietary intake and excretion. When Na^+ accumulates faster than it is excreted, ECF volume expands. Conversely, when Na^+ is lost faster than it is ingested, ECF volume contracts. Diuretics produce a transient natriuresis, leading to reduced total body content of Na^+ and, consequently, reduced volume of the ECF. The effect is moderated, however, after 1–2 days, when a new equilibrium is attained and a new balance between intake and excretion is achieved, and body weight stabilizes. This "braking" phenomenon, in which there is refractoriness to the effects of the diuretic, is not a true "tolerance" but results from activation of compensatory salt-retaining mechanisms. Specifically, contraction of the ECF volume activates the sympathetic nervous system, leading to increased release of angiotensin II, aldosterone, and antidiuretic

hormone that may cause a compensatory increase in Na^+ reabsorption (Chapter 39). Moreover, continued delivery of Na^+ to more distal nephron segments induced by loop diuretics, and its compensatory reabsorption, may lead to structural hypertrophy of these cells, thereby enhancing Na^+ reabsorption.

The therapeutic applications of these compounds are presented in the Therapeutic Overview Box.

MECHANISMS OF ACTION

All diuretics promote natriuresis and diuresis to reduce ECF volume; however, their mechanisms and sites of action differ. The primary sites of action of the five classical types of diuretics are depicted in Fig. 38.1. Prototypes of these classes with their mechanisms of action are listed in Table 38.1. Also listed is a novel class of agents, the vasopressin (antidiuretic hormone) receptor antagonists, which block V_2 vasopressin receptors expressed in high density only in the kidney. Knowledge of the mechanisms and sites of action of these agents is important in selecting the appropriate drug and anticipating and preventing complications. In addition, because each class exerts effects at specific targets, a combination of two or more drugs will often result in additive or synergistic effects to affect the reabsorption or excretion of Na^+, Cl^-, HCO_3^-, water, and, to some extent, K^+, H^+, and organic ions. Further, combining two diuretics with different mechanisms may offset the deleterious effects due to significant losses of one electrolyte. For example, hypokalemia (increased excretion of K^+) could be offset by coadministering a K^+-sparing diuretic, which preserves K^+. To understand the mechanisms and consequences of the actions of the diuretics, a basic knowledge of renal physiology is essential.

THERAPEUTIC OVERVIEW

Goal: To Increase Excretion of Salt and Water

Thiazide Diuretics
Hypertension
Chronic heart failure (mild)
Renal calculi (nephrolithiasis)
Nephrogenic diabetes insipidus
Chronic renal failure (as an adjunct to loop diuretic)
Osteoporosis

Loop Diuretics
Hypertension, in patients with impaired renal function
Chronic heart failure (moderate to severe)
Acute pulmonary edema
Chronic or acute renal failure
Nephrotic syndrome
Hyperkalemia
Chemical intoxication (to increase urine flow)

K⁺-Sparing Diuretics
Chronic liver failure
Chronic heart failure, when hypokalemia is a problem

Carbonic Anhydrase Inhibitors
Cystinuria (to alkalinize tubular urine)
Glaucoma (to decrease intraocular pressure)
Periodic paralysis that affects muscle membrane function
Acute mountain sickness (to counteract respiratory alkalosis)
Metabolic alkalosis

Osmotic Diuretics
Acute or incipient renal failure
Reduce intraocular or intracranial pressure (preoperatively)
Acute cerebral edema

Vasopressin Receptor Antagonists
Syndrome of inappropriate antidiuretic hormone, chronic heart failure

Renal Function and Regulation
Renal Epithelial Transport and Nephron Function

At a normal human glomerular filtration rate (GFR) of approximately 180 L/day and a normal plasma Na⁺ concentration of 140 mmol/L, 25,200 mmol of Na⁺ are filtered each day. To maintain Na⁺ balance, the kidney must reabsorb more than 99% (24,950 mmol) of the filtered load of Na⁺ by employing different reabsorption mechanisms at distinct segments of the nephron. Specifically, renal epithelial cells transport solute and water from the apical cell membrane to the basolateral cell membrane. The polarization of structures that differentiate the apical membrane from the basolateral membrane allows the vectorial transport of solute and water (Fig. 38.2). The basolateral cell membrane expresses the ubiquitous Na⁺/K⁺-adenosine triphosphatase (ATPase), referred to as the Na⁺ pump, that exchanges three Na⁺ ions for two K⁺ ions. This results in decreased intracellular Na⁺, providing a chemical gradient and an electronegative cell interior that attracts Na⁺ entry from the lumen through the apical membrane (a potential difference of approximately 60 mV). The concentration gradient then favors passive efflux of the K⁺ that entered the cell to the intercellular space. Because the ECF concentration of K⁺ is low relative to Na⁺, recycling of K⁺ between the cell and interstitial fluid is necessary to maintain the Na⁺ pump.

The transport of Na⁺ across the apical cell membrane adjacent to the tubular fluid is achieved by passive diffusion via proteins that form a pore or channel (see Fig. 38.2A) and two types of carrier-mediated transport: (1) a cotransport (symport) pathway (see Fig. 38.2B) that transports two or three species in the same direction (e.g., Na⁺ and another solute species such as Cl⁻ or amino acids) and (2) a counter-transport (antiport) pathway (see Fig. 38.2C) that transports Na⁺ and another solute species (H⁺) in opposing directions. In general, the low

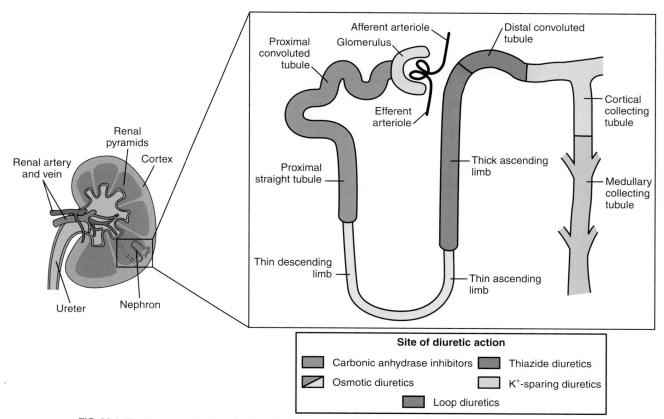

FIG. 38.1 The Nephron, Depicting Its Location, Segments, and the Sites of Action of Different Classes of Diuretics.

TABLE 38.1   Sites and Mechanisms of Action of Diuretics

Prototype		Sites of Action	Mechanism
Osmotic			
Mannitol		Proximal tubule	↓ Na⁺ resorption by osmotic action
		Descending loop of Henle	↑ Medullary blood flow
		Collecting duct	Washout of medullary tonicity
Vasopressin Receptor Antagonists			
Conivaptan, tolvaptan		Throughout kidney	Blocks vasopressin action on V₂ receptors
Carbonic Anhydrase Inhibitors			
Acetazolamide		Proximal tubule	Inhibits carbonic anhydrase and increases HCO₃⁻ excretion
Thiazide Diuretics			
Hydrochlorothiazide		Distal convoluted tubule	Inhibits luminal cotransport (Na⁺, Cl⁻)
Loop Diuretics			
Type I	Ethacrynic acid	Cortical and medullary thick ascending loop of Henle	Inhibits luminal cotransport (Na⁺, K⁺, 2Cl⁻)
Type II	Furosemide	Cortical and medullary thick ascending loop of Henle	Inhibits luminal cotransport (Na⁺, K⁺, 2Cl⁻)
K⁺-Sparing Diuretics			
Spironolactone		Cortical collecting tubule	Competes for aldosterone receptor
Triamterene		Cortical collecting tubule	Inhibits luminal Na⁺ channels

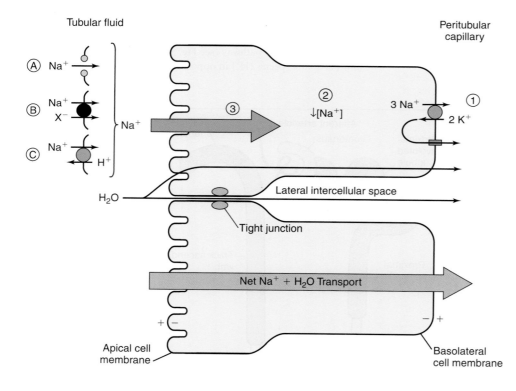

FIG. 38.2 Polarized Renal Epithelial Cells. Distinct transporters are present in apical cell and basolateral cell membranes to mediate the net transepithelial transport of Na⁺ and water. Operation of the basolateral cell membrane Na⁺/K⁺-ATPase (1) initiates the movement of Na⁺ and water by decreasing the intracellular Na⁺ concentration (2) and maintaining a negative interior potential in the cell. Na⁺ enters the cell from the lumen (3) down an electrochemical gradient via three types of transport mechanisms: channel A, symport; B, in which X may be glucose, amino acids, or PO₄, and C, antiport.

intracellular Na⁺ concentration as a consequence of the action of the Na⁺/K⁺-ATPase pump provides the electrochemical gradient for Na⁺ entry.

This transepithelial transport causes the osmolality of the lateral intercellular spaces to increase as a result of the accumulation of solute, producing an osmotic gradient that permits water to flow by two routes (see Fig. 38.2):

- Transcellular water flow in segments that are permeable to water

- Paracellular water flow (between cells, through tight junctions) in which solute is carried as a result of solvent drag

In the primary pathway of water flow, water moves from lumen to cell to interstitial fluid to capillary as a direct result of the transepithelial osmotic gradient.

Tubular Reabsorption: Transport by the Proximal Tubule

The GFR of healthy adults ranges from 1.7–1.8 mL/min/kg, and approximately two-thirds of the water and NaCl filtered at the glomerulus

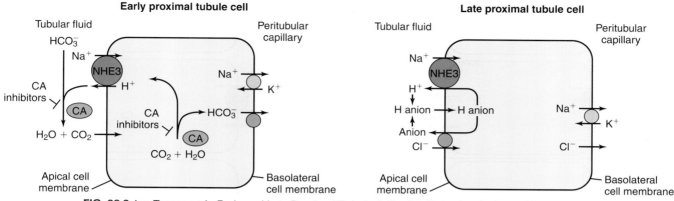

FIG. 38.3 Ion Transport in Early and Late Proximal Tubule Cells. *CA*, Carbonic anhydrase; *NHE3*, the Na⁺/H⁺ exchange protein.

is reabsorbed by the proximal tubule. HCO_3^-, glucose, amino acids, and other organic solutes are also reabsorbed. When GFR increases, salt and water excretion increase, but fractional reabsorption in the proximal tubule does not change. This is termed **glomerulotubular balance**, which moderates but does not entirely eliminate the effects of alterations in the GFR on salt and water excretion.

The transport of Na^+, HCO_3^-, and Cl^- is important to the action of several diuretics that act on the proximal tubule. Na^+ is reabsorbed primarily with HCO_3^- in the early proximal tubule, whereas Na^+ is reabsorbed primarily with Cl^- in the late proximal tubule (Fig. 38.3). At the apical cell membrane of the early proximal tubule, Na^+ entry is coupled with H^+ efflux via the Na^+/H^+ antiporter (NHE3), which is a protein containing 10–12 transmembrane-spanning domains and a hydrophilic C-terminal domain and is subject to regulation by a variety of factors, including angiotensin II, which increases its activity. The H^+ extruded from the cell combines with HCO_3^- to form carbonic acid (H_2CO_3), which rapidly forms CO_2 and water in the presence of the enzyme carbonic anhydrase. The CO_2 diffuses into the cell, is rehydrated to form H_2CO_3, and because the concentration of cellular H^+ is low, the reaction proceeds as follows: $CO_2 + H_2O \rightarrow H_2CO_3 \rightarrow H^+ + HCO_3^-$. Thus a constant supply of H^+ is furnished for countertransport with Na^+. The HCO_3^- that accumulates is cotransported with Na^+ across the basolateral cell membrane into the interstitial fluid and, subsequently, into the blood. Although the cytoplasmic hydration reaction occurs spontaneously, the rate is inadequate to allow reabsorption of the HCO_3^- load filtered (approximately 4000 mEq/day). However, little or none of the filtered HCO_3^- is excreted because of the presence of carbonic anhydrase. The net effect of coupling of the Na^+/H^+ antiporter to the carbonic anhydrase-mediated hydration and rehydration of CO_2 is preservation of HCO_3^- and reabsorption of Na^+, which is transferred from the interstitial fluid into peritubular capillaries.

In the late proximal tubule (see Fig. 38.3), Na^+ is reabsorbed primarily with Cl^-. Reabsorption is secondary to activation of both the NHE3, which couples inward Na^+ transport with outward H^+ transport, and a Cl^- base (formate) exchanger that transports Cl^- from lumen to cell in exchange for a base. The parallel operation of both exchangers results in net Na^+ and Cl^- absorption by the late proximal tubule. Passive transport of Na^+ and Cl^- also occurs between cells through the paracellular pathway.

Reabsorptive transport systems of the proximal tubule deliver large amounts of fluid and solutes to the interstitial space, which raises pressure in the interstitium. For reabsorption to continue, pressure must be decreased. The permeable peritubular capillary can easily carry away reabsorbed fluids and solutes. Pushed by interstitial pressure and pulled

TABLE 38.2 Summary of Reabsorption in the Proximal Tubule[a]

Component	mEq/day		
	Filtered	**Reabsorbed**	**Entering Loop**
Na^+	25,200	17,640	7560
Cl^-	19,440	13,414	6026
K^+	810	405	405
HCO_3^-	4320	3825	495
H_2O	180 L	126 L	54 L

[a]Representative values for a 70-kg human.

by the oncotic pressure of intracapillary proteins (higher in postglomerular than in preglomerular capillaries), filtered fluid and solutes return to the blood.

In summary, the proximal tubule reabsorbs approximately 70% of filtered water, Na^+, and Cl^-; 85% of filtered HCO_3^-; and 50% of filtered K^+ (Table 38.2). These percentages are relatively constant regardless of the actual filtered amounts. As a result, minor fluctuations in GFR do not influence fluid and electrolyte reabsorption or excretion very much. The driving force for reabsorption of water and electrolytes is the Na^+/K^+-ATPase. Passive movements of other ions and water are initiated and sustained by active transport of Na^+ across basolateral cell membranes. Osmotic equilibrium with plasma is maintained to the end of the proximal tubule. Filtered HCO_3^- is not reabsorbed directly from the lumen; rather, it is combined with H^+ to form H_2CO_3, which is then converted to CO_2 and water in the vicinity of the brush border membranes, where large concentrations of carbonic anhydrase are located. The direction of this reaction is established by the high concentration of carbonic acid in luminal fluid resulting from the secretion of H^+. Carbonic anhydrase in the cytoplasm catalyzes the formation of H_2CO_3. Cellular H^+ is then exchanged for luminal Na^+, and the filtered HCO_3^- is indirectly reabsorbed across the basolateral cell membranes.

Tubular Reabsorption: Transport by the Loop of Henle

Diuretics have no noticeable actions in the descending limb of the loop of Henle. The epithelial cells of this segment of the loop permit water to diffuse from the lumen to the medullary interstitium, but they lack specialized transport systems (molecular targets for diuretics) and are relatively impermeable to Na^+ and Cl^-.

In contrast, the thick ascending limb and its transport functions are an important site of action of the **loop** (also called **high-ceiling**)

Thick ascending limb cell

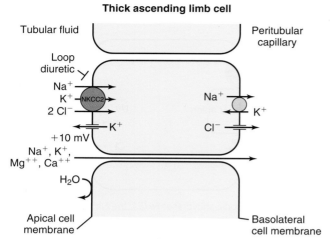

FIG. 38.4 Ion Transport by Thick Ascending Limb Cells. This segment, also referred to as the diluting segment, is impermeable to water, and thus the tubular lumen concentration of ions decreases.

Distal convoluted tubule cell

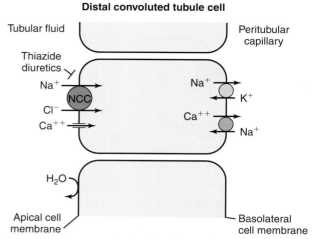

FIG. 38.5 Ion Transport by the Distal Convoluted Tubule Cell. As in the case for the thick ascending limb, this segment is relatively impermeable to water.

diuretics (Fig. 38.4). Approximately 25%–35% of filtered Na^+ and Cl^- is reabsorbed in the loop of Henle. The Na^+/K^+-ATPase in the basolateral membrane provides the gradient for Na^+ and Cl^- absorption. Na^+ entry across the apical membrane is mediated by an electroneutral transport protein that binds one Na^+, one K^+, and two Cl^- ions and is referred to as the $Na^+/K^+/2Cl^-$ (NKCC2) cotransporter. Although the ascending limb is highly permeable to Na^+, K^+, and Cl^-, it is impermeable to water. The continuous reabsorption of these ions without reabsorption of water dilutes the luminal fluid, thus the name "diluting segment." Na^+ entry down an electrochemical gradient drives the uphill transport of K^+ and Cl^-. This system depends on the simultaneous presence of all three ions in the luminal fluid. Once inside the cell, K^+ passively reenters the lumen (K^+ recycling) via conductive K^+ channels in the apical membrane, while Cl^- exits the cell via conductive Cl^- channels in the basolateral membrane. Depolarization of the basolateral membrane occurs as a consequence of Cl^- efflux, creating a lumen-positive (relative to the interstitial fluid) transcellular potential difference of approximately 10 mV. This drives paracellular cation transport, including Na^+, Ca^{++}, and Mg^{++}. Inhibition of the NKCC2 cotransporter not only results in excretion of Na^+ and Cl^- but also in excretion of other divalent cations, such as Ca^{++} and Mg^{++}.

Based on its molecular structure, the NKCC2 cotransporter belongs to a family of protein transporters referred to as electroneutral Na^+/Cl^- cotransporters, which also includes the Na^+/Cl^- cotransporter (NCC) that is sensitive to thiazide diuretics. These proteins have a structure similar to NHE3 and appear to be up regulated by reduction of intracellular Cl^- activity and cell shrinkage. Individuals with Bartter syndrome type I (a renal tubular disorder) appear to have mutations in the gene encoding the NKCC2 transporter, while types II and III of this syndrome present with mutations in K^+ and Cl^- channel proteins, respectively. The well-recognized countercurrent mechanism in the renal medulla depends on the activity of this cotransport system, and drugs that inhibit this pathway diminish the ability of the kidney to excrete urine that is either more concentrated or more dilute than plasma.

In summary, fluid (water) is reabsorbed from the lumen of the descending limb of the loop as it progresses deeper into the medullary areas of higher osmotic pressure. Electrolyte concentrations increase to a maximum at the bend and gradually decrease as the NKCC2 cotransport mechanism and Na^+ pump work in tandem to reabsorb Na^+, K^+, and Cl^-. The thick ascending limb reabsorbs 25% of filtered

NaCl and 40% of filtered K^+, but not water, whereas the entire loop reabsorbs 15% of the fluid.

Tubular Reabsorption: Transport by the Distal Convoluted Tubule

In contrast to the proximal tubule and loop of Henle, there is less reabsorption of water and electrolytes in the distal convoluted tubule. It reabsorbs approximately 10% of the filtered load of NaCl. Similar to the thick ascending limb, this segment is impermeable to water, and the continuous reabsorption of NaCl further dilutes tubular fluid. NaCl entry across the apical membrane is mediated by the electroneutral NCC cotransporter that is sensitive to thiazide diuretics (Fig. 38.5). Unlike the NKCC2 cotransporter of the thick ascending limb, this cotransporter does not require participation of K^+. As in other segments, the basolateral Na^+/K^+-ATPase provides the low intracellular Na^+ concentration that facilitates downhill transport of Na^+. The distal tubule has no pathway for K^+ recycling, so the transepithelial voltage is near zero, and the reabsorption of Ca^{++} and Mg^{++} is not driven by electrochemical forces. Instead, Ca^{++} crosses the apical membrane via a Ca^{++} channel and exits the basolateral membrane via the Na^+-Ca^{++} exchanger. Thus by inhibiting the NCC cotransporter, thiazide diuretics indirectly affect Ca^{++} transport through changes in intracellular Na^+. Another mechanism leading to increased Ca^{++} reabsorption by thiazide diuretics is an increase in the intracellular concentrations of Ca^{++}-binding proteins. These two processes lead to hypercalcemia in patients treated with thiazide diuretics, which is therapeutically beneficial in postmenopausal women and in individuals prone to Ca^{++} stone formation (less Ca^{++} will reach the collecting duct). On the other hand, hypercalcemia might become clinically troubling in the presence of digoxin due to the increased potential for the development of tachyarrhythmias.

Recently, inactivating mutations have been identified in the human gene encoding the NCC transporter in patients with Gitelman syndrome, characterized by hypotension, hypokalemia, hypomagnesemia, and hypercalcemia, similar to the effects of thiazides. Pseudohypoaldosteronism type II is an autosomal dominant disease characterized by hypertension, hyperkalemia, and sensitivity to thiazide diuretics. It has been suggested that an activating mutation of the NCC cotransporter is responsible. Recently, two protein kinases have also been linked to the pathogenesis of this syndrome. They are found in the distal nephron and are thought to control the activity of the cotransporters.

Tubular Reabsorption: Transport by the Collecting Tubule

The collecting tubule is the final site of Na^+ reabsorption, and approximately 3% of filtered Na^+ is reabsorbed by this segment. Although the collecting tubule reabsorbs only a small percentage of the filtered load, two characteristics are important for diuretic action. First, this segment is the site of action of aldosterone, a hormone controlling Na^+ reabsorption and K^+ secretion (Chapter 39). Second, virtually all K^+ excreted results from its secretion by the collecting tubule. Thus the collecting tubule contributes to the hypokalemia produced by diuretics.

The collecting tubule is composed of two cell types with separate functions. Principal cells are responsible for the transport of Na^+, K^+, and water, whereas intercalated cells are primarily responsible for the secretion of H^+ or HCO_3^-. Intercalated cells are of two types, A and B, the former responsible for secretion of H^+ via an H^+-ATPase (primary active ion pump) in the apical cell membrane, and the latter responsible for secretion of HCO_3^- via a $Cl^--HCO_3^-$ exchanger in the apical membrane. In contrast to more proximal cells, the principal cells do not express transport systems in the apical membrane but express separate channels that permit selective conductive transport of Na^+ and K^+ (Fig. 38.6). Na^+ is reabsorbed through a conductive Na^+ channel. The low intracellular Na^+, as a result of the basolateral Na^+/K^+-ATPase, generates a favorable electrochemical gradient for Na^+ entry through epithelial Na^+ channels (ENaCs). Because Na^+ channels are present only in the apical cell membrane of principal cells, Na^+ conductance causes depolarization, resulting in asymmetrical charge distribution across the cell that creates a lumen-negative transepithelial potential difference. This difference, together with a high intracellular-to-lumen K^+ gradient, provides the driving force for K^+ secretion.

The molecular identity of this amiloride-sensitive Na^+ channel has recently been determined with the cloning of ENaC. The channels are composed of three subunits, α, β, and γ, with 30% homology between them. It has been proposed that ENaC is a heterotetrameric protein, αβαγ, regulated by several factors including hormones (e.g., vasopressin, oxytocin), signaling elements (e.g., G-proteins and cAMP), and intracellular ion concentrations (Na^+, H^+, and Ca^{++}). These factors alter Na^+ reabsorption by either increasing the number of channels expressed at the cell surface or by increasing the probability of opening of the conducting channels rather than increasing single-channel conductance levels.

Mutations of ENaC could result in either gain of function (e.g., Liddle syndrome) associated with hypertension and hypokalemia or loss of function (e.g., pseudohypoaldosteronism) associated with

hypotension and hyperkalemia. The amount of Na^+ and K^+ in the urine is tightly controlled by the adrenal cortical hormone aldosterone, which acts through receptors on principal cells. Aldosterone penetrates the principal cell basolateral membrane and binds to a cytosolic mineralocorticoid receptor (Fig. 38.7), where activation causes the receptor-aldosterone complex to translocate to the nucleus to induce formation of specific messenger ribonucleic acids (mRNAs), encoding proteins that enhance Na^+ conductance in apical cell membranes and Na^+/K^+-ATPase activity in basolateral cell membranes. As a result, transepithelial Na^+ transport is increased, further depolarizing the apical membrane. An increase in the lumen-negative potential, in turn, enhances K^+ secretion through K^+ channels in the apical membrane. The final equilibration steps occur in medullary collecting tubules, where small amounts of NaCl and K^+ are reabsorbed. In the presence of antidiuretic hormone, water is transported out of the lumen into the interstitium. The direction of water movement is determined by the medullary tonicity established by the countercurrent mechanism. A quantitative summary of the fractional reabsorption of water and Na^+ of each tubule segment is shown in Fig. 38.8.

Tubular Secretion and Bidirectional Transport of Organic Acids and Bases

Except for osmotic agents, vasopressin antagonists, and competitive aldosterone inhibitors, all diuretics in clinical use release or accept an H^+ at the pH of body fluids and are subsequently secreted into the proximal tubular lumen. Thus these drugs exist as both uncharged molecules and charged organic ions so that H^+ concentrations in body fluids determine the nature of drug transport and action (Chapter 3).

The proximal tubular secretion of organic anions and cations into tubular fluid illustrates the influence of electrical charge on drug delivery to their sites of action and on their rapid decline in plasma. Two generic systems for transporting organic ions from blood to urine reside in the proximal tubule. One transports organic acids (anions as the A^- form of acid HA), and the other transports organic bases (cations as BH^+ form) of base B (Chapter 3). For transport, at least one step is active and against the concentration gradient, although energy is furnished indirectly. In addition, transport is saturable and susceptible to competitive inhibition by other organic ions. The lack of specific structural requirements supports the idea that these two mechanisms underlie the urinary excretion of many endogenous and

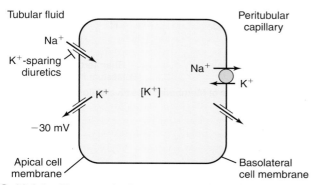

FIG. 38.6 Ion Transport by Principal Cells of the Collecting Tubule. The principal cell contains both Na^+ and K^+ channels in the apical cell membrane. The Na^+ channel depolarizes the membrane and provides an asymmetrical transepithelial voltage profile that favors K^+ secretion.

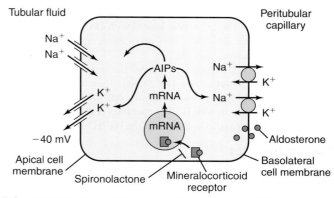

FIG. 38.7 Effects of Aldosterone. The principal cell is the primary target for aldosterone, which binds to cytoplasmic receptors, causing them to translocate into the nucleus and initiate synthesis of new proteins (aldosterone-induced proteins [AIPs]). AIPs induce newly synthesized Na^+ channels and Na^+/K^+-ATPase and increase the translocation of existing transporters from the cytosol to the surface membrane.

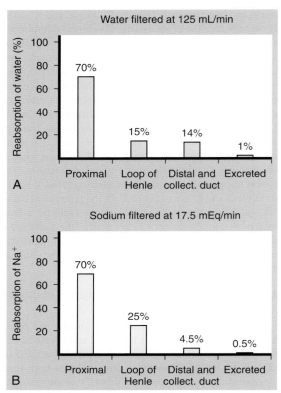

FIG. 38.8 Summary of Renal Reabsorption of Filtered H_2O (A) and Na^+ (B) in a 70-kg Human.

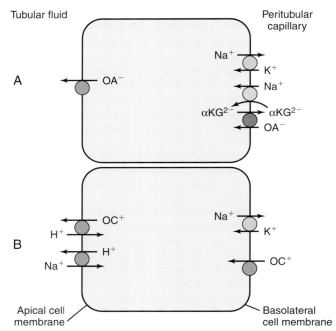

FIG. 38.9 Transport of Organic Anions (A) and Cations (B). *OA⁻*, Organic anion; *OC⁺*, organic cation; *αKG2⁻*, α-ketoglutarate.

environmental chemicals. Many of these are solutes of low molecular weight that bind to plasma proteins and thus are not filtered through glomerular membranes. In addition to most of the diuretics, organic acids and bases that are secreted include acetylcholine and choline, bile acids, uric acid, para-aminohippuric acid, epinephrine, norepinephrine, histamine, antibiotics, and morphine.

The tubular transport of organic acids and bases is illustrated in Fig. 38.9. Organic anions (OA^-) are taken up by the basolateral cell membrane through indirect coupling to Na^+ (see Fig. 38.9A). The Na^+/K^+-ATPase maintains a steep inward Na^+ gradient, which provides energy for entry of Na^+-coupled dicarboxylate (α-ketoglutarate). The operation of a parallel dicarboxylate/OA^- exchange drives the uphill movement of OA^- into the cell. The cell is now loaded with OA^-, which enters the lumen by facilitated diffusion. This mechanism may involve anion exchange or conductive transport.

Organic cations (OC^+) gain entry from the interstitial fluid across basolateral cell membranes (see Fig. 38.9B). Their entry is aided by carrier-facilitated diffusion. Once inside the cell, OC^+ enter the lumen through countertransport with H^+. The operation of this cation exchange is dependent on the parallel operation of the Na^+/H^+ antiporter, NHE3.

Osmotic Diuretics

These nonelectrolyte agents include mannitol, urea, glycerol, and isosorbide. The structure of mannitol is shown in Fig. 38.10. These agents all undergo free glomerular filtration and exhibit limited tubular reabsorption. They are also pharmacologically inert and are usually resistant to metabolic alteration. Osmotic diuretics are unique because they do not interact directly with receptors or other renal transport mechanisms. Their activity depends entirely on the osmotic pressure they exert in solution.

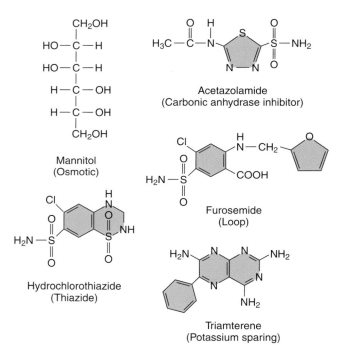

FIG. 38.10 Structures of Members of the Five Major Classes of Diuretic Drugs.

Na^+ is a major determinant of how much water will be reabsorbed from the proximal renal tubule, and concomitant with Na^+ reabsorption, water diffuses passively to maintain a constant concentration of Na^+. A selective decrease in water reabsorption without a change in the reabsorption of Na^+ could be achieved if the tubular fluid contained a nonelectrolyte, nonreabsorbable agent such as mannitol. Thus because of a relatively larger volume of tubular water, the net Na^+ concentration will be less than that of extracellular fluid. This will limit Na^+ and water reabsorption and may facilitate the movement of Na^+ back to the tubular fluid because of the abnormal gradient established in that direction. Further, mannitol diffuses from the blood into the interstitial space, where the increased osmotic pressure draws water from the cells to increase ECF volume. This increases medullary renal blood flow, which reduces the medullary osmotic gradient created by countercurrent forces. Thus the NaCl concentration in the thick ascending limb is reduced, indirectly diminishing the efficiency of the NKCC2 cotransport system and decreasing the transport of Na^+ and water. Ascending limb cells are an important site of natriuretic action. The overall consequence is an increase in urine flow associated with a relatively smaller increase in Na^+ excretion. Overzealous administration of mannitol may result in hypernatremia, hyperkalemia, and volume depletion.

Vasopressin Receptor Antagonists

The "vaptans" represent a relatively new class of diuretics that promote water excretion by inhibiting V_2 receptors on the basolateral membrane of the principal cell of the collecting duct. V_2 receptors are G-protein–coupled receptors (GPCRs) whose activation by vasopressin leads to an increase in cAMP and the phosphorylation of aquaporin-2 (AQP-2), causing AQP-2 vesicles to translocate to the apical membrane. This promotes water reabsorption, leading to an increase in the osmolality of the tubular fluid. Conivaptan and tolvaptan are V_2 receptor antagonists that prevent this effect and block water reabsorption, leading to the excretion of a dilute urine and increasing Na^+ in the circulation. Conivaptan is less selective than tolvaptan and interacts with both V_{1a} and V_2 receptors.

Carbonic Anhydrase Inhibitors

Acetazolamide, whose structure is shown in Fig. 38.10, is the prototypical carbonic anhydrase inhibitor. Carbonic anhydrase is a metalloenzyme in high concentrations in renal proximal tubule cells, ciliary processes of the eye, red blood cells, choroid plexus, intestine, and pancreas. There are thirteen mammalian isozymes, of which only two are relevant to its action in the proximal tubule. Type IV is expressed in basolateral and apical cell membranes, and type II is expressed in cytoplasm. Carbonic anhydrase catalyzes the hydration of CO_2 and dehydration of carbonic acid. The prevailing direction of the reaction is established by pH; normally CO_2 is hydrated, resulting in H^+ generation. The H^+ is then exchanged for Na^+, which enters the cell.

Acetazolamide inhibition of carbonic anhydrase reduces the H^+ concentration in the tubule lumen and decreases the availability of H^+ for Na^+/H^+ exchange. This results in an increase in HCO_3^- and Na^+ in the proximal portion of the lumen (see Figs. 38.1 and 38.3). Although some HCO_3^- is reabsorbed at other tubular sites, approximately 30% of the filtered load appears in the urine after carbonic anhydrase inhibition. A hyperchloremic metabolic acidosis results from HCO_3^- depletion, which renders subsequent doses of acetazolamide ineffective.

Thiazide Diuretics

Thiazide diuretics, such as hydrochlorothiazide (see Fig. 38.10 for structure), were developed to identify compounds that increase the excretion of Na^+ and Cl^- rather than Na^+ and HCO_3^-, as occurs with carbonic anhydrase inhibitors. The major site of action of the thiazides is the distal convoluted tubule (see Figs. 38.1 and 38.5), where they inhibit electroneutral NaCl absorption by binding to the NCC cotransporter expressed in the distal convoluted tubules.

Thiazide diuretics inhibit Na^+ and Cl^- transport in distal tubules, increasing delivery to more distal portions of the nephron, where a small fraction of excess Na^+ is reabsorbed and replaced with K^+. Because about 15% of the glomerular filtrate reaches the distal tubule, the maximum effect of the thiazides is more limited than with drugs acting in the thick ascending limb. The distal tubule is relatively impermeable to water; thus thiazide diuretics also reduce urinary dilution.

In addition to enhancing Na^+ and Cl^- excretion, thiazide diuretics influence the urinary excretion of other ions. Chlorothiazide can inhibit HCO_3^- transport in the proximal tubule as a consequence of carbonic anhydrase inhibition; most other thiazides are only weak carbonic anhydrase inhibitors. Chlorthalidone also inhibits vascular carbonic anhydrase isozymes, leading to enhanced generation of nitric oxide (NO) and improved endothelial function. Thiazide diuretics decrease Ca^{++} excretion at the proximal and distal tubules, in contrast to enhanced Ca^{++} secretion caused by loop diuretics. Sustained decreases in Ca^{++} excretion resulting from the long-term administration of thiazide diuretics are accompanied by mild elevations in serum Ca^{++}. Thiazide diuretics also enhance Mg^{++} excretion through unknown mechanisms, and long-term use can lead to hypomagnesemia. Thiazides, particularly at higher doses, can reduce ECF volume and uric acid excretion, which can lead to hyperuricemia.

Loop (High-Ceiling) Diuretics

Loop diuretics generate larger responses than those produced by the thiazides. Acting on the thick ascending limb, loop diuretics can inhibit the reabsorption of as much as 25% of the glomerular filtrate (Fig. 38.11) and are often effective when thiazides do not suffice. Despite their efficacy, loop diuretics are remarkably safe when used properly.

Four loop diuretics are available in the United States: ethacrynic acid, furosemide, torsemide, and bumetanide. Ethacrynic acid and furosemide are prototypes of loop I and II drugs, respectively. Bumetanide is considerably more potent and differs pharmacokinetically but is otherwise similar to the older drugs. Ethacrynic acid reacts with sulfhydryl groups, but this reaction may not have a bearing on diuresis because several chemically similar natriuretic compounds do not share sulfhydryl group reactivity. Ethacrynic acid also inhibits Na^+/K^+-ATPase but only in high concentrations.

Furosemide, whose structure is shown in Fig. 38.10, inhibits the reabsorption of Na^+ and Cl^- in the thick ascending limb by competing with Cl^- for a binding site on the NKCC2 cotransporter. Because the

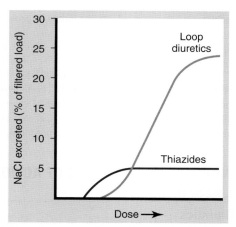

FIG. 38.11 Dose-Response Curves Comparing Na^+ Excretion After Administration of Thiazides or Loop Diuretics.

loop of Henle is responsible for accomplishing the countercurrent multiplication that generates a concentrated medullary interstitium, loop diuretics prevent formation of a concentrated urine. Loop diuretics also enhance Ca^{++} and Mg^{++} excretion in addition to the increased Na^+ and Cl^- excretion. Because transepithelial Na^+ and Cl^- transport through the NKCC2 cotransporter creates a lumen-positive potential, furosemide inhibits this transporter and reduces the gradient for passive Mg^{++} and Ca^{++} absorption through paracellular pathways.

Under Na^+-replete conditions, loop diuretics increase GFR and redistribute blood from medulla to cortex. The increase in GFR results in part from release of the vasodilatory prostaglandin PGI2 (prostacyclin). GFR is also controlled by tubuloglomerular feedback, which relies on a unique anatomical arrangement where a segment of nephron is juxtaposed between afferent and efferent arterioles of the glomerulus. This segment, the macula densa, lies between the cortical thick ascending limb and the distal convoluted tubule. The apical cell membrane of macula densa cells expresses a furosemide-sensitive NKCC2 cotransporter. Tubular fluid flow is monitored by macula densa cells, which cause afferent arterioles to constrict and GFR to decrease. There is evidence that Na^+ and Cl^- transport by the NKCC2 cotransporter is the critical sensing step because furosemide inhibits tubuloglomerular feedback and increases GFR. Loop diuretics reach their sites of action by first entering the tubular fluid through proximal tubular secretion. Drugs that block tubular secretion (e.g., probenecid) influence the temporal response to diuretics but do not abolish their effects.

Potassium-Sparing Diuretics

The K^+-sparing diuretics comprise three pharmacologically distinct groups: aldosterone (mineralocorticoid) receptor antagonists, pteridines, and pyrazinoylguanidines. Their site of action is the collecting tubule, where they interfere with Na^+ reabsorption and indirectly with K^+ secretion (see Figs. 38.1 and 38.6). Their diuretic activity is weak because fractional Na^+ reabsorption in the collecting tubule usually does not exceed 3% of the filtered load. For this reason, K^+-sparing drugs are ordinarily used in combination with thiazides or loop diuretics to restrict K^+ loss and sometimes augment diuretic action.

Spironolactone and its major and longer acting metabolite canrenone and the aldosterone analogue eplerenone bind to mineralocorticoid receptors in the kidney and elsewhere, acting as competitive inhibitors of aldosterone (Chapter 39). Aldosterone antagonists decrease Na^+ conductance at the apical membrane of principal cells, thereby reducing the lumen-negative potential. This results in a decrease in the electrical gradient for K^+ secretion.

Triamterene (see Fig. 38.10 for structure) and amiloride are structurally different from spironolactone but have the same functional effects. Both drugs are organic bases secreted into the lumen by proximal tubular cells, and both block the apical membrane Na^+ channel of principal cells and reduce Na^+ conductance (see Fig. 38.7). Similar to spironolactone, these drugs eliminate the lumen-negative potential, which decreases Ca^{++} and H^+ excretion, and reduce the electrochemical gradient for K^+ secretion. Amiloride also blocks Na^+/H^+ exchange, Na^+/Ca^{++} exchange, and Na^+/K^+-ATPase, but it blocks the Na^+ channel only at therapeutic doses. In addition, amiloride decreases Ca^{++} and H^+ excretion as a consequence of a decreased lumen-negative potential.

RELATIONSHIP OF MECHANISMS OF ACTION TO CLINICAL RESPONSE

Osmotic Diuretics

Mannitol is the osmotic agent of choice because its properties best satisfy the requirements of an efficient osmotic diuretic. It is nontoxic,

freely filtered through glomeruli, essentially nonreabsorbable from tubular fluid, and not readily metabolized. Urea, glycerol, and isosorbide are less efficient because they penetrate cell membranes. Consequently, as urea, glycerol, or isosorbide is reabsorbed, luminal concentrations decrease, and the tendency to retain filtered fluid diminishes. Mannitol may also produce a modest excretion of Mg^{++}, HCO_3^-, PO_4^{-3}, Ca^{++}, and K^+, which may account for the mild hyperkalemia observed in patients treated with mannitol.

Mannitol does not increase GFR or renal blood flow in humans. Mannitol has been administered prophylactically to prevent acute renal failure associated with severe trauma, cardiovascular and other complicated surgical procedures, or therapy with cisplatin and other nephrotoxic drugs. However, in cases of severe renal ischemia resulting from nephrotoxic agents, the tubular epithelium damage produce by the agents may cause the diuretics to lose their effectiveness as they become reabsorbable.

Because osmotic drugs reduce the volume and pressure of the aqueous humor by extracting fluid from it, they are used for the short-term treatment of acute glaucoma. Similarly, infusions of mannitol are used to lower the elevated intracranial pressure caused by cerebral edema associated with tumors, neurosurgical procedures, or similar conditions. Reduction of the pressure and volume of cerebrospinal fluid (CSF) occurs by increasing the osmolality of plasma and enhancing the diffusion of water from CSF to plasma. However, osmotic diuretics (mannitol) should be avoided if there is evidence of hemorrhagic stroke (compromised blood-brain barrier) to avoid counterintuitive entry of the drug and administered fluids into the CNS. Osmotic agents redistribute body fluids, increase urine flow rate, and accelerate renal elimination of filtered solutes, which are often the goals for treatment for many clinical disorders. Mannitol is occasionally used to promote renal excretion of bromides, barbiturates, salicylates, or other drugs after overdoses.

Vasopressin Receptor Antagonists

Conivaptan and tolvaptan antagonize the action of vasopressin at receptors in the vasculature, central nervous system, and kidney. These agents are approved for use in the treatment of hyponatremia in patients with syndrome of inappropriate antidiuretic hormone (SIADH) and as an adjunct in patients with congestive heart failure in which water retention occurs due to excessive vasopressin secretion.

Carbonic Anhydrase Inhibitors

Acetazolamide has limited use as a diuretic. It is used primarily to reduce intraocular pressure in glaucoma and to treat metabolic alkalosis because of its ability to enhance HCO_3^- excretion (produces metabolic acidosis). It is also used prophylactically to treat acute mountain sickness and to induce urinary alkalization to enhance renal excretion of uric acid and weak acids (e.g., aspirin), but these effects are of relatively short duration and require bicarbonate infusion to maintain continuing diuresis. The popularity of carbonic anhydrase inhibitors as diuretics has waned because tolerance develops rapidly, increased urinary excretion of HCO_3^- results in the development of systemic acidosis, and more effective and less toxic agents have been developed. Nevertheless, acetazolamide is administered for short-term therapy, especially in combination with other diuretics, to patients who are resistant to other agents.

Thiazide Diuretics

In general, thiazide diuretics are used for the treatment of hypertension, chronic heart failure, and other conditions in which a reduction in ECF volume is beneficial. Many large clinical studies have clearly defined the efficacy and tolerability of these agents in the treatment of hypertension. One trial showed no difference in mortalities and cardiac-related events between hypertensive patients taking thiazides and patients treated with β-adrenergic receptor–blocking drugs. As a result, this class of diuretics is recommended as monotherapy or in combination with other agents as first-line agents in the treatment of hypertension. The blood pressure reduction in patients with hypertension results in part from contraction of the ECF volume (Chapter 37). This occurs acutely, leading to a decrease in cardiac output with a compensatory elevation in peripheral resistance. Vasoconstriction then subsides, enabling cardiac output to return to normal. Thereafter, a reduction in vascular resistance ensues and mediates the long-term antihypertensive effect of this class of drugs. Augmented synthesis of vasodilator prostaglandins (prostacyclin; PGI_2) has been reported and may be a crucial factor for long-term maintenance of a lower pressure, even though ECF volume tends to return toward normal.

In addition to their use in the treatment of edematous disorders and hypertension, thiazide diuretics are also used in other disorders. Because they decrease renal Ca^{++} excretion, they are used in the treatment of Ca^{++} nephrolithiasis and osteoporosis. Thiazide diuretics are also used in the treatment of nephrogenic diabetes insipidus, where tubules are unresponsive to vasopressin, and patients undergo a water diuresis. Often the volume of dilute urine excreted is large enough to lead to intravascular volume depletion if it is not offset by an adequate intake of fluid. Chronic administration of thiazides increases urine osmolality and reduces flow. The mechanism hinges on excretion of Na^+ and its removal from the ECF, which contracts ECF volume. When Na^+ transport in the distal convoluted tubule is inhibited, the proximal tubule avidly reabsorbs Na^+, which decreases urine flow rate and increases urine osmolality. Drug therapy in this instance is most effective when used in combination with dietary salt restriction.

Loop Diuretics

Loop (high-ceiling) diuretics are very efficacious at low dosages. NaCl losses are equivalent to those obtained with thiazides; at high doses, massive amounts of salt are excreted. The magnitude of responses to loop diuretics is limited by both the existing salt and water balance and the delivery of drug to its site of action. Contraction of ECF volume lessens the response by enhancing proximal and distal tubular reabsorption of Na^+. Renal insufficiency causes less drug to reach the NKCC2 transporter because glomeruli, proximal tubular pathways, or both have been compromised.

The value of loop diuretics in pulmonary edema may be attributed in part to their stimulation of prostaglandin (prostacyclin; PGI_2) synthesis in kidney and lung. Furosemide and ethacrynic acid increase renal blood flow for brief intervals, promoting the urinary excretion of prostaglandin E. Intravenous (IV) injection of furosemide also reduces pulmonary arterial pressure and peripheral venous compliance. Indomethacin, an inhibitor of prostaglandin synthesis (Chapter 29), interferes with these actions.

Common indications for loop diuretics overlap those of the thiazides, with some major differences. For example, the greater efficacy of loop agents often evokes a diuresis in edemas that are cardiovascular, renal, or hepatic in origin. On the other hand, it has been reported that thiazides and related drugs, especially longer acting agents, are more efficacious than loop agents in reducing blood pressure. Loop diuretics increase Ca^{++} excretion and therefore are used to lower serum Ca^{++} concentrations in patients with hypercalcemia. Loop diuretics also increase K^+ excretion and are useful in treating acute and chronic hyperkalemia.

Potassium-Sparing Diuretics

Spironolactone and eplerenone are most effective in patients with primary hyperaldosteronism (adrenal adenoma or bilateral adrenal hyperplasia) or secondary hyperaldosteronism (chronic heart failure, cirrhosis, nephrotic syndrome). These drugs prevent binding of aldosterone to a cytosolic receptor in principal cells of the collecting tubule. They can be added to drug regimens, including thiazide or loop diuretics, to further reduce ECF volume and prevent and correct hypokalemia. They are especially appropriate for the treatment of cirrhosis with ascites, a condition often associated with secondary hyperaldosteronism. This class is as effective, if not more so, than loop or thiazide diuretics in this setting because thiazide and loop diuretics are highly protein bound and enter the tubular fluid primarily by proximal tubular secretion. Tubular secretion of these agents in patients with cirrhosis and ascites decreases as a result of competition with toxic organic metabolites. Because thiazide and loop diuretics act at the apical cell membrane, decreased tubular secretion and lower concentrations inside the tubules reduce their effectiveness. Inhibitors of aldosterone, on the other hand, do not depend on filtration or secretion because they gain access to their receptors from the plasma side. A combination of a loop diuretic with spironolactone can be used to increase natriuresis when the diuretic effect of an aldosterone inhibitor alone is inadequate.

Although their natriuretic action is weak, these agents lower blood pressure in patients with mild or moderate hypertension and are often prescribed for this purpose. Evidence has suggested that the addition of spironolactone to "standard-of-care" treatment for heart failure reduces morbidity and mortality. Eplerenone and spironolactone are currently approved as antihypertensive medications as well as in the management of postmyocardial infarction heart failure.

Triamterene and amiloride are generally used in combination with K^+-wasting diuretics, especially when it is clinically important to maintain normal serum K^+ (e.g., patients with dysrhythmias, receiving a cardiac glycoside, or with low serum K^+). Fixed-combination preparations are generally not appropriate for initial therapy but may be more expedient once the dosage is demonstrated to be optimal. Because the site and mechanism of action of these drugs differ from those of thiazides and loop agents, they are sometimes administered together to increase the response in patients who are refractory to a single drug.

PHARMACOKINETICS

The pharmacokinetic parameters of the diuretic agents are summarized in Table 38.3.

Mannitol is not readily absorbed from the gastrointestinal (GI) tract and is administered by the IV route. It distributes in ECF and is excreted almost entirely by glomerular filtration, with approximately 90% appearing in the urine within 24 hours. Less than 10% is reabsorbed by the renal tubule, and an equal amount is metabolized in the liver.

Isosorbide and glycerol are administered orally to reduce intraocular pressure before ophthalmological surgical procedures.

Urea is administered IV as an aqueous solution containing dextrose, or invert sugar, and is rarely given by mouth because it induces nausea and emesis. Urea, glycerol, and isosorbide are metabolized extensively.

Conivaptan is only available in an IV formulation and therefore is restricted for use only in controlled hospital settings. Tolvaptan is available in an oral formulation and can be used to treat SIADH on an outpatient basis.

The several thiazides differ considerably with respect to their pharmacokinetics and pharmacodynamics. Hydrochlorothiazide, the most commonly prescribed compound in the United States, has a bioavailability of approximately 70%. It has a large apparent volume of distribution and a rapid onset of action. Unlike hydrochlorothiazide, GI absorption of chlorothiazide is dose dependent. As a group, thiazide diuretics have longer half-lives than loop diuretics and are mostly prescribed once a day. Indapamide, chlorthalidone, and polythiazide

TABLE 38.3 Pharmacokinetic Parameters

Drug	Administration	Onset (hrs)	t$_{1/2}$ (hrs)	Disposition
Carbonic Anhydrase Inhibitors				
Acetazolamide	Oral	1	5	R
Methazolamide	Oral	2–3	14	R
Vasopressin Receptor Antagonists				
Conivaptan	IV	12	5	M, B (main)
Tolvaptan	Oral	2–4	12	M, R, B
Thiazide Diuretics				
Chlorothiazide	Oral	1–3	6–12	R (main), B
	IV	0.25	2	R (main), B
Hydrochlorothiazide	Oral	1	8–12	R (main), B
Chlorthalidone	Oral	2–4	24	R (main), B
Metolazone	Oral	1	12–24	R (main), B
Indapamide	Oral	1–2	18–36	R (main), B
Loop Diuretics				
Furosemide	Oral	1	2	R (40%), M
	IV	5–10 min	2	R (40%), M
Ethacrynic acid	IV	0.25	3	R (main), M[a]
Bumetanide	Oral	0.5–1	4–6	M[a]
	IV	0.25	0.5–1	M[a]
Torsemide	Oral	1	3–4	R, M (80%)
	IV	10 min	3–4	R, M (80%)
K$^+$-Sparing Diuretics				
Spironolactone	Oral	1–2 days	2–3 days	R, M, B
Eplerenone	Oral	1–2 hrs	4–6 hrs	R, M, B
Triamterene	Oral	2	12–16	R, M, B
Amiloride	Oral	2	24	R, M, B

[a]Active metabolite.
B, Biliary excretion; *M,* metabolized; *R,* renal excretion (parent drug).

have the longest half-lives. Plasma protein binding varies from 10% to 95%. Free drug enters the tubular fluid by filtration and organic acid secretion and reaches its site of action via the distal convoluted tubular fluid.

The highly lipid-soluble members of the thiazide family possess larger apparent volumes of distribution and lower renal clearances. Indapamide, **bendroflumethiazide**, and polythiazide are primarily metabolized in the liver, and the major route of elimination is by glomerular filtration and proximal tubular secretion of unchanged drug.

Differences in the chemical structure of the loop diuretics influence oral bioavailability, renal elimination/metabolism, and duration of action. The prototype (gold standard for loop diuretics) **furosemide** achieves approximately 60% oral bioavailability and essentially exhibits the highest renal elimination rate (needed for its diuretic activity). On the other hand, compared to furosemide, **torsemide** exhibits better oral bioavailability (80%) and substantially lower renal elimination (20%). Collectively, these differences explain the higher efficacy of furosemide as a diuretic at the expense of a shorter half-life than torsemide. The over twofold longer duration of action of torsemide qualifies it to be prescribed as antihypertensive medication (Chapter 37). Furosemide is practically insoluble in lipid and almost totally bound to plasma proteins. It is excreted unchanged and as a glucuronide by the kidneys. A significant proportion of bumetanide and torsemide is metabolized in the liver.

Ethacrynic acid, administered IV, has a rapid onset and is rapidly excreted. It is conjugated with glutathione, forming an ethacrynic acid-cysteine adduct that is more potent than the parent drug. Because ethacrynic acid is poorly lipid soluble, its apparent volume of distribution is small. Plasma protein binding is extensive, and the compound and its metabolites are excreted in urine by filtration and proximal tubule secretion. Elimination by the intestine is augmented through biliary transport, and this accounts for approximately one-third of the administered dose. Ethacrynic acid achieves much higher oral bioavailability (nearly 100%) and a slightly higher renal elimination rate compared to furosemide. It must be remembered that furosemide is available in a parenteral form, which can help achieve 100% bioavailability, if needed, in emergency situations.

Acetazolamide is well absorbed from the GI tract. More than 90% of the drug is plasma protein bound. Because it is relatively insoluble in lipid, acetazolamide does not readily penetrate cell membranes or cross the blood-brain barrier. The highest concentrations are found in tissues that contain large amounts of carbonic anhydrase, such as the renal cortex and red blood cells. Renal effects are noticeable within 30 minutes and are usually maximal at 2 hours. Acetazolamide is excreted rapidly by glomerular filtration and proximal tubular secretion; methazolamide is absorbed more slowly.

The pharmacokinetics of **spironolactone** are presented in Chapter 39. **Triamterene** has good bioavailability and is metabolized in the liver to an active metabolite, which is excreted in the urine. The half-life of this active metabolite increases in renal insufficiency but is unchanged in liver disease.

Amiloride is not metabolized and is excreted in the urine; renal insufficiency increases its half-life.

PHARMACOVIGILANCE: ADVERSE EFFECTS AND DRUG INTERACTIONS

The repeated and continuous use of diuretics is frequently associated with shifts in acid-base balance, and changes in serum electrolytes include K^+ depletion and hyperuricemia. Patients at risk include the elderly, those with severe disease, those taking cardiac glycosides, and the malnourished. Such changes are difficult to avoid in most patients unless counteractive measures are taken. Supplemental intake of K^+ (dietary or oral KCl) or concomitant use of K^+-sparing with thiazide or loop diuretics is often used to circumvent this problem.

Paradoxical diuretic-induced edema may occur in patients with hypertension if diuretics are abruptly withdrawn after long-term use. This occurs because long-term use results in persistently elevated plasma renin activity and a secondary aldosteronism. If it is necessary to discontinue diuretic therapy, a stepwise reduction over a few weeks combined with a reduction in Na^+ intake is recommended. Alternatively, renin- or angiotensin-converting enzyme inhibitors or angiotensin-receptor blockers can be administered to circumvent this clinical problem (Chapter 39).

Osmotic Diuretics

Acute expansion of ECF volume engendered by osmotic diuretics increases the workload of the heart. Patients in cardiac failure are especially susceptible, and pulmonary edema may develop. Therefore they should not be treated with these drugs. Underlying heart disease in the absence of frank heart failure, though not an absolute contraindication, is a serious risk factor. Mannitol is sometimes given to restore urine flow in patients in oliguric or anuric states induced by extrarenal factors (e.g., hypovolemia, hypotension). In these cases, the response to a test dose should be evaluated before therapeutic quantities are administered.

Severe volume depletion and hypernatremia may result from prolonged administration of mannitol unless Na^+ and water losses are replaced. Mild hyperkalemia is often observed, but intolerable K^+ elevations are not likely except in patients with diabetes, adrenal insufficiency, or severely impaired renal function.

Vasopressin Receptor Antagonists

Any agent that blocks the effects of vasopressin can lead to hypernatremia and nephrogenic diabetes insipidus. Therefore it is important to monitor serum Na^+. Tolvaptan can cause hypotension and produce an elevation in liver function tests. As would be predicted, antagonists of vasopressin will increase thirst, and both agents can produce dry mouth.

Carbonic Anhydrase Inhibitors

Among the side effects of carbonic anhydrase inhibitors are metabolic acidosis, drowsiness, fatigue, central nervous system depression, and paresthesia. Hypersensitivity reactions are rare.

Thiazide Diuretics

Thiazides (and loop diuretics), whose action is exerted proximal to the K^+ secretory sites, increase the excretion of K^+. The fraction of patients in whom hypokalemia develops or who show evidence of K^+

depletion while undergoing long-term treatment is variable. Some younger people with hypertension may have no effect or become only slightly hypokalemic. Mild hypokalemia should be avoided in cirrhotic patients, those taking cardiac glycosides, diabetics, and the elderly. Disturbances in insulin and glucose metabolism can often be prevented if K^+ depletion is avoided. Thiazide diuretics, particularly high doses, also produce clinically significant reductions in plasma Na^+ (hyponatremia) in some patients. Although the magnitude of the effect is variable, values of less than 100 mEq/L have been reported, which can be life-threatening.

Although Mg^{++} is primarily reabsorbed in the proximal tubule, thiazides and loop diuretics can accelerate its excretion. Mg^{++} depletion in patients on long-term diuretic therapy is occasionally reported and is considered by some to be a risk factor for ventricular dysrhythmias. Addition of K^+-sparing diuretics reportedly prevents Mg^{++} loss.

Thiazides increase the serum concentration of uric acid by increasing proximal tubular reabsorption and reducing tubular secretion. Hyperuricemia develops in more than 50% of patients on long-term thiazide therapy. In most, the elevation is modest and does not precipitate gout unless the patient has primary disease or a gouty diathesis. Currently, there is no reason to believe that the risk of hyperuricemia outweighs the benefits of thiazide therapy in most patients.

Long-term treatment with thiazide diuretics can result in small increases in serum lipid and lipoprotein concentrations. Low-density lipoprotein cholesterol and triglyceride concentrations may increase during short-term therapy, but total cholesterol and triglyceride concentrations usually return to baseline values in studies of more than 1 year. This action may be linked to glucose intolerance and may be a consequence of K^+ depletion. These side effects are more evident when high doses of thiazides are used.

Because most complications of thiazide therapy are direct manifestations of their pharmacological effects, adverse events are usually predictable. However, many adverse reactions have no apparent relationship to the known pharmacology of the drugs. Although relatively uncommon, these hazards are usually more serious. Thiazides also reduce the clearance of lithium and, as a rule, should not be administered concomitantly. Similarly, because thiazides decrease Mg^{++} and K^+ and increase serum Ca^{++}, the potential for development of a negative drug-drug interaction with digoxin exists that should be monitored. Although not absolutely contraindicated, their use in pregnant women is not recommended unless the anticipated benefit justifies the risk. Thiazides cross the placenta and appear in breast milk. Anuria and a known hypersensitivity to sulfonamides are absolute contraindications.

Loop Diuretics

Loop diuretics also increase excretion of K^+, Ca^{++}, Mg^{++}, and H^+, and their use is associated with all the electrolyte-depletion phenomena associated with thiazide use. Similarly, carbohydrate intolerance and hyperlipidemia have also been observed.

Vertigo and deafness sometimes develop in patients receiving large IV doses of loop diuretics; the coadministration of an aminoglycoside antibiotic produces additive effects. Higher rates of ototoxicity are associated with ethacrynic acid, limiting its use. Additional drug interactions occur with indomethacin (decreased activity), warfarin (displacement from plasma protein), digoxin (electrolyte imbalances), and lithium (decreased clearance and increased risk of toxicity). All diuretics are contraindicated in anuric patients.

Potassium-Sparing Diuretics

The most serious adverse effect of spironolactone therapy is hyperkalemia. Serum K^+ should be monitored periodically even when the drug is administered with a K^+-wasting diuretic. Gynecomastia and decreased

TABLE 38.4   **Potential Drug-Drug Interactions**

Diuretic	Drug Class or Agent	Problem
Thiazide diuretics	β-adrenergic receptor blockers	Increase in blood glucose, urates, and lipids
	Chlorpropamide	Hyponatremia
Thiazides and loop diuretics	Digitalis glycosides	Hypokalemia resulting in increased digitalis binding and toxicity
	Adrenal steroids	Enhanced hypokalemia
Loop diuretics	Aminoglycosides	Ototoxicity, nephrotoxicity
K⁺-sparing diuretics	Angiotensin-converting enzyme inhibitors	Hyperkalemia, cardiac effects

libido and impotence may occur in men, possibly as a consequence of the binding of canrenone to androgen receptors. Menstrual irregularities, hirsutism, or swelling and breast tenderness may develop in women. Triamterene and amiloride may cause hyperkalemia, even when a K⁺-wasting diuretic is part of the therapy. The risk is highest in patients with limited renal function. Additional complications include elevated serum blood urea, nitrogen and uric acid, glucose intolerance, and GI tract disturbances. Triamterene may contribute to, or initiate, the formation of renal stones, and hypersensitivity reactions may occur in patients receiving it, and the drug is a weak folic acid antagonist. Some drug-drug interactions involving diuretics are presented in Table 38.4.

Diuretic Resistance

During therapy with a loop diuretic, a patient may no longer respond to a previously effective dose. Chronic use of loop diuretics is associated with an adaptive response by nephron segments distal to their site of action. Distal tubule cells after chronic loop diuretic administration are characterized by cellular hypertrophy, hyperplasia, increased activity, and expression of Na⁺/Cl⁻ cotransporter and increased Na⁺/K⁺-ATPase activity. This adaptation is thought to be due to higher rates of solute delivery to distal nephron segments and to an increase in aldosterone. The net result is a reduction of the magnitude of natriuresis normally expected from loop diuretic administration, due to a compensatory increase in Na⁺ reabsorption by distal tubule cells. Additional factors may contribute to resistance, including a high NaCl intake, progressive renal failure, concomitant use of nonsteroidal antiinflammatory agents (NSAIDs), reduced GI absorption stemming from edema of the bowel, or hypoalbuminemia and albuminuria. Solutions include combined use of a loop and another diuretic, especially a thiazide.

Adverse reactions associated with the use of the diuretics are summarized in the Clinical Problems Box.

NEW DEVELOPMENTS

Novel agents that antagonize water transport are currently being developed. Water excretion can be enhanced by agents that inhibit water channels. Our understanding of membrane water transport has advanced significantly with the molecular characterization of the water transport proteins, the **aquaporins**. Indeed, the vasopressin V₂ receptor antagonists,

or "vaptans," represent a relatively new class of diuretics whose mechanism of action results in blocking the phosphorylation of aquaporin-2 (AQP-2), promoting diuresis. These agents are in various stages of development as therapeutics for the treatment of congestive heart failure, cirrhosis, and nephrotic syndrome, as well as other conditions characterized by ECF volume expansion resulting from NaCl and water retention. Lixivaptan and satavaptan are currently in late clinical trials and will be available as oral formulations within the near future.

Recent clinical studies have targeted the natriuretic peptide family in mediating natriuresis in heart failure (Chapter 44). The renal hemodynamic effects of A and B natriuretic peptides include increased GFR, afferent arteriolar dilation, and efferent arteriolar constriction. In addition, they have direct effects to block Na⁺ transport in the inner medullary collecting duct and block aldosterone release. Nesiritide, a recombinant human B natriuretic peptide, is currently used for the treatment of fluid retention in congestive heart failure.

Another molecular target is the Na⁺-HCO₃⁻ symporter in the proximal convoluted tubule. Selective adenosine A₁ receptor antagonists have been identified that inhibit this symport. cAMP inhibits the Na⁺-HCO₃⁻ symporter at this site, thereby reducing the reabsorption of Na⁺ and HCO₃⁻. Notably, A₁-adenosine receptor activation by endogenous adenosine reduces cAMP formation, which results in enhancement of tubular reabsorption of Na⁺-HCO₃⁻. Therefore selective pharmacological blockade of the adenosine A₁ receptor at this site will result in the opposite effects, inhibition of Na⁺ and Na⁺-HCO₃⁻ reabsorption. Rolofylline was developed and evaluated in clinical trials but discontinued due to central nervous system toxicity and alterations in GFR; other agents are currently being evaluated.

Inhibitors of the Na⁺-glucose cotransporter 2 (SGLT2) are approved for use in the treatment of diabetes mellitus (Chapter 53), and two of these agents have diuretic effects; they not only increase water excretion but also the excretion of glucose and sodium. There is some interest in pursuing this molecular target.

CLINICAL RELEVANCE FOR HEALTHCARE PROFESSIONALS

The goal of antihypertensive therapy is to reduce end-organ damage associated with chronic elevated blood pressure. However, the effects of therapy on other cardiovascular risk factors must also be considered, since end-organ damage is not related exclusively to blood pressure. For example, thiazide and other K⁺-losing diuretics produce a modest elevation of low-density lipoprotein and total triglycerides that may be responsible for less effectiveness in reducing the incidence of coronary heart disease. Thiazide diuretics also increase insulin resistance, which is recognized as a risk factor for coronary artery disease.

Healthcare professionals who need to initiate antihypertensive therapy in diverse populations of patients must be aware of the recent recommendations of JNC-8 and consider comorbidities that may exist in patients to select appropriate regimens. Due to the prevalence of hypertension in the population, all healthcare professionals should be aware of the major side effects associated with the diuretics, in particular those agents that alter the baroreceptor reflex, which could lead to orthostatic hypotension upon transitioning from a supine position to standing. Caution must also be observed in patients exiting aquatherapy or terminating aerobic exercise without an appropriate cool-down period. Cardiac output may be reduced in patients receiving one or more of several of these agents. Drug-induced electrolyte alterations could lead to reduced skeletal muscle function and an increased risk of cardiac dysfunction.

CLINICAL PROBLEMS

Osmotic Diuretics

Acute increase in ECF volume and serum K^+ concentration, nausea and vomiting, headache

Vasopressin Receptor Antagonists

Nephrogenic diabetes insipidus, hypernatremia

Carbonic Anhydrase Inhibitors

Metabolic acidosis, drowsiness, fatigue, central nervous system depression, paresthesia

Thiazides

Depletion phenomena (hypokalemia, dilutional hyponatremia, hypochloremic alkalosis, hypomagnesemia), retention phenomena (hyperuricemia, hypercalcemia), metabolic changes (hyperglycemia, hyperlipidemia, insulin resistance), hypersensitivity (fever, rash, purpura, anaphylaxis), and azotemia in patients with poor renal function

Loop Diuretics

Hypokalemia; hyperuricemia; metabolic alkalosis; hyponatremia; hearing deficits, particularly with ethacrynic acid; watery diarrhea with ethacrynic acid

K^+-Sparing Diuretics

Aldosterone inhibitors: hyperkalemia, gynecomastia, hirsutism, menstrual irregularities

Triamterene: hyperkalemia, megaloblastic anemia in patients with cirrhosis

Amiloride: hyperkalemia, increase in blood urea nitrogen, glucose intolerance in diabetes mellitus

TRADE NAMES

In addition to generic and fixed-combination preparations, the following trade-named materials are some of the important compounds available in the United States.

Osmotic Diuretics

Isosorbide dinitrate (Dilatrate-SR, Isochron)
Mannitol (Osmitrol)

Vasopressin Receptor Antagonists

Conivaptan (Vaprisol)
Tolvaptan (Samsca)

Carbonic Anhydrase Inhibitors

Acetazolamide (Diamox)
Methazolamide (Neptazane)

Thiazide Diuretics

Bendroflumethiazide (Naturetin)
Benzthiazide (Aquatag, Proaqua, Exna)
Chlorothiazide (Diuril)
Chlorthalidone (Hygroton)
Cyclothiazide (Anhydron)
Hydrochlorothiazide (Esidrix, Hydrodiuril)
Hydroflumethiazide (Diucardin, Saluron)
Indapamide (Lozol)
Methyclothiazide (Enduron)
Metolazone (Diulo, Zaroxolyn)
Polythiazide (Renese)
Trichlormethiazide (Metahydrin, Naqua)

Loop Diuretics, Types I and II

Bumetanide (Bumex)
Ethacrynic acid (Edecrin)
Furosemide (Lasix)
Torsemide (Demadex)

K^+-Sparing Diuretics

Amiloride hydrochloride (Midamor)
Eplerenone (Inspra)
Spironolactone (Aldactone)
Triamterene (Dyrenium)

Others

Nesiritide (Natrecor)
Quinethazone (Hydromox)

SELF-ASSESSMENT QUESTIONS

1. The loop diuretics have their principal diuretic effect on the:
   A. Ascending limb of the loop of Henle.
   B. Distal convoluted tubule.
   C. Proximal convoluted tubule.
   D. Distal pars recta.
   E. Collecting duct.

2. When assessing a patient who has been taking a loop diuretic on a long-term basis, which potential side effect is MOST important?
   A. Disturbed sensory perception, visual.
   B. Disturbed sensory perception, auditory.
   C. Impaired physical mobility.
   D. Altered mucous membranes.

3. Spironolactone:
   A. Competes for aldosterone receptors.
   B. Inhibits the excretion of K^+.
   C. Acts at the late distal tubule.
   D. Is characterized by B and C.
   E. Is characterized by all of the above.
4. Potential side effects of the thiazide diuretics include:
   A. Hypokalemia, hyperglycemia, and hyperlipidemia.
   B. Hypokalemia, ototoxicity, and hyperuricemia.
   C. Hypokalemia, alkalosis, nausea, and vomiting.
   D. Increase in blood urea nitrogen, hyperkalemia, and metabolic acidosis.
   E. Hypermagnesemia, hypercalcemia, and fever.

5. A patient has been diagnosed with uncomplicated primary hypertension. Of the choices below, what type of drug or combination of drugs would be preferable?
   A. A direct-acting vasodilator.
   B. Two types of β blockers, a cardioselective and a nonselective one.
   C. An ACE inhibitor and an angiotensin receptor blocker.
   D. A thiazide diuretic.

FURTHER READING

Kurtz TW. Chlorthalidone: don't call it "thiazide-like" anymore. *Hypertension.* 2010;56(3):335–337.

Roush GC, Sica DA. Diuretics for hypertension: a review and update. *Am J Hypertens.* 2016;29:1130–1137.

Supuran CT. Carbonic anhydrases: novel therapeutic applications for inhibitors and activators. *Nat Rev Drug Discov.* 2008;7:168–181.

Wang DJ, Gottlieb SS. Diuretics: still the mainstay of treatment. *Crit Care Med.* 2008;36(1 suppl):S89–S94.

WEBSITES

http://www.mayoclinic.org/diseases-conditions/high-blood-pressure/in-depth/diuretics/art-20048129
This website is from the Mayo Clinic and has valuable information for clinicians, as well as patients and their families, on diuretics.

Drugs Affecting the Renin-Angiotensin-Aldosterone System

Abdel A. Abdel-Rahman

MAJOR DRUG CLASSES

Renin inhibitors
Angiotensin-converting enzyme inhibitors
Angiotensin receptor blockers
Aldosterone (mineralocorticoid) receptor antagonists

ABBREVIATIONS

ACE	Angiotensin-converting enzyme
AT_1 and AT_2	Angiotensin receptor type 1 and type 2
ARB	Angiotensin receptor blocker
DRI	Direct renin inhibitor
MR	Mineralocorticoid receptor
CNS	Central nervous system
Epi	Epinephrine
NE	Norepinephrine
RAAS	Renal-angiotensin-aldosterone system

THERAPEUTIC OVERVIEW

The renin-angiotensin-aldosterone system (RAAS) plays a major role coordinating renal and cardiovascular functions and is pivotal in the homeostatic control of blood volume, electrolyte balance, and vascular resistance. The components of the RAAS include the principal enzymes **renin** and **angiotensin-converting enzyme (ACE)**, the primary signaling molecule **angiotensin II**, and the angiotensin receptors AT_1 and AT_2. The pathways involved in the RAAS are shown in Fig. 39.1.

Renin is a proteolytic enzyme stored in, and released from, juxta-glomerular cells in the kidneys in response to sympathetic activation, systemic hypotension, and decreased tubular Na^+. A decrease in arterial pressure produces a decrease in renal perfusion pressure and baroreflex-mediated sympathetic activation of **renal β_1-adrenergic receptors**, inducing the release of **renin** into the blood. Renin catalyzes the first and rate-limiting step in the RAAS, the conversion of the circulating glycoprotein angiotensinogen, which is continuously synthesized by the liver, to the decapeptide **angiotensin I**. Angiotensin I is hydrolyzed by ACE1 present in endothelial cell membranes, especially in the lung, to the octapeptide **angiotensin II**, which activates AT_1 and AT_2. Activation of AT_1 **receptors** mediates potent vasoconstriction, sympathoexcitation, renal sodium resorption, left ventricular hypertrophy, and **aldosterone** release, while activation of AT_2 **receptors** leads to vasodilation, natriuresis, and reduced left ventricular mass.

Angiotensin I also serves as a substrate for several peptidases, whereas angiotensin II serves as a substrate for ACE2 and peptidases, generating **angiotensin (1–7)**, another biologically active peptide that activates the G-protein–coupled receptor (GPCR) Mas. Mas activation leads to the generation of nitric oxide (NO), inhibition of cyclooxygenase-2 (COX-2), and vasodilation.

There are four classes of drugs that inhibit the RAAS at different molecular targets. These include **renin inhibitors**, **ACE inhibitors**, **angiotensin receptor blockers (ARBs)**, and **aldosterone (mineralo-corticoid) receptor antagonists (MRAs)**. These classes of drugs and their therapeutic uses are shown in the Therapeutic Overview Box.

THERAPEUTIC OVERVIEW

Class	Indications
Renin inhibitors	Hypertension
Angiotensin-converting enzyme inhibitors	Hypertension, heart failure, post myocardial infarction, diabetes, chronic renal disease, recurrent stroke prevention
Angiotensin receptor blockers	Hypertension, heart failure, diabetes, chronic renal disease
Aldosterone receptor antgonists	Hypertension, heart failure, post myocardial infarction, edema, primary hyperaldosteronism

MECHANISMS OF ACTION

Renin Inhibitors

The **β-adrenergic receptor antagonists** inhibit renin release by competitively antagonizing the effects of norepinephrine (NE) and epinephrine (Epi) on β_1 receptors in the heart and renin-secreting cells of the kidney. The pharmacology of these compounds is discussed in Chapter 12. Some of these compounds, such as **propranolol** and **pindolol**, are nonselective and antagonize both β_1 and β_2 receptors, whereas others, like **atenolol**, are selective for the β_1 receptor subtype. Regardless of their cardioselectivity, these drugs inhibit renin release, an important mechanism of action for their therapeutic use in both hypertension and heart failure (Chapters 37 and 44, respectively).

In 2007, the first and only available direct renin inhibitor (DRI), **aliskiren**, was approved by the United States Food and Drug Administration for the treatment of hypertension. Aliskiren binds renin in the

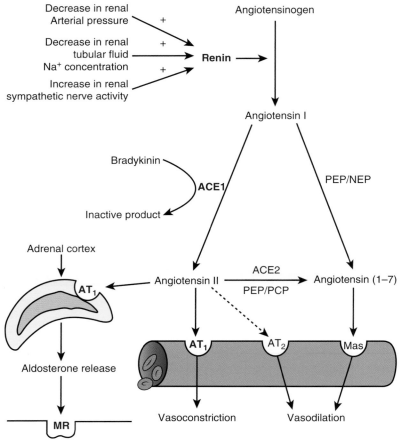

FIG. 39.1 Pathways in the Renin-Angiotensin-Aldosterone System (RAAS). The sites of drug action are bold and dark blue. *ACE,* Angiotensin-converting enzyme; *AT₁,* angiotensin receptor type 1; *AT₂,* angiotensin receptor type 2; *MR,* aldosterone (mineralocorticoid) receptor; *NEP,* neutral endopeptidase 24.11 (neprilysin); *PCP,* prolylcarboxypeptidase; *PEP,* prolyl endopeptidase.

plasma with high affinity to prevent the formation of angiotensin I and, hence, angiotensin II (see Fig. 39.1). At the cellular level, the DRIs dampen AT_1 and aldosterone receptor signaling, leading to reductions in total peripheral resistance and vascular and cardiac hypertrophy.

Angiotensin-Converting Enzyme Inhibitors

The ACE inhibitors, such as captopril, enalapril, and lisinopril, are the oldest classical RAAS inhibitors and reversibly inhibit the second metabolic step in the RAAS—namely, the conversion of angiotensin I to angiotensin II (see Fig. 39.1). As a consequence of ACE inhibition, the reduction in circulating, as well as tissue-formed, angiotensin II, dampens AT_1 receptor signaling in different tissues, reducing vascular tone and inflammation, as well as the release of aldosterone from the adrenal cortex. This latter effect, in concert with inhibition of direct AT_1 receptor–dependent Na^+ reabsorption, results in a natriuretic effect. The reduction in angiotensin II formation also compromises its AT_2 receptor–mediated vasodilation. In addition, ACE inhibitors also lead to the preservation of the vasodilating peptide bradykinin, which is also catabolized by ACE1 (see Fig. 39.1). Although bradykinin is a potent vasodilator contributing to the natriuretic effects of the ACE inhibitors, it has protussive and inflammatory effects and is responsible for the dry cough and angioedema associated with use of the ACE inhibitors.

A comparison of the effects of activation of AT_1 and AT_2 receptors is shown in Table 39.1.

TABLE 39.1 Effects of AT₁ Versus AT₂ Activation

	AT₁	AT₂
Vasculature	Vasoconstriction	Vasodilation
Proliferation/hypertrophy	Left ventricular hypertrophy	Decreased ventricular mass
Sodium reabsorption/ excretion	Antinatriuresis	Natriuresis

Angiotensin Receptor Blockers

As their name implies, the ARBs, such as losartan and valsartan, antagonize the effects of angiotensin II at the AT_1 receptor. The ARBs block vascular, adrenal, and neuronal AT_1 receptors, which mediate increases in vascular resistance, aldosterone release, and sympathetic activity, respectively. The ARBs do not lead to bradykinin accumulation because ACE activity is preserved or even increased as a compensatory mechanism to generate more angiotensin II. As a consequence, the accumulated angiotensin II activates vascular AT_2 receptors, leading to vasodilation. It also serves as a substrate for ACE2 and several peptidases, leading to the formation of angiotensin (1–7), which activates the Mas receptor, leading to vasodilation and antiinflammation.

Aldosterone (Mineralocorticoid) Receptor Antagonists

Spironolactone and eplerenone are the two currently available MRAs. Spironolactone is a nonselective competitive antagonist that also blocks androgen and glucocorticoid receptors, whereas eplerenone is selective for the mineralocorticoid receptor (MR). These drugs reduce aldosterone-mediated vascular and cardiac hypertrophy, leading to their antihypertensive and salutary cardiac effects. Further, blockade of the aldosterone receptor in the nephron leads to the loss of water and Na^+ while preserving K^+ (Chapter 38), an action that might modestly contribute, but does not fully explain, the antihypertensive effect of the MRAs.

RELATIONSHIP OF MECHANISMS OF ACTION TO CLINICAL RESPONSE

Renin Inhibitors

The antihypertensive effects of the renin inhibitors are more pronounced in high-renin hypertension than in normal- or even low-renin hypertension. The classification of high- or low/normal-renin hypertension is based on the relative activity of the RAAS in hypertensive individuals. While still considered a subtype of essential or primary hypertension (unknown etiology), classifying hypertension as high or low/normal renin has clinical and therapeutic ramifications. Assays that accurately determine the level and activity of plasma renin indicate high-renin hypertension if the ratio of plasma aldosterone levels to plasma renin activity exceeds an arbitrary normal value.

Aliskiren reduces renin levels and activity and, when used as monotherapy, produces a modest decrease in blood pressure in patients with mild to moderate hypertension. It has additive effects with the thiazide diuretics, the ARBs, and the calcium-channel blockers and is a good choice for adjunctive therapy with these other antihypertensive medications.

Angiotensin-Converting Enzyme Inhibitors

The ACE inhibitors are also particularly effective antihypertensive drugs in individuals with high-renin hypertension. ACE inhibitors also reduce blood pressure in hypertensive individuals with normal- or even low-renin hypertension, although to a lesser extent than in those with high-renin hypertension. It is important to note that the diagnosis of high- or low-renin hypertension is based on circulating renin activity and does not take into consideration the potential of enhanced tissue (cardiovascular and neuronal) RAAS activity. Other mechanisms might also contribute to the antihypertensive action of these drugs in these populations. The ACE inhibitors decrease the production of angiotensin II and increase the accumulation of angiotensin I, which can elevate the levels of angiotensin (1–7) and activate Mas receptors.

It must be emphasized that even in clinical instances where the RAAS drugs cause little or even no reduction in blood pressure, such drugs still confer renal and cardioprotection. For this reason, ACE inhibitors are particularly useful for treating hypertension associated with other risk factors, such as heart failure, post myocardial infarction, diabetes, kidney disease, and stroke (Chapter 36).

Angiotensin Receptor Blockers

Similar to ACE inhibitors, the ARBs are also effective in treating hypertension of all forms, as well as being especially effective in hypertensive patients with other comorbidities, such as diabetes, heart failure, post myocardial infarction, and stroke. ARBs are used as a monotherapy or combined with other antihypertensive medications.

Aldosterone (Mineralocorticoid) Receptor Antagonists

MRAs are used as a monotherapy or combined with other antihypertensive medications such as ACE inhibitors or β-adrenergic receptor antagonists. They are particularly effective as K^+-sparing diuretics and are the only diuretics that improve symptoms and lower the risk of death and hospitalization for individuals with heart failure (Chapter 38).

PHARMACOKINETICS

Pharmacokinetic parameters for drugs affecting the RAAS are summarized in Table 39.2. The pharmacokinetics for the β-adrenergic receptor blocking drugs are discussed in Chapter 12.

The renin inhibitor aliskiren is an orally active nonpeptide drug with poor absorption (approximately 2.5% bioavailability). Peak plasma levels are reached within 1–3 hours, and approximately 25% of the absorbed dose is excreted unchanged in the urine. The remainder is excreted unchanged in the feces with minimal to no metabolism.

ACE inhibitors are administered orally and have a rapid onset of action, within minutes for captopril and hours for the prodrug enalapril. These drugs are subject to both metabolism and renal excretion, and several agents are prodrugs that require biotransformation to an active compound.

The ARBs are also administered orally and typically are >90% bound to plasma proteins. These drugs differ with respect to plasma half-lives and selectivity for the AT_1 receptor, as well as metabolism and excretion.

Spironolactone is 80%–90% absorbed, and food increases bioavailability. It is rapidly metabolized by cytochrome P450s to both canrenone and 7α-methylspironolactone and is extensively (>90%) bound to plasma proteins. Spironolactone and its metabolites are more than 90% bound to plasma proteins and are excreted primarily in the urine and secondarily in bile. The onset of action for spironolactone is very slow, with a peak response 36–48 hours after the initial dose.

Spironolactone has been reported to induce cytochrome P450s. Eplerenone is rapidly absorbed, and moderately (33%–60%) protein bound, primarily to α1-acid glycoprotein. It is metabolized by CYP3A4 but does not have any active metabolites.

PHARMACOVIGILANCE: ADVERSE EFFECTS AND DRUG INTERACTIONS

All RAAS drugs should be avoided in patients with either unilateral or bilateral renal artery stenosis. While inhibitors of the RAAS confer renal protection in hypertension and diabetes, these drugs cause counterintuitive renal failure in patients with solo or bilateral renal artery stenosis. In these individuals, glomerular filtration becomes heavily dependent on the angiotensin II–mediated constriction of the efferent glomerular arterioles via activation of the AT_1 receptor in these vascular beds. This intrarenal adjustment requires up regulation of the intrarenal synthesis of angiotensin II to activate the AT_1 receptor. Therefore medications that inhibit angiotensin II formation or block the AT_1 receptor will interfere with this self-protecting effect and result in reduced glomerular filtration and kidney failure. The acute renal failure due to the reduction of renal angiotensin II production is attributed to a disproportionate dilation of efferent renal blood vessels compared with afferent vessels.

Agents that interact with the RAAS system are also contraindicated during the second and third trimesters of pregnancy because of the risk of fetal hypotension, anuria, and renal failure, sometimes associated with fetal malformations or death. Recent evidence has also emerged that implicates first-trimester exposure to ACE inhibitors as a teratogenic risk. Therefore after pregnancy has been established, discontinuance or substitution with another antihypertensive agent is mandatory.

Renin Inhibitors

Adverse effects associated with the use of β-blockers are discussed in Chapter 12.

TABLE 39.2   Selected Pharmacokinetic Parameters

Agent	Plasma $t_{1/2}$ (hrs)	Disposition	Remarks
Direct Renin Inhibitors			
Aliskiren	24	M (75%), R (25%)	Poor bioavailability (2.5%) and absorption reduced by high-fat meals
Angiotensin-Converting Enzyme Inhibitors			
Captopril	1–2	M (50%), R (50%)	Absorption reduced by food
Enalapril[a]	11	Active metabolite	
Lisinopril	12–24	R (mainly)	No biotransformation required
Benazepril[a]	10–11	M, R (90%)	
Fosinopril[a]	11–12	M (50%)	
Quinapril[a]	2	M, R (95%)	
Ramipril[a]	3–17	M, R (60%)	
Angiotensin Receptor Blockers			
Losartan	2–3	M (90%)	
Valsartan	6	M	Highly selective for AT_1 receptor
Candesartan[a]	9–12	M, R (26%)	Given as prodrug; low bioavailability
Telmisartan	24	M, F	
Aldosterone (Mineralocorticoid) Receptor Antagonists			
Spironolactone[a]	1.3	M, R (90%)	Its metabolite canrenone is available in Europe.
Eplerenone	4–6	M, R (60%)	

[a]Prodrugs metabolized to active compounds.
F, Fecal elimination; *M*, metabolized; *R*, renal elimination; $t_{1/2}$, half-life.

Aliskiren administration produces a compensatory increase in renin release (i.e., hyperreninemia), though this effect is not clinically significant. Since aliskiren does not interfere with the ACE-induced catabolism of bradykinin, the hyperkalemia, cough, or angioedema produced by aliskiren is considerably blunted compared with that seen with ACE inhibitors. There is a low potential for drug-drug interactions with aliskiren because it is not metabolized.

ACE Inhibitors

The most frequent side effect of the ACE inhibitors is the development of a dry, nonproductive cough, which occurs in about 10%–20% of patients. Bradykinin and substance P seem to be responsible for both the cough and angioedema following ACE inhibition. Angioedema occurs more with ACE inhibitors than with either aliskiren or ARBs. Other adverse effects common to these agents include acute renal failure (particularly in patients with renal artery stenosis), hyperkalemia, and angioedema. Hyperkalemia is more likely to occur in patients with renal insufficiency or diabetes. Patients taking ACE inhibitors, especially captopril, may experience alterations in taste, and skin rashes and fever can also occur. The lowered blood pressure may lead to orthostatic hypotension.

Important drug-drug interactions occur with many ACE inhibitors. These interactions include those with K^+ supplements or K^+-sparing diuretics, which can result in clinically serious hyperkalemia. In addition, nonsteroidal antiinflammatory drugs may impair the hypotensive effects of the ACE inhibitors by abrogating bradykinin-mediated vasodilation, which is, at least in part, prostaglandin mediated.

Angiotensin Receptor Blockers

The adverse effects associated with the ARBs are somewhat similar to those described for ACE inhibitors, including the hazards of use during pregnancy. ARBs can produce kidney failure, especially in patients with renal artery stenosis. Although angioedema may occur in a small percentage of patients, ARBs can be used in patients who have ACE inhibitor–mediated angioedema because only about 8% of patients with ACE inhibitor–induced angioedema show similar responsiveness to ARBs. ARBs are most commonly used in patients who have had adverse reactions to ACE inhibitors. Combinations of ACE inhibitors and ARBs or aliskiren, which had once been considered useful for more complete inhibition of the RAAS, are not recommended due to toxicity demonstrated in recent clinical trials.

NEW DEVELOPMENTS

Current drugs affecting the RAAS are based on inhibiting the synthesis of angiotensin II or disrupting its signaling at the AT_1 receptor. However, recent evidence suggests that other members of the RAAS family, in particular angiotensin (1–7), the enzyme ACE2, and the Mas receptor, constitute viable molecular targets for new therapeutics. Angiotensin (1–7) and activation of Mas lead to reductions in vascular tone and inflammation and consequently blood pressure. In addition, recent findings also suggest that the AT_1 receptor might mediate vasoconstriction in a ligand-independent manner, as a consequence of shear stress. The molecular mechanisms and clinical ramifications of these signaling pathways need to be elucidated to help develop new therapeutics for the treatment of hypertension and other cardiovascular diseases.

CLINICAL RELEVANCE FOR HEALTHCARE PROFESSIONALS

Many individuals are maintained chronically on several antihypertensive medications to control their blood pressure. It is critical that all healthcare professionals are aware of the adverse effects associated with the use of these compounds and advise patients to be aware of the development of skin rashes, allergic reactions, and fevers. The potential to alter

CLINICAL PROBLEMS

Class	Adverse Effects
Renin Inhibitors	
Angiotensin-converting enzyme inhibitors	Hyperkalemia, dry cough, angioedema
Angiotensin receptor blockers	Hyperkalemia
Aldosterone receptor antgonists	Diarrhea, gynecomastia, hyperkalemia, metbolic acidosis

electrolytes, especially potassium, needs to be monitored, as does renal function. Hyperkalemia can lead to muscle cramping and increase the risk of cardiac dysfunction. It can also impact the nature and outcome of therapy sessions where aerobic activity is emphasized. Patients taking ACE inhibitors, especially captopril, may also experience orthostatic hypotension, so care needs to be exercised in moving a patient from a reclining to an upright position. In addition, patients who experience some orthostatic hypotension may not be able to participate in certain exercise programs as part of therapy.

TRADE NAMES

In addition to generic and fixed-combination preparations, the following trade-named materials are some of the important compounds available in the United States.

Renin Inhibitor
Aliskiren (Tekturna)

Angiotensin-Converting Enzyme Inhibitors
Benazepril (Lotensin)
Captopril (Capoten)
Enalapril (Vasotec)
Fosinopril (Monopril)
Lisinopril (Prinivil, Zestril)
Moexipril (Univasc)
Perindopril (Aceon)
Quinapril (Accupril)

Ramipril (Altace)
Trandolapril (Mavik)

Angiotensin Receptor Blockers
Candesartan (Atacand)
Eprosartan (Teveten)
Irbesartan (Avapro)
Losartan (Cozaar)
Olmesartan (Benicar)
Telmisartan (Micardis)
Valsartan (Diovan)

Aldosterone Receptor Antagonists
Spironolactone (Aldactone)
Eplerenone (Inspra)

SELF-ASSESSMENT QUESTIONS

1. Which one of the following pharmacological effects is shared between lisinopril, eplerenone, and aliskiren?
   A. Reduced vascular aldosterone receptor signaling.
   B. Reduced renin activity.
   C. Reduced vascular angiotensin AT_2 receptor signaling.
   D. Reduced angiotensin II synthesis.
   E. Reduced formation of angiotensin (1–7).
2. A 32-year-old hypertensive woman just found out she was pregnant. Which one of the following antihypertensive drugs is contraindicated in pregnant hypertensive women?
   A. Diltiazem.
   B. Nebivolol.
   C. Enalapril.
   D. Hydrochlorothiazide.
   E. Alpha-methyldopa.
3. Which one of the following statements best describes the basis for the hyperkalemia associated with the reduction in blood pressure caused by administration of either propranolol or losartan?

A. Losartan reduces potassium entry into skeletal muscle.
B. Propranolol increases potassium entry into skeletal muscles.
C. Both drugs reduce aldosterone secretion.
D. Both drugs block the aldosterone receptor.
E. Both drugs block epithelial Na^+ channels.

4. A 52-year-old man was precribed an antihypertensive drug to control his blood pressure, but after several months, he stopped taking his medication because he developed a dry, nonproductive cough. Which one of the following drugs was he prescribed?
   A. Lisinopril.
   B. Clonidine.
   C. Propranolol.
   D. Prazosin.
   E. Eplerone.

FURTHER READING

Anguiano L, Riera M, Pascual J, et al. Circulating angiotensin converting enzyme2 activity as a biomarker of silent atherosclerosis in patients with chronic kidney disease. *Atherosclerosis*. 2016;253:135–143.

ALLHAT Collaborative Research Group. Major outcomes in high-risk hypertensive patients randomized to angiotensin-converting enzyme inhibitor or calcium channel blocker vs diuretic. The antihypertensive and lipid-lowering treatment to prevent heart attack trial (ALLHAT). *JAMA*. 2002;288:2981–2997.

Atlas SA. The renin-angiotensin-aldosterone system: pathophysiological role and pharmacologic inhibition. *J Manag Care Pharm*. 2007;13(8 suppl 8):9–20.

James P, Oparil S, Carter B, Cushman W, et al. 2014 Evidence-based guideline for the management of high blood pressure in adults: report from the panel members appointed to the Eighth Joint National Committee. *JAMA*. 2014;507–520.

Whelton PK, Carey RM, Aronow WS. 2017 ACC/AHA/AAPA/ABC/ACPM/AGS/APhA/ASH/ASPC/NMA/PCNA Guideline for the Prevention, Detection, Evaluation, and Management of High Blood Pressure in Adults: A Report of the American College of Cardiology/American Heart Association Task Force on Clinical Practice Guidelines. *J Am Coll Cardiol*. 2017;S0735-1097(17)41519-1. doi:10.1016/j.jacc.2017.11.006.

WEBSITES

http://www.pathwaymedicine.org/raas-system

This is a Pathway Medicine website that covers the essential aspects of the renin-angiotensin-aldosterone system.

https://www.merckmanuals.com/professional/cardiovascular-disorders/hypertension/overview-of-hypertension

This is the Merck Manual website on hypertension and includes evidence-based guidelines for its management.

http://www.onlinejacc.org/content/accj/early/2017/11/04/j.jacc.2017.11.006.full.pdf

This link connects to the full article in the J. Am Col Cardiol by Whelton et al.

Calcium Channel Blockers

Kelly D. Karpa

MAJOR DRUG CLASSES
Dihydropyridines
Benzothiazepines
Phenylalkylamines

ABBREVIATIONS	
Ca^{++}	Calcium
CCBs	Calcium-channel blockers
IP_3	Inositol triphosphate
SA	Sinoatrial
VGCC	Voltage-gated calcium channels

THERAPEUTIC OVERVIEW

Calcium is an essential signaling molecule involved in a variety of cellular functions, ranging from muscle contraction to gene expression. The intracellular concentration of Ca^{++} is tightly regulated by two major classes of calcium channels: ligand-gated Ca^{++} channels, such as inositol triphosphate (IP_3) receptors, ryanodine receptors, and store-operated channels, and voltage-gated Ca^{++} channels (VGCCs). Activation of VGCCs is required for key cellular functions, including neurotransmitter release, hormone secretion, and excitation-contraction coupling.

VGCCs are classified into at least five types based on electrophysiological and pharmacological properties. The three best characterized channels include the L-type (long-lasting, large channels), T-type (transient, tiny channels), and N-type (present in neuronal tissue and distinct from the others in terms of kinetics and inhibitor sensitivity). Only L-type Ca^{++} channels, which are enriched in cardiac and vascular muscle, are targeted by the currently available Ca^{++} channel blockers (CCBs).

Under normal circumstances, the primary modulator of Ca^{++} channels is membrane potential. At rest, membrane potential ranges from -30 to -100 mV, depending on cell type, and Ca^{++} channels are closed. Free intracellular Ca^{++} (0.1 μM) is more than 10,000 times lower than extracellular Ca^{++} (1–1.5 mM), providing a gradient that serves as a large driving force for Ca^{++} to enter cells when provided an opportunity. This gradient is maintained by a membrane that is largely impermeable to Ca^{++} and contains active transport systems that pump Ca^{++} out of cells. When cellular membranes depolarize, the VGCCs open, and Ca^{++} enters cells. This is followed by relatively slow inactivation of L-type Ca^{++} channels, during which time they become impermeable to Ca^{++}. Channels must transition from the inactivated state to the resting conformation before they can open again.

VGCCs play an important role in the muscle excitation-contraction-relaxation cycle. At rest, when intracellular Ca^{++} is low, regulatory proteins prevent actin and myosin filaments from interacting with each other, and muscle is relaxed. When intracellular Ca^{++} concentrations increase (by influx or release from internal stores), Ca^{++} occupies binding sites on Ca^{++}-binding regulatory proteins, such as troponin C (in cardiac and skeletal muscle) and calmodulin (in vascular smooth muscle). These Ca^{++}-bound proteins interact with other cytosolic elements (e.g., troponin I in cardiac and skeletal muscle and myosin light-chain kinase in smooth muscle), allowing cross-bridge formation between actin and myosin, which underlies and initiates contraction. When Ca^{++} channels inactivate, Ca^{++} is pumped out of the cell, activation of contractile proteins is reversed, actin dissociates from myosin, and the muscle relaxes.

Depolarization of vascular smooth muscle cells depends primarily on the influx of Ca^{++}, which is the first step in elevating intracellular Ca^{++}. A second mechanism for raising intracellular Ca^{++} is the agonist-induced production of IP_3 leading to the release of Ca^{++} from the sarcoplasmic reticulum. A third mechanism that increases intracellular Ca^{++} involves receptor-operated channels that open and permit extracellular Ca^{++} entry in response to receptor occupancy.

The CCBs inhibit the voltage-gated inward movement of Ca^{++} through L-type Ca^{++} channels. For this reason, these agents have also been called Ca^{++} entry blockers (CEBs) or Ca^{++} channel antagonists (CCAs). The CCBs are used for the treatment of hypertension, supraventricular arrhythmias, and myocardial ischemia and angina, as well as for the relaxation of uterine smooth muscle in premature labor.

Indications for the use of the CCBs and their primary effects are shown in the Therapeutic Overview Box.

THERAPEUTIC OVERVIEW	
Goals	Decrease blood pressure
	Treat atrial tachyarrhythmias
	Treat symptoms of ischemic heart disease
	Treat premature labor
Drug therapy	Vasodilation
	Slow ventricular response to atrial tachyarrhythmias
	Decrease workload of the heart by slowing heart rate and decrease demand for oxygen
	Decrease uterine contractions

MECHANISMS OF ACTION

VGCCs are composed of a single large subunit (i.e., α subunit) that contains four domains of homologous sequences arranged in tandem to form a pore in the membrane. The CCBs bind most effectively to the inactivated state of the channel. Because the channel can transition to the inactivated state only after opening, and channel opening depends on membrane depolarization, drug binding is "use dependent," a characteristic similar to that for many sodium-channel antagonists such as the local anesthetics (Chapter 27). In addition, the binding of CCBs is also frequency dependent, and binding CCBs to the channel reduces the frequency of channel opening in response to depolarization. These drugs also dissociate relatively rapidly from their binding sites on Ca^{++} channels. If the time between sequential membrane depolarizations is relatively long, most drugs will dissociate from the channel, resulting in little inhibition of Ca^{++} flux. However, if the frequency is rapid, the channels will cycle more frequently, drug will bind to or remain bound to the channel, and blockade of the channel will persist. Therefore inhibition is directly proportional to depolarization rate—that is, it will be frequency dependent.

Differences in the frequency and use dependence and tissue selectivity among the CCBs likely results from the differential sensitivity for each class toward specific sequences and domains within the α1 subunit of the channel. The pore-forming α1 subunit of L-type VGCCs, which is uniquely sensitive to the CCBs, is referred to as Ca_V1. There are four isoforms of this subunit ($Ca_V1.1$–$Ca_V1.4$) that share a common topology consisting of four homologous domains (domains I–IV), with each domain composed of six putative transmembrane segments (S1–S6).

CCBs are classified according to their chemical structure. The dihydropyridines include amlodipine, clevidipine, felodipine, isradipine, nicardipine, nifedipine, nimodipine, and nisoldipine. The nondihydro-pyridines include the phenylalkylamines, such as verapamil, and the benzothiazepines, such as diltiazem. The structures of representative compounds are shown in Fig. 40.1. The dihydropyridines, such as amlodipine, bind to transmembrane segments in both domains III and IV, whereas the phenylalkylamine verapamil binds to transmembrane segment 6 of domain IV (IVS6). The benzothiazepines, such as diltiazem, bind to the cytoplasmic loop that connects domains III and IV. These differences in molecular target sites may be responsible for the differential effects that these three major families of agents have on cardiac versus vascular tissue VGCCs. Verapamil exhibits more frequency dependence than nifedipine; the frequency dependence of diltiazem is intermediate.

These differences in pharmacodynamics also underlie the clinical utility of the drugs as they define tissue selectivity.

RELATIONSHIP OF MECHANISMS OF ACTION TO CLINICAL RESPONSE

The dihydropyridines, such as amlodipine, are arterial vasodilators that preferentially block Ca^{++} channels in vascular smooth muscle relative to channels in cardiac muscle. By blocking Ca^{++} entry, activation of calmodulin, the ubiquitous intracellular Ca^{++} receptor, is dampened, resulting in decreased activation of calmodulin-dependent myosin light-chain kinase (MLCK), decreasing smooth muscle contraction (Fig. 40.2A). As a consequence of this action, the dihydropyridines are useful for treating hypertension. They reduce arterial muscle tone, decrease peripheral resistance, and alleviate vasospasms in coronary and peripheral arteries. As arterial pressure and afterload are reduced, this also decreases the workload of the heart, thus reducing the demand for oxygen, providing antianginal effects. Thus the dihydropyridines also have utility in treating myocardial ischemia. At therapeutic doses, the dihydropyridines do not have negative inotropic effects and do not directly affect the function of nodal tissues in the heart.

The nondihydropyridines verapamil and diltiazem have direct actions on the heart, in addition to their effects on vascular smooth muscle. In cardiac myocytes, Ca^{++} entry interacts with the ryanodine receptor to increase Ca^{++}-induced Ca^{++} release from the sarcoplasmic reticulum (see Fig. 40.2B). The Ca^{++} binds to troponin C, leading to a conformational change that promotes myosin-actin interactions and muscle contraction. The sinoatrial (SA) and atrioventricular (AV) nodes have a high expression of L-type Ca^{++} channels that depend on extracellular Ca^{++} for depolarization. These channels are responsible for both the magnitude and frequency of cardiac contraction. In the absence of these currents, arising from either channel mutations or pharmacological blockade, spontaneous SA node pacemaker frequency is slow and irregular, resting heart rate is reduced, and diastolic depolarization is prolonged. The nondihydropyridines slow phase IV depolarization and conduction at the AV node. Thus these compounds have negative chronotropic, dromotropic, and inotropic effects and are sometimes used to treat supraventricular arrhythmias (Chapter 45). Their ability

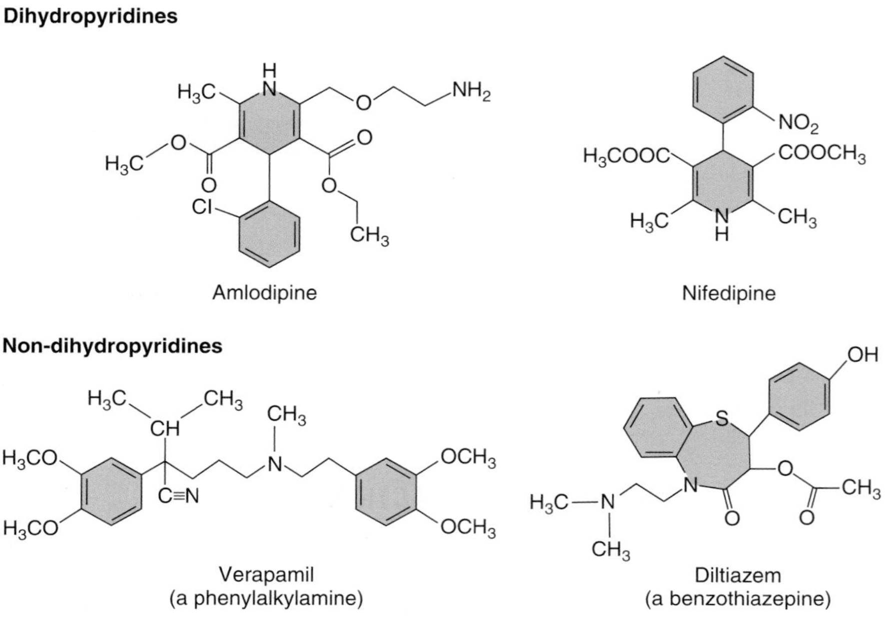

Dihydropyridines

Amlodipine

Nifedipine

Non-dihydropyridines

Verapamil
(a phenylalkylamine)

Diltiazem
(a benzothiazepine)

FIG. 40.1 Representative Structures of Ca^{++}-Channel Blockers.

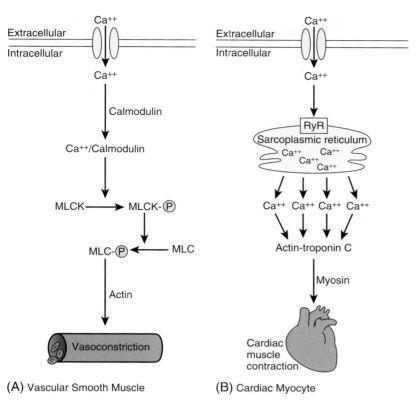

FIG. 40.2 (A) Processes involved in Ca^{++}-mediated contraction of vascular smooth muscle. Ca^{++} entry through L-type Ca^{++} channels leads to calmodulin activation, which phosphorylates myosin light-chain kinase (MLCK), leading to the phosphorylation of myosin light chain (MLC), promoting interactions with actin, and resulting in vasoconstriction. (B) In cardiac myocytes, Ca^{++} entry through L-type Ca^{++} channels stimulates ryanodine receptors (RyR) on the sarcoplasmic reticulum to release Ca^{++}, which interacts with troponin C to promote actin-myosin interactions, leading to contraction.

TABLE 40.1	Pharmacokinetic Properties of Calcium-Channel Blockers			
Drug	**Oral Bioavailability (%)**	**Protein Binding (%)**	**Metabolism**	**Elimination t$_{1/2}$ (hrs)**
Amlodipine	64–90	93	Hepatic	30–50
Clevidipine	NA	>99.5	Plasma esterases	0.25
Diltiazem	40	70–80	Hepatic	3–10[a]
Felodipine	20	>99	Hepatic	11–16
Isradipine	15–24	>95	Hepatic	8
Nicardipine	35	>95	Hepatic	2–9[a]
Nifedipine	49–89	92–98	Hepatic	2–5
Nimodipine	13	>95	Hepatic	1–2
Nisoldipine	5	>99	Hepatic	9–18
Verapamil	20–35	90	Hepatic	3–12[a]

[a]Depends upon immediate or extended-release formulation. *NA*, Not applicable; *t$_{1/2}$*, half-life.

to slow AV nodal conduction velocity and refractoriness makes them useful for controlling the ventricular rate in response to atrial tachyarrhythmias. In addition, by decreasing heart rate and reducing oxygen consumption, the direct cardiodepressant effects of these drugs also make them useful for treating angina pectoris (Chapter 43).

PHARMACOKINETICS

Most of the CCBs are available as oral formulations except clevidipine, which is only available as an intravenous emulsion. In addition to their oral formulations, nicardipine, verapamil, and diltiazem may also be administered intravenously. The intravenous formulations are particularly useful in situations of supraventricular tachycardia and hypertensive urgencies or emergencies where rapid blood pressure reduction is required.

Oral bioavailability following absorption varies among drugs (Table 40.1), and most CCBs are highly protein bound. With the exception of clevidipine, which undergoes rapid hydrolysis by esterases, thereby accounting for its short half-life, CCBs are metabolized by the liver, with half-lives that range from hours to days, depending upon the product and formulation.

PHARMACOVIGILANCE: ADVERSE EFFECTS AND DRUG INTERACTIONS

Most adverse effects caused by the CCBs can be attributed to an extension of their pharmacological action to produce vasodilation—that is, flushing, headache, dizziness, and hypotension. In addition, ankle edema can be a limiting factor for continuing therapy. The dihydropyridines can worsen angina, likely due to a baroreceptor-mediated reflex increase in

CLINICAL PROBLEMS

Dihydropyridines	Hypotension, heart failure, flushing, headaches, dizziness, peripheral edema, angina (with short-acting drugs because of reflex tachycardia), gingival hyperplasia
Nondihydropyridines (benzothiazepines and phenylalkylamines)	Heart block, bradycardia, heart failure, edema, constipation, gingival hyperplasia

TRADE NAMES

In addition to generic and fixed-combination preparations, the following trade-named materials are some of the important compounds available in the United States.

Amlodipine (Norvasc)
Clevidipine (Cleviprex)
Diltiazem (Cardizem)
Felodipine (Plendil)
Isradipine (Dynacirc)
Nicardipine (Cardene)
Nifedipine (Procardia, Adalat)
Nimodipine (Nimotop)
Nisoldipine (Sular)
Verapamil (Calan, Isoptin, Verelan)

heart rate when arterial pressure decreases. This seems most problematic with short-acting nifedipine.

Constipation is also a frequent complaint, particularly with verapamil, due to inhibition of Ca^{++}-mediated contractility of intestinal smooth muscle. Because of direct effects on the heart, verapamil (and to a lesser extent, diltiazem) can lead to bradycardia, AV blockade, and a decrease in left ventricular function. Generally, the CCBs are not used in patients with heart failure, due to a lack of benefit and/or worse outcomes associated with negative inotropic actions.

As a class, the CCBs have been associated with gingival hyperplasia, and thus good oral hygiene is recommended. Considerations that are unique with intravenous clevidipine stem from its formulation as an emulsion. Patients with allergies to soy or egg products, as well as those with defective lipid metabolism, are not candidates for this medication.

The concomitant use of the CCBs with other drugs that lower blood pressure can enhance hypotensive effects. Furthermore, bradycardia and signs of heart failure have been reported when β-adrenergic receptor blockers have been used in combination with nondihydropyridine CCBs. With the exception of clevidipine, the CCBs are all substrates for hepatic cytochrome P450s, especially CYP3A4. Thus other medications that inhibit or induce CYP3A4 can lead to drug-drug interactions and affect the metabolism of the CCBs. Further, nicardipine, verapamil, and diltiazem are inhibitors of P-glycoprotein, resulting in increased plasma concentrations of drugs that are substrates for this efflux pump. For some CCBs, significantly elevated plasma levels can arise from the ingestion of grapefruit juice, which competitively inhibits CYP3A4. Studies have shown that plasma concentrations of verapamil can increase by 8- to 24-fold when taken in conjunction with grapefruit juice (Chapter 3).

Adverse effects associated with the use of the CCBs are summarized in the Clinical Problems Box.

NEW DEVELOPMENTS

The CCBs currently used to treat cardiovascular conditions primarily affect the $Ca_V1.2$ and $Ca_V1.3$ channels but do not discriminate between them (e.g., the drugs are nonselective). Because $Ca_V1.3$ affects heart rate but not ventricular excitation-contraction coupling, selective blockers of this isoform would be advantageous for the treatment of cardiac ischemia without the negative inotropic effects associated with inhibition of the $Ca_V1.2$ isoform. The differential tissue selectivity and use and frequency dependence also suggest that it may be possible to develop agents that are more tissue selective by focusing on the specific sequences and domains in the pore-forming α1 subunit.

CLINICAL RELEVANCE FOR HEALTHCARE PROFESSIONALS

The clinical relevance of this class of agents to specific groups of healthcare providers is related at least in part to the specific agent and healthcare field. For example, dentists and dental hygienists need to be aware that patients taking verapamil are at increased risk of developing gingival hyperplasia. For physical therapists, the ability of patients to respond effectively to therapy depends to a large degree on which medication is being prescribed. For example, verapamil has significant potential to produce cardiac depression, while dihydropyridines produce substantial vasodilation leading to orthostatic hypotension; both situations may affect the ability of patients to complete their therapy.

SELF-ASSESSMENT QUESTIONS

1. A 65-year-old patient with recent onset of atrial tachycardia is started on a calcium-channel blocker that slows conduction at sinoatrial and atrioventricular nodes. Which of the following medications was initiated?
   A. Amlodipine.
   B. Clevidipine.
   C. Diltiazem.
   D. Felodipine.
   E. Nifedipine.

2. Which of the following dihydropyridine calcium-channel blockers has the greatest likelihood of preventing calmodulin activation in a patient taking the medication on an outpatient basis to manage symptoms associated with stable ischemic heart disease?

   A. Amlodipine.
   B. Clevidipine.
   C. Diltiazem.
   D. Verapamil.
   E. Metoprolol.

3. A 62-year-old woman taking medications for ischemic heart disease develops gingival hyperplasia. Which of the following drugs is the most likely culprit?
   A. Nitroglycerin.
   B. Ranolazine.
   C. Metoprolol.
   D. Verapamil.
   E. Clopidogrel.

4. A 60-year-old female tells her pharmacist that she has noticed swelling in her ankles recently. The pharmacist reviews her chart and notes that the patient takes several medications. Which of the following is most likely contributing to her current complaint?
A. Spironolactone.
B. Diltiazem.
C. Aliskiren.
D. Nifedipine.
E. Verapamil.

5. An athletically active 63-year-old woman with hypertension controlled by verapamil develops congestive heart failure. Verapamil should no longer be used by this woman because it:
A. May increase heart rate during exercise.
B. Increases sympathetic activity during exercise.
C. Induces coronary steal phenomenon.
D. Has negative inotropic effects.
E. May increase blood pressure during exercise.

FURTHER READING

Fihn SD, Gardin JM, Abrams J, et al. 2012 ACCF/AHA/ACP/AATS/PCNA/ SCAI/STS guideline for the diagnosis and management of patients with stable ischemic heart disease: a report of the American College of Cardiology Foundation/American Heart Association Task Force on Practice Guidelines, and the American College of Physicians, American Association for Thoracic Surgery, Preventive Cardiovascular Nurses Association, Society for Cardiovascular Angiography and Interventions, and Society of Thoracic Surgeons. *Circulation*. 2012;126(25):e354–e471.

Whelton PK, Carey RM, Aronow WS. 2017 ACC/AHA/AAPA/ABC/ACPM/ AGS/APhA/ASH/ASPC/NMA/PCNA Guideline for the Prevention, Detection, Evaluation, and Management of High Blood Pressure in Adults: A Report of the American College of Cardiology/American Heart Association Task Force on Clinical Practice Guidelines. *J Am Coll Cardiol*. 2017;S0735-1097(17):41519–1. doi:10.1016/j.jacc.2017.11.006.

Yancy CW, Jessup M, Bozkurt B, et al. 2013 ACCF/AHA guideline for the management of heart failure: a report of the American College of Cardiology Foundation/American Heart Association Task Force on Practice Guidelines. *Circulation*. 2013;128(16):e240–e327.

Zamponi GW, Striessnig J, Koschak A, Dolphin AC. The physiology, pathology, and pharmacology of voltage-gated calcium channels and their future therapeutic potential. *Pharmacol Rev*. 2015;67:821–870.

WEBSITES

http://www.mayoclinic.org/diseases-conditions/high-blood-pressure/ in-depth/calcium-channel-blockers/art-20047605
This is the Mayo Clinic website on calcium-channel blockers.
http://www.onlinejacc.org/content/accj/early/2017/11/04/j.jacc. 2017.11.006.full.pdf
This is the link to the 2017 evidence-based guideline for the management of high blood pressure in adults.

Vasodilators for Hypertensive Crises, Pulmonary Hypertension, and Erectile Dysfunction

David A. Tulis and David S. Middlemas

MAJOR DRUG CLASSES

Nitric oxide–based vasodilators
    Nitrates
    Phosphodiesterase type 5 inhibitors
Potassium-channel activators
Prostacyclin analogues
Endothelin-receptor antagonists
Other vasodilators

ABBREVIATIONS

BPH	Benign prostatic hyperplasia
cGMP	Cyclic guanosine monophosphate
ED	Erectile dysfunction
ET-1	Endothelin-1
IV	Intravenous
NO	Nitric oxide
PAH	Pulmonary arterial hypertension
PDE5	Phosphodiesterase type 5
PGI$_2$	Prostacyclin
PH	Pulmonary hypertension
PKG	Cyclic guanosine monophosphate–dependent protein kinase

THERAPEUTIC OVERVIEW

Drugs that produce vasodilation are used to treat a wide variety of clinical disorders, including hypertension, myocardial ischemia, and heart failure, and include agents in many pharmacological classes. Commonly used agents for the treatment of hypertension include drugs that decrease sympathetic tone (Chapter 37), diuretics (Chapter 38), drugs affecting the renin-angiotensin-aldosterone system (Chapter 39), and calcium-channel blockers (Chapter 40). Drugs for the treatment of myocardial ischemia and angina pectoris are discussed in Chapter 43, while those for the treatment of heart failure are discussed in Chapter 44. This chapter covers vasodilators that have specific utility for the treatment of hypertensive crises, pulmonary hypertension (PH), and erectile dysfunction (ED).

Hypertensive Crises

As defined by the American Heart Association, hypertensive crises can manifest as hypertensive urgency or hypertensive emergency. Hypertensive urgency occurs when systolic blood pressure reaches or exceeds 180 mm Hg and diastolic pressure reaches or exceeds 120 mm Hg and can be associated with severe headaches, shortness of breath, nosebleeds, and/or heightened anxiety without detectable associated organ damage. In comparison, a hypertensive emergency, which is usually symptomatic and can be life threatening, occurs when systolic pressure exceeds 180 mm Hg or diastolic pressure exceeds 120 mm Hg and can manifest as loss of memory or consciousness, seizures, cerebral and/or myocardial infarction, aortic and/or other vascular rupture or hemorrhage, pulmonary edema, congestive heart failure, preeclampsia and eclampsia, and/or significant and progressive damage to the brain, heart, vasculature, eyes, and/or kidneys.

A hypertensive crisis is due to abrupt increases in peripheral vascular resistance that can damage the intimal endothelial lining of arterioles, with fibrinoid necrosis and platelet and fibrin deposition, leading to a loss of homeostatic vessel autoregulation. These alterations can quickly lead to positive feedback, exacerbating the immediate elevation in blood pressure. This type of crisis occurs most frequently in individuals with a history of hypertension and/or those who abruptly discontinue current antihypertensive medications. Hypertensive crises may also be attributed to autonomic hyperactivity, collagen-vascular diseases, head trauma, acute glomerulonephritis, stimulant drug use, neoplasias such as pheochromocytoma, preeclampsia or eclampsia, and renovascular hypertension. In both hypertensive urgencies and emergencies, the goal is to reduce blood pressure as fast as possible and restore normal blood pressure profiles. Vasodilators commonly used to treat hypertensive crises must rapidly decrease blood pressure and include agents that increase nitric oxide (NO), activate K$^+$ channels, or block Ca^{++} channels, the latter discussed in Chapter 40.

Pulmonary Hypertension

PH and pulmonary arterial hypertension (PAH), the latter due to the pathological narrowing of pulmonary arteries, are disorders characterized by high blood pressure in the pulmonary circulation. The conditions that lead to PH are not well understood, but it is often associated with chronic renal disease. If left untreated, patients with PH or PAH will ultimately develop heart failure. The goal of treatment is to reduce the time to develop heart failure and other consequences of poor cardiac activity produced by high vascular resistance. PH may be treated with several classes of vasodilators, including synthetic prostacyclin (PGI$_2$) analogues, endothelin-1 (ET-1) receptor antagonists, and the phosphodiesterase type 5 (PDE5) inhibitor sildenafil.

Erectile Dysfunction

Although not a life-threatening disorder, ED, the inability to attain or maintain an erection, is a common medical problem affecting nearly

20 million men in the United States. The disorder can be chronic and unrelenting, with a complex etiology involving the nervous and endocrine systems and blood vessels. ED involves a lack of sufficient blood flow to the penis and may be secondary to hormonal imbalances, atherosclerosis, heart disease, diabetes, metabolic syndrome, or other medical conditions. The pharmacological treatment of erectile dysfunction involves increasing blood flow to the penis using a specific class of vasodilators, the PDE5 inhibitors.

Another male-related issue is benign prostatic hyperplasia (BPH), a noncancerous enlargement of the prostate gland characterized by the proliferation of both smooth muscle and epithelial cells. The nonmalignant enlargement of the prostate may cause lower urinary tract symptoms (LUTS), including impaired urethral function, leading to urinary retention. BPH affects 25% of men by age 55 and is thought to be part of the normal aging process. Several drugs are used for the treatment of BPH including α-adrenergic antagonists that relax smooth muscle in the prostate and neck of the bladder (Chapter 12), 5α-reductase inhibitors that block hormonal changes that mediate prostate growth (Chapter 52), and the PDE5 inhibitor tadalafil.

The Therapeutic Overview Box lists the common clinical problems and related goals for vasodilator pharmacotherapy.

THERAPEUTIC OVERVIEW

Clinical Problem	Goals of Drug Intervention
Hypertensive crises (urgencies, emergencies)	Rapid reduction of blood pressure
Hypertension (essential)	Maintenance of reduced blood pressure
Angina pectoris	Vasodilate coronary arteries and increase coronary artery blood flow
Congestive heart failure	Reduce myocardial insufficiency, myocardial oxygen consumption; increase cardiac output
Pulmonary hypertension	Reduce blood pressure
Coronary artery insufficiency	Increase coronary artery blood flow
Coronary artery vasospasm	Increase coronary artery relaxation
Peripheral vascular disease	Increase blood flow to ischemic tissues
Erectile dysfunction/impotence	Increase penile corpus cavernosum blood flow and flow-mediated erection

MECHANISMS OF ACTION

Most vasodilators act at discrete sites in the biochemical cascade, mediating vascular smooth muscle contraction/relaxation. These mechanisms are depicted in Fig. 41.1.

Nitric Oxide–Based Vasodilators

NO activates soluble guanylyl cyclase, generating cGMP. Cyclic GMP activates distinct serine/threonine protein kinases including cGMP-dependent protein kinase (PKG) and decreases intracellular Ca^{++}. PKG stimulates downstream signaling cascades, including that of myosin light-chain phosphatase, which dephosphorylates actin-myosin cross-bridges and inhibits vascular smooth muscle contraction. NO serves as the distal mediator for several endogenous transmitters that cause vascular smooth muscle relaxation to decrease blood pressure, many of which rely on an intact and functional adjacent endothelial layer to elicit these responses. Bradykinin, histamine, adenosine triphosphate (ATP) and adenosine diphosphate (ADP), substance P, and acetylcholine act on vascular endothelial cells to liberate NO.

Nitrates

Sodium nitroprusside, whose structure is shown in Fig. 41.2, reacts with sulfhydryl groups in compounds such as cysteine and glutathione to form radical intermediates and, through an electron transfer mechanism, results in the release of NO. Sodium nitroprusside acts on both arteriolar and venous (arterial > venous) tissues, leading to direct vasodilation. Additional mechanisms posited for the actions of sodium nitroprusside include decreased Ca^{++} influx, stimulation of intracellular Ca^{++} sequestration into the sarcoplasmic reticulum, decreased Ca^{++} sensitivity of the contractile proteins, and reduced phosphatidylinositol hydrolysis.

Phosphodiesterase Type 5 Inhibitors

The PDEs are a superfamily of enzymes that hydrolyze the cyclic nucleotides cAMP and cGMP; PDE5 is selective for cGMP, is expressed by many cells throughout the body, and is the predominant PDE expressed in the penile corpus cavernosum, where it plays a major role in normal physiological processes underlying sexual arousal–induced erection. This process involves the neurogenic-induced activation of guanylyl cyclase, increasing levels of cGMP, dilating the blood vessels of the corpus cavernosum.

Sildenafil, tadalafil, and vardenafil are competitive reversible inhibitors of PDE5 that bind to the catalytic site of the enzyme, preventing the catabolism of cGMP, thereby prolonging its actions promoting vasodilation. In males, sexual stimulation activates the synthetic enzyme nitric oxide synthase (NOS), leading to the increased synthesis and release of NO, which activates soluble guanylyl cyclase and the synthesis of cGMP. In the presence of a PDE5 inhibitor, blood flow to the penis is increased, leading to an erection.

PDE5 is also expressed in the smooth muscle cells in the prostate and lower urinary tract, and a PDE5 inhibitor will relax smooth muscle in the prostate and bladder and increase blood perfusion, promoting voiding; tadalafil is currently the only agent in this class approved for the treatment of BPH.

In pulmonary arteries, PDE5 leads to vasoconstriction, and thus the PDE5 inhibitors increase pulmonary arterial vasodilation and inhibit vascular remodeling. This decreases pulmonary arterial pressure and pulmonary vascular resistance. Sildenafil is the only agent of this class currently approved for the treatment of PH.

K+ Channel Activators

Adenosine triphosphate–sensitive K^+ channels (K_{ATP}) in vascular smooth muscle cells are tonically active and play an important role in regulating vasoconstriction/vasodilation. These channels are activated by several endogenous compounds, including calcitonin gene–related peptide, vasoactive intestinal polypeptide, PGI_2, and adenosine. The induced membrane hyperpolarization closes voltage-gated Ca^{++} channels, reducing intracellular Ca^{++} and causing vasodilation.

Minoxidil is a prodrug that is metabolized to minoxidil sulfate, which activates K_{ATP} in vascular smooth muscle cells, resulting in smooth muscle relaxation. Minoxidil primarily affects arterioles without marked venous actions. It reduces elevated systolic and diastolic blood pressure by decreasing peripheral vascular resistance.

Prostacyclin Analogues

PGI_2 is a prostanoid derived from the metabolism of arachidonic acid (Chapter 29) that plays a major role in smooth muscle function, inflammation, and homeostasis. PGI_2 is synthesized by and released from endothelial cells and activates the IP prostanoid receptor, a G-protein–coupled receptor (GPCR), leading to increased cAMP, decreased intracellular Ca^{++}, and smooth muscle relaxation, thereby counteracting

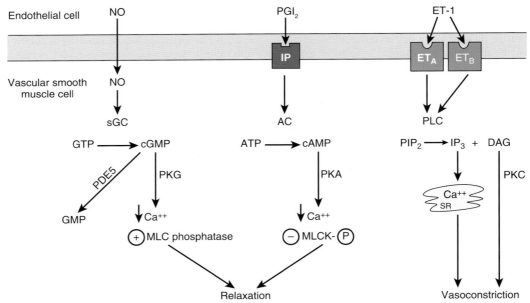

FIG. 41.1 Biochemical Cascade Mediating Vascular Smooth Muscle Contraction/Relaxation. Nitric oxide (NO) activates soluble guanylyl cyclase (sGC) to promote the synthesis of cGMP, activating cGMP-dependent protein kinase (PKG). This decreases intracellular Ca^{++} and increases the activity of myosin light-chain (MLC) phosphatase, which dephosphorylates actin-myosin cross-bridges and inhibits vascular smooth muscle contraction, thereby promoting relaxation. Prostacyclin (PGI_2), formed from the metabolism of arachidonic acid in endothelial cells, activates the IP prostanoid receptor, increasing adenylyl cyclase (AC) activity, promoting the formation of cAMP. cAMP activates cAMP-dependent protein kinase (PKA), which phosphorylates MLC kinase (MLCK) at a site that desensitizes the enzyme, preventing the phosphorylation of MLC and actin-myosin cross-bridge formation, promoting relaxation. Endothelin-1 (ET-1) stimulates ET_A and ET_B receptors, leading to the activation of phospholipase C (PLC), promoting the release of IP_3. IP_3 enhances Ca^{++} release from the sarcoplasmic reticulum (SR), while diacylglycerol (DAG) activates protein kinase C (PKC), both of which promote vasoconstriction.

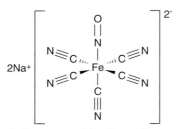

FIG. 41.2 Structure of Sodium Nitroprusside.

the vasoconstrictor effects of thromboxane A_2 ($TBXA_2$). PGI_2 also prevents platelet aggregation, again counteracting the proaggregation effects of $TBXA_2$.

Epoprostenol, iloprost, and treprostinil are synthetic PGI_2 analogues. As for PGI_2, activation of prostanoid IP receptors by these agents leads to vasodilation of pulmonary and systemic vascular smooth muscle, as well as inhibition of platelet aggregation. These agents are approved for use in PAH.

Endothelin Receptor Antagonists

The endothelins, ET-1, ET-2, and ET-3, are expressed by many cells throughout the body. ET-1 is widely expressed throughout the body, ET-2 is produced mainly within the kidneys and gastrointestinal tract, with smaller amounts in the myocardium, placenta, and uterus, while ET-3 is present in the circulation, brain, gastrointestinal tract, lungs,

and kidneys. ET-1 is the only ET expressed by endothelial cells, is a potent vasoconstrictor, and plays an important role in vascular physiology and disease including hypertension, cardiac hypertrophy, coronary artery disease, and PH. ET-1 is not stored in secretory granules but is synthesized on demand, within minutes, in response to stimuli such as hypoxia and ischemia.

The ETs bind to two types of receptors (ET_A and ET_B), both of which are G-protein–coupled receptors (GPCRs). ET_A receptors are expressed on vascular smooth muscle and mediate the vasoconstrictor actions of ET-1; ET_B receptors are also present and may contribute to the vaso-constricting effects of ET-1. The activation of ET receptors by ET-1 leads to the stimulation of phospholipase C and production of inositol 1,4,5-triphosphate (IP_3) and diacylglycerol (DAG), both of which contribute to vasoconstriction.

Bosentan, ambrisentan, and macitentan are endothelin receptor antagonists used for the treatment of PH and PAH. Ambrisentan is a selective antagonist of ET_A receptors, whereas bosentan and macitentan are nonselective and competitively inhibit both ET_A and ET_B receptors. As endothelin receptor antagonists, these agents prevent endogenous ET-1 from activating its receptor, leading to vasodilation.

Others

Hydralazine belongs to the hydrazinophthalazine class of drugs and was one of the first antihypertensive agents. Even though a defined mechanism of action has yet to be solidified, current theories contend that hydralazine may act through reduction of intracellular Ca^{++} mobilization from the sarcoplasmic reticulum, through K^+ channel induction (leading to hyperpolarization) and possibly via the stimulation of endothelium-dependent NO synthesis. Studies also suggest that cAMP may be involved. Ultimately, hydralazine decreases intracellular Ca^{++} and has a direct vasodilatory effect, primarily on arterioles with little impact on veins, minimizing orthostatic hypotension and increasing cardiac output. As a result, blood pressure is rapidly decreased, with diastolic pressure reduced more than systolic pressure. Hydralazine does not have a direct effect on the heart.

RELATIONSHIP OF MECHANISMS OF ACTION TO CLINICAL RESPONSE

Nitric Oxide–Based Vasodilators

Sodium nitroprusside is the drug of choice for rapid pharmacologic treatment of hypertensive crises due to its potency, efficacy, and fast action.

The PDE5 inhibitors are used primarily for erectile dysfunction, but specific PDE5 inhibitors are also approved for other indications. Sildenafil is approved for use in PH by increasing pulmonary artery vasodilation, whereas tadalafil is approved for the treatment of BPH by relaxing smooth muscle in the prostate and bladder.

K⁺ Channel Activators

Minoxidil produces greater vasodilation than hydralazine but can also cause more significant adverse effects and is reserved for patients who are unresponsive to safer drugs. Minoxidil decreases forearm and renal vascular resistance, leading to increased forearm blood flow with maintained renal blood flow and glomerular filtration rate. Because the predominant site of minoxidil is arterial without venodilation, postural hypotension is unusual following its administration. Minoxidil is also used topically to promote the survival and viability of hair cells or hair follicles in androgenetic alopecia, an action that may involve its vasodilating effect but has also been attributed to altering signal transduction pathways that enhance proliferative and antiapoptotic factors.

Prostacyclin Analogues

Epoprostenol is administered both short term and long term. For the latter, it is administered through a surgically placed central venous catheter. When administered intravenously (IV) to patients with idiopathic PAH, epoprostenol improved survival and increased exercise capacity. Similar results were obtained in patients with PAH associated with connective tissue disease.

Endothelin Receptor Antagonists

The ET-1 receptor antagonists are approved for use as a single agent for the treatment of PAH to improve exercise ability and delay clinical worsening. Patients with PAH have been shown to express elevated levels of ET-1 in vascular endothelial cells of pulmonary arteries. Thus the endothelin receptor antagonists, such as macitentan, that prevent the binding of ET-1 to both ET_A and ET_B receptors, improve survival in patients with PH. It is unclear whether blocking both receptor subtypes is important for the treatment of PAH, as the older agent ambrisentan is selective for ET_A. However, the density of ET_A receptors in pulmonary arterial smooth muscle cells is greater than that of ET_B receptors. For patients with PH, the combination of an ET-1 receptor antagonist and the PDE5 inhibitor tadalafil also improves exercise ability and reduces the risks of disease progression and hospitalization.

Others

The decreased peripheral vascular resistance following hydralazine administration is accompanied by a reflex-mediated increased heart rate, cardiac output, and stroke volume in hypertensive patients. Patients with congestive heart failure also exhibit increased cardiac output as a consequence of the decreased systemic vascular resistance. The reflex-sympathetic discharge also typically leads to increased renin release, increasing the production of angiotensin II, resulting in increased aldosterone with consequent Na^+ reabsorption. A diuretic is often administered concurrently.

PHARMACOKINETICS

Sodium nitroprusside is generally administered parenterally, and hypotensive effects can be realized almost immediately (and, in turn, its effects dissipate almost as quickly following cessation of dosing). The biological half-life of sodium nitroprusside is about 2 minutes, and it is metabolized to yield five cyanide groups, which are converted to thiocyanate by the liver and excreted via the urine over several days.

The PDE5 inhibitors are orally available, and most of them have serum half-lives in the range of about 2–4 hours, rendering them suitable for on-demand use once in 24 hours. In contrast, tadalafil has a half-life of about 17.5 hours, prolonging its effects to 1–2 days. Because of this, a low dose of tadalafil, administered once daily, is indicated for the treatment of either BPH or ED. The PDE5 inhibitors are metabolized by CYP3A4.

Minoxidil is rapidly and completely absorbed following oral administration, with maximal vascular dilation within 2–3 hours, although residual vasodilation may persist through several days following the initial dose and should be monitored closely. Minoxidil has a biological half-life between 3–4 hours and is extensively metabolized (90%) by the liver and excreted as glucuronides in the urine. Little to no accumulation and the absence of tolerance or refractoriness has been reported with various dosing regimens of minoxidil.

Epoprostenol is unstable at room temperature and needs to be kept cold at all times, even during infusion. It is administered by continuous infusion through an implanted central venous catheter with a half-life of about 3–5 minutes. Treprostinil, which is chemically stable at room temperature, is available for both IV and subcutaneous administration. The drug has a long terminal half-life of about 4 hours but a relatively short effective half-life of 10 minutes following IV and 60 minutes following subcutaneous administration. Clearance is decreased in patients with hepatic disease. Iloprost is available for IV and inhalation administration, with a plasma half-life of 20–30 minutes. The inhaled preparation leads to pulmonary vasodilation for 1–2 hours.

Ambrisentan, bosentan, and macitentan are available as oral preparations with relatively good bioavailability (bosentan is only 50% bioavailable). All compounds are highly protein bound (>98%) and are metabolized by the liver (mainly by CYP3A4). Macitentan is highly lipophilic and exhibits greater penetration into tissues than ambrisentan. It also exhibits slower receptor dissociation kinetics than the other available agents. Maximum plasma levels of macitentan are achieved in about 8 hours after oral dosing, and the drug has a half-life of 15–16 hours, with an active metabolite (~20%) with a very long (48 hours) half-life. Macitentan and its metabolites are excreted in both the urine and feces.

Hydralazine is rapidly acting (<10 minutes) following parenteral administration. Following oral dosing, hydralazine is readily absorbed but undergoes extensive first-pass metabolism by acetylation. Hydralazine exhibits slightly delayed kinetics, with effects beginning within 45 minutes after ingestion and lasting 6 hours. The biological half-life of hydralazine is 2–8 hours, and it undergoes extensive hepatic metabolism and is excreted mainly as metabolites in the urine. Hydralazine is metabolized and inactivated through acetylation. Thus individuals who are rapid acetylators eliminate the drug more rapidly, while those who are slow acetylators inactivate the drug slowly, resulting in accumulation in the body and pronounced/excessive vascular dilation and exaggerated side effects. Indeed, large differences in the therapeutic and adverse event profile have been observed in the patient population, underscoring the importance of pharmacogenetics (Chapter 4).

PHARMACOVIGILANCE: ADVERSE EFFECTS AND DRUG INTERACTIONS

Despite the beneficial, rapid antihypertensive actions of these vasodilatory pharmacotherapies during episodes of hypertensive crisis, they can elicit some potentially significant adverse effects and contraindications that warrant attention. One primary concern among vasodilators is that during vascular relaxation and reduced peripheral vascular resistance, baroreceptor-mediated reflex activation of the sympathetic nervous system can ensue, leading to unwanted cardiac (tachycardia, increased contractility, increased cardiac output) and/or renal (increased release of renin and fluid retention) effects. In patients with coronary artery disease, this may overload the heart and lead to angina pectoris and/or myocardial stress/infarction. To counteract potentially adverse reflex sympathetic stimulation, β-adrenergic receptor antagonists and/or diuretics are often administered concomitant with vasodilators. Orthostatic (postural) hypotension should also be monitored as a general side effect of antihypertensive therapies and systemic vascular relaxation, and the patient should be monitored for light-headedness and dizziness and the dose(s) adjusted accordingly. Although unusual, if used to combat pregnancy-induced hypertension, vasodilators may interrupt labor by relaxing uterine smooth muscle as an off-target effect. Also, despite the use of these agents during acute hypertensive crises, their prolonged use can result in aldosterone-mediated Na^+ and water retention and blood volume expansion, thereby offsetting the beneficial capacities of the vasodilator. In addition to these generalized adverse effects, more specific limitations, as well as contraindications, for the vasodilators are discussed below.

Nitric Oxide–Based Vasodilators

Given the unique mode of action of sodium nitroprusside via generation of vasoactive NO and the many potential off-target effects of NO on the vasculature and other tissues, there are many possible limitations and precautions to its use during hypertensive crises and other disorders. The most common adverse effect of sodium nitroprusside is hypotension and dysrhythmias resulting from direct vasodilation. Another concern associated with sodium nitroprusside is the potential toxic effects of its cyanide/thiocyanate metabolites. Each molecule of sodium nitroprusside reacts with hemoglobin to yield one molecule of cyanmethemoglobin and four cyanide ions. Normally, cyanide is converted to thiocyanate by a mitochondrial transferase present in excess in the body, and thiocyanate is eliminated in the urine. Although thiocyanate toxicity is not common, it can result in tinnitus, nausea, abdominal pain, and mental status alterations. Although cyanide toxicity is very rare, cyanide can react with ferric iron in methemoglobin, cytochrome oxidase, and other enzymes to produce methemoglobinemia, abnormal oxygen utilization, coma, metabolic acidosis, or respiratory arrest and death.

Another possible drawback to the use of sodium nitroprusside is its dilatory effect on venous tissues, which can lead to peripheral blood pooling and reduced venous return and ventricular pressures, which could present a caveat for patients with impaired myocardial function. Some other commonly observed adverse effects include palpitations, apprehension and anxiety, confusion, somnolence, body rash, thyroid suppression, oliguria, and renal azotemia. Less common side effects can include abdominal pain, chest discomfort, and retching. The incidence of adverse events and toxicity is usually manifest by individuals who have taken the drug for a prolonged period or those with renal or hepatic impairment. Sodium nitroprusside is contraindicated for use in patients with liver disease or those with low levels of thiosulfate, compensatory hypertension (as a result of arteriovenous stenting or aortic coarctation), or inadequate cerebral perfusion or severe renal dysfunction.

Phosphodiesterase 5 Inhibitors

PDE5 inhibitors are contraindicated in patients taking nitrates for angina, such as nitroglycerin, isosorbide dinitrate, and isosorbide mononitrate, or inhaled amyl nitrate (poppers). Combination administration of a PDE5 inhibitor with a nitrate may cause a substantial and threatening drop in blood pressure. Therefore nitrates should not be administered to patients who have taken sildenafil, vardenafil, or avanafil within 24 hours and tadalafil within 36–48 hours. PDE5 inhibitors are not contraindicated with other drugs that lower blood pressure, such as α-adrenergic receptor–blocking drugs, but patients should be advised to use caution, as orthostatic hypotension and syncope may ensue.

Changes in color perception (shift to blue) may arise from inhibition of PDE6 expressed in the retina; PDE6 is inhibited less potently than PDE5 by these inhibitors. Other adverse effects include headache, flushing, nasal congestion, dyspepsia, and myalgia, which may be due to vasodilation in other parts of the body. Sildenafil and vardenafil are differentially affected by fatty food, but tadalafil and avanafil are less affected. Because these drugs are metabolized by CYP3A4, coadministration of CYP3A4 inhibitors is contraindicated, as levels of the PDE5 inhibitors may increase 10-fold. Moderate potency CYP3A4 inhibitors, such as cimetidine and grapefruit juice, may increase the serum levels of PDE5 inhibitors modestly, about 1.5-fold.

K+ Channel Activators

One specific yet potentially serious side effect associated with use of minoxidil is pericardial effusion, or fluid buildup, beneath the pericardium as a result of fluid retention. This could lead to cardiac tamponade, a compression of the heart, which reduces cardiac function. If cardiac tamponade occurs, the use of minoxidil should be stopped immediately, and the patient may have to undergo pericardiocentesis or surgical drainage. Other specific adverse effects of minoxidil include breast tenderness, glucose intolerance, thrombocytopenia, and skin reactions. While the use of minoxidil for hypertensive crises is acute, prolonged (>4 weeks) use can result in hypertrichosis, or excessive hair growth of the face, arms and legs, and back. While largely cosmetic and benign in nature, this often leads to cessation of use of minoxidil for alternate agents. Minoxidil should not be taken with guanethidine, as this may cause exaggerated hypotension and should not be used in patients with pheochromocytoma (adrenal gland tumor).

Prostacyclin Analogues

Several events have been associated with the central catheter administration of epoprostenol, such as sepsis, cellulitis, hemorrhage, and pneumothorax. Treprostinil, which can be administrated subcutaneously, often leads to injection site pain. Other adverse effects associated with long-term administration of epoprostenol and treprostinil include jaw pain, headache, nausea, diarrhea, photosensitivity, flushing of the skin, and muscle or joint pain. The most common adverse effect of iloprost is flushing.

Endothelin Receptor Antagonists

The endothelin receptor antagonists are generally well tolerated. All effects are consistent with the mechanism of action of these agents and include hypotension, headache, nasal congestion, and peripheral edema. Macitentan and ambrisentan can lead to anemia in a small percentage of individuals, whereas anemia associated with bosentan occurs in about

50% of all patients. Because all of these agents are metabolized by CYP3A4 and CYP2C9, the potential for drug-drug interactions exists.

Others

Some common side effects associated with hydralazine use can include headaches, palpitations, flushing, joint and muscle aches, diarrhea and other gastrointestinal disturbances, and edema. Uncommon or rare side effects can include an autoimmune response similar to lupus erythematosus (most often in patients who are slow acetylators, i.e., they inactivate hydralazine slowly), proteinuria, glomerulonephritis, hepatitis, appetite and weight loss, anxiety and tremor, peripheral neuritis, acute renal dysfunction and/or failure, and hallucinations. Hydralazine can be used with a β-adrenergic receptor blocker to offset potential reflex sympathetic activation and with a diuretic to offset Na⁺ and water retention and blood volume expansion. These represent situations of concurrent yet beneficial drug administration. Conversely, caution is warranted when using hydralazine with other vascular relaxants, as excessive and possibly dangerous hypotension could result. Hydralazine is contraindicated in patients with preexisting autoimmune disorders, tachycardia, and/or heart failure (or other forms of myocardial insufficiency), pulmonary hypertension (with isolated right heart dysfunction or failure), or dissecting aortic aneurysm.

NEW DEVELOPMENTS

Many vasodilators act directly on the smooth muscle layer of blood vessels to control excitation-contraction coupling and calcium-mediated muscle contraction, thereby regulating vascular resistance and, in turn, blood pressure; however, the adjacent vascular endothelium plays key roles in the maintenance and regulation of vascular function and warrants heightened attention as a potential therapeutic target. The intimal endothelial and underlying medial smooth muscle cell layers communicate closely to control vascular function, yet only a small (but significant) proportion of vasodilators (namely, sodium nitroprusside via actions of NO) act predominantly on the vascular endothelium to elicit relaxation. Considering its crucial functions in the regulation of vascular contraction/dilation and growth, as well as the maintenance of a nonthrombogenic interface between luminal blood and the vessel wall, the vascular endothelium represents an emerging pharmacotherapeutic target of particular interest.

During episodes of vascular trauma and/or disease, vascular smooth muscle superoxide anion production is increased, which can rapidly offset the actions of NO and limit the beneficial effects of sodium nitroprusside. Identifying agents capable of controlling superoxide anion production that could be used concomitantly with NO-mediated vascular therapy warrants attention.

CLINICAL RELEVANCE FOR HEALTHCARE PROFESSIONALS

The use of vasodilators to control blood pressure is only becoming commonplace as a mechanism of long-term blood pressure management and usually in the context of managing blood pressure in patients suffering from heart failure. Therefore healthcare professionals who practice in critical care settings will need to be familiar with the adverse effects of many of these compounds, including the potential for sodium

nitroprusside to produce cyanide poisoning if continued for significant periods. Similarly, individuals who practice in the emergency department will need to be cognizant of the potential drug-drug interactions between nitrates and PDE5 inhibitors. Of particular importance, healthcare professionals should recognize the potential for nearly all of the agents to produce orthostatic hypotension upon transitioning from a supine position to standing or reflex tachycardia, which poses a problem with patients with some cardiac tissue damage.

CLINICAL PROBLEMS

Drug	Adverse Effects
All vasodilators	Orthostatic hypotension, tachycardia
Nitroprusside	Headache, tolerance, thiocyanate accumulation, cyanide toxicity
Phosphodiesterase type 5 inhibitors	Color vision, headache, flushing, nasal congestion, dyspepsia, myalgia
Minoxidil	Pericardial effusion, breast tenderness, glucose intolerance, thrombocytopenia, excessive hair growth
Prostacyclin analogues	Jaw pain, headache, nausea, diarrhea, photosensitivity, muscle or joint pain
Endothelin receptor antagonists	Hypotension, headache, nasal congestion, peripheral edema
Hydralazine	Headaches, palpitations, flushing, joint and muscle aches, lupus-like effects

TRADE NAMES

In addition to generic and fixed-combination preparations, the following trade-named materials are some of the important compounds available in the United States.

Nitric Oxide–Based Vasodilators
Sodium nitroprusside (Nitropress, Nipride, RTU)
Sildenafil (Revatio, Viagra)
Tadalafil (Cialis, Adcirca)
Vardenafil (Levitra, Staxyn)
Avanafil (Stendra)

K⁺ Channel Activators
Minoxidil (Loniten [systemic], Rogaine [topical])

Prostacyclin Analogues
Epoprostenol (Flolan, Veletri)
Iloprost (Ventavis)
Treprostinil (Remodulin, Orenitram, Tyvaso)

Endothelin Receptor Antagonists
Bosentan (Tracleer)
Macitentan (Opsumit)
Ambrisentan (Letairis)

Others
Hydralazine (Apresoline)

SELF-ASSESSMENT QUESTIONS

1. The vasodilatory action of which of the following agents involves activation of potassium channels in vascular smooth muscle?
   A. Diltiazem.
   B. Hydralazine.
   C. Sodium nitroprusside.
   D. Minoxidil.
   E. All are correct.
2. The actions of sodium nitroprusside during episodes of hypertensive crisis:
   A. Are dependent upon activation of endothelial nitrous oxide.
   B. Occur rapidly and reversibly.
   C. Can be associated with cyanide/thiocyanate toxicity.
   D. B and C are correct.
   E. All are correct.
3. Common adverse effects associated with the use of vasodilators can include:
   A. Reflex activation of the sympathetic nervous system.
   B. Dizziness and light-headedness.
   C. Sodium and water retention.
   D. Orthostatic hypotension.
   E. All are correct.
4. A 63-year-old male patient is prescribed a phosphodiesterase-5 inhibitor for erectile dysfunction. A serious drug-drug interaction with nitroglycerin could cause:
   A. Hypotension.
   B. Hypertension.
   C. Hyperglycemia.
   D. Hypoglycemia.
   E. Nephrotoxicity.
5. A 66-year-old male presents with an enlarged prostate on a digital rectal examination during his annual routine medical examination. In further discussion on his overall wellness, he complains of having difficulty with urine flow and erectile dysfunction. An appropriate treatment would be:
   A. A daily oral dose of sildenafil.
   B. Topical minoxidil administration.
   C. A daily oral low dose of tadalafil.
   D. Oral tadalafil as needed.
   E. Oral sildenafil as needed.

FURTHER READING

Brozovich FV, Nicholson CJ, Degen CV, et al. Mechanisms of vascular smooth muscle contraction and the basis for pharmacologic treatment of smooth muscle disorders. *Pharmacol Rev.* 2016;68(2):476–532.

Pak KJ, Hu T, Fee C, et al. Acute hypertension: a systematic review and appraisal of guidelines. *Ochsner J.* 2014;14(4):655–663.

WEBSITES

http://www.heart.org/HEARTORG/Conditions/HighBloodPressure/AboutHighBloodPressure/Hypertensive-Crisis_UCM_301782_Article.jsp#.WXjddFGQyUk

This website is maintained by the American Heart Association and contains information on hypertensive crises.

http://sites.jamanetwork.com/jnc8/

This site is maintained by the Journal of the American Medical Association, with evidence-based guidelines for the treatment of hypertension.

http://www.acc.org/latest-in-cardiology/ten-points-to-remember/2015/09/15/15/19/2015-esc-ers-guidelines-for-the-diagnosis-and-treatment-of-ph

This website is maintained by the American College of Cardiology, with guidelines for the diagnosis and treatment of pulmonary hypertension.

https://auanet.org/guidelines/erectile-dysfunction-(2005-reviewed-and-validity-confirmed-2011)

This website is maintained by the American Urological Association and contains guidelines for the management of erectile dysfunction.

Drug Therapy for Hyperlipidemias and Atherosclerotic Cardiovascular Disease

Michael T. Piascik and Robert W. Hadley

MAJOR DRUG CLASSES

HMG-CoA reductase inhibitors
PCSK9 inhibitors
Cholesterol uptake inhibitors
Bile acid sequestrants
MTTP inhibitors
ApoB-100 synthesis inhibitors
Fibrates
Niacin

ABBREVIATIONS

ASCVD	Atherosclerotic cardiovascular disease
HDL or HDL-C	High-density lipoprotein or high-density lipoprotein cholesterol
HMG-CoA	Hydroxy-3-methyl-glutaryl coenzyme A
IDL	Intermediate-density lipoprotein
LDL or LDL-C	Low-density lipoprotein or low-density lipoprotein cholesterol
MTTP	Microsomal triglyceride transfer protein
PCSK9	Proprotein convertase subtilisin/kexin type 9
PPAR-α	Peroxisome proliferator–activated receptor-α
$t_{1/2}$	Half-life for drug elimination
VLDL	Very low-density lipoprotein

THERAPEUTIC OVERVIEW

The antihyperlipidemics are drugs used to treat abnormal blood lipid levels. The blood lipids of most clinical interest are cholesterol and triglycerides. These lipids have poor water solubility and are transported in large complexes termed lipoproteins—that is, high-density lipoprotein (HDL), low-density lipoprotein (LDL), and very low-density lipoprotein (VLDL). Abnormally elevated levels of plasma lipids are termed hyperlipidemias, with hypercholesterolemia and hypertriglyceridemia referring to elevated levels of cholesterol or triglycerides, respectively. A mixed hyperlipidemia refers to an elevation of both types of lipids. The term hyperlipoproteinemia refers to elevated levels of a specific lipoprotein, such as LDL. Hyperlipidemias often require treatment due to their clinical consequences. Over the long term, moderate hypertriglyceridemia is associated with the development of atherosclerotic cardiovascular disease (ASCVD). The main concern with severe hypertriglyceridemia is the increased the risk of acute pancreatitis.

Pathophysiology

Atherosclerosis is a systemic arterial disease that develops secondary to endothelial injury. The vast majority of deaths from cardiovascular disease have been attributed to atherosclerosis and its complications. Major complications of ASCVD include myocardial infarction, angina pectoris, sudden cardiac death, chronic heart failure, ischemic stroke, and claudication (exercise-induced leg pain). Both hypercholesterolemia and hypertriglyceridemia are associated with the progression of atherosclerosis. Cholesterol levels are particularly important; for every 1% lowering of cholesterol, there is approximately a 2% reduced risk of coronary artery disease. LDL-cholesterol (LDL-C) is the specific lipoprotein most closely associated with the development of ASCVD, as its small size contributes to its ability to penetrate the blood vessel wall and its atherogenicity. In contrast, HDL-C is antiatherogenic, as it participates in the removal of cholesterol from the periphery through a phenomenon known as reverse cholesterol transport.

Atherosclerosis is primarily an inflammatory response to injury. At least six major processes occur in the development of atherosclerotic plaques (atheromas):

1. Endothelial injury facilitating entry of monocytes and adherence of platelets.
2. Transport of LDL particles into the subendothelial space followed by their oxidation.
3. Conversion of monocytes to macrophages that ingest oxidized LDL and transform into foam cells that then coalesce into fatty streaks.
4. T lymphocytes mediate inflammatory responses.
5. Smooth muscle cells and fibroblasts provide a matrix skeleton of collagen, fibrin, and calcification.
6. Spontaneous death or digestion of foam cells with release of cholesterol and other lipids to form a lipid pool.

Buildup of plaques over decades leads to the gradual narrowing of coronary and other conduit arteries (Fig. 42.1), resulting in various chronic ischemic syndromes such as angina. Acute ischemic events (e.g., myocardial infarctions) are most often associated with the rupture or fissure of a plaque, leading to the sudden occlusion of a blood vessel by a thrombus. Characteristics of plaques vulnerable to sudden rupture include a thin fibrous cap, increased macrophages and T lymphocytes, few smooth muscle cells and collagen fibers, and a large lipid core.

One hyperlipidemia of special interest is familial hypercholesterolemia, which is an inherited autosomal dominant disorder caused by defects in LDL receptors. The heterozygous form of familial hypercholesterolemia is uncommon (0.2% of the general population), while the homozygous form is very rare but produces particularly severe disease. Total serum cholesterol can range up to 500 mg/dL for heterozygotes and up to 1000 mg/dL for homozygotes. These individuals are very likely to develop premature ASCVD; novel drugs such as lomitapide

337

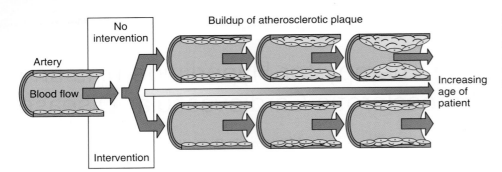

No intervention

Buildup of atherosclerotic plaque

Artery

Blood flow

Intervention

Increasing age of patient

FIG. 42.1 Atherosclerosis Prevention. Intervention involves (1) diet to decrease cholesterol and fats, (2) cessation of smoking, (3) drugs to reduce serum cholesterol levels, (4) control of blood pressure, (5) control of diabetes, and (6) regular exercise.

and mipomersen have been developed specifically for the treatment of the disorder.

Atherogenic or diabetic dyslipidemia refers to three observations commonly seen in patients with metabolic syndrome or type 2 diabetes mellitus: increased serum triglycerides; decreased HDL-C; and smaller, more atherogenic LDL-C particles. Patients with diabetes are considered high risk for developing early ASCVD and are often aggressively treated with antihyperlipidemics. Patients with diabetes are also at risk of developing end-organ damage, such as retinopathy or nephropathy, due to microvascular disease, which can be reduced by antihyperlipidemic therapy.

Antihyperlipidemics

Drug therapy can lead to specific changes in patients' lipid panels, including elevating HDL-C or lowering total serum cholesterol, LDL-C, or triglycerides. Most often, the ultimate goal is to improve clinical outcomes, such as preventing ASCVD. For moderate hypertriglyceridemia, the goal is long-term reduction of ASCVD, with statin therapy most effective. For severe or very severe hypertriglyceridemia, episodes of acute pancreatitis become more worrisome, with the fibrates recommended; however, both niacin and omega-3 fatty acids are also used. Indications for the use of the antihyperlipidemics are presented in the Therapeutic Overview Box.

THERAPEUTIC OVERVIEW

The goals of drug therapy are to reduce:

- The risk of myocardial infarction, stroke, or revascularization procedures in patients with coronary heart disease or those without established disease but who have risk factors;
- Total cholesterol, LDL-C, or triglycerides or to increase HDL-C in patients with primary hyperlipidemias or mixed hyperlipidemias;
- Triglycerides and prevent acute pancreatitis with severe hypertriglyceridemia; and
- LDL-C in patients with heterozygous or homozygous familial hypercholesterolemia.

MECHANISMS OF ACTION

Antihyperlipidemics mainly target cholesterol, triglycerides, and their associated lipoproteins. Altering lipid levels is often not the end goal of therapy but is a means to prevent or treat ASCVD or acute pancreatitis. The preeminent use of antihyperlipidemics is to lower LDL-C to slow the progression, and perhaps enhance the regression, of atheromas. To understand the mechanisms of action of the antihyperlipidemics, it is essential to understand cholesterol balance and the transport of lipids by lipoproteins.

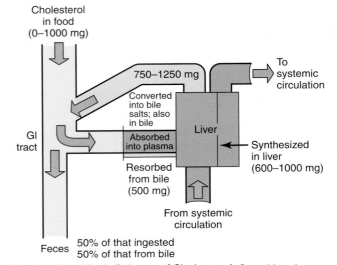

Cholesterol in food (0–1000 mg)

750–1250 mg

To systemic circulation

Converted into bile salts; also in bile

GI tract

Absorbed into plasma

Liver

Synthesized in liver (600–1000 mg)

Resorbed from bile (500 mg)

From systemic circulation

Feces 50% of that ingested 50% of that from bile

FIG. 42.2 Total Body Balance of Cholesterol. Quantities shown are approximate daily amounts.

Cholesterol Balance

The dynamics of cholesterol ingestion, synthesis, and elimination are depicted in Fig. 42.2. Dietary intake of cholesterol can vary from zero to 1000 mg/day, with 30%–75% of that amount absorbed. Hepatic synthesis is the most important endogenous source of cholesterol, with approximately 600–1000 mg synthesized each day. Synthesis, which is depicted in Fig. 42.3, involves a reaction between acetyl-CoA and acetoacetyl-CoA to produce hydroxy-3-methyl-glutaryl coenzyme A (HMG-CoA). HMG-CoA is reduced to mevalonate, catalyzed by the enzyme HMG-CoA reductase, representing the rate-limiting step for cholesterol biosynthesis. This enzyme is a major drug target and inhibited by the statins.

The liver is also the primary organ for cholesterol excretion. Approximately 750–1250 mg of cholesterol is secreted into the bile per day. One-half to two-thirds of biliary cholesterol is reabsorbed, and the remainder is excreted in the stool. Cholesterol is also converted to bile acids, which are secreted into the intestine to emulsify ingested fats. Most of the bile acids are reabsorbed and recycled, the latter normally limiting the amount of bile acids that need to be synthesized. This cycle is the major drug target of the bile acid sequestrants.

Lipoproteins and Lipids

The principal route by which dietary fat is transported is referred to as the exogenous pathway (Fig. 42.4). Cholesterol and triglycerides are transported in lipoproteins, which have a lipid core encased in a phospholipid coat, and contain various apolipoproteins. The chylomicrons

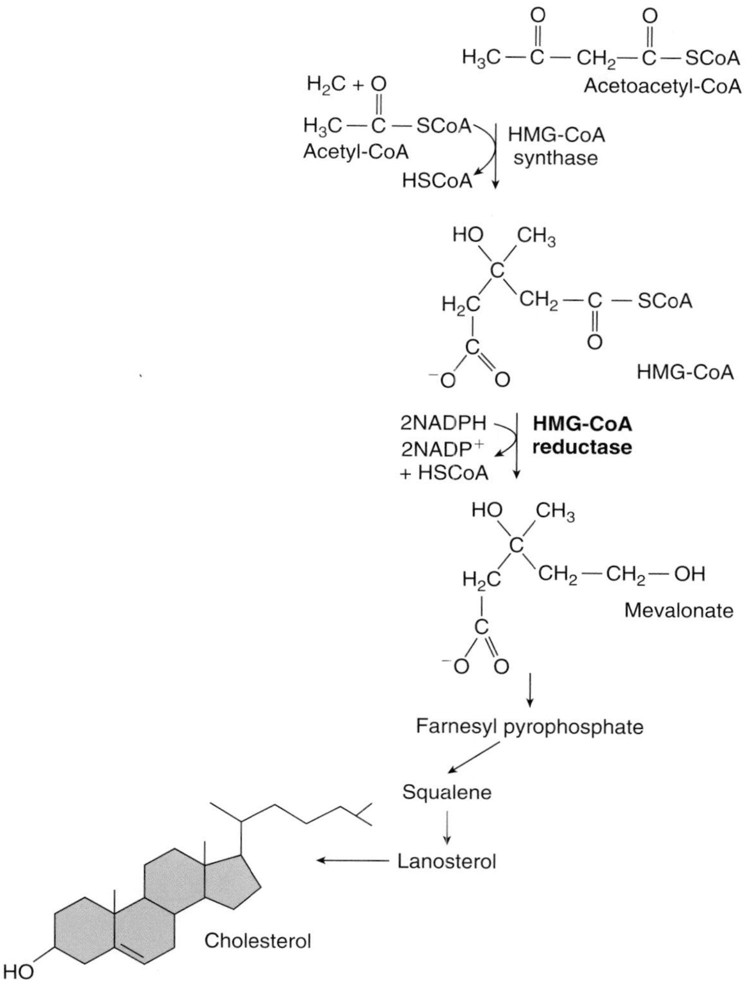

FIG. 42.3 Sequence for the Biosynthesis of Cholesterol From Acetyl-CoA.

are the largest plasma lipoproteins and are synthesized in the intestine, principally to transport dietary fats to the liver. Key apolipoproteins associated with chylomicrons are ApoB-48 and ApoA-I. In addition, ApoC-II also plays a significant role promoting chylomicron catabolism by binding to and activating lipoprotein lipase, an enzyme on vascular endothelium that removes triglycerides from the lipoprotein. Once these lipids are removed, the chylomicron remnants are cleared from circulation by specific hepatic remnant receptors.

The endogenous pathway involves the hepatic synthesis of triglycerides and cholesterol ester and their transport via VLDL particles (see Fig. 42.4). These particles are synthesized in the liver, are much smaller than chylomicrons, and are particularly enriched in triglycerides, although they also carry cholesterol. VLDL triglycerides are synthesized by the liver or released by adipose tissue and transported to the liver. VLDL particles contain several apolipoproteins, including ApoB-100 and ApoC-II. The drugs lomitapide and mipomersen interfere with the incorporation of both triglycerides and ApoB-100 into VLDL particles.

VLDL particles are metabolized in muscle and adipose tissue by the endothelial enzyme lipoprotein lipase, releasing free fatty acids. Lipoprotein lipase converts VLDL into smaller intermediate-density lipoprotein (IDL) particles, some of which are removed from the circulation by the same hepatic remnant receptors that clear chylomicron remnants. Other IDL particles continue to lose triglycerides via both lipoprotein lipase and hepatic lipase, resulting in even smaller particles known as LDLs. LDL particles contain 50%–60% cholesterol, less than

10% triglyceride, and ApoB-100 and are highly atherogenic because they readily cross the vascular endothelium, where they can be oxidized and trapped in the blood vessel wall. Lipoprotein lipase is a target for drugs like niacin and the fibrates, which promote VLDL catabolism.

The LDL apolipoprotein ApoB-100 binds to LDL receptors on hepatocyte cell membranes, and the complex is endocytosed. The LDL particles separate from the receptors in the endosomes, and the receptors are either recycled to the cell membrane or are bound by the enzyme proprotein convertase subtilisin/kexin type 9 (PCSK9), leading to lysosomal degradation. PCSK9 is the target of the PCSK9 inhibitors. It is important to note that the transcription of LDL receptors in hepatocytes increases with low levels of intracellular cholesterol, a compensatory mechanism that results in the increased LDL receptor–mediated uptake of LDL-C from the blood. This effect contributes to the cholesterol-lowering ability of several antihyperlipidemics.

HDL is the major vehicle for the transport of cholesterol from peripheral tissues to the liver for use or excretion. Higher levels of HDL are associated with decreased ASCVD, coronary events, strokes, and deaths. VLDL and IDL exchange their triglycerides for cholesterol from HDL, a process facilitated by the cholesterol ester transfer protein, and return the cholesterol to the liver. These two mechanisms contribute to the antiatherosclerotic process known as reverse cholesterol transport. Various treatment strategies designed to raise HDL levels have been developed with the goal of preventing ASCVD. Unfortunately, drugs that elevate HDL levels, such as cholesterol ester transfer protein

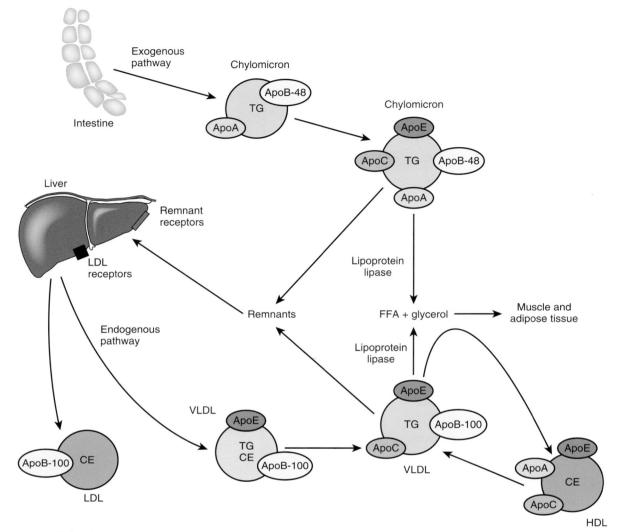

FIG. 42.4 Lipoprotein metabolism depicts (1) the exogenous pathway where ingested free fatty acids are converted to triglycerides, combined with ApoB-48, and covered by phospholipid to form chylomicrons in intestinal lymph and (2) the endogenous pathway where triglycerides synthesized in the liver combine with ApoB-100 to form VLDLs in the liver. Not shown is ApoC-II, which promotes chylomicron catabolism by binding to and activating lipoprotein lipase. *CE,* Cholesterol ester; *FFA,* free fatty acids; *HDL,* high-density lipoproteins; *LDL,* low-density lipoproteins; *TG,* triglycerides; *VLDL,* very low-density lipoproteins.

inhibitors, have not yet succeeded at decreasing cardiovascular events or mortality in clinical trials.

Drug Classes
HMG-CoA Reductase Inhibitors
Statins are usually the drugs of choice to lower LDL-C. The statins have a common structural feature of a side chain that either ends in a carboxylic acid or contains a lactone that is converted in vivo to a carboxylic acid (Fig. 42.5). This essential feature of the statins resembles HMG-CoA and renders the statins competitive antagonists of HMG-CoA reductase, the critical enzyme in hepatic cholesterol biosynthesis (see Fig. 42.3). As a consequence, the statins lead to decreased hepatic and serum cholesterol, the former likely contributing to the statin-induced decreased triglycerides as well, because cholesterol is an essential component in the hepatic assembly of VLDL particles. In addition, because decreased intracellular cholesterol induces increased transcription of hepatocyte LDL-receptors, the statins increase the hepatic clearance of LDL particles, removing them from the blood and reducing cholesterol and LDL-C.

Finally, statins are thought to have substantial pleiotropic effects, which are lipid-independent mechanisms that protect against ASCVD and other disorders. The mechanisms underlying these effects are less well defined than the effects of statins on lipids. However, many pleiotropic effects are thought to be due to the decreased availability of isoprenoids such as farnesyl pyrophosphate, whose synthesis is also reduced following inhibition of HMG-CoA reductase (see Fig. 42.3). These isoprenoids are used in protein prenylation, a process that "anchors" cell-signaling proteins to membranes and specific locations in cells. Reduced protein prenylation has the potential to disrupt certain cell signaling pathways, particularly those that involve small GTPases like Rho and Rac. These pleiotropic mechanisms may be responsible for some of the clinical benefits of the statins, possibly including improved endothelial function and antiinflammatory and antioxidant effects.

PCSK9 Inhibitors
PCSK9 inhibitors are used to produce a large decrease in LDL-C in patients at high risk of ASCVD, when statins alone are either insufficient

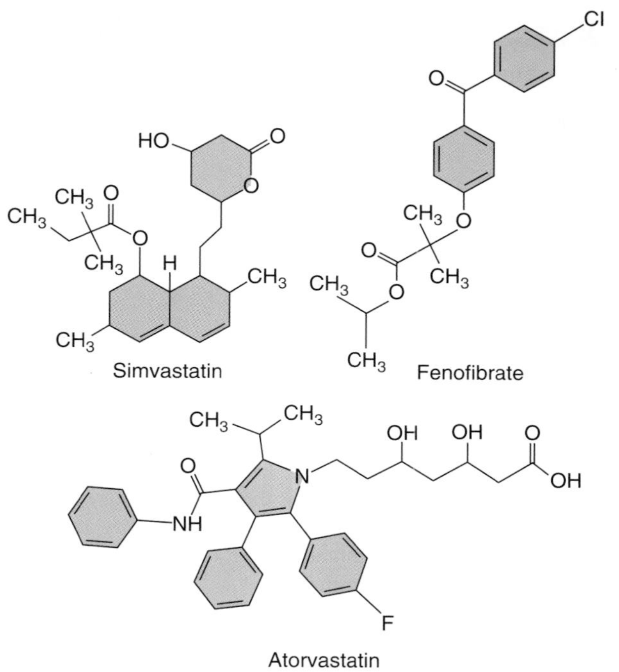

Simvastatin

Fenofibrate

Atorvastatin

FIG. 42.5 Structures of Selected Antihyperlipidemics.

7α-hydroxylase (CYP7A1), which catalyzes the first and rate-limiting step in bile acid synthesis. Because cholesterol is a bile acid precursor, increased synthesis decreases the hepatic cholesterol pool, leading to increased LDL-receptor expression and increased LDL-C uptake, lowering LDL-C levels.

MTTP Inhibitors

The incorporation of triglycerides into VLDL particles requires the hepatic endoplasmic reticulum protein, microsomal triglyceride transfer protein (MTTP). Inhibition of MTTP prevents the assembly of VLDL particles, which leads to decreased levels of other ApoB-containing lipoproteins, most importantly LDL. Lomitapide binds to and inhibits MTTP, thereby decreasing LDL-C. Lomitapide is used in patients with familial hypercholesterolemia.

ApoB-100 Synthesis Inhibitors

ApoB-100 is a key LDL apolipoprotein that binds LDL receptors on hepatocyte cell membranes, leading to endocytosis of the LDL receptor complex. Mipomersen is a phosphorothioate antisense oligo-nucleotide designed to be complementary to human ApoB-100 mRNA, to which it binds, targeting ApoB-100 mRNA for degradation by RNase H. The loss of ApoB-100 mRNA decreases ApoB-100 protein levels, preventing the endocytosis of the LDL receptor complex and thus decreasing LDL-C. Mipomersen is used in patients with familial hypercholesterolemia.

Fibrates

Peroxisome proliferator-activated receptor-α (PPAR-α) is a nuclear receptor that alters the expression levels of various proteins, most importantly in muscle and hepatic tissues. PPAR-α forms a heterodimer with another nuclear receptor, the retinoid X receptor, and the complex can bind to specific response elements (peroxisome proliferator response elements) in the promoter region of several genes. Fibrates activate PPAR-α, enabling the heterodimer to alter the expression of genes that contain these response elements.

In the liver, fibrates increase the expression of β-oxidation enzymes, leading to increased fatty acid metabolism rather than their use for triglyceride synthesis. In peripheral tissues like skeletal muscle, fibrates increase the expression of endothelial lipoprotein lipase, which accelerates the removal of triglycerides from VLDL particles. The catabolism of VLDL is also enhanced by a fibrate-mediated decreased expression of ApoC-III, a VLDL apolipoprotein that inhibits VLDL binding to lipoprotein lipase. The most important effect of drugs like fenofibrate on blood lipids is a profound drop in triglyceride levels due to both decreased incorporation of triglycerides into VLDL particles in the liver and increased removal of triglycerides from VLDL in peripheral tissues, such as skeletal muscle blood vessels. Fibrates also produce a modest increase in HDL levels, which may be attributed to increased expression of specific HDL apolipoproteins, such as ApoA-I and ApoA-II.

Niacin

Niacin is only active as an antihyperlipidemic when it is administered as nicotinic acid, not as nicotinamide, and only at much higher doses than is required as a vitamin. The most prominent effect of niacin on lipids is a large decrease in triglyceride and VLDL levels, likely due to both decreased hepatic triglyceride and VLDL synthesis and increased VLDL clearance and triglyceride metabolism by peripheral lipoprotein lipase. Niacin also produces a modest decrease in LDL-C and a sizeable increase in HDL-C levels. These may be secondary to the decrease in VLDL synthesis because VLDL is a precursor to LDL particles, and VLDL particles are required for cholesterol ester transfer protein to remove cholesterol from HDL particles.

or cannot be tolerated. This large drop in LDL-C is mediated by increased hepatic uptake of LDL particles. Alirocumab and evolocumab are monoclonal antibodies that bind PCSK9. As mentioned, PCSK9 promotes the lysosomal degradation of LDL receptors in hepatocyte endosomes. By binding to PCSK9, the antibodies prevent the effects of PCSK9, increasing both the number of LDL-receptors on the hepatocyte cell membrane and LDL-C uptake.

Cholesterol Uptake Inhibitors

When dietary or biliary cholesterol reaches the intestinal lumen, it binds to the intestinal transport protein Niemann-Pick C1-like 1 (NPC1L1) localized to the apical membrane of small intestinal enterocytes, increasing cholesterol transport and absorption. The transport inhibitor ezetimibe binds to and inhibits NPC1L1, thereby preventing the delivery of dietary and biliary cholesterol to the liver. An additional indirect effect of ezetimibe is to increase LDL uptake as a consequence of the increased number of hepatocyte membrane LDL-receptors secondary to decreased delivery of dietary and biliary cholesterol. Thus the main beneficial effect of ezetimibe is a significant drop in blood levels of LDL-C.

Bile Acid Sequestrants

Bile acid sequestrants are high-molecular-weight resins with numerous positively charged moieties. Their structure enables them to bind negatively charged bile acids with relatively high affinity. The sequestrants can bind other hydrophobic, negatively charged molecules as well, although colesevelam is more selective for bile acids than the older agents, cholestyramine and colestipol.

The sequestrants are taken orally with a meal to ensure that they are present in the gastrointestinal tract when the gallbladder contracts. The unabsorbable sequestrants complex bile acids and are eliminated from the body in the feces, interrupting normal enterohepatic recirculation, during which up to 95% of bile acids are reabsorbed in the jejunum and ileum and returned to the liver. Low hepatic levels of bile acids lead to increased transcription of the hepatic enzyme cholesterol

TABLE 42.1   Effect of Selected Antihyperlipidemics on Serum Lipid Values

Drug	Dose	LDL-C (vs. placebo)	Triglycerides	HDL-C
Atorvastatin	80 mg/day	↓60%	↓37%	↑5%
Pravastatin	80 mg/day	↓37%	↓19%	↑3%
Rosuvastatin	40 mg/day	↓63%	↓28%	↑10%
Alirocumab[a]	75–150 mg/2 weeks	↓54%	–	–
Colesevelam	4.5 g/day	↓18%	↑9%	↑3%
Ezetimibe	10 mg/day	↓18%	↓8%	↑1%
Fenofibric acid	135 mg/day	↓21% to ↑45%	↓29–55%	↓11%–23%
Lomitapide[a]	Up to 60 mg/day	↓40%	↓45%	↓7%
Mipomersen[a]	200 mg/week	↓21%	↓18%	↑11%
Niacin (extended release)	2 g/day	↓16%	↓38%	↑22%

Most studies involved monotherapy of patients with primary hyperlipidemias, but [a] indicates familial hypercholesterolemia patients treated with multiple drugs.

RELATIONSHIP OF MECHANISMS OF ACTION TO CLINICAL RESPONSE

HMG-CoA Reductase Inhibitors

The statins provide the largest decrease in LDL-C (except possibly for the PCSK9 inhibitors), a substantial decrease in serum triglycerides, and a modest increase in HDL levels (Table 42.1). Because individual statins exhibit significant differences in their maximal efficacy to low LDL-C, they have been classified as those used for high-intensity therapy (defined in practice guidelines as dropping LDL-C by at least 50%) and those used for moderate-intensity therapy (lowers LDL-C between 30% and 50%). All seven available statins can be used at doses effective for moderate-intensity therapy, while only higher doses of atorvastatin or rosuvastatin qualify as high intensity.

The statins are regarded as the drugs of choice for treating hypercholesterolemia because of the magnitude of their effect on LDL-C and because the statins are the best-established drugs for preventing cardiovascular events (e.g., infarct, ischemic stroke). Many clinical trials have established the efficacy of statins for both primary prevention (avoiding an initial event such as a myocardial infarction) and for secondary prevention (avoiding a cardiovascular event in patients who have already experienced one). The statins are also effective at preventing cardiovascular events in patients whose LDL-C is not substantially elevated but are considered at elevated risk for other reasons, such as elevated C-reactive protein, a vascular marker of inflammation.

Practice guidelines also recommend the statins as the drug of choice for treating moderate hypertriglyceridemia, although other drug classes produce larger decreases in serum triglycerides. The reason for this is that the goal of treating moderate hypertriglyceridemia is to decrease the incidence of cardiovascular events such as myocardial infarctions, and clinical trials have established long-term statin therapy as the most effective approach. Treatment of severe hypertriglyceridemia differs in that the triglyceride level must be lowered as much as possible to prevent acute pancreatitis, so drugs with a stronger effect on triglycerides are preferred.

PCSK9 Inhibitors

Initial enthusiasm for the use of the PCSK9 inhibitors has been high, tempered mainly by the absence of long-term clinical outcome and safety studies and the high cost of monoclonal antibodies. The principal benefit of these agents on lipid profiles is to lower total serum cholesterol and LDL-C, where they appear as efficacious as high-intensity statin therapy, even in patients taking multiple antihyperlipidemics (see Table 42.1). The PCSK9 inhibitors are currently used only for high-risk hypercholesterolemia patients, such as those with heterozygous familial hypercholesterolemia or established ASCVD (e.g., history of myocardial infarctions). These drugs are intended to be adjuncts to dietary changes and maximum tolerable statin therapy.

Cholesterol Uptake Inhibitors

The major benefit of ezetimibe on lipid profiles is a useful drop in LDL-C, which is not as extensive as that following moderate-intensity statins like pravastatin (see Table 42.1). Ezetimibe can be used alone for hypercholesterolemia with statin-intolerant patients. However, it may be most useful as adjunctive therapy when statins do not produce a large enough drop in LDL-C. The 2014 IMPROVE-IT clinical trial demonstrated that adding ezetimibe to simvastatin for patients with established coronary heart disease had a small but significant benefit on clinical outcomes (evaluated using a composite measure of death, myocardial infarction, ischemic stroke, and coronary revascularization). Ezetimibe was the first drug proven to improve clinical outcomes when added to statin therapy.

Bile Acid Sequestrants

The bile acid sequestrants were the drugs of choice for hypercholesterolemia decades ago but have largely been displaced by the statins. The best use of these compounds currently may be as add-on therapy for hypocholesterolemia in patients who require larger drops in LDL-C. However, patient adherence to sequestrant therapy is often limited by inconvenient dosing and gastrointestinal discomfort. The sequestrants should also be avoided in patients with mixed hyperlipidemias, as they often cause a rise in serum triglyceride levels. One notable advantage of colesevelam is that it can also be used as adjunct therapy in type 2 diabetes mellitus, as it has shown the ability to improve glycemic control and reduce glycosylated hemoglobin.

MTTP and ApoB-100 Synthesis Inhibitors

The use of both lomitapide and mipomersen is limited to homozygous familial hypercholesterolemia. Although these drugs produce a substantial decrease in LDL-C, even in patients who are taking other antihyperlipidemics, the incidence of serious hepatic adverse effects limits their use to patients at very high risk of cardiovascular disease.

Fibrates

Fenofibrate may be the most effective drug at lowering serum triglycerides (see Table 42.1). It can also lower LDL-C in patients with primary hypercholesterolemia. However, it can increase LDL-C in patients with hypertriglyceridemia because of the fibrate-induced conversion of numerous VLDL particles to LDL. Practice guidelines recommend fibrates as adjunct or second-line drugs for most uses due to the failure of fibrates to decrease mortality when added to statin therapy in clinical trials like the 2010 ACCORD clinical trial. However, fenofibrate may be useful in protecting diabetics from the retinopathy and nephropathy caused by microvascular disease. Fenofibrate is also particularly useful in the treatment of severe hypertriglyceridemia, when triglycerides must be lowered to prevent acute pancreatitis.

Niacin

Niacin can lead to a substantial fall in triglycerides, a significant drop in LDL-C, and the largest available increase in HDL levels. However, whether niacin can improve clinical outcomes (e.g., mortality) remains mostly unproven, particularly when patients are already being treated with a statin. As a result, niacin is regarded as an adjunct or second-line drug for most uses. An exception is severe hypertriglyceridemia, where niacin is one recommended option to quickly lower triglycerides to avoid acute pancreatitis.

PHARMACOKINETICS

HMG-CoA Reductase Inhibitors

Statins have many similar pharmacokinetic properties, but there are clear differences in elimination that are critical to understanding the clinical use of each statin. All of the statins available in the United States are administered orally once a day (Table 42.2). The shorter duration agents (e.g., pravastatin) are administered in the evening to ensure that peak blood levels occur while the patient is fasting, and hepatic cholesterol synthesis would be at its peak. The time of administration for the longer duration agents (e.g., atorvastatin or rosuvastatin) is more flexible. These longer acting statins are also the most effective at lowering LDL-C and are the statins recommended for high-intensity statin therapy.

Lovastatin and simvastatin are prodrugs that contain a lactone, which must be hydrolyzed to an active acid metabolite before being able to inhibit HMG-CoA reductase. Other statins are administered as free acids. (Compare simvastatin to atorvastatin in Fig. 42.5.)

The distinctions among statin elimination pathways account for clinically relevant differences concerning drug interactions. The

liver predominantly eliminates all of the statins, although renal elimination makes a moderate contribution to pravastatin clearance. Oxidation by hepatic CYP3A4 is the most important elimination mechanism for atorvastatin, lovastatin, and simvastatin. Fluvastatin is also eliminated by hepatic oxidation, but CYP2C9 is the most important enzyme. Pitavastatin is eliminated by hepatic glucuronidation and biliary/fecal excretion. Rosuvastatin's main elimination mechanism is biliary/fecal excretion. Pravastatin is eliminated by multiple processes, including hepatic isomerization and hydroxylation, as well as renal elimination.

Most statins are transported into hepatocytes by the OATP1B1 anionic transporter before they are metabolized or excreted. Multiple OATP1B1 genotypes exist in humans, some of which have decreased activity. These genotypes are more common in East Asian populations, and patients with these genotypes are more likely to experience elevated blood levels and statin-induced myopathy with standard doses. Atorvastatin, pitavastatin, and simvastatin are most likely to require dosage adjustment in these patients, while fluvastatin is the least affected by transporter genotype.

PCSK9 Inhibitors

These drugs are monoclonal antibodies that are self-administered as subcutaneous injections every 2 weeks using prefilled pens or syringes. The drugs are slowly absorbed into blood and lymph from the injection site. Alirocumab has a long half-life ($t_{1/2}$) of 17–20 days and is eliminated by proteolysis and cellular uptake.

Cholesterol Uptake Inhibitors

Ezetimibe is administered orally once a day and is eliminated by hepatic glucuronidation and fecal excretion. Its duration of action is extended by enterohepatic recirculation. Ezetimibe is available by itself or combined with simvastatin.

Bile Acid Sequestrants

These compounds are very large molecules that are not absorbed into the blood after oral administration. The three sequestrants are available in various oral dosage forms such as tablets or packets of loose drug that can be mixed with drinks or applesauce. Dosage varies for each drug but usually entails taking several grams of the drug at least twice a day with meals. Patient adherence with the drug regimen is often impacted by the inconvenience of administration. The drugs are eliminated in feces.

MTTP and ApoB-100 Synthesis Inhibitors

Lomitapide is administered orally 2 hours after the evening meal because taking the drug with food increases the likelihood of gastrointestinal adverse effects. Lomitapide dosing is complicated and must be carefully adjusted for each patient to minimize hepatic adverse effects. The drug undergoes extensive hepatic metabolism, mostly by CYP3A4.

Mipomersen is an unabsorbable antisense oligonucleotide and is administered by a weekly subcutaneous injection. Mipomersen is metabolized by tissue endonucleases to form shorter oligonucleotides, which are metabolized further by exonucleases. The $t_{1/2}$ of mipomersen is approximately 1–2 months in humans.

Fibrates

The related drugs fenofibrate and fenofibric acid are available in several oral dosage forms, which differ considerably in their pharmacokinetics. The drugs are not bioequivalent, and their dosages differ. The oral bioavailability of the original fenofibrate formulation was limited by poor water solubility, and as a consequence, it was necessary to take the drug with food to improve absorption. Improved fenofibrate tablets decreased the particle size of the drug, which both enhanced oral

TABLE 42.2 Pharmacokinetic Summary of Selected Antihyperlipidemics

Drug	Administration	$t_{1/2}$	Major Elimination Route(s)
Atorvastatin	Oral (daily)	14 hrs	H (CYP3A4)
Pravastatin	Oral (daily)	2 hrs	H (multiple mechanisms), R
Rosuvastatin	Oral (daily)	19 hrs	F
Alirocumab	SQ (every 2 weeks)	20 days	Proteolysis
Colesevelam	Oral (1–2 times a day)	N/A	F
Ezetimibe	Oral (daily)	22 hrs	H (glucuronidation)
Fenofibric acid	Oral (daily)	20 hrs	H (glucuronidation), R
Lomitapide	Oral (daily)	40 hrs	H (CYP3A4)
Mipomersen	SQ (weekly)	1–2 mo	Endonucleases and exonucleases
Niacin (extended release)	Oral (daily)	1 hr	H (multiple mechanisms), R

F, Fecal excretion; H, hepatic metabolism; R, renal excretion; SQ, subcutaneous; $t_{1/2}$, half-life.

bioavailability and allowed the drug to be taken without food. These fenofibrate products are referred to as "micronized" or "nanocrystallized." Fenofibric acid is the active metabolite of fenofibrate and has improved oral bioavailability relative to fenofibrate products. Fenofibrate or fenofibric acid is administered once a day. In comparison to fenofibrate, gemfibrozil has a much shorter $t_{1/2}$, 2 versus 20 hours, with hepatic glucuronidation the principal elimination pathway for both. Gemfibrozil is orally administered twice a day.

Niacin

Niacin is administered orally in several different dosage forms. Immediate-release niacin is available without a prescription in the United States and causes a rapid rise in niacin blood levels but has to be administered two to three times a day due to a short $t_{1/2}$. The extended-release form of niacin is administered once a day but is only available by prescription. Additional dosage forms of niacin are available without a prescription, some of which are sustained-release products, but are only labeled for use as dietary supplements. Niacin is eliminated through both renal excretion and various hepatic metabolic pathways.

PHARMACOVIGILANCE: ADVERSE EFFECTS AND DRUG INTERACTIONS

HMG-CoA Reductase Inhibitors

Statins have well-known adverse effects, but the incidence is low, and most patients tolerate statins very well. Skeletal muscle myopathy is their most important adverse effect and can lead to discontinuation of therapy. Myopathy is evaluated by assessing patient symptoms and measuring serum creatine kinase levels, which increase upon significant muscle damage. Myopathy ranges from myalgia (muscle pain or weakness without elevated creatine kinase) to myositis (symptoms accompanied by significantly elevated creatine kinase) to rhabdomyolysis, a rare but serious event in which muscle necrosis releases both potassium (a potential cause of cardiac arrhythmias) and myoglobin (a potential cause of renal damage) into the blood. An older statin, cerivastatin, and the 80-mg dose of simvastatin were discontinued in the United States due to a high incidence of rhabdomyolysis. Certain risk factors increase the incidence of rhabdomyolysis, including higher doses of statins, hepatic dysfunction, specific hepatic OATP1B1 drug transporter genotypes, and drug interactions that slow statin elimination. Inhibitors of OATPB1 are also well known to increase statin blood levels and drug-induced myopathy. The official prescribing information for all statins recommends against their use with OATPB1 inhibitors such as gemfibrozil and cyclosporine.

Statins frequently cause a modest asymptomatic increase in serum hepatic transaminase levels. Patients usually tolerate this well, and it may not be cause for discontinuation. However, discontinuation may be necessary if transaminase levels increase further or if the patient has signs and symptoms consistent with hepatotoxicity (e.g., malaise, jaundice). Practice guidelines recommend that baseline measurements of hepatic transaminase levels be taken before starting statin therapy and repeated if hepatotoxicity is suspected.

The statins can increase blood glucose levels and moderately increase the incidence of type 2 diabetes mellitus. As a result, patients on statins should be screened for new-onset diabetes. The development of diabetes during statin therapy is not usually a cause for discontinuation of drug therapy, as statins are considered the drug of choice in preventing cardiovascular events in these patients. Other interventions (e.g., diet and weight loss, exercise, etc.) should be emphasized instead. Use of the statins during pregnancy or nursing is contraindicated, as various statin-induced abnormalities, including skeletal defects, have been observed in fetal animals.

As mentioned, elimination among the statins differs considerably, causing differential susceptibility of individual statins to drug interactions. CYP3A4 inhibitors increase blood levels and the risk of myopathy and rhabdomyolysis of several statins, particularly atorvastatin, lovastatin, and simvastatin. Coadministration of statins with strong enzyme inhibitors (e.g., azole antifungals, macrolide antibiotics, ritonavir) should be avoided, while more moderate CYP3A4 inhibitors can be coadministered if the statin dose is kept low. Pravastatin, pitavastatin, and rosuvastatin are statins whose elimination least depends on CYP450 isozymes. The inhibition of CYP3A4 by cyclosporine contributes to its interactions with some statins.

PCSK9 Inhibitors

Conclusions about the long-term safety of these drugs are constrained by the limited size and duration of the clinical studies carried out to date. Reports of adverse effects have mostly been related to injection site reactions such as itching or swelling, as well as an increased incidence of nasopharyngitis and influenza. The PCSK9 inhibitors are much less susceptible to drug interactions, as their elimination does not involve hepatic CYP450 isozymes or glucuronidation.

Cholesterol Uptake Inhibitors

Ezetimibe has a low incidence of serious adverse effects. Guidelines suggest that it is reasonable to obtain baseline hepatic transaminase levels to allow hepatotoxicity monitoring.

Bile Acid Sequestrants

A major advantage of the sequestrants is a very low incidence of serious adverse effects, as the drugs are not systemically absorbed. The sequestrants are contraindicated if the patient has a significant bowel obstruction. Drug interactions occur exclusively in the gastrointestinal tract with other orally administered drugs. Lipid-soluble or negatively charged drugs or nutrients (e.g., warfarin, oral contraceptives, vitamin K) can form unabsorbable complexes with the sequestrants. Colesevelam is purported to be more selective for binding bile acids than cholestyramine or colestipol and thus has less potential for drug interactions. Drug interactions can be minimized by administering susceptible drugs either 1 hour before or 2–4 hours after the sequestrant is taken.

MTTP and ApoB-100 Synthesis Inhibitors

The most important adverse effects of lomitapide drug are accumulation of hepatic fat (steatosis) and the induction of hepatotoxicity. These adverse effects are the subject of a boxed warning in official prescribing information and limit drug use. Lomitapide is contraindicated in patients with significant hepatic dysfunction, and hepatic enzyme levels need to be monitored closely. Patient use of alcohol should be limited to one drink per day. Diarrhea, nausea, and vomiting are very common and can sometimes be severe. Use of lomitapide is contraindicated during pregnancy, as it may cause harm to the fetus.

Lomitapide is both a substrate and moderate inhibitor of CYP3A4. Concurrent use of lomitapide and moderate to strong CYP3A4 inhibitors (e.g., verapamil, clarithromycin) is contraindicated, and the dose of drug should be reduced when combined with weak inhibitors. Grapefruit juice also must be avoided. Lomitapide can slow elimination of other drugs metabolized by CYP3A4, such as warfarin. In addition, lomitapide is an inhibitor of the drug transporter p-glycoprotein, which may slow the clearance of certain drugs (e.g., digoxin).

Like lomitapide, the most important adverse effects of mipomersen are drug-induced hepatic steatosis and hepatotoxicity, the subjects of the boxed warning in the prescribing information. Mipomersen also resembles lomitapide in having similar requirements for hepatic enzyme monitoring and restrictions on alcohol use. Injection site reactions such as pain, erythema, and inflammation occur in most patients, and the appearance of influenza-like symptoms (e.g., fever, chills, myalgia, fatigue) is also common.

Fibrates

The most important adverse effects of the fibrates are myopathy, hepatotoxicity, and increased biliary excretion of cholesterol. The fibrates should be avoided with biliary tract disease, as cholelithiasis can occur. Serum hepatic transaminases should be measured periodically. Gemfibrozil is a troublesome antihyperlipidemic because it elevates blood levels of many statins and increases the likelihood of stain-induced myopathy. This renders gemfibrozil difficult to include in combined antihyperlipidemic therapy. These drug interactions are often due to inhibition of the hepatic drug transporter OATPB1, which is involved in the elimination of many statins. Gemfibrozil can also increase blood levels of other coadministered drugs by inhibiting hepatic glucuronidase. Fenofibrate causes fewer drug interactions, although it is known to enhance the anticoagulant effects of warfarin.

Niacin

A mixture of irritating and serious adverse effects hinders the use of nicotinic acid. Niacin's best known adverse effect is flushing over the face and upper body accompanied by a burning or tingling sensation. The flushing is generally regarded as harmless except that it can significantly impact the patient's adherence to niacin therapy. The flushing is caused by prostaglandin-induced cutaneous vasodilation mediated by DP1 receptors. Prostaglandin production and flushing can be reduced by coadministration of aspirin. Flushing can also be made more tolerable by starting the patient at a low dose and then gradually titrating the dose upward. Upper gastrointestinal irritation is another problem seen with niacin therapy. Niacin has also been reported to increase serum uric acid levels, decrease insulin sensitivity, and induce hepatotoxicity. These adverse effects often warrant monitoring of a patient's uric acid levels, fasting blood glucose, hemoglobin A1C, and serum hepatic transaminases. Niacin is involved in fewer pharmacokinetic drug interactions than other antihyperlipidemics, but there have been some reports of drug-induced myopathy when coadministered with statins.

The adverse effects associated with the use of the antihyperlipidemic drugs are summarized in the Clinical Problems Box.

NEW DEVELOPMENTS

The identification of PCSK9 as a molecular target for therapeutic agents in the management of hyperlipidemia has provided a novel mechanism that is currently reserved for use for severe hyperlipidemia but may offer some utility in other forms of the disease. Efforts to target diacyl glycerolacyltransferase 1 (DGAT-1), an enzyme responsible for catalyzing the final step in triglyceride synthesis, have not proven to be clinically useful at this point. However, this enzyme remains a potential target for treating obesity and dyslipidemias.

CLINICAL RELEVANCE FOR HEALTHCARE PROFESSIONALS

Guidelines most relevant to the treatment of noninherited hypercholesterolemia were published jointly by the American College of Cardiology and the American Heart Association in 2013 and use LDL-C levels and other risk factors to recommended drug therapies for ASCVD. The guidelines focus largely on the use of statins, as the strongest evidence for improving clinical outcomes has been obtained using these drugs. For patients who cannot tolerate or have an inadequate response to

TABLE 42.3 Recommendations for Reducing ASCVD

Patient Group	Statin Therapy
Primary Prevention	
LDL-C >190 mg/dL	High intensity
Primary Prevention	
40–75 years old	
LDL-C 70–189 mg/dL	Moderate or high
if 10-year risk of cardiovascular event ≥7.5%	intensity
Primary Prevention	
40–75 years old	
LDL-C 70–189 mg/dL	
Diabetes mellitus	
if 10-year risk of cardiovascular event ≥7.5%	High intensity
if 10-year risk of cardiovascular event <7.5%	Moderate intensity
Secondary Prevention	
A history of ASCVD and <75 years old	High intensity
A history of ASCVD and >75 years old	Moderate intensity

High-intensity therapy may be achieved with high doses of atorvastatin (40–80 mg) or rosuvastatin (20–40 mg). Moderate-intensity therapy may be achieved with the recommended dose of any available statin.

statins, other antihyperlipidemics may be considered; ezetimibe is often the preferred nonstatin. These guidelines are summarized in Table 42.3.

The antihyperlipidemics include many of the most commonly prescribed drugs in Western nations. Thus knowledge of the basic and clinical pharmacology of these drugs, particularly the statins, is essential to all healthcare professionals for the assessment and initiation of drug therapy of common hyperlipidemias. Awareness of the prominent adverse effects of the statins (e.g., myopathy) is also particularly important for physical therapists, as patients taking statins and other antihyperlipidemic agents may have increased risk for myalgia, arthralgia, and muscle weakness that could be significant enough to interfere with therapy.

CLINICAL PROBLEMS

Drug Class	Common or Important Adverse Effects
HMG-CoA reductase inhibitors	Myopathy/rhabdomyolysis, increased incidence of diabetes mellitus, occasional hepatotoxicity, contraindicated in pregnancy
PCSK9 inhibitors	Injection site reactions, nasopharyngitis
Cholesterol uptake inhibitors	Occasional hepatotoxicity
Bile acid sequestrants	Gastrointestinal bloating, constipation
MTTP inhibitors	Significant hepatic steatosis, contraindicated in pregnancy
ApoB-100 synthesis inhibitors	Significant hepatic steatosis or hepatotoxicity, injection site reactions
Fibrates	Cholelithiasis/gallstones, occasional myopathy
Niacin	Flushing and burning sensations, gastrointestinal irritation, decreased insulin sensitivity, hepatotoxicity

HMG-CoA, Hydroxy-3-methyl-glutaryl coenzyme A; *MTTP,* microsomal triglyceride transfer protein.

TRADE NAMES

In addition to generic and fixed-combination preparations, the following trade-named materials are some of the important compounds available in the United States.

HMG-CoA Reductase Inhibitors
Atorvastatin (Lipitor)
Fluvastatin (Lescol)
Lovastatin (Altoprev)
Pitavastatin (Livalo)
Pravastatin (Pravachol)
Rosuvastatin (Crestor)
Simvastatin (Zocor)

PCSK9 Inhibitors
Alirocumab (Praluent)
Evolocumab (Repatha)

Cholesterol Uptake Inhibitors
Ezetimibe (Zetia)

Bile Acid Sequestrants
Cholestyramine (Prevalite)
Colesevelam (Welchol)
Colestipol (Colestid)

MTTP Inhibitors
Lomitapide (Juxtapid)

ApoB-100 Synthesis Inhibitors
Mipomersen (Kynamro)

Fibrates
Fenofibrate (Tricor, Trilipix)
Gemfibrozil (Lopid)

Niacin
Niacin (Niaspan)

SELF-ASSESSMENT QUESTIONS

1. A 59-year-old male patient has been treated for hypercholesterolemia for 10 years and also suffered a myocardial infarction 3 months ago. The patient's current LDL-C level is 170 mg/dL. Which of the following drugs is the most appropriate treatment for this patient?
   A. Alirocumab.
   B. Ezetimibe.
   C. Fenofibrate.
   D. Pravastatin.
   E. Rosuvastatin.

2. A 42-year-old woman presents to the emergency department with epigastric pain and vomiting. Her lipid panel indicates a serum triglyceride level of 1470 mg/dL. Which of the following antihyperlipidemic mechanisms of action would be most useful in treating this patient?
   A. Activation of PPAR-α.
   B. Bile acid sequestration.
   C. Inhibition of intestinal cholesterol absorption.
   D. MTTP inhibition.
   E. PCSK9 inhibition.

3. A patient with familial hypercholesterolemia who is at severe risk for adverse cardiovascular events is receiving lomitapide. Which one of the following mechanisms best describes the substantial reduction in LDL-C caused by lomitapide?

   A. Inhibition of LDL receptor recycling in the liver.
   B. Prevention of ApoB-containing lipoprotein assembly in hepatocytes.
   C. Activation of PPAR-alpha.
   D. Inhibition of bile acid synthesis.
   E. Inhibition of NPC1L1, which facilitates intestinal cholesterol absorption.

4. A 48-year-old female patient's recent medical history includes hypercholesterolemia and a myocardial infarction. The patient is taking the maximum tolerated dose of rosuvastatin, but her LDL-cholesterol is still 160 mg/dL. Choose the best drug to add to rosuvastatin therapy.
   A. Colesevelam.
   B. Fenofibrate.
   C. Mipomersen.
   D. Nicotinic acid.
   E. Ezetimibe.

FURTHER READING

Berglund L, Brunzell JD, Goldberg AC, et al. Evaluation and treatment of hypertriglyceridemia: an Endocrine Society clinical practice guideline. *J Clin Endocrinol Metab.* 2012;97(9):2969–2989.

Stone NJ, Robinson JG, Lichtenstein AH, et al. 2013 ACC/AHA guideline on the treatment of blood cholesterol to reduce atherosclerotic cardiovascular risk in adults. A report of the American College of Cardiology/American Heart Association Task Force on Practice Guidelines. *Circulation.* 2014;129:S1–S45.

WEBSITES

https://www.acc.org/clinical-topics/dyslipidemia?w_nav=MN#sort=%40fwhatstrendingscore86069%20descending

The American College of Cardiology maintains a website with the most up-to-date information on dyslipidemias and their treatment.

https://www.ncbi.nlm.nih.gov/pubmedhealth/PMHT0022430/

The United States National Library of Medicine maintains a website on hypercholesterolemia for researchers, clinicians, and consumers, with links to many resources.

Drug Therapy for Myocardial Ischemia and Angina Pectoris

J. West Paul, Jr.

MAJOR DRUG CLASSES

Organic nitrates
Funny channel inhibitors

ABBREVIATIONS

GTN	Glyceryl trinitrate, nitroglycerin
ISDN	Isosorbide dinitrate
ISMN	Isosorbide mononitrate
NO	Nitric oxide
PETN	Pentaerythritol tetranitrate

THERAPEUTIC OVERVIEW

Myocardial ischemia results from the inadequate delivery of oxygen to the heart to meet the oxygen demand of myocardial cells. Myocardial ischemia is a complex process involving a sequence of events that can lead to myocardial death (infarct) if left uninterrupted. Angina pectoris and its equivalents are symptoms of the underlying pathology in the myocardium and coronary vessels. Classic angina pectoris, characterized by crushing or gripping left sternal pain, is not always described in patients with acute coronary syndromes (ACS). Women, in particular, may not present with classic angina pectoris but may frequently present with equivalents such as jaw pain, left arm pain, upper back pain, and even nausea or may have no particular pain symptoms at all. The worsening or alleviation of this discomfort is often used as a clinical gauge of the ongoing oxygen mismatch and is often used to titrate medications for the treatment of ACS, the latter referring to any situation in which there is a blockage of blood supply to heart muscle.

Pathophysiology

Coronary artery narrowing is a chronic process that leads to a gradual physical reduction in blood flow. Central to coronary artery narrowing is cholesterol plaque deposition and subsequent endothelial damage through a cyclical pattern of plaque rupture and repair. As the artery continues to narrow (often eccentrically promoting blood flow disruption and thrombogenesis), multiple mechanisms promote further damage and trigger host responses that produce both structural changes within the arterial wall and intimal surface changes, resulting in an increased propensity for clot formation. The coagulation cascade plays an integral role in both initial coronary artery thrombosis and clot propagation (Chapter 46).

As plaques rupture, several mechanisms are activated to repair the break in endothelial integrity. One of the most detrimental early steps is the rapid activation and subsequent aggregation of platelets at the site of injury. Both tissue factors and activated platelets trigger the coagulation cascade to further stabilize and enlarge the area of thrombosis (Chapter 46, Fig. 46.2). In addition, as clot formation continues to narrow the coronary artery lumen, inflammatory mediators and other biochemical events stimulate arterial contraction and vasospasm, decreasing coronary artery blood flow and further limiting myocardial blood supply and oxygen delivery.

Last, with increased ischemia, there is increased pain with the concordant physiological response of increasing sympathetic tone, resulting in increased heart rate (myocardial work) and blood pressure (afterload), both of which increase myocardial oxygen demand. The events leading to cardiac ischemia and approaches to interfere at each step are summarized in the Therapeutic Overview Box.

THERAPEUTIC OVERVIEW

Events Leading to Myocardial Ischemia
Atherosclerosis-mediated narrowing of coronary artery
Plaque rupture
Increased platelet aggregation
Activation of coagulation cascade
Clot formation
Coronary vasospasm
Ischemia

Interventions
HMG-CoA reductase inhibitors to reduce plaque burden
Aspirin, clopidogrel, or GPIIb/IIA inhibitors (abciximab, eptifibatide, and tirofiban) to inhibit platelet aggregation
Heparin, fondaparinux, or the hirudins (desirudin and lepirudin) to inhibit the coagulation cascade
Fibrinolytics (reteplase and tenecteplase) to clear occluded arteries
β-adrenergic receptor blockers to decrease heart rate and ventricular contractility
Ca++-channel blockers to increase coronary blood flow and decrease blood pressure

MECHANISMS OF ACTION

Organic Nitrates

Nitrovasodilators are organic nitrates that provide a source of nitric oxide (NO), which activates soluble guanylyl cyclase in vascular smooth muscle, causing an increase in intracellular cGMP, resulting in smooth muscle relaxation (Chapter 41, Fig. 41.1). Unlike nitrovasodilators that spontaneously release NO, such as nitroprusside (Chapter 41), the organic nitrates require enzymatic cleavage. Based on activation mechanisms and vasodilator potency, this group of compounds may be categorized as high-potency agents, including nitroglycerin (glyceryl trinitrate, GTN) and pentaerythritol tetranitrate (PETN), or low-potency agents, including isosorbide mononitrate (ISMN) and isosorbide dinitrate (ISDN). The structures of these agents are shown in Fig. 43.1. Further, evidence suggests that the high-potency compounds are bioactivated to release NO by vascular mitochondrial aldehyde dehydrogenase 2, while the low-potency agents are activated by cytochrome P450s (Fig. 43.2).

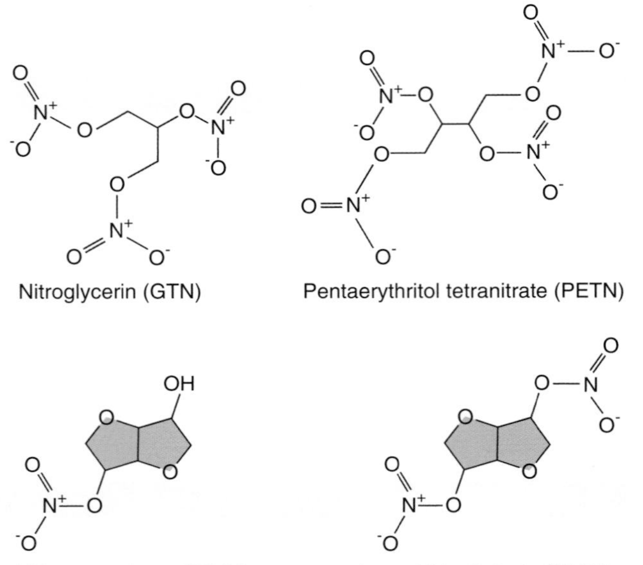

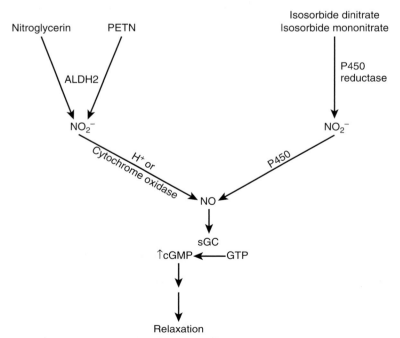

FIG. 43.1 Chemical Structures of the Organic Nitrates.

Nitroglycerin (GTN)

Pentaerythritol tetranitrate (PETN)

Isosorbide mononitrate (ISMN)

Isosorbide dinitrate (ISDN)

Funny Channel Inhibitors

The funny channel is a critical component of the electrical conduction system of the heart and an integral part of sinoatrial (SA) node myocyte membranes. SA node myocytes self-generate repetitive action potentials and, as such, exhibit phase 4 diastolic (pacemaker) depolarization, during which time the membrane voltage slowly depolarizes until threshold is reached for firing another action potential. Thus diastolic depolarization mediates the repetitive activity. The funny current (I_f) is an inward current that plays a major role in pacemaker activity and rate modulation. It is regulated by intracellular levels of cAMP and is a basic mechanism involved in the autonomic regulation of heart rate, with sympathetic activation increasing rate and parasympathetic activation decreasing rate. Blockade of I_f leads to a negative chronotropic effect without additional cardiovascular side effects, indicating that I_f is highly selective as a pacemaker generator and rate controller.

Ivabradine is a recently developed open channel blocker that interacts at a binding site within the channel pore in a concentration-dependent manner to disrupt current flow. Ivabradine gains access to the pore from inside the cell, and its action is voltage dependent, with greater blockade at depolarized voltages. The current evidence suggests that it is highly selective for this ionic current and without effects on any other cardiac ion channel, dampening the steepness of diastolic depolarization without affecting any other action potential parameters. By lowering heart rate, ivabradine decreases myocardial oxygen demand, mitigating ischemia and reducing angina episodes.

RELATIONSHIP OF MECHANISMS OF ACTION TO CLINICAL RESPONSE

The key to successful treatment of myocardial ischemia is early pharmacological intervention and treatment and, when indicated, percutaneous or surgical intervention. Following diagnosis of an acute myocardial event, patients should be supplemented with oxygen and administered

FIG. 43.2 Enzymatic Mechanisms Mediating the Bioactivation of the Organic Nitrates. *ALDH2,* Aldehyde dehydrogenase 2; *cGMP,* cyclic guanosine monophosphate; *GTP,* guanosine triphosphate; *NO,* nitric oxide; *PETN,* pentaerythritol tetranitrate; *sGC,* soluble guanylyl cyclase.

antiplatelet medications and anticoagulants to interrupt the cascade of events leading to worsening ischemia and myocardial damage. Medications to reduce myocardial oxygen demand and increase oxygen delivery, such as β-adrenergic receptor blockers and nitrates, should also be initiated and titrated to reduce pain and blood pressure to an acceptable level while preventing hypotension. If pain relief is not provided, then the addition of analgesics such as morphine sulfate (Chapter 28) is recommended because they have both analgesic and anxiolytic effects, as well as hemodynamic properties that may be beneficial. Morphine should not be used in patients with concomitant heart failure, and nonsteroidal antiinflammatory agents other than aspirin should never be used due to an increased risk of adverse cardiac events.

Much of the therapy relies on agents that have been discussed in other chapters in this text. HMG-CoA reductase inhibitors (statins) lower LDL cholesterol (Chapter 42) and, in acute ischemia, stabilize and reduce plaque burden and the chronic cycle of plaque rupture and repair. They also reduce circulating inflammatory mediators that can lead to further thrombosis and ischemia. Thus early initiation of statins in clinical presentations of acute ischemia with long-term use at discharge after an acute myocardial ischemic event is recommended.

Inhibition of both platelet aggregation and the coagulation pathway is also key for preventing clot propagation and the worsening of myocardial ischemia. Platelet aggregation can be inhibited by aspirin (Chapter 29), clopidogrel, and the GPIIb/IIIa inhibitors abciximab, eptifibatide, and tirofiban (Chapter 46), while the coagulation cascade, which plays an integral role in both initial coronary artery thrombosis as well as clot propagation, can be inhibited by heparin, fondaparinux, or the hirudins (Chapter 46). Once an occlusive arterial clot forms, neither antiplatelet agents nor anticoagulants significantly reduce clot burden or open the blockage. In this case, fibrinolytics, such as recombinant forms of tissue plasminogen activator and urokinase plasminogen activator, can be used acutely to open up occluded coronary arteries in a limited time frame (Chapter 46).

β-Blockers decrease heart rate and ventricular contractility, reducing myocardial oxygen demand (Chapter 12). In addition, chronic treatment reduces blood pressure, further reducing myocardial oxygen demand and improving symptomatic angina. Their use can decrease infarct size and improve exercise tolerance in chronic angina pectoris.

The Ca^{++}-channel blockers verapamil and diltiazem increase coronary blood flow and decrease blood pressure (afterload), thus improving vasospasm, as well as reducing myocardial oxygen demand (Chapter 40). These agents are used only if β-blockers are contraindicated and cannot be used in patients with severe left ventricular dysfunction and AV node heart block. Verapamil and diltiazem are especially useful in the treatment of Prinzmetal angina, in which ischemia is produced through coronary artery vasoconstriction.

Angiotensin-converting enzyme (ACE) inhibitors reduce both morbidity and mortality in patients with acute and chronic myocardial ischemia but have their maximal benefits in patients with reduced ventricular function. The short-acting ACE inhibitors such as captopril and enalapril should be used in the first 24 hours, and blood pressure, renal function, and potassium levels should be monitored at initiation and with chronic use.

Organic Nitrates

The **nitrates** are mainstays of antianginal therapy and have been used effectively for approximately 100 years to vasodilate coronary arteries, redistribute blood flow in the heart, and/or reduce cardiac oxygen demand. The nitrates do not provide a permanent beneficial effect on the underlying pathological condition but afford temporary symptomatic and pain relief, alleviating detrimental physiological responses to ongoing pain. Nitrates have important uses in the management of coronary

artery disease and are also effective in hypertension (Chapter 41) and heart failure (Chapter 44).

The goal of therapy in coronary artery disease is to reduce pain and increase exercise tolerance, which can be accomplished by administration of the organic nitrates. The pharmacological properties of these compounds that make them useful depend on the underlying cause of the angina. If pain is associated with atherosclerosis, the chief benefit arises from actions on the peripheral circulation and not on coronary vessels. Nitrates produce vasodilation of the venous vasculature. Dilation of venous capacitance vessels diminishes venous return to the heart, reducing ventricular volume and pressure. This decreases ventricular wall tension, a major contributor to the oxygen demands of the heart. Thus by decreasing preload on the heart, oxygen needs diminish, and demand is consistent with supply.

Other consequences of organic nitrate administration also contribute to the beneficial effect in angina. For example, nitrates cause relaxation of resistance vessels of the arterial circulation, which decreases afterload placed on the heart, or the impedance against which the heart must pump. Reducing afterload decreases the oxygen demands of the heart similar to reducing preload. The nitrate effect on resistance vessels generally requires somewhat higher concentrations than those needed for venodilation.

Another beneficial feature of the organic nitrate actions in angina is redistribution of blood flow to the subendocardial regions of the heart, which are especially vulnerable to ischemia. Perfusion of the subendocardial region occurs most prominently during early diastole. Later in diastole, as the ventricle fills, subendocardial arteries are constricted because of pressure in the ventricles, with the subsequent decrease in perfusion of these arteries. By decreasing preload, nitrates reduce ventricular filling pressure and increase the time available for endocardial perfusion. Further, the organic nitrates are useful in the management of angina pectoris caused by coronary artery spasm because they can dilate constricted coronary vessels.

Funny Channel Inhibitors

Ivabradine is currently the only commercially available funny channel inhibitor for the treatment of stable angina and can be used specifically to slow the heart. It was approved in 2015 for the treatment of angina, ischemic heart disease, and heart failure. Evidence indicates that ivabradine reduces angina episodes and provides patients with a higher exercise capacity. Because the action of ivabradine is rate dependent, it exhibits increased activity at higher heart rates. The bradycardic effects of ivabradine are dose dependent and linear, with a plateau effect, lessening the risk of serious sinus bradycardia.

PHARMACOKINETICS

Both **GTN** and **ISDN** are available in several preparations, with the choice depending on the pharmacokinetic profile desired. **GTN** is available as sublingual or oral tablets; as an aerosol spray, transdermal patch, or rectal ointment; or for intravenous administration. Sublingual GTN is the mainstay of therapy in anginal attacks and is also used prophylactically. Peak plasma concentrations are achieved in 1–2 minutes, with a duration of action of 30–60 minutes, depending on patient activity. There is minimal first-pass effect with sublingual administration. The GTN aerosol spray is as rapid and effective as the sublingual tablets.

Absorption is much slower with topical ointments and transdermal patches, and plasma concentrations attained with transdermal preparations are lower and more variable than those obtained with ointments. The transdermal patches are not as effective as the oral, timed-release preparations. Because of tolerance, transdermal patches left in place for 24 hours are ultimately ineffective for the treatment of angina, even if the dose is increased. However, patches that deliver 10 mg or more can be effective if the patches are removed for 10–12 hours daily. GTN is rapidly metabolized in the liver to inorganic nitrite and to denitrated metabolites.

ISDN is available as a tablet, slow-release tablet, and spray, while ISMN is available as a tablet only. The absorption of ISDN is nearly complete after oral dosing with extensive first-pass metabolism. Maximal serum levels are reached in about an hour. ISDN is metabolized both hepatically and nonhepatically and converted to both active and inactive metabolites. Both the 5-mononitrate and 2-mononitrate metabolites are biologically active, with the former characterized by a half-life of 5 hours, which may account for its longer duration of action than GTN.

PETN is available orally. It has an onset of about 10–20 minutes, with an 8- to 12-hour duration of action, and an elimination half-life of 4–5 hours. It is metabolized by the liver to several inactive metabolites, which are excreted in the urine.

Ivabradine has relatively poor absorption, with 40% bioavailability. It should be taken with food, which slows the rate of absorption but increases total systemic absorption by 20%–30%. It is 70% bound to plasma proteins and has a half-life of 2 hours. Ivabradine is metabolized extensively by oxidation in both the gastrointestinal tract and liver by CYP3A4 to its *N*-desmethyl derivative, which is an active metabolite also metabolized by CYP3A4. Metabolites are excreted in both the urine and feces.

PHARMACOVIGILANCE: ADVERSE EFFECTS AND DRUG INTERACTIONS

The primary adverse effects associated with nitrate therapy include headache, orthostatic hypotension, and tachycardia, but the extent of these effects differs among the nitrates. Vascular headaches, which may be severe, are the most commonly reported side effect. Headaches are most frequent following the use of GTN but may decrease in severity and frequency upon continued use. In contrast, headaches associated with the administration of ISDN recur with each daily dose, especially at higher doses; headaches following the use of ISMN and PETN are rare.

Transient lightheadedness and orthostatic hypotension may occur following the administration of GTN and PETN but is infrequent with ISDN and ISMN. Orthostatic hypotension can be minimized by careful adjustment of dose and by having the patient avoid the upright position when taking rapid-acting preparations. For some patients, it might be severe enough to discontinue the drug.

Both rebound hypertension and angina have been reported after acute withdrawal. Physical dependence has been observed in munitions workers exposed continuously to very high concentrations of nitrates. In these individuals, withdrawal from the industrial environment may result in angina, but this phenomenon is not commonly observed in patients taking therapeutic doses of nitrates. It can occur, however, in individuals who have been taking large doses for a prolonged period.

Tolerance to the vascular effects of nitrates does occur, and cross-tolerance exists between GTN and other nitrate esters. These alterations have been attributed to numerous mechanisms including, but not limited to, inhibition of aldehyde dehydrogenase 2, increased vascular superoxide production and oxidative stress, and desensitization of soluble guanylyl cyclase. Tolerance can be reduced by a short period of nitrate abstention, and GTN seems to elicit tolerance to a greater extent than the other organic nitrates.

The vasodilating effects of the nitrates are additive with other antihypertensives, possibly leading to hypotension. A significant drug-drug interaction occurs with the phosphodiesterase type 5 (PDE5) inhibitors. In patients currently taking these drugs for erectile dysfunction

or benign prostatic hypertrophy (Chapter 41), the administration of an organic nitrate (especially intravenously) can cause a severe drop in blood pressure sufficient to cause mortality. If nitrates are medically necessary in a life-threatening situation, at least 24 hours after the administration of sildenafil or vardenafil or 48 hours after tadalafil must elapse before the nitrate can be administered.

Nitrates can be reduced to nitrites, which, in turn, can oxidize the ferrous iron of hemoglobin, converting it to methemoglobin, reducing oxygen delivery to tissues. Although the induction of methemoglobinemia is extremely rare following the use of therapeutic doses of the nitrates, it may be observed in accidental poisoning or overdose.

Ivabradine has been promoted as a "pure" heart rate–lowering drug, producing a more favorable side effect profile than other agents that effectively lower heart rate, such as the nondihydropyridine Ca^{++}-channel blockers and β-adrenergic receptor blockers. To date, the most common side effect reported has been visual disturbances (phosphenes) that have been attributed to the blockade of funny channels in the retina. Further, because laboratory animal studies suggest that ivabradine may cause fetal toxicity and teratogenic effects, effective contraception is recommended for women while using ivabradine.

Although both ivabradine and its active metabolite are substrates for CYP3A4, their affinity for the enzyme is relatively weak, and thus it is unlikely that the metabolism of other drugs is affected. However, inhibitors or inducers of CYP3A4 may affect plasma levels of ivabradine and should not be coadministered.

Although serious adverse effects associated with the use of ivabradine have not yet been reported, there is evidence from laboratory studies suggesting that the drug blocks the hERG channel, which is the potassium channel required for repolarization of cardiac action potentials. Inhibition of this current could lead to QT interval prolongation. Although no clinical trials have reported induction of *torsades de pointes*, the drug was approved in the United States in 2015; postmarketing surveillance will be critical.

NEW DEVELOPMENTS

The management of myocardial ischemic events has evolved over the past several years, but many of the targets have remained constant. The current approaches employ multiple agents with many different targets. However, recent success with agents that improve myocardial efficiency (e.g., ranolazine) have opened up additional areas for consideration. The matricellular proteins (e.g., osteopontin and tenascin C) represent de-adhesion cellular proteins that are being explored as potential targets. Evidence that osteopontin levels are elevated in response to mechanical stress but not under normal physiological conditions suggests that the protein may represent an inducible target that would only be useful under conditions of myocardial ischemia and stress. Similarly, tenascin C is an extracellular matrix protein that may be involved in the ventricular remodeling associated with inflammation, ischemia, reperfusion, and hypertension.

Razolidine represents a new development in the pharmacological management of ischemic events in the heart. The success achieved with ranolazine has also identified new potential molecular targets, including partial fatty acid oxidase (pFOx) and the late sodium current induced under conditions of myocardial ischemia.

Since the first description of I_f, its role in underlying generation of pacemaker activity and rate control has been investigated in detail in a variety of conditions and established on the basis of several experimental findings. Recently, practical developments of the concept of I_f-dependent pacemaking have shown that the properties of funny channels can be exploited in clinically relevant applications. Thus use of "heart rate–reducing" drugs, such as ivabradine, which acts by selective inhibition

CLINICAL PROBLEMS

Organic Nitrates
Headache, orthostatic hypotension, reflex tachycardia, tolerance

Funny Channel Inhibitors
Visual disturbances (phosphenes)

TRADE NAMES

In addition to generic and fixed-combination preparations, the following trade-named materials are some of the important compounds available in the United States.
Organic nitrates
    Nitroglycerin
        Sublingual (Nitrostat, NitroQuick, GoNitro)
        Intravenous (Nitro-Bid IV)
        Oral (Glyceryl trinitrate)
        Rectal (Rective)
        Transdermal (Nitro-Dur)
        Aerosol (NitroMist)
    Isosorbide dinitrate (Dilatrate-SR, Isordil, Isordil Titradose, ISDN)
    Isosorbide mononitrate (Imdur, Monoket, ISMN)
    Pentaerythritol tetranitrate (PETN)
Ivabradine (Corlanor)

of the I_f current, allows pharmacologically controlled slowing of cardiac rate, an important tool in the therapeutic approach to ischemic heart disease and other diseases whose prognoses are ameliorated by slowing heart rate. Furthermore, certain HCN4 protein mutations are associated with inheritable cardiac arrhythmias such as sinus bradycardia, suggesting the existence of a general mechanism for rhythm disorders based on altered function of funny channels. Finally, exporting funny channels to silent cardiac tissue through either gene- or cell-based protocols represents a viable tool for the future development of biological pacemakers eventually able to replace electronic ones. Further knowledge of the molecular details of funny channel structure and function will likely allow in the future a more efficient and clinically relevant approach to cardiac rate control.

Typically, given their exclusive role in pacemaking, funny channels are ideal targets of drugs to control cardiac rate. Molecules able to bind specifically to and block these channels can be used as pharmacological tools for heart rate reduction with little or no adverse cardiovascular side effects.

CLINICAL RELEVANCE FOR HEALTHCARE PROFESSIONALS

The development of tolerance to nitrovasodilators is an area that can impact all healthcare professionals because patients will not receive the relief needed to maintain the activities of daily living and aerobic exercises that are appropriate for rehabilitation from an ischemic event. Certainly the need to increase activity levels slowly is one concern that transcends healthcare professional careers. The orthostatic hypotension that accompanies the reduced blood pressure also places additional burden on healthcare providers who may require positional change as part of their procedures. In addition, nitrovasodilators also induce a reflex tachycardia that may interfere with patients' ability to perform certain activities and participate in specific types of exercises.

SELF-ASSESSMENT QUESTIONS

1. A patient asks how nitroglycerin works to relieve anginal pain. The correct answer would be that nitroglycerin:
   A. Constricts coronary arteries to increase blood flow to the heart.
   B. Increases the oxygen demand in the cardiac muscle.
   C. Increases ventricular filling to improve cardiac output.
   D. Promotes vasodilation, which reduces preload and oxygen demand.

2. An overweight man in his early 40s comes into the ED complaining of chest pain and shortness of breath. After a complete examination, he is placed on nitroglycerin and diltiazem to prevent angina. Which one effect is most likely caused by both of these drugs?
   A. Increased cGMP levels.
   B. Decreased cAMP levels.
   C. Relaxation of vascular smooth muscle.
   D. Decreased heart rate.
   E. Inhibition of sodium influx.

3. Explaining the pharmacology of nitroglycerin to a junior colleague, you point out that while the mechanism is not completely understood, it has been established that the primary enzyme responsible for the development of tolerance to nitroglycerin is:
   A. Nitrate reductase.
   B. Alcohol dehydrogenase.
   C. Aldehyde dehydrogenase.
   D. CYP3A4.
   E. Dihydrofolate reductase.

4. Sublingual nitroglycerin can be used in lower dosages than with other routes because:
   A. It does not need to be absorbed into the bloodstream.
   B. It bypasses the liver.
   C. The potency is 100 times higher.
   D. It is not catabolized down by gastric acids.

5. A 56-year-old male complains of mild, intermittent chest pain and shortness of breath that is exacerbated by exercise. After a thorough cardiac workup, you decide to start the patient on nitroglycerin to relieve these symptoms. Which of the following best explains the mechanism of action of nitroglycerin?
   A. It activates phospholipase C to increase intracellular calcium.
   B. It produces reactive nitrogen species (ONO^-) that activate adenylyl cyclase.
   C. It produces nitric oxide (NO) that activates guanylyl cyclase.
   D. It inhibits of calcium influx through L-type calcium channels.
   E. It activates muscarinic receptors on endothelial cells to reduce blood pressure.

FURTHER READING

Okamoto H, Imanaka-Yoshida K. Matricellular proteins: new molecular targets to prevent heart failure. *Cardiovasc Ther*. 2012;30(4):e198–e209.

Jain A, Elgendy IY, Al-Ani M, et al. Advancements in pharmacotherapy for angina. *Expert Opin Pharmacother*. 2017;18(5):457–469.

Mengesha HG, Weldearegawi B, Petrucka P, et al. Effect of ivabradine on cardiovascular outcomes in patients with stable angina: meta-analysis of randomized clinical trials. *BMC Cardiovasc Disord*. 2017;17(1):105.

WEBSITES

http://dx.doi.org/10.1161/CIR.0b013e3182742c84

This website provides a direct link to the 2013 ACCF/AHA Guideline for the Management of ST-Elevation Myocardial Infarction: Executive Summary. A Report of the American College of Cardiology Foundation/American Heart Association Task Force on Practice Guidelines.

http://dx.doi.org/10.1016/j.jacc.2016.03.513

This website provides a direct link to the 2016 ACC/AHA Guideline Focused Update on Duration of Dual Antiplatelet Therapy in Patients with Coronary Artery Disease: A Report of the American College of Cardiology/American Heart Association Task Force on Clinical Practice Guidelines.

http://circ.ahajournals.org/content/130/25/e344

This website provides a direct link to the 2014 AHA/ACC Guideline for the Management of Patients with Non–ST-Elevation Acute Coronary Syndromes: A Report of the American College of Cardiology/American Heart Association Task Force on Practice Guidelines.

Treatment of Heart Failure

Michael T. Piascik and Robert W. Hadley

MAJOR DRUG CLASSES
Inhibitors of the renin-angiotensin-aldosterone system
β-Adrenergic receptor antagonists
Cardiac glycosides
Diuretics
Positive inotropes
Vasodilators

ABBREVIATIONS	
ACE	Angiotensin-converting enzyme
ACCF/AHA	American College of Cardiology Foundation/American Heart Association
ARB	Angiotensin receptor blocker
ARNI	Angiotensin receptor/neprilysin inhibitor
BNP	B-type natriuretic peptide
EF	Ejection fraction
HF	Heart failure
HFpEF	Heart failure with preserved ejection fraction
HFrEF	Heart failure with reduced ejection fraction
LV	Left ventricle
NO	Nitric oxide
PDE3	Phosphodiesterase type 3
RAAS	Renin-angiotensin-aldosterone system
SNS	Sympathetic nervous system

THERAPEUTIC OVERVIEW

According to the American College of Cardiology Foundation/American Heart Association (ACCF/AHA), heart failure (HF) is a complex syndrome resulting from structural or functional impairments involving ventricular filling or ejection of blood. As a result, the heart cannot provide adequate perfusion of peripheral organs to meet their metabolic requirements. Depending on the specific pathophysiology, patients with HF may experience fatigue, dyspnea, exercise intolerance, pulmonary congestion, and/or systemic edema. While some patients may experience a decrease in functional capacity, not all develop edema or signs of fluid retention.

HF is a progressive disorder that can develop as a consequence of other cardiovascular comorbidities such as coronary artery disease, diabetes, hypertension, myocardial infarction, and metabolic syndrome. HF can also occur as a result of structural heart disease or other factors such as dilated cardiomyopathies, drug abuse or toxicity, pericardial constriction or tamponade, restrictive cardiomyopathies, or valvular heart disease.

Epidemiological data from 2012 indicated that the lifetime risk for developing HF was 20% for Americans over 40, and it has been estimated that 5.7 million people in the United States have HF. Despite improvement in outcomes for other cardiovascular diseases such as hypertension, the prognosis for HF continues to be bleak, with a 5-year mortality rate of 50%.

Pathophysiology

HF is classified according to ejection fraction (EF), which is defined as the fraction of end diastolic volume ejected during each systole. A normal value for EF ranges from 55% to 75%. Patients with HF may exhibit a preserved (>50%) EF (HFpEF) or a reduced (≤40%) EF (HFrEF). There is an equal distribution of these two types in the HF patient population.

HFpEF is primarily a problem of ventricular relaxation (diastolic dysfunction) and was previously termed diastolic HF. HFpEF may result from impaired early diastolic relaxation and/or increased stiffness of the ventricular wall. HFpEF is characterized by normal or near-normal EF and cardiac output. Hypertension, valvular disease, or congenital abnormalities lead to the development of diastolic dysfunction, with hypertrophied, thickened, or poorly compliant ventricular walls impeding filling of the left ventricle (LV). In this case, ventricular filling can be achieved only at greater-than-normal filling pressures. Patients with HFpEF often present with systemic edema because the elevated LV diastolic pressure is transmitted from the pulmonary circulation to systemic veins.

HFrEF is characterized by a systolic dysfunction and was previously termed systolic HF. HFrEF occurs as a result of pathologic insults to the LV. For example, damage from chronic coronary artery disease or following a myocardial infarction results in impaired myocyte function, loss of myocytes, or fibrotic scarring. This results in decreased myocardial contractility and cardiac output. The chronic pressure overload caused by untreated long-standing hypertension or aortic stenosis results in an increase in afterload. The chronic elevation in afterload ultimately decreases cardiac output. In the setting of HFrEF, there is tonic activation of both the sympathetic nervous system (SNS) and the renin-angiotensin-aldosterone system (RAAS), which results in pathologic remodeling of the left ventricle involving alterations in cardiac gene expression. In HFrEF, the heart becomes large and dilated, with an increase in chamber size and thinning of the LV wall. The symptoms of HFrEF are dyspnea, orthopnea, fatigue, and pulmonary edema.

The decrease in cardiac output and resultant fall in blood pressure trigger a complex and well-orchestrated series of compensatory circulatory changes that maintain cardiac output and tissue perfusion for a period of time. Initially, the increase in left ventricular end diastolic

353

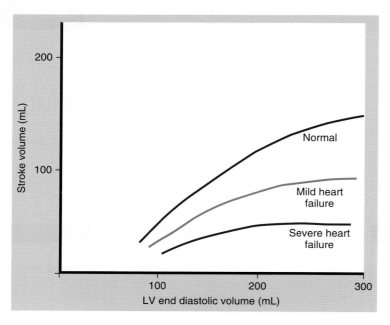

FIG. 44.1 The Frank-Starling Ventricular Function Curve. This curve depicts the relationship between left ventricular (LV) end diastolic volume and stroke volume (or cardiac output). In the normal heart, greater filling of the LV results in an increase in stroke volume, whereas in the failing heart, this relationship is compromised. In heart failure, there is incomplete LV emptying and an increase in LV end diastolic volume. However, because of the Frank-Starling mechanism, this elevated end diastolic volume cannot fully augment stroke volume, leading to less stroke volume than in the normal heart. In severe heart failure, the heart functions on a relatively flat curve, and increasing LV end diastolic volume can no longer augment stroke volume. The significant accumulation of fluid leads to pulmonary congestive symptoms.

pressure/volume increases the stretch on the ventricular myocardium and via the Frank-Starling mechanism (Fig. 44.1) and induces an increase in stroke volume and cardiac output. However, this compensatory mechanism has limits. As the LV enlarges, it can no longer function effectively as a pump, and the Frank-Starling curve flattens at higher-end diastolic volumes; cardiac output can no longer be augmented via this mechanism. In addition to the Frank-Starling mechanism, neurohumoral systems are activated to compensate for these deleterious circulatory events. As cardiac output falls, the baroreceptors sense the hemodynamic changes and initiate countermeasures to maintain support of the circulatory system.

Activation of the SNS leads to activation of myocardial β_1-adrenergic receptors to increase contractility and heart rate in an attempt to maintain adequate cardiac output. There is also enhanced sympathetic tone that activates vascular α_1-adrenergic receptors to maintain systemic blood pressure (Chapters 36 and 37). Ultimately, these responses are maladaptive and actually exacerbate HF. The increase in vascular tone increases peripheral vascular resistance and the afterload on the failing heart, which further impairs its ability to produce an adequate cardiac output. The tonic activation of myocardial β_1-adrenergic receptors stimulates maladaptive LV remodeling, which makes this chamber less efficient as a pump. The prolonged elevation of sympathetic tone also leads to desensitization and down regulation of myocardial β_1 receptors, thus depriving the failing heart of a vital inotropic receptor system.

The tonic engagement of the RAAS (Chapter 39) also triggers a series of compensatory circulatory responses. The fall in renal perfusion pressure secondary to a decrease in cardiac output triggers the release of renin, which ultimately results in increased circulating levels of angiotensin II, stimulating the release of aldosterone from the adrenal gland. Angiotensin II increases peripheral vascular resistance to maintain blood pressure, while aldosterone acts in the renal collecting duct to promote Na^+ reabsorption, which will expand plasma volume. The expanded plasma volume will help maintain cardiac output and blood pressure. In addition, circulating levels of vasopressin (antidiuretic hormone) increase, which promotes water retention in the distal nephron. These alterations ultimately contribute to the downward progression of cardiac function, exacerbating the degree of HF. The increase in peripheral vascular resistance increases afterload, exerting negative

consequences on cardiac function, and the fluid retention will further volume overload an LV already incapable of producing a sufficient cardiac output. Finally, angiotensin II and aldosterone are both potent stimulators of cardiac remodeling. Thus all the compensatory neurohumoral mechanisms engaged to support the failing myocardium actually contribute to the downward spiral of HF.

The management of HF is multifaceted and often involves a combination of interventions to relieve symptoms and improve hemodynamics, leading to improved quality of life, a reduction in hospitalization, and decreased mortality. For acute HF, the short-term aim is to stabilize the patient by achieving an optimal hemodynamic status and providing symptomatic treatment through use of intravenous interventions.

Cardiac and vascular changes associated with HF, the goals of treatment, and drugs used for both acute and chronic HF are shown in the Therapeutic Overview Box.

MECHANISMS OF ACTION

Inhibitors of the Renin-Angiotensin-Aldosterone System

The pharmacology of the angiotensin-converting enzyme (ACE) inhibitors, angiotensin receptor blockers (ARBs), and other agents that affect the RAAS are discussed in Chapter 39. In the setting of HF, the maladaptive cardiovascular actions described occur through AT_1 receptor activation (Chapter 39, Fig. 39.1). Thus blocking the formation of angiotensin II with ACE inhibitors or blocking AT_1 receptors with ARBs represents an effective approach. The currently available ARBs are selective for AT_1 receptors; they do not affect AT_2 receptors. This selectivity is highly beneficial for HF because activation of AT_2 receptors leads to vasodilation, reduces hyperplasia and hypertrophy of vascular smooth muscle and cardiomyocytes, and increases the levels of bradykinin and subsequent release of nitric oxide (NO).

The elevated circulating angiotensin II levels in patients with HF also lead to the increased production of aldosterone, which is an important mediator in the progressive development of HF. Aldosterone binds mineralocorticoid receptors in renal epithelial cells, promoting the reabsorption of Na^+ in exchange for K^+, expanding plasma volume. Further, activation of cardiac mineralocorticoid receptors promotes maladaptive cardiac remodeling and hypertrophic growth. Thus the

Problem

Impaired left ventricle function
Decreased left ventricle compliance
Reduced force of contraction
Decreased cardiac output
Increased total peripheral resistance
Inadequate organ perfusion
Activation of neurohumoral systems
Ventricular remodeling
Development of systemic and/or pulmonary edema
Decreased exercise tolerance
Ischemic heart disease
Sudden death

Goals

Improve patient survival
Decrease hospitalizations
Alleviation of symptoms, improve quality of life
Treat underlying comorbidities
Arrest ventricular remodeling

Nondrug Therapy

Reduce cardiac work, restrict sodium, treat sleep disorders, promote weight
    loss, engage in regular physical activity

Drug Therapy

Acute heart failure
    Intravenous diuretics, inotropic agents, phosphodiesterase type 3 inhibitors,
        vasodilators
Chronic heart failure
    Angiotensin converting enzyme inhibitors, β-adrenergic receptor blockers,
        angiotensin receptor blockers, the angiotensin receptor/neprilysin inhibitor,
        aldosterone receptor antagonists, digoxin, diuretics, vasodilators

mineralocorticoid receptor antagonists spironolactone and eplerenone block the deleterious effects of aldosterone and provide therapeutic benefit in the overall treatment of HF.

A unique approach to inhibiting the RAAS for HF uses a newly developed drug combination of an ARB and a neprilysin (neutral endopeptidase 24.11) inhibitor, termed an angiotensin receptor/ neprilysin inhibitor (ARNI). Neprilysin catabolizes B-type natriuretic peptide (BNP), a hormone produced by the heart in response to changes in intracardiac pressure, such as atrial or ventricular stress. BNP activates guanylyl cyclase, increasing cGMP levels, which decreases sympathetic tone and vascular resistance (Chapter 41, Fig. 41.1). BNP also decreases hypertrophic responses and induces natriuresis and diuresis (Fig. 44.2). Sacubitril is a prodrug that is metabolized to LBQ657, which is a neprilysin inhibitor. Inhibition of neprilysin increases BNP levels, promoting effects favorable in the setting of HF (especially HFrEF). In addition to inhibiting BNP catabolism, sacubitril also inhibits the metabolism of angiotensin I to angiotensin (1–7), leading to increased levels of both angiotensin I and angiotensin II (Chapter 39, Fig. 39.1). The presence of the ARB in this drug combination selectively blocks AT_1 receptor activation by angiotensin II, furthering the beneficial effects of AT_2 receptor activation as discussed.

β-Adrenergic Receptor Antagonists

These drugs inhibit the adverse effects of the SNS in patients with HF. Whereas cardiac adrenergic drive initially serves as a compensatory mechanism to support the failing heart, long-term activation leads to a down regulation of β_1 receptors and an uncoupling from adenylyl cyclase, thereby reducing myocardial contractility. The tonic stimulation of β_1-adrenergic receptors also contributes to maladaptive cardiac remodeling. The beneficial effects of β-receptor antagonists are due in part to blockade of these negative effects on the myocardium. There is also evidence that the combination α,β-receptor blocker approved for the treatment of HF, carvedilol, has antioxidant actions and decreases oxidative stress generated by reactive oxygen species by mechanisms unrelated to α,β-receptor blockade.

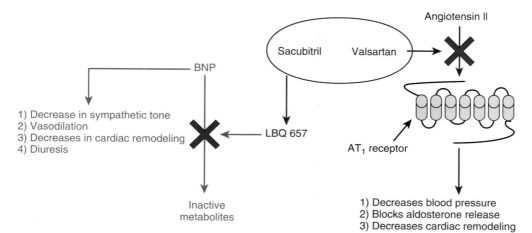

FIG. 44.2 Mechanism of Action of the Combination Valsartan/Sacubitril. Valsartan is an AT_1 receptor antagonist that inhibits the negative effects of angiotensin II on the failing heart. Sacubitril is a prodrug metabolized to LBQ 657 that inhibits the endopeptidase neprilysin, blocking the catabolism of B-type natriuretic peptide (BNP). Inhibition of neprilysin allows the accumulation of BNP, with resultant beneficial actions in heart failure. These dual actions mediate the therapeutic efficacy of this drug combination in heart failure.

Cardiac Glycosides

Digoxin, which is the only cardiac glycoside still available for clinical use, inhibits sarcolemmal Na^+, K^+-ATPase, leading to increased intracellular Na^+, which promotes Ca^{++} influx though Na^+/Ca^{++} exchange. The increased intracellular Ca^{++} results in increased Ca^{++} release following depolarization, increasing the force of myocardial contraction. Digoxin also increases vagal tone, leading to a decrease in conduction velocity and an increase in the effective refractory period, thereby slowing heart rate.

Diuretics

Furosemide is the most frequently used loop diuretic, although **bumetanide** and **torsemide** are also available. These agents compete with Cl^- for a binding site on the Na^+, K^+, Cl^- cotransporter protein (NKCC2) in the thick ascending limb of the loop of Henle, thereby inhibiting the reabsorption of Na^+ and Cl^- (Chapter 38).

Positive Inotropes
Dopamine and Dobutamine

Dopamine is a positive inotrope with dose-dependent actions. At low doses (1–2 µg/kg/min), it activates DA_1 receptors in renal vascular beds to increase renal blood flow, producing a diuretic effect. At moderate doses (2–10 µg/kg/min), it activates cardiac β_1-adrenergic receptors to elicit a positive inotropic action, whereas at higher doses, it activates vascular α_1-adrenergic receptors, producing vasoconstriction and an increase in afterload, the latter undesirable effects that would exacerbate HF.

Dobutamine activates β_1 receptors and is devoid of activity at DA_1 receptors. It has complex actions on the vasculature because it activates both α_1 and β_2 receptors, but the net effect is vasodilation and decreased peripheral vascular resistance.

Phosphodiesterase Type 3 Inhibitors

Inamrinone (previously named amrinone) and **milrinone** are positive inotropic agents that inhibit cAMP-dependent phosphodiesterase type 3 (PDE3) expressed in the heart and blood vessels, leading to increased cAMP levels. Increased cAMP levels in the heart promote the protein kinase A–mediated phosphorylation of Ca^{++} channels, enhancing Ca^{++} influx and leading to a positive inotropic action similar to that of the catecholamines. Increased cAMP levels in the vasculature lead to vasodilation, decreasing the afterload on the failing heart. Milrinone is a derivative of inamrinone with 20–30 times the ionotropic potency of inamrinone. The unique feature of the PDE3 inhibitors is that they act downstream of β_1 receptors and therefore do not lead to receptor down regulation.

Vasodilators

Vasodilators used for the treatment of chronic HF include the antihypertensive agent hydralazine (Chapter 41) and isosorbide dinitrate, used in the treatment of ischemic heart disease (Chapter 43). **Hydralazine** produces selective arterial vasodilation by several mechanisms, including increasing NO and cGMP, and/or activating outward K^+ channels to hyperpolarize the arterial smooth muscle cell membrane (Chapter 41), decreasing the afterload on the failing myocardium. **Isosorbide dinitrate** is metabolized to NO, which increases vascular cGMP levels, but in contrast to hydralazine, isosorbide dinitrate is a venous selective vasodilator, decreasing the preload on the failing heart.

Vasodilators used for the treatment of decompensated acute heart failure to provide rapid reduction in preload and afterload include **nitroprusside** and **nitroglycerin**. **Nitroprusside** spontaneously decomposes to NO, leading to increased levels of cGMP (Chapter 41), and is a very potent, balanced vasodilator, relaxing both venous and arterial smooth muscle. **Nitroglycerin**, which is enzymatically converted to NO, reduces preload and decreases LV end diastolic pressure (Chapter 43). Similarly, **nesiritide**, which is recombinant human BNP, decreases sympathetic tone, leading to vasodilation.

RELATIONSHIP OF MECHANISMS OF ACTION TO CLINICAL RESPONSE

Historically, the treatment of HF focused on treating symptoms with positive inotropic agents and vasodilators to decrease preload and afterload on the failing heart. Currently, the focus is on blocking the cardiac remodeling associated with HF, improving quality of life, reducing hospitalizations, and prolonging survival. The ACCF/AHA have derived a series of evidence-based guidelines for HF therapy based on the stages of HF (A–D), as shown in Table 44.1. These guidelines focus on the treatment of HFrEF because most clinical trials have been carried out with patients with this form of HF; no guidelines are available for HFpEF.

Inhibitors of the Renin-Angiotensin-Aldosterone System

Drugs that interfere with the activity of the RAAS are particularly effective in HF treatment. **ACE inhibitors** have actions at several levels in the cardiovascular system that are beneficial. The vascular actions of ACE inhibitors decrease preload and afterload and systemic arterial blood pressure. These drugs also block the effects of sustained neurohumoral activation of the RAAS and inhibit maladaptive cardiac and vascular smooth muscle growth responses. These beneficial effects have been demonstrated at all levels of HF severity. The ACCF/AHA treatment guidelines indicate that ACE inhibitors are drugs of first choice in Stage B HF, and if patients cannot tolerate an ACE inhibitor, an **ARB** should be considered as an alternative. Although clinical trials indicate that the ARBs have beneficial effects similar to the ACE inhibitors, the evidence is stronger and more complete for the ACE inhibitors. There is no evidence to suggest that the combination of both an ACE inhibitor and an ARB is more beneficial than either drug alone. Treatment should begin at low doses, and if no adverse effects are observed, doses should be increased to maximally effective doses.

Sustained activation of the RAAS leads to an angiotensin II–mediated increase in aldosterone release, with resultant increases in plasma Na^+ content and volume and activation of cardiac remodeling. Aldosterone concentrations are elevated as much as 20-fold in patients with HF. Mineralocorticoid receptor antagonists are recommended currently for use in patients who, despite being treated with an ACE inhibitor or ARB and a β-blocker, still present with HF symptoms. The administration of **spironolactone** or **eplerenone** to patients who were receiving an ACE inhibitor exhibited a greater reduction in mortality than patients who did not receive the aldosterone antagonists. Mineralocorticoid receptor antagonists have been shown to benefit patients who recently suffered a myocardial infarction and have a decreased EF. Current guidelines recommend using these drugs in patients with preserved renal function and normal K^+ levels. Plasma K^+ must be monitored carefully, and caution should be exercised in patients taking K^+ supplements or using other K^+-sparing diuretics because of the risk of hyperkalemia.

The combination of **valsartan/sacubitril** is a first-in-class drug combination. BNP has several beneficial effects in HF patients, including decreasing sympathetic tone on the failing heart, blocking pathologic cardiac remodeling, and promoting diuresis, all of which are beneficial in the volume-overloaded patient. Recent trials have shown that this drug combination was more effective than an ACE inhibitor alone at decreasing hospitalizations and mortality in HFrEF. However, because

TABLE 44.1 **ACCF/AHA Classification of Heart Failure Stages: Symptoms, Treatment Goals, and Interventions**

Patient Population/Symptoms	Treatment Goals	Interventions
Stage A: High Risk for HF, Without Structural Disease or HF Symptoms		
Comorbid or history of hypertension, diabetes, metabolic syndrome	• Prevent progression to HF	• Treat comorbid disorders • Lifestyle modifications
Stage B: Structural Heart Disease, Without Signs or HF Symptoms		
Acute coronary syndromes or post infarction with reduced EF; loss of viable myocardial muscle	• Prevent the onset of HF • Block cardiac remodeling • Decrease adverse neurohumoral effects • Improve quality of life • Decrease mortality	• ACE inhibitors or ARBs and • β-adrenergic receptor antagonists
Stage C: Structural Disease With Prior or Current HF Symptoms		

Diagnostic evidence of structural heart disease with dyspnea, fatigue, systemic and/or pulmonary edema	• Manage contributing factors
	• Control of symptoms
	• Prevent further deterioration of myocardial performance
	• Decrease hospitalization
	• Reduce mortality
		• ACE inhibitors or ARBs
		   and
		• β-adrenergic receptor antagonists
		   and
		   one or more
		• Aldosterone receptor antagonist
		• An ARNI (requires stopping ACE inhibitor or ARB)
		• Loop diuretic
		• Vasodilator
		• Digoxin

Stage D: HF Refractory to Treatment, Requires Specialized Interventions (End-Stage HF)		
Dyspnea and fatigue at rest or minimal exertion, pulmonary and/or systemic congestion and frequent hospitalizations	• Rapid reduction of symptoms	• Intravenous loop diuretics (for fluid overload) • Vasodilators (to decrease preload and afterload) • Positive inotropes (to increase contractility) • Mechanical circulatory support such as left-ventricular assist devices or transplantation

clinical experience with this combination is lacking, current recommendations are for use only in advanced stages of HF. If patients are receiving an ACE inhibitor or an ARB, these drugs should be withdrawn prior to initiation of therapy with valsartan/sacubitril.

β-Adrenergic Receptor Antagonists

There is overwhelming evidence to support the use of β-adrenergic receptor blockers in HF. The β-blockers improve symptoms, decrease hospitalizations, and improve survival. These agents act at several levels to interfere with maladaptive responses, including blockade of the adverse cardiac remodeling characteristic of HF. They also lower the work of the heart, decrease heart rate, have antiarrhythmic actions, and have the ability to resensitize receptors that have been down regulated by the sustained increase in catecholamine levels. The decrease in oxygen consumption and antiarrhythmic actions of the β-blockers render them particularly effective in treating HFrEF following a myocardial infarction. Currently, only three agents, bucindolol, carvedilol, and metoprolol succinate (the sustained-release salt form of metoprolol) have been shown to be effective. Thus it cannot be determined at this time whether the efficacy of β-blockers for HF is a class effect. Because bucindolol and metoprolol are selective β₁-blockers, while carvedilol is a nonselective antagonist, it is not clear whether selective blockade of the β₁-receptor underlies the benefit in HF. In addition, carvedilol has actions unrelated to β-receptor antagonism, including an antioxidant effect leading to decreased reactive oxygen species, which could contribute to its efficacy.

Treatment with β-blockers should begin with low doses because patients might experience a temporary worsening of symptoms due to decreases in heart rate and stroke volume. Once patients tolerate the drug, doses can be increased to maximally tolerated levels. In the long term, there will be improvement in systolic function.

Cardiac Glycosides

Cardiac glycosides have a rich history in HF treatment, and these agents were once considered the cornerstones of therapy. However, their use has been supplanted by safer, more effective agents. Digoxin is the only orally active agent available. Its unique mechanism of action bypasses the β-adrenergic receptor system, which could be down regulated as a result of HF. Digoxin augments the contraction of the failing heart, leading to an increase in cardiac output, which is of obvious benefit in the HF patient. In addition, the slowing of ventricular rate allows improved filling and increased EF or stroke volume. The enhanced cardiac output also decreases the neurohumoral tone on the cardiovascular system. As many HF patients develop atrial fibrillation, digoxin-induced slowing of the heart rate provides an additional benefit. There is evidence that digoxin can reduce symptoms and hospitalizations, but there is no evidence that it improves patient survival or blunts cardiac remodeling. Therefore the major use of digoxin is to provide relief of symptoms. Because digoxin has a narrow margin of safety, blood levels should not exceed 1.0 mg/mL. Higher doses do not provide additional therapeutic efficacy and only increase the likelihood of toxicity.

Diuretics

Loop diuretics are effective in providing symptomatic relief of pulmonary and systemic edema in advanced forms of HF, but there is no evidence that they decrease mortality. These agents are used in volume-overloaded patients presenting with dyspnea and peripheral and/or pulmonary edema. In addition to reducing the systemic edema and pulmonary congestion that often occurs as HF progresses, the diuretic-induced volume reduction has a positive effect on cardiac performance. Furosemide is most often used with bumetanide and torsemide as alternatives. These agents can be used to reduce volume overload in both chronic HF and acute decompensated HF.

Positive Inotropes
Dopamine and Dobutamine

Dopamine and dobutamine are positive inotropes administered intravenously for the acute management of symptoms associated with severe forms of HF. Dopamine is useful because it both maintains renal perfusion and increases cardiac output. However, at doses higher than those needed to activate myocardial β_1 receptors, dopamine activates vascular α_1-adrenergic receptors, producing vasoconstriction and an increase in afterload, undesirable effects that would exacerbate HF. Thus dosing may be difficult because an infusion rate has to be achieved that produces the desired actions without producing vasoconstriction. Dobutamine also activates myocardial β_1 receptors to increase cardiac output, but it can decrease the afterload on the failed heart by β_2-receptor–mediated vasodilation. This action would augment stroke volume and improve organ perfusion.

Phosphodiesterase Type 3 Inhibitors

The PDE3 inhibitors inamrinone and milrinone increase cardiac output and decrease preload and afterload. These drugs are useful in patients taking β-blockers who require inotropic support. Milrinone is often preferred for short-term parenteral inotropic support in patients with severe cardiac decompensation. Milrinone also decreases plasma fibrinogen and increases fibrinolytic activity, leading to decreased blood viscosity.

Vasodilators

The vasodilator combination of hydralazine and isosorbide dinitrate has long been used in HF, although it has been supplanted by the ACE inhibitors, ARBs, and β-blockers. Nonetheless, this drug combination decreases mortality in HF patients. The combined hemodynamic actions of these drugs to reduce both afterload by arterial vasodilation (hydralazine) and preload by venous vasodilation (isosorbide dinitrate) reduces cardiac filling pressures and improves myocardial performance and cardiac output. Current recommendations of this drug combination are for patients who present with HF symptoms despite being treated with an ACE inhibitor or ARB and a β-blocker or for individuals who cannot tolerate an ACE inhibitor or ARB.

The combination of hydralazine and isosorbide dinitrate is particularly effective in increasing survival in African-Americans with HF, an ethnic group who do not respond as well to ACE inhibitors or ARBs as do other ethnic groups. Therefore African-Americans currently receiving an ACE inhibitor or ARB and a β-blocker who present with HF symptoms should be given a combination of hydralazine and isosorbide dinitrate. The drugs can be given as two individual medications or in a fixed-dose combination.

Nitroprusside, nitroglycerin, and nesiritide are administered intravenously and used exclusively in the treatment of decompensated acute heart failure to provide rapid reduction in preload and afterload. Vasodilators should be given in doses that reduce peripheral resistance but do not cause a sharp decrease in blood pressure to avoid increasing end-organ damage.

Nitroprusside is unstable in solution and must be reconstituted immediately before use. Vascular effects are seen within minutes of beginning the infusion and include relaxation of both venous and arterial smooth muscle, thereby reducing resistance to ventricular ejection and increasing venous capacitance. These changes reduce the effect of volume overload on the failing cardiovascular system. In the presence of increased peripheral vascular resistance and with relatively high doses administered intravenously, nitroglycerin also elicits a vasodilator effect on the arterial circulation.

Nesiritide has beneficial hemodynamic actions, including arterial and venous dilation, enhanced Na^+ excretion, and suppression of the RAAS and SNS. It alleviates the symptoms of acute decompensated heart failure and is useful in augmenting the effects of loop diuretics in patients who fail to respond with an adequate diuresis. However, there is no evidence of a survival benefit in patients suffering from acute decompensated heart failure.

PHARMACOKINETICS

The pharmacokinetics of many of the compounds used for HF are presented in chapters corresponding to their main classification (drugs affecting the RAAS are discussed in Chapter 39, β-receptor blockers and sympathomimetics in Chapters 11 and 12, diuretics in Chapter 38, hydralazine and nitroprusside in Chapter 41, and isosorbide dinitrate and nitroglycerin in Chapter 43).

Angiotensin Receptor Blocker/Neprilysin Inhibitor

This complex formulation consists of six molecules each of valsartan and sacubitril. Sacubitril is a prodrug converted to the active enzyme inhibitor LBQ657 by esterases. Both sacubitril and LBQ657 are highly bound to plasma proteins (>90%), with half-lives of 1–4 hours for sacubitril and 9–11 hours for LBQ657. About 50%–70% of sacubitril is excreted as its active metabolite in the urine and 40%–50% in feces.

Digoxin

Digoxin may be administered orally or intravenously. It is 70%–80% absorbed following oral administration, primarily in the proximal part of the small intestine. Digoxin is 25% protein bound with a peak effect in 6 hours, and a plasma half-life of 36–48 hours. Digoxin is metabolized by the liver but not appreciably by cytochrome P450s. The drug is excreted mainly by the kidneys, with 50%–70% unchanged and the remainder as glucuronide- and sulfate-conjugated metabolites.

Phosphodiesterase Type 3 Inhibitors

Inamrinone and milrinone are administered parenterally. Inamrinone has a half-life of 2–4 hours, is metabolized by the liver, and is renally excreted as both the parent molecule and metabolites. Milrinone has a half-life of 30–60 minutes and is also metabolized by the liver and renally excreted. The elimination half-lives of both inamrinone and milrinone are approximately doubled in HF patients.

Nesiritide

When administered intravenously to patients with HF, as an infusion or bolus injection, nesiritide exhibits a biphasic pattern of disposition. The mean terminal elimination half-life is approximately 18 minutes. Nesiritide is cleared by three mechanisms—namely, binding to cell surface natriuretic peptide receptor C with subsequent internalization and lysosomal proteolysis, hydrolysis by endopeptidases on the vascular luminal surface, and renal filtration.

PHARMACOVIGILANCE: ADVERSE EFFECTS AND DRUG INTERACTIONS

The adverse effects associated with ACE inhibitors, ARBs, and aldosterone antagonists are discussed in Chapter 39, those of the β-receptor blockers and sympathomimetics in Chapters 11 and 12, diuretics in Chapter 38, hydralazine and nitroprusside in Chapter 41, and isosorbide dinitrate and nitroglycerin in Chapters 43. However, in the context of HF, several adverse effects are notable, particularly those involving the loop diuretics and positive inotropes.

The loop diuretics can lead to excessive diuresis, resulting in an excessive reduction in preload that could ultimately decrease filling pressure to the point that cardiac output decreases. Another concern with the use of these potent diuretics is that they can induce hypokalemia and increase the arrhythmic risk.

The major concerns with positive inotropic agents (dopamine, dobutamine, and PDE3 inhibitors) are the production of tachycardia and genesis of arrhythmias, which can increase mortality. Further, sustained infusion of dopamine or dobutamine could lead to further desensitization and down regulation of myocardial β$_1$ receptors, with a resultant decrease in therapeutic action. In addition, the effectiveness of these agonists could be significantly reduced in patients treated with β-receptor blockers.

The most common adverse effects associated with the ARNI sacubitril/valsartan include hypotension, hyperkalemia, cough, dizziness, and renal failure.

Cardiac Glycosides

Toxic effects of digoxin include visual disturbances with the appearance of yellow-green haloes around objects, nausea and vomiting, and arrhythmias. Hypokalemia can potentiate the toxic actions of digoxin. Therefore caution should be used when digoxin is administered with the loop diuretics, which can cause hypokalemia. Drugs such as verapamil and amiodarone block the renal elimination of digoxin and thus increase the likelihood of toxicity. One of the major drawbacks of digoxin is its very narrow therapeutic index.

NEW DEVELOPMENTS

In 2016, two new drugs were approved for the treatment of HF, the ARNI valsartan/sacubitril and ivabradine, the latter which decreases heart rate and is discussed in somewhat greater detail in Chapter 45.

The combination valsartan/sacubitril was the first ARNI developed and has proven beneficial, leading to more studies of similar combinations. Ivabradine was approved in April 2015 for HFrEF patients in sinus rhythm with a resting heart rate ≥70 beats per minute and who are not taking β-blockers or are already receiving the maximum β-blocker dose.

One area of drug development that requires more attention is treatment of patients with HF who have a preserved ejection fraction. Although about 50% of HF patients present with HFpEF, treatment guidelines are not available for this group of patients—that is, no therapy has been specifically approved for HF with preserved ejection fraction. Drugs such as ACE inhibitors, ARBs, or β-blockers do not decrease morbidity or mortality in HFpEF. Therefore the major therapeutic goal for these patients has been to treat the underlying comorbidities such as hypertension, coronary artery disease, hyperlipidemias, and atrial fibrillation. Diuretics are recommended to treat volume overload, and there is some evidence that mineralocorticoid receptor antagonists may have some benefit in HFpEF. Further studies are undoubtedly needed.

CLINICAL RELEVANCE FOR HEALTHCARE PROFESSIONALS

Many healthcare professionals may treat individuals with HF who are on multidrug regimens. Thus it is imperative for all practitioners to be aware of limitations associated with both the patient's condition and the medications. Physical therapists work with HF patients to improve exertion tolerance, endurance, and improved quality of life that may engage multiple modalities. The drugs improve cardiac function so that patients can participate in rehabilitation, but the drugs may also produce adverse effects that negatively impact outcomes. Physical therapists need to be aware of the potential for orthostatic hypotension that accompanies many of these agents, monitor participation in hydrotherapy, and provide adequate time for cool down from exercise. Dental professionals must also be aware of orthostatic hypotension, which could be problematic in patients changing position in the dental chair.

SELF-ASSESSMENT QUESTIONS

1. A 63-year-old African-American female is being treated with lisinopril and carvedilol for Stage B heart failure characterized by a reduced EF. Despite this drug therapy, she begins to develop HF symptoms and is prescribed an additional drug combination, which has proven to be particularly effective in African-Americans. Which of the following was the patient mostly likely prescribed?
   A. Digoxin/furosemide.
   B. Eplerenone/losartan.
   C. Hydralazine/isosorbide dinitrate.
   D. Valsartan/nitroprusside.
   E. Milrinone/valsartan/sacubitril.

2. Recent clinical trials have shown that a fixed combination of valsartan and sacubitril is more effective than lisinopril in decreasing mortality in patients with heart failure with reduced ejection fraction. Which one of the following correctly describes the mechanisms of action exhibited by this drug combination?
   A. Blockade of angiotensin converting enzyme and the β-adrenergic receptor.
   B. Inhibition of the aldosterone receptor and the angiotensin-converting enzyme.
   C. Blockade of the β-adrenergic receptor and the AT_1 receptor.
   D. Blockade of the AT_1 receptor and neprilysin.

3. A 65-year-old female with an ejection fraction of 35% is prescribed metoprolol succinate and a second medication to slow the progression of heart failure and prevent the development of heart failure symptoms. After 3 weeks of therapy, she calls the office and complains of a bothersome and persistent cough, which you attribute to the second medication. Which one of the following is the most likely cause of her symptoms?
   A. Furosemide.
   B. Losartan.
   C. Digoxin.
   D. Lisinopril.

4. A patient is admitted to the coronary intensive care unit in acute decompensated congestive heart failure. The patient is treated with intravenous furosemide to reduce the level of edematous fluid. In addition, an infusion of dobutamine is given to increase the inotropic state of the heart. At which one of the following receptors does dobutamine act to produce this positive inotropic action?
   A. α_1-Adrenergic.
   B. β_1-Adrenergic.
   C. β_2-Adrenergic.
   D. DA_1.

5. Which one of the following agents inhibits phosphodiesterase type 3?
   A. Digoxin.
   B. Dobutamine.
   C. Milrinone.
   D. Propranolol.

FURTHER READING

McMurray JJV. Neprilysin inhibition to treat heart failure: a tale of science, serendipity and second chances. *Eur J Heart Failure.* 2015;17:242–247.

Sica DA, Gehr TWB, Frishman WH. Use of diuretics in the treatment of heart failure in older adults. *Heart Fail Clin.* 2017;13(3):503–512.

Suthahar N, Meijers WC, Sillje HHW, de Boer RA. From inflammation to fibrosis-molecular and cellular mechanisms of myocardial tissue remodeling and perspectives on differential treatment opportunities. *Curr Heart Fail Rep.* 2017;4:235–250.

Yamamoto K. Pharmacological treatment of heart failure with preserved ejection fraction. *Yonago Acta Med.* 2017;60(2):71–76.

WEBSITES

http://circ.ahajournals.org/content/128/16/e240
This is a direct link to the 2013 American College of Cardiology Foundation/American Heart Association Guideline for Management of Heart Failure.

http://www.hfsa.org/accahahfsa-guideline-management-heart-failure-update/
This website, maintained by the Heart Failure Society of America, provides a link to the 2016 update of the 2013 ACCF/AHA Guideline for Management of Heart Failure.

https://www.cdc.gov/heartdisease/
This website is maintained by the United States Centers for Disease Control and Prevention and contains information on heart disease for both healthcare professionals and the public.

Antiarrhythmic Drugs

David A. Taylor and Stephanie W. Watts

MAJOR DRUG CLASSES

Membrane stabilizers
β-Adrenergic receptor antagonists
Action potential–prolonging agents
Calcium-channel blockers

THERAPEUTIC OVERVIEW

The heart is a four-chambered pump that circulates blood to the body in quantities sufficient to provide adequate O_2 and nutrients to maintain aerobic metabolism. To function efficiently, the heart needs to contract sequentially (atria and then ventricles) and in a synchronized manner. In addition, there must be adequate time between contractions for chamber filling (diastole). This need for relaxation distinguishes cardiac from smooth and skeletal muscle, both of which can produce tetanic contractions. To function efficiently, the heart needs an electrical system that allows for the rapid and organized generation and propagation of electrical impulses such that the electrical signals can be converted into mechanical energy.

Electrical activation originates in specialized pacemaker cells of the sinoatrial (SA) node, located in the high right atrium near the junction with the superior vena cava that exhibit unique actions potentials as illustrated in Fig. 45.1. After exiting the SA node, the electrical signal assumes a more characteristic shape (Fig. 45.1) and spreads rapidly throughout the atrium, leading to atrial contraction. However, the atria are electrically isolated from the ventricles by the fibrous atrioventricular (AV) ring (AV node), with electrical activity propagation between atrium and ventricles occurring solely through the AV node, which displays another uniquely shaped action potential (Fig. 45.1). The AV node delays electrical impulse passage from the atrium to ventricles, providing additional filling time before ventricular contraction that leads to blood ejection, as well as serving as a frequency regulator to prevent excessive ventricular rate. The system serves as a conduit for electrical activity to rapidly invade the ventricle to produce syncytial activation of myocardial cells (Fig. 45.1). The signal then rapidly spreads throughout the ventricles using the His-Purkinje system, allowing a synchronized contraction. The movement of electrical activity between the various areas of the heart is also clearly associated with specific components of the electrocardiogram (ECG) as illustrated in Fig. 45.1.

When orderly propagation of the electrical signal is perturbed, the function of the heart may be adversely affected. Slowed electrical conduction through some cardiac regions, as occurs with first-degree heart block or bundle branch block in the ventricles, is generally well tolerated. Other abnormalities may lead to clinical symptoms, and in its most extreme form, cardiovascular collapse. Abnormalities in heart rhythm are called arrhythmias or dysrhythmias and may result in abnormally fast or slow heart rates. Options for the clinical management of

ABBREVIATIONS

ATP	Adenosine triphosphate
AV	Atrioventricular
CCB	Calcium-channel blocker
CNS	Central nervous system
ECG	Electrocardiogram
GI	Gastrointestinal
IV	Intravenous
NAPA	N-Acetylprocainamide
NE	Norepinephrine
SA	Sinoatrial
$t_{1/2}$	Half-life

arrhythmias have been rapidly expanding and include drugs, mechanical assist devices such as pacemakers and defibrillators, and transcatheter therapies such as radiofrequency ablation.

Currently available antiarrhythmic drugs work by one of two mechanisms. They either directly alter the function of ion channels that participate in a normal heartbeat, or they interfere with neuronal control of rate and/or conduction. Although antiarrhythmic drugs are intended to restore normal sinus rhythm, suppress initiation of abnormal rhythms, or both, their use is hampered by the potential risk for the development of new arrhythmias, which may be life-threatening. In the most famous example, the Cardiac Arrhythmia Suppression Trial (CAST) demonstrated that even though ventricular arrhythmias predictive of sudden death could be suppressed by Na^+-channel–blocking drugs (e.g., lidocaine), their use was associated with an increased incidence of sudden death.

Antiarrhythmic drugs are used for all types of tachycardias and are ineffective for long-term therapy of symptomatic bradycardia. Although mechanical therapies are preferred for many patients, drugs continue to be used as adjunctive therapy, and their complex interactions with these mechanical devices must be appreciated. A summary of the agents used for specific arrhythmias is presented in the Therapeutic Overview Box.

MECHANISMS OF ACTION

An understanding of the mechanisms by which antiarrhythmic drugs act requires an understanding of normal cardiac electrophysiology because many channels, pumps, and ion exchangers are targets for these drugs.

Cardiac Electrophysiology
Resting Membrane Potential
Cardiac myocytes, like other excitable cells, maintain a transmembrane electrical gradient, with the interior of the cell negative with respect to the exterior. This transmembrane potential is created by an unequal

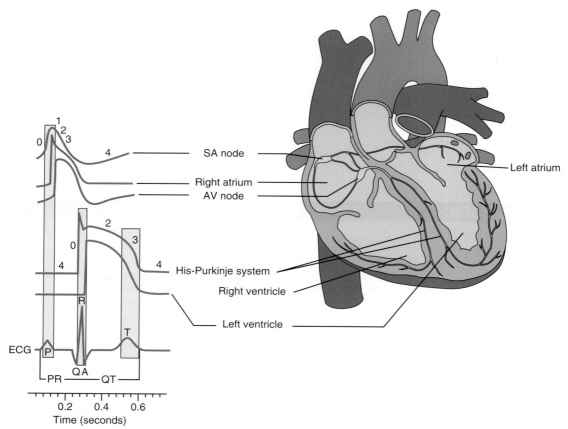

FIG. 45.1 The image of the heart depicts the atria and ventricles and electrical system, including the SA node where the impulse is initiated, the AV node that dampens the signal from the atria before it enters the ventricles, and the His-Purkinje network that transmits the impulse to the ventricles. The relationship of the electrical activity from specific areas of the heart to the coordinated activity monitored through the electrocardiogram (ECG) is also shown. The parameters that are identified (P wave/atrial depolarization, PR interval/passage from atrium to ventricle, and QT interval/depolarization and repolarization of the ventricle) are used to assess normal and abnormal electrical activity and the effect of antiarrhythmic drugs.

THERAPEUTIC OVERVIEW

Goal: To treat abnormal cardiac impulse formation or propagation
Effects: Modify ion fluxes, block Na⁺, K⁺, or Ca⁺⁺ channels; modify
β-adrenergic receptor–activated processes

Drug Action	Uses
Membrane stabilizers	Paroxysmal supraventricular tachycardia, atrial fibrillation or flutter, ventricular tachycardia; digoxin-induced arrhythmias
β-adrenergic receptor blockade	Paroxysmal supraventricular tachycardia, atrial or ventricular premature beats, atrial fibrillation or flutter
Prolong action potentials and repolarization	Ventricular tachycardia, atrial fibrillation or flutterᵃ
Ca⁺⁺-channel blockade	Paroxysmal supraventricular tachycardia, atrial fibrillation or flutter
Other	
Adenosine	Paroxysmal supraventricular tachycardia
Digitalis glycosides	Atrial fibrillation or flutter with increased ventricular rate

ᵃOnly amiodarone is widely used for all.

TABLE 45.1   Typical Ion Concentrations

Ion	Extracellular	Intracellular	Approximate Equilibrium Potential (mV)ᵃ
Na⁺	145 mM	10 mM	+50
K⁺	4 mM	140 mM	−90
Ca⁺⁺	2 mM	10⁻⁷ M	+140

ᵃCalculated from the Nernst equation.

distribution of ions between the intracellular and extracellular compartments (Table 45.1). Ions can permeate the sarcolemmal membrane only through selective channels or via pumps and exchangers that have selectivity for specific ion species. The resting potential is an active, energy-dependent process, relying on these channels, pumps, and exchangers and large intracellular immobile anionic proteins. Critical components include the Na⁺/K⁺-adenosine triphosphatase (ATPase) and the inwardly rectifying K⁺ channel (Iₖ). The Na⁺/K⁺-ATPase exchanges three Na⁺ ions from inside for two K⁺ ions outside the cell, resulting in a net outward flow of positive charge.

The unequal distribution of these ions across the membrane leads to both electrical and chemical forces causing ions to move into or out of the cell. If a membrane is permeable to only a single ion, then for that ion, there is an "equilibrium potential" at which there is no net driving force. This can be calculated using the Nernst equation:

$$E_x = RT/F \ln[X]_0/[X]_i \qquad \textbf{(Eq. 45.1)}$$

where R = the gas constant, T = absolute temperature, F = the Faraday constant, and X is the ion in question. Because the usual intracellular and extracellular concentrations of K^+ are 140 and 4 mM, respectively, its equilibrium potential is approximately −94 mV. At rest, the plasma membrane is nearly impermeable to Na^+ and Ca^{++} but highly permeable to K^+. Therefore the resting potential of most cardiac myocytes approaches the equilibrium potential for K^+ (−80 to −90 mV). However, the cellular membrane is a dynamic entity, with constantly changing permeability to various ions, leading to changes in membrane potential. The theoretical membrane potential at any given moment can be calculated based on knowledge of ion concentrations and permeability.

Action Potentials

The cardiac action potential of nonpacemaker cells is divided into five phases, as illustrated in Fig. 45.2. The injection of current into a

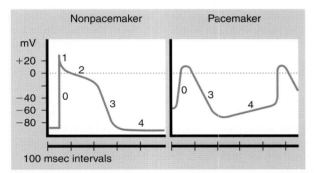

FIG. 45.2 Phases of the Cardiac Action Potential in a Nonpacemaker Cell *(Left)* Versus a Pacemaker Cell *(Right)*. Numbers refer to phases. **Nonpacemaker cell**: 0, rapid depolarization: 1, initial repolarization; 2, action potential plateau; 3, repolarization; 4, resting potential. **Pacemaker cell**: 0, rapid depolarization; 3, plateau and repolarization; 4, slow diastolic depolarization (pacemaker potential).

cardiac myocyte, or local current flow from an adjoining cell, causes the cell to depolarize (become less negative). If the membrane potential reaches a critical level (i.e., **threshold**), voltage-gated Na^+ channels open (Fig. 45.3). Electrochemical gradients allow Na^+ to permeate the cell, making the membrane potential less negative. During **phase 0**, there is **rapid depolarization** of the membrane potential, producing an action potential in which Na^+ influx is the dominant conductance, and the membrane potential approaches the equilibrium potential for Na^+ (+64 mV). However, Na^+ channels open for only a very short time and close quickly as they cycle into an **inactivated** state in which they are unable to open and participate in another action potential. Therefore if a significant percentage of Na^+ channels are in the inactivated state, the cell is refractory to further stimulation. The **maximal rate of depolarization** defines how fast electrical impulses can be passed from cell to cell, which determines conduction velocity. Slowing of conduction by inhibition of Na^+ channels is the basis for the action of **Class I antiarrhythmic drugs**. Action potentials in normal cardiac cells are referred to as **fast responses** because their rate of depolarization is extremely rapid as the membrane potential moves toward the sodium equilibrium potential.

However, in the specialized cells of the heart (e.g., **pacemaker cells**), like those in the SA and AV nodes and the specialized conducting tissues, the resting membrane potential is much less negative, and many Na^+ channels are inactivated and do not participate in initiation of the action potential. In these cells, phase 0 is mediated almost entirely by increased conductance of Ca^{++} through voltage-gated Ca^{++} channels. These "**slow**" action potentials exhibit a much slower rate of depolarization. These specialized cells do not display a true "resting" potential because the membrane spontaneously depolarizes, which permits the generation of electrical impulses and also speeds the conduction of electrical activity between the atrium and the ventricle.

The voltage and time dependence of currents through individual ion channels are unique. Na^+ channels open at more negative voltages than Ca^{++} channels, and ionic current kinetics are quite different. Physical structures, known as **activation** and **inactivation gates**, help regulate the flow of ions. These gates function to create Na^+ channels that exist in one of three distinct states during the cardiac action potential, as shown in Fig. 45.3. At normal resting potentials, most Na^+ channels are in a **resting** state, available for activation. Upon depolarization to

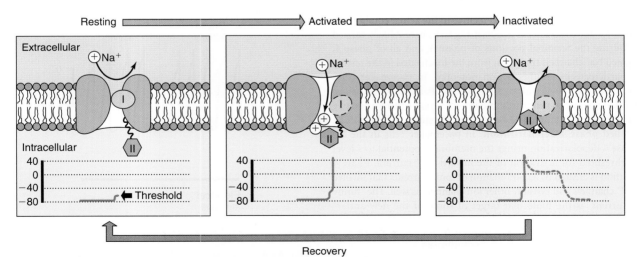

FIG. 45.3 Postulated Conformational Arrangements of Cardiac Na^+ Channels Compatible With the Concept of Resting, Activated, and Inactivated States. Transitions among resting, activated, and inactivated states are dependent only on membrane potential and time. Activation gate is shown as I and inactivation gate as II. Membrane potentials typical for each state are shown under each channel schema as a function of time.

threshold, most channels become activated, allowing Na⁺ to flow into the cell and causing a rapid depolarization. Na⁺ channels quickly become inactivated, limiting the time for Na⁺ entry to a few milliseconds or less. The inactivation threshold for sodium channels is also voltage dependent.

Near the end of phase 0, an overshoot of the action potential occurs. This is the most positive potential achieved and represents an abrupt transition between the end of depolarization and the onset of repolarization, known as phase 1, or initial rapid repolarization. This phase of initial repolarization is caused by two factors: inactivation of the inward Na⁺ current and activation of a transient outward current, which possesses both a K⁺ and Cl⁻ component.

Phase 2, or the plateau phase of the cardiac action potential, is one of its most distinguishing features of nonpacemaker cardiac cells. In contrast to action potentials in nerves and other cells (Chapter 27), the cardiac action potential has a relatively long duration of 200–500 msec, depending on the cell (Fig. 45.2). The plateau results from a voltage-dependent decrease in K⁺ conductance (through a channel known as the inward rectifier) and is maintained by the influx of Ca⁺⁺ through Ca⁺⁺ channels that inactivate slowly at more positive membrane potentials. During this phase, another outward K⁺ current, the delayed rectifier, is slowly activated, which nearly balances the maintained influx of Ca⁺⁺. As a result, there is only a small change in potential during the plateau because net current flow across the membrane is small.

As the plateau phase transitions to repolarization, the voltage-activated Ca⁺⁺ channels close, leaving the outward hyperpolarizing K⁺ current unopposed, known as phase 3 repolarization. The hyperpolarizing current during phase 3 is carried through three distinct K⁺ channels: the slowly activating delayed rectifier (I_{Ks}), the rapidly activating delayed rectifier (I_{Kr}), and the ultra-rapidly activating delayed rectifier (I_{Kur}). The importance of these currents to ventricular repolarization is underscored by the clinical significance of abnormalities of these channels. The potentially lethal long QT syndrome results from abnormalities in the ion channels responsible for repolarization, causing a delay in repolarization and producing an arrhythmic substrate in ventricles.

In normal cardiac cells, phase 4 is characterized by a return of the membrane to its resting potential. Atrial and ventricular myocytes maintain a constant resting potential awaiting the next depolarizing stimulus, established by a voltage-activated K⁺ channel, I_{K1}. The resting potential remains slightly depolarized relative to the actual equilibrium potential of K⁺ due to an inward depolarizing leak current likely carried by Na⁺. During the terminal portions of phase 3, and all of phase 4, voltage-gated Na⁺ channels transition from the inactivated to the resting state to participate in another action potential. In pacemaker cells, however, there is a slow depolarization during diastole, which brings the membrane potential near threshold for activation of a regenerative inward current, which initiates a new action potential (see Fig. 45.2). This is called phase 4 depolarization. In pacemaker cells in the SA node, phase 4 depolarization brings the membrane potential to a level near the threshold for activation of the inward Ca⁺⁺ current. Phase 4 depolarization is created by a combination of ionic currents that involve Na⁺ and K⁺ channels and possibly other ion channels as well. The "funny sodium current" is the molecular target of some of the new antiarrhythmic drugs (see New Developments).

Mechanisms Underlying Cardiac Arrhythmias

Arrhythmias result from disorders of impulse formation, conduction, or both. Several factors may contribute to the development of abnormal rhythms, such as ischemia with resulting pH and electrolyte abnormalities, excessive myocardial fiber stretch, excessive discharge of or sensitivity to autonomic transmitters, and exposure to chemicals or toxic substances. Disorders of impulse formation can involve either a change in pacemaker activity (e.g., sinus bradycardia or tachycardia) or the development of an ectopic pacemaker. Ectopic activity may arise as a consequence of the emergence of a latent pacemaker because many cells of the conduction system are capable of rhythmic spontaneous activity. Normally these latent pacemakers are prevented from spontaneously discharging because of the dominance of the rapidly firing SA node pacemaker cells. Under some conditions, however, they may become dominant because of abnormal slowing of SA node cells or abnormal acceleration of latent pacemaker cells. Such ectopic activity may also result from injury due to ischemia or hypoxia, causing depolarization. Two areas of cells with different membrane potentials may result in current flow between adjacent regions (injury current), which can depolarize normally quiescent tissue to a point where ectopic activity is initiated. Finally, development of oscillatory afterdepolarizations occurring between phase 2 and phase 3 (called early afterdepolarization) can initiate spontaneous activity in normally quiescent tissue. Other afterdepolarizations can occur at the end of phase 3 (Fig. 45.4) and, if large enough in amplitude, reach threshold and initiate a burst of spontaneous activity when the cell has returned to rest. This type of activity is termed delayed afterdepolarization and is thought to be due to intracellular Ca⁺⁺ accumulation. Toxic concentrations of digitalis or norepinephrine (NE) can initiate such effects. This mechanism has also been proposed to explain ventricular arrhythmias in patients with the long QT syndrome.

Disorders of impulse conduction can result in either bradycardia, such as the rhythm that develops with AV block, or tachycardia, such as when a reentrant circuit develops. Fig. 45.5 shows an example of a hypothetical reentrant circuit. For a reentrant circuit to develop, a region of unidirectional block must exist, and the conduction time around the alternative pathway must exceed the refractory period of the tissue adjacent to the block. Before the development of a unidirectional block (see Fig. 45.5A), impulse propagation initially branches as a result of the anatomical properties of the circuit. Some of these impulses collide and extinguish on the other side of the branch point. If an area of unidirectional block develops, impulses around the branch do not collide and become extinguished but may excite tissue and cells proximal

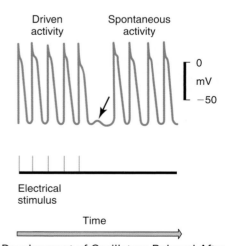

FIG. 45.4 Development of Oscillatory Delayed Afterdepolarization *(Arrow)* **That Leads to Use-Driven Spontaneous Activity, as Observed With Cardiac Glycosides.** First five action potentials were elicited by electrical stimuli *(bottom trace)*, followed by an afterdepolarization, which was subthreshold initially but attained threshold subsequently, leading to spontaneous discharges.

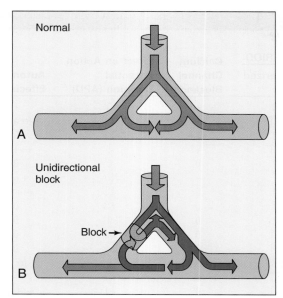

FIG. 45.5 Hypothetical Reentrant Circuit. *A,* Normally electrical excitation branches around the circuit and becomes extinguished due to collision of action potentials in their refractory period. *B,* An area of unidirectional block develops in one of the branches, allowing excitation of the blocked area by an impulse traveling from the opposite direction. This leads to reexcitation of adjacent tissue if it is not refractory, and reentrant activity will begin to propagate.

TABLE 45.2 Classification of Antiarrhythmic Agents

Class I (Na⁺-channel blockers)	Class II (β-adrenergic receptor blockers)	Class III (action potential–prolonging agents)	Class IV (CCBs)
IA	Propranolol	Bretylium	Verapamil
- Quinidine	Metoprolol	Amiodarone	Diltiazem
- Procainamide	Nadolol	Sotalol	
- Disopyramide	Atenolol	Dofetilide	
IB	Acebutolol	Ibutilide	
- Lidocaine	Pindolol		
- Phenytoin	Sotalol		
- Tocainide	Timolol		
- Mexiletine	Esmolol		
IC			
- Flecainide			
- Propafenone			

to the site of block, establishing a circular pathway for continuous reentry (see Fig. 45.5B). Clinical examples include AV reentrant tachycardia (Wolff-Parkinson-White syndrome), AV nodal tachycardia, atrial flutter, and incisional/scar (atrial or ventricular) tachycardia. A long reentry pathway, slow conduction, and a short effective refractory period all favor reentrant circuits.

Mechanisms of Action of Antiarrhythmic Drugs

Antiarrhythmic drugs affect normal cardiac function and therefore have the potential for many serious adverse effects. In the most dramatic example, antiarrhythmic drugs have the potential to actually be proarrhythmic. Therefore treatment of a tachycardia, which is a nuisance clinically but not life-threatening, may initiate a life-threatening ventricular arrhythmia—truly a case of the cure being worse than the disease. Such potentially serious side effects require vigilance to ensure proper dosing, proper serum levels, a thorough knowledge of drug-drug interactions, and close follow-up with the patient.

There is no universally accepted classification scheme for antiarrhythmic agents. The most commonly used scheme, the Vaughan-Williams classification, is based on the presumed primary mechanism of action of individual drugs (Table 45.2). This scheme classifies agents that stabilize the membrane through blockade of voltage-gated Na⁺ channels in Class I, those with sympathetic blocking actions in Class II, those that prolong action potential duration and refractoriness in Class III, and those with Ca⁺⁺-channel–blocking (CCB) properties in Class IV. However, while this is a simplistic and easily understandable classification, the actual classification is complicated by the fact that many drugs have multiple actions that span different classes. As shown in Table 45.3, these drugs often have effects on multiple targets. Although this scheme is useful in learning the properties of antiarrhythmic agents, all classifications are of limited use for treatment of arrhythmias because of their complex pathophysiology.

Class I Antiarrhythmic Agents: Membrane Stabilizers

Class I agents are subdivided into three groups based on their effects (Table 45.4). Class IA agents slow the rate of rise of phase 0 of the action potential (and slow conduction velocity) and prolong the ventricular refractory period, although they do not alter resting potential. They are also defined on the basis of recovery from drug-induced blockade and directly decrease the slope of phase 4 depolarization in pacemaker cells, especially those arising outside the SA node. Class IB drugs slow conduction and shorten the action potential in normal cardiac tissue. The IB agents preferentially act on depolarized myocardium, as they preferentially bind to Na⁺ channels in the inactivated state. Drugs in Class IC markedly depress the rate of rise of phase 0 of the action potential. They shorten the refractory period in Purkinje fibers, although not altering the refractory period in adjacent myocardium.

Class IA

Quinidine was one of the first antiarrhythmic agents used clinically. It has a wide spectrum of activity and has been used to treat both atrial and ventricular arrhythmias. However, its use has significantly diminished because of its high incidence of development of new arrhythmias and availability of newer and more effective agents. Quinidine shares most properties with quinine (Chapter 63). In addition to blocking voltage-gated Na⁺ channels, quinidine inhibits the delayed rectifier K⁺ channel. The effect of quinidine on the heart depends on the dose and level of parasympathetic input. A slight increase in heart rate is seen at low doses due to muscarinic cholinergic receptor blockade, whereas higher concentrations depress spontaneous diastolic depolarization in pacemaker cells, overcoming the anticholinergic actions and leading to a slowing of heart rate.

Quinidine administration results in a dose-dependent depression of responsiveness in atrial and ventricular muscle fibers. The maximum rate of phase 0 depolarization and its amplitude are depressed equally at all membrane potentials. Quinidine also decreases excitability, actions that are often referred to as local anesthetic or membrane-stabilizing properties. Quinidine prolongs repolarization in cardiac Purkinje fibers and ventricular muscle, resulting in a prolongation of action potential duration. An increased refractoriness known as post-repolarization refractoriness has been observed in which the inactivated drug-bound

TABLE 45.3   Antiarrhythmic Drug Actions[a]

Drug	Vaughn-Williams Class	SODIUM-CHANNEL BLOCKADE		EFFECT ON REFRACTORY PERIOD		Calcium-Channel Blockade	Effect on Action Potential Duration (APD)	Autonomic Effects
		Normal Cells	Depolarized Cells	Normal Cells	Depolarized Cells			
Adenosine	Other	0	0	0	0	+	0	+
Amiodarone	Multiple	+	+++	↑↑	↑↑	+	↓↓	+ (α and β)
Diltiazem	IV	0	0	0	0	+++	↓↓	0
Disopyramide	IA	+	+++	↑	↑↑	+	↓	++ (M₂)
Dofetilide	III	0	0		?	0	0	0
Dronedarone	Multiple	+	+	↑	↑	+	N/A	+ (β₁)
Esmolol	II	0	+	0	0	0	↓↓	+++ (β₁)
Flecainide	IC	+	+++	0	↑	0	↓↓	0
Ibutilide	III	0	0	↑	?	0	0	0
Lidocaine	IB	+	+++	↓	↑↑	0	↓↓	0
Mexiletine	IB	+	+++	0	↑↑	0	↓↓	0
Procainamide	IA	+	+++	↑	↑↑↑	0	↓	+ (α, M₂)
Propafenone	IC	+	++	↑	↑↑	+	↓↓	+
Propranolol	II	0	+	↓	↑↑	0	↓↓	+++ (β₁)
Quinidine	IA	+	++	↑	↑↑	0	↓↓	+ (α, M₂)
Sotalol	Multiple	0	0	↑↑	↑↑↑	0	↓↓	++
Verapamil	IV	0	+	0	↑	+++	↓↓	+

M₂, Cardiac muscarinic receptor blockade; *α and β*, α- and β-adrenergic receptor blockade.

TABLE 45.4   Differences Among Class I Antiarrhythmic Drugs

Class	Phase "0" Depression	Repolarization	Action Potential Duration
IA	Moderate	Prolonged	Increased
IB	Weak	Shortened	Decreased
IC	Strong	No effect	No effect

channels display a prolonged return to the resting state. The indirect anticholinergic properties of quinidine are not a factor in its actions on ventricular muscle and Purkinje fibers.

Procainamide, like quinidine, increases the effective refractory period and decreases conduction velocity in the atria, His-Purkinje system, and ventricles. Although having weaker anticholinergic actions than quinidine, it also has variable effects on the AV node. Procainamide increases the threshold for excitation in atrium and ventricle and slows phase 4 depolarization, a combination that decreases abnormal automaticity. Procainamide is used in the treatment of atrial arrhythmias, such as premature atrial contractions, paroxysmal atrial tachycardia, and atrial fibrillation of recent onset, in addition to being effective for most ventricular arrhythmias. Because of proarrhythmic risks, treatment should be limited to hemodynamically significant arrhythmias. Long-term therapy is complicated by the need for frequent dosing and side effects discussed below.

Disopyramide suppresses atrial and ventricular arrhythmias and has a longer duration of action than other drugs in its class. Although effective in treating atrial arrhythmias, disopyramide is only approved to treat ventricular arrhythmias in the United States. Despite prominent anticholinergic effects, disopyramide has a pronounced negative inotropic effect, which is so prominent it has been used in therapy of hypertrophic cardiomyopathy. The electrophysiological effects of disopyramide are nearly identical to those of quinidine and procainamide. However, its anticholinergic effects are far more prominent and limit its utility. Disopyramide blocks voltage-gated Na⁺ channels, thereby depressing action potentials. It also reduces conduction velocity and increases the refractory period in atria. Post-repolarization refractoriness does not occur. Interestingly, abnormal atrial automaticity may be abolished at concentrations of disopyramide that fail to alter conduction velocity or refractoriness. Conduction velocity slows, and the refractory period increases in the AV node via a direct action, which is offset to a variable degree by its anticholinergic actions. Action potential duration is prolonged, which results in an increase in refractory period of the His-Purkinje and ventricular muscle tissue. Slowed conduction in accessory pathways has been demonstrated. Like quinidine, the effect of disopyramide on conduction velocity depends on extracellular K⁺ concentrations. Hypokalemic patients may respond poorly to its antiarrhythmic action, whereas hyperkalemia may accentuate its actions.

Class IB

Lidocaine is a local anesthetic (Chapter 27) that has long been used to treat arrhythmias. Unlike quinidine, lidocaine rapidly blocks both activated and inactivated Na⁺ channels, though there is some preference for the inactivated state. Blockade of Na⁺ channels in the inactivated state leads to greater effects on myocytes with long action potentials, such as Purkinje and ventricular cells, compared with atrial cells. The rapid kinetics of lidocaine at normal resting potentials result in recovery from block between action potentials, with no effect on conduction velocity. In partially depolarized cells (such as those injured by ischemia or in cardiac glycoside toxicity), lidocaine significantly depresses membrane responsiveness, leading to conduction delay and block. Lidocaine also elevates the ventricular fibrillation threshold.

Mexiletine is a derivative of lidocaine that is orally active. Its actions and side effects are similar to those of lidocaine. As with other members of Class IB, mexiletine slows the maximal rate of depolarization of the cardiac action potential and exerts a negligible effect on repolarization. Mexiletine also blocks the Na^+ channel with rapid kinetics, making it more effective in control of rapid, as opposed to slow, ventricular tachyarrhythmias, and ineffective in treating atrial arrhythmias.

Phenytoin is an anticonvulsant (Chapter 21) that has been used as an antiarrhythmic agent for decades, though it is rarely used now for this purpose. Its actions are similar to those of lidocaine. It depresses membrane responsiveness in the ventricular myocardium and His-Purkinje system to a greater extent than in the atrium.

Class IC

Flecainide was initially developed as a local anesthetic and was subsequently found to have antiarrhythmic effects. Flecainide blocks Na^+ channels, causing slowing of conduction in all parts of the heart, most notably in the His-Purkinje system and ventricles. It has minor effects on repolarization. Flecainide also inhibits abnormal automaticity.

Propafenone also results in conduction slowing due to Na^+ channel blockade. Propafenone is also a weak β-adrenergic receptor antagonist (Class II) with a much lower potency than propranolol, as well as an L-type Ca^{++} channel blocker (Class IV).

Moricizine possesses actions that most closely resemble those of the Class IC agents. It is used to treat life-threatening ventricular arrhythmias. Moricizine reduces automaticity by altering the threshold and is effective against ectopic foci by virtue of its ability to reduce afterdepolarizations (an action that resembles that of Class IB agents). The slope of phase 0 is reduced, and an increase in PR and QRS intervals is observed (an action similar to the Class 1A agents). Of particular importance is the fact that moricizine does not possess negative inotropic activity.

Class II Antiarrhythmics: β-Adrenergic Receptor Antagonists

The antiarrhythmic properties of β-adrenergic receptor antagonists result primarily from blockade of myocardial $β_1$-adrenergic receptors, even though many of these agents also possess direct membrane-stabilizing effects at higher concentrations, which would lead to blockade of Na^+ channels. Propranolol is the prototypical β-adrenergic receptor blocker and, in addition to blocking $β_1$ receptors in the heart, also has direct membrane-stabilizing effects in the atrium, ventricle, and His-Purkinje system. It causes a slowing of SA nodal and ectopic pacemaker automaticity and decreases AV nodal conduction velocity by virtue of its ability to block intrinsic sympathetic activity. There is little change in action potential duration and refractoriness in the atrium, ventricle, or AV node. The β-adrenergic receptor antagonists currently used for arrhythmias (Table 45.2) may be differentiated by their pharmacokinetics, selectivity for $β_1$ receptors, lipophilicity, and intrinsic sympathomimetic effects. Esmolol is an important agent in this class because it has an extremely short duration of action, which makes it ideal for emergency management of sympathetically mediated arrhythmias. A more complete discussion of these drugs is provided in Chapter 12.

Class III Antiarrhythmics: Drugs That Prolong Action Potentials

Amiodarone is a Class III agent that prolongs action potentials as a result of blockade of several types of K^+ channels. However, amiodarone has an extremely complex spectrum of actions that likely contributes to the extensive use of this antiarrhythmic agent. Amiodarone also blocks both Na^+ and Ca^{++} channels (Class I and IV effects) and is a noncompetitive α- and β-adrenergic receptor antagonist (Class II effect). Due to its broad spectrum of actions, amiodarone is useful for both ventricular (for which it is approved) and supraventricular arrhythmias (e.g., atrial fibrillation),

and it is less likely to induce *torsades de pointes* than those agents that selectively block K^+ channels. Amiodarone decreases automaticity in the SA node and in ectopic pacemakers but does not affect automaticity in other parts of the heart. Conduction velocity in the AV node and the effective refractory period of the AV node are prolonged by virtue of the Ca^{++}-channel–blocking activity of the drug. Conduction velocity in the His-Purkinje system and the ventricle is slowed, and the ventricular fibrillation threshold is elevated. A metabolite, desethylamiodarone, also possesses antiarrhythmic activity that is due to K^+-channel blockade. Desethylamiodarone also binds to thyroid hormone receptors, leading to an inhibition of thyroid hormone gene expression. The acute effects of amiodarone administration also differ from the effects seen with chronic use, which may in part be explained by its complex pharmacokinetics and the creation of active metabolites.

Dronedarone is a structural analogue of amiodarone in which the iodine substitutions have been removed and a methanesulfonyl group added to the benzofuran ring. The molecule was developed in an effort to reduce the impact of amiodarone on thyroxine levels and to improve the pharmacokinetic profile. These alterations appear to have succeeded in that effort. Like amiodarone, dronedarone blocks multiple channels and is a β-adrenergic receptor–blocking agent. However, the success of dronedarone in treating arrhythmias does not parallel that of amiodarone, and the agent has a box warning against use in patients with acute decompensated or advanced (Class IV) heart failure.

Sotalol prolongs the action potential by inhibiting the delayed rectifier K^+ channel. Sotalol is available as either the isolated *d*-isomer or as the racemic *d,l*-mixture. In addition to its ability to prolong action potentials, *d,l*-sotalol is a nonselective β-adrenergic receptor antagonist (Class II effect) most evident at low doses, with the action potential prolonging the effects predominating at high doses. The *d*-isomer, which is a pure Class III agent, is devoid of β-adrenergic receptor antagonist activity and was thought to selectively block myocardial K^+ channels involved in initiating action potential repolarization. However, clinical development of *d*-sotalol was halted when it was shown to be associated with increased mortality in patients after infarction.

Ibutilide is structurally related to sotalol and, like other Class III agents, leads to action potential prolongation. However, in addition to blocking the delayed rectifier K^+ channel, ibutilide is unique because it activates a slow inward Na^+ channel, both of which act in concert to delay repolarization.

Dofetilide is a "pure" Class III agent that selectively blocks the rapid component of the delayed rectifier K^+ current (I_{Kr}). At clinically relevant concentrations, dofetilide does not affect any other K^+, Na^+, or Ca^{++} channels and has no antagonist action at adrenergic receptors. The increase in effective refractory period is observed in both atria and ventricles. Dofetilide is approved for use in atrial arrhythmias. Its effects are dependent on the concentration of extracellular K^+ and are exaggerated by hypokalemia, which is important in patients receiving diuretics. Conversely, hyperkalemia decreases its effects, which may limit its efficacy in conditions such as myocardial ischemia.

Bretylium is a unique Class III agent that was first introduced for the treatment of essential hypertension but was subsequently shown to suppress ventricular fibrillation associated with acute myocardial infarction. Bretylium selectively accumulates in sympathetic ganglia and postganglionic adrenergic neurons, where it inhibits NE release. Bretylium has been demonstrated experimentally to increase action potential duration and effective refractory period without changing heart rate.

Class IV Antiarrhythmics: Calcium-Channel Blockers

CCBs, represented by verapamil, diltiazem, and the dihydropyridines such as nifedipine, are used for the treatment of several cardiovascular disorders, including arrhythmias. However, only verapamil and diltiazem are used for the treatment of arrhythmias because the dihydropyridines possess some preference for vascular smooth muscle Ca^{++} channels. Verapamil and diltiazem slow the rate of AV conduction in patients with atrial fibrillation or slow ectopic atrial pacemakers. CCBs have also been used for treating idiopathic left ventricular tachycardia arising from the posterior fascicle. These agents and their use are discussed extensively in Chapter 40.

Nonclassified Antiarrhythmics

Adenosine is an endogenous nucleoside produced by the metabolism of adenosine triphosphate and is an agonist at adenosine A_1 receptors in the heart, which are G-protein–coupled receptors (G_i) that increase K^+ conductance and decrease Ca^{++} channel activity, leading to hyperpolarization. These receptors are located on myocytes in the atria and at the SA and AV nodes, and stimulation leads to hyperpolarization of the resting potential. Effects include a decrease in the slope of phase 4 spontaneous depolarizations and shortening of action potential duration. However, the effects are most dramatic in the AV node and result in transient conduction block leading to asystole. This effect terminates atrial tachycardias, which use the AV node as one limb of a reentrant circuit. There is no effect on the ventricular myocardium because this K^+ channel is not expressed in the ventricle.

Digoxin is discussed in detail in Chapter 44.

Magnesium is useful in patients with digitalis-induced arrhythmias if hypomagnesemia is present and is a drug of choice for patients with *torsades de pointes* even if magnesium levels are normal. The mechanism of action is not well established and could involve an interaction with Na^+, K^+-ATPase, and Na^+, K^+, or Ca^{++} channels.

Ivabradine and ranolazine are novel agents discussed in greater detail in New Developments. Ivabradine is a novel agent that selectively blocks the *funny* sodium channel specifically expressed in the SA node. It slows diastolic depolarization and reduces heart rate without a negative inotropic effect and without altering intracardiac conduction or ventricular repolarization. It also possesses antianginal activity in patients with coronary artery disease. Ranolazine blocks several species of ion channels.

RELATIONSHIP OF MECHANISMS OF ACTION TO CLINICAL RESPONSE

Class I Antiarrhythmics

Quinidine has potent anticholinergic properties that cause effects opposite to those due to its direct effects in parasympathetically innervated regions of the heart. After initial administration, there may be a small SA nodal tachycardia and an increase in AV nodal conduction velocity (decrease in PR interval) as a result of its indirect anticholinergic effects. These are usually followed by direct effects, including a decrease in heart rate and a slowing of AV nodal conduction velocity (increase in PR interval). At therapeutic concentrations, the QRS complex often shows slight widening as a result of a decrease in ventricular conduction velocity. The QT interval is lengthened because of the prolonged action potential in the ventricular myocardium.

Procainamide and disopyramide depress automaticity in SA nodal cells and ectopic pacemakers. Procainamide has much less of an anticholinergic effect than quinidine. Therefore its effects on heart rate and AV nodal conduction velocity are more direct and usually involve a decrease in heart rate and a slight prolongation of the PR interval. Disopyramide, however, has similar, if not more, potent anticholinergic properties than quinidine. Therefore it has the same indirect and direct effects on heart rate and AV conduction velocity as quinidine. When disopyramide is administered for the treatment of atrial flutter or

fibrillation, a digitalis glycoside will often be coadministered to minimize its anticholinergic properties. Procainamide and disopyramide block Na^+ channels and slightly prolong the QRS complex. However, the major metabolite of procainamide, *N*-acetylprocainamide (NAPA), is a potent Class III agent and prolongs the QT interval during oral therapy. Therefore a widening of the QRS complex and a lengthening of the QT interval are also observed after administration of these agents. Both compounds are broad-spectrum antiarrhythmics used to treat supraventricular and ventricular arrhythmias.

Lidocaine has little effect on automaticity within the SA node over a relatively large concentration range, and hence heart rate remains relatively normal. Conversely, lidocaine suppresses automaticity in ectopic ventricular pacemakers and Purkinje fibers. Shortening of the action potential and effective refractory period is possible and is more prominent in Purkinje fibers than in the ventricular myocardium. Lidocaine has little effect on AV nodal conduction and at therapeutic concentrations has minimal effect on the resting electrocardiogram. Lidocaine is used exclusively for ventricular arrhythmias, especially those associated with acute myocardial infarction. It has no efficacy in the treatment of supraventricular arrhythmia, such as atrial flutter or fibrillation. Lidocaine is also used for the treatment of digitalis-induced arrhythmias.

Phenytoin depresses the automaticity of both SA nodal cells and ectopic pacemakers. Though devoid of anticholinergic properties, it increases AV nodal conduction velocity by an unknown mechanism. Phenytoin results in small decreases in the PR and QT intervals on the electrocardiogram. Its use is limited to the management of postoperative arrhythmias and digitalis toxicity in pediatric patients.

Flecainide and propafenone depress SA nodal automaticity and slow AV nodal conduction. They may produce conduction block in patients with preexisting AV nodal conduction disturbances, and at therapeutic concentrations they prolong the PR and QRS intervals. Both drugs also cause conduction slowing in accessory pathways, contributing to their effectiveness in treating AV reentrant tachycardia. Drugs in Class IC should be used with extreme caution in patients with structural heart disease and anyone with concerns about myocardial ischemia.

Class II Antiarrhythmics

The β-adrenergic receptor blockers at therapeutic doses prolong the PR interval with occasional shortening of the QT interval. These drugs are reasonably efficacious in suppressing ventricular ectopic pacemakers and are first-line therapy for most supraventricular and ventricular arrhythmias. They decrease overall mortality rate after a myocardial infarction. Agents such as metoprolol and acebutolol (but not propranolol) have a greater selectivity for β_1 receptors than for β_2 receptors (Chapter 12). There are also differences between these compounds on cardiac channels and their intrinsic sympathomimetic activities. Esmolol, a short-acting agent, may be used for acute conversion or ventricular rate control.

Class III Antiarrhythmics

Amiodarone profoundly depresses SA nodal automaticity and ectopic pacemakers. Effects on the electrocardiogram include prolongation of the PR, QRS, and QT intervals. Amiodarone has become the most widely used agent because of its effectiveness in suppressing ventricular and supraventricular arrhythmias refractory to other drugs. However, its systemic toxicity and highly variable half-life ($t_{1/2}$) make it necessary to use extreme caution during therapy.

Dronedarone is approved by the United States Food and Drug Administration only for use in the treatment of atrial flutter and fibrillation. However, the drug increases the risk of death, stroke, and heart failure, leading to a box warning. The drug does not appear to be an effective replacement for amiodarone.

Sotalol is marketed as the racemic mixture. At low doses, its predominant antiarrhythmic effect results from β-adrenergic receptor blockade. At higher doses, its effects on K⁺ channels predominate, thereby increasing atrial and ventricular refractoriness. Sotalol prolongs repolarization and increases the QT interval. The risk for a drug-induced, potentially life-threatening ventricular arrhythmia (torsades de pointes) is 3%–5% and necessitates initiation of therapy in an inpatient setting. Like amiodarone, sotalol has a profound effect on SA node activity and can magnify SA node dysfunction. It is used in the treatment of supraventricular arrhythmias and ventricular arrhythmias but should be reserved for use in life-threatening arrhythmias only because of its high risk of ventricular proarrhythmias.

Ibutilide is used for conversion of atrial fibrillation or flutter. It is an alternative to electrical cardioversion and is effective in 60%–80% of patients. Like other QT-prolonging drugs, its use is associated with a relatively high incidence of torsades de pointes.

Bretylium is used in the emergency treatment of ventricular fibrillation.

Class IV Antiarrhythmics

CCBs are most effective in treating supraventricular arrhythmias, which involve reentry and may also be effective in treating arrhythmias resulting from enhanced automaticity. The ability of these drugs to slow AV nodal conduction velocity and refractoriness makes them useful for controlling ventricular rate. CCBs are rarely used to treat ventricular arrhythmias, although they may be effective for treating a form of idiopathic fascicular ventricular tachycardia.

Nonclassified Antiarrhythmics

Digoxin slows conduction velocity and increases the refractory period in the AV node. These actions are useful in the treatment of supraventricular tachycardias, such as atrial flutter and fibrillation, by slowing conduction through the AV node and helping control ventricular rate.

Adenosine is useful for terminating reentrant supraventricular tachycardias that involve the AV node, where it causes conduction block. Adenosine has a serum $t_{1/2}$ of approximately 5 seconds, limiting its clinical usefulness to bolus intravenous (IV) therapy.

PHARMACOKINETICS

The pharmacokinetics of the β-adrenergic receptor blockers are discussed in Chapter 12 and those of the CCBs in Chapter 40.

Quinidine is readily absorbed from the gastrointestinal (GI) tract. It is metabolized in the liver and excreted by the kidneys. Therefore both hepatic and renal functions must be assessed in patients to prevent the accumulation of toxic concentrations in plasma.

Procainamide is metabolized in the liver by acetylation to NAPA, which has Class III actions and a longer serum $t_{1/2}$ than procainamide. In the United States, approximately half of the population (90% of Asians) are homozygous for the N-acetyltransferase gene and are termed rapid acetylators (Chapter 4). These individuals have a higher concentration of plasma NAPA than procainamide at steady state. When its concentration exceeds 5 ng/mL, NAPA can contribute to the antiarrhythmic actions of procainamide because of its Class III actions that prolong repolarization. Concentrations greater than 20 ng/mL have been associated with adverse effects, including the life-threatening arrhythmia torsades de pointes.

Lidocaine is inactive when administered orally because of a high first-pass metabolism. It is therefore usually given by IV administration for acute treatment of ventricular cardiac arrhythmias. Because most of the drug is metabolized, liver function is important. The main route of metabolism is N-dealkylation, which produces metabolites with only mild antiarrhythmic activity but potent central nervous system (CNS) toxicity.

Mexiletine does not have a large first-pass effect, with a bioavailability in the range of 90%–100%. However, its $t_{1/2}$ is approximately 35% less in smokers than nonsmokers, likely due to induction of hepatic enzymes. Other inducers, such as barbiturates, phenytoin, and rifampin, also increase the metabolism of mexiletine. Antacids, cimetidine, and narcotic analgesics slow its absorption from the GI tract.

The long plasma $t_{1/2}$ of phenytoin shows considerable variation, which can be influenced markedly by drugs that alter hepatic microsomal drug metabolism.

Therapy with several antiarrhythmic drugs is complicated by the fact that they are predominantly metabolized by a specific cytochrome P450 that exhibits genetic polymorphisms, with a bimodal pattern of distribution in Caucasians. Seven percent of Caucasians (1% of Asians and African-Americans) are homozygous for mutations that result in low levels of, or no, active enzyme. These individuals, usually termed poor metabolizers, show a very slow elimination of many drugs, including several antiarrhythmics (e.g., flecainide, mexiletine, propafenone, disopyramide, metoprolol, and timolol). They also show greater β-adrenergic receptor blockade when given normal doses of β-adrenergic receptor antagonists. These patients also exhibit higher plasma concentrations of flecainide or mexiletine and exhibit greater Na⁺ channel blockade when given usual doses. Because these individuals are not identified routinely before initiation of therapy, all patients must be started at low doses.

The pharmacokinetics of amiodarone are extremely complex. When administered orally, it displays very low bioavailability (20%–50%). It is a highly lipid-soluble drug that is sequestered in tissues, which creates a very high volume of distribution (approximately 60 L/kg). It is also highly bound to plasma proteins, which leads to an extraordinarily variable $t_{1/2}$ (12–103 days). Due to its long $t_{1/2}$, drug therapy with amiodarone is usually initiated with a loading dose. It is metabolized by N-deethylation by cytochrome P450s (CYP3A4) to N-desethylamiodarone, which is biologically active. Serum concentrations of this potentially active metabolite are highly variable and may relate to the large variability in CYP3A4 activity among individuals. Due to its metabolism by CYP3A4, levels of amiodarone can be significantly modified in the presence of other inhibitors (e.g., cimetidine) or inducers (e.g., rifampin) of the enzyme. Furthermore, amiodarone can influence the plasma levels of a number of other agents due to inhibition of several other cytochrome P450 enzymes. Amiodarone is eliminated by biliary excretion with negligible excretion in urine. Amiodarone and its metabolite cross the placenta and appear in breastmilk.

Dronedarone, like amiodarone, is a substrate and an inhibitor of CYP3A, which limits the use of other agents that inhibit the enzyme, such as azole antifungal agents and protease inhibitors. Dronedarone is poorly absorbed following oral administration (4%), but absorption is increased in the presence of food, especially foods high in fat.

Ibutilide has a highly variable pharmacokinetic profile. Because of extensive first-pass metabolism, ibutilide must be given IV. It is progressively oxidized to yield eight metabolites, one of which has antiarrhythmic effects.

Dofetilide is available for either oral or IV use.

Adenosine is taken up by erythrocytes and vascular endothelial cells and metabolized to inosine and adenosine monophosphate. Hepatic and renal dysfunction do not affect its metabolism. Its actions are potentiated by nucleoside transport blockers, such as dipyridamole, and antagonized by methylxanthines, such as caffeine and theophylline.

TABLE 45.5   Selected Pharmacokinetic Parameters

Drug	Plasma Protein Bound (%)	$t_{1/2}$ (hrs unless noted)	Disposition	Therapeutic Serum Concentration (µg/mL)
Class IA				
Quinidine (O, IV)	80	5–7	M/R (50%)	2–5
Procainamide (O, IV)	15	2.5–5	M (20%)/R (50%)	4–10
Disopyramide (O)	35–65	4.5	M (30%)/R (50%)	2–5
Class IB				
Lidocaine (IV)	80	1–2	M (90%)/R (10%)	1–5
Mexiletine (O)	50–60	9–11	M/R (20%)[a]	0.5–2
Phenytoin (O, IV)	70–95	22	M (90%)/R	10–20
Class IC				
Flecainide (O)	40	13	M (60%)/R (30%)[a]	0.2–1
Propafenone (O)	–	2–32	M[a]	0.2–1
Class III				
Amiodarone (O, IV)	96	20–100 days	M/bile	1–2.5
Dronedarone	>98	26	M (extensive)	0.85–1.7
Sotalol (O)	0	10–15	R	1–4
Ibutilide (IV)	40	3–6	M/R	–
Dofetilide	60–70	7–10	M (minimal)/R	–

[a]Polymorphic metabolism. Class II and IV drugs are covered in Chapters 12 and 40, respectively.

IV, Intravenous; *M*, hepatic metabolism; *O*, oral; *R*, renal elimination as unchanged drug (% by this pathway if known); *RBCs*, metabolized by red blood cells.

Pharmacokinetic parameters of selected antiarrhythmic drugs are summarized in Table 45.5.

PHARMACOVIGILANCE: ADVERSE EFFECTS AND DRUG INTERACTIONS

Class I Antiarrhythmics

The use of quinidine is limited by adverse side effects that are generally dose related and reversible. Common effects include diarrhea, upper GI distress, and lightheadedness. The most worrisome side effects are related to cardiac toxicity and include AV and intraventricular conduction block, ventricular tachyarrhythmias, and depression of myocardial contractility. "Quinidine syncope" is a loss of consciousness resulting from ventricular tachycardia that may be fatal. This devastating side effect is more common in women and may occur at therapeutic or subtherapeutic concentrations. Quinidine is a potent inhibitor of CYP2D6 and CYP3A4 and interacts with many other drugs.

Procainamide administration may result in hypotension, AV or intraventricular block, ventricular tachyarrhythmias, and complete heart block. If severe depression of conduction (severe prolongation of the QRS interval) or repolarization (severe prolongation of the QT interval) occurs, the dose must be decreased or the drug discontinued. Long-term treatment is problematic because of induction of a lupus-like syndrome. Increased antinuclear antibody titers are present in greater than 80% of patients treated for more than 6 months, whereas 30% of patients develop a clinical lupus-like syndrome. Symptoms may disappear within a few days of cessation of therapy, although clinical tests remain positive for several months. Prolonged administration should be accompanied by hematological studies because agranulocytosis may occur. Procainamide has little potential to produce CNS toxicity.

The negative inotropic effects of disopyramide may precipitate heart failure in patients with or without preexisting depression of left ventricular function. Parasympatholytic effects, including urinary retention, dry mouth, blurred vision, constipation, and worsening of preexisting glaucoma (Chapter 8), may require discontinuation of therapy. Disopyramide should not be used in patients with uncompensated congestive heart failure, glaucoma, hypotension, urinary retention, and baseline prolonged QT interval.

Lidocaine does not have negative hemodynamic effects at therapeutic concentrations and is well tolerated, even in significant ventricular dysfunction. However, excessively rapid injection or high doses may cause asystole. Most toxic side effects are caused by its actions on the CNS and include drowsiness, tremor, nausea, hearing disturbances, slurred speech paresthesias, disorientation, and at high doses, psychosis, respiratory depression, and convulsions (Chapter 27).

Mexiletine and tocainamide have similar actions and side effects as lidocaine, but pharmacokinetic differences allow their oral use. At higher concentrations, mexiletine may produce reversible nausea and vomiting and CNS effects (dizziness/lightheadedness, tremor, nervousness, coordination difficulties, change in sleep habits, paresthesias/numbness, weakness, fatigue, tinnitus, and confusion/clouded sensorium). Most effects are manageable with downward dose titration. Mexiletine can inhibit ventricular escape rhythms and is contraindicated in the presence of preexisting second- or third-degree AV block, unless the patient has an indwelling pacemaker.

Phenytoin at high levels can produce adverse CNS effects, including vertigo, nystagmus, ataxia, tremors, slurring of speech, and sedation. Because of its long $t_{1/2}$ and the nonlinear relationship between dose and clearance, considerable variations in response to an oral dose are typical. Rapid IV administration may produce transient hypotension from peripheral vasodilation and direct negative inotropic effects (Chapter 21).

The side effects of flecainide include dizziness, blurred vision, headache, and nausea. Data from the Cardiac Arrhythmia Suppression

Trial suggest that all Class IC drugs carry an added proarrhythmic risk, and their use has been reserved for life-threatening arrhythmias, particularly in structural heart disease. Flecainide may also slow conduction in a reentrant circuit without terminating it. This may lead to accelerating the ventricular rate during atrial flutter because fewer atrial beats are blocked as a result of the slower cycle length, and it may also lead to converting a rapid but self-limited AV-reentrant (accessory pathway–mediated) tachycardia into a slower but persistent arrhythmia.

Propafenone may cause new or worsen existing arrhythmias. Similar to flecainide, most of the proarrhythmic events occur during the first week of therapy, although late events have been observed, suggesting that an increased risk is present throughout treatment. Agranulocytosis has been reported in patients receiving propafenone, though it is generally seen within the first 2 months of therapy and resolves upon discontinuation. Liver metabolism necessitates careful administration to patients with hepatic dysfunction. Also, a small segment of the population has a genetic abnormality of CYP2D6, which is responsible for the metabolism of propafenone.

Class II Antiarrhythmics

The β-adrenergic receptor antagonists should be used with caution when combined with other drugs that also slow AV nodal conduction velocity because their effects may be synergistic. These agents are generally contraindicated in patients with existing AV nodal conduction disturbances, congestive heart failure, or bronchial asthma. Their toxicity and side effects are described in Chapter 12.

Class III Antiarrhythmics

Amiodarone therapy is fraught with multiple complications, both cardiac and systemic, after IV or oral administration. Major side effects of IV administration include hypotension, heart block, and bradycardia. The most feared noncardiac complication is pulmonary fibrosis, which has an insidious onset and may occur as early as 7 weeks or as late as years after starting treatment. It is more frequent in patients receiving doses exceeding 400 mg/day but has been reported in a patient taking 200 mg/day. Close monitoring of pulmonary status is required during chronic amiodarone therapy because this is a potentially fatal condition that may not resolve with discontinuation. Other serious side effects include thyroid abnormalities, photosensitivity, rash, slate-blue skin discoloration, severe nausea, and chemical hepatitis. Although amiodarone prolongs the QT interval dramatically, the risk of *torsades de pointes* is relatively low compared with other Class III agents. Amiodarone magnifies any sinus node dysfunction and may require pacemaker placement if ongoing therapy is necessary. Dronedarone appears to negatively influence cardiac function and increases the risk of stroke, heart failure, and death, which has prompted a box warning against using it in patients with acute decompensated or advanced heart failure.

Sotalol has fewer systemic side effects than amiodarone but a higher incidence of ventricular arrhythmias. In patients with a history of ventricular tachycardia, the use of sotalol was associated with a 4% risk of *torsades de pointes*; the risk in patients with no history of ventricular arrhythmias was approximately 1%. Because of this risk, therapy should be initiated as an inpatient. Sotalol is contraindicated in patients with asthma as a consequence of its nonselective β-adrenergic receptor–blocking action. Sotalol exacerbates sinus node dysfunction and may aggravate second- and third-degree AV block with suppression of ectopic ventricular pacemakers. Therefore its use for patients with such conditions should be restricted unless a functioning pacemaker is present. Other contraindications include congenital or acquired long QT syndromes, cardiogenic shock, and uncontrolled congestive heart failure.

Dofetilide prolongs repolarization and the QT interval, which increases the risk of *torsades de pointes*. The risk of *torsades de pointes*

in patients treated for atrial fibrillation is 0.8%. Dofetilide should not be used in patients with a prolonged QT interval at baseline. A clinical trial evaluating the use of dofetilide in patients after myocardial infarction demonstrated no increased mortality, different from results from trials with sotalol, flecainide, and encainide.

Bretylium is not considered a first-choice antiarrhythmic agent because of its toxicity and side effects. It is primarily used to stabilize cardiac rhythm in patients with ventricular fibrillation or recurrent tachycardia resistant to other treatments. Its most severe side effect is persistent hypotension caused by peripheral vasodilation due to adrenergic nerve blockade. Also, catecholamine release can transiently enhance ectopic pacemaker activity and cause increases in myocardial O_2 consumption in patients with ischemic heart disease. Nausea and vomiting are also common side effects.

Nonclassified Antiarrhythmics

Adenosine leads to transient AV block, which is generally well tolerated. Prolonged AV block and asystole may be observed and can be quite dramatic when used for the first time. Adenosine shortens the refractory period of atrial myocytes, which may lead to initiation of atrial fibrillation. In patients with Wolff-Parkinson-White syndrome, this may result in rapid conduction across the accessory pathway, which is not blocked by adenosine, and ventricular fibrillation occurs. Adenosine may also trigger bronchospasm in patients with asthma, which may last up to 30 minutes. Heart transplantation patients have also been documented to have a prolonged effect from adenosine.

Major problems associated with the use of the antiarrhythmic agents are summarized in the Clinical Problems Box.

NEW DEVELOPMENTS

Antiarrhythmic therapy is changing rapidly. Increasingly, mechanical therapy via transcatheter methods such as radiofrequency ablation, or implanted devices such as pacemakers and defibrillators, are being used to control abnormal heart rhythms. Antiarrhythmic drug therapy is being used in conjunction with these therapies, and an appreciation of the interactions between drugs and devices is important. Antiarrhythmic drugs can dramatically affect the performance of implanted devices. Certain compounds may increase the amount of energy devices need to either pace or defibrillate the heart. Amiodarone, flecainide, lidocaine, propafenone, and mexiletine all lead to increased defibrillation thresholds, whereas sotalol and dofetilide cause them to decrease.

Two new drugs that have been introduced that are approved for use in other disorders but are also used for the management of cardiac arrhythmias are ivabradine and ranolazine. Ivabradine selectively blocks the funny sodium current (I_f) that is expressed only in the SA node. This current plays an important role in pacemaker activity and is therefore a logical target. Ivabradine blocks the open state of the current, much like Class IA and IC agents, and slows pacemaker activity by decreasing the slope of the diastolic depolarization. Unlike many agents that decrease cardiac rate, ivabradine does not produce a negative inotropic effect, nor does it modify conduction or ventricular repolarization. The agent has shown some efficacy in the management of angina through its ability to reduce rate without significantly modifying other characteristics of cardiac function. The drug appears to be well tolerated, with inappropriate sinus tachycardia being one uncommon adverse effect. Since I_f is involved in the retina, there have been some reports of visual disturbances. Ranolazine is approved for use in the management angina, but has clear antiarrhythmic properties that result from blockade of both Na^+ and K^+ currents. It elicits mixed effects on action potential duration and may be useful in patients with long QT syndrome, as it appears to shorten action potential duration and QT interval in an

CLINICAL PROBLEMS

Quinidine	Diarrhea, precipitates arrhythmias; *torsades de pointes*, elevates digoxin concentrations, vagolytic effects
Procainamide	Arrhythmias, granulocytopenia, fever, rash, lupus-like syndrome
Disopyramide	Precipitates congestive heart failure, anticholinergic effects
Lidocaine	CNS effects (dizziness, seizures), first-pass metabolism
Phenytoin	CNS effects, hypotension
Mexiletine	CNS effects
Flecainide	Negative inotropic effect, proarrhythmogenic, CNS side effects
Propafenone	CNS effects, proarrhythmogenic
β-adrenergic receptor blockers	Negative inotropic and chronotropic effects; precipitates congestive heart failure, AV conduction block
Amiodarone	Hypotension, pneumonitis, bradycardia; precipitates congestive heart failure, photosensitivity, thyroid abnormalities
Dronedarone	Increase in serum creatinine, increased risk of stroke and heart failure, increased risk of death
Sotalol	Modest negative inotropic and chronotropic effects, *torsades de pointes*
Dofetilide	*Torsades de pointes*
Ibutilide	*Torsades de pointes*
Bretylium	Hypotension, nausea
Verapamil	Hypotension, negative inotropic and chronotropic effects
Adenosine	Atrial fibrillation, bronchospasm, prolonged AV block, asystole, flushing

TRADE NAMES

In addition to generic and fixed-combination preparations, the following trade-named materials are some of the important compounds available in the United States.

Membrane Stabilizers
Disopyramide (Norpace, Norpace CR)
Flecainide (Tambocor)
Lidocaine (Xylocaine)
Mexiletine (Mexitil)
Procainamide (Pronestyl, Procan SR)
Propafenone (Rythmol)
Quinidine sulfate; quinidine gluconate
Quinidine polygalacturonate (Cardioquin)

β-Adrenergic Receptor Blockers
Acebutolol (Sectral)
Esmolol (Brevibloc)
Propranolol (Inderal)

Action Potential–Prolonging Agents
Amiodarone (Cordarone)
Dofetilide (Tikosyn)
Dronedarone (Multaq)
Ibutilide (Corvert)
Sotalol (Betapace)

Calcium-Channel Blockers
Diltiazem (Cardizem)
Verapamil (Calan, Isoptin)

Nonclassified Agents
Adenosine (Adenocard)
Magnesium sulfate

animal model of long QT syndrome. The mechanism of action in the treatment of angina is to switch the fuel preference of the heart from fatty acids to glucose by partial inhibition of fatty acid oxidase. The exact relationship between this enzyme inhibition and inhibition of Na^+ and K^+ currents is unclear.

All antiarrhythmic drugs interact either directly or indirectly with ion channels that participate in the normal action potential and therefore interfere with the normal function of the heart. Identification of ion channels that may participate only in pathological states would make ideal drug targets. One possibility is the ATP-gated K^+ channel. This is a large conductance K^+ channel in many tissues, including the heart, pancreas, and vasculature. It is normally tonically inhibited by physiological intracellular concentrations of ATP. When intracellular ATP falls and the ATP/ADP ratio is altered, the channel opens, leading to rapid repolarization and a shortened refractory period, predisposing the tissue to reentrant arrhythmias. The ability to block this channel, which does not participate in the normal action potential, is an attractive target. Similarly, the ultra-rapidly activating component of the inward rectifier K^+ channel (I_{Kur}) has been identified in the human atrium only and not the ventricles. If it were possible to target channels in the atrium, the risk of ventricular proarrhythmic activity would be abolished and make drug therapy much safer. Another potential molecular target that has recently emerged is the cystic fibrosis transmembrane conductance regulator (CFTR). The CFTR is a chloride channel whose genetic expression is altered in cystic fibrosis. The CFTR Cl^- channel has recently been identified in the heart, where it participates in modulating action

potential duration and membrane potential during sympathetic stimulation. The toxicities associated with this family of drugs would certainly support an increased emphasis in developing newer and safer agents with specific cardiac targets.

CLINICAL RELEVANCE FOR HEALTHCARE PROFESSIONALS

Physicians, physician assistants, and nurse practitioners who prescribe antiarrhythmic drugs should be well versed in the adverse effects of these agents. The potential for significant adverse effects with these agents requires referral to a cardiologist for appropriate therapy. For patients who currently receive an antiarrhythmic agent, the sympatholytic activity and potential for developing new arrhythmias must always be considered.

Physical therapists, occupational therapists, and other healthcare professionals working with patients being treated with antiarrhythmic drugs should also be aware of the major side effects associated with these agents. These agents have the potential to produce new and life-threatening arrhythmias in patients who are performing procedures that elevate sympathetic tone. In addition, many of the agents possess some ability to produce orthostatic hypotension, which interferes with a patient's ability to move from a sitting or supine position to standing. Patients receiving β-adrenoceptor–blocking agents may also display hypoglycemia during aerobic exercise, and the elevation in heart rate often used to assess the condition will be prevented in these patients. Cardiac output may be reduced in patients receiving one or more of several of the agents used as many of them possess significant negative inotropic activity.

Antiarrhythmic drugs pose a significant potential issue for dentists, since many of the drugs produce hematological problems that could cause excessive bleeding, especially in the oral cavity. In addition, transitioning from supine to upright is also a concern for dentists. Some agents (especially Class 1A) possess antimuscarinic activity, which causes dry mucous membranes and low saliva production, which can be problematic for individuals who work on the oral cavity.

SELF-ASSESSMENT QUESTIONS

1. Which electrophysiological actions does amiodarone possess?
   A. Class I.
   B. Class II.
   C. Class III.
   D. Class IV.
   E. All of the above.

2. During reperfusion following coronary artery bypass graft surgery, a patient develops a rapid and irregular supraventricular tachycardia, and the attending surgeon calls for an IV infusion of a short-duration β-adrenergic receptor blocker to achieve better rate control. The drug most likely is:
   A. Metoprolol.
   B. Sotalol.
   C. Esmolol.
   D. Propranolol.
   E. Carvedilol.

3. A patient with ventricular tachycardia is placed on a drug that dissociates very slowly from sodium channels and lengthens the QT interval. This drug is most likely:
   A. Flecainide.
   B. Lidocaine.
   C. Disopyramide.
   D. Mexiletine.
   E. Quinidine.

4. You have decided to use high-dose, intravenous amiodarone on a patient to treat her ventricular tachyarrhythmia. Of the following clinical variables, which should be monitored very closely in this patient throughout this intervention?
   A. Blood pressure.
   B. Pulse.
   C. PR interval.
   D. QT interval.
   E. Respirations.

5. A patient in the coronary care unit develops episodes of paroxysmal AV nodal reentrant tachycardia (PSVT). Which one of the following agents would generally be considered a first-line drug for promptly stopping the arrhythmia?
   A. Adenosine.
   B. Quinidine.
   C. Procainamide.
   D. Amiodarone.
   E. Propafenone.

FURTHER READING

Bengel P, Ahmad S, Sossalla S. Inhibition of late sodium current as an innovative antiarrhythmic strategy. *Curr Heart Fail Rep*. 2017;14(3): 179–186.

Jazwinska-Tarnawska E, Orzechowska-Juzwenko K, Niewinski P, et al. The influence of CYP2D6 polymorphism on the antiarrhythmic efficacy of propafenone in patients with paroxysmal atrial fibrillation during 3 months propafenone prophylactic treatment. *Int J Clin Pharmacol Ther*. 2001;39(7):288–292.

Patel PA, Ali N, Hogarth A, Tayebjee MH. Management strategies for atrial fibrillation. *J Roy Soc Med*. 2017;110(1):13–22.

WEBSITES

http://www.heart.org/HEARTORG/Conditions/Arrhythmia/PreventionTreatmentofArrhythmia/Medications-for-Arrhythmia_UCM_301990_Article.jsp#.WWUKhlGQyUk

This website is maintained by the American Heart Association and presents an overview of medications to treat arrhythmias and has links to other resources.

http://www.aafp.org/afp/2003/1201/p2189.html

This website from the American Family Physician has guidelines for the use of amiodarone.

Anticoagulant, Fibrinolytic, and Antiplatelet Agents

Frank Herrmann, Paul T. Kocis, Kelly D. Karpa, and Kent E. Vrana

---

MAJOR DRUG CLASSES

Anticoagulants
Antiplatelet drugs
Fibrinolytics

ABBREVIATIONS

aPTT	Activated partial thromboplastin time
DOAC	Direct oral anticoagulant
GP IIb/IIIa	Glycoprotein $\alpha_{IIb}\beta_{IIIa}$–integrin $\alpha_{IIb}\beta_{IIIa}$ receptor complex
INR	International normalized ratio
IV	Intravenous
LMWHs	Low-molecular-weight heparins
PAR-1	Protease-activated receptor-1
PT	Prothrombin time
$t_{1/2}$	Half-life
t-PA	Tissue plasminogen activator
TXA$_2$	Thromboxane A$_2$
u-PA	Urokinase plasminogen activator
vWF	von Willebrand factor

THERAPEUTIC OVERVIEW

Modification of the balance between coagulation and fibrinolysis, which is critical to prevent hemorrhage and thrombosis, is necessary and routine for many patients undergoing surgery or for the prevention and treatment of thromboembolic events and disease. The primary reasons for intervention are to inhibit blood coagulation; stimulate lysis of an already formed, but unwanted, thrombus; or inhibit platelet function.

Procedures such as orthopedic joint replacement and cardiopulmonary bypass, in which blood comes into contact with foreign materials, initiate coagulation and thrombus formation. In these settings, the prophylactic administration of anticoagulants diminishes unwanted thrombus formation. In situations where a thrombus has already formed, such as deep vein thrombosis, acute myocardial infarction, and pulmonary embolism, rapid activation of the fibrinolytic system to lyse the thrombus and initiation of anticoagulation therapy to minimize further clot formation are effective. In addition, for cardiovascular disease and stroke, clinical evidence supports the use of medications that inhibit platelet function.

Therapeutic uses of agents for preventing or lysing thrombi are summarized in the Therapeutic Overview Box.

MECHANISMS OF ACTION

The interactions among the coagulation, fibrinolytic, and platelet systems are summarized in Fig. 46.1. Endothelial cells in the blood vessel lumen normally present a nonthrombogenic surface. When the endothelium is damaged, two processes occur. Blood comes into contact with thrombogenic substances within the subendothelium that activate platelets, and the subendothelium tissue factor (a cell-surface glycoprotein that is normally shielded from the blood) is exposed to plasma factor VII that initiates coagulation (the extrinsic pathway). The coagulation process occurs by the sequential conversion of a series of inactive proteins into catalytically active proteases (Fig. 46.2). A catalytically active complex of tissue factor and plasma factor VII converts factor X to its enzymatically active form (Xa). In turn, factor Xa, in the presence of factor Va and a phospholipid surface (usually that of activated platelets), converts prothrombin to thrombin. Thrombin removes small peptides from fibrinogen, converting it to a fibrin monomer that spontaneously polymerizes to form a clot.

THERAPEUTIC OVERVIEW

Anticoagulation	
Unfractionated heparin, low-molecular-weight heparins (LMWHs), fondaparinux (heparin pentasaccharide), coumarin, direct thrombin inhibitors, factor Xa inhibitors	Arterial thrombosis, atrial fibrillation, cardiomyopathy, cerebral emboli, orthopedic surgery, vascular prostheses, heart valve disease, venous thromboembolism
Fibrinolysis	
Streptokinase, urokinase, tissue plasminogen activator and its derivatives	Acute myocardial infarction, deep venous thrombosis, pulmonary embolism
Platelet Aggregation Inhibition	
Aspirin	Cerebrovascular accident, stroke, coronary artery bypass surgery, coronary angioplasty/stenting or thrombolysis, myocardial infarction, transient ischemic attack
Clopidogrel, cangrelor, prasugrel, ticagrelor	Coronary artery disease, cerebrovascular accident, stroke, peripheral arterial disease, stents
Glycoprotein IIb/IIIa inhibitors	Acute coronary syndromes, coronary artery stent
Vorapaxar (PAR-1 antagonist)	Myocardial infarction, peripheral arterial disease
Phosphodiesterase inhibitors (dipyridamole, cilostazol)	Cardiac valve replacement, transient ischemic attack, ischemic stroke, intermittent claudication

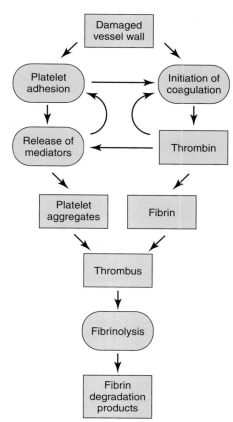

FIG. 46.1 Involvement of Thrombin and Platelets and Their Interaction in Thrombosis.

Fibrin is stabilized by factor XIIIa (transglutaminase) that introduces covalent bonds between fibrin molecules.

In addition to clotting fibrinogen, thrombin activates platelets and converts factors V and VIII to their active forms (Va and VIIIa). Factor VIIIa participates with activated platelets in the generation of factor Xa by an alternative route (the intrinsic pathway). This involves factor IX that is activated by the factor VIIa–tissue factor complex or by factor XIa. In vitro, upon contact of blood with a glass surface, the contact phase of coagulation involving factor XII, prekallikrein, and high-molecular-weight kininogen leads to activation of factor XI (the contact phase). The relevance of this pathway to initiation of coagulation in vivo is not clear because people with defects in these proteins seldom demonstrate excessive bleeding.

Most enzymes involved in coagulation are trypsin-like serine proteases with considerable homology. Plasma contains many inhibitors that regulate the coagulation cascade (Table 46.1). These proteins prevent inappropriate clotting and also prevent appropriate localized activation of the coagulation cascade from progressing to systemic coagulation. Anticoagulant medications function by either blocking thrombin formation or inhibiting the activity of thrombin after it is formed.

Parenteral Anticoagulants

Heparin is a linear polysaccharide with alternating residues of glucosamine and either glucuronic or iduronic acid (Fig. 46.3) derived from animal sources. The amino group of glucosamine is either acetylated or sulfated, and there is a variable degree of sulfation (≤40%) on the hydroxyl groups, rendering heparin a heterogeneous compound. Unfractionated heparin represents a collection of large and varied polysaccharides (molecular weight as high as 30 kDa, composed of well over a hundred sugar units) with limited bioavailability. Low-molecular-weight heparins (LMWHs) have an average size of approximately 5 kDa and have been size-selected to provide a more predictable pharmacokinetic profile.

Heparin acts by increasing the activity of antithrombin, a plasma glycoprotein that inhibits serine protease–clotting enzymes. Heparin binds to antithrombin, causing a conformational change that renders the reactive site on antithrombin more accessible to serine proteases, inactivating thrombin (factor IIa) and factors IXa and Xa (see Fig. 46.2); LMWHs inhibit mainly factor Xa. After the binding of antithrombin to thrombin, the heparin molecule is released and can bind to another antithrombin molecule. Although low doses of heparin act primarily by neutralizing factor Xa, at high doses it prevents thrombin-induced platelet activation and prolongs bleeding time. Although the heparin-antithrombin complex is a very efficient inhibitor of free thrombin, clot-bound thrombin is resistant to inhibition.

Fondaparinux is a synthetic pentasaccharide corresponding to the minimal five-residue active oligosaccharide of heparin required for anticoagulation. Fondaparinux binds to antithrombin and selectively catalyzes inactivation of factor Xa. Because of its short chain length, it does not promote thrombin inhibition, making it an antithrombin-dependent selective factor Xa inhibitor. Fondaparinux is used to prevent and treat deep venous thrombosis and does not affect platelet function.

Several other parenterally administered agents inhibit thrombin directly, including the hirudins, argatroban, and bivalirudin (see Fig. 46.2). Hirudin is a 65-amino-acid leech salivary gland protein that directly inhibits thrombin activity by blocking the active site of thrombin, as well as another site that mediates fibrinogen binding. Recombinant hirudins include desirudin and lepirudin, while analogues include bivalirudin. These compounds are used primarily in patients intolerant of heparin. Argatroban is a synthetic, direct-acting thrombin inhibitor derived from L-arginine that reversibly binds to the active site of thrombin. Argatroban is used as an alternative to the hirudin analogues.

Oral Anticoagulants

The oral anticoagulants, typified by warfarin and the coumarins (see Fig. 46.3), represent a very important class of agents whose action involves inhibition of vitamin K activity. A subset of blood coagulation factors (II, VII, IX, X) and anticoagulant proteins C and S are activated via the γ-carboxylation of several glutamic acid residues that mediate their Ca^{++}-dependent binding to phospholipid surfaces, critical for assembly of complexes necessary to generate thrombin. This activation requires vitamin K as a cofactor, and carboxylation of these vitamin K–dependent coagulation factors leads to the concomitant oxidation of vitamin K to its corresponding epoxide. The regeneration of vitamin K necessary to sustain the carboxylation reaction is mediated by vitamin K epoxide reductase, an enzyme inhibited by warfarin and the coumarins. Thus these epoxide reductase antagonists block recycling of the oxidized form of vitamin K to the reduced form required for cofactor function. Because these compounds inhibit the synthesis of clotting factors but have no direct effect on previously synthesized factors, plasma levels of preexisting vitamin K–dependent factors must decline before the anticoagulant effect of these agents becomes apparent, typically requiring several days. The first to decline is factor VII, followed by other factors with longer half-lives (Table 46.2).

Proteins C and S, which are also vitamin K dependent, inhibit excessive coagulation in the activated state. This mechanism involves the binding of thrombin to thrombomodulin, an endothelial cell-surface protein, which results in a different proteolytic specificity than free thrombin. In this state, thrombin does not cleave fibrinogen or activate platelets. Rather, it activates protein C, which, in combination with protein S,

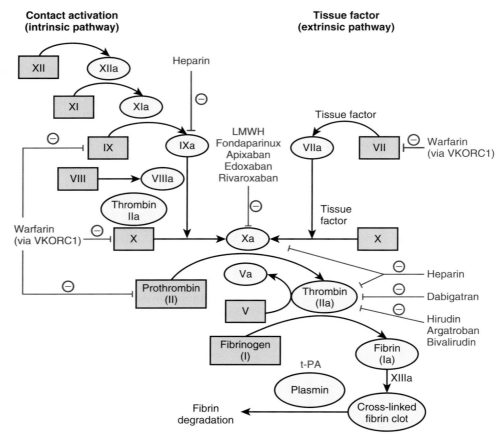

FIG. 46.2 A Simplified Model of the Coagulation Cascade Depicting Sites of Drug Action. Reactions fall into two pathways that occur preferentially on surfaces. The vascular subendothelium or nonvascular tissue provides the surface for the extrinsic pathway, while foreign surfaces, such as glass and collagen, activate the contact phase (intrinsic pathway). Activated platelets contribute to both pathways. In each, a multicomponent complex is assembled comprising an enzyme, its substrate (a proenzyme), and a cofactor. This complex affects conversion of proenzymes (rectangle) to their corresponding active forms (oval) at a rate thousands of times faster than that of the enzymes alone. Ultimately, thrombin cleaves two small peptides from fibrinogen, allowing its polymerization to fibrin. Thrombin also converts factor XIII to an active transglutaminase (XIIIa). This enzyme stabilizes fibrin by introducing Glu-Lys isopeptide bonds between adjacent fibrin molecules. Fibrin and fibrinogen are both substrates for the thrombolytic enzyme plasmin.

TABLE 46.1 Plasma Protease Inhibitors That Regulate Blood Coagulation and Fibrinolysis

Name	Principal Target
α_1-Protease inhibitor	Elastase
α_1-Antichymotrypsin	Cathepsin G_1
Antithrombin	Thrombin, Xa, IXa
α_2-Macroglobulin	Plasmin, kallikrein, and other proteases
C1 inhibitor	Complement, XIIa
α_2-Antiplasmin	Plasmin
Heparin cofactor II	Thrombin, Xa
Plasminogen activator inhibitor-1 (PAI-1)	t-PA, u-PA

proteolytically inactivates clotting factors Va and VIIIa (Fig. 46.4), thereby providing feedback inhibition to down regulate blood clotting after vascular injury. Genetic deficiency of protein C or protein S can cause thromboembolic disease.

Dabigatran, apixaban, edoxaban, and rivaroxaban are known as direct oral anticoagulants (DOACs), a nomenclature recommended by the Society for Thrombosis and Haemostasis. These compounds have simplified mechanisms of action compared to the complexities of the coumarin derivatives (warfarin) by acting on a single factor within the coagulation cascade and without the need for cofactors (see Fig. 46.2). Dabigatran is a synthetic, reversible, direct oral thrombin inhibitor that blocks the effects of free and clot-bound thrombin, preventing the formation of fibrin from fibrinogen, thereby decreasing thrombin-induced platelet aggregation. Apixaban, edoxaban, and rivaroxaban are factor Xa inhibitors. These agents bind directly and reversibly to

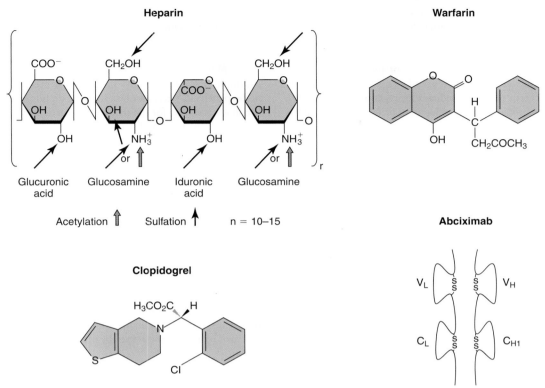

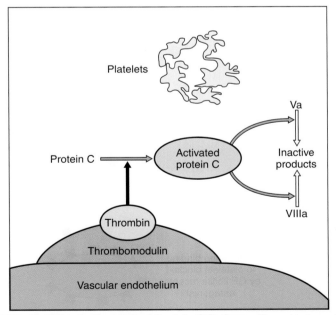

FIG. 46.3 Structures of Selected Anticoagulants. *Top left:* Structure of a repeating unit in heparin. There is considerable variation in the extent of sulfation of different hydroxyl groups. *Lower right:* Abciximab is a Fab fragment of a chimeric human-murine monoclonal antibody. The variable (V) and constant (C) regions of the light (L) and heavy (H1) chains are shown (note that this is a large recombinant protein). For comparison, both the small molecule structures for warfarin and clopidogrel are also shown.

TABLE 46.2 **Rates of Disappearance (Half-Lives) of Vitamin K–Dependent Proteins From Blood**	
Protein	**Time**
Coagulation Factors	
Factor VII	5 hours
Factor IX	15 hours
Factor X	1 day
Prothrombin	2–3 days
Anticoagulant Proteins	
Protein C	6 hours
Protein S	10 hours

the activated form of factor X (factor Xa) and inhibit both free and clot-bound factor Xa, as well as prothrombinase (factor Xa and factor Va complex) activity. As a consequence, thrombin production and activity decrease.

Antiplatelet Drugs

The activation and subsequent aggregation of platelets is a major component of arterial thrombosis and may be involved in initiation of venous thrombosis. Interaction of platelets with vessel wall collagen appears to be a key step. Disruption of platelet membrane phospholipids leads to the formation and release of **thromboxane A₂ (TXA₂)** from

FIG. 46.4 The Anticoagulant Protein C Pathway. Thrombin bound to thrombomodulin on the surface of vascular endothelial cells has a proteolytic selectivity different from that of free thrombin. Rather than cleaving fibrinogen, it cleaves protein C to activated protein C, which then cleaves factors Va and VIIIa to yield inactive products. This process is accelerated in the presence of protein S and platelets. Both protein C and protein S are vitamin K dependent and are affected by warfarin.

arachidonic acid (Chapter 29). TXA$_2$ is a potent aggregating agent and vasoconstrictor. Platelet activation also causes the secretion of adenosine diphosphate from storage granules. Both TXA$_2$ and adenosine diphosphate, which act through specific receptors, cause activation of integrin $\alpha_{IIb}\beta_{IIIa}$ receptors on the platelet surface that bind fibrinogen and other adhesive proteins, including **von Willebrand factor (vWF)**. Fibrinogen binding to its integrin receptor mediates aggregation, whereas vWF binding is involved primarily in the adhesion of platelets to extracellular matrices in the vessel wall. Thrombin, generated locally on the surface of activated platelets, greatly amplifies the response by causing further activation and mediator secretion (see Figs. 46.1 and 46.2). Although TXA$_2$, adenosine diphosphate, and thrombin all increase cytoplasmic Ca^{++}, the mechanism by which thrombin activates its receptor is unique. Thrombin cleaves the *N*-terminal sequence of its platelet receptor (PAR-1), forming a new *N*-terminus that serves as a "tethered ligand" and binds to and activates the receptor to induce transmembrane signaling. Platelet activation is inhibited by elevations of intracellular cyclic adenosine monophosphate (cAMP), and agents that increase this second messenger inhibit aggregation. The most active agent is **prostacyclin**, released by cells of the blood vessel wall (Chapter 29). Other mediators from endothelial cells may also contribute.

The major therapeutic approach to reducing platelet aggregation is through inhibition of cyclooxygenase. **Aspirin** irreversibly inhibits platelet cyclooxygenase by acetylating a serine residue near the active site of the enzyme, thereby blocking TXA$_2$ formation (Chapter 29). Aspirin also blocks the synthesis of the endogenous vasodilator and platelet inhibitor prostacyclin, although at standard doses, this prothrombotic effect is insignificant.

Clopidogrel (Fig. 46.3), which is a prodrug metabolized by cytochrome CYP2C19 to its active metabolite, irreversibly blocks activation of the platelet P2Y receptor by adenosine diphosphate. Clopidogrel has become a mainstay for the treatment of patients with coronary artery disease (Chapter 43) and is commonly administered to patients with peripheral arterial occlusive disease and cerebrovascular disease. It is routinely administered with aspirin, particularly to patients who have received coronary artery stents.

Dipyridamole is a phosphodiesterase inhibitor that blocks the uptake of adenosine into vascular and blood cells and stimulates prostacyclin synthesis, enhancing its platelet-inhibitory and vasodilatory actions. At therapeutic doses, dipyridamole does not prolong bleeding time or inhibit ex vivo platelet aggregation. **Aggrenox** is a combination antiplatelet agent consisting of dipyridamole and aspirin that is useful for the secondary prevention of stroke.

The fibrinogen cross-linking of platelets, which is the final common pathway of aggregation (Fig. 46.5), can be blocked by inhibitors of the **glycoprotein IIb/IIIa integrin αIIbβIIIa receptor complex (GP IIb/IIIa)**. The GP IIb/IIIa inhibitors, which include **abciximab**, **eptifibatide**, and **tirofiban**, are administered by intravenous (IV) infusion, primarily

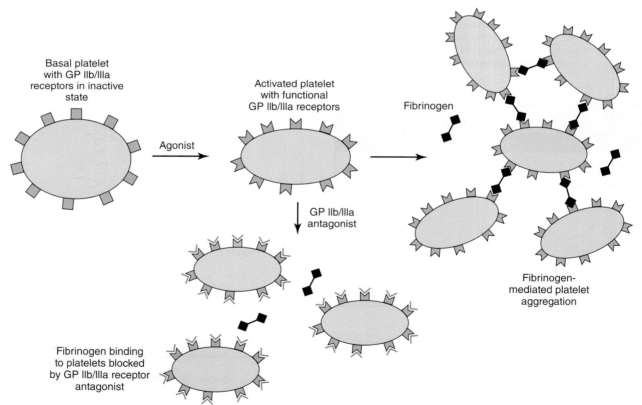

FIG. 46.5 Inhibition of Platelet Aggregation by Glycoprotein (GP) IIb/IIIa Receptor Antagonists. The GP IIb/IIIa receptors on unstimulated platelets exist in an inactive conformation that does not support fibrinogen binding. Activation of platelets by agonists, such as adenosine diphosphate (ADP), epinephrine, thrombin, and thromboxane A$_2$, converts the GP IIb/IIIa receptors to an active conformation capable of binding fibrinogen, which leads to the formation of platelet aggregates. Blocking GP IIb/IIIa receptors with antagonists, such as abciximab, eptifibatide, and tirofiban, prevents fibrinogen from cross-linking activated platelets, thereby inhibiting thrombus growth.

to prevent platelet-dependent thrombosis during the treatment of acute coronary artery syndromes and after implantation of intracoronary stents. Abciximab is the Fab fragment of a chimeric human-murine monoclonal antibody (see Fig. 46.3) that binds to both the GP IIb/IIIa receptor on platelets and the vitronectin receptor ($\alpha_V\beta_3$) on platelets, vascular endothelial cells, and vascular smooth muscle cells. Platelet function gradually recovers after abciximab infusion is stopped. Plasma drug levels fall quickly, though platelet-bound abciximab can be detected for up to 15 days. Eptifibatide is a cyclic heptapeptide containing six amino acids and one mercaptopropionyl (des-amino cysteinyl) residue. Inhibition of platelet aggregation by eptifibatide is reversible after the drug is stopped due to dissociation from the platelet surface. Tirofiban is a nonpeptide antagonist of the platelet GP IIb/IIIa receptor. Platelet inhibition after tirofiban is reversible after infusion is stopped.

Vorapaxar exhibits a unique antiplatelet mechanism by antagonizing PAR-1 on platelets, inhibiting thrombin-induced and thrombin receptor agonist peptide (TRAP)-induced platelet aggregation. While indicated in patients following myocardial infarction and with peripheral artery disease, it is contraindicated in patients with a history of stroke, transient ischemic attacks, or intracranial hemorrhage. Currently, vorapaxar is used in combination with aspirin and/or clopidogrel; it has not been used as a sole antiplatelet agent.

Fibrinolytics

Fibrin clots are lysed mainly through the proteolytic action of plasmin, the enzyme produced by the proteolytic activation of plasminogen by plasminogen activators (see Fig. 46.2 and Fig. 46.6). Plasmin formed by the action of plasminogen activators attacks not only fibrin but also several other proteins, including fibrinogen, factor V, and factor VIII. A minor aspect of clot lysis may result from the release of proteolytic enzymes, such as elastase, from leukocytes.

The two major classes of endogenous plasminogen activators are tissue plasminogen activator (t-PA) and urokinase plasminogen activator (u-PA). Recombinant forms of these proteins were originally used as clot-dissolving medications, but they are no longer commonly used in the United States. Rather, modified versions of t-PA that have deletions or mutations to prolong their half-lives ($t_{1/2}$), such as reteplase and tenecteplase, are primarily utilized.

Streptokinase, a protein produced by streptococci, is also used as a thrombolytic agent. Streptokinase complexes with and activates free plasminogen molecules to form plasmin. The recombinant forms of t-PA have advantages over streptokinase because of their selectivity in binding to the fibrin clot. In addition, streptokinase is also highly

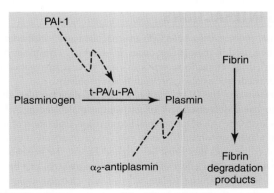

FIG. 46.6 Key Components of the Fibrinolytic System. *Dotted lines* depict inhibition of tissue plasminogen activator (t-PA) and urokinase plasminogen activator (u-PA) by plasminogen activator inhibitor-1 (PAI-1) and the inhibition of plasmin by α_2-antiplasmin.

immunogenic and cannot be used repeatedly; it is no longer readily available in the United States.

RELATIONSHIP OF MECHANISMS OF ACTION TO CLINICAL RESPONSE

Anticoagulants and Antiplatelet Drugs

Anticoagulant and antiplatelet compounds are commonly used to prevent thromboembolic disease. Heparin is effective for the prevention and treatment of venous thrombosis and pulmonary embolism. For prophylaxis, it is administered by subcutaneous injection once or twice daily at a dose that does not affect in vitro clotting times, as measured by the activated partial thromboplastin time (aPTT). A higher dose is required for the treatment of ongoing thrombotic processes. If unfractionated heparin is used, its anticoagulant effect must be monitored, such as by aPTT. The anticoagulant response varies significantly among patients with thromboembolic disease, and the risk of bleeding is increased as the dose increases. For this reason, the aPTT is used to monitor the degree of anticoagulation. Because of their shorter chain lengths, LMWHs have a greater affinity for inhibiting factor Xa than thrombin. Consequently, at standard clinical doses, they produce only a mild prolonging of the aPTT. Self-administered LMWHs can be used to provide full anticoagulation in the outpatient setting without monitoring. Because they are excreted from the blood by the kidneys, their dosing must be adjusted in patients with renal insufficiency.

Oral coumarin anticoagulants are effective for the primary and secondary prevention of arterial and venous thromboembolism. The one-stage prothrombin time (PT), a rapid test that permits assessment of the functional levels of five coagulation factors (fibrinogen, prothrombin, and factors V, VII, and X), is used to measure their anticoagulant effects. Because different clinical laboratories use different thromboplastins, a formula was developed to transform the PT, which is measured in seconds, to an index that allows comparison and standardization of results from different laboratories. This index, the international normalized ratio (INR), is used routinely to report PT results. Warfarin therapy prolongs the PT and increases the INR.

The DOACs are indicated for the primary and secondary prevention of thrombosis, as well as for the treatment of venous thromboembolism. The aPTT and PT will increase when these agents are utilized; however, the use of these tests is neither beneficial nor necessary in treatment. The only necessary form of clinical monitoring is renal function testing once or twice yearly. Platelet function can be assessed by measurement of bleeding time, which involves incising the forearm skin under standardized conditions and measuring the time required for bleeding to stop. Platelet aggregation in vitro can be monitored optically using an aggregometer.

If a patient has an acute thrombus or is at high risk of forming one within a few days, heparin or the LMWHs will be used because their antithrombotic effects are immediate, whereas that of warfarin is delayed. The rapid onset of action of the DOACs also provides a good alternative to the bridging of parenteral agents (heparin, LMWHs) to warfarin. If long-term anticoagulation is necessary, warfarin can be started as soon as therapeutic anticoagulation with heparin (or LMWHs) is achieved. After therapeutic anticoagulation with warfarin is achieved, heparin is often continued for 1–2 days. This overlap is commonly used because the antithrombotic effect of warfarin can lag behind laboratory measurements of warfarin anticoagulation. If warfarin is started for prophylaxis of thrombosis, and the short-term risk is not high (e.g., a patient with atrial fibrillation being started on warfarin to lower stroke risk), heparin may be unnecessary. Most experts recommend that loading doses of warfarin should not be used. That is, the patient should be started on the anticipated maintenance dose. During the first week of warfarin therapy, the coagulation response should be checked at least twice. Depending on the rapidity and stability of this measure, the time interval between subsequent determinations is gradually increased.

Clinical trials have shown that aspirin reduces the incidence of myocardial infarction and death from cardiac causes by 30%–50% in patients with unstable angina (Chapter 43). Aspirin also significantly reduces the incidence of a first myocardial infarction in men with stable angina and is effective as an antithrombotic agent after coronary angioplasty/stenting or bypass grafting. Aspirin is effective in the secondary prevention of myocardial infarction and is also recommended for use in patients with transient ischemic attacks. There are, of course, adverse effects of long-term aspirin therapy (Chapter 29).

PHARMACOKINETICS

The principal pharmacokinetic parameters and routes for administration of the anticoagulants, antiplatelet drugs, and fibrinolytics are driven by bioavailability. Heparin is administered by IV infusion or subcutaneously because it is large and not orally bioavailable and exhibits an immediate anticoagulant effect. Heparin is not bound to plasma albumin, and the $t_{1/2}$ of LMWHs is longer than that of the naturally occurring unfractionated compound. Thus LMWHs are effective when administered by subcutaneous injection once or twice daily. Due to different mechanisms of action, the anticoagulant effect of warfarin typically occurs within 3–7 days, whereas the direct oral anticoagulants act within 1–4 hours of oral administration.

The DOACs have predictable responses using fixed doses without coagulation monitoring. Absorption after oral administration is rapid but subject to the effects of the P-glycoprotein efflux system, the ATP-dependent drug transporter pump found in the small intestine. Metabolism occurs in the liver; however, the DOACs have reduced drug-drug interactions compared to warfarin because they are subject to a more limited impact by the cytochrome P450 enzyme system. Larger doses of rivaroxaban must be administered with food to maintain its high bioavailability. Because renal excretion is the major route of elimination for DOACs, dose reductions are necessary in patients with moderate kidney dysfunction; DOAC use is contraindicated in cases of severe kidney impairment.

Aspirin is hydrolyzed in plasma to salicylic acid, with a $t_{1/2}$ of 15–20 minutes, as discussed in Chapter 29. However, because aspirin is a covalent, irreversible inhibitor of cyclooxygenase, the antithrombotic effect of aspirin persists for at least 2 days for new platelets to form to restore TXA_2 concentrations; circulating platelets (lacking nuclei) cannot synthesize cyclooxygenase.

Reteplase and tenecteplase have a prolonged $t_{1/2}$, which enables them to be administered as a bolus rather than a continuous infusion to patients with acute myocardial infarction.

Warfarin is a racemic mixture with S-warfarin more potent than R-warfarin. The full anticoagulant effect of warfarin is typically reached within 4–7 days, with its efficacy and metabolism determined by genetic variants in *VKORC1* and *CYP2C9*. VKORC1 is a vitamin K epoxide reductase that converts vitamin K epoxide back to vitamin K. This rate-limiting enzyme in vitamin K cycling is inhibited by warfarin, leading to its anticoagulant effect. A *VKORC1* polymorphism accounts for approximately 25% of the variance in stabilized warfarin dosing and is the single greatest predictor of warfarin dosing. This single-nucleotide polymorphism (SNP) results in a guanine (G) being substituted with an adenine (A) at position −1639 (1639 nucleotides upstream of the transcription start site; reported as −1639G>A). The "A" allele expresses less VKORC1; consequently, less warfarin is required to inhibit this variant if one or two copies are carried by the patient.

The "A" allele is quite common, ranging from 90% in Asians to 40% in Caucasians to 14% in African-Americans.

S-warfarin is primarily metabolized in the liver by CYP2C9. The *CYP2C9* gene has more than 30 known genetic variant alleles. The normal *CYP2C9*1* allele (the wild-type or common gene variant) is classified as the normal metabolizer. The next most common variants, *CYP2C9*2* and *CYP2C9*3* (the "star 2" and "star 3" alleles), change single amino acids in the protein and impair the metabolism of S-warfarin by about 30%–40% and 80%–90%, respectively. Therefore less warfarin is required because it will be metabolized more slowly by *2 or *3. The *CYP2C9*2* variant is not very common (10%–20% in Caucasians, 1%–3% in Asians, and <6% in African-Americans). Similarly, the *3 allele is less than 10% in most populations and extremely rare in African-Americans.

When combined, *VKORC1* and *CYP2C9* variants affect the efficacy and metabolism of warfarin. Indeed, according to prescribing guidelines approved by the United States Food and Drug Administration, a patient with two copies of the *VKORC1 G>A* variant (lower *VKORC1* expression) and two copies of *CYP2C9*3* (slow metabolizer of warfarin) requires as little as one-tenth the amount of warfarin as a patient with wild-type alleles for these two genes. Because of genetic variations in metabolism, drug interactions, and differences in vitamin K intake, significant variations among individuals exist in the time required for a maximal effect and in the doses required for maintenance. Thus careful monitoring of PT is necessary.

Pharmacogenomics also affect the efficacy of clopidogrel, which is a thienopyridine prodrug metabolized by CYP2C19 to an active metabolite that irreversibly inhibits platelet aggregation. The *CYP2C19* genotype has been linked to clinical outcomes among clopidogrel-treated acute coronary syndrome (ACS) patients undergoing percutaneous coronary intervention (PCI). Patients are genotypically categorized as either ultrarapid metabolizer (UMs), extensive metabolizers (EMs), intermediate metabolizers (IMs), or poor metabolizers (PMs).

The UMs (*CYP2C19*17*, a gain-of-function variant) represent about 3%–21% of patients and leads to normal or enhanced platelet inhibition following clopidogrel. The EMs (*CYP2C19*1*, the normal allele) include about 35%–50% of patients and also exhibit normal platelet inhibition. In contrast, IMs *(CYP2C19*2)* have the most common loss-of-function variant and represent 15% of Caucasians and Africans and 29%–55% in Asians, while the PMs (*CYP2C19*3* through **8*) are rare (<1%), except for the *3 allele that occurs in 2%–9% of Asians. All IMs and PMs exhibit reduced platelet inhibition in response to clopidogrel because of insufficient conversion to its active metabolite.

PHARMACOVIGILANCE: ADVERSE EFFECTS AND DRUG INTERACTIONS

The major problem associated with anticoagulant and antiplatelet agents, even when used in therapeutic doses, is bleeding. Thrombocytopenia (heparin), drug interactions (warfarin), and platelet aggregation caused by other medications also pose significant problems.

Warfarin and the DOACs have similar bleeding profiles, although warfarin has a decreased risk of gastrointestinal bleeding, while the DOACs lessen the risk of intracranial hemorrhage. Utilization of multiple anticoagulants concomitantly, as in cases of coronary stent placement, poses bleeding risks that must be weighed against the benefits.

The anticoagulant effect of unfractionated heparin can be rapidly reversed with protamine sulfate, a positively charged molecule that binds avidly to the negatively charged heparin. Rapid reversal of the effect of warfarin can be achieved only by transfusion of plasma containing clotting factors or prothrombin complex concentrates (PCC). Oral or IV use of vitamin K_1 (phytonadione) also provides an antidote for

BOX 46.1 Drug Interactions With Warfarin

Decreased Anticoagulation

Increased warfarin metabolism by cytochrome P450: barbiturates, carbamazepine, griseofulvin, rifampin

Reduced warfarin absorption: cholestyramine

Increased Anticoagulation

Inhibition of warfarin clearance: disulfiram, amiodarone, metronidazole, sulfinpyrazone

Displacement of warfarin from plasma albumin: salicylates, chloral hydrate

Increased clearance of clotting factors: thyroid hormones

Functional Synergism

Inhibition of coagulation: heparin, thrombolytic agents

Inhibition of platelet function: aspirin and other nonsteroidal antiinflammatory medications, clopidogrel, glycoprotein IIb/IIIa inhibitors

patients who have been over-anticoagulated with warfarin. The monoclonal antibody fragment idarucizumab binds specifically to dabigatran and its metabolites, thus neutralizing its effects immediately after IV administration.

Transient thrombocytopenia is a well-recognized, usually asymptomatic complication of heparin therapy. Thrombocytopenia induced by heparin is generally considered clinically significant if the platelet count falls to less than 100×10^9/L. Heparin-induced thrombocytopenia can be mediated by immune and nonimmune mechanisms, with the immune form involving formation of complexes of heparin, platelet factor 4, and immunoglobulin. Its incidence ranges from 0.3%–3% in patients exposed to unfractionated heparin for greater than 4 days and is less common with the LMWHs than with unfractionated heparin. It is associated with arterial or venous thrombosis in a small but significant subset of patients and occasionally can be extremely serious and even fatal. Platelet counts should be monitored at regular intervals in patients receiving heparin for prolonged periods. When heparin is discontinued, the platelet count usually returns to normal within 4 days.

Heparin does not cross the placenta and does not produce untoward effects in the fetus, whereas warfarin crosses the placenta and is a teratogen. Characteristic abnormalities associated with warfarin embryopathy include nasal bridge deformities and abnormal bone formation. Fetal risk from warfarin exposure is greatest during weeks 6–12 of development. Any woman with a possibility to become pregnant should be advised of warfarin's potential teratogenic effects and instructed to contact her healthcare provider immediately if she believes that she may be pregnant.

Because warfarin treatment often extends over months or years, the possibility of drug-drug interactions due to alterations in plasma protein binding and renal elimination is high. Common warfarin-drug interactions are listed in Box 46.1. The long-term use of warfarin is also complicated by the need for routine INR laboratory monitoring and dosage adjustment, which is unnecessary with the use of fixed-dose DOACs. Drug interactions with DOACs are limited compared to the numerous interactions with warfarin. Warfarin is widely known for dietary interactions with foods containing high concentrations of vitamin K. While the DOACs have numerous benefits compared to the intricacies of warfarin therapy, the DOACs come at a significant economic cost compared to the much less expensive warfarin, an effective product first introduced in 1954.

Common adverse effects associated with the use of these compounds are shown in the Clinical Problems Box.

CLINICAL PROBLEMS

Heparin

Bleeding, thrombocytopenia, hypersensitivity, transient hypercoagulability when discontinued

Warfarin

Bleeding, drug interactions, some patients are resistant

Direct Oral Anticoagulants (DOACs)

Bleeding, contraindicated in patients with mechanical prosthetic valves

Streptokinase

Bleeding, immunogenic

Urokinase and Recombinant Tissue Plasminogen Activator

Bleeding, hypersensitivity reactions

Aspirin

Dose-dependent gastrointestinal upset, hypersensitivity reactions, Reye syndrome in children, exacerbation of gout

Platelet Inhibitors

Bleeding, rash, gastrointestinal disturbances

Glycoprotein IIB/IIIA Inhibitors

Bleeding, thrombocytopenia

Directly Acting Thrombin Inhibitors

Bleeding

Fondaparinux

Bleeding, thrombocytopenia

NEW DEVELOPMENTS

Although the fibrinolytics currently available for the treatment of stroke have yielded success with a limited number of patients, their narrow therapeutic window and frequent occurrence of side effects have led to concerted efforts to develop newer compounds with better benefit/risk ratios. The newer agents, such as reteplase, have both pharmacokinetic and pharmacodynamic advantages relative to t-PA, and newer developments offer hope for the future, particularly for those patients who do not reach a healthcare professional until hours after the stroke has occurred. Similarly, thrombolytics to treat acute myocardial infarction have their limitations, particularly as related to their ability to achieve complete reperfusion without significant bleeding. The new antiplatelet medications in combination with fibrinolytics and anticoagulants may yield faster lysis of clots and greater flow rates than using a single approach. Given the successes achieved with the DOACs, the development of improved versions continues. Currently, three new DOACs that may have improved pharmacokinetic profiles are in early clinical trials. Future work will focus on reversal agents for oral factor Xa inhibitors. Andexanet alfa (a modified factor Xa that binds to the Xa inhibitor with a higher affinity than factor Xa itself) is currently under investigation as an antidote to the factor Xa inhibitors and the LMWHs.

CLINICAL RELEVANCE FOR HEALTHCARE PROFESSIONALS

Many patients are prescribed anticoagulants as an addition to other types of therapies and interventions. One obvious concern for all healthcare professionals working with patients receiving anticoagulants is the potential risk for bleeding. Healthcare providers such as dentists need to ensure that patients receiving these medications are monitored closely. Therefore it is helpful to assess baseline clotting values prior to initiation of treatment, if possible. In addition, physical and occupational therapists may engage individual therapy sessions that involve aerobic or high-impact activities. Patients receiving anticoagulants are at risk for developing myalgia and arthralgia that could compromise the outcome of any given session and may not appear for 1–2 days after the session. Furthermore, these patients are at risk for significant bruising that could result from some activities. It is important for all healthcare professionals to be aware of these issues as well as potential drug-drug interactions. Last, to help prevent potential adverse events, genotype-guided dosing of both warfarin and clopidogrel should be used to improve treatment outcomes. Although this guided treatment approach has not been adopted universally, it is being used at many academic-associated institutions.

TRADE NAMES

In addition to generic and fixed-combination preparations, the following trade-named materials are available in the United States.

Anticoagulants
Heparin Na+ (Heparin Sodium)
Low-molecular-weight heparins
   Dalteparin (Fragmin)
   Enoxaparin (Lovenox)
Bivalirudin (Angiomax)
Dipyridamole (Persantine)
Fondaparinux (Arixtra)
Lepirudin (Refludan)
Warfarin Na+ (Coumadin)
Direct Oral Anticoagulants
   Apixaban (Eliquis)
   Dabigatran (Pradaxa)
   Edoxaban (Savaysa)
   Rivaroxaban (Xarelto)

Anticoagulation Reversal
Vitamin K_1, phytonadione (AquaMEPHYTON [inj.]; Mephyton [oral])

Fibrinolytics
Recombinant tissue plasminogen activator (Activase)
Reteplase (Retavase)
Streptokinase (Streptase, Kabikinase)
Tenecteplase (TNKase)
Urokinase (Abbokinase)

Platelet Function Inhibitors
Abciximab (ReoPro)
Cilostazol (Pletal)
Clopidogrel (Plavix)
Eptifibatide (Integrilin)
Prasugrel (Effient)
Ticagrelor (Brilinta)
Tirofiban (Aggrastat)
Vorapaxar (Zontivity)

SELF-ASSESSMENT QUESTIONS

1. Heparin:
   A. Has thrombolytic activity.
   B. Has most prolonged activity when given orally.
   C. Acts by binding to antithrombin.
   D. Inhibits the aggregation of platelets caused by TXA_2.
   E. Acts by blocking hepatic vitamin K regeneration.
2. Warfarin:
   A. Acts rapidly when given orally.
   B. Is potentiated by barbiturates.
   C. Is antagonized by protamine sulfate.
   D. Affects the activity of clotting factors.
   E. Is potentiated by platelet factor 4.
3. The risk of bleeding in patients receiving heparin is increased by aspirin because aspirin:
   A. Inhibits heparin anticoagulant activity.
   B. Inhibits platelet aggregation.
   C. Displaces heparin from plasma protein-binding sites.
   D. Inhibits prothrombin formation.
   E. Causes thrombocytopenia.

4. Aspirin can:
   A. Prevent the formation of TXA_2.
   B. Prolong whole blood clotting time.
   C. Shorten bleeding time.
   D. Inhibit fibrinolysis.
   E. Inhibit the effects of warfarin.
5. A 35-year-old female developed deep vein thrombosis (DVT) following an extended car trip and was taken to the emergency department. Which one of the following agents was administered upon her arrival?
   A. Abciximab.
   B. Heparin.
   C. Idarucizumab.
   D. Ticagrelor.
   E. Tissue plasminogen activator.

FURTHER READING

Ieko M, Naitoh S, Yoshida M, Takahashi N. Profiles of direct oral anticoagulants and clinical usage—dosage and dose regimen differences. *J Intensive Care.* 2016;4:19. doi:10.1186/s40560-016-0144-5.

Martínez-Sánchez P, Díez-Tejedor E, Fuentes B, et al. Systemic reperfusion therapy in acute ischemic stroke. *Cerebrovasc Dis.* 2007;24:143–152.

Massicotte A. A practice tool for the new oral anticoagulants. *Can Pharm J (Ott).* 2014;147:25–32.

McRae SJ, Ginsberg JS. New anticoagulants for venous thromboembolic disease. *Curr Opin Cardiol.* 2005;20:502–508.

Mukherjee D, Eagle KA. The use of antithrombotics for acute coronary syndromes in the emergency department: considerations and impact. *Prog Cardiovasc Dis.* 2007;50:167–180.

Rao PSS, Burkhart T. Advances in oral anticoagulation therapy – What's in the pipeline? *Blood Rev.* 2017;http://dx.doi.org/10.1016/j.blre.2017.02.002.

WEBSITES

https://ashp.org/Pharmacy-Practice/Resource-Centers/Anticoagulation
This site is maintained by the American Society of Health-System Pharmacists and has an excellent description of the use of agents in both ambulatory and acute settings.

http://www.aafp.org/afp/2013/0415/p556.html
This site from the American Association of Family Physicians provides guidelines for outpatient anticoagulation.

https://www.acc.org/clinical-topics/anticoagulation-management#sort=%40fwhatstrendingscore86069%20descending
This site is maintained by the American College of Cardiology and has links to numerous resources.

47

Drug Therapy for Hemophilia and the Deficiency Anemias

David A. Taylor and Pamela Potter

THERAPEUTIC OVERVIEW

Hemophilia

Hemophilia is a rare genetic disorder that occurs almost exclusively in males and is characterized by a decrease in the ability of blood to clot normally. The majority of cases are inherited through a defective maternal gene, with only about 30% of cases attributed to spontaneous gene mutations. Individuals with hemophilia have a deficiency in the intrinsic pathway for blood coagulation (Chapter 46, Fig. 46.2). Hemophilia A is due to a deficiency in the activated form of factor VIII, while hemophilia B is attributed to a deficiency in the activated form of factor IX, both of which lead to impaired fibrin production. Platelet aggregation is unaffected.

The magnitude of impairment is a function of the nature of the mutation, which leads to different degrees of hemophilia ranging from mild to severe. The severe form of hemophilia is most prevalent in individuals with hemophilia A, with nearly 60% of patients exhibiting serious bleeding tendencies, particularly in the joints (most often the knees, but also in the elbows, ankles, shoulders, and hips) and soft tissues, including muscle. These individuals can experience life-threatening hemorrhage in response to very minor trauma. In patients with hemophilia B, severe bleeding occurs in less than 50% of the patients.

The primary approach to treating hemophilia is replacement therapy with the appropriate factor. For some patients with mild hemophilia A, bleeding tendencies can be reduced by treatment with desmopressin, a drug that promotes the release of factor VIII from the vascular endothelium. In cases where additional clotting might be required, antifibrinolytic agents (i.e., drugs that inhibit the breakdown of fibrin) can be used as adjunctive therapy.

Anemias

Anemia, which is the most common blood condition in the United States, is defined as a decrease in the number, size, or hemoglobin content of red blood cells (RBCs), resulting in a decrease in the oxygen-carrying capacity of the blood and leading to extreme fatigue and weakness, pale skin with cold extremities, dizziness, exercise intolerance, shortness of breath, and tachycardia.

Iron deficiency anemia is the most common type of anemia worldwide, and it is estimated that approximately 5% of the United States population is iron deficient. Iron deficiency anemia is characterized by reduced hemoglobin synthesis and microcytic and hypochromic RBCs. The most common causes of iron deficiency anemia include chronic blood loss from gastrointestinal (GI) or uterine origins, a lack of dietary iron, an inability to absorb iron, and pregnancy-associated blood volume expansion and increased fetal RBC synthesis. In addition, premature or low-birth-weight infants may not get enough iron in their formula or breastmilk, and children may be at risk during growth spurts.

Megaloblastic macrocytic anemia most often results from deficiencies of vitamin B_{12} or folate. An inadequate absorption of vitamin B_{12} may occur in older people and in individuals treated chronically with proton pump inhibitors. Efficient absorption of vitamin B_{12} requires the presence of intrinsic factor, which is a substance secreted by the parietal cells of the stomach. Vitamin B_{12} is complexed with intrinsic factor and delivered to the ileum, where it interacts with specific receptors that enable the complex to be absorbed by cells in the intestinal wall. The absence of intrinsic factor leads to significant reductions in vitamin B_{12} absorption and results in pernicious anemia, characterized by large ovoid RBCs. Symptoms of megaloblastic macrocytic anemia attributed to vitamin B_{12} deficiency include memory loss and paresthesia.

Folic acid deficiency may occur in individuals who abuse alcohol, have hepatic disease or malabsorption syndromes, or who are on renal dialysis. Folic acid deficiency can also result from a lack of dietary intake; some drugs, in particular, methotrexate, trimethoprim, pyrimethamine, and phenytoin; and pregnancy, which increases the need for folate. A deficiency in folic acid during this time is a major cause of neural tube defects in developing fetuses. In contrast to the symptoms of anemia as a consequence of vitamin B_{12} deficiency, anemia due to a folate deficiency is not accompanied by neurological abnormalities.

Anemia may also occur in patients with chronic kidney failure due to decreased EPO production or may be drug induced following treatment for human immunodeficiency and other viral diseases, especially following the use of zidovudine and ribavirin, and from cancer chemotherapy. Drug-induced anemia and that associated with kidney disease are treated with erythropoietin or erythropoietin stimulating agents (ESAs).

Treatment involves vitamin or folic acid supplementation or correction of the underlying cause. Agents used for the treatment of hemophilias and specific anemias are presented in the Therapeutic Overview Box.

MECHANISMS OF ACTION

Antihemophilic Agents

The cofactors that need to be replaced in the treatment of hemophilia are part of the intrinsic clotting cascade described in Chapter 46. There are some specific agents used in hemophiliac patients that have mechanisms of action that are slightly different but are still intimately involved in the process of blood clotting.

Factor VIII and IX Concentrates and Releasers

Factor VIII or factor IX concentrates replace the deficient factor, depending upon the form of hemophilia expressed in the patient. These factors may be derived from human plasma or may be genetically engineered using DNA technology.

Desmopressin is an analogue of antidiuretic hormone that stimulates the release of factor VIII from vascular endothelial cells, leading to increases in the circulating levels of factor VIII. It can also be used to stop episodes of trauma-induced bleeding.

Antifibrinolytic Agents

The antifibrinolytic agents (aminocaproic acid and tranexamic acid) interfere with the normal process by which fibrin is broken down. Specifically, the drugs prevent the formation of plasmin from its precursor, plasminogen. Plasmin is responsible for dissolving the fibrin meshwork in a clot, which permits the clot to dissolve (Chapter 46, Fig. 46.2). Inhibition of plasmin production prolongs the length of time that the clot exists.

Agents for Deficiency Anemias

Iron

Iron is a mineral that is an essential part of heme proteins including hemoglobin and myoglobin, as well as cytochrome P450. It is also a vital part of many metalloproteins such as ferritin and serves as a cofactor for many reactions such as those involving catalases and lipoxygenases.

Nearly 80% of the iron in the body is present in hemoglobin; thus it is not surprising that nutritional deficiency of iron can lead to dysfunction of the oxygen-carrying capacity of RBCs. Iron needed for hemoglobin synthesis is provided by the catabolism of hemoglobin and from dietary sources. Iron absorption and recycling in response to the need for hemoglobin is regulated by the peptide hepcidin, which is produced

by the liver. Dietary iron in the form of heme is found in meats and fish, while nonheme iron is in plants and other foods. Nonheme iron must be reduced from the ferric (Fe^{3+}) to the ferrous (Fe^{2+}) form to be absorbed by the gastrointestinal (GI) microvilli via the divalent metal transporter 1 (DMT1). Heme iron can be absorbed directly into the cytoplasm by the heme carrier protein (HCP1) or can be taken up into intestinal enterocytes via receptor-mediated endocytosis. The absorbed iron, and that liberated from heme, is oxidized to Fe^{3+} in epithelial cells and transported into the blood via the ferroportin transmembrane protein or stored as ferritin in a complex with apoferritin. Once iron enters the blood, it binds to transferrin and is transported to either erythrocyte precursor cells in the bone marrow for hemoglobin synthesis or to the liver for storage. The total body iron content is carefully regulated by uptake such that when iron levels are high uptake decreases, and when iron levels are low, uptake increases.

Vitamin B$_{12}$ and Folic Acid

Vitamin B$_{12}$ is essential for the synthesis of both methionine and tetrahydrofolate, providing methyl groups for protein and DNA synthesis, while folic acid plays a major role in the synthesis, repair, and methylation of DNA. As shown in Fig. 47.1, vitamin B$_{12}$ is a cofactor in the conversion of homocysteine to methionine, transferring a methyl group from N^5-methyltetrahydrofolate to homocysteine, converting N^5-methyltetrahydrofolate, a major storage form of dietary folate, to tetrahydrofolate (THF) in the folic acid cycle. These reactions lead to the formation of deoxythymidine monophosphate (dTMP) from deoxyuridine monophosphate (dUMP), a necessary step in DNA synthesis. Thus both vitamin B$_{12}$ and folate are essential nutrients. Vitamin B$_{12}$ is also known as cobalamin, and cyanocobalamin is a synthetic form of vitamin B$_{12}$.

RELATIONSHIP OF MECHANISMS OF ACTION TO CLINICAL RESPONSE

Antihemophilic Agents

The management of hemophilia depends upon the type and magnitude of the disorder. In patients with hemophilia type A, treatment involves factor VIII replacement, while for patients with hemophilia type B, factor IX is replaced. As indicated in Table 47.1, both factor concentrates are available in two formulations based upon their derivation. Recombinant preparations are produced in cell culture, are very safe, and considered to be the agents of choice. The treatment schedule follows one of two courses depending on the need. Prophylactic treatment is used to maintain plasma factor VIII levels above 1% of normal in patients who have the severe form of the disease to reduce or prevent joint disease and is continued indefinitely. Secondary prophylaxis is employed for defined periods of time to manage bleeding that has continued for a short period, and individuals need regular treatments. The second primary form of treatment is "on-demand" therapy, which is short-term treatment of active bleeding.

Desmopressin is useful only in hemophilia A because it causes the release of factor VIII from endothelial cells. The absence of any release of factor IX makes desmopressin ineffective in hemophilia B.

The use of the antifibrinolytic agents aminocaproic acid and tranexamic acid is limited to special circumstances where additional clotting is needed (e.g., tooth extractions). When used as a liquid, these agents inhibit an enzyme in the saliva that lyses clots.

Agents for Deficiency Anemias

Iron is used either by itself or as a supplement to erythropoietin stimulating agents (Chapter 70) for the treatment of iron deficiency anemia. Oral iron therapy often corrects the anemia within 1–2 months if there

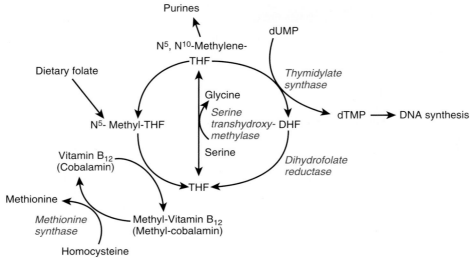

FIG. 47.1 The Roles of Vitamin B$_{12}$ and Folic Acid in DNA Synthesis. Abbreviations: *dTMP*, Deoxythymidine monophosphate; *dUMP*, deoxyuridine monophosphate, *THF*, tetrahydrofolate.

TABLE 47.1   Summary of Factor VIII and IX Concentrates

Preparation	Factor VIII	Factor IX
Recombinant Formulations		
First generation	Recombinate	
Second generation	Helixate FS, Kogenate FS	
Third generation	Advate, Xyntha	BeneFix
Plasma-Derived Preparations		
Ultrapure	Hemofil-M, Monoclate-P, Wilate[b,c]	AlphaNine SD, Bebulin VH,[a] Mononine, Profilnine SD[a]
Intermediate and high purity	Alphanate,[b] Koate-DVI,[b] Humate-P[b]	

[a]Contains factors II, VII, and X, in addition to factor IX.
[b]Contains von Willebrand factor in addition to factor VIII.
[c]Approved only for von Willebrand disease.

is sufficient GI absorption. If not, or if higher amounts of iron are needed, iron can be administered parenterally. The duration of treatment is governed by the rate of recovery of hemoglobin and the need to restore iron stores in the body, which can take 3–6 months. If the iron deficiency is a result of acute bleeding, treatment may be shorter. Some patients with chronic iron deficiency may need continuous low-dose treatment. The preparation of choice is oral ferrous sulfate.

Microcytic anemia, characterized by a decrease in erythrocyte mean cell volume and hemoglobin concentration, is also treated with iron supplementation. Causes of iron deficiency include inadequate levels of iron in the diet, especially during certain life stages in which iron needs are increased, such as infancy, growth spurts in children, menarche, pregnancy, and lactation. Patients with chronic kidney disease develop anemia due to a lack of erythropoietin and, when they are treated, require iron supplementation as well. Malabsorption after gastrectomy or in patients with severe bowel disease can also lead to iron deficiency. Blood loss in patients with heavy menstrual bleeding, colon cancer, or other GI bleeding can also lead to anemia.

The inability to absorb sufficient vitamin B$_{12}$ can result in pernicious anemia, which is most common in aged people. Vitamin B$_{12}$ deficiency

may also occur in vegetarians because plants do not contain vitamin B$_{12}$. Vitamin B$_{12}$ deficiency often has a slow and insidious onset because the liver contains a 3- to 5-year supply of the vitamin. Patients with pernicious anemia exhibit decreased erythrocyte production and hemoglobin levels, as well as neurological impairments, including paresthesias and weakness. In pernicious anemia, injectable forms of vitamin B$_{12}$ are required, including hydroxocobalamin and cyanocobalamin, which are administered frequently until the deficiency is reversed and then once a month for maintenance therapy.

Parenteral iron therapy is often used in patients with chronic renal disease, and many patients on dialysis require frequent iron infusions. **Iron dextran** is approved for replacement therapy in iron deficiencies of all causes and is currently the most commonly employed form of parenteral iron. **Sodium-ferric gluconate complex (SFGC)**, **iron sucrose**, and **ferumoxytol** are formulations of iron delivered parenterally and limited for use by patients with iron deficiency who have chronic renal disease; SFGC is only available for patients with chronic renal disease who are concurrently undergoing dialysis and receiving erythropoietin.

Vitamin B$_{12}$ and/or folic acid deficiency also results in megaloblastic anemia. Megaloblastic anemia stems from decreased synthesis of purines and thymidine, reducing the ability of hematopoietic cells to synthesize DNA. Disruption of DNA replication results in production of abnormally large cells (megaloblasts), which are released from the bone marrow in an immature state in attempts to compensate for anemia. Diagnostic tests to determine the cause of megaloblastic anemia include measurement of serum or red blood cell folate, vitamin B$_{12}$ levels, and serum and urine levels of methylmalonic acid and serum homocysteine, which become elevated in vitamin B$_{12}$ deficiency. Lack of folic acid and vitamin B$_{12}$ can also lead to increases in homocysteine, which may contribute to cardiovascular disease. Megaloblastic anemia is treated with vitamin B$_{12}$ or folic acid supplementation.

Because the requirement for folic acid increases in pregnancy, folic acid supplements are routinely used during this time to reduce the incidence of neural tube defects in the fetus.

Further, all enriched grain products in the United States and Canada are supplemented with folic acid, which has decreased both neural tube defects in infants and elevated levels of homocysteine in adults.

Because folic acid treatment alone will reverse the hematological effects of vitamin deficiency but could exacerbate the neurological symptoms associated with vitamin B$_{12}$ deficiency, it should never be used alone unless the deficit is clearly identified to be one of folic acid. Folic acid preparations exist in two different forms, one of which (folinic acid or leucovorin) is used for rescue therapy in patients receiving cancer chemotherapy.

PHARMACOKINETICS

Antihemophilic Agents

Factor VIII concentrate is a powder that is dissolved in a sterile solution immediately prior to intravenous administration. The powder is made using recombinant DNA technology or by purification from human plasma. Factor VIII concentrates must be infused every other day due to the relatively short half-life.

Factor IX concentrate is also a powder that is dissolved in a sterile solution immediately prior to intravenous administration, similar to factor VIII concentrate. Prophylactic therapy with factor IX concentrates require only two infusions per week due to the long half-life.

Desmopressin is administered intravenously or as a nasal spray.

Aminocaproic acid is available as an intravenous or oral formulation, the latter as a pill or liquid, whereas tranexamic acid is approved for use as an intravenous formulation for bleeding associated with dental extractions. It is available in an oral formulation but only approved for oral use in the management of heavy cyclic menstrual bleeding.

Agents for Deficiency Anemias

Iron supplements may be taken orally or by injection. Oral iron preparations include various ferrous salts that vary in the amount of elemental iron present (Table 47.2); all are available as standard tablets and enteric-coated and sustained-release formulations. They are well absorbed from the GI tract, although the enteric-coated and sustained-release formulations have a more variable rate of iron release. Ferrous salts are generally taken at doses that deliver 100–200 mg of elemental iron per day, until the anemia is corrected, and then at doses that deliver 60 mg of elemental iron daily for 3–6 months. Food reduces the bioavailability of iron by 30%–50%, and antacids decrease absorption, which occurs primarily in the upper part of the small intestine. Although the oral salts taken with meals reduces significant GI side effects, it is recommended that they are taken between meals to attain a better absorption of the iron. Carbonyl iron is a form of elemental iron created as microparticles, which confers good bioavailability. It is available in tablet, chewable tablets, or a suspension form.

Parenteral iron is used in patients who are unable to absorb or tolerate oral iron supplementation or in patients in whom oral iron is insufficient

to correct the anemia. Four forms of parenteral iron preparations are available. Ferumoxytol is a superparamagnetic form of iron oxide that is coupled to nanoparticles. This formulation is more convenient than the others because it can be given more rapidly and only requires two doses given over 3–8 days versus more doses given over weeks for the other forms.

Vitamin B_{12} and folic acid are available in a variety of preparations. Hydroxocobalamin and cyanocobalamin are injected intramuscularly for the treatment of vitamin B_{12} deficiency. Hydroxocobalamin is preferred because it is highly protein bound and has a long duration of action due to its persistence in the circulation. Cyanocobalamin is also available as an oral preparation, as well as a nasal gel or spray, the latter providing passive diffusion through the nasal mucosa, bypassing concerns about oral absorption. Both hydroxocobalamin and cyanocobalamin are converted to cobalamin (vitamin B_{12}) in the body.

Folic acid is available in both an oral form and as a solution for injection, the latter usually reserved for individuals who have severely impaired GI absorption. Folic acid is well absorbed orally, with peak effects 1 hour following administration. The treatment of folic acid deficiency is usually accomplished through dietary modifications.

PHARMACOVIGILANCE: ADVERSE EFFECTS AND DRUG INTERACTIONS

Antihemophilic Agents

Factor VIII and IX concentrates are generally safe. The potential for the development of viral infections with plasma-derived forms has declined substantially, though some risk for the development of human adenovirus and parvovirus B19 infections, as well as prion-induced Creutzfeldt-Jakob disease (CJD), still exists. The possibility of viral infection with factor concentrates created using recombinant technology is extraordinarily low to nonexistent. For prophylactic therapy used to prevent bleeding in severe hemophiliacs, there is a risk associated with the need for a central venous access device due to the repeated infusions that are necessary. These devices carry a risk of infection and thrombosis even though they greatly facilitate prophylactic therapy.

Desmopressin is an analogue of antidiuretic hormone whose primary adverse effects of fluid retention and hyponatremia are predicted.

The antifibrinolytics (aminocaproic acid and tranexamic acid) produce some intravascular thrombosis due to inhibition of plasminogen activator. In addition, both aminocaproic acid and tranexamic acid have the capacity to produce some hypotension, myopathy, abdominal discomfort, diarrhea, vomiting, and nasal stuffiness.

Agents for Deficiency Anemias

The most common side effects of oral iron supplementation are GI symptoms, which are dose related. Heartburn, upper abdominal and gastric discomfort, nausea, and either diarrhea or constipation are frequently reported. Decreasing the dose, or starting with a lower dose and titrating up slowly, may improve these adverse effects. Hemochromatosis (iron overload) is rare, even at very high doses in most people. The oral iron preparations should not be used in patients with peptic ulcer disease, regional enteritis, or ulcerative colitis, as these disorders are significantly exacerbated by these agents. Oral iron preparations may turn stools dark green or black in color, which can be unsettling to patients, but is not indicative of GI bleeding. Iron preparations given as a solution may also stain teeth, which can be prevented by dilution, using some form of administration that avoids the teeth (e.g., medicine droppers or straws), or oral rinsing after treatment.

Iron poisoning may occur with ingestion of large amounts (2–10 g), especially in children. Symptoms may begin within 30 minutes and include abdominal pain, diarrhea, and vomiting. The stomach lining is frequently damaged, and vomit may contain blood. Pallor, cyanosis,

TABLE 47.2 Comparison of Common Oral Iron Preparations		
Preparation	% Elemental Iron	Dose Delivering 100 mg of Iron (mg)
Ferrous Iron Salts		
Ferrous sulfate	20	500
Ferrous sulfate (dried)	30	330
Ferrous fumarate	33	300
Ferrous gluconate	11.6	860
Ferrous aspartate	16	625
Carbonyl (Elemental) Iron		
Tablets	100	100
Film-coated tablets		
Chewable tablets		
Suspension		

CLINICAL PROBLEMS

Hemophilia

Preparation	Adverse Effects
Plasma-derived factor VIII and IX concentrates	Risk of viral infection (hepatitis A, parvovirus B19)
	Risk of prion-induced Creutzfeldt-Jakob disease
Recombinant factor VIII and IX concentrates	–
Desmopressin	Fluid retention, hyponatremia
Antifibrinolytic agents	Intravascular thrombosis, hypotension, myopathy

Deficiency Anemias

Oral iron	GI symptoms, hemochromatosis, poisoning, drowsiness, pallor, cyanosis, acidosis, cardiovascular collapse
Parenteral iron	Anaphylaxis, headache, fever, urticaria, arthralgias, exacerbation of rheumatoid arthritis, hypotension, circulatory failure
Vitamin B$_{12}$	Anaphylaxis, angioedema, vascular thrombosis
Folic acid	Allergic reactions, nausea, flatulence, bad taste in mouth

drowsiness, acidosis, and cardiovascular collapse may occur, leading to death. Depending on the iron concentration and estimation of the number and location of iron pills in the GI tract by X-ray, treatment may consist of inducing vomiting, treatment with the iron chelator deferoxamine, and supportive therapy.

Parenteral iron therapy may cause hypersensitivity reactions, headache, fever, urticaria, arthralgias, and exacerbation of rheumatoid arthritis. Fatal anaphylactic reactions have been observed with **parenteral iron dextran**, which appear to be the result of the dextran. Even though it is a rare event, caution should be used whenever this agent is employed, and epinephrine and resuscitation devices need to be present. The risk of anaphylaxis is low with the other formulations, but sodium-ferric gluconate has been associated with transient flushing and hypotension and severe pain in a number of body regions, including the back, chest, and groin. These effects can be minimized by very slow infusions or by preceding the infusion or injection with a very small dose. Iron sucrose has been observed to produce cramps and hypotension as well as heart failure and sepsis. While the latter two are rare, it is recommended that facilities for resuscitation be easily available. Ferumoxytol is generally well tolerated but has been associated with nausea, vomiting, dizziness, hypotension, and headache, with only a very small percentage of patients exhibiting anaphylactic-type reactions. Due to its formulation, it may interfere with magnetic resonance imaging.

Vitamin B$_{12}$ (cyanocobalamin) is relatively nontoxic and is very well tolerated with hypokalemia as a natural consequence of the increased production of RBCs, which incorporate potassium in significant amounts. Anaphylactic reactions or angioedema to injection have been described, as well as peripheral vascular thrombosis. Pulmonary edema and exacerbation of heart failure may ensue as a consequence of increased blood volume, but all of these reactions are very rare. The most common side effects are arthralgia, dizziness, and nasal congestion.

Folic acid is considered to be nontoxic when used for short periods of time. Nausea, flatulence, and bad taste in the mouth have been reported, with the most severe effect the possibility of an allergic reaction. There has been some suggestion that long-term treatment with high doses may be associated with an increased risk of colorectal or prostatic cancer.

TRADE NAMES

In addition to generic and fixed-combination preparations, the following trade-named materials are some of the important compounds available in the United States.

Factor VIII Concentrates
First generation (Recombinate)
Second generation (Helixate FS, Kogenate FS)
Third generation (Advate)

Factor IX Concentrates
Third generation (BeneFix)
Desmopressin (DDAVP, Stimate)

Antifibrinolytic Agents
Aminocaproic acid
Tranexamic acid (Cyklokapron)

Agents for Patients With Inhibitors
Factor VIIa (NovoSeven RT)
Anti-inhibitor coagulant complex (AICC) (Feiba NF)

Oral Iron Preparations
Ferrous sulfate (Feosol, FeroSul, Slow FE)
Ferrous gluconate (Fergon, Floradix)
Ferrous fumarate (Ferro-Sequels, Hemocyte)
Ferrous aspartate (FE Aspartate)
Ferrous bisglycinate (Ferrochel)
Ferric ammonium citrate (Iron Citrate)
Carbonyl iron (Feosol, Ircon, Icar)
Heme-iron polypeptide (Proferrin)
Polysaccharide iron complex (Niferex-150 Forte, Ferrex 150)
Iron sucrose tablet (Velphoro)

Parenteral Iron Preparations
Iron dextran (INFeD, Dexferrum)
Sodium-ferric gluconate complex (SFGC) (Ferrlecit)
Iron sucrose (Venofer)
Ferumoxytol (Feraheme)

Vitamin B$_{12}$
Cyanocobalamin (Nascobal)
Hydroxocobalamin (Cyanokit)

Folic Acid
Oral tablet (Folacin)

NEW DEVELOPMENTS

Management of patients who develop resistance to the factor concentrates continues to be evaluated. Current solutions involve immune tolerance therapy (ITT). However, when ITT fails, the patients must be treated with drugs (factor VIIa) or the antiinhibitor coagulant complex (AICC). Efforts to develop novel factor concentrates with a reduced propensity for antibody development would be valuable. In addition, efforts to develop gene therapy products and protocols that may offer hope of providing a cure are continuing.

CLINICAL RELEVANCE FOR HEALTHCARE PROFESSIONALS

All healthcare professionals who manage patients with hemophilia must be alert to the possibility of hemorrhage. This is especially pertinent for any type of procedure, including minor surgeries or dental procedures that could lead to excessive gingival or postextraction bleeding. If necessary, coagulant agents may be employed prior to the procedure to reduce the risk of hemorrhage. It is especially important to remember to select appropriate analgesic medications that do not interfere with platelet aggregation. For patients with hemophilia, care must be exercised by physical therapists to monitor activity and prevent incidents that could lead to excessive bleeding. In addition, wound care may be problematic in this patient population.

For patients who present with anemia, it is essential to identify the source and type of the anemia (e.g., microcytic vs. megaloblastic) to reach the appropriate decision regarding pharmacological treatment. Dental management of patients with anemia is important since the gums are frequently one of the first soft tissues to exhibit demonstrable effects of anemia. Physical therapists, occupational therapists, and other healthcare professionals working with patients with anemia should recognize that these patients may have reduced aerobic capacity and immune responses that may present as exercise intolerance or inability to fight infection.

SELF-ASSESSMENT QUESTIONS

1. A dialysis patient with chronic kidney disease presents with iron deficiency anemia. You choose to administer ferumoxytol, which:
   A. Must be administered slowly to avoid gastrointestinal side effects.
   B. Produces fewer antimuscarinic side effects than other parenteral iron products.
   C. Can be administered rapidly to reduce both side effects and the time required for therapy.
   D. Generates less free iron than other parenteral iron products, thereby reducing toxicity.
   E. Is the newest parenteral iron preparation, which means it must be the best.

2. A patient has undergone gastric bypass surgery, and the surgeon reminds the patient that a monthly injection of vitamin B_{12} will be necessary to avoid developing anemia. Which one of the following statements is true about vitamin B_{12}?
   A. Loss of vitamin B_{12} from the body is a rapid process.
   B. The vitamin B_{12} molecule contains copper.
   C. Vitamin B_{12} is not required for fatty acid metabolism.
   D. Deficiency of vitamin B_{12} results in impaired DNA replication.
   E. Neurologic deficits resulting from vitamin B_{12} deficiency can be resolved by the administration of vitamin B_6.

3. A patient with hemophilia A needs a small procedure that might cause some bleeding. A drug that could be given to prevent bleeding problems in this patient is:
   A. Tolvaptan.
   B. Lanreotide.
   C. Somatostatin.
   D. Desmopressin.
   E. Somatropin.

4. The most common side effect of oral iron preparations involves:
   A. The hematopoietic system.
   B. The pulmonary system.
   C. The gastrointestinal system.
   D. The kidneys.
   E. The liver.

5. A 35-year-old female is complaining that she feels tired all time and cannot do her regular exercise because she becomes short of breath. She also is having frequent headaches and has a 6-month history of strong, irregular menstrual bleeding. Laboratory tests reveal low hemoglobin and hematocrit and decreased mean corpuscular volume and mean corpuscular hemoglobin. Her serum iron was at the lowest end of normal, her serum ferritin was slightly below normal, and her total iron-binding capacity was greater than normal. Based on her symptoms and laboratory results, the patient should be treated with:
   A. Cyanocobalamin.
   B. Ferumoxytol.
   C. Ferrous sulfate.
   D. Folic acid.
   E. Iron dextran.

6. The patient in the question above is likely to complain about which of the following side effects, and what can be done to reduce it?
   A. Abdominal discomfort; decrease the initial dose and work up slowly.
   B. Bone pain; treat with acetaminophen.
   C. Nasal congestion; treat with inhaled alpha agonists.
   D. Venous thrombosis; reverse anemia only to a hemoglobin level of 10 g/dL.
   E. Tachycardia; reduce dose and give more frequently.

FURTHER READING

Pasca S, Milan M, Sarolo L, Zanon E. PK-driven prophylaxis versus standard prophylaxis: when a tailored treatment may be a real and achievable cost-saving approach in children with severe hemophilia A. *Thromb Res.* 2017;157:58–63.

Short MW, Domagalski JE. Iron deficiency anemia: evaluation and management. *Am Fam Physician.* 2013;87(2):98–104.

WEBSITES

https://www.hemophilia.org/Researchers-Healthcare-Providers
This website is maintained by the National Hemophilia Foundation and contains information on bleeding disorders for healthcare professionals including guidelines for the management of hemophilia.
https://www.cdc.gov/ncbddd/hemophilia/
This website is maintained by the Centers for Disease Control and Prevention and provides links to numerous resources for healthcare professionals, patients, and their families on hemophilia.
http://www.hematology.org/Patients/Anemia/
This is the website for the American Society of Hematology and contains valuable information on all blood disorders and their treatment.

SECTION 7

Endocrine Pharmacology

48

Introduction to Endocrine Pharmacology

Shelley Tischkau

INTRODUCTION

The endocrine system is a complex communication system responsible for maintaining homeostasis throughout the body, and it is vital to individual and species survival and propagation, as well as adaptation to the environment. The system consists of a diverse group of ductless glands that secrete chemical messengers called hormones into circulation. The secreted hormones are transported in the bloodstream to target organs, where they act to regulate cellular activities. For a hormone to elicit a response, it must interact with specific receptors on the cells of the target organ, much like the interaction between neurotransmitters and receptors involved in the process of neurotransmission in the central and peripheral nervous systems. Receptors play a key role in the mechanisms of action of endocrine hormone systems; key receptor mechanisms pertinent to endocrine systems are summarized in Chapter 2.

In general, all endocrine systems share several common features. At the uppermost level, the secretion of each hormone is controlled tightly by input from higher neural centers in response to alterations in plasma levels of the hormone or other substances. The second component is the gland itself, where hormone synthesis and secretion occur in specialized cells. After synthesis, hormones are typically packaged and stored for later release as needed. Signals from the nervous system or special releasing hormones, or both, bring about secretion of stored hormone.

HORMONES

Hormones are chemically and structurally diverse compounds and can be divided into three main classes based on chemical composition: the amino acid analogues, the peptides, and the steroids. The amino acid analogues, often termed amine hormones, are all derived from tyrosine and include epinephrine (Epi) and the iodothyronines or thyroid hormones. The peptide hormones are subclassified on the basis of size and glycosylation state and may be single- or double-chain peptides. The steroid hormones are all derived from cholesterol and may be subclassified as adrenal steroids or sex steroids, the former synthesized primarily in the adrenal cortex and the latter synthesized in the ovaries or testes. The major endocrine glands and their associated hormones are listed in Box 48.1.

Hormones are generally distinguished from other types of modulatory factors (i.e., neurotransmitters) by a longer duration of effect and more extensive circulation in the body. While in the circulation, a hormone is frequently associated with one or more types of transport proteins from which it must dissociate to interact with responsive receptors. In addition, availability to tissues is dependent upon membrane exclusion mechanisms, susceptibility to tissue modification, and, ultimately, the rate of renal or hepatic metabolism, inactivation, and excretion. As mentioned, hormones exert their effects by binding to and activating

ABBREVIATIONS	
DHEA	Dehydroepiandrosterone
DNA	Deoxyribonucleic acid
Epi	Epinephrine
GnRH	Hypothalamic gonadotropin-releasing hormone

receptors on target cells. These receptors can be located on the cell surface, as for peptide hormones, or within the cell, as in the case of steroids and thyroid hormones. After receptor activation, intracellular signaling pathways (e.g., second messenger systems or ligand-activated transcription factors) are modulated, which acutely or chronically alter cellular physiology and potentially whole organism physiology.

All secreted steroids are synthesized from cholesterol, which can be synthesized de novo or derived from circulating lipoproteins. Similar metabolic pathways mediate steroid synthesis in all organs (Fig. 48.1). The organ-specific formation of secreted steroids depends on the presence of specific catalytic enzymes (Table 48.1). A review of the normal biochemistry and physiology describing synthesis and function of endogenous hormones in normal activity will serve as a basis for understanding the pharmacologic agents and their roles in therapeutic interventions. A summary of strategies to manage the levels and action of hormones is presented in Box 48.2.

The action of steroids is mediated largely by altering gene transcription through interaction with the promoter deoxyribonucleic acid (DNA) of genes. Steroid receptors are dimeric and coupled with accessory proteins until activated by ligands outside the nucleus. The steroid-receptor complex is phosphorylated and translocated into the nucleus through a nuclear pore, facilitated by the importin protein. The interaction with the gene promoter region occurs through steroid-specific palindromic nucleotide sequences within the receptor. The interaction of DNA and the steroid-receptor complex is dependent on steroid structural differences, the amino acid sequence of the DNA-binding domain, the nucleotide sequence of the DNA-binding site, and the architecture of the gene promoter. The structures of the primary circulating steroids are shown in Fig. 48.2.

NEW DEVELOPMENTS

There is a significant role for the use of long-acting depot forms of GnRH analogues to treat androgen-dependent neoplasms, such as prostate cancer, and to use GnRH agonist therapy to manage male and female infertility. Further, the ability of GnRH analogues to diminish gonadotropic hormones suggests a potential adjunct role in female and male contraception.

BOX 48.1 Major Endocrine Glands and Their Hormones

Adrenal
Cortisol, corticosterone, aldosterone

Ovaries, Testes
Estradiol, progesterone, testosterone

Thyroid
Thyroid hormones

Pancreas
Insulin, glucagon, somatostatin, pancreatic polypeptide

Pituitary
Antidiuretic hormone, oxytocin, adrenocorticotropic hormone, thyroid-stimulating hormone, luteinizing hormone, follicle-stimulating hormone, growth hormone, prolactin, gonadotropin-releasing hormone, luteinizing-hormone-releasing hormone, thyrotropin-releasing hormone, prolactin-inhibiting factor

Parathyroid
Parathyroid hormone, calcitonin

BOX 48.2 Strategies to Manage the Levels and Action of Hormones

Mechanisms to Increase Hormone Levels and Activity
Increase endogenous hormone synthesis, release, and transport
Reduce endogenous hormone metabolism and excretion
Increase peripheral activation of circulating hormone (if required)
Hormone replacement therapy

Mechanisms to Decrease Hormone Levels and Activity
Lower endogenous hormone synthesis, release, or both
Reduce peripheral conversion to activated forms
Promote hepatic/renal metabolism/excretion
Decrease receptor activity by reducing receptor number or affinity for hormone or use competitive receptor antagonists
Suppress response of target tissue to receptor-hormone interaction by interfering with generation of second messengers
Modify tissue metabolism to blunt the effects of hormone excess

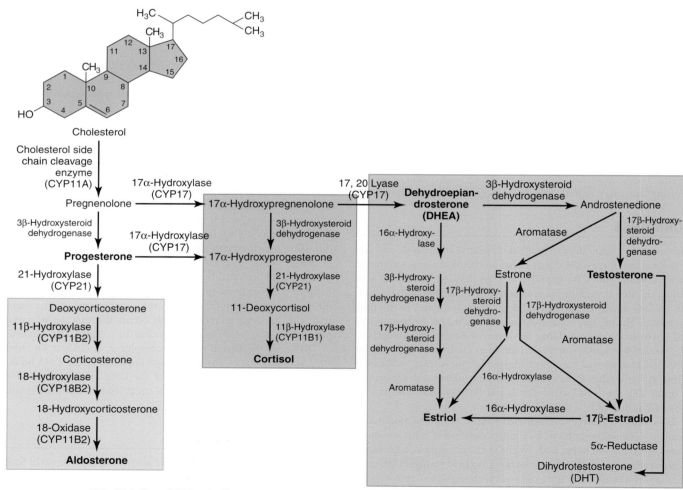

FIG. 48.1 Steroid Metabolism. The biosynthesis of the steroids is illustrated. The enzymes with the prefix CYP represent the mitochondrial cytochrome P450 mixed-function oxidases, and the numbers indicate the site of steroid hydroxylation. The other enzymes are located primarily at the endoplasmic reticulum or both endoplasmic reticulum and mitochondria. The steroids indicated in bold are the primary secreted steroids.

TABLE 48.1   Enzymes Present in Different Tissues Mediating the Organ- or Tissue-Specific Formation of Steroid Hormones

Tissue	CYP11A	CYP11B	CYP17	CYP21	Aromatase[a]	5α-Reductase[a]
Adrenal glands						
Zona glomerulosa	+	++	−	+	−	−
Zona fasciculata	+	+	+	+	−	−
Zona reticularis	+	+	+	+	−	−
Testes						
Sertoli cells	−	−	−	−	+	−
Leydig cells	+	−	+	−	−	−
Ovary						
Glomerulosa	+	−	−	−	+	−
Theca	+	−	+	−	−	−
Corpus luteum	+	−	−	−	+	−
Adipose tissue	−	−	−	−	+	−
Prostate	−	−	−	−	−	+

[a]Aromatase and 5α-reductase can also metabolize circulating steroids.

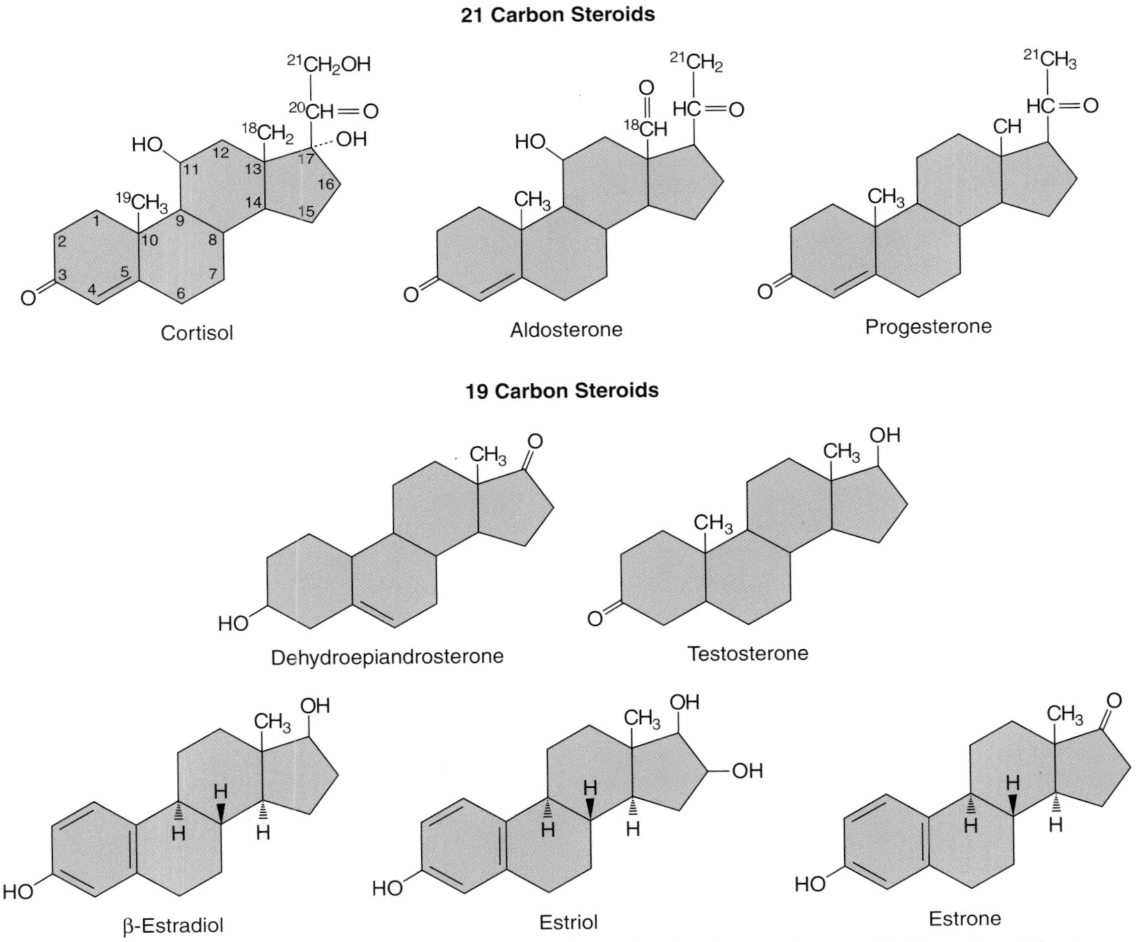

FIG. 48.2 Structures of the Primary Circulating Steroids. Steroids may be classified broadly as 19- or 21-carbon steroids on the basis of the number of carbon atoms in the steroid structure. The 19-carbon forms, testosterone and the estrogens, are released from gonadal tissues; although DHEA is formed in these tissues, its release is normally less than that from the adrenal gland. Progesterone is released from the corpus luteum and placenta. Cortisol, DHEA, and aldosterone are released primarily from the zona fasciculata, zona reticularis, and zona glomerulosa, respectively. Note that the numbering system shown for cortisol applies to all steroids.

CLINICAL RELEVANCE FOR HEALTHCARE PROFESSIONALS

The role of the endocrine system as a response system to input from external and internal stimuli is analogous to the nervous system. The endocrine system responds to these stimuli to help maintain homeostasis in the body, similar to the responses of the nervous system but usually by slower mechanisms that are more diffuse in their effects. Effects of specific endocrine hormone systems, such as the adrenocortical hormones, or pituitary or hypothalamic hormones, will be addressed in each of the subsequent chapters. All healthcare professionals must be cognizant of the mechanisms by which hormones affect changes in body functions, such as alterations in calcium regulation that may impact bone structure and strength, and they must be vigilant in understanding effects, adverse effects, and potential interactions that may influence patient responses to their interventions. For example, glucocorticoid effects on the immune system that may impact resistance to infection is an example of a global effect that will impact all healthcare provider-patient interactions. These potential issues will be addressed in more detail in the chapters dealing with each endocrine system.

49

Treatment of Hypothalamic and Pituitary Disorders

Shelley Tischkau

MAJOR DRUG CLASSES

Hypothalamic hormones and analogues
Pituitary hormones and analogues

ABBREVIATIONS

ACTH	Adrenocorticotropic hormone
AVP	Arginine vasopressin, antidiuretic hormone
CNS	Central nervous system
CRH	Corticotropin-releasing hormone
DA	Dopamine
Epi	Epinephrine
FSH	Follicle-stimulating hormone
GH	Growth hormone
GHRH	Growth hormone-releasing hormone
GI	Gastrointestinal
GnRH	Gonadotropin-releasing hormone
hCG	Human chorionic gonadotropin
hGH	Human growth hormone
hMG	Human menopausal gonadotropin
IGF-1	Insulin-like growth factor-1
IM	Intramuscular
IV	Intravenous
LH	Luteinizing hormone
SC	Subcutaneous
SRIF	Somatostatin, somatotropin-release–inhibiting hormone
TRH	Thyrotropin-releasing hormone
TSH	Thyroid-stimulating hormone

THERAPEUTIC OVERVIEW

In general, all endocrine systems share several common features. At the uppermost level, the secretion of hormones is controlled tightly by input from higher neural centers in response to alterations in plasma levels of the hormone or other substances. The second component is the gland itself, where hormone synthesis occurs in specialized cells. Hormones are packaged and stored and secreted as needed by signals from the nervous system, special releasing hormones, or both.

Pharmacology of Hypothalamic and Pituitary Hormones

The hypothalamus and pituitary gland work in concert to regulate endocrine systems throughout the body. Peptides and biogenic amines synthesized and secreted by specialized neurons within the hypothalamus are transported to the anterior pituitary by the **hypothalamic-hypophyseal portal circulation**, where they act through specific receptors to stimulate or inhibit hormone secretion (Fig. 49.1). **Anterior pituitary hormones** trigger peripheral endocrine organs to produce hormones, which have individual functions and provide feedback to the hypothalamus and pituitary to regulate the synthesis and release of their tropic hormones.

Hypothalamic **gonadotropin-releasing hormone (GnRH)** stimulates the secretion of **luteinizing hormone (LH)** and **follicle-stimulating hormone (FSH)** by the pituitary. These hormones promote **gametogenesis** and gonadal hormone production by the ovaries and testes. **Growth hormone-releasing hormone (GHRH)** stimulates and **somatostatin (SRIF; somatotropin-release inhibiting factor)** inhibits the production of **growth hormone (GH)**, which has numerous effects on growth and metabolism. Hypothalamic **dopamine (DA)** tonically inhibits the secretion of **prolactin**, the hormone primarily responsible for lactation and suppression of fertility while nursing. **Thyrotropin-releasing hormone (TRH)** stimulates secretion of **thyroid-stimulating hormone (TSH)**, which in turn controls thyroid function. **Corticotropin-releasing hormone (CRH)** stimulates the secretion of **adrenocorticotropic hormone (ACTH)**, which promotes the secretion of **cortisol** by the adrenal cortex.

Unlike the anterior pituitary, the posterior pituitary (or **neurohypophysis**) consists of neurons with cell bodies in the hypothalamus. These cells synthesize **oxytocin** and **arginine vasopressin (AVP; antidiuretic hormone)**, which are transported by carrier proteins (neurophysins) through axons to the posterior pituitary for storage and release into the systemic circulation.

GnRH, SRIF, DA, LH/FSH, GH, and AVP are used **therapeutically**, whereas GHRH, TRH, CRH, TSH, and ACTH are used primarily for **diagnostic** purposes. A summary of the hypothalamic and pituitary hormones and analogues and their therapeutic uses is presented in the Therapeutic Overview Box.

MECHANISMS OF ACTION

Hypothalamic Hormones

Gonadotropin-Releasing Hormone

Most **GnRH**-positive neurons in humans are located in the medial basal hypothalamus between the third ventricle and the median eminence. Projections from these neurons terminate in the median eminence, in contact with the capillary plexus of the hypothalamic-hypophyseal portal circulation. This allows GnRH to reach the circulation without passing through a blood-brain barrier. GnRH is formed from a larger prohormone, prepro-GnRH, and transported in secretory granules to nerve terminals for storage, degradation, or release into pituitary portal blood vessels.

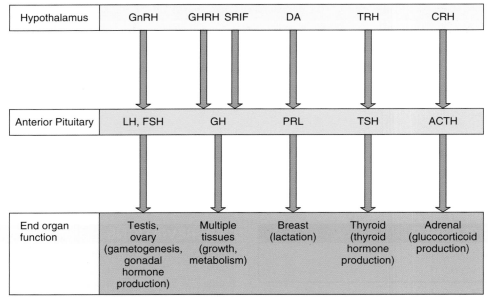

FIG. 49.1 Relationships Among Hypothalamic Releasing and Inhibiting Factors, the Anterior Pituitary Hormones Controlled by Hypothalamic Hormones, and Their Respective Target Organs or Tissues. *ACTH,* Adrenocorticotropic hormone; *CRH,* corticotropin-releasing hormone; *DA,* dopamine; *FSH,* follicle-stimulating hormone; *GH,* growth hormone; *GHRH,* growth hormone–releasing hormone; *GnRH,* gonadotropin-releasing hormone; *LH,* luteinizing hormone; *PRL,* prolactin; *SRIF,* somatotropin-release–inhibiting factor (somatostatin); *TRH,* thyrotropin-releasing hormone; *TSH,* thyroid-stimulating hormone.

THERAPEUTIC OVERVIEW

Hypothalamic Hormones
GnRH
   Replacement therapy for idiopathic hypogonadotropic hypogonadism

GnRH Analogues
   Prostate and breast cancer
   Idiopathic precocious puberty
   Endometriosis
   Fertility/contraception

Dopamine Agonists
   Pathological hyperprolactinemia
   Acromegaly
   Parkinson's disease

Somatostatin and Analogues
   Acromegaly
   Carcinoid and vasoactive intestinal peptide-secreting tumors

Pituitary Hormones
LH and FSH
   Infertility in women
   Infertility in men with hypogonadotropic hypogonadism

GH Agonists
   Adult GH deficiency
   Growth failure

AVP Agonists and Antagonists
   Diabetes insipidus
   Syndrome of inappropriate antidiuretic hormone

GnRH-receptor interaction initiates secretion of LH and FSH. The GnRH receptor gene is a 327–amino acid protein with seven transmembrane domains lacking a typical intracellular C-terminus of a G-protein–coupled receptor. Microaggregation stimulates up regulation of GnRH receptors followed by internalization of the hormone-receptor complex. Receptor activation results in increased intracellular Ca^{++}.

GnRH, whose structure is shown in Fig. 49.2, is released in a pulsatile manner by the "hypothalamic GnRH pulse generator" and is essential for normal function. GnRH secretion is increased by norepinephrine, epinephrine (Epi), neuropeptide Y, galanin, and *N*-methyl-D-aspartic acid, and decreased by endogenous opioids, progesterone, and prolactin; estradiol also inhibits GnRH secretion except for a brief period of stimulation, which results in the midcycle LH surge.

Continuous administration of GnRH leads to both a desensitization and down regulation of GnRH receptors on pituitary gonadotrophs. GnRH analogues can be either agonists or antagonists, with agonists leading to a transient increase in gonadotropin release and decreased receptor expression, like GnRH. These analogues have been synthesized by selective amino acid substitution in the GnRH peptide, decreasing susceptibility to enzymatic degradation, resulting in prolonged biological activity.

Growth Hormone–Releasing Hormone and Somatostatin

As mentioned, GHRH and SRIF regulate the secretion of GH in opposite directions. GHRH is a 44–amino acid peptide synthesized by the arcuate nucleus of the hypothalamus and released in a pulsatile manner. It is transported to the anterior pituitary by the hypothalamo-hypophyseal portal system, where it interacts with its receptors to regulate GH secretion. SRIF is a cyclic peptide processed from a preprohormone into two molecular forms: SRIF-14 and SRIF-28, in which the 14–amino acid sequence at the carboxyl terminal of SRIF-28 is identical to SRIF-14. In addition to its presence in the hypothalamus, SRIF is widely distributed throughout the central nervous system (CNS) as a neurotransmitter

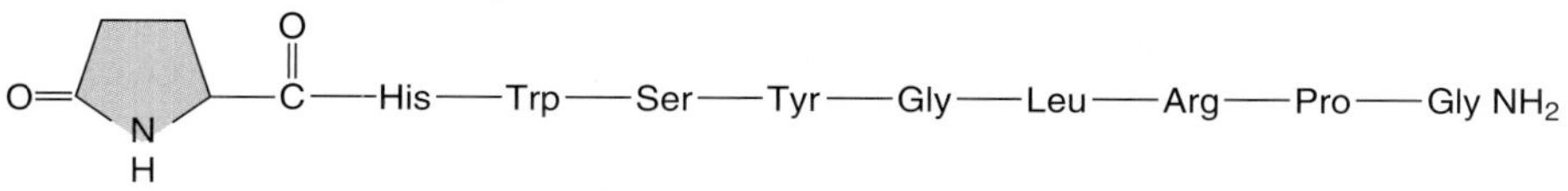

O=⬠(N-H)—C(=O)—His—Trp—Ser—Tyr—Gly—Leu—Arg—Pro—Gly NH₂

FIG. 49.2 Structure of Gonadotropin-Releasing Hormone (GnRH).

and a neuromodulator, the gastrointestinal (GI) tract, pancreas, thyroid, thymus, heart, skin, and eye. SRIF has multiple actions, including inhibition of GI hormone secretion, pancreatic exocrine secretion, pancreatic endocrine secretion, GI motility, gastric emptying, gallbladder contraction, and decreased GI absorption and mesenteric blood flow. The five somatostatin receptor subtypes (SSTR1–SSTR5) are G-protein–coupled receptors and differ in tissue distribution and signaling pathways. SRIF-14 and SRIF-28 bind all five receptor subtypes. Binding of SRIF to SSTR2 and SSTR5 suppresses both GH and TSH secretion.

Dopamine

DA is synthesized by the tuberoinfundibular neurons of the hypothalamus and transported to the anterior pituitary gland via the hypothalamic-hypophyseal portal system. DA acts at DA type 2 (D_2) receptors on the pituitary lactotrophs to inhibit prolactin secretion. Prolactin is the only anterior pituitary hormone under tonic inhibition by a hypothalamic hormone.

Pituitary Hormones
Luteinizing Hormone and Follicle-Stimulating Hormone

The gonadotropins LH and FSH are structurally similar, each with two polypeptide subunits, an identical 89–amino acid α-chain, and a unique 115–amino acid β-chain, which confer receptor specificity. After synthesis, both subunits are glycosylated. Specifically, two complex carbohydrates are attached to the FSH-β subunit and one to the LH-β subunit. A terminal sialic acid, found on approximately 1% and 5% of LH and FSH carbohydrate molecules, respectively, prolongs the metabolic clearance of glycoproteins and results in a longer half-life for FSH than for LH. There is no evidence that other molecular forms of LH and FSH, such as prohormones and fragments, circulate in the plasma. The pituitary gonadotropes secrete LH and FSH.

Gonadotropins bind with high affinity to membrane glycoprotein receptors in the testes and ovaries encoded by homologous genes and characterized by seven transmembrane-spanning domains. A large N-terminal region forms the binding site for the specific gonadotropin. The activation of LH and FSH receptors is associated with distinctive Ca^{++} signaling properties and increased 3′–5′ cyclic adenosine monophosphate (cAMP) production that increases phosphorylation of proteins involved in steroidogenesis through activation of cAMP-dependent protein kinase.

In addition to regulating estrogen production, gonadotropins have multiple effects on ovarian follicles. FSH directly stimulates follicular growth and maturation and enhances granulosa cell responsiveness to LH. LH is essential for the breakdown of the follicular wall, resulting in ovulation, and for the subsequent resumption of oocyte meiosis. By contrast, testicular steroidogenesis requires only LH. The Leydig cells, approximately 10% of testicular volume, are stimulated to produce testosterone by LH binding to surface receptors. FSH binds to Sertoli cells and, with testosterone, is essential for mediating cellular maturation and spermatid differentiation, the first step of spermatogenesis. The Sertoli cell is necessary for maintenance of seminiferous tubule function and germ cell development.

Growth Hormone

GH, a 191–amino acid polypeptide belonging to a family of structurally similar hormones, including prolactin and chorionic somatomam-

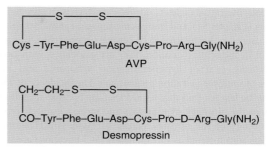

FIG. 49.3 Amino Acid Sequences of Arginine Vasopressin (AVP) and 1-Desamino-8-D-Arginine-Vasopressin (Desmopressin).

motropin (also known as human placental lactogen), is synthesized by somatotropes of the anterior pituitary. The precise signaling mechanism by which GH exerts its intracellular effects likely involves its interaction with specific plasma membrane receptors and activation of the JAK-STAT) family of nuclear transcription factors (Chapter 2, Fig. 2.8). Most actions of GH are mediated through stimulation of **insulin-like growth factor-1 (IGF-1)** produced in liver, cartilage, bone, muscle, and kidney. Other direct effects of GH on tissue include DNA and RNA synthesis, plasma protein synthesis, and amino acid transport and incorporation into proteins.

Arginine Vasopressin

AVP, a polypeptide that functions as the primary antidiuretic hormone in humans, is synthesized primarily in the magnocellular neuronal systems of the supraoptic and paraventricular nuclei of the hypothalamus. The AVP precursor molecule contains a signal peptide, a neurophysin, and a glycosylated moiety, in addition to the AVP sequence. After translation of the messenger RNA to form a preprohormone (166 amino acids), the signal peptide is cleaved, forming a prohormone; the structure of AVP is shown in Fig. 49.3. The prohormone is stored in neurosecretory granules that travel down the supraoptico-hypophyseal tract to the posterior pituitary. The primary stimuli for AVP release are hyperosmolarity and volume depletion; nausea, emesis, and hypoglycemia may also stimulate AVP release.

AVP acts via V1 and V2 receptors in smooth muscle and renal collecting tubules, respectively. V1 receptors mediate vasoconstriction, while V2 receptors mediate antidiuretic effects. Specifically, AVP binding to V2 receptors activates adenylyl cyclase and results in fusion of the water channel, **aquaporin-2**, with the luminal membrane to allow water reabsorption.

RELATIONSHIP OF MECHANISMS OF ACTION TO CLINICAL RESPONSE

Hypothalamic Hormones
Gonadotropin-Releasing Hormone and Analogues

GnRH and analogues approved by the United States Food and Drug Administration (FDA) are used for several disorders, each of which requires different administration strategies. GnRH has been used successfully to induce ovulation in women with **primary hypothalamic (or central) amenorrhea**, characterized by abnormal functioning of the GnRH pulse generator, resulting in inadequate gonadotropin secretion, failure of ovarian follicular development, and amenorrhea. Because the pituitary is intrinsically normal and will release LH and FSH in response to GnRH, pulsatile administration of GnRH can compensate for the underlying defect. A portable infusion pump that administers GnRH intravenously (IV) at 90-minute intervals frequently restores LH, FSH, estradiol, and progesterone profiles to those observed in normal spontaneous menstrual cycles. Clomiphene, which is an estrogen receptor antagonist (Chapter 51), and human menopausal gonadotropin (hMG) are also used for the treatment of central amenorrhea, but although successful in inducing ovulation, they are associated with two major complications, ovarian hyperstimulation syndrome and increased incidence of multiple-gestation pregnancies. The incidence of complications may be less for pulsatile GnRH therapy because it maintains the integrity of the pituitary-ovarian axis and more accurately reproduces the physiology of the normal menstrual cycle. GnRH agonists and antagonists administered as subcutaneous (SC) injections are frequently used for in vitro fertilization approaches to prevent premature LH surges in women undergoing controlled ovarian hyperstimulation.

Faulty GnRH secretion in men is referred to as idiopathic hypogonadotropic hypogonadism. Long-term pulsatile administration of GnRH for at least 3 months demonstrated significant increases of serum testosterone concentrations and testicular size. Mature spermatogenesis was achieved in 50% of patients, and men with unfused epiphyses experienced linear bone growth. Idiopathic or surgically induced hypogonadotropic hypogonadism is treated with testosterone to promote masculinization and to preserve bone mineral density. Human chorionic gonadotropin (hCG) and hMG are used to promote spermatogenesis and restore fertility in male hypogonadotropic hypogonadism.

Because of the association of orchiectomy and regression of prostate cancer, methods to induce androgen deprivation, including orchiectomy, estrogen therapy, and administration of GnRH analogues and antiandrogens, are used in treating metastatic hormone-dependent prostate cancer. Orchiectomy, an effective and relatively safe surgical procedure that significantly lowers testosterone levels (90%), is less desirable in men with cancer because of the emotional impact. Estrogen, an alternative treatment, suppresses LH secretion that decreases serum androgen levels in men, but it has been linked with an increased incidence of deep venous thrombosis and gynecomastia.

Long-acting GnRH agonists, used to down regulate pituitary gonadotropin receptors and suppress LH (Fig. 49.4), reduce serum testosterone concentrations comparable to those with orchiectomy. However, continuous GnRH agonist therapy will initially increase LH secretion from the pituitary, causing a transient increase in serum testosterone that occurs approximately 72 hours after initiating therapy

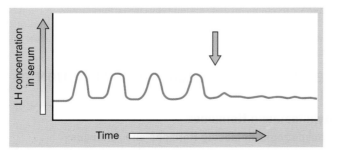

FIG. 49.4 Luteinizing Hormone (LH) Serum Concentration Profile in a Normal Subject, Showing Initial LH Pulses Resulting From Gonadotropin-Releasing Hormone (GnRH) Pulse Generator. Administration of a long-acting GnRH agonist (orange arrow) down regulates receptors and leads to decreased LH secretion.

and can exacerbate symptoms of metastatic prostate cancer, such as bone pain and ureteral obstruction. Coadministration of the antiandrogen flutamide with a GnRH agonist can prevent these negative effects. Pituitary gonadotroph desensitization occurs 1–2 weeks after starting the GnRH agonist, with castrate levels of testosterone seen in 2–4 weeks. GnRH antagonists can also dramatically reduce serum testosterone. Unlike agonists, GnRH antagonists suppress pituitary gonadotrophs immediately, avoiding the undesired transient increases in LH secretion and serum testosterone concentrations and obviating the need for coadministration of an antiandrogen.

GnRH agonists and antagonists have also been used in premenopausal women with hormone-dependent metastatic breast cancer as an alternative to oophorectomy to decrease serum estrogen to menopausal levels. Breast cancer "flare" reactions have occurred in some women treated with continuous GnRH agonists and are likely related to a transient increase in gonadotropin secretion from the pituitary. Comparison of the GnRH agonist goserelin with oophorectomy in premenopausal women with estrogen-receptor-positive or progesterone-receptor-positive metastatic breast cancer indicated that response rates, failure-free survival, and overall survival were equivalent.

GnRH analogue therapy is approved as a means of obtaining a medical oophorectomy for treatment of endometriosis and uterine leiomyomas. Treatment with GnRH agonists for 6 months has been shown to be as effective as danazol in reducing the size of endometrial implants and decreasing clinical symptoms, including pelvic pain, dysmenorrhea, and dyspareunia. In addition, GnRH agonists have been used for treatment of hirsutism and other manifestations of hyperandrogenism in women who have failed conventional therapies (oral contraceptives or antiandrogens). In addition, several GnRH agonists are used to treat idiopathic precocious puberty.

Somatostatin and Analogues

The short half-life and requirement for continuous IV administration limit the usefulness of SRIF. The analogues octreotide and lanreotide, however, have many uses, including treatment for excessive GH secretion. Gigantism occurs if GH hypersecretion is present before epiphyseal closure during puberty, and acromegaly occurs if hypersecretion develops after puberty. Excessive GH secretion has many deleterious effects, such as tissue growth stimulation and altered glucose and fat metabolism.

Generally, patients with gigantism or acromegaly are treated by transsphenoidal resection of the GH-secreting adenoma. Medical therapy for nonsurgical treatment of acromegaly includes DA agonists, pegvisomant (a GH receptor antagonist), or SRIF analogues, the latter of which bind to pituitary SRIF receptors and block GH secretion. SSTR2 and SSTR5 are the main SRIF receptors found in GH-secreting pituitary tumors and are the receptors for which octreotide and lanreotide have the highest affinity. Several studies show that long-acting SRIF analogues are useful as adjunct therapy in acromegaly. Improvement in symptoms can be seen even without normalization of serum GH and IGF-1 levels, most likely because even small reductions in GH secretion will result in a clinical response. Such therapy can also lead to tumor shrinkage in 30% of patients treated for acromegaly.

SRIF analogues have also been approved for use in the treatment of carcinoid syndrome and vasoactive intestinal peptide tumors. In addition, because most neuroendocrine tumors express SRIF receptors, radiolabeled SRIF analogues have been used to image these tumors (scintigraphy) and to deliver isotopes to the tumors to inhibit their growth.

Dopamine Agonists

Pathologic hyperprolactinemia, most commonly caused by a prolactin-secreting pituitary adenoma, results in suppression of gonadotropin secretion, with resulting sex steroid deficiency. Women with hyperprolactinemia commonly present with oligomenorrhea, amenorrhea, or infertility. Men with hyperprolactinemia commonly present with decreased libido, erectile dysfunction, and other signs of low testosterone, including osteoporosis. DA agonists, used to treat hyperprolactinemia caused by both prolactinomas and lactotroph hyperplasia, bind to D_2 receptors on the lactotrophs, decrease prolactin synthesis and secretion, and decrease the size of the lactotrophs, shrinking the prolactinoma. Decreases in prolactin concentration occur within 2–3 weeks of initiating therapy, but significant abatement of the clinical signs and symptoms of the intracranial tumor may be noted within days. A significant reduction of tumor size may be seen within 6 weeks of initiating therapy. With reduction of the serum prolactin concentration to normal, galactorrhea is abolished and gonadal function restored. Patients who do not respond to one DA agonist may respond to another. Women with pathological hyperprolactinemia requiring treatment with a DA agonist who desire pregnancy should be treated with bromocriptine because this drug has not been reported to lead to birth defects.

DA agonists also inhibit GH secretion and can be used in the treatment of acromegaly, with bromocriptine less effective than cabergoline. The combination of a DA agonist with an SRIF analogue may be effective when neither agent alone is adequate.

Pituitary Hormones
Luteinizing Hormone and Follicle-Stimulating Hormone
Ovulation may be induced by hMG, purified urinary FSH, and recombinant FSH. hMG consists of a purified preparation of LH and FSH extracted from the urine of postmenopausal women. Administered either SC or intramuscularly (IM), hMG is indicated for ovulation induction in women with amenorrhea caused by hypogonadotropic hypogonadism (including hypothalamic amenorrhea) or normogonadotropic amenorrhea, including women with polycystic ovary syndrome who have failed to ovulate with clomiphene. In a recent study, the use of gonadotropins for ovulation induction in women with polycystic ovary syndrome was successful in approximately 70% of patients, with 40% achieving pregnancy. Multiple-gestation births occur in approximately 10% to 15% of patients receiving gonadotropins.

The gonadotropins, both urinary and recombinant, can be used to induce spermatogenesis in the treatment of male-factor infertility. Men with hypogonadotropic hypogonadism caused by hypothalamic or pituitary disease are candidates for treatment with hCG, hMG, or both. Because hCG has LH biological activity, it is used to stimulate testosterone production from Leydig cells and subsequently spermatogenesis. If the onset of hypogonadism occurs after puberty, Sertoli cells will have already been primed by FSH, and hCG alone could be effective. Onset before puberty will likely require FSH in addition to LH, and treatment with hMG (containing both) is indicated.

Growth Hormone
GH promotes linear growth by causing generation of IGF-1 and influences all aspects of metabolism. GH is anabolic, lipolytic, and diabetogenic, promoting insulin resistance. The use of recombinant human GH (hGH) to treat GH deficiency is effective in children and stimulates the incorporation of amino acids into muscle protein and promotes long bone growth. In GH-deficient adults, hGH produces maximum size, decreases adipose mass, and increases muscle mass compared with untreated GH-deficient adults.

Arginine Vasopressin
Three forms of AVP are approved for clinical use: native AVP, vasopressin tannate, and desmopressin. Clinical indications include diabetes insipidus,

GI variceal hemorrhage, nocturnal enuresis, bleeding diatheses, and cardiac arrhythmia. Central (or neurogenic) diabetes insipidus results from inadequate secretion of AVP from the posterior pituitary and responds to AVP with an increase in urine osmolality. In contrast, patients with nephrogenic diabetes insipidus, resulting from failure of the kidney to respond to secreted AVP, exhibit no change in urine osmolality following the administration of AVP.

AVP is also used for the treatment of certain bleeding disorders, such as mild hemophilia A and mild to moderate von Willebrand disease. AVP increases circulating concentrations of factor VIII (antihemophilic factor), perhaps by stimulating its release from cells in the vascular endothelium. Desmopressin is used for the treatment of acute bleeding in patients with platelet dysfunction caused by uremia and is preferred to AVP because of its lack of vasopressor activity.

PHARMACOKINETICS

The pharmacokinetic parameters for the hypothalamic and pituitary hormones and analogues are summarized in Table 49.1.

Hypothalamic Hormones
Gonadotropin-Releasing Hormone and Analogues
Continuous SC infusions of GnRH in hypogonadotropic patients produce steady-state concentrations that are one-third less than those achieved with the IV route. Therefore SC administration results in delayed and prolonged absorption and lower serum concentrations. In patients receiving SC pulsatile GnRH therapy, these characteristics cause significant dampening of plasma GnRH concentration peaks. The lack of a pulsatile change in GnRH concentrations may lead to desensitization and diminished pituitary responsiveness, which likely explains the decreased success rate for induction of ovulation associated with SC as compared with IV administration.

Initially, GnRH agonists were administered daily either intranasally or by SC injection. More recently, long-acting depot formulations have been developed. For example, a long-acting suspension of leuprolide can be administered either SC or IM every 1, 3, or 4 months, depending on dose. Leuprolide is also available as an SC implant, which releases leuprolide acetate every day for 1 year. Similarly, goserelin is administered as an SC implant every 28 days or every 3 months. Triptorelin can be administered as a short-acting SC injection or as a long-acting IM formulation in biodegradable polymer microspheres that last for a month. Nafarelin is administered intranasally.

GnRH is not significantly bound to plasma proteins. Renal excretion represents its primary route of elimination, and thus renal insufficiency decreases the overall clearance rate. Moderate abnormalities of hepatic function do not affect GnRH clearance.

Somatostatin and Analogues
SRIF is inactivated rapidly by peptidases and cannot be administered orally. Although the IV administration of native SRIF results in a prompt decline in serum GH concentrations, continuous IV infusion makes it unsuitable for therapeutic use. Octreotide and lanreotide, two cyclic octapeptide SRIF analogues, are more potent inhibitors of GH, glucagon, and insulin secretion because of their increased duration of action. Octreotide can be administered by SC injection three times a day or as a long-acting release formulation dispersed in microspheres of a biodegradable polymer available for monthly administration.

Dopamine Agonists
DA is a sympathomimetic commonly used to treat certain cardiac and renal morbidities. Because of its vasoconstrictor properties, it is

TABLE 49.1   Pharmacokinetic Parameters

Drugs	Administration	Absorption	$t_{1/2}$	Disposition
Hypothalamic Hormones and Analogues				
GnRH	IV, SC	–	2–8 min	R, M
GnRH agonists	SC, intranasal, depot[a]	–	3 hr	–
Bromocriptine	Oral	Fair (28%)	6 hr[b]	M, B
Octreotide	SC	–	80–90 min	–
Pituitary Hormones and Analogues				
LH	IM, SC	Good	30–60 min	M
FSH	IM, SC	Good	4–5 hr	–
GH	IM, SC	–	19–25 min	–
Vasopressin	IM, SC	Good	3–15 min	M
Vasopressin tannate	IM	Erratic	–	M
Desmopressin	IV, SC, oral, intranasal	Good	75 min	M
Clomiphene	Oral	Good	5 days	B (main)

[a]Depot preparations are long acting.
[b]90% bound to serum albumin.
B, Excreted in bile; M, metabolized; R, renal excretion as unchanged drug.

not administered SC or IM. Required continuous IV infusion with a short half-life makes it unsuitable for treatment of hyperprolactinemia, although it effectively decreases serum prolactin levels. Bromocriptine, a long-acting agonist, reaches peak plasma levels in 1 hour, has a half-life of about 6 hours, and is heavily bound to serum albumin (>90%). An intravaginal route can be used effectively to avoid drug sensitivity. Bromocriptine is metabolized by the liver and excreted in bile (84.6% within 120 hours). Cabergoline is another long-acting dopamine agonist with a high affinity for D_2 receptors. After a single oral dose, mean peak plasma levels are observed within 2 to 3 hours, with a significant fraction undergoing first-pass metabolism. The elimination half-life is 63 to 69 hours, allowing twice-weekly administration.

Pituitary Hormones
Luteinizing Hormone and Follicle-Stimulating Hormone
The absorption characteristics and subsequent metabolism of the gonadotropins LH and FSH have not been elucidated, but the liver appears to be the major route of clearance after the enzymatic removal of sialic acid. The estimated half-life of LH is shorter than that of FSH because the latter has a higher sialic acid content and consequently a decreased hepatic uptake. The clearance of LH is approximately 30 mL/min in women and 50 mL/min in men. The clearance of FSH is approximately 15 mL/min in women and has not been determined in men.

Growth Hormone
Endogenous GH has a short half-life. GH produced from recombinant DNA, which is administered three to six times per week, has a mean half-life of approximately 4 hours and is metabolized by both liver and kidney.

Arginine Vasopressin
AVP, vasopressin tannate, and desmopressin circulate unbound to plasma proteins. All are metabolized in liver and kidney and may be inactivated initially by cleavage of the C-terminal glycinamide. A small amount of AVP is excreted intact in urine. The duration of action of the three preparations differs. When administered SC, AVP is effective for only 2–8 hours. After IM administration, vasopressin tannate is often absorbed erratically, with a duration of action of 48–96 hours; desmopressin has a longer half-life than AVP.

PHARMACOVIGILANCE: ADVERSE EFFECTS AND DRUG INTERACTIONS
Hypothalamic Hormones
GnRH is generally well tolerated, but occasionally nausea, lightheadedness, headache, and abdominal discomfort are reported. SC administration is associated with antibody formation in a few patients. GnRH agonist and antagonist therapy is associated with hot flashes/flushes, decreased libido, fatigue, and decreased bone mineral density.

GI side effects, such as nausea, vomiting, diarrhea, and abdominal cramps, have been reported after treatment with native SRIF. Alterations in blood glucose and hypothyroidism caused by SRIF inhibition of TSH may also be manifest. After discontinuing an IV infusion of SRIF, rebound hypersecretion of GH, insulin, and glucagon can occur. Side effects of SRIF analogues are similar to those of the native peptide. In addition, patients may develop gallbladder sludge or cholelithiasis.

When a DA agonist is first administered, patients may experience nausea, vomiting, dizziness, or orthostatic hypotension (Chapter 15). These effects can be minimized if therapy is begun with low doses and administered with food and at bedtime, with gradual increased frequency as appropriate. A few patients experience headache, fatigue, abdominal cramping, nasal congestion, drowsiness, or diarrhea.

Pituitary Hormones
The major adverse reactions of hMG include multiple-gestation pregnancy and ovarian hyperstimulation syndrome. Ovarian enlargement and extravascular accumulation of fluid resulting in ascites, pleural and pericardial effusions, renal failure, and hypovolemic shock are potentially life-threatening. Ovarian enlargement can be classified as mild, moderate, or severe; the incidence of massive ovarian enlargement of greater than 12 cm is rare (<2%).

Administration of hGH can result in the formation of anti-GH antibodies and may include hyperglycemia, peripheral edema, arthralgias, paresthesias, and carpal tunnel syndrome. Benign intracranial hypertension (pseudotumor cerebri) has rarely been associated with children receiving hGH therapy. A dosage appropriate for size and age must be used to prevent gigantism because improper management or unsupervised use can lead to excessive serum GH concentrations. Because hGH is potentially diabetogenic, care must be given when administering to a patient with a personal or family history of abnormal glucose tolerance.

CLINICAL PROBLEMS

Hypothalamic Hormones and Analogues

GnRH	Breast tenderness, decreased sex drive; hot flashes/sweating; impotence
	Occasional nausea or vomiting, headache, abdominal discomfort, difficulty sleeping
	Anaphylaxis (rare) with IV use
	Localized problems at injection site
Somatostatin analogues	Hyperglycemia, loose stools, gallstones
Dopamine agonists	Nausea, orthostatic hypotension initially
	Confusion, headache, dizziness, drowsiness, faintness

Pituitary Hormones and Analogues

LH and FSH	Multiple gestation pregnancy
	Gynecomastia in men
	Occasional febrile reactions
GH	Antibodies
	Blurred vision, unusual tingling feelings, dizziness, nervousness, severe headache, altered heartbeat
	Abuse in athletics
AVP	Nausea, vertigo, headache
	Anaphylaxis
	Angina, myocardial infarction

TRADE NAMES

In addition to generic and fixed-combination preparations, the following trade-named materials are some of the important compounds available in the United States.

Hypothalamic Hormones and Analogues

GnRH Analogues
Buserelin (Suprefact)
Gonadorelin (Factrel)
Goserelin (Zoladex)
Histrelin (Supprelin)
Leuprolide (Lupron, Lupron Depot, Viadur)
Nafarelin (Synarel)
Triptorelin (Trelstar Depot, Trelstar LA)
Cetrorelix (Cetrotide)
Ganirelix (Antagon)

Dopamine Agonists
Bromocriptine (Parlodel)
Cabergoline (Dostinex)

Somatostatin Analogue
Octreotide (Sandostatin, Sandostatin LAR)
Lanreotide (Somatuline LA)
Vapreotide (Sanvar IR)

Pituitary Hormones and Analogues

LH and FSH Analogues and Related Compounds
Clomiphene (Clomid, Milophene, Serophene)
Human chorionic gonadotropin (Ovidrel)
LH-FSH (Pergonal, Repronex)
Urofollitropin (Bravelle, Fertinex, Follistim, Gonal-F, Metrodin)

Growth Hormone Receptor Agonist
Human recombinant GH (Genotropin, Humatrope, Norditropin, Nutropin, Protropin, Saizen, Serostim)

Growth Hormone Receptor Antagonist
Pegvisomant (Somavert)

AVP Analogues
Desmopressin (DDAVP, Stimate nasal spray)
Vasopressin (Pitressin)

ADH Receptor Antagonists
Conivaptan (Vaprisol)
Tolvaptan (Samsca, Jinarc)

Nonspecific adverse reactions to AVP include nausea, vertigo, headache, and anaphylaxis. Other signs and symptoms may relate directly to specific pressor and antidiuretic effects. Vasoconstriction may be mild, leading to skin blanching or abdominal cramping, or may be life-threatening, leading to angina or myocardial infarction. All preparations should be used with caution in patients with coronary artery disease; desmopressin has lower pressor effects and may be a drug of choice. All vasopressins may cause water retention and hyponatremia. Signs and symptoms of hyponatremia include drowsiness, listlessness, weakness, headaches, seizures, and coma.

Simultaneous administration of AVP with carbamazepine, chlorpropamide, clofibrate, fludrocortisone, and tricyclic antidepressants may potentiate AVP effects, while lithium carbonate, heparin, and alcohol may inhibit AVP effects.

Side effects and clinical problems associated with the use of the hypothalamic and pituitary hormones and their analogues are summarized in the Clinical Problems Box.

NEW DEVELOPMENTS

There is a significant role for the use of long-acting depot forms of GnRH analogues to treat androgen-dependent neoplasms such as prostate cancer and to use GnRH agonist therapy to manage male and female infertility. Further, the ability of GnRH analogues to diminish gonadotropic hormones suggests a potential adjunct role in female and male contraception. Development of recombinant analogues, largely replacing naturally occurring purified hormones, is continuing and should be beneficial in clinical therapy.

CLINICAL RELEVANCE FOR HEALTHCARE PROFESSIONALS

Hypothalamic and pituitary hormones function to regulate the endocrine system, providing trophic factors to stimulate the release of hormones by target glands in response to stimulus input and feedback systems.

These trophic factors and the hormones released by target glands, in concert with the nervous system, are an intimate part of the body's regulatory ability to maintain a homeostatic balance. Alterations of any of these regulatory factors can put patients at risk during various healthcare encounters. For example, alteration of hypothalamic function can increase sensitivity to Epi, resulting in increased risk of arrhythmias, increased sweating, and tremors. Use of Epi in dental practice, if systemically absorbed, could induce an arrhythmia. Tremors and increased sweating could be mistaken for some other issue by nurses or physician assistants or produce an altered response to physical therapy interventions. Therefore awareness of the endocrine status of a patient, and any therapeutic intervention, can provide the healthcare practitioner important information relevant to care being administered.

SELF-ASSESSMENT QUESTIONS

1. A young man with central diabetes insipidus was given desmopressin rather than arginine vasopressin because desmopressin:
   A. Has greater affinity for the vasopressin receptor.
   B. Has an increased duration of action.
   C. Is less likely to form autoantibodies because it is a synthetic compound.
   D. More effectively controls polyuria, polydipsia, and dehydration.
   E. Reduces the incidence of cardiovascular side effects.

2. A 28-year-old woman wanted to get pregnant, but she was infertile as a consequence of central amenorrhea. The best treatment for her condition is:
   A. Clomiphene.
   B. Human menopausal gonadotropin.
   C. Pulsatile GnRH.
   D. Bromocriptine.
   E. Octreotide.

3. A 78-year-old man with prostate cancer elects not to have surgery. His physician may produce a functional orchiectomy by administering:
   A. A GnRH analogue.
   B. A DA agonist.
   C. A GH agonist.
   D. An SRIF analogue.
   E. A GnRH antagonist.

4. A 27-year-old man with acromegaly, who is not a surgical candidate, has been experiencing metabolic issues. His physician likely prescribes which of the following to treat his condition?
   A. An SRIF analogue.
   B. A GnRH agonist.
   C. A DA receptor agonist.
   D. Human recombinant GH.
   E. An AVP receptor antagonist.

5. A 6-year-old female was diagnosed with precocious puberty. To prevent further development, her endocrinologist prescribed which of the following?
   A. A GnRH analogue.
   B. An SRIF analogue.
   C. A DA receptor agonist.
   D. A GH antagonist.
   E. Human recombinant GH.

FURTHER READING

Anonymous. Cool.Click: A needle-free device for growth hormone delivery. *Med Lett.* 2001;43:2–3.

Anonymous. Pegvisomant (Somavert) for acromegaly. *Med Lett.* 2003;45:55–56.

Anonymous. Growth hormone for normal short children. *Med Lett.* 2003;45:89–90.

WEBSITES

https://www.endocrine.org/
The Endocrine Society maintains an excellent website with numerous resources, including continually updated pages on Clinical Practice Guidelines for the treatment of endocrine disorders.

https://www.aace.com/publications/guidelines
The American Association of Clinical Endocrinologists also maintains an excellent website containing Clinical Practice Guidelines and other resources.

Treatment of Adrenocorticosteroid Disorders

Gerald B. Call

MAJOR DRUG CLASSES	
Glucocorticoids	
Mineralocorticoids	
Steroidogenesis inhibitors	
Corticosteroid receptor antagonists	

ABBREVIATIONS	
ACTH	Adrenocorticotropic hormone
CRH	Corticotropin-releasing hormone
GR	Glucocorticoid receptor
GI	Gastrointestinal
HPA	Hypothalamic-pituitary-adrenal
MR	Mineralocorticoid receptor

THERAPEUTIC OVERVIEW

The adrenocorticosteroids produced by the adrenal gland cortex include the **glucocorticoids** and the **mineralocorticoids**. Glucocorticoids are synthesized and secreted in response to adrenocorticotropic hormone (ACTH) synthesized by the anterior pituitary (Chapter 49). ACTH is a tropic hormone that directly controls the size of the adrenal cortex in a concentration-dependent manner. Disruption of plasma ACTH concentrations may lead to adrenal cortex atrophy (low levels) or promote adrenal cortex hyperplasia (high levels). Because the steroids do not accumulate significantly, the actions of ACTH are primarily at the level of biosynthesis regulation. Further, ACTH pulses exhibit greater frequency and magnitude in the early morning compared with the afternoon, leading to circadian alterations in corticosteroid synthesis.

Cortisol, the primary endogenous glucocorticoid in humans, is involved in the regulation of intermediary metabolism, the stress response, some aspects of central nervous system function, and the regulation of immunity. The main therapeutic uses of the glucocorticoids are (1) **replacement therapy** for patients exhibiting inadequate endogenous cortisol production; (2) **antiinflammatory** or **immunosuppressant** agents; and (3) adjuvants in the treatment of myeloproliferative diseases and other malignant conditions.

Aldosterone, the main mineralocorticoid, is involved primarily with electrolyte regulation and balance; therefore, its synthesis is primarily regulated by angiotensin II (Chapter 39) and potassium levels. The major therapeutic use of the synthetic mineralocorticoids is replacement for patients with **primary adrenal insufficiency** or **isolated aldosterone deficiency**.

When corticosteroids are in excess, as occurs with corticotroph adenomas or adrenalcortical tumors secreting excessive ACTH or cortisol, respectively, **steroidogenesis inhibitors** may be required. Similarly, drugs that antagonize corticosteroid receptors may be warranted when corticosteroids are overproduced.

A summary of the use of the glucocorticoids, mineralocorticoids, and other agents for the treatment of adrenocorticosteroid disorders is presented in the Therapeutic Overview Box.

THERAPEUTIC OVERVIEW

Glucocorticoids
Replacement therapy in adrenal insufficiencies
Antiinflammatory and immunosuppressive action
Myeloproliferative diseases

Mineralocorticoids
Replacement therapy in primary adrenal insufficiencies
Hypoaldosteronism

Steroidogenesis Inhibitors
Adrenocortical hyperfunction

Corticosteroid Receptor Antagonists
Glucocorticoid excess
Mineralocorticoid excess

MECHANISMS OF ACTION

Corticosteroid Biosynthesis

The biosynthetic pathways and structures for cortisol and aldosterone are shown in Chapter 48, Figs. 48.1 and 48.2. The synthesis of cortisol is initiated by ACTH activation of its receptor, the melanocortin type 2 receptor (MC2R), which is a G-protein–coupled receptor (GPCR), resulting in increased cyclic adenosine monophosphate (cAMP). ACTH-stimulated increases in cAMP accelerate transcription rates of the genes coding for the cholesterol side-chain cleavage enzyme, CYP11A1, and most other enzymes in the cortisol biosynthetic pathway. The rate-limiting step in overall steroid synthesis is the cholesterol transport process through the outer mitochondrial membrane, regulating its availability to CYP11A1, which is located on the inner mitochondrial membrane.

Serum concentrations of ACTH are increased in response to metabolic stresses, such as severe trauma, illness, burns, hypoglycemia, hemorrhage, fever, exercise, and psychological stresses, such as anxiety and depression.

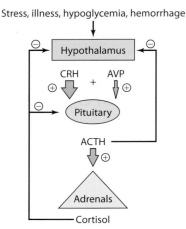

Stress, illness, hypoglycemia, hemorrhage

FIG. 50.1 Regulatory Mechanisms in the HPA. *ACTH*, Adrenocorticotropic hormone; *AVP*, arginine vasopressin; *CRH*, corticotropin-releasing hormone.

These stresses induce physiological changes by altering the release of the hypothalamic peptides, **corticotropin-releasing hormone (CRH)**, and, to a lesser extent, **arginine vasopressin (AVP)**, both of which promote ACTH release. This hypothalamic-pituitary-adrenal (HPA) axis is also sensitive to feedback inhibition by circulating cortisol, which acts directly on the hypothalamus to inhibit CRH release and on the pituitary to decrease ACTH synthesis and secretion and suppress the pituitary response to CRH. Because this negative feedback can last for weeks after cessation of glucocorticoid therapy, cessation from treatment must be approached cautiously. HPA axis regulation is depicted in Fig. 50.1.

Corticosteroid Receptors

All natural and synthetic corticosteroids act by binding to specific receptors that are members of the nuclear receptor superfamily, leading to alterations in gene transcription (Chapter 2). The mineralocorticoid receptors (MRs), expressed predominantly in the kidney, have high affinity for both mineralocorticoids and glucocorticoids, while the glucocorticoid receptors (GRs), expressed in virtually all cells, are specific for glucocorticoids. Although aldosterone and cortisol have a similar affinity for MRs, cortisol is converted by 11β-hydroxysteroid dehydrogenase 2 in MR-expressing cells to cortisone, an inactive metabolite with virtually no MR affinity. Inhibition of this enzyme by compounds like licorice can evoke inappropriate cortisol activation of the MR, resulting in hypertension. Additionally, supraphysiological glucocorticoid levels can overwhelm 11β-hydroxysteroid dehydrogenase 2, allowing activation of the MR by glucocorticoids.

Glucocorticoids

As a consequence of GR activation, the glucocorticoids have metabolic, antiinflammatory, and immunosuppressant actions. Glucocorticoids decrease glucose uptake in many tissues and stimulate liver glucose production, possibly to protect the brain and heart. They also disrupt lipid metabolism and facilitate the lipolytic effects of other agents to increase gluconeogenesis, again as a possible protection of the heart and brain. The metabolic effects of the glucocorticoids include:

- Increased glycogenolysis and gluconeogenesis
- Increased protein catabolism and decreased protein synthesis, causing muscle wasting in striated muscle
- Decreased osteoblast formation and activity
- Decreased Ca^{++} absorption from the gastrointestinal (GI) tract
- Decreased thyroid-stimulating hormone secretion

The glucocorticoids also inhibit the synthesis of inflammatory response mediators and phagocytosis both locally and systemically. The antiinflammatory actions of these compounds include:

- Decreased production of prostaglandins, cytokines, and interleukins
- Decreased proliferation and migration of lymphocytes and macrophages

In addition, the glucocorticoids increase circulating neutrophils, inhibit macrophage antigen processing, suppress T-helper cell function, and induce eosinopenia and lymphopenia. Even with increases in neutrophils, glucocorticoids decrease their accumulation at inflammatory sites. This action, along with the suppression of the phagocytic, bactericidal, and antigen-processing activity of these cells, compromises the immune system.

Glucocorticoids can have profound direct and indirect effects on the central nervous system. The indirect effects occur through actions on blood pressure, plasma glucose levels, and other similar actions, while the direct effects include altered mood, behavior, and neural excitability, with frank psychosis in some patients receiving these agents.

Glucocorticoids also regulate growth and development, particularly in fetal tissues, where it induces surfactant synthesis in the lungs before birth. As a result, cortisol can lessen the severity of respiratory distress syndrome due to insufficient surfactant secretion in preterm infants.

Mineralocorticoids

Aldosterone, the major mineralocorticoid produced by the adrenal cortex, acts primarily at the distal portion of the convoluted renal tubule to promote the reabsorption of Na^+ and the excretion of K^+ to maintain homeostasis. Adrenal secretion of aldosterone is controlled by the renin-angiotensin system, specifically angiotensin II, and the circulating concentrations of K^+.

MRs are expressed both in epithelial tissue where electrolyte transport occurs, such as distal nephrons, salivary glands, colon, and sweat glands, and in nonepithelial cells, such as the hippocampus, cardiomyocytes, adipocytes, and vasculature.

The structures of the principal synthetic glucocorticoids and mineralocorticoids are shown in Fig. 50.2.

Steroidogenesis Inhibitors and Corticosteroid Receptor Antagonists

Drugs that inhibit steroid biosynthesis include mitotane, metyrapone, and ketoconazole. **Mitotane** is an adrenotoxic agent with an active metabolite that is cytotoxic to adrenal cells by an unknown mechanism of action. **Metyrapone** is a selective inhibitor of CYP11B1, which catalyzes the conversion of 11-deoxycortisol to cortisol, while the antifungal drug **ketoconazole** inhibits CYP17 at low doses, thereby decreasing the hydroxylation of progesterone and pregnenolone, and it also inhibits CYP11A1 at higher doses, decreasing the conversion of cholesterol to pregnenolone (Chapter 48, Fig. 48.1).

Mifepristone is an antagonist at GRs with an 18-fold higher affinity for the receptor than cortisol. It is also a high-affinity antagonist at the progesterone receptor. **Spironolactone** is a diuretic that competitively inhibits the action of aldosterone at MRs.

RELATIONSHIP OF MECHANISMS OF ACTION TO CLINICAL RESPONSE

Therapeutic properties of clinically useful glucocorticoids and mineralocorticoids are summarized in Table 50.1.

Glucocorticoids

Hydrocortisone and **cortisone** are used primarily for replacement therapy in patients with primary or secondary adrenal insufficiency because they

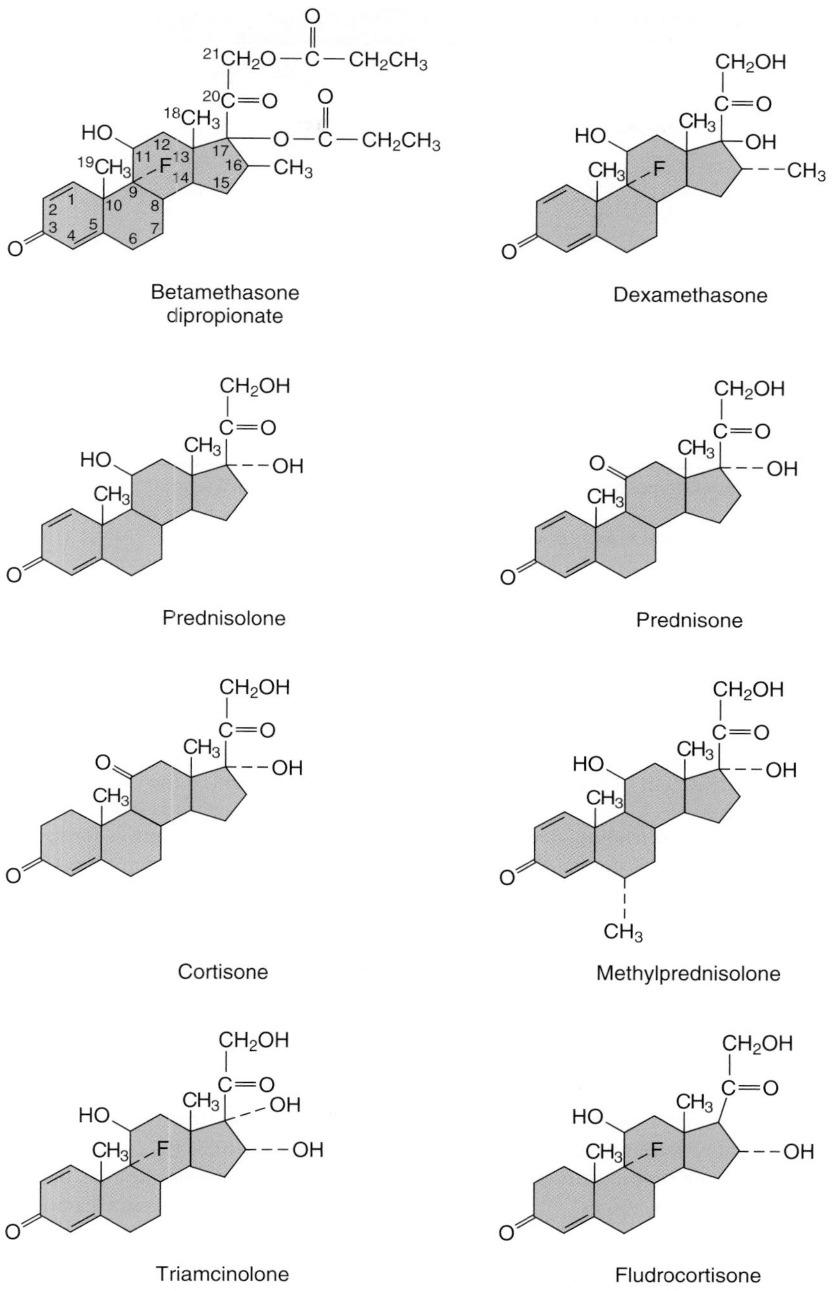

FIG. 50.2 Structures of Representative Glucocorticoids and Mineralocorticoids.

have equal glucocorticoid and mineralocorticoid effects, allowing them to fulfill both needs. If adequate glucocorticoid levels are achieved but more mineralocorticoid effects are required, fludrocortisone is supplemented. Primary adrenal insufficiency (Addison's disease) is most commonly caused by a polyglandular autoimmune syndrome but may also result from tuberculosis or other infections, adrenal hemorrhage, metastatic neoplasia, drugs, and congenital adrenal disorders. Secondary causes of adrenal insufficiency include adrenal suppression occurring after the administration of exogenous glucocorticoids (very common) or after treatment of Cushing syndrome, or diseases of the hypothalamus or pituitary gland leading to ACTH deficiency.

Plasma cortisol concentrations should be measured in patients with suspected acute adrenal insufficiency, and, if low, patients should be treated immediately with intravenous hydrocortisone. A further test

is required to confirm a diagnosis in patients with suspected chronic adrenal insufficiency, in which a synthetic polypeptide subunit of ACTH (cosyntropin) is administered intravenously. If the problem is at the secondary or pituitary level (low ACTH secretion), a response will occur; failure to respond indicates a primary adrenal insufficiency. In either situation, cortisol replacement should be initiated.

Glucocorticoids are also used for the treatment of congenital adrenal hyperplasia, which can result from alterations in any of the steps in steroid synthesis, leading to diminished cortisol secretion and consequent stimulation of synthesis and release of ACTH. The cornerstone for treatment is administration of glucocorticoids to suppress ACTH secretion, thereby decreasing growth stimulation of the adrenal gland.

Prednisone, prednisolone, and methylprednisolone have considerable antiinflammatory activity and relatively low mineralocorticoid

TABLE 50.1   Therapeutic Properties of Corticosteroids

Drugs	Antiinflammatory	Salt-Retaining	Duration of Action[a]
Glucocorticoids			
Hydrocortisone (Cortisol)	1	1	S
Cortisone	0.8	0.8	S
Prednisone	4	0.3	I
Prednisolone	4	0.3	I
Methylprednisolone	5	0	I
Triamcinolone	5	0	I
Betamethasone	25–40	0	L
Dexamethasone	30	0	L
Mineralocorticoids			
Fludrocortisone	10	250	I
Aldosterone (for reference)	0.25	500	S

Relative therapeutic potencies of common corticosteroids for both their glucocorticoid (antiinflammatory) and mineralocorticoid (salt-retaining) effects.
[a]S, Short, 10–90 minutes; I, intermediate, several hours; L, long, 5 hours or more.

activity, ideal characteristics for long-term antiinflammatory and immunosuppressant regimens. Prednisone and its derivatives are the most commonly used glucocorticoids for the treatment of several autoimmune diseases, including collagen diseases, vasculitis syndromes, GI inflammatory diseases, and renal autoimmune diseases. Intermediate-acting glucocorticoids are also used for treatment of bronchial asthma and chronic obstructive pulmonary disease.

Alternate day–therapy glucocorticoid administration, developed to reduce adverse effects, involves administration of double the normal daily dose of an intermediate-acting glucocorticoid, such as prednisone, every other day. However, alternate-day therapy can become problematic, with some patients finding this approach intolerable because of fluctuations of hormone levels and inconvenience.

Dexamethasone and betamethasone have minimal to no mineralocorticoid activity and maximal antiinflammatory activity. Their primary use is to induce strong antiinflammatory therapy acutely. They should not be used long term because of their bone demineralization properties and growth suppression in children. Dexamethasone is also used as a diagnostic agent to cause negative feedback of the HPA axis in Cushing syndrome in the dexamethasone suppression test because it does not cross-react with cortisol and its metabolites.

Mineralocorticoids

Aldosterone, the most potent endogenous corticosteroid for fluid and electrolyte regulation, is not used therapeutically to replace a loss of mineralocorticoid activity because of its short duration of action. Fludrocortisone (9α-fluorohydrocortisone) is the mineralocorticoid drug of choice for the treatment of primary adrenocortical insufficiency, aldosterone insufficiency, salt-losing congenital adrenal hyperplasia, and idiopathic orthostatic hypotension. The benefits include enhanced reabsorption of Na^+ from renal tubules with excretion of K^+ and H^+ to promote fluid and electrolyte balance.

Steroidogenesis Inhibitors and Corticosteroid Receptor Antagonists

Mitotane, metyrapone, and ketoconazole are typically used to control hypercortisolemia associated with Cushing syndrome not due to the excessive administration of corticosteroids. Following administration of these agents, plasma levels of 11-deoxycortisol or ACTH are determined. The lack of a change in 11-deoxycortisol or ACTH is indicative of adrenal insufficiency. Mitotane is also the drug of choice for patients with inoperable adrenocortical carcinoma. Metyrapone is the drug of choice in this group for pregnant women.

For patients with Cushing syndrome who are glucose intolerant or who have type 2 diabetes, mifepristone is used. Mifepristone is the first oral drug approved by the United States Food and Drug Administration to control hyperglycemia in Cushing syndrome.

Spironolactone is effective for lowering blood pressure in patients with primary hyperaldosteronism (Chapter 39).

PHARMACOKINETICS

Glucocorticoids

Glucocorticoids are administered through most routes, but local administration is preferred to minimize adverse effects associated with systemic actions. Circulating cortisol is 80%–90% bound to plasma proteins with high affinity to corticosteroid-binding globulin (CBG, transcortin), 5%–10% loosely bound to albumin, and 3%–10% as the free, active fraction. CBG can also bind synthetic glucocorticoids such as prednisone and prednisolone, but not dexamethasone, resulting in almost 100% of plasma dexamethasone bioactive. Elevated concentrations of estrogen, such as occurs in pregnancy, contraceptive use, or hormone replacement therapy, increase the biosynthesis of CBG in the liver, requiring increased plasma cortisol concentrations to maintain an appropriate bioactive fraction.

Most glucocorticoids are absorbed rapidly and readily from the GI tract and from synovial and conjunctival spaces because of their lipophilic character, but they are absorbed very slowly through the skin. Different structural modifications of some topical glucocorticoids can alter lipophilicity and solubility, changing systemic absorption characteristics that may result in systemic effects following excessive and prolonged local application. The presence of the hydroxyl group at position 11 (see Fig. 50.2) confers glucocorticoid activity on both cortisol (hydrocortisone) and prednisolone. Cortisone and prednisone are 11-ketocorticoids and must be hydroxylated by 11β-hydroxylase to be activated, primarily in the liver, suggesting that 11-ketocorticoids should be avoided in patients with abnormal liver function.

The addition of a fluorine atom at position 9 enhances glucocorticoid and mineralocorticoid activity, such as with fludrocortisone, dexamethasone, and triamcinolone, and enhances activity at GR and MR, with

MR activity more greatly enhanced. However, the addition of a methyl group at position 16, as present in betamethasone and dexamethasone (see Fig. 50.2), increases GR activation and virtually eliminates MR activation, yet does increase the duration of action of these compounds. Prednisone, prednisolone, and methylprednisolone have intermediate plasma half-lives, whereas betamethasone and dexamethasone are long-acting analogues.

The liver and kidney are the major sites of glucocorticoid inactivation, which typically involves reduction of the double bond at position 4/5, reduction of the keto group at position 3, hydroxylation at position 6, and side-chain cleavage. Approximately 30% of inactivated cortisol is metabolized to tetrahydrocortisol-glucuronide and tetrahydrodeoxycortisol-glucuronide and excreted in the urine. Inducers of hepatic drug metabolism, such as rifampin, may accelerate the hepatic biotransformation of the glucocorticoids and necessitate an increase in dose. Hypothyroidism may decrease glucocorticoid metabolism.

Mineralocorticoids

Aldosterone does not bind to a specific plasma protein but binds weakly to several different plasma proteins from which it dissociates rapidly. The half-life of aldosterone is very short (a few minutes), and without ongoing secretion from the adrenals, its rapid clearance from plasma effectively limits its biological effects.

Steroidogenesis Inhibitors and Corticosteroid Receptor Antagonists

Mitotane is 40% absorbed following oral administration and is distributed throughout the body with fat as the primary site. It is metabolized to a water-soluble compound that is excreted in the urine and bile and has a median half-life of 53 days.

Metyrapone is absorbed rapidly following oral administration, reaching peak plasma levels in approximately an hour. It is reduced to metyrapol, which is an active alcohol metabolite, and both parent and metyrapol are excreted as glucuronides.

The pharmacokinetics of ketoconazole are presented in Chapter 62, those of mifepristone in Chapter 51, and those of spironolactone in Chapter 39.

PHARMACOVIGILANCE: ADVERSE EFFECTS AND DRUG INTERACTIONS

Glucocorticoids

Excessive levels of glucocorticoids, whether due to overtreatment or an endogenous source, can result in suppression of the HPA axis leading to various complications and disturbances in many systems. Fluid and electrolyte abnormalities, GI disorders, hyperglycemia, hypertension, bone and muscle abnormalities, visual problems, lipid redistribution, and behavioral problems are all possible manifestations of excess glucocorticoid levels. Further, altered immune responses predispose the patient to increased susceptibility to infection or reactivation of latent infections, a very dangerous complication of long-term glucocorticoid treatment.

A major side effect of glucocorticoids, especially when given for prolonged periods, is their detrimental action on bone leading to osteoporosis. Patients at the highest risk of acquiring glucocorticoid-induced osteoporosis are children and postmenopausal women. Glucocorticoids cause osteoporosis by disrupting the regulation of Ca^{++} metabolism at several levels: (1) by decreasing the intestinal absorption and renal reabsorption of Ca^{++}; (2) by exerting a direct catabolic action on bone by inhibiting osteoblastic activity; and (3) by blocking the protective effect of calcitonin (Chapter 55). Therefore many patients

starting long-term glucocorticoid therapy who are at risk for osteoporosis are routinely given drugs to prevent osteoporosis.

Excessive exposure to glucocorticoids leads to Cushing syndrome, characterized by hypertension, truncal obesity, diabetes, hirsutism, acne, moon facies, proximal muscle weakness, wide purple stria over the skin, and behavioral abnormalities. The syndrome results most commonly from the exogenous administration of glucocorticoids, but there are also endogenous causes. Fig. 50.3 illustrates changes in the HPA axis accompanying the different Cushing syndromes—namely, pituitary ACTH-dependent Cushing syndrome (also known as Cushing disease), ectopic ACTH syndrome, and cortisol-secreting adrenal adenomas or carcinomas. A high-dose dexamethasone suppression test is used to differentiate between pituitary ACTH-dependent Cushing disease and other causes of Cushing syndrome.

The rapid withdrawal of corticosteroids, especially when prolonged therapy has suppressed the HPA axis, typically leads to several issues. Acute adrenal insufficiency is the most serious problem that may occur, while the possible return or "flare-up" of the underlying disease is the most frequent problem. Although patient response to withdrawal is variable, established protocols for corticosteroid withdrawal should be followed to minimize issues. Other characteristics of withdrawal syndrome may include fever, myalgia, arthralgia, malaise, and, in rare circumstances, even pseudotumor cerebri.

In most children, linear growth rate is impaired with long-term glucocorticoid therapy. Although long-term administration causes a decreased secretion of growth hormone, the inhibitory effect of glucocorticoids on growth is thought to be due to inhibition of the effects of insulin-like growth factor-1 (IGF-1).

Mineralocorticoids

Excessive exposure to mineralocorticoids occurs occasionally in patients with adrenal tumors, manifest as a syndrome of hypertension, hypokalemia and metabolic alkalosis, and mild hypernatremia. In the absence of a surgical cure, an important inhibitor is spironolactone, which is also used clinically as a diuretic and an antihypertensive agent. Spironolactone binds to the MR and acts as a competitive antagonist to aldosterone.

Steroidogenesis Inhibitors and Corticosteroid Receptor Antagonists

The steroidogenesis inhibitors all lead to fatigue, GI upset, headaches, muscle aches, hypertension, and hypokalemia. Mitotane contains a boxed warning for drug discontinuation following shock or severe trauma because its primary action is adrenal suppression. Long-term use can be neurotoxic.

The adverse effects associated with the use of ketoconazole are presented in Chapter 62, those for mifepristone in Chapter 51, and those for spironolactone in Chapter 39.

The clinical problems associated with the use of the corticosteroids are summarized in the Clinical Problems Box.

NEW DEVELOPMENTS

During the past 10 years, much effort has been expended on identifying drugs for treating disorders involving excess cortisol production. The approval of mifepristone for Cushing syndrome in patients with glucose intolerance represents a major step forward. One of the newest agents approved for patients with Cushing syndrome resulting from an inoperable pituitary tumor is pasireotide, a somatostatin analogue. Further studies will undoubtedly identify the role of many peptides regulating cortisol production, leading to the development of newer and perhaps more efficacious therapeutic agents.

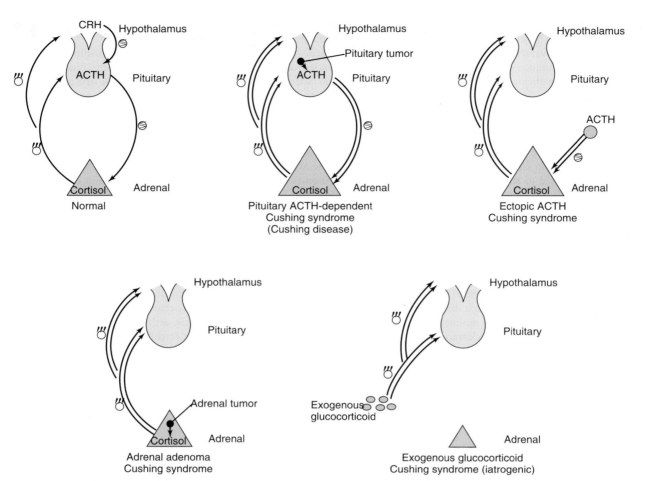

FIG. 50.3 Hypercortisolemia and Its Impact on Normal Feedback Mechanisms in Cushing Syndrome, Pituitary ACTH-Dependent Cushing Syndrome, Ectopic ACTH Syndrome, Adrenal Adenoma, and Exogenous Steroid Administration. +, stimulation; −, inhibition. *CRH*, Corticotropin-releasing hormone; *ACTH*, adrenocorticotropic hormone.

CLINICAL PROBLEMS

The most common side effects resulting from high concentrations of corticosteroids maintained for a long time include:

- Development of cushingoid habitus (truncal obesity, moon facies, buffalo hump), salt retention, and hypertension (i.e., iatrogenic Cushing syndrome)
- Suppression of the immune system (rendering the patient vulnerable to common and opportunistic infections)
- Osteoporosis (rendering the patient vulnerable to fractures)
- Peptic ulcers (resulting in gastric hemorrhages or intestinal perforation)
- Suppression of growth in children
- Behavioral problems
- Reproductive problems
- Prolonged suppression of the HPA axis

CLINICAL RELEVANCE FOR HEALTHCARE PROFESSIONALS

Healthcare providers need to be aware of the adverse effects of the glucocorticoids, especially their possible impact on several organ systems. These agents may lead to increased ocular pressure and cataracts, increased central adiposity with decreased muscle mass, and decreased wound healing. The long-term use of these compounds may cause bone mineral density loss leading to osteoporosis, increased glucose intolerance leading to type 2 diabetes mellitus, iatrogenic adrenal insufficiency, and psychological changes. When withdrawing a patient from long-term therapy, the dose should be tapered gradually over a time frame that is directly proportional to the therapeutic dose and administration duration to avoid potential adrenal crisis. It is also important to note that most adverse effects manifest with long-term administration, whereas psychological effects can occur acutely.

For patients with adrenal insufficiency, it is important to increase their glucocorticoid dose during times of stress to maintain well-being or avoid acute adrenal crisis. A small dose increase may be necessary for mild to moderate stress, while a larger dose may be needed for major stress such as trauma or surgery. Although it has been a common practice to increase the glucocorticoid dose in adrenal insufficiency patients with any dental procedure, recent literature indicates that an adrenal crisis is rare in dental patients. This suggests that an increased glucocorticoid dose is needed only in adrenal insufficiency patients undergoing moderate or major procedures or have other precipitating risk factors (e.g., poor health status, pain, infection, lengthy procedures, use of a barbiturate anesthetic). The increased dose should be given the day of the procedure and for at least one day following to avoid the possibility of an adrenal crisis.

TRADE NAMES

In addition to generic and fixed-combination preparations, the following trade-named materials are some of the important compounds available in the United States.

Glucocorticoids
Betamethasone (Celestone)
Cortisone
Dexamethasone (Decadron)
Hydrocortisone, Cortisol (Cortef)
Methylprednisolone (A-Methapred, Medrol)
Prednisolone (Orapred)
Prednisone (Deltasone)
Triamcinolone (Kenalog)

Mineralocorticoids
Fludrocortisone (Florinef)

Steroidogenesis Inhibitors
Ketoconazole (Nizoral)
Metyrapone (Metopirone)
Mitotane (Lysodren)

Corticosteroid Receptor Antagonists
Mifepristone, RU-486 (Mifeprex)
Spironolactone (Aldactone)

SELF-ASSESSMENT QUESTIONS

1. Which of the following moieties on the cortisol molecule must be present for maximal activation of the glucocorticoid receptor?
   A. Hydroxyl group at carbon 11.
   B. Hydroxyl group at carbon 17.
   C. Hydroxyl group at carbon 21.
   D. Keto group at carbon 3.
   E. Keto group at carbon 20.
2. Addition of which moiety virtually eliminates MR activation?
   A. Hydroxyl group at carbon 11.
   B. Hydroxyl group at carbon 17.
   C. Keto group at carbon 3.
   D. Methyl group at carbon 16.
   E. Methyl group at carbon 20.
3. A 48-year-old man with adrenal insufficiency was prescribed a glucocorticoid and instructed to take it every other day. What is the primary advantage of this dosing schedule?
   A. It reduces adverse effects.
   B. It is advantageous to achieve elevated and sustained immuno-suppression.
   C. It minimizes effects following abrupt withdrawal.
   D. It leads to stabilized hormone levels.
   E. It prevents activation of mineralocorticoid receptors.
4. The corticosteroid with high antiinflammatory activity and minimal effects on blood pressure after acute administration is:
   A. Cortisone.
   B. Hydrocortisone.
   C. Dexamethasone.
   D. Prednisone.
   E. Fludrocortisone.
5. What is the major concern with a 72-year-old woman using prednisone for knee problems for a prolonged period of time?
   A. Hypertension.
   B. Precipitation of a stroke.
   C. Renal insufficiency.
   D. Hepatic necrosis.
   E. Osteoporosis.

FURTHER READING

Arnaldi G, Angeli A, Atkinson AB, et al. Diagnosis and complications of Cushing syndrome: a consensus statement. *J Clin Endocrinol Metab.* 2003;88:5593–5602.

Findling JW, Raff H. Differentiation of pathologic/neoplastic hypercortisolism (Cushing's syndrome) from physiologic/non-neoplastic hypercortisolism (formerly known as pseudo-Cushing's syndrome). *Eur J Endoc.* 2017;176:R205–R216.

Liu D, Ahmet A, Ward L, et al. A practical guide to the monitoring and management of the complications of systemic corticosteroid therapy. *Allergy Asthma Clin Immunol.* 2013;9:30.

Hajar T, Leshem YA, Hanifin JM, et al., the National Eczema Association Task Force. A systematic review of topical corticosteroid withdrawal ("steroid addiction") in patients with atopic dermatitis and other dermatoses. *J Am Acad Dermatol.* 2015;72(3):541–549.e2.

Rhen T, Cidlowski JA. Antiinflammatory action of glucocorticoids—new mechanisms for old drugs. *N Engl J Med.* 2005;353:1711–1723.

Speiser P, White PC. Congenital adrenal hyperplasia. *N Engl J Med.* 2003;349:776–788.

Khalaf MW, Khader R, Cobetto G, et al. Risk of adrenal crisis in dental patients: results of a systematic search of the literature. *J Am Dent Assoc.* 2013;144:152–160.

WEBSITES

http://www.mayoclinic.org/steroids/art-20045692
This site is maintained by the Mayo Clinic and has information on the benefits and risks of prescribing prednisone.
https://www.rheumatology.org/practice-quality/clinical-support/clinical-practice-guidelines/glucocorticoid-induced-osteoporosis
This website is maintained by the American College of Rheumatology and contains the latest guidelines for preventing and treating glucocorticoid-induced osteoporosis.

Female Hormone Regulation

Julia Ousterhout

THERAPEUTIC OVERVIEW

The two major classes of female sex hormones are the estrogens and the progestogens, the latter a generic term for progestational agents and representing both endogenous progesterone and the synthetic progestins. The endogenous 19-carbon steroids in humans that have estrogenic activity are 17β-estradiol, estrone, and estriol. The principal estrogen synthesized in the ovaries is 17β-estradiol, which is the primary circulating form in young women. The major circulating estrogen in postmenopausal women is estrone, which is synthesized in adipose tissue. During pregnancy, the placenta synthesizes large amounts of estrone and estriol. The most important endogenous progestogen is progesterone, although several hydroxyprogesterone metabolites have weak progestational activities.

The estrogens and progesterone serve important functions including the development of female secondary sex characteristics; the progressive maturation of the fallopian tubes, uterus, vagina, and external genitalia in the control of the ovulatory-menstrual cycle; maintenance of pregnancy; regulation of bone homeostasis; and modulation of many metabolic processes.

Several menstrual cycle disorders are treated with estrogens, progestins, or both. In females with primary ovarian failure, estrogens and progestins are administered to optimize normal development of secondary sex characteristics and induce menses. An important pharmacological use of estrogens and progestins, especially in combination, is as contraceptives. Estrogens and progestins act predominantly at the pituitary-hypothalamic axis to decrease production of the gonadotropins, follicle-stimulating hormone (FSH), and luteinizing hormone (LH). Inhibition of the midcycle LH surge prevents ovulation. Conversely, antiestrogens have been developed to aid in the treatment of infertility by inducing an increase in circulating FSH and LH, which leads to ovulation. Estrogen alone or combined with a progestin has been used extensively in the treatment of symptoms arising at menopause due to a deficiency of estrogen.

Some forms of cancer, such as breast and endometrial cancer, are estrogen dependent for growth. The antiestrogens and aromatase inhibitors are used for the former, while the progestins are used for the treatment of the latter.

In addition to estrogen and the progestogens and agents affecting the regulation of these hormones, oxytocin (OT) is a peptide hormone released from the posterior pituitary that plays a role in uterine contraction during labor and nipple stimulation for breastfeeding. The uterotonic or oxytocic drugs act like OT to stimulate uterine smooth muscle and are used to induce or augment labor during late gestation, to prevent or arrest postpartum hemorrhage from uterine atony, and to induce abortion during the first half of pregnancy. In contrast, the tocolytic drugs relax uterine smooth muscle and are used to prevent or arrest preterm labor, reverse inadvertent overstimulation, facilitate intrauterine manipulations, and relieve painful contractions during menstruation (dysmenorrhea).

The major therapeutic uses of estrogens, progestins, other synthetic agonists and antagonists, and inhibitors of estrogen biosynthesis are summarized in the Therapeutic Overview Box.

MECHANISMS OF ACTION

Estrogen and Progesterone Synthesis and Transport

Estrogens and progesterone are produced by steroidogenesis in various tissues (Chapter 48). The ovaries are the predominant source of these steroids in nonpregnant, premenopausal women. A significant amount of estrogenic activity is also found in liver and adipose tissue through the conversion of androgens to estrone. In men, small amounts of estradiol are produced in the testes or from extragonadal conversion

Fertility Control
Combination contraception (estrogens plus progestins)
Progestin-only contraception (progestins)
Emergency contraception (progestins)

Infertility Treatment
Ovulation induction (clomiphene, gonadotropins, GnRH analogues)

Replacement Therapy
Acute symptoms of menopause (estrogens, estrogens plus progestins)
Prevention of osteoporosis (estrogens, raloxifene)
Ovarian failure (estrogens plus progestins)

Cancer Chemotherapy
Breast cancer treatment (antiestrogens, aromatase inhibitors)
Breast cancer prevention (antiestrogens)
Advanced endometrial cancer (progestins)

Other Uses
Dysfunctional uterine bleeding (progestins, estrogens plus progestins)
Endometriosis (estrogens plus progestins, progestins, GnRH analogues, NSAIDs)
Luteal phase dysfunction (progesterone)
Prevention of preterm birth (hydroxyprogesterone)

Uterine Stimulation	Uterine Relaxation
Pregnancy termination	Arrest of preterm labor
Cervical ripening	Facilitation of intrauterine manipulation
Induction of labor	Reversal of pharmacological uterine
Augmentation of labor	hyperstimulation
Postpartum uterine atony	Relief of dysmenorrhea

of androgens to estrogens. Certain brain areas in males and females may also produce estrogens.

Steroid hormones are highly hydrophobic molecules that must be transported by serum proteins to their target tissues. Circulating estrogens are specifically bound by sex hormone–binding globulin (SHBG) and progesterone by corticosteroid-binding globulin (CBG). These are relatively high-affinity, low-capacity interactions compared with those of albumin. The concentrations of the binding globulins are hormonally regulated, and the synthesis of both globulins increases in response to estrogen administration; serum albumin concentrations are unaffected. Synthetic ligands show variable affinities for these serum proteins.

The Menstrual Cycle

During the menstrual cycle, the pituitary gonadotropins FSH and LH regulate the synthesis and release of estrogen and progesterone from the ovaries. Periodic release of hypothalamic gonadotropin-releasing hormone (GnRH), in turn, regulates FSH and LH synthesis and release. GnRH concentrations are regulated through negative and positive feedback by the steroid hormones. Estrogens and progesterone also act directly on the pituitary gonadotrophs to decrease FSH and LH concentrations. In addition, an ovarian protein, inhibin, negatively affects FSH synthesis. The pathways for the integrated control of hormone regulation are shown in Fig. 51.1A.

The ovarian and endometrial changes that occur during the normal human menstrual cycle are shown in Fig. 51.2. The ovarian cycle is divided into the follicular (preovulatory) phase, when ovarian follicles mature, ovulation, when the ovum is released, and the luteal (postovulatory) phase, when the corpus luteum is formed. The follicle is the basic reproductive unit of the ovary and consists of an oocyte surrounded by granulosa cells. At the onset of a menstrual cycle, FSH accelerates maturation of several follicles and increases aromatase activity, which stimulates conversion of androgens to estradiol. Under negative feedback

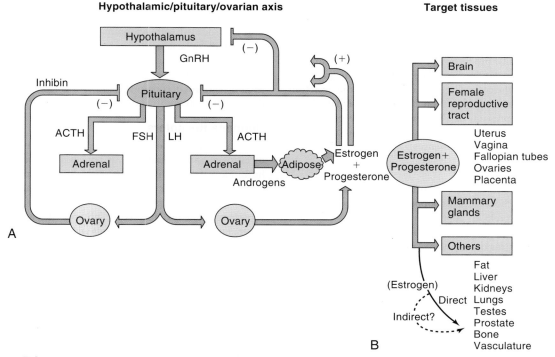

FIG. 51.1 Feedback Loops and Target Tissues. (A) Negative and positive feedback actions of estrogens and progesterone on the hypothalamic-pituitary-ovarian axis. (B) Other target tissues for these steroid hormones.

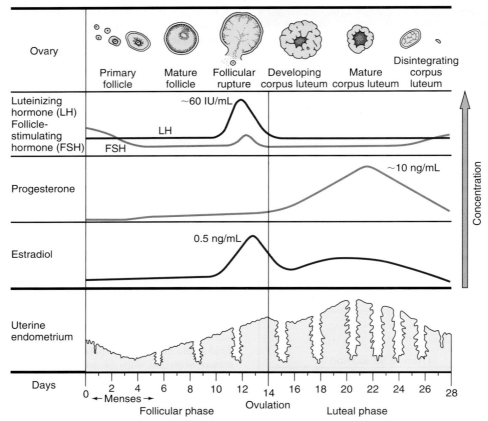

FIG. 51.2 Ovulatory and Menstrual Cycle. Ovarian and uterine alterations that occur with the cyclical hormonal changes during the normal human menstrual cycle. Note the increase in LH, FSH, and estradiol concentrations before ovulation during the follicular phase. Progesterone rises and peaks in the midluteal phase, concomitant with reductions in LH, FSH, and estradiol concentrations.

from estrogens, FSH levels decrease, but the dominant follicle becomes more sensitive to circulating gonadotropins. In the late follicular phase, estradiol levels increase rapidly and initiate a midcycle LH surge. Increased LH levels promote follicular production of progesterone, and ultimately, follicular rupture and ovulation occur. After ovulation, the granulosa and theca cells become the corpus luteum, and progesterone secretion prepares the endometrium for implantation. If fertilization and implantation do not occur, suppression of FSH and LH release promotes a decline in progesterone and estrogen levels that results in breakdown and shedding of the endometrium (**menses**).

Pregnancy

During **pregnancy**, the placenta secretes chorionic gonadotropin into the maternal circulation. The chorionic gonadotropin concentration rises rapidly after implantation and peaks in approximately 6–8 weeks. Chorionic gonadotropin maintains the corpus luteum and stimulates progesterone production, which initially maintains placental implantation and pregnancy. Sometime after the fifth week of pregnancy, the fetal-placental unit becomes the major source of circulating progesterone and estrogens, especially estriol.

Menopause

As women age, the number and size of follicles in the ovaries diminish, predominantly as a result of atresia. Eventually, normal menstrual cycles cease entirely (**menopause**). Without estrogen and progesterone to suppress the hypothalamic-pituitary axis, FSH and LH concentrations increase. Although adrenal androgens, predominantly androstenedione, can be converted to estrone by peripheral tissues, circulating estrogen

concentrations fall to extremely low levels in postmenopausal women. This is associated with symptoms of estrogen deficiency, which may occur rapidly or be delayed (e.g., osteopenia). The major acute symptoms include vasomotor instability (hot flushes and night sweats) and vulvovaginal atrophy. Other symptoms possibly related to decreased estrogen levels include loss of concentration, loss of libido, weight gain, depression, thinning hair, joint discomfort, and sleep disruption.

Hormone Receptors

The molecular basis for steroid hormone action, including the actions of estrogen and progesterone, is reviewed in Chapter 2. Free steroid hormone passively diffuses into cells but accumulates only in cells expressing the specific cytoplasmic steroid–binding proteins. Both ERs and progesterone receptors (PGRs) are members of the nuclear receptor superfamily. The two distinct ER subtypes **ERα** and **ERβ** are products of separate genes, but estrogen binds with high affinity to both receptor subtypes. These receptor subtypes have different ligand-binding domains and tissue distributions, and they apparently mediate different functions. ERα is highly expressed in the reproductive tract and breast, where it mediates many of the effects of estrogen on sexual development and reproductive function. ERβ is highly expressed in the ovaries, with lower expression in other organs. Only one gene encodes the PGR, but two protein isoforms, **PGR-A** and **PGR-B**, are produced by differential processing. The biological activities of the PGR isoforms are distinct, and their ratios vary in different tissues. However, they have the same ligand-binding domain, and reproductive effects of progesterone involve both isoforms.

The classical mechanism of action of nuclear steroid hormones is that the hormone-receptor complex can act as a steroid-activated transcription factor (Chapter 2).

Receptor expression influences tissue responses and is strongly affected by the hormonal environment. PGRs are expressed in response to estrogen exposure, and high concentrations of progesterone decrease ER concentrations, which, in turn, leads to decreased PGR levels. Furthermore, each hormone can directly regulate its own receptor concentration (down or up). Some steroid hormone receptors, including those for estrogen and progesterone, are located on the plasma membrane of cells. Activation of these membrane receptors results in more rapid responses than those produced by activation of nuclear receptors.

Estrogen Receptor Ligands

Compounds with estrogenic activity can be classified as either steroidal or nonsteroidal. Steroidal estrogens can be subdivided into natural and synthetic forms. The biosynthetic pathways and structures of the three endogenous human estrogens (17β-estradiol, estrone, and estriol) are shown in Chapter 48 (Figs. 48.1 and 48.2). Estradiol is the most potent of the three natural estrogens, and estriol is the least potent. Synthetic hormones that are used therapeutically generally have a heterocyclic structure resembling endogenous steroids. Endogenous human estrogens have a low bioavailability if administered orally as a result of poor absorption and rapid inactivation by first-pass hepatic metabolism. Estrogen conjugates are formed by enzymatic addition of sulfate or glucuronic acid, which enhances their excretion. The endogenous pool of estrogenic steroids represents a balance among the three naturally occurring estrogens. Conjugated estrogens derived from pregnant mares' urine are effective if administered orally and are used in the treatment of menopausal symptoms. The synthetic estrogens ethinyl estradiol and mestranol have an ethinyl group at C17, which slows hepatic inactivation. Mestranol, the three-methyl ether of ethinyl estradiol, is activated by hepatic conversion to ethinyl estradiol. The ethinylated compounds are used mainly in combination oral contraceptives.

Several nonsteroidal synthetic compounds, called selective estrogen receptor modulators (SERMs), are partial agonists/antagonists that can interact with estrogen receptors (ERs) with some tissue selectivity. The idea that the SERMs act as agonists in some tissues and as antagonists in others is based on the presence or absence of coregulator proteins in specific tissues that function as either coactivators to facilitate gene transcription or as corepressors to prevent gene transcription. Clomiphene has two stereoisomers that have weak agonist and antagonist properties and is used to treat infertility by blocking the negative feedback effects of estrogen and inducing ovulation. Tamoxifen has antiestrogenic activity in the breast and is used to treat or prevent breast cancer in women whose tumors express ERs (Chapter 69). However, a major concern with tamoxifen is the significantly increased risk of endometrial cancer and venous thrombosis related to its estrogenic activity. Raloxifene has agonist activity in bone and is used to prevent or treat osteoporosis in postmenopausal women (Chapter 55). Unlike tamoxifen, raloxifene displays little estrogenic activity in the uterus and does not increase the risk of endometrial cancer. Other ligands for ERs include fulvestrant, a pure receptor antagonist that has no partial agonist activity. By binding to the ER, fulvestrant increases receptor turnover, resulting in down regulation of the ER protein, thereby preventing estrogen-regulated gene transcription. Fulvestrant is used for the treatment of postmenopausal women with locally advanced or metastatic breast cancer.

Progesterone Receptor Ligands

The progestin derivatives are classified on the basis of their structure at positions C21 or C19 (19-nortestosterone). The C21 derivatives include the natural progestogens, progesterone, and 17α-hydroxyprogesterone,

which are derived from pregnenolone (Chapter 48, Fig. 48.1). Synthetic C21 compounds in the pregnane family include medroxyprogesterone acetate, megestrol acetate, and hydroxyprogesterone caproate. Synthetic 19-nortestosterone derivatives are similar to testosterone but lack the C19 methyl group. They may have an ethinyl group at C17α, which slows hepatic inactivation following oral administration. These compounds are divided into the estranes and 13-ethyl gonanes, which are components of most oral and some long-acting contraceptives. The estranes include norethindrone, norethindrone acetate, norethynodrel, and ethynodiol diacetate. The 13-ethyl gonanes include levonorgestrel, desogestrel, and norgestimate. Progestins that are structurally related to testosterone but not ethinylated include dienogest and drospirenone, an analogue of spironolactone that binds to mineralocorticoid receptors and has antimineralocorticoid properties. In addition to their progestational activity, progestins may also possess variable amounts of estrogenic, antiestrogenic, androgenic, or antiandrogenic activities, which contribute to their pharmacological effects. Danazol is a 19-nortestosterone derivative that has significant progestational and androgenic activity, whereas mifepristone is a 19-norsteroid analogue that blocks PGRs and glucocorticoid receptors and is useful as an antiprogestin.

Estrogen priming is necessary for PGR expression in almost all progesterone-responsive tissues, including the uterus. Progesterone concentrations rise rapidly in the luteal phase of the menstrual cycle, resulting in modulation of the action of estrogen on the uterus. Progesterone antagonizes estrogen-induced proliferation in the endometrium and initiates secretory changes in preparation for embryo implantation. In the absence of pregnancy, plasma progesterone concentrations decrease, resulting in sloughing of the endometrial lining. Progesterone is responsible for increasing basal body temperature observed in the luteal phase. Progesterone is important in mammary glandular development and stimulating the development of lobules and alveoli. It induces differentiation of estrogen-prepared ductal tissue and supports the secretory function of the breast during lactation. Progesterone promotes maintenance of pregnancy and inhibits uterine contractions. Progesterone may affect carbohydrate metabolism and increase Na^+ and water elimination by competitive antagonism of aldosterone interaction with mineralocorticoid receptors. Progesterone has little effect on protein metabolism or plasma lipoprotein concentrations, but synthetic progestins with androgenic activity may decrease high-density lipoprotein (HDL) concentrations and increase low-density lipoprotein (LDL) concentrations.

Drugs Affecting Uterine Function

Changes in plasma estrogen and progesterone concentrations throughout the menstrual cycle and during pregnancy can significantly alter uterine responses to drugs through alterations in receptor density, coupling to effector mechanisms, or other processes. Anatomically, the uterus (Fig. 51.3) consists of a body (fundus) and an outflow tract (cervix) through which the fetus and placenta must pass during parturition. The fundus is composed principally of smooth muscle (myometrium) surrounding the uterine cavity, which is lined with a specialized endometrium containing stromal cells and glandular epithelium. During pregnancy, the myometrium undergoes massive hypertrophy and hyperplasia, predominantly under the influence of estrogen. The endometrium is also a target for estrogen and progesterone, which produce sequential changes throughout the menstrual cycle. The pregnant endometrium is termed the decidua. As pregnancy progresses, the fetus grows in a gestational sac composed of two types of fetal tissues—the inner amnion and the outer chorion. As the fetus develops, the amniochorial layer becomes fused with the maternal decidua.

The timing of parturition is a complex and coordinated event involving hormonal interactions between fetal tissues and maternal

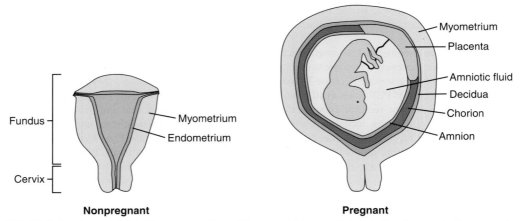

FIG. 51.3 Anatomy of the Nonpregnant and Pregnant Uterus. Note relative changes in the muscular layer (myometrium) and the lining (endometrium), which becomes the decidua during pregnancy. The gestational sac is composed of an epithelial cell layer (amnion) and the chorion, which is a continuation of the placental trophoblast that extends from the edge of the placenta and surrounds the entire developing conceptus. There is growing evidence that in late pregnancy, paracrine interactions involving the fetal membranes (amnion and chorion), endometrium (decidua), and myometrium may be major regulators of uterine activity.

systems. Changes in the intrauterine environment and the maternal immune system may be important regulators of human parturition. For successful parturition, the cervix must first undergo progressive changes, called remodeling, during which the connective tissue of the cervix transforms from a rigid into a soft and pliable structure. During ripening, the cervix becomes thin (effacement), and it begins to open (dilation). Active labor contractions ensue to continue the process of dilating the cervix and pushing the fetus through the maternal pelvis. These processes must be well coordinated to ensure normal progressive labor. Evolution of the uterus from its quiescent state to a sensitive contractile organ at the onset of labor involves two distinct phases: activation and stimulation. As term approaches the myometrium acquires an increased number of OT and PG receptors, ion channels, and gap junctions. Gap junctions are important in efficient cell-to-cell signal transmission essential for the generation of strong, coordinated contractions characteristic of active labor. Following activation, the "primed" uterus can be stimulated to contract by the action of uterotonic agents, such as PGs and OT. After delivery, the uterus undergoes involution, mediated primarily by OT.

In most species, a large increase in the maternal serum estrogen/progesterone ratio stimulates increased uterine contractility and labor onset. This "progesterone withdrawal" is thought to be a critical step in transformation of the uterus from its quiescent state during pregnancy into an active state during parturition. In humans, however, there are no significant changes in the estrogen/progesterone ratio in maternal serum before labor onset. Fetal membranes and the maternal decidua can synthesize and metabolize steroid hormones, suggesting the possible existence of a paracrine system within the pregnant human uterus. Evidence suggests that there is an increase in the estrogen/progesterone ratio in these tissues and an increase in the local synthesis of PGs and OT at the onset of human labor. It has also been speculated that a functional progesterone withdrawal may result from local progesterone metabolism, a change in the ratio of PGR isoforms, and altered expression of PGR coregulators. Thus the hormonal mechanisms involved in human parturition may be similar to those in animals, albeit occurring in a more localized manner.

Uterine Stimulants

The myometrium is an electrically excitable tissue that undergoes spontaneous changes in the membrane potential, which can result in bursts of action potentials that elicit phasic contractions. The frequency and configuration of action potentials change with gestation and hormonal status. The molecular mechanisms that underlie myometrial contraction are similar in most respects to those of other smooth muscles. The final common denominator of the contractile response is the interaction of phosphorylated myosin light chains (MLCs) with actin. Phosphorylation of MLCs is regulated by the balance of activity between MLC kinase (MLCK) and MLC phosphatase (MLCP), which is regulated in turn by Ca^{++}-calmodulin and other intracellular messengers (Fig. 51.4). Uterine stimulants such as OT and $PGF_{2\alpha}$ bind to specific G-protein–coupled membrane receptors that activate G_q and membrane phospholipase C (Chapter 2). This leads to the release of Ca^{++} from the sarcoplasmic reticulum and an influx of Ca^{++} through L-type Ca^{++} channels. The resultant increase in intracellular free Ca^{++} increases MLCK activity and uterine contraction. Relaxation of the myometrium occurs when intracellular Ca^{++} levels fall, which decreases MLCK activity, and the MLCs undergo dephosphorylation by MLCP.

The most potent and specific compound used clinically to stimulate uterine motility is OT, which is commonly used to induce or augment labor in late gestation. This nonapeptide hormone is synthesized in the hypothalamus and stored in the posterior pituitary, where it is released into the circulation in response to various stimuli. OT is also synthesized locally by intrauterine tissues and the fetus. OT has long been used to stimulate uterine contractions that are indistinguishable from those occurring during normal spontaneous labor. Although circulating levels of OT do not change significantly during pregnancy or prior to the onset of labor in humans, there is a marked increase in the concentration of OT receptors in the uterus at the time of parturition, suggesting that OT plays an important functional role in mediating this event. Moreover, OT acts indirectly to increase PG synthesis at labor onset.

The prostaglandins (PGs), principally PGE_2 and $PGF_{2\alpha}$, are also used clinically. Because the uterus is always responsive to PGs, they can stimulate contractions at any stage of gestation. PGE_2 also appears to be important in stimulating processes that result in ripening of the cervix prior to labor induction by OT. PGs have a critical role in the process of labor, and the rate of intrauterine synthesis of PGs increases several-fold at parturition. PGs increase myometrial sensitivity to OT by increasing gap junction formation and/or OT receptor concentrations. Because PGs are known to stimulate uterine activity at any time during gestation, they are effective abortifacients.

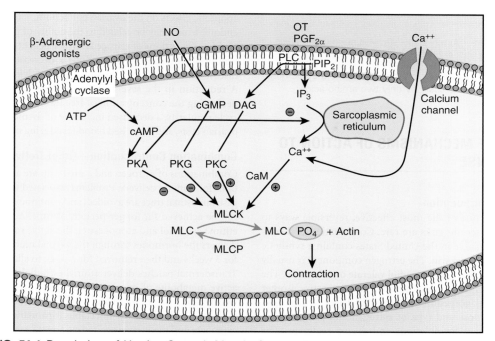

FIG. 51.4 Regulation of Uterine Smooth Muscle Contractility. The major uterine stimulants are OT and PGF$_{2\alpha}$, which have specific G-protein–coupled receptors on the cell surface linked to membrane phospholipase C (PLC). This enzyme hydrolyzes phosphatidylinositol-4,5-bisphosphate (PIP$_2$) to produce inositol trisphosphate (IP$_3$) and diacylglycerol (DAG). IP$_3$ stimulates the release of Ca^{++} from the sarcoplasmic reticulum, and membrane depolarization increases Ca^{++} influx through L-type Ca^{++} channels. The increased intracellular Ca^{++} binds to and activates calmodulin (CaM), which activates myosin light-chain kinase (MLCK). This enzyme phosphorylates myosin light chains (MLC), which stimulate the myosin-actin interaction that results in contraction. DAG stimulates protein kinase C (PKC), which may contribute to the activation of MLCK. Uterine contractions may be suppressed by pharmacologically inhibiting any of the steps in this pathway. Uterine relaxation may result from stimulation of β$_2$ receptors, which increases the production of cyclic AMP (cAMP). This activates protein kinase A (PKA), which phosphorylates and inactivates MLCK. The rise in cAMP also increases Ca^{++} reuptake into the sarcoplasmic reticulum. Nitric oxide (NO) stimulates soluble guanylyl cyclase, which increases the production of cyclic GMP (cGMP). This activates protein kinase G (PKG), which may have an effect similar to that of PKA. Stimulation of these inhibitory pathways may promote uterine quiescence. Other signaling pathways and mechanisms may also exist.

In addition, the **ergot alkaloids** can cause intense tonic myometrial contractions, which are undesirable during labor but are useful for treating postpartum hemorrhage. Ergot alkaloids, such as methylergonovine, are generally reserved for women who do not respond to OT or PGs. **Ergot alkaloids** are produced by a fungus that grows on rye plants. The mechanism of action of ergot alkaloids in the uterus is unclear, but the uterus is more sensitive to ergot alkaloids at term than earlier in pregnancy. Most evidence suggests their contractile effects are mediated by interaction with α_1 adrenergic receptors (Chapter 11), but they also bind to serotonin and dopamine receptors.

Last are the **PGR antagonists**, of which mifepristone is the prototype. Mifepristone is particularly useful in combination with a PG for termination of early pregnancy, when uterine quiescence is dependent principally on progesterone. Administration of **PGR antagonists** (antiprogestins) during early pregnancy causes uterine contractions leading to abortion. The molecular mechanisms of antiprogestins may include sensitization of the myometrium to PGs as well as production of a functional progesterone withdrawal.

Uterine Relaxants

Several classes of pharmacological agents are used to relax the uterus, including β$_2$-adrenergic receptor agonists such as ritodrine or terbutaline (Chapter 11); nonsteroidal antiinflammatory drugs (Chapter 29); magnesium sulfate; calcium-channel blockers; principally nifedipine (Chapter 40); and nitric oxide donors such as nitroglycerin (Chapter 41). Uterine relaxants suppress myometrial contractions via signaling pathways involved in smooth muscle relaxation or by inhibiting the synthesis or actions of known uterine stimulants (Fig. 51.5). As in many other smooth muscles, β$_2$-adrenergic receptor stimulation causes relaxation by activation of adenylyl cyclase, which results in a signaling cascade that ultimately inhibits MLCK activity (Chapters 11 and 41). Nitrates or other **nitric oxide donors** activate guanylyl cyclase, which also results in inactivation of MLCK in smooth muscles (Chapter 41). Nonsteroidal antiinflammatory drugs (NSAIDs) inhibit PG synthesis by inhibiting cyclooxygenase (COX, Chapter 29). Both COX-1 and COX-2 catalyze PG generation in the pregnant uterus, but the increased PG generation noted at parturition appears to result predominantly from COX-2. The mechanism of action of **magnesium sulfate** as a tocolytic agent is unclear but may be related to its actions as a divalent cation to compete with Ca^{++} in myometrial cells. Magnesium acts both extracellularly and intracellularly to decrease the availability of Ca^{++} for contraction. **Calcium-channel blockers** inhibit uterine contractions by blocking Ca^{++} influx through L-type Ca^{++} channels in smooth muscle cells (Chapter 40). The resulting decrease in intracellular free Ca^{++} inhibits calcium-dependent MLCK phosphorylation, leading to myometrial relaxation.

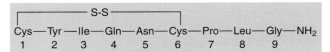

FIG. 51.5 Amino acid sequence of oxytocin (OT). OT is a cyclic nona-peptide that differs from vasopressin by only two amino acids.

RELATIONSHIP OF MECHANISMS OF ACTION TO CLINICAL RESPONSE

Birth Control

Combination Oral Contraception

Oral contraceptives are one of the most effective, reversible ways to prevent pregnancy, and serious risks are rare. Combination oral contraceptives currently available in the United States contain a synthetic estrogen and a synthetic progestin. The estrogen component is usually ethinyl estradiol or, less commonly, estradiol valerate or mestranol. The progestins include norethindrone, norgestrel and its active isomer levonorgestrel, desogestrel, norgestimate, ethynodiol diacetate, dienogest, and drospirenone. The dose and type of estrogen and progestin are available in many different formulations and dosing regimens. The most commonly used oral contraceptives consist of a combination preparation taken for 21 days followed by 7 days without any steroids to induce withdrawal bleeding. Monophasic oral contraceptives contain fixed doses of estrogen and progestin in each active pill. Multiphasic oral contraceptives vary the dose of one or both hormones during the pill cycle and may have a lower total hormone dose per cycle. The dosage may be altered two, three, or four times during the cycle; these are referred to as biphasic, triphasic, or quadriphasic regimens, respectively. Newer regimens include fewer hormone-free days per cycle, or extended cycles (e.g., 91 days) with fewer withdrawal bleeds per year. Extended-cycle regimens may have advantages for women with conditions that improve with menstrual suppression, such as dysmenorrhea and endometriosis.

Combination oral contraceptives prevent pregnancy by inhibiting ovulation, presumably as a result of the negative feedback effects of the estrogen and progestin on the hypothalamic-pituitary axis to suppress gonadotropin synthesis and release. There is no increase in the FSH concentration in the early follicular phase, and the midcycle peaks of FSH and LH are not observed in patients taking combination oral contraceptives. The lower concentration of FSH results in decreased ovarian function with minimal follicular development. In addition, lower concentrations of endogenous steroids are secreted during both phases of the menstrual cycle. Oral contraceptives also act directly on the cervix and uterus. The cervical mucus of oral contraceptive users is usually thicker and less abundant than that normally seen in the postovulatory phase. This may also aid in preventing pregnancy by inhibiting sperm penetration. In addition, the endometrium may be prevented from developing into the appropriate state for implantation. The risk of pregnancy is substantially increased if two or more doses are missed during a cycle. Therefore a high compliance rate is needed to ensure adequate contraception, especially with low-dose preparations.

Combination oral contraceptives confer several well-documented health benefits beyond the control of fertility, including a decreased risk of ovarian and endometrial cancers. The relative risk of these cancers is approximately half that in oral contraceptive users as compared with nonusers. This protective effect continues for 10–20 years after discontinuance of oral contraceptives. The protective effect on the ovaries may be a combination of ovulation inhibition and progestin-mediated apoptotic effects on the ovarian epithelium. The protective effect on the endometrium may be related to the ability of progestins to oppose the proliferative actions of estrogens. Other benefits of long-term combination oral contraceptive use include a decreased risk of benign breast disease and a reduction in the risk of pelvic inflammatory disease. A reduction in the severity of acne is also observed, presumably by decreasing the concentration of free testosterone. Increased menstrual cycle regularity, a decreased incidence of dysmenorrhea and functional ovarian cysts, and decreased blood loss during menses are other benefits.

Combination Contraception—Other Delivery Forms

Combinations of estrogen and a progestin are also available in formulations for nonoral delivery. Problems associated with absorption from the gastrointestinal tract are avoided, and continuous serum hormone levels can be achieved for longer periods of time. A vaginal ring containing ethinyl estradiol and etonogestrel, the active metabolite of desogestrel, delivers the hormones through the vaginal mucosa. The ring is inserted for 3 weeks and then removed for 1 week to allow withdrawal bleeding. Transdermal patches deliver ethinyl estradiol and norelgestromin, the active metabolite of norgestimate, through the skin. They are applied weekly for 3 weeks, with no patch worn the fourth week to allow withdrawal bleeding. An injectable formulation containing estradiol cypionate and medroxyprogesterone acetate can be used monthly. These contraceptive methods have the same mechanism of action to inhibit ovulation and a similar efficacy to that of combination oral contraceptives.

Progestin-Only Contraception

Progestin-only formulations of hormonal contraceptives were developed to avoid the adverse effects of estrogens in combination contraceptives. Progestin-only contraceptives suppress FSH/LH concentrations and inhibit ovulation to variable degrees, but they have additional contraceptive actions. Progestins modify cervical secretions, with the scant, thick cervical mucus preventing sperm penetration. Progestins also cause endometrial atrophy, which makes conditions less favorable for implantation. Menstrual cycles that are quite variable in duration likely contribute to prevention of pregnancy as well.

A progestin-only oral contraceptive (the mini-pill) is taken daily and contains one of the synthetic progestins, usually norgestrel or norethindrone. Major problems with this approach are a slightly higher failure rate and a much higher incidence of menstrual disturbances, including irregular bleeding and amenorrhea. To avoid the inconvenience of taking a pill daily and to achieve continuous doses of steroid, several other methods of progestin-only administration have been developed. A depot formulation of medroxyprogesterone acetate injected intramuscularly (IM) or subcutaneously provides effective contraception for 3 months. Implants containing etonogestrel or levonorgestrel are placed subdermally, usually in the upper arm. Progestin-releasing intrauterine devices (IUDs) deliver low, continuous doses of the steroid locally instead of systemically. The progestin-induced endometrial atrophy decreases bleeding, which is a significant problem associated with non–steroid-containing IUDs. The major benefits of implants and IUDs are that they are effective for 3–5 years, and normal menstrual cycles and fertility return rapidly after removal. Problems include irregular uterine bleeding and the need for surgical insertion and removal.

Emergency Contraception

Large doses of a progestin alone or an estrogen in combination with a progestin may prevent pregnancy after unprotected intercourse or suspected contraceptive failure. However, to prevent pregnancy, these compounds should be taken within 3 days (72 hours) of coital exposure. The high hormone doses act primarily by inhibiting or delaying ovulation. The most commonly used regimen consists of levonorgestrel alone, which is available without a prescription. Several existing combination oral contraception formulations can also be used for emergency contraception. Ulipristal acetate, a partial agonist at PGRs, is more effective than levonorgestrel and can be taken up to 5 days (120 hours) after unprotected intercourse. This product is available by prescription only in the United States, but it is available without a prescription in Europe. Contraindications for use of conventional oral contraceptives do not apply to short-term use of emergency contraceptives.

Infertility

Infertility occurs in about 10%–15% of couples, with multifactorial causes. Approximately one-third of cases are due to problems with ovulation or other female factors. Agents that can be used to induce ovulation include gonadotropins, GnRH analogues, and clomiphene citrate. Clomiphene has both agonist and antagonist properties on ERs and is used to treat ovulatory failure in women with normal hypothalamic and pituitary function. This agent acts by blocking ERs in the hypothalamus, relieving estrogen-induced negative feedback on GnRH release. Clomiphene administration for 5 days at the beginning of the menstrual cycle increases FSH and LH release, which stimulates the ovaries and promotes follicular development and ovulation. Clomiphene is most effective in women with normal concentrations of estrogen before therapy and is not useful in women with primary ovarian or pituitary dysfunction. Gonadotropins may be used for ovulation induction in women who fail to respond to clomiphene. GnRH analogues are used occasionally for stimulating gonadotropin production in the treatment of infertility.

Menopausal Hormone Therapy

Menopause, the natural cessation of menses, results from ovarian failure after depletion of functional ovarian follicles. The resultant decreased estrogen and progesterone production leads to physiological and psychological changes. The increase in vasomotor symptoms, genitourinary atrophy, osteoporosis, and cardiovascular disease in postmenopausal women has long been presumed to result from the loss of estrogen. There is a substantial decrease in vasomotor symptoms, genitourinary atrophy, and osteoporosis in women who begin estrogen therapy during or shortly after menopause. Although controversy exists, estrogen remains the most effective treatment for the acute symptoms of menopause. It is used for moderate to severe symptoms of vulvovaginal atrophy and moderate to severe vasomotor symptoms, such as hot flushes (also called "hot flashes") and night sweats. The most commonly used preparation is a mixture of conjugated estrogens taken orally, but other oral estrogen products are available. Transdermal and vaginal delivery routes for estrogens are also effective. Vaginal estrogen alone is recommended when treatment is only for symptoms of genitourinary atrophy. Women with an intact uterus who take systemic estrogen should also take a progestin to oppose the proliferative actions of estrogen on the endometrium. It is currently recommended that hormone therapy for postmenopausal women be used for the shortest period of time and at the lowest dose possible to relieve symptoms.

Estrogen is very effective at reducing the risk of osteoporosis by inhibiting bone resorption (Chapter 55). Because raloxifene is an agonist in bone but an antagonist in the breast, it has been approved for the prevention and treatment of postmenopausal osteoporosis and prevention of breast cancer in postmenopausal women at high risk. A combination of conjugated estrogens and the estrogen agonist/antagonist bazedoxifene was recently approved for the treatment of vasomotor symptoms and prevention of osteoporosis in postmenopausal women with an intact uterus. While bazedoxifene inhibits the stimulating effects of estrogen on the endometrium and breast, this combination has not been shown to reduce the risk of breast cancer.

For many years, estrogen was believed to reduce the risk of cardiovascular disease in women. Before menopause, the incidence of coronary artery disease is lower in women than in men of the same age, but after menopause, the incidence increases with age and eventually equals that in men. The increased risk may be associated with changes in lipoproteins (lower HDL concentrations and higher LDL concentrations) following menopause. Oral estrogen therapy exerts beneficial effects on lipoproteins by increasing HDL concentrations and lowering LDL concentrations. Data from observational studies had suggested that the risk of atherosclerotic cardiovascular disease was reduced as much as 50% in postmenopausal women who used estrogen with or without a progestin. Randomized placebo-controlled clinical trials were conducted to determine the benefits and risks of estrogen therapy alone or estrogen plus a progestin. The Heart and Estrogen/Progestin Replacement Study (HERS) found that combination therapy did not reduce cardiovascular events in postmenopausal women with established coronary artery disease, and the Women's Health Initiative (WHI) study showed an increase in the risk of cardiovascular disease in women without preexisting disease. The cardiovascular risks and benefits of menopausal estrogen therapy may depend on a woman's age, with those under 60 deriving some benefit and those over 60 experiencing an increased risk of coronary artery disease. Recently, the Early versus Late Intervention Trial with Estradiol (ELITE) examined the hypothesis that the cardiovascular effects of postmenopausal hormone therapy varied with the timing of therapy initiation (the hormone-timing hypothesis). Oral estradiol therapy was associated with less progression of subclinical atherosclerosis, measured by the rate of change in carotid artery intima-media thickness, compared with placebo when therapy was initiated within 6 years after menopause but not when it was initiated 10 or more years after menopause. The relevance of these results to the occurrence of clinical coronary heart disease events is unknown.

Other Uses of Hormone Therapy

Hormone therapy is useful for treating several conditions characterized by a deficiency or excess of estrogen and/or progesterone including primary ovarian failure, dysfunctional uterine bleeding, and luteal phase deficiency. Estrogen therapy initiated near the time of puberty helps to stimulate normal sexual development in girls with primary ovarian failure from multiple causes. This can be followed by cyclical administration of estrogen and a progestin to establish regular menses. Dysfunctional uterine bleeding occurs during anovulatory menstrual cycles and is often characterized by heavy, prolonged bleeding. When progesterone levels are insufficient to counteract estrogen-induced endometrial proliferation, the endometrium undergoes spontaneous sloughing at irregular intervals. High-dose progestin therapy can be used to stop an episode of prolonged bleeding but should be followed by long-term cyclical therapy to ensure the occurrence of regular withdrawal bleeding. Luteal phase deficiency also results from insufficient progesterone. Ovulation is normal, but the corpus luteum functions subnormally, with inadequate amounts of progesterone produced to maintain pregnancy. The most popular method of treating this condition is natural progesterone supplementation.

Endometriosis results from implantation and proliferation of ectopic endometrial cells outside the uterus, where they continue to respond to steroid hormones. Clinically, patients with endometriosis experience dysmenorrhea, dyspareunia, chronic pelvic pain, and reduced fertility. Since endometriosis is estrogen dependent, the goal of therapy is to induce an estrogen-poor environment and alleviate symptoms by inhibiting the growth of endometrial tissue. Treatment options for endometriosis include combination oral contraceptives, progestins, danazol, and GnRH analogues. Combinations of an estrogen and a progestin suppress ovarian function through negative feedback effects on gonadotropin release. Progestins and estrogen-progestin combinations reduce endometriosis by decidualization and subsequent atrophy of endometrial tissue. Danazol interacts with both androgen receptors and PGRs to inhibit gonadotropin release, but it also inhibits steroidogenic enzymes in the ovary that are responsible for estrogen production, creating a hypoestrogenic and hyperandrogenic environment. Chronic treatment with GnRH analogues causes down regulation of GnRH receptors, leading to decreased FSH/LH secretion (Chapter 49). The main side effects of GnRH agonists result from the hypoestrogenic state they produce, which can be minimized by add-back therapy with hormone replacement. NSAIDs are often used alone or combined with hormonal therapies to treat dysmenorrhea and pelvic pain.

Cancer Chemotherapy

Endocrine therapies are useful for the adjuvant treatment of several types of cancers (Chapter 69). Since estrogens, and in some cases, progesterone, promote proliferation of breast cancer cells, current adjuvant treatment strategies focus on preventing activation of ERs by estrogens or inhibiting estrogen biosynthesis. After completion of chemotherapy, and during or after radiation therapy, an **antiestrogen** is often used to prevent recurrence of breast cancer in women whose tumors express ERs. Tamoxifen is a partial agonist/antagonist that acts in the breast by competing with endogenous estrogens for binding to ERs. Tamoxifen is approved for adjuvant therapy of ER-positive breast cancer in premenopausal or postmenopausal women. It can also be used as a breast cancer preventative in women at high risk, depending on such factors as age and family history of breast cancer. Raloxifene, another partial agonist/antagonist at ERs, was approved more recently for the prevention of breast cancer in high-risk women, but it is not used for adjuvant therapy. Fulvestrant, a pure antagonist at ERs, is used for the treatment of ER-positive advanced or metastatic breast cancer in postmenopausal women whose disease has progressed on prior antiestrogen therapy.

A reduction in circulating estrogen levels can be achieved by inhibiting peripheral aromatization of adrenal androgens by the aromatase enzyme, which converts androstenedione to estrone and testosterone to estradiol (Chapter 48, Fig. 48.1). Several drugs are now available that specifically inhibit this enzyme, including the steroidal androstenedione derivative, exemestane, and two nonsteroidal triazole derivatives, anastrozole and letrozole. Exemestane binds irreversibly to the aromatase enzyme, causing permanent inactivation, whereas anastrozole and letrozole bind in a competitive, reversible manner. These **aromatase inhibitors** are used for adjuvant therapy of ER-positive breast cancer in postmenopausal women and as first-line treatment in advanced disease (Chapter 69). Since the primary site of estrogen production in premenopausal women is in the ovaries and aromatase inhibitors are not capable of completely inhibiting ovarian estrogen synthesis, these drugs should be used with ovarian ablation therapy to lower estrogen levels in premenopausal women. Women treated with adjuvant endocrine therapy should be treated for a minimum duration of 5 years, but recent clinical studies have shown that therapy for an additional 5 years further reduces the risk of breast cancer recurrence.

Endocrine therapy may be useful for the adjuvant treatment of advanced endometrial carcinoma in women whose tumors are positive for ERs and PGRs. Progestins likely act through the PGR to down regulate the ER and induce formation of 17β-hydroxysteroid dehydrogenase, which increases estradiol metabolism. In addition, progestins may have direct cellular actions, leading to decreased cell division. Synthetic progestins, such as medroxyprogesterone acetate or megestrol acetate, are effective when administered alone or in sequence with an antiestrogen. The aromatase inhibitors are not effective in the treatment of endometrial cancer.

Drugs Affecting Uterine Function

The use of **uterotonic** drugs that stimulate uterine contractions to terminate early pregnancy is increasingly replacing surgical procedures and their attendant complications. In addition, the use of **oxytocic** drugs to induce or augment labor and to prevent or treat postpartum hemorrhage has reduced some of the complications associated with labor and delivery that contribute to maternal morbidity and mortality. Although treatment goals may be similar for each of these situations, the specific drugs used differ because of subtle differences in uterine environment and physiological status. Uterine contractions during labor are naturally **phasic**, allowing for resumption of normal utero-fetal-placental hemodynamics between contractions. Thus drugs used to induce labor or augment slowly progressing labor should mimic the physiological process as much as possible. However, to prevent or stop postpartum hemorrhage, stimulation of **tonic** contractions is necessary to avert excessive blood loss.

Induction/Augmentation of Labor

Induction of labor must include **ripening of the cervix** if this has not occurred naturally. Oxytocic drugs stimulate contractions but often must be administered for a prolonged time if the cervix is unripe. Preinduction use of **PGE** preparations will facilitate labor in such instances. Whereas the uterine contractile effects of OT are immediate, it takes several hours for cervical ripening by PGE. Mechanical devices are also used to ripen the cervix, and their effects may be partially mediated by induction of PGE_2 synthesis. In the presence of a ripe cervix, IV infusion of **OT** is the best way to stimulate or augment uterine contractions. Care must be taken to avoid **overstimulation**, and two types of stimulants should generally not be used together.

Early Pregnancy Termination

There are few OT receptors in the myometrium in early pregnancy, and OT is of little use in stimulating activity at this time. The **antiprogestin** mifepristone can disrupt embryonic and placental development. However, when given alone, there is a high rate of incomplete abortion that may still require surgical completion. When given in combination with a **PG analogue**, mifepristone is very successful in inducing abortion in pregnancies at less than 8 weeks' gestation. Surgical abortion is usually preferred beyond 8 weeks' gestation. Administration of PGs locally is also efficacious, particularly after 18 weeks of gestation.

Treatment of Preterm Labor

Preterm parturition may result from premature activation of physiological processes that normally occur at term or may result from pathological processes such as intrauterine infection, inflammation, or overdistention. Activation of the immune response results in production of inflammatory cytokines and PGs that can initiate uterine contractions and weaken the amniotic membranes. The main method for delaying preterm birth involves inhibition of myometrial contractions. However, the lack of understanding of the precise mechanisms involved in initiation of parturition has hindered development of more effective tocolytic agents. While the drugs currently used do cause myometrial relaxation, none of them has specific effects on uterine smooth muscle. Vascular relaxation, subsequent decreases in blood pressure, and tachycardia, along with the development of tachyphylaxis, limit the duration of successful treatment with many of these drugs.

There is still much controversy about the use of tocolytic drugs, particularly concerning their effectiveness and risk/benefit ratio. The ultimate goal of preventing preterm birth is to eliminate the risks of neonatal complications and death. The goal is to delay delivery by at least 48 hours so that antenatal administration of glucocorticoids to the mother can accelerate fetal pulmonary maturation to reduce neonatal respiratory distress syndrome and provide time for safe transport to a facility with an appropriate level of neonatal care in the event of preterm delivery.

Several classes of drugs can be used to reduce the strength and frequency of uterine contractions, especially during late pregnancy when the fetus may be too premature to thrive outside the uterus. These drugs are administered to inhibit acute preterm labor before 37 weeks of gestation and delay delivery. However, most uterine relaxants are nonspecific and may cause relaxation of other smooth muscle beds, including blood vessels.

Although progesterone does not stop acute preterm labor, it has been used for maintenance tocolytic therapy following arrest of premature labor. Supplementation with progesterone or hydroxyprogesterone caproate starting at 16–24 weeks of gestation reduces the risk of recurrent spontaneous preterm birth. Progesterone therapy helps to maintain uterine quiescence and delay cervical ripening.

Treatment of Dysmenorrhea

The most common form of dysmenorrhea is primary dysmenorrhea, consisting of crampy, lower abdominal pain during menses and in the absence of underlying pathology. Uterine spasms result from the release of PGs from degenerating endometrial cells. NSAIDs such as ibuprofen are extremely effective in preventing or ameliorating this condition (Chapter 29), and oral contraceptives may be used to inhibit ovulation and cause thinning of the endometrium, reducing the incidence of dysmenorrhea.

PHARMACOKINETICS

Estrogens, Progestogens, SERMs, and Aromatase Inhibitors

The pharmacokinetic parameters of selected estrogens, progestogens, SERMs, and aromatase inhibitors are summarized in Table 51.1.

Estrogens

Estrogens are well absorbed from the GI tract and skin and mucous membranes and after parenteral injection. Because unconjugated natural estrogens are rapidly metabolized in the GI tract and liver following oral administration, their delivery by other routes (transdermal, vaginal, or IM) will delay inactivation and produce more constant blood levels. Estradiol is rapidly cleared from the blood and converted to estrone. Estrone is converted to estrone sulfate, which is excreted or hydrolyzed back to estrone. Micronized estradiol, steroidal estrogens that contain an ethinyl group at C17, conjugated estrogens, and nonsteroidal estrogens are active orally. Once absorbed, estrogens are metabolized in the liver and excreted primarily as polyhydroxylated forms conjugated with sulfate or glucuronide. Conjugated estrogens are distributed into the bile, hydrolyzed and reabsorbed from the GI tract, and recirculated to the liver (enterohepatic recirculation). Approximately 20% of the estrogen is excreted in the feces, with the remainder in the urine. The synthetic steroidal estrogens, ethinyl estradiol and mestranol, are metabolized more slowly than estradiol and consequently have much longer half-lives.

Progestogens

Orally administered progesterone is almost completely inactivated in the liver; thus synthetic modifications are necessary to produce orally active compounds. Progesterone can be administered parenterally but has an elimination half-life of only a few minutes because it is converted in the liver to pregnanediol, which is conjugated with glucuronic acid and excreted mainly in the urine. Micronized preparations of progesterone are available for oral or vaginal administration. Hydroxyprogesterone acetate or caproate is administered weekly by IM injection. Medroxyprogesterone acetate can be administered orally on a daily basis or by IM or subcutaneous injections every 3 months, whereas megestrol acetate is administered orally. The 19-nortestosterone derivatives are all orally active. The plasma half-lives of the C21 derivatives and the 19-nortestosterone compounds are longer than those of progesterone. Most of them are metabolized in the liver, conjugated with sulfate or glucuronide, and excreted in the urine or feces.

Other Estrogen Receptor Ligands

Clomiphene citrate is well absorbed following oral administration. Clomiphene undergoes hepatic metabolism and may enter the enterohepatic circulation, with approximately 50% excreted in the feces within 5–7 days. Tamoxifen is administered orally and undergoes extensive hepatic metabolism, enterohepatic recirculation, and excretion primarily by the biliary route into the feces. The antiestrogenic action of tamoxifen is likely due to its active metabolites. Genetic polymorphisms affect the extent of metabolism and may contribute to the variable efficacy of tamoxifen in the treatment of breast cancer. Raloxifene is administered orally and is extensively conjugated to glucuronides in the liver before elimination primarily in the feces. Bazedoxifene is administered orally, undergoes glucuronidation, and is excreted mainly in the feces. Fulvestrant is

TABLE 51.1 Selected Pharmacokinetic Parameters: Estrogens, Progestogens, SERMs, and Aromatase Inhibitors			
Drug	**Route of Administration**	**Elimination $t_{1/2}$**	**Disposition**
Estradiol	Oral (esters), IM, topical, transdermal	Variable	M, R, B
Ethinyl estradiol	Oral	6–20 hr	M, R
Progesterone	Oral, IM, vaginal	5–20 min (oral)	M, R
Medroxyprogesterone	Oral, IM	12–17 hr (oral)	M, R
Levonorgestrel	Oral	17–27 hr	M, R
Norethindrone	Oral	8 hr	M, R
Danazol	Oral	9 hr	M, R
Clomiphene	Oral	5–7 days	M, R
Tamoxifen	Oral	5–7 days	M, B
Raloxifene	Oral	32 hr	M
Fulvestrant	IM	40 days	M
Anastrozole	Oral	50 hr	M, B

B, Biliary excretion; *IM*, intramuscular; *M*, metabolism; *R*, renal excretion.

TABLE 51.2	**Selected Pharmacokinetic Parameters: Drugs Affecting Uterine Function**		
Drug	**Route of Administration**	**Elimination $t_{1/2}$**	**Disposition**
Oxytocin	IV, IM	3–6 min	M, R
PGE$_2$	Intracervical, intravaginal, IV	Variable	M
Misoprostol	Oral, rectal, intravaginal	20–40 min	M, R
Methylergonovine	Oral, IM, IV	30 min–3 hr	M
Mifepristone	Oral	20–30 hr	M, B
Indomethacin	Oral, rectal	4–5 hr	M, R, B
Magnesium sulfate	IV, IM	—	R
Nifedipine	Oral	2–3 hr	M, R

B, Biliary excretion; *IM,* intramuscular; *IV,* intravenous; *M,* metabolism; *R,* renal excretion.

administered monthly by IM injection. Fulvestrant is metabolized in the liver, undergoes glucuronidation, and is eliminated primarily in the feces. Fulvestrant is highly bound to lipoproteins and has a long half-life.

Aromatase Inhibitors

Aromatase inhibitors are well absorbed after oral administration, extensively metabolized in the liver, and excreted either in the urine or feces. Elimination half-lives vary from 24 hours for exemestane to about 50 hours for anastrozole.

Drugs Affecting Uterine Function

During pregnancy, several important maternal adaptations can influence the pharmacokinetic profile of a drug, including increased blood flow or more efficient mucosal absorption that can affect drug absorption; increased maternal blood volume that can increase the initial volume of distribution; increased blood flow to maternal liver and kidney that may increase metabolism, excretion, or both; and an increased concentration of plasma-binding proteins that may decrease metabolism and excretion. In addition, the placenta may be a site of drug metabolism or maternal drug disposal secondary to fetal transfer, with subsequent transfer back into the maternal compartment. Pharmacokinetic parameters of selected drugs affecting the uterus are summarized in Table 51.2.

Uterine Stimulants

OT is a peptide that is administered IV by infusion to induce or augment labor. OT is rapidly inactivated by the liver and excreted by the kidney; consequently, it has a short half-life. In concentrations used to induce or augment labor, OT produces clonic uterine activity. The infusion rate is increased at intervals until the frequency and amplitude of contractions are satisfactory. For prophylaxis or treatment of postpartum hemorrhage, OT can be administered IM or IV in large doses, which result in tonic, sustained contractions. Carbetocin, a long-acting synthetic OT agonist, has similar pharmacological properties to those of natural OT. It is available in many countries (but not in the United States) for the prevention of uterine atony and hemorrhage. A potential advantage of carbetocin over OT is its longer duration of action.

PG preparations are used extensively in late gestation to ripen the cervix before induction of labor or to induce labor. Misoprostol, a methylated analogue of PGE$_1$, can be administered orally or vaginally. Methylated PGs are more resistant to metabolism, are more efficacious, and have longer actions than nonethylated PGs. After oral administration, misoprostol is converted to an active metabolite, misoprostol acid. Plasma concentrations of misoprostol acid peak in approximately 30 minutes. The drug is primarily metabolized in the liver. Dinoprostone, a synthetic analogue of PGE$_2$, is administered as an intracervical gel or as a vaginal insert or suppository. Once the cervix is ripe, it is common to switch to IV OT to induce labor. OT induction that follows PG use for cervical ripening should be delayed for at least 6 hours following PGE$_2$ gel administration or at least 30 minutes after removal of the vaginal insert. Carboprost tromethamine, or methyl-PGF$_{2\alpha}$, can be administered IM to contract the uterus and produce vasoconstriction to control postpartum hemorrhage.

Ergot alkaloids can be given orally, IM, or IV to produce a tonic uterine contraction that controls postpartum hemorrhage. Administration of ergot alkaloids is usually delayed until after delivery of the placenta. Methylergonovine has a rapid onset of action and a longer duration of action than OT, but it is reserved for women who have not responded to OT or PGs.

The antiprogestin mifepristone is used primarily for early termination of pregnancy (<70 days' gestation). Plasma concentrations peak 1–2 hours after oral administration, and the drug is highly bound to plasma proteins. The unbound drug is extensively metabolized and excreted mainly in the bile. Mifepristone is generally followed by the administration of misoprostol 24–48 hours later. This sequential treatment increases the efficiency of induction of uterine contractions compared with the use of mifepristone or PG analogues alone. Mifepristone and misoprostol are also effective for termination of pregnancy in the second trimester, albeit with increased chances of serious complications such as uterine rupture or hemorrhage.

Uterine Relaxants

Terbutaline and other β$_2$-adrenergic receptor agonists used to treat asthma have also been used to suppress preterm labor (Chapter 11). Terbutaline can be administered subcutaneously by intermittent injection or IV by infusion pump, with the dose carefully titrated to uterine activity. Maternal and fetal cardiovascular and metabolic parameters should be monitored carefully to avoid the predictable side effects of these agents. These drugs often lose their effectiveness as a consequence of tachyphylaxis.

Indomethacin is the most commonly used NSAID for tocolysis. A loading dose may be administered orally or rectally, followed by repeated oral administration of a lower dose every 4–6 hours. Indomethacin is highly bound to plasma proteins and undergoes extensive metabolism by the liver. It is excreted in the urine and feces and has a half-life of 4–5 hours.

For tocolysis, magnesium sulfate is administered IV as a loading dose, followed by a continuous infusion. The infusion rate should be titrated based on assessment of contraction frequency and maternal toxicity. Since magnesium is excreted by the kidney, its dose should be adjusted in patients with impaired renal function.

An initial loading dose of nifedipine is usually administered orally, followed by additional oral doses every 3–8 hours. The half-life of nifedipine is approximately 2–3 hours, and the duration of a single dose is up to 6 hours. Nifedipine is almost completely metabolized by the liver and excreted by the kidney.

PHARMACOVIGILANCE: ADVERSE EFFECTS AND DRUG INTERACTIONS

Estrogens

Adverse effects of estrogen therapy are related to dose. Low doses may lead to changes in vaginal bleeding patterns, nausea, occasional vomiting, abdominal cramps, bloating, diarrhea, appetite changes, fluid retention, dizziness, headache, breast discomfort, weight gain, mood changes, ocular changes, allergic rash, and changes in some serum proteins. The more serious side effects occasionally encountered with estrogen usage include endometrial cancer, thromboembolic disorders, and gallbladder disease. The incidence of endometrial cancer is increased as much as 24-fold in those exposed to prolonged (>5 years) unopposed estrogens, but this increased risk can be eliminated by using a progestin in combination. The risk of venous thromboembolism increases two- to threefold with estrogens and is greatest among older smokers. An increased risk of ovarian cancer has been reported with postmenopausal estrogen use, particularly of long duration. Studies of estrogen-only therapy show little, if any, increased risk of breast cancer, and any increased risk was associated with prolonged use and higher doses. Oral estrogens should be used with caution or avoided in women with hypertriglyceridemia, active gallbladder disease, or known thrombophilias, such as factor V Leiden.

Progestins

Progestin-only oral contraceptives and implants are associated with an increased incidence of ectopic pregnancy upon contraceptive failure. Adverse effects of progestin-only therapy include breakthrough bleeding, spotting, changes in menstrual flow, amenorrhea, edema, weight changes, nausea, bloating, headache, allergic rash, mood changes, and changes in lipoprotein concentrations (decreased HDL, increased LDL). Drospirenone may cause less fluid retention and bloating, but it can cause hyperkalemia due to renal retention of potassium. Glucose intolerance may occur in some women receiving progestins, especially those who are already diabetic or have a history of gestational diabetes. The most common side effects of depot medroxyprogesterone acetate and contraceptive implants are menstrual abnormalities, characterized by irregular bleeding early in the treatment, followed by amenorrhea in a majority of patients after 2 years of treatment. The return of fertility can be delayed for 6–12 months after the last injection of medroxyprogesterone. There may also be a reversible reduction in bone mineral density with depot medroxyprogesterone. In addition, the surgical insertion and removal of implants and IUDs can be associated with patient discomfort and possible infection.

The use of danazol is associated with multiple antiestrogenic and androgenic side effects, including weight gain, muscle cramps, decreased breast size, deepening of the voice, edema, amenorrhea, emotional lability, flushing, sweating, acne, mild hirsutism, oily skin and hair, altered libido, nausea, headache, dizziness, insomnia, rash, increased LDL and decreased HDL concentrations, and increased hepatic enzyme activities. Most of these effects are reversed on cessation of the drug. Danazol is contraindicated in pregnant women or in breastfeeding mothers.

Combination Oral Contraceptives

Many of the mild side effects of combination oral contraceptives result from an excess or deficiency of either estrogen or progestin. These effects can often be managed by adjusting the estrogen/progestin balance or by using a formulation with a different progestin. Several clinical studies have supported an association between combined oral contraceptive use and thromboembolic disease in the absence of other predisposing factors. The risk of thromboembolic events is greater in women who smoke, are over 35 years of age, and take higher doses of estrogen. The risk of venous thromboembolism also depends on the type of progestin used. However, the risk of thromboembolic disease rapidly returns to normal after oral contraceptive use is discontinued. Combination oral contraceptives can cause a small increase in both systolic and diastolic blood pressure in some patients. Nearly all recent studies have shown no increased risk of myocardial infarction or ischemic stroke without other major risk factors. However, compared with nonusers, there is a substantial increased risk of myocardial infarction and ischemic stroke in women who use combination oral contraceptives and have one or more of these risk factors: smoking, uncontrolled hypertension, diabetes, and hypercholesterolemia. The cardiovascular risks increase with age.

Multiple studies have shown no change in the incidence of breast cancer in women who take combination oral contraceptives, although a few studies showed an increased risk for some women, specifically those who have the *BRCA1* gene mutation. Given the relatively small number of breast cancer patients in the age group of women using contraception, the number of increased cases is actually small. Women who are positive for human papillomavirus and use oral contraceptives may be at increased risk for cervical cancer, if they have used these drugs for more than 5 years.

Oral contraceptives are contraindicated in women with a current or past history of thrombophlebitis or thromboembolic disorders; cerebrovascular or coronary artery disease; a known or suspected pregnancy; undiagnosed abnormal genital bleeding; a known or suspected carcinoma of the breast, uterus, cervix, vagina, or other estrogen-dependent neoplasm; hepatic adenoma or carcinoma; and cholestatic jaundice of pregnancy or jaundice after previous oral contraceptive use. Oral contraceptives should be used with caution in patients with liver or renal disease, asthma, migraine headaches, diabetes, hypertension, or congestive heart failure and in patients receiving medications that can interfere with their effectiveness. Women who smoke and use oral contraceptives should be advised to use alternative methods of birth control after 35 years of age.

Several drugs can increase the risk of contraceptive failure by inducing the hepatic metabolism of oral contraceptives. Examples include barbiturates, rifampin, ritonavir, phenylbutazone, phenytoin, carbamazepine, oxcarbazepine, and topiramate. Contraceptive failure has also been reported with concurrent use of some antibiotics including penicillins and tetracyclines. Oral contraceptives can impair the hepatic metabolism of some drugs, such as theophylline, tricyclic antidepressants, and benzodiazepines; can decrease the effectiveness of warfarin by increasing levels of clotting factors; and can counteract the effects of hypoglycemic agents by increasing levels of glucose.

Combination Menopausal Hormone Therapy

Results from the Women's Health Initiative (WHI) clinical trial indicated that the most serious risks for users of estrogen plus progestin therapy were an increase in venous thromboembolic disease, stroke, nonfatal myocardial infarction and fatal coronary heart disease, and breast cancer. Much of the increased relative risk of cardiovascular disease was observed in the first year, but the overall rates of cardiovascular disease were low. An increase in the risk of breast cancer was observed for users of estrogen plus progestin but not estrogen alone. The difference between the hormone-treated and placebo groups became evident only after 4 years. Based on these findings, it is currently recommended that combined estrogen/progestin therapy for acute symptoms of menopause be used for the shortest duration possible. The treatment of patients should be governed by the age and particular risk profile of the individual. Use is contraindicated in women with abnormal genital bleeding, a history of breast cancer or other estrogen-dependent neoplasia, venous or arterial thromboembolic disease, or liver dysfunction.

Other Estrogen Receptor Ligands and Aromatase Inhibitors

The frequency and severity of the adverse effects of clomiphene citrate are dose related and include vasomotor symptoms that resemble those in menopausal patients. Other common side effects include abdominal discomfort, GI disturbances, abnormal uterine bleeding, breast tenderness, headache, and dizziness. Visual problems occur occasionally. Other high-dose side effects include ovarian enlargement or cyst formation, ovarian hyperstimulation syndrome, and depression. There is a 5%–8% incidence of multiple gestations, particularly twins, in women taking clomiphene, as compared with a 1% incidence in the general population. Clomiphene is contraindicated in patients with ovarian cysts, pregnancy, a history of liver disease, abnormal uterine bleeding, and thyroid or adrenal dysfunction.

The side effects of tamoxifen include an increased risk of endometrial cancer, pulmonary thromboembolism, deep vein thrombosis, and stroke. Less serious adverse effects include vasomotor symptoms, irregular menses, vaginal discharge, hair loss, vision changes, nausea, and vomiting. Although the teratogenic effects of tamoxifen in humans are unknown, pregnancy should be avoided in women taking tamoxifen because numerous defects have been demonstrated in animals. Tamoxifen is contraindicated in women using anticoagulation therapy or with a history of deep vein thrombosis or pulmonary embolus. The serious side effects of raloxifene also include an increase in the risk of pulmonary thromboembolism, deep vein thrombosis, and stroke. Less serious side effects of raloxifene include vasomotor symptoms. Raloxifene is contraindicated in women who are lactating, pregnant, or have a history of venous thromboembolic events.

Common adverse effects of aromatase inhibitors include fatigue, nausea, headache, vasomotor symptoms, and muscle or joint pain. Estrogen deficiency may also result in a loss of bone mineral density. Compared with tamoxifen, the aromatase inhibitors are associated with a higher risk of osteoporotic fractures, cardiovascular disease, and hypercholesterolemia. By contrast, they are associated with a lower risk of venous thromboembolism and endometrial cancer. The adverse effects of fulvestrant are similar to those of the aromatase inhibitors.

Drugs Affecting Uterine Function

Regardless of whether drugs are given to stimulate or relax the pregnant uterus, most will cross the placenta and may have adverse effects on the fetus. Many agents affect fetal cardiovascular function, subsequently requiring special vigilance to avoid detrimental outcomes for either the mother or the fetus.

Uterine Stimulants

The major side effect of uterine stimulants is uterine tachysystole, also referred to as hyperstimulation. This is characterized by frequent (<2-minute interval) contractions or a prolonged tetanic contraction usually accompanied by maternal pain and often fetal bradycardia. Hyperstimulation produced by OT administered IV is easily reversed by reducing the infusion rate or discontinuing the drug. Because OT has a short half-life, normal uterine tone returns within a few minutes. Maternal side effects from OT administration are dose related and include cardiovascular instability (hypotension, tachycardia, myocardial ischemia, arrhythmias), nausea, vomiting, headache, and flushing. High doses of OT can result in cross-stimulation of vasopressin receptors, leading to an antidiuretic effect. This can cause water intoxication with severe hyponatremia if large volumes of fluid are infused.

Side effects of PGs include uterine tachysystole, fever, chills, nausea, vomiting, and diarrhea. The frequency of these side effects depends on the type of PG, dose, and route of administration. PGE_2 preparations for cervical ripening may be associated with an increased incidence of uterine rupture during labor in women who have had a previous cesarean section. PGE_2 should not be used in patients with a history of asthma, glaucoma, or myocardial infarction. Unexplained vaginal bleeding, chorioamnionitis, ruptured membranes, and previous caesarean section are relative contraindications to the use of PGs for cervical ripening.

Because ergot alkaloids can cause vasoconstriction, a serious risk of IV administration is hypertension. Hypertension may be associated with nausea, vomiting, and headache. Myocardial ischemia and infarction also have been reported. Ergot alkaloids are contraindicated in women with hypertension, a history of migraine, or Raynaud phenomenon.

Mifepristone is usually well tolerated but is associated occasionally with prolonged uterine bleeding. Other common side effects include uterine cramping and abdominal pain, which are expected with abortion. Transient headache and GI disturbances may occur with concomitant misoprostol. Since mifepristone is a glucocorticoid receptor antagonist, it is contraindicated in patients with either chronic adrenal failure or who are on concurrent long-term corticosteroid therapy. Mifepristone should not be used by women with hemorrhagic disorders or who are on anticoagulant therapy or medications that interfere with hemostasis, since this may lead to excessive bleeding during pregnancy termination.

Uterine Relaxants

Most tocolytic agents lack specificity for the uterus and produce predictable side effects stemming from their actions on other tissues. For example, selective β2-adrenergic receptor agonists may lead to cardiovascular complications in the mother or fetus as a consequence of peripheral vasodilation, which commonly results in hypotension. Maternal tachycardia may arise as a compensatory mechanism and from a direct action of the drug on the heart. β_2-adrenergic receptor agonists also increase hepatic glycogenolysis, resulting in maternal hyperglycemia, stimulating insulin secretion. As glucose is driven into cells by insulin, K^+ also accumulates intracellularly, resulting in maternal hypokalemia. The cardiovascular side effects, particularly in the face of hypokalemia, may trigger cardiac dysrhythmias, which can lead to heart failure. Infusion of β_2-adrenergic receptor agonists IV, especially in combination with glucocorticoids (which have salt-retaining properties), may cause excessive fluid retention, which can result in a potentially fatal pulmonary edema. Fluid balance should be monitored closely when these drugs are used in pregnant women. Tachycardia, hyperglycemia, and hyperinsulinemia may also develop in the fetus. Neonatal hypoglycemia may result from prolonged hyperinsulinemia. Maternal contraindications for β_2-adrenergic receptor agonists include tachycardia-sensitive cardiac disease and poorly controlled hyperthyroidism or diabetes mellitus.

Maternal side effects of indomethacin are primarily related to the GI tract and include nausea, esophageal reflux, gastritis, and vomiting. Concerns have been raised about the use of NSAIDs to arrest preterm labor because of potential adverse effects on the fetus, such as premature closure of the ductus arteriosus. Although this effect may be greater in term fetuses, it can be seen throughout the third trimester. Fetal renal toxicity is also frequent and commonly manifests as a reduction in fetal urine output, resulting in reduced amniotic fluid volume (oligohydramnios). Maternal contraindications for NSAIDs include platelet dysfunction or bleeding diathesis, hepatic or renal dysfunction, GI ulcerative disease, and hypersensitivity to aspirin.

Magnesium sulfate commonly causes diaphoresis and flushing. Other maternal side effects include nausea, headache, lethargy, and hypotension. High doses may cause obtundation, a loss of deep tendon reflexes, respiratory depression, and myocardial depression. Signs of magnesium toxicity in the fetus include neuromuscular and respiratory depression. Continuous administration for more than 7 days may cause fetal bone abnormalities. Magnesium is contraindicated in women with myasthenia gravis and should be avoided in women with known myocardial compromise or cardiac conduction defects.

Calcium-channel blockers in the dihydropyridine class, such as nifedipine, are peripheral vasodilators. Maternal side effects include nausea, flushing, headache, dizziness, and palpitations. Vasodilation may trigger a reflex increase in heart rate and stroke volume, which generally maintain blood pressure. However, hypotension can occur, so calcium-channel blockers are contraindicated in women with hypotension. The fetal effects of calcium-channel blockers are related to their maternal effects, which can lead to hypoperfusion of the uterus and placenta.

Potential problems associated with some of the important drugs are briefly summarized in the Clinical Problems Box.

NEW DEVELOPMENTS

Until recently, most oral contraceptives contained the synthetic estrogen, ethinyl estradiol, in combination with one of a variety of synthetic progestins. However, combination oral contraceptives still exert some unwanted metabolic effects, including changes in lipid profiles, carbohydrate metabolism, and coagulation factors. A new approach is to balance the actions of the estrogen and progestin in a more natural way by using a combination of 17β-estradiol or estradiol valerate with a "purer" progestin that does not interact with other steroid hormone receptors. It remains to be determined whether this approach will improve the safety of hormonal contraception.

Major concerns still exist about the overall safety of hormone administration after menopause. Although the Women's Health Initiative and Heart and Estrogen/Progestin Replacement Study (HERS) reported an increased risk of cardiovascular events in postmenopausal women, especially aged women, using combined estrogen/progestin therapy, many questions were not addressed, including the relationship of risk to the dose and types of hormones used, oral versus alternative routes of administration, or whether the timing of initiation of estrogen therapy (at the time of menses cessation vs. years later) affects the risk profile. A formulation that combines estrogen therapy with a partial estrogen agonist/antagonist, instead of a progestin, is now available for controlling vasomotor symptoms and preventing osteoporosis. However, the long-term risks associated with this combination remain to be determined.

Identifying more selective receptor modulators that are capable of exerting agonistic or antagonistic activity in a tissue-specific manner is an important focus of drug development. The ideal agent for postmenopausal women would be an agent that reduces vasomotor symptoms and acts as an agonist in bone but as an antagonist in the breast and uterus, with no increased cardiovascular risks. The development of new agents and regimens for the adjuvant treatment and prevention of breast cancer is also important. While treatment of breast cancer with drugs that selectively block ERs or inhibit estrogen synthesis has been a major advance, there are large variations in the therapeutic efficacy and side effects of these drugs that may result from genetic differences between individuals or their tumors. A better understanding of genetic polymorphisms in the target receptors, the aromatase enzyme, and drug metabolizing enzymes may allow for the development of more individualized recommendations for therapy.

The search for novel agents and treatment regimens to promote uterine quiescence and prevent preterm labor continues. PG receptor antagonists with specificity for the $PGF_{2\alpha}$ receptor are effective in inducing

uterine quiescence in animal models, but effects in humans have not yet been examined. Sildenafil, which inhibits the breakdown of cGMP by phosphodiesterase-5, has also shown promise in reducing uterine contractility in animal models. In a small randomized trial, women with preeclampsia who took the drug had longer pregnancy durations than those given a placebo.

TRADE NAMES

In addition to generic and fixed-combination preparations, the following trade-named materials are some of the important compounds available in the United States.

Estrogens
Conjugated equine estrogens (Premarin)
Conjugated synthetic estrogens (Cenestin, Enjuvia)
Esterified estrogens (Menest)
Estradiol (Alora, Climara, Estraderm, Estrace, Estring, EstroGel, Femring)
Estradiol cypionate (Depo-estradiol, Depogen)
Estropipate (Ogen, Ortho-Est)

Antiestrogens
Clomiphene (Clomid, Serophene)
Fulvestrant (Faslodex)
Raloxifene (Evista)
Tamoxifen (Nolvadex)

Progestogens
Danazol (Danocrine)
Etonogestrel (Implanon)
Hydroxyprogesterone caproate (Makena)
Levonorgestrel (Mirena, Next Choice, Plan B)
Medroxyprogesterone (Depo-Provera, Provera)
Megestrol (Megace)
Norethindrone (Micronor, Nor-QD)
Norgestrel (Ovrette)
Progesterone (Crinone, Prometrium)
Ulipristal (Ella)

Combination Oral Contraceptives
Estradiol valerate, dienogest (Natazia)
Ethinyl estradiol, desogestrel (Cyclessa, Desogen, Mircette, Ortho-Cept)

Ethinyl estradiol, drospirenone (Yasmin, Yaz)
Ethinyl estradiol, ethynodiol (Demulen)
Ethinyl estradiol, levonorgestrel (Alesse, Aviane, Levlen, Levora 28, Lybrel, Nordette, Seasonale, Tri-Levlen, Triphasil, Trivora)
Ethinyl estradiol/norgestimate (Ortho-Cyclen, Ortho Tri-Cyclen)
Ethinyl estradiol/norgestrel (Lo/Ovral, Ovral, Ogestrel)
Ethinyl estradiol/norethindrone (Brevicon, Estrostep, Loestrin, Norinyl 1+35, Tri-Norinyl, Ortho-Novum, Ovcon)
Mestranol/norethindrone (Necon 1/50, Norinyl 1+50)

Combination Menopausal Hormone Therapy
Conjugated estrogens/bazedoxifene (Duavee)
Conjugated estrogens/medroxyprogesterone (Prempro)
Estradiol/norethindrone acetate (Activella)
Ethinyl estradiol/norethindrone acetate (Femhrt)

Aromatase Inhibitors
Anastrozole (Arimidex)
Exemestane (Aromasin)
Letrozole (Femara)

Uterine Stimulants
Carboprost tromethamine (Hemabate)
Dinoprostone, PGE_2 (Cervidil, Prepidil, Prostin E_2)
Methylergonovine (Methergine)
Mifepristone (Mifeprex)
Misoprostol (Cytotec)
Oxytocin (Pitocin, Syntocinon)

Uterine Relaxants
Indomethacin (Indocin)
Nifedipine (Adalat, Procardia)
Terbutaline (Brethine)

CLINICAL RELEVANCE FOR HEALTHCARE PROFESSIONALS

Because hormonal contraception and menopausal hormone therapy are utilized by otherwise healthy individuals, it is imperative for all healthcare providers to understand the benefits as well as potential adverse events and risks associated with the use of these compounds. Healthcare professionals should be aware of variations in sex hormone levels during different life stages—that is, changes that may occur at the onset of puberty, during the menstrual cycle, during pregnancy, and during and after menopause. Practitioners should also keep in mind that drug metabolism changes during the developmental life cycle as well. It is important to ensure that patients are aware of possible adverse events and potential drug-drug interactions associated with hormonal therapy.

SELF-ASSESSMENT QUESTIONS

1. A postmenopausal 72-year-old woman with breast cancer was taking anastrozole to suppress the conversion of androgens to estrogens. Which enzyme does anastrozole inhibit?
   A. Aromatase.
   B. Desmolase.
   C. 17α-hydroxylase.
   D. 17β-hydroxysteroid dehydrogenase.
   E. 5α-reductase.

2. Which of the following best explains why raloxifene is an estrogen agonist in bone but an estrogen antagonist in the breast? Raloxifene:
   A. Has different affinities for ER subtypes in bone and breast tissues.
   B. Produces distinct conformational changes in ERs in different tissues.
   C. Causes increased turnover of ERs in the breast.
   D. Is more readily transported into bone cells.
   E. Is more rapidly inactivated in the breast.

3. A 25-year-old woman went to her gynecologist to request an oral contraceptive. Which of the following conditions is an absolute contraindication for the use of these drugs?
   A. Concurrent use of ampicillin.
   B. Diabetes mellitus type 1.
   C. Medical history of a deep venous thrombosis.
   D. Recent abortion using mifepristone.
   E. Smoking one or more packs of cigarettes per day.

4. A 32-year-old woman was given a prescription for a combination oral contraceptive containing both an estrogen and a progestin. The combination of these two hormones is better than an estrogen-only contraceptive because the addition of the progestin reduces which adverse effect of estrogen-only administration?
   A. Breast cancer.
   B. Endometrial cancer.
   C. Myocardial infarction.
   D. Stroke.
   E. Thromboembolic disorders.

5. A pregnant patient at term presents for induction of labor. The best pharmacological approach would be administration of:
   A. PGE until the woman is in active labor.
   B. PGE with concurrent intravenous infusion of oxytocin.
   C. Oxytocin intramuscularly.
   D. PGE until the cervix has ripened followed by oxytocin.
   E. Ergonovine intramuscularly.

6. A 30-year-old pregnant woman presents to the emergency room with severe abdominal cramping and moderate uterine bleeding; she is at approximately 8 weeks of gestation. Because oxytocin administration was ineffective to control the bleeding, ergot alkaloids were administered. Which of the following is correct concerning the use of ergot alkaloids in spontaneous abortion?
   A. Oral administration of ergot alkaloids is the most effective means for providing immediate relief.
   B. Ergot alkaloids are used to treat oxytocin toxicity.
   C. Ergot alkaloids commonly cause maternal hypotension.
   D. Large doses of ergot alkaloids act to reduce bleeding by causing sustained contraction of the uterus.
   E. PGs are more effective than ergot alkaloids for the management of severe uterine bleeding.

FURTHER READING

Arrowsmith S, Wray S. Oxytocin: its mechanism of action and receptor signaling in the myometrium. *J Neuroendocrinol*. 2014;26:356–369.

Bahamondes L, Bahamondes MV, Shulman LP. Non-contraceptive benefits of hormonal and intrauterine reversible contraceptive methods. *Human Reprod Update*. 2015;21:640–651.

Chabbert-Buffet N, Gerris J, Jamin C, et al. Toward a new concept of "natural balance" in oral estroprogestin contraception. *Gynecol Endocrinol*. 2013;29:891–896.

De Leo V, Musacchio MC, Cappelli V, et al. Hormonal contraceptives: pharmacology tailored to women's health. *Human Reprod Update*. 2016;22:634–646.

Hale GE, Shufelt CL. Hormone therapy in menopause: an update on cardiovascular disease considerations. *Trends Cardiovasc Med*. 2015;25:540–549.

Stuenkel CA, Davis SR, Gompel A, et al. Treatment of symptoms of the menopause: an Endocrine Society clinical practice guideline. *J Clin Endocrinol Metab*. 2015;100:3975–4011.

Suhag A, Saccone G, Berghella V. Vaginal progesterone for maintenance tocolysis: a systematic review and meta-analysis of randomized trials. *Am J Obstet Gynecol*. 2015;213:479–487.

WEBSITES

https://www.cdc.gov/reproductivehealth/contraception/index.htm
   The United States Centers for Disease Control and Prevention maintains an excellent website with guidelines for the use of oral contraceptives, as well as information and links to numerous resources on maternal and fetal health.

https://www.acog.org/
   The American Congress of Obstetricians and Gynecologists maintains a very comprehensive website and guidelines for numerous aspects of women's healthcare.

Androgens, Antiandrogens, and Their Clinical Uses

David S. Middlemas

MAJOR DRUG CLASSES

Androgens
Antiandrogens
Androgen receptor antagonists
GnRH analogues

ABBREVIATIONS

AR	Androgen receptor
ARI	α-Reductase inhibitors
BPH	Benign prostatic hyperplasia
DHEA	Dehydroepiandrosterone
DHT	Dihydrotestosterone
FSH	Follicle-stimulating hormone
GnRH	Gonadotropin-releasing hormone
HDL	High-density lipoprotein
HRT	Hormone replacement therapy
LDL	Low-density lipoprotein
LH	Luteinizing hormone
LUTS	Lower urinary tract symptoms
PEDs	Performance-enhancing drugs
SHBG	Sex hormone–binding globulin

THERAPEUTIC OVERVIEW

Androgens are produced primarily by the testes, ovaries, and adrenal glands and are involved in several diverse functions. Androgens stimulate virilization and spermatogenesis, are precursor steroids for estradiol production (Chapter 48), stimulate body hair and bone growth, promote a positive nitrogen balance, increase muscle development, and stimulate erythropoiesis.

Androgens are approved for hormone replacement therapy (HRT) in men with diagnosed testosterone deficiency and are effective treatment for primary hypogonadism (congenital or acquired) caused by testicular failure and hypogonadotropic hypogonadism (congenital or acquired) caused by deficiency of some related hormone activity or pituitary-hypothalamic injury. Androgens are also approved to treat delayed puberty, muscle wasting in both sexes due to chronic disease or malnutrition, and certain types of breast cancers in females.

The androgens act by binding to the androgen receptor (AR), and the antiandrogens or AR antagonists prevent androgens from activating their receptors. These compounds are used in males for the treatment of benign prostatic hyperplasia (BPH), prostate cancer, and male androgenic alopecia. These agents are also used in females for the treatment of acne, hirsutism, and hyperandrogenism and are part of the HRT regimen for transgender patients.

The agents used for the treatment of erectile dysfunction, which affects more than 18 million men in the United States, are vasodilators and are discussed in Chapter 41.

The principal therapeutic considerations pertaining to the androgens and related drugs are summarized in the Therapeutic Overview Box.

MECHANISMS OF ACTION

Androgen Synthesis

Androgens are synthesized from cholesterol in testicular Leydig cells, the adrenal cortex, and ovarian theca cells (Chapter 48, Fig. 48.1). The precursor cholesterol is synthesized in the Leydig cells from acetate or is supplied by plasma low-density lipoproteins (LDL) and high-density lipoproteins (HDL) via the LDL receptor–mediated endocytosis pathway (Chapter 42). Unlike the peptide hormones, the intracellular storage of steroid hormones that can be mobilized and secreted is minimal.

THERAPEUTIC OVERVIEW

Androgens
Primary hypogonadism (congenital or acquired)
Hypogonadotropic hypogonadism (congenital or acquired)
Constitutional delay of growth and puberty

Antiandrogens and Androgen Receptor Antagonists
Virilization in women
Precocious puberty in boys
Prostate cancer, benign prostatic hyperplasia

The regulation of testosterone synthesis and secretion is depicted in Fig. 52.1. The gonadotropin luteinizing hormone (LH), which is produced by the anterior pituitary gland, is the principal regulator of testosterone synthesis and secretion and stimulates the production of testosterone by Leydig cells. During puberty in males, the secretion of LH follows a diurnal rhythm, with elevated concentrations of LH and testosterone at night. In adult men, the diurnal rhythm for LH is less demonstrable, with approximately 25% higher levels of testosterone in the early morning than in the late afternoon. LH secretion fluctuates every 1–2 hours, resulting from intermittent stimulation of gonadotrophs by gonadotropin-releasing hormone (GnRH). GnRH secretory episodes, in turn, are coupled to excitatory discharges of a neural oscillator system. Intermittent GnRH secretion is required for the pituitary to function normally. Consequently, testosterone is released into the circulation in a fluctuating manner in response to the pulsatile stimulation of Leydig cells by LH.

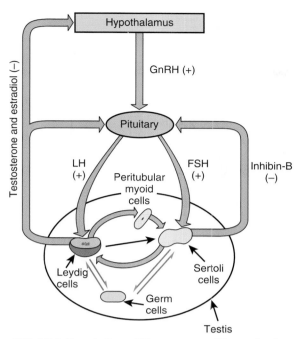

FIG. 52.1 Regulation of Testosterone Biosynthesis.

After puberty, the adult adrenal gland can also produce androgens, including dehydroepiandrosterone (DHEA), from which androstenedione, testosterone, estrone, estradiol, and estriol are derived (Chapter 48, Fig. 48.1). The adrenal production and secretion of these hormones into the circulation increase between 7 and 10 years of age and decline in the elderly and during severe illness.

Testosterone and Dihydrotestosterone

The Leydig cell has cell surface LH rceptors, which are G-protein-coupled and associated with G_s. Activation of these receptors leads to the stimulation of adenylyl cyclase, which evokes rapid testosterone synthesis, mediated primarily by the steroidogenic acute regulatory protein (StAR). Testosterone synthesis regulatory factors produced in the seminiferous tubules by germ cells and Sertoli cells or peritubular myoid cells maintain the serum concentration of testosterone in normal adult men between 280 and 300 ng/dL at the lower level and 1000 and 1100 ng/dL at the upper level. HRT may be warranted if testosterone levels are below the lower limits.

The Sertoli cells are somatic cells within the seminiferous tubules. Follicle-stimulating hormone (FSH) is the major regulator of Sertoli cell function, promoting tight junctions between Sertoli cells at the base of seminiferous tubules to form a blood-testis barrier that creates a pharmacological sanctuary in this tissue. Sertoli cells secrete proteins important in spermatogenesis, such as androgen-binding protein, transferrin, and inhibin B.

The testes are stimulated by gonadotropins released by the pituitary, but the testes, in turn, regulate LH and FSH secretion via negative feedback inhibition (see Fig. 52.1). Testosterone suppresses gonadotropin secretion by slowing the pulsatile release of GnRH. Also, inhibin B selectively reduces FSH synthesis and secretion. Testosterone is required for the normal development of the internal ducts of the male reproductive tract, with its metabolite dihydrotestosterone (DHT) responsible for stimulating the development of male external genitalia during the first trimester of fetal life. DHT is formed from testosterone by the action of the enzyme 5α-reductase.

The increase in circulating androgen concentrations that occurs during puberty in males promotes adult male secondary sex characteristics including testicular enlargement, scrotum darkening and rugation, growth of beard and body hair, stimulation of sebaceous glands, and growth of the penis, prostate, seminal vesicles, and larynx (leading to lowering of voice pitch). Physical stature changes including increased muscle mass, linear growth, skeleton maturation, and expression of male characteristics, including libido enhancement, also occur. These processes fail to develop completely if androgen action is impaired. Testosterone is also an important spermatogenic hormone stimulating Sertoli and myoid cells via activation of ARs. Androgen deficiency may be associated with hypospermatogenesis, and hypogonadal men are often infertile.

Endogenous or exogenous testosterone is bound to sex hormone binding–globulin (SHBG) in the circulation, with only a small fraction (1%–3%) unbound and available for entering target tissues and altering gene activity. There is evidence that SHBG binds androgen target cells and may play a role in the action of testosterone. SHBG formation is increased by estrogens and thyroxine and decreased by androgens, growth hormone, and insulin. The higher levels of estrogen in women lead to two- to threefold higher levels of SHBG than in men. Also, patients with hyperthyroidism exhibit elevated SHBG levels. Obesity is associated with lower levels of SHBG, perhaps because of hyperinsulinemia and insulin resistance.

Depending on the tissue, intracellular testosterone or the active metabolite DHT can interact directly with ARs. When testosterone enters cells in the prostate gland or any tissue with significant 5α-reductase activity, nearly 90% of it is metabolized to DHT. There are two isoenzymes of 5α-reductase encoded by two different genes. Type I 5α-reductase is expressed primarily in the liver and skin, sebaceous glands, and most hair follicles, whereas type II predominates in genital skin, beard, and scalp hair follicles and the prostate gland. An insufficient conversion of testosterone to DHT, caused by a rare mutation of the type II 5α-reductase gene, may result in a female or ambiguous genital phenotype in patients with a male genotype, stressing the importance of this enzyme in the normal development of male external genitalia. The distribution of the isozymes has been exploited to develop tissue-specific inhibitors of 5α-reductase activity.

Androgen binding to ARs and the events that follow are similar to those of other steroid hormones (Chapter 2). Ligand binds to the AR in the cytoplasm, the androgen-receptor complex translocates to the nucleus where it binds to DNA response elements, multiple coactivator proteins are recruited, and transcription is stimulated, leading to the increased synthesis of tissue-specific proteins (Fig. 52.2). Although most actions of the androgens are mediated by transcriptional activity of the receptor, testosterone also activates the mitogen-activated protein kinase pathway in an AR-dependent manner that is rapid and independent of AR-DNA interactions. Androgen regulation of target tissues may be positive, as in the stimulation of androgen-dependent proteins within the prostate gland, or negative, as in the inhibition of pituitary gonadotropin α-subunit gene expression and GnRH release by the hypothalamus. Negative regulation is less well understood, but in certain cases has been explained by AR binding to, and interfering with, the action of stimulatory transcription factors.

Antiandrogens and Androgen Receptor Antagonists

The actions of the androgens can be prevented by inhibiting their synthesis, blocking the AR, blocking GnRH receptors at the pituitary to prevent LH secretion, or through feedback inhibition at the level of the hypothalamus to decrease GnRH release.

Testosterone synthesis inhibitors include drugs that inhibit CYP17A, which has 17α-hydroxylase and 17,20-lyase activity and is required for the synthesis of testosterone from cholesterol in the adrenals, testes,

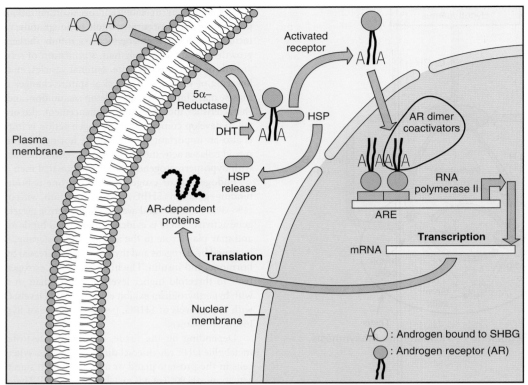

FIG. 52.2 Activation of Androgen Receptors and Downstream Consequences. *A*, Androgen; *ARE*, androgen response element; *DHT*, dihydrotestosterone *HSP*, heat shock protein complex.

and prostate (Chapter 48, Fig. 48.1). These drugs include ketoconazole, aminoglutethimide, and abiraterone. The synthesis of DHT from testosterone can be inhibited by the 5α-reductase inhibitors (ARIs). These compounds include finasteride, which is a selective competitive inhibitor of the type II isoenzyme responsible primarily for testosterone conversion to DHT in the prostate and the increased prostatic volume, and dutasteride, which is a competitive inhibitor of types I and II 5α-reductase.

The AR antagonists used clinically in humans in the United States are the nonsteroidal compounds flutamide, bicalutamide, nilutamide, and enzalutamide. These compounds competitively block androgen binding to the receptor.

Gonadotropin-Releasing Hormone Analogues

GnRH antagonists, such as degarelix, block GnRH binding to its receptors at the pituitary, thereby decreasing both LH and FSH release, leading to decreased testosterone and estradiol synthesis. The GnRH agonists leuprolide and goserelin decrease testosterone levels through negative feedback inhibition. Leuprolide is a synthetic nonapeptide, while goserelin is a synthetic decapeptide analogue of GnRH. These drugs act at pituitary GnRH receptors to produce an initial stimulation of LH and FSH release, stimulating testosterone and estradiol synthesis in a nonpulsatile, nonphysiological manner, disrupting normal feedback systems; upon continued administration, they decrease the secretion of both LH and FSH and reduce testosterone and estradiol biosynthesis.

RELATIONSHIP OF MECHANISMS OF ACTION TO CLINICAL RESPONSE

Testosterone deficiency may result from a disorder intrinsic to the testes or from insufficient stimulation of the testes by pituitary gonadotropins.

These conditions, primary testicular failure and hypogonadotropic hypogonadism, respectively, may be congenital or acquired. The goal of therapy is to stimulate development of body and male characteristics, including libido. Although testosterone treatment stimulates the expression of secondary sex characteristics in males with primary testicular failure, they remain infertile.

Age-related decline in testicular function, with decreased testosterone produced, may be treated with testosterone. The risks and benefits of HRT for healthy older men are difficult to assess, although a family or personal history of prostate cancer or BPH may increase these risks. Testosterone is also used in boys to treat congenital microphallus, to stimulate sexual development, to increase the height of short teenagers with constitutional delay of puberty, and to treat low testosterone levels in cryptorchidism (failure of one or both testes to descend) in prepubertal boys. However, premature closure of the epiphyseal plates with resultant growth arrest and unacceptable virilization may occur if treatment is not carefully monitored. Androgens have been used to increase libido and sexual function, mood, and well-being in women, but the Endocrine Society does not recommend it. Danazol, a weak androgen, has been used to treat endometriosis.

BPH results from proliferation of epithelial and smooth muscle cells within the transition zone of the prostate, producing prostatic enlargement, which may cause lower urinary tract symptoms (LUTS) including outlet obstruction. Pharmacological symptomatic relief of BPH includes the use of competitive α-adrenergic receptor antagonists and vasodilators. Disease modification of LUTS secondary to BPH may occur with ARIs. Competitive α-adrenergic receptor antagonists with more selective actions that decrease adverse effects, like tamsulosin, terazosin, and silodosin, are commonly used for symptomatic relief for LUTS. The ARIs finasteride and dutasteride may improve symptoms and act as disease-modifying drugs, decreasing the progression of

LUTS secondary to BPH, and are indicated for symptomatic relief in prostate enlargement. The vasodilator tadalafil is also effective for this condition (Chapter 41). Finasteride is also approved and effective for male androgenetic alopecia via enzyme inhibition in the scalp; visible improvement is observed in about half of treated men. The vasodilator minoxidil may also be effective for this condition (Chapter 41).

Androgen deprivation therapy is used for androgen-dependent prostate cancers, and may be accomplished using the GnRH antagonists, such as degarelix, the AR antagonists such as flutamide, enzalutamide, bicalutamide, and nilutamide, and the testosterone synthesis inhibitors such as abiraterone. The GnRH agonists, including leuprolide and goserelin, which are effective through negative feedback regulation of testosterone synthesis via the hypothalamic-pituitary axis (Fig. 52.1), may also be used. GnRH agonists are often coadministered with an AR antagonist, such as flutamide, to prevent an initial flare of symptoms. Other drugs approved to treat metastatic castration-resistant prostate cancer include the CYP17 inhibitors ketoconazole, aminoglutethimide, and abiraterone acetate.

Testosterone, antiandrogens, and GnRH analogues are all used in conjunction with psychological counseling for sex affirmation changes in transgender patients. Testosterone is used predominantly to alter secondary sexual characteristics in individuals assigned as female at birth, while the antiandrogens are used to block male characteristics in individuals assigned as male at birth. GnRH analogues are used to delay puberty.

Androgens are abused as performance-enhancing drugs (PEDs) and are classified by the United States Drug Enforcement Administration as Schedule III. It should be noted that the abuse of androgens typically involves supraphysiological doses and complex administration schedules. Although clinical trials with these doses are limited, there is no doubt

that all of the androgenic drugs are anabolic, enhancing muscle mass, strength, and athletic performance. Although some of the drugs, notably the 17α-methylated androgens, have a high myotrophic index, defined as the ratio of myotrophic effects to androgenic effects in an in vitro rat model, there is no clear clinical evidence that these androgens are more anabolic than testosterone. Androgens used as PEDs that are commonly abused for their anabolic activity include **nandrolone**, **oxandrolone**, **oxymetholone**, and **stanozolol**; testosterone and testosterone derivatives are also used.

PHARMACOKINETICS

Androgens

The hepatic metabolism of testosterone is shown in Fig. 52.3. Nearly half of hepatic testosterone is metabolized to the 17-ketosteroids, 5α-androsterone and etiocholanolone, both of which are excreted in the urine. In addition, testosterone is also conjugated and excreted as glucuronides and sulfates. Although DHT and estradiol represent minor (5%) metabolites (Chapter 48, Fig. 48.1), they are highly biologically active. Circulating levels of DHT are approximately 10% that of testosterone, and estradiol levels in men approximate those in women in the early follicular phase of the menstrual cycle. Estradiol plays a role in bone matrix regulation in males and females and contributes to negative feedback control of GnRH and gonadotropins.

The pharmacokinetic properties of the androgens available for clinical use are listed in Table 52.1. Testosterone is not administered orally because it rapidly undergoes first-pass metabolism. Transdermal delivery of testosterone produces stable physiological drug concentrations by avoiding first-pass hepatic metabolism. Formulations include gels,

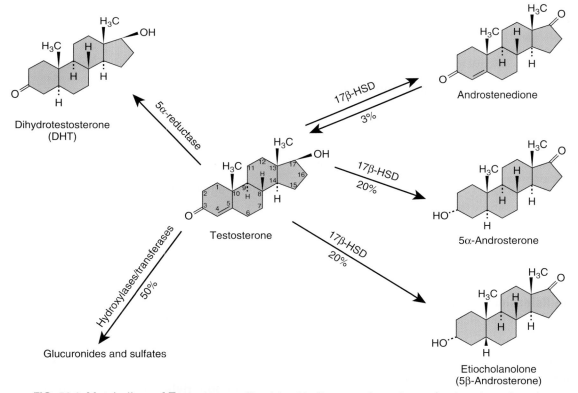

FIG. 52.3 Metabolism of Testosterone. The right side illustrates the pathways for the primary hepatic metabolism of testosterone via 17β-hydroxysteroid dehydrogenase (17β-HSD) to 5α-androsterone and etiocholanolone and the relative percentages of metabolites. The left side depicts the metabolism of testosterone to DHT via the action of 5α-reductase, the pathway inhibited by the 5α-reductase inhibitors (ARIs) finasteride and dutasteride.

TABLE 52.1 Pharmacokinetic Parameters

Drug	Route of Administration	Duration
Testosterone propionate	IM	Short-acting (1 day, 2–3 days)
Testosterone cypionate	IM	Long-acting (1–2 days, 10–14 days)
Testosterone enanthate	IM	Long-acting (1–2 days, 10–14 days)
Methyltestosterone	Oral, buccal	Short-acting (1–2 hours, 4–5 hours)
Fluoxymesterone	Oral	Short-acting (1 hour, 2–3 days)
Danazol	Oral	Short-acting (2 hours, 2–3 days)
Nandrolone	IM	Long-acting (5–7 days, 3–4 weeks)

IM, Intramuscularly.

transdermal patches, and a buccal tablet placed on the surface of the gums. Caution most be exercised with the placement of gels on the patient's body to avoid transfer to women or children.

The synthetic 17α-alkylated androgens methyltestosterone and oxandrolone are less extensively metabolized by the liver and are orally available. Methyltestosterone has a relatively short duration of action. These drugs are used only after sexual maturation because they lack the potency to facilitate sexual development.

Testosterone esterified at the 17β-hydroxyl position (e.g., as the propionate, cypionate, enanthate, or undecanoate) and contained in an oil suspension is administered by intramuscular injection. Esterification increases lipid solubility and decreases hepatic metabolism, prolonging the duration of action. The testosterone esters are administered every 2–4 weeks and are converted to free testosterone.

Antiandrogens and Androgen Receptor Antagonists

The ARI finasteride is orally available, with absorption unaffected by food. Plasma concentrations peak in approximately 1–2 hours, and the drug is metabolized extensively by hepatic CYP3A4 to weakly active metabolites that are excreted in the urine. The parent compound is also excreted in the feces. Dutasteride takes 2–3 hours to reach peak plasma levels following oral administration, and food decreases absorption. Dutasteride is metabolized by CYP3A4 and CYP3A5, and both the parent and metabolites are excreted primarily in the feces.

The AR antagonist flutamide is completely absorbed following oral administration with one metabolite biologically active. Metabolites are excreted in the urine. Bicalutamide is well absorbed after oral administration, unaffected by the presence of food, and highly protein bound (>95%).

Gonadotropin-Releasing Hormone Analogues

The pharmacokinetics of the GnRH analogues are presented in Chapter 49.

PHARMACOVIGILANCE: ADVERSE EFFECTS AND DRUG INTERACTIONS

Androgens

Many side effects of androgens are dose related and occur when target tissues are stimulated excessively. The testosterone esters lead to high levels of testosterone and estradiol within the first few days after injection

that may produce acne, polycythemia, and gynecomastia and are associated with mood swings in some patients. Testosterone can also lead to priapism (sustained erection over 4 hours) and prostatic enlargement. Androgens in high doses also decrease HDL concentrations and may be atherogenic. Weight gain and sodium retention may occur during androgen therapy, though the mechanism is unclear. Long-term androgen treatment suppresses gonadotropin secretion, decreases testis size, and depresses spermatogenesis. For this reason, testosterone has been evaluated as a male contraceptive. Occasionally, gynecomastia develops in patients treated with testosterone, which may result from metabolism to estradiol. Obstructive sleep apnea may be exacerbated in susceptible men treated with testosterone, and androgens should not be used in men with suspected prostate or breast cancer.

All of the drugs are clinically androgenic, with adverse effects including virilization in women, particularly when being abused at supraphysiological levels. The testosterone precursor androstenedione is classified as Schedule III and banned by most major sports organizations. It is controversial whether consumption of DHEA enhances athletic performance. However, adverse effects, especially cardiovascular and hepatic risk, and an unfair competitive advantage from using anabolic androgenic steroids prompted a ban from most major sports organizations and the Olympics.

The 17α-alkylated androgens are associated with hepatotoxicity, especially when abused at supraphysiological levels, and may lead to a rise in serum transaminase concentrations and the development of jaundice in 1%–2% of patients as a result of intrahepatic cholestasis. Peliosis hepatis and hepatocellular carcinoma have both been observed in a few patients treated with very high doses of alkylated androgens. The 17α-methylated androgens produce greater suppression of HDL cholesterol concentrations than testosterone because of their oral route of administration, thereby exposing the liver to high drug concentrations; in addition, they are not converted to estrogens. Danazol may produce acne, oily skin, decreased breast size, hirsutism, and decreased HDL cholesterol in women.

Use of multiple androgens in doses that far exceed physiological concentrations may suppress gonadotropin secretion and reduce testicular function, including spermatogenesis. Recovery of normal function may take several years. These drugs also cause increased concentrations of LDL cholesterol and decreased HDL synthesis and serum levels and may increase the risk of atherosclerosis. Long-term, high-dose androgen treatment may also increase the risk of BPH and cause prostate cancer as men age.

Antiandrogens and Androgen Receptor Antagonists

The most common side effects associated with the use of drugs that antagonize or inhibit the effects of the androgens include impotence, loss of sex drive, inability to achieve orgasm, and other sexually related issues. In addition, the ARIs may lead to increased breast size or breast tenderness. Because dutasteride and finasteride are metabolized by CYP3A4, drug levels will increase with the concomitant use of CYP3A4 inhibitors. In addition, studies have shown that the calcium-channel blockers verapamil and diltiazem decrease the clearance of dutasteride, resulting in increased blood levels.

The AR antagonist flutamide has been reported to lead to hepatic failure and hypersensitivity reactions, although these appear to be rare events.

Gonadotropin-Releasing Hormone Analogues

The adverse effects and drug interactions of the GnRH analogues are presented in Chapter 49.

The potential problems associated with the use of the androgens are summarized in the Clinical Problems Box.

CLINICAL PROBLEMS

Growth acceleration in children
Priapism
Masculinization in women
Jaundice
Edema
Acne
Hypertension
Weight gain
Suppression of spermatogenesis
Lipid disturbances
Fetal masculinization during pregnancy

TRADE NAMES

In addition to generic and fixed-combination preparations, the following trade-named materials are some of the important compounds available in the United States.

Androgens
Danazol (Danocrine)
Fluoxymesterone (Halotestin)
Methyltestosterone (Android, Metandren, Testred, Virilon)
Nandrolone (Deca-Durabolin, Durabolin)
Oxandrolone (Anavar)
Oxymetholone (Anadrol)
Stanozolol (Winstrol)
Testosterone cypionate (Depo-testosterone, Virilon IM)
Testosterone gel (AndroGel, Testim)
Testosterone enanthate (Delatestryl)
Transdermal testosterone (Androderm, Testoderm)

Antiandrogens and Androgen Receptor Antagonists
5α-Reductase Inhibitors
Finasteride (Propecia, Proscar)
Dutasteride (Avodart)

GnRH Agonists
Degarelix (Firmagon)

Androgen Receptor Antagonists
Flutamide (Eulexin)
Bicalutamide (Casodex)

Long-Acting GnRH Analogues
Leuprolide (Lupron Depot)
Goserelin (Zoladex)

NEW DEVELOPMENTS

Anabolic pharmacological strategies may be used to offset the protein catabolism associated with long-term corticosteroid use and in some critically ill patients. Several small clinical trials have shown positive effects using oxandrolone for chronic catabolic disorders, treating patients with AIDS-associated wasting, Duchenne muscular dystrophy, amyotrophic lateral sclerosis, and chronic pulmonary obstructive disease.

CLINICAL RELEVANCE FOR HEALTHCARE PROFESSIONALS

Androgens and antiandrogens can have profound effects on skeletal muscle biology. Therefore all healthcare professionals, including dentists, physical and occupational therapists, physician assistants, nurses, nutritionists, and others should be aware of potential body changes and adverse effects of these drugs. Healthcare providers may recognize androgen abuse in patients exhibiting active truncal acne, prominent muscularity, and testicular atrophy and thus can play a direct role in deterring androgen abuse. Awareness of the baseline status of individuals and changes that occur during therapy interventions can allow the healthcare provider to monitor such changes and provide guidance regarding the use of such drugs.

SELF-ASSESSMENT QUESTIONS

1. BPH can be characterized by frequent urinary urgency, diminished urinary stream, urinary retention, and prostate-specific antigen levels within normal limits for age. Finasteride reduces the size of the prostate by:
   A. Inhibiting the interaction of the DHT-androgen receptor complex with promoter DNA.
   B. Decreasing the formation of gonadotropins.
   C. Antagonizing 5α-reductase, reducing formation of DHT.
   D. Decreasing gonadal androgen production.
   E. Competitively antagonizing the androgen receptor.

2. A 67-year-old male was diagnosed with androgen-dependent prostate cancer. The drug of choice for treatment of this individual is:
   A. Testosterone.
   B. Dihydrotestosterone.
   C. Flutamide.
   D. Nandrolone.
   E. Minoxidil.

3. A 72-year-old man presents with fatigue, lack of interest in activities, and poor libido. Blood tests reveal normal fasting blood glucose, HbA1C, and TSH. His testosterone level was 97 ng/dL. An appropriate treatment is:
   A. Metformin.
   B. Levothyroxine.
   C. Insulin.
   D. Testosterone.
   E. Sildenafil.

FURTHER READING

Gormley GJ, Stoner E, Bruskewitz RC, et al. The effect of finasteride in men with benign prostatic hyperplasia. *N Engl J Med*. 1992;327:1185–1191.

Hembree WC, Cohen-Kettenis P, Delemarre-van de Waal HA, et al. Endocrine treatment of transsexual persons: an Endocrine Society clinical practice guideline. *J Clin Endocrinol Metab*. 2011;94(9):3132–3154.

Testosterone Therapy in Adult Men with Androgen Deficiency Syndromes. An Endocrine Society clinical practice guideline. *J Clin Endocrinol Metab*. 2010;95(6):2536–2559.

WEBSITES

https://www.endocrine.org/education-and-practice-management/clinical-practice-guidelines

This page is maintained by the Endocrine Society and is an excellent resource. It contains clinical practice guidelines for the use of testosterone therapy in adult men with androgen deficiency and the endocrine treatment of transsexual individuals, in addition to numerous other links.

Drug Therapy for the Management of Diabetes

Julio A. Copello

MAJOR DRUG CLASSES

Insulin

Insulin Secretagogues

Sulfonylureas and meglitinides (K_{ATP} channel inhibitors)

Gliptins (dipeptidyl peptidase-IV inhibitors)

Incretin analogues (glucagon-like peptide-1 receptor agonists)

Drugs That Decrease Insulin Resistance

Biguanides

Thiazolidinediones (peroxisome proliferator–activated receptor agonist)

Amylin analogues

Other Antihyperglycemic Agents

D_2 dopamine receptor agonists

Bile acid sequestrants

Gliflozins (sodium-glucose cotransport 2 inhibitors)

α-Glucosidase inhibitors

ABBREVIATIONS

Akt	Protein kinase B
DM	Diabetes mellitus
DPP-IV	Dipeptidyl peptidase-IV
GI	Gastrointestinal
GIP	Glucose-dependent insulinotropic polypeptide
GLP-1	Glucagon-like peptide-1
GLUT	Glucose transporter
GS	Glycogen synthase
HbA1c	Glycated hemoglobin
IR	Insulin receptor
IRS	Insulin receptor substrate
K_{ATP}	ATP-sensitive K^+ channel
PPAR	Peroxisome proliferator–activated receptor
SC	Subcutaneous
SGLT2	Sodium-glucose cotransporter 2
SUR1	Sulfonylurea subunit of the ATP-sensitive K^+ channel

THERAPEUTIC OVERVIEW

Diabetes mellitus (DM) includes a group of common metabolic disorders characterized by fasting hyperglycemia and/or abnormal postprandial glucose management. Patients with DM exhibit differences in onset and time course of disease progression, vascular complications, and severity, including the magnitude of declining pancreatic insulin secretion, the incapacity of glucose usage in tissues, and exacerbation of hepatic gluconeogenesis. DM has a multifactorial etiology including environmental, developmental, genetic, age, ethnicity, and race factors, all of which influence disease severity. According to the National Institutes of Health (NIH), the incidence of DM in the United States increased from ~4.5% in 2000 to ~9.3% in 2014, reflecting increases in obesity, sedentary lifestyle, and environmental stress. Complications of DM are also on the rise and represent the leading cause for new cases of blindness in adults, renal failure, and nontraumatic amputations. Additionally, DM is a major risk factor for reduced longevity, neuropathy, heart disease, and stroke.

Pathophysiology

Normally, blood glucose is maintained within a relatively narrow range (70–100 mg/dL, or 0.39–0.55 mM), with the 3-month average blood glucose reflected by the amount of glycated hemoglobin A1c (HbA1c), which is about 5% for the normal population, 5.7%–6.4% for the prediabetic state, and ≥6.5% for diabetics. Increased plasma glucose levels stimulate pancreatic insulin secretion, promoting the uptake and

storage of glucose, amino acids, and fatty acids in liver, skeletal muscle, and adipose tissue and inhibiting gluconeogenesis in the liver and fatty acid release from adipose tissue. These alterations result in the transfer of nutrients from the blood into tissues to meet the energy and metabolic demands of the body. Hyperglycemia occurs when insulin secretion is insufficient or tissue responses are inadequate.

Different pharmacological strategies exist for treating and managing the two primary types of DM, type 1 and type 2. Type 1 DM is caused primarily by a T cell–mediated autoimmune response that destroys insulin-producing pancreatic β cells, causing irreversible complete or major insulin deficiency. Tissue responsiveness to insulin is not usually affected in DM type 1. Type 2 DM, the more common disorder, is associated with genetic and metabolic defects that impact glucose metabolism, insulin secretion, or insulin action in tissues. Type 2 DM progresses very slowly from impaired glucose tolerance to insulin-independent type 2 DM to insulin-requiring type 2 DM, leading to hyperglycemia and other symptoms. Fig. 53.1 illustrates changes in plasma glucose and insulin levels after an oral glucose tolerance test administered to normal individuals (A), individuals with type 1 and type 2 DM (B and C), and individuals with impaired glucose tolerance (D).

The management of diabetes is individualized and considers patient characteristics, severity of the disease, tissue responsiveness, and insulin preparations available. Pharmacological management of hyperglycemia for patients with minimal insulin resistance involves stimulation of endogenous insulin secretion, but the long-term use of these agents could induce β-cell dysfunction, leading to dependence on exogenous

433

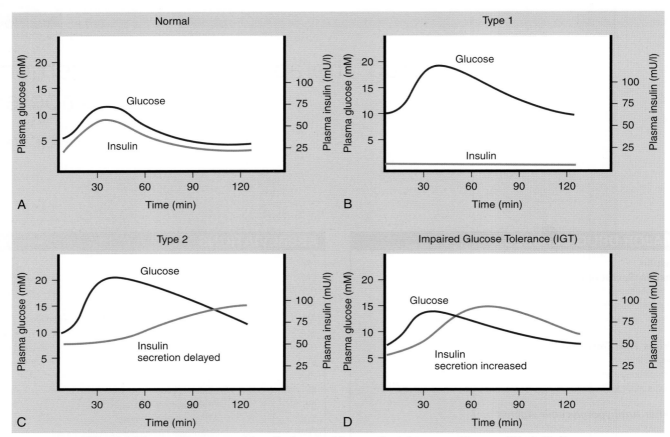

FIG. 53.1 Plasma Glucose and Insulin Levels After an Oral Aqueous Glucose (75-g) Challenge Following an 8-Hour Fast. Subjects were grouped based on a diagnosis of normal (A); type 1 diabetes mellitus (B); type 2 diabetes mellitus (C); and impaired glucose tolerance (D). (A) Nondiabetic individuals display a peak glucose concentration of 10–15 mM by 30 minutes and normoglycemia (5 mM) in 90–120 minutes; the insulin concentration follows a similar response. (B) At all time points, patients with type 1 diabetes mellitus exhibit greatly elevated plasma glucose levels compared with normal, with plasma insulin levels essentially undetectable. In clinical practice, patients with suspected type 1 diabetes mellitus are not usually subjected to oral glucose tolerance tests. Diagnosis of insulinopenia, which is accompanied by elevated blood glucose levels, is adequate information to initiate insulin treatment. (C) Hyperglycemia at all time points is also characteristic of type 2 diabetes mellitus. However, plasma insulin levels exhibit an extended delay, although nearly normal levels can be observed. In type 2 diabetes mellitus with insulin resistance, plasma glucose concentrations can remain elevated in spite of nearly normal levels of insulin. (D) For patients with impaired glucose tolerance, blood glucose at 30–60 minutes is higher than normal and may remain elevated at 120 minutes. Because of β cell compensation for impaired glucose, the plasma insulin concentrations are higher than normal, both in the fasting state and after glucose is administered. For many patients, this is a temporary situation, and depending on the cause, the outcome can return to normal, remain unchanged, or mimic type 2 diabetes mellitus.

insulin. For the patient with type 2 DM who exhibits primarily insulin resistance, management includes reducing glucose intake through diet, weight loss, easing insulin resistance with drugs such as metformin, and, when needed, insulin supplementation. For the patient with both reduced insulin secretion and insensitivity to exogenous insulin, combination therapy involving drugs that affect insulin levels and resistance, along with diet, weight loss, and exercise provide the best management. Epidemiological studies indicate that the continuous and steady control of blood glucose levels has a significant positive impact on patient outcomes. New drug classes and therapeutic concepts have improved the consistency of blood glucose control, reducing pathological sequelae of this disease. A summary of the types of diabetes and their management is presented in the Therapeutic Overview Box.

MECHANISMS OF ACTION

Insulin

Insulin is formed by the β cells of the pancreatic islets of Langerhans from the primary precursor **preproinsulin**, which contains 110 amino acids. A 24-residue signal peptide directs this precursor to the rough endoplasmic reticulum, where it is cleaved to form **proinsulin**, the secondary insulin precursor. Proinsulin contains an amino terminal B chain, a carboxy terminal A chain, and the C peptide that connects the two. Endopeptidases in the endoplasmic reticulum cleave the C peptide, generating mature insulin, composed of a 21–amino acid A chain with an intramolecular disulfide bond, and a 30–amino acid B chain that is covalently linked to the A chain by two disulfide bonds (Fig. 53.2).

Active insulin is complexed with Zn^{++}, aggregates into dimers and hexamers, and is packaged with the C peptide and islet amyloid polypeptide (amylin) in the Golgi apparatus into secretory granules. Upon an appropriate stimulus, insulin, amylin, and the C peptide are released into the circulation. Amylin contributes to glycemic control by slowing

gastric emptying and promoting satiety, thereby preventing postprandial blood glucose spikes; the C peptide has no established biological action and is mostly excreted into the urine.

Insulin release is controlled primarily by glucose but is affected by many factors (Box 53.1). When blood glucose levels increase, more glucose is taken up and metabolized by the pancreatic β cell. Glucose is metabolized by glycolysis, generating adenosine triphosphate (ATP), which increases the ATP/ADP ratio (Fig. 53.3). This change inhibits the ATP-sensitive potassium channel (K_{ATP}) composed of four inward-rectifying subunits ($K_{ir}6.2$) forming the pore and four modulatory sulfonylurea subunits (SUR1) with ATPase activity. Inhibition of K_{ATP} decreases outward K^+ currents in β cells, partially depolarizing the cell membrane and activating Ca^{++} entry via L-type voltage-gated Ca^{++} channels. The increased intracellular Ca^{++} stimulates granule exocytosis that releases equimolar amounts of insulin and C peptide, in addition to small concentrations of proinsulin and amylin into the blood.

The released insulin rapidly reaches the liver, muscles, and adipose tissue and activates glucose uptake. The cellular effects of insulin are initiated by binding to and activating the insulin receptor (IR), which is a tyrosine kinase receptor composed of 2 α-subunits and 2 β-subunits (Fig. 53.4). The binding of insulin to the extracellular α-subunits results in a conformational change of the β-subunits, leading to phosphorylation of tyrosine residues on the β-subunit. The activated IR can phosphorylate the phosphotyrosine-binding domains of the scaffolding proteins, insulin receptor substrate, IRS-1 or IRS-2, which serves as a docking site for common signal transduction intermediates. The

THERAPEUTIC OVERVIEW

Type 1 Diabetes Mellitus
Medical nutrition counseling; exercise

Insulin

Drugs to control insulin resistance (amylin analogues, α-glucosidase inhibitors, others)

Management of Diabetic Ketoacidosis
Fluid replacement; insulin; Na^+, K^+, bicarbonate, and glucose

Type 2 Diabetes Mellitus
Medical nutrition counseling; exercise

Insulin

Insulin secretagogues (sulfonylureas, meglitinides, gliptins, incretin analogues)

Agents that decrease insulin resistance (biguanides, thiazolidinediones, amylin analogues)

Other antihyperglycemic agents (D_2 dopamine receptor agonists, bile acid sequestrants, gliflozins)

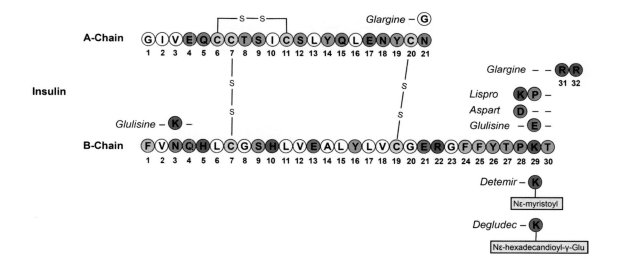

FIG. 53.2 Primary Structures of Insulin and Glucagon. The amino acid sequences of the 21–amino acid A chain and the 30–amino acid B chain of human insulin and the 29 amino acids in human glucagon are shown. The single-letter code for the amino acids is consistent with accepted nomenclature. Color code for amino acids is based on the characteristics of the side chain as follows: white (small and/or hydrophobic), orange (aromatic and hydrophobic), brown (proline), pink (methionine), yellow (cysteine), purple (polar, hydroxyl group), aqua (polar, amide group), red (electrically charged, acidic), and green (electrically charged, basic). The two interchain disulfide bridges and the intrachain disulfide in the A chain of insulin are indicated. Residues in all recombinant human insulins (glargine, lispro, aspart, glulisine, detemir, and degludec) that differ from those in unmodified human insulin are shown above or below the A- and B-chain sequences. Also depicted are the groups that acylate the ε-amino of lysine (K29) in insulin detemir and degludec.

BOX 53.1   Some Factors That Control the Release of Endogenous Insulin

Stimulants

Elevated Plasma Levels of Nutrients

Glucose

Other monosaccharides

Amino acids

Fatty acids

Ketone bodies

Neural and Humoral Elements

β-Adrenergic receptor stimulation

Parasympathetic stimulation

Glucagon and glucagon-like peptide 1

Cholecystokinin

Vasoactive intestinal peptide

Gastric inhibitory polypeptide

Gastrin

Secretin

Drugs

β-Adrenergic receptor agonists

Cholinergic (muscarinic) agonists

Inhibitors

Decreased blood glucose

Somatostatin

α-Adrenergic receptor agonists

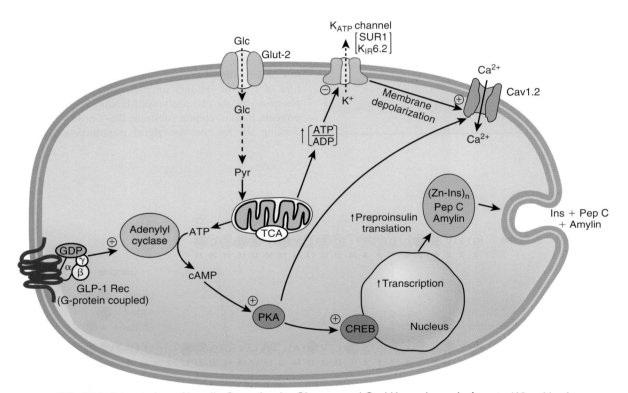

FIG. 53.3 Stimulation of Insulin Secretion by Glucose and Oral Hypoglycemic Agents. When blood glucose (Glc) increases, more Glc enters the pancreatic β cell via the glucose transporter, GLUT2. The Glc is phosphorylated and subsequently metabolized via the tricarboxylic acid (TCA) cycle, increasing the ATP/ADP ratio. This results in inhibition of the inwardly rectifying ATP-sensitive K^+ channel (K_{ATP}), resulting in membrane depolarization, triggering activation of voltage-gated Ca^{++} channels. The rise in intracellular Ca^{++} stimulates exocytosis of secretory granules containing insulin (Ins), peptide C (Pep C), and amylin. The sulfonylureas and meglitinides bind to sites on the K_{ATP} to inhibit channel conductance, resulting in membrane depolarization and Ca^{++} entry, promoting insulin release. The incretins bind to their receptors, leading to the increased cAMP-mediated phosphorylation of both K_{ATP} and the calcium channel Cav1.2, resulting in decreased K_{ATP} activity, prolonged Ca^{++} channel openings, and less depolarization required for Ca^{++} entry. Increased cAMP also results in increased synthesis of insulin and the triggering of other pathways that synergize the effects of plasma glucose on insulin release (not shown).

activation of **phosphatidylinositol 3-kinase (PI 3-kinase)** by IRS proteins mediates the acute metabolic effects of insulin. The phospholipid products generated through this pathway promote activation of several protein kinases, including protein kinases B (Akt) and C, which phosphorylate effectors that promote the insertion of the glucose transporter 4 (GLUT4) in muscle and adipose tissue cell membranes. By activating Akt, insulin promotes the translocation of GLUT4 from intracellular vesicles to the plasma membrane (Fig. 53.5); an atypical protein kinase C is involved to a lesser extent. Increasing glucose transporters at the cell surface increases glucose uptake into the cell.

Akt also regulates the activity of glycogen synthase (GS), the enzyme that promotes the storage of glucose as glycogen in liver and skeletal muscle, a critical component of the action of insulin to lower blood glucose concentrations. GS activity is regulated by phosphorylation/dephosphorylation mechanisms with phosphorylation by glycogen synthase kinase (GSK-3) inactivating and dephosphorylation by the protein phosphatase PP1G–activating GS (see Fig. 53.5). Akt phosphorylates and inactivates GSK-3, thereby tipping the balance to favor activation of GS by PP1G. In addition, by stimulating glucose transport via GLUT4, Akt increases intracellular glucose 6-phosphate, an allosteric activator of GS. Akt also increases the synthesis of triglycerides from free fatty acids in adipose tissue and stimulates protein synthesis.

Overall, activation of insulin receptors promotes glucose removal from the blood, either for use or storage, and affects carbohydrate, lipid, and protein metabolism, detailed in Box 53.2. Insulin affects hepatic metabolism by activating hepatic glucose storage as glycogen and metabolic glucose utilization by various paths, including glycolysis and the Krebs cycle. Insulin inhibits glycogenolysis and gluconeogenesis, which decrease glucose production and release to the blood.

Insulin decreases serum lipid concentrations, especially triglycerides, by promoting the hepatic synthesis of triglycerides from plasma free fatty acids or newly synthesized acetyl coenzyme A from plasma glucose.

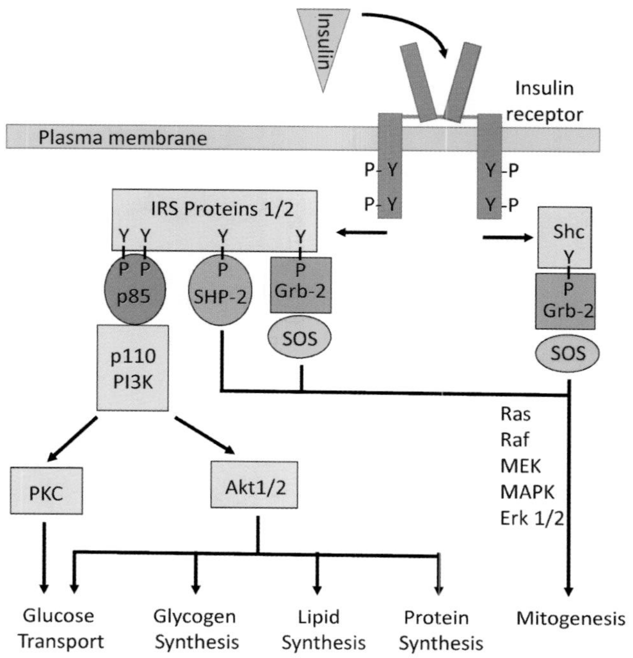

FIG. 53.4 Major Signal Transduction Pathways Mediating the Effects of Insulin. Insulin binding to its receptor results in autophosphorylation on tyrosine (Y) residues and the phosphorylation of the adapter proteins, insulin receptor substrate (IRS) proteins 1 and 2. This creates docking sites for downstream effectors, which bind to phosphotyrosine-containing sites. Phosphoinositide 3-kinase (PI3K) binds phosphorylated IRS proteins through SH domains in its p85 regulatory subunit. Binding activates the p110 catalytic subunit, generating phospholipid products that activate several downstream protein kinases, including protein kinase B (Akt) and some isoforms of protein kinase C. These downstream kinases phosphorylate regulatory proteins that lead to the activation of glucose transport and increases in the rates of synthesis of glycogen, lipid, and protein.

BOX 53.2 Actions of Insulin

Carbohydrate Metabolism
Increases glucose uptake
Increases glycogen synthesis and decreases glycogenolysis
Increases glycolysis and decreases gluconeogenesis
Increases glucose oxidation

Lipid Metabolism
Increases fatty acid transport
Increases triglyceride synthesis (includes fatty acid and glycerol synthesis and esterification)
Decreases lipolysis

Protein Metabolism
Increases amino acid transport
Increases protein synthesis (including messenger ribonucleic acid transcription and translation)
Decreases protein degradation

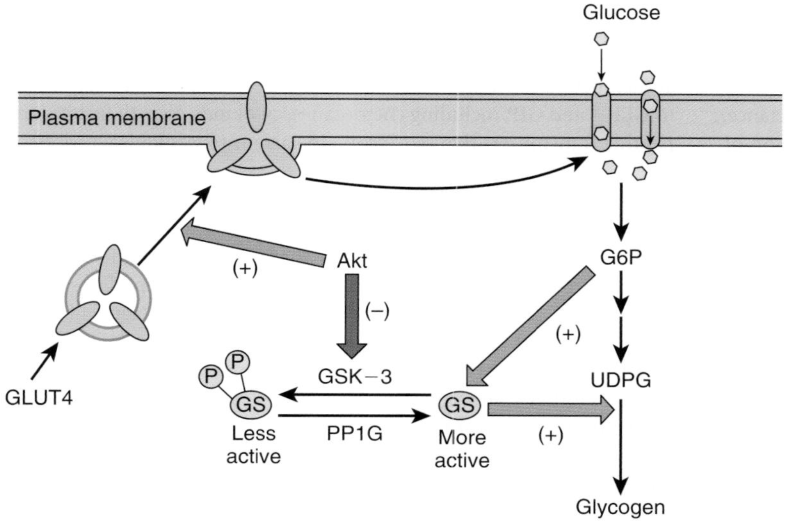

FIG. 53.5 Consequences of Akt Activation by Insulin. The activation of Akt by insulin promotes the translocation of glucose transporter (GLUT4)-containing vesicles to the plasma membrane. Following vesicle fusion, the number of GLUT4 molecules at the cell surface increases, resulting in more glucose transport into the cell. Insulin-stimulated Akt activation also phosphorylates and inactivates glycogen synthase kinase-3 (GSK-3), favoring dephosphorylation by protein phosphatase (PP1G), leading to activation of glycogen synthase (GS) and the synthesis of glycogen from uridine diphosphoglucose (UDPG). Concurrently, glucose that enters cells is phosphorylated to glucose 6-phosphate (G6P), which has two functions—namely, it serves as the source of UDPG, the substrate for GS, and acts as a positive allosteric modulator of GS, both of which promote glycogen synthesis.

Glucagon

Glucagon, a single-chain polypeptide (see Fig. 53.2), is synthesized and secreted by the α cells of pancreatic islets. Sometimes referred to as a **counterregulatory hormone**, glucagon increases glucose levels. The major physiological role of glucagon is to maintain blood glucose during fasting. Glucagon secretion is inhibited by hyperglycemia and stimulated by activation of class B G-protein–coupled receptors expressed in pancreatic α cells, liver, kidney, adipose tissue, and brain, to increase cAMP or activate the phospholipase C inositol phosphate pathway and increase inositol triphosphate and intracellular Ca^{++}, depending on the tissue. Through these signal transduction cascades, glucagon increases glycogenolysis and gluconeogenesis while inhibiting glycolysis and glycogenesis. Glucagon also stimulates lipolysis in adipocytes and has chronotropic and inotropic effects in the heart.

Incretins

The **incretins** are hormones released from endocrine cells in the epithelium of the small intestine in response to food that act on pancreatic β cells to regulate insulin secretion. The two primary incretin hormones in humans are **glucose-dependent insulinotropic polypeptide (GIP,** also known as **gastric inhibitory peptide)** and **glucagon-like peptide-1 (GLP-1)**. The incretins bind to specific G-protein–coupled receptors, which are expressed in pancreas, adipose tissue, and brain. In the pancreas, the incretins increase cAMP to promote glucose dependent insulin secretion from β cells and promote the growth and mass of β cells. They also impair glucagon secretion from pancreatic α cells, particularly when circulating glucose levels are high.

GLP-1 delays gastric emptying and promotes the feeling of satiety through central mechanisms. It also decreases blood pressure and increases thermogenesis and lipolysis in adipose tissue via release of atrial natriuretic peptide. Endogenous incretins are rapidly catabolized by **dipeptidyl peptidase-IV (DPP-IV)**, an ectoenzyme expressed at high levels in endothelium and T-lymphocyte cell membranes.

Insulin Secretagogues

Four classes of drugs promote insulin secretion: **sulfonylureas**, **meglitinides**, **gliptins**, and **incretin analogues**. Structures of representative compounds in each class are shown in Fig. 53.6. The effectiveness of all of these agents depends on functioning pancreatic β cells. These agents are not beneficial for patients exhibiting severe insulin deficiency.

Sulfonylureas and Meglitinides

The sulfonylureas and meglitinides have a common mechanism of action to promote insulin release by binding to SUR1 of K_{ATP} channels (see Fig. 53.3). Although these drug classes bind to different sites on the channel subunit, they both inhibit ATP-sensitive potassium conductance, resulting in partial depolarization of the membrane and activation of voltage-sensitive Ca^{++} channels. Ca^{++} entry increases cytosolic Ca^{++}, which promotes the exocytosis of the secretory granules containing insulin. **Tolbutamide, tolazamide,** and **chlorpropamide** are first-generation sulfonylureas, whereas **glyburide, glipizide,** and **glimepiride** are second-generation agents and are more effective than the first-generation compounds at 10–100 times lower doses. **Repaglinide** and **nateglinide** are meglitinides, with weak binding affinity, dissociating rapidly with a short-lived effect.

Gliptins

The gliptins are competitive inhibitors of DPP-IV, the enzyme that inactivates endogenous incretin hormones, leading to a two- to threefold increase in postprandial and fasting plasma levels of GIP and GLP-1.

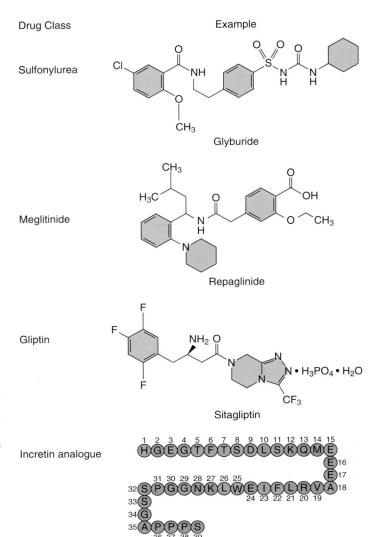

FIG. 53.6 Structures of Representative Insulin Secretagogues.

As a result, insulin release increases, and glucagon levels decrease in a glucose-dependent manner. All agents in this group, including **sitagliptin, saxagliptin, linagliptin,** and **alogliptin,** exhibit selectivity for DPP-IV at therapeutic concentrations. DPP-IV has several substrates in addition to GLP-1 and GIP, including chemokines, cytokines, growth factors, and peptide transmitters that participate in various physiological processes.

Incretin Analogues

The incretin analogues **liraglutide, dulaglutide,** and **albiglutide** are synthetic analogues of human GLP-1 that have been engineered to be resistant to degradation by DPP-IV and neutral endopeptidases and to reside in the circulation for a prolonged period. These agents bind to and activate the GLP-1 receptor on pancreatic β cells similar to the incretins. Both cAMP-dependent and -independent pathways induce insulin synthesis and enhance the response to glucose challenges by accelerating glucose uptake and intensifying the intracellular calcium response, significantly increasing the amount of insulin released to the blood. As incretins, these agents also decrease glucagon secretion by pancreatic α cells in the fed state and have extrapancreatic effects that

Drug Class   Example

Biguanide

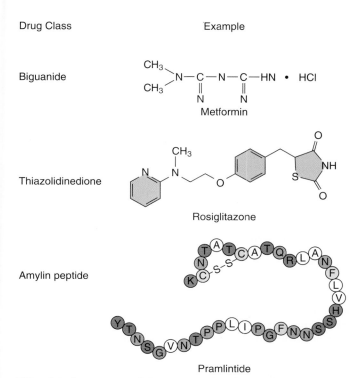

Metformin

Thiazolidinedione

Rosiglitazone

Amylin peptide

Pramlintide

FIG. 53.7 Structures of Representative Drugs That Decrease Insulin Resistance.

result in a mild decrease in blood pressure, slowed gastric emptying, and enhanced sensation of satiety.

Drugs That Decrease Insulin Resistance

Drugs that decrease insulin resistance are used to improve glucose management by the body and/or to synergize with the action of insulin. These drugs include the biguanides, the thiazolidinediones, and amylin analogues. Structures of representative agents in each class are shown in Fig. 53.7.

Biguanides

Metformin, a biguanide, decreases hepatic gluconeogenesis primarily through inhibition of the mitochondrial respiratory chain complex 1, decreasing cAMP-mediated signaling in response to glucagon. Metformin synergizes with insulin to promote glucose uptake and utilization by skeletal muscle and adipose tissue. The ability of metformin to increase insulin sensitivity may involve IRS signaling pathways to modulate lipid metabolism. In addition, metformin has shown to increase glucose transport in skeletal muscle and adipocytes by promoting translocation of GLUT4 to the cell membrane.

Thiazolidinediones

The thiazolidinediones rosiglitazone and pioglitazone lower blood glucose by improving insulin sensitivity. These agents activate the peroxisome proliferator–activated receptor type γ (PPAR-γ), which is expressed at high levels in adipose tissue, the main tissue target of the thiazolidinediones. Activation of PPAR-γ leads to dissociation of transcriptional repressors, attraction of transcriptional activators, and activation of insulin-responsive genes. Activation of PPAR-γ in adipocytes results in cell differentiation, facilitating the utilization of glucose for glycerol synthesis and storage of fatty acids as triglycerides. Circulating insulin decreases with the thiazolidinediones, leading to an increase in insulin sensitivity.

Amylin Analogues

Pramlintide is a synthetic analogue of human amylin, a peptide hormone synthesized by pancreatic β cells that is cosecreted with insulin (1:20 ratio) in response to elevated blood glucose. Amylin binds to neuronal receptor complexes in the hypothalamus, medulla, and other brain regions to affect neural transmission to the periphery, resulting in inhibition of glucagon secretion from pancreatic α cells, which decreases liver gluconeogenesis and glycogenolysis and improves insulin sensitivity within peripheral tissues. Pramlintide has a similar centrally mediated mechanism and delays gastric emptying without altering nutrient absorption and suppresses appetite, leading to weight loss.

Other Antihyperglycemic Agents

In addition to drugs that promote the release of insulin or decrease insulin resistance, several other groups of drugs decrease plasma glucose and are used for the treatment of type 2 DM. These drugs include the dopamine D2 receptor agonists, bile acid sequestrants, gliflozins, and α-glucosidase inhibitors.

D₂ Dopamine Receptor Agonists

Bromocriptine, an ergot derivative, is a D₂ receptor agonist used for several disorders, including syndromes of prolactin excess, acromegaly, and Parkinson disease (Chapter 15). Doses of bromocriptine much lower than those used for the treatment of Parkinson disease have moderate antihyperglycemic efficacy. Although the mechanism mediating this effect is not well understood, it has been attributed to a circadian-related inhibition of noradrenergic and serotonergic activity within the central nervous system, resulting in decreased postprandial hyperglycemia. Its action appears unrelated to alterations in either insulin release or sensitivity.

Bile Acid Sequestrants

Colesevelam is a bile acid sequestrant known for its ability to bind intestinal bile acids, leading to decreased LDL cholesterol (Chapter 42). Although the mechanisms mediating the ability of colesevelam to improve glycemic control are not well understood, it is likely related to activation of the bile acid receptor TGR5. The binding of colesevelam to bile acids increases the activation of these receptors, which increases the secretion of GLP-1 and other incretins, leading to decreased hepatic gluconeogenesis. Colesevelam, like the D2 agonists, does not alter insulin secretion or sensitivity.

Gliflozins

The gliflozins, including canagliflozin, dapagliflozin, and empagliflozin, are selective inhibitors of the sodium-glucose cotransporter 2 (SGLT2) in the kidneys. This cotransporter in proximal convoluted tubules reabsorbs virtually all of the glucose filtered by the glomerulus. By competitively inhibiting glucose binding to the transport sites on SGLT2, the gliflozins induce a large increase in glucose excretion in the urine. In addition, the presence of high glucose levels in the renal tubules induces osmotic diuresis, which decreases Na⁺ reabsorption and increases urine volume. Thus the SGLT2 inhibitors lead to plasma volume depletion. They also lead to mild decreases in triglycerides, cholesterol, and uric acid levels.

α-Glucosidase Inhibitors

Acarbose and miglitol are synthetic oligosaccharides that competitively inhibit α-glucosidases, enzymes in the gastrointestinal (GI) tract that degrade complex carbohydrates. By slowing down the generation of monosaccharides (which are more readily absorbed than complex carbohydrates), these inhibitors blunt the rise in blood glucose concentrations after a meal, leading to small decreases in blood glucose levels.

RELATIONSHIP OF MECHANISMS OF ACTION TO CLINICAL RESPONSE

Hyperglycemia in DM promotes many cellular pathways, including hyperglycation of proteins, increased production of reactive oxygen species, and hyperlipidemia, all of which induce a detrimental inflammatory state in the microvasculature. Epidemiological studies have determined that an increase in the incidence of retinopathy is detected first when fasting blood glucose reaches a sustained level of 126 mg/dL, a critical point for diagnosing DM. Higher glycated hemoglobin (HbA1c) values in DM patients are associated with increased retinopathy, with correlations established between the severity of hyperglycemia and most other complications. Pharmacotherapy that reduces blood glucose to near-normal levels clearly reduces the severity and rate of progression of vascular complications, including atherosclerosis, cardiovascular disease, stroke, nephropathy, retinopathy, and neuropathy.

Alterations in Diabetes

Insulin

Altered glucose and insulin metabolism in DM type 2 or prediabetic stages are commonly associated with excess abdominal fat, dyslipidemia, and/or hypertension; the coexistence of these symptoms is referred to as metabolic syndrome. The causal role of certain of these elements to the genesis of type 2 DM is uncertain, but there is no doubt that concurrent obesity, hypertension, and dyslipidemia cooperatively promote the development of vascular complications in DM. Consequently, DM therapy should not be circumscribed to the control of blood glucose but also needs to attack all other comorbidities that place type 2 DM patients at an exacerbated risk of developing vascular complications. Promoting weight loss and aggressively treating hypertension, heart disease, hyperlipidemia, and prothrombotic state in such individuals is important to decrease the risk of cardiovascular disease.

Insulin is also critical in preventing ketoacidosis, or the overproduction of ketone bodies (acetoacetate, acetone, and β-hydroxybutyrate) synthesized in the liver from acetyl coenzyme A. The hepatic release of ketone bodies into the blood peaks during fasting, as these energy-rich compounds are provided to peripheral tissues as an alternative to glucose and are crucial for the survival of brain cells under hypoglycemic conditions. Severe ketosis does not develop in nondiabetic individuals, however, because only a small amount of insulin is needed to reduce lipolysis in adipocytes. This reduces the supply of free fatty acids for acetyl coenzyme A formation in the liver. When insulin concentrations are decreased, as occurs in diabetes or fasting, production of ketone bodies is favored. Severe ketoacidosis correlates with marked insulin deficiency and occurs most often in patients with type 1 DM. Acetone is volatile and is excreted by the lungs, accounting for the "fruity" acetone breath of people with severe ketosis. Except for acetone, all ketone bodies are organic acids, explaining the occurrence of metabolic acidosis with anion gap. Long-lasting diabetic ketoacidosis is also associated with severe fluid depletion, partly because of the osmotic diuresis caused by increased glucose and ketone bodies in the urine; fluid loss also occurs with vomiting. Unconsciousness, referred to as diabetic coma, followed by cardiovascular collapse and death, could occur if appropriate therapy with insulin and rehydration is not instituted. Recommended therapy involves the intravenous infusion of insulin until ketosis has subsided with replacement of fluids, electrolytes, and glucose as required to prevent hypoglycemia.

Postprandial high insulin levels increase protein synthesis in various cells by stimulating several steps in the synthetic pathway, including transcription, rate of amino acid uptake, and translation of messenger ribonucleic acid into protein. Insulin also potently slows proteolysis. In contrast, during fasting periods when insulin levels are low, net intracellular protein degradation occurs. Muscle wasting is a consequence of untreated type 1 DM that is corrected by insulin treatment.

Glucagon

Glucagon levels may be inappropriately elevated and contribute to hyperglycemia in both type 1 and type 2 diabetics. Glucagon can be used as a drug to increase blood glucose concentrations in patients with severe hypoglycemia who are unable to take glucose orally. Its major clinical use, however, is in radiology; when administered with a radiopaque substance, glucagon relaxes GI smooth muscles for better visualization of tumors and other GI disorders. Occasionally, glucagon can be used to stimulate cardiac function after an overdose of a β-adrenergic receptor antagonist.

Incretin

Individuals with type 2 diabetes typically have decreased incretin activity. The secretion of GIP is near normal, but its ability to decrease insulin secretion is reduced, while the secretion of GLP-1 is impaired, but its insulinotropic action and glucagon suppression are maintained, albeit lower than in healthy individuals. Restoring incretin activity and promoting the health and function of the islets has become the focus of type 2 diabetes drug development (i.e., GLP-1 analogues and DPP-IV inhibitors).

Insulin Secretagogues

Sulfonylureas and Meglitinides

The sulfonylureas and meglitinides lower blood glucose by promoting insulin release from pancreatic β cells and are effective for the management of type 2 DM if the patient does not exhibit severe insulin deficiency. The sulfonylureas are also effective in individuals with neonatal diabetes due to a mutation in the *ABCC8* and *KCNJ11* genes, which encode K_{ATP} channels that do not inactivate in response to glucose and changes in the ATP/ADP ratio.

Increasing insulin plasma levels is essential for the hypoglycemic actions of the sulfonylureas early in therapy. However, after prolonged treatment with sulfonylureas, the magnitude of insulin release returns to pretreatment values, despite persistence of the hypoglycemic effect of the drug. This indicates that long-term therapy increases insulin sensitivity in target tissues by activating glucose transport and metabolic enzymes in liver, skeletal muscle, and adipose cells.

Gliptins and Incretin Analogues

The gliptins and the incretin analogues are efficient insulin secretagogues developed as adjunct therapy. Exenatide and human GLP-1 derivatives have shown beneficial effects, including weight loss (a desirable outcome for overweight patients with type 2 DM), mild antihypertensive action, and central effects that may synergize insulin action and decrease postprandial glucose levels.

Drugs That Decrease Insulin Resistance

Biguanides

Metformin acts in part by enhancing insulin sensitivity, inhibiting hepatic glucose output, and increasing glucose transport in an insulin-independent manner. Metformin decreases elevated blood glucose in type 2 DM and has been proven to decrease the incidence of long-term diabetic complications. At therapeutic doses in type 2 DM patients, metformin is similar in long-term efficacy to the sulfonylureas in maintaining lower levels of blood glucose. However, a single dose of a sulfonylurea or meglitinide has a greater acute hypoglycemic effect than metformin. In general, metformin, unlike K_{ATP} inhibitors, rarely causes hypoglycemia. Additionally, metformin produces a mild weight loss or is weight neutral, unlike the K_{ATP} inhibitors, insulin, or the thiazolidinediones, all of which are associated with significant weight gain. The addition of metformin to insulin therapy in type 1 DM patients is also moderately effective in counteracting insulin resistance in both adults and adolescents. Additionally, metformin can decrease vascular inflammation and/or produce cardioprotection in ischemia (common comorbidities in diabetic patients) and has additional benefits in lipid disorders, including an improvement in markers of metabolic syndrome and a reduction in cancer incidence. Metformin is often one of the preferred drugs in the treatment of type 2 DM.

Thiazolidinediones

Rosiglitazone and pioglitazone increase insulin sensitivity in muscle, liver, and adipose tissue, enhancing the action of insulin on glucose, lipid, and protein metabolism. By decreasing the amount of insulin necessary to control blood glucose, the thiazolidinediones may also exert protective effects on β cells. Rosiglitazone and pioglitazone synergize with the sulfonylureas and insulin to decrease blood glucose in type 2 DM. However, in monotherapy, thiazolidinediones are less effective than sulfonylureas in lowering blood glucose levels. Consequently, thiazolidinediones are commonly used in combination therapy. In type 1 DM, thiazolidinediones are completely ineffective if used without insulin. In contrast to the immediate effects of most drugs described, the effects of the thiazolidinediones are manifest after days to weeks of treatment, as changes in the patterns of synthesis and expression of endogenous proteins are required.

Amylin Analogues

Pramlintide inhibits glucagon secretion, which promotes hepatic insulin sensitivity by increasing glucose use. It also decreases gastric emptying and appetite. Pramlintide is used as adjunctive treatment of patients with both type 1 and 2 DM who fail to achieve full glycemic control with insulin and other agents. Pramlintide induces mild reductions of HbA1c, total cholesterol, and triglycerides.

Other Antihyperglycemic Agents

D$_2$ Receptor Agonists

Bromocriptine inhibits central mechanisms that induce hyperglycemia. It can be used as monotherapy to treat type 2 DM and in combination with sulfonylureas. However, decreased D2 receptor activity induces metabolic changes that mimic type 2 DM, including excessive adrenergic and serotoninergic tone that increases liver glucose and triglyceride production in addition to promoting insulin resistance. In practice, bromocriptine use is reserved for subjects with poor glycemic control who are already on high-dose insulin therapy and do not respond well to other antidiabetic drugs.

Bile Acid Sequestrants

Colesevelam improves glycemic control by increasing GLP-1 levels and decreasing gluconeogenesis by a indirect action in the liver. It also induces a mild decrease in plasma cholesterol levels, which is important to counteract atherogenesis in type 2 DM. Colesevelam, added to type 2 DM therapy, improves basal and postprandial glycemic control.

Gliflozins

The gliflozins promote substantial glucose elimination in the urine (equivalent to a 200- to 360-kCal reduction of daily caloric intake), which significantly decreases plasma glucose levels in an insulin-independent manner and reduces HbA1c. Because the effects are independent of insulin, these agents are effective for decreasing blood glucose in types 1 and 2 DM. They also decrease body weight and

slightly improve plasma lipid profiles, both of which are associated with a decrease in cardiovascular risk and renoprotection.

α-Glucosidase Inhibitors

Miglitol delays glucose absorption, which blunts postprandial blood glucose levels; fasting blood glucose is unaffected. The reduction of blood glucose produced by these inhibitors is small and has only minor effects on hyperglycemia associated with diabetes. However, these agents can act as fine tuners for combination therapy regimens.

PHARMACOKINETICS

Human and Recombinant Insulin

Proteolytic degradation in the GI tract prohibits the oral administration of insulin; subcutaneous (SC) injection is the most common route of administration for maintenance, while intravenous administration is common for the emergency treatment of diabetic coma and ketoacidosis. Recently, insulin infusion pumps and inhaled recombinant human insulin formulations are being used increasingly for rapid-acting postprandial supplementation.

Human insulin and various recombinants with different pharmacokinetics are used for therapy of DM (Table 53.1). These different insulin preparations address the several physiological functions of insulin, such as the maintenance of relatively constant and low plasma glucose levels during fasting to meet cellular requirements, as well as managing glucose storage after rapid increases due to nutritional intake. Individual insulins, with differing pharmacokinetics, can be divided into four categories: rapid acting, regular, intermediate acting, and long acting (see Table 53.1). Rapid-acting preparations with short durations are commonly used with meals to maximize the storage of nutrients, whereas longer acting forms that have flat activity peaks are used to maintain baseline levels. Current therapies frequently use "biphasic insulin," a combination of intermediate/long-acting and regular/rapid-acting insulin to improve control of blood glucose by reducing the incidence of hypoglycemia and hyperglycemia.

Insulin preparations contain monomers and dimers through interactions of C terminal B-chain residues, which are stabilized by hydrogen

TABLE 53.1 Pharmacokinetic Parameters[a] of Selected Human Insulin Preparations			
Insulin Preparation	Onset (min)	Peak (hrs)	Duration (hrs)
Rapid Acting			
Lispro	10–20	0.5–1.5	3–5
Aspart	10–20	0.6–1.0	3–5
Glulisine	15–30	0.6–2.0	2–4
Regular Insulin			
U-100 regular	30–60	2	4–6 (dose dependent)
U-500 regular	30–60	2–5	5–14 (dose dependent)
Intermediate Acting			
NPH	2–4	4–12	10–16
Long Acting			
Glargine	3–4	Flat response	24
Detemir	3–4	4–9	6–24 (dose dependent)
Degludec	1–2	6–9	30–40

[a]Following subcutaneous administration.

TABLE 53.2   Pharmacokinetic Properties of Commonly Used Insulin Secretagogues

Drug	Administration	$t_{1/2}$ (hrs)	Plasma Protein Binding	Duration (hrs)	Metabolite Activity	Elimination
Second-Generation Sulfonylureas						
Glipizide	Oral	3–7	>90%	24	None	90% M, R
Glyburide	Oral	10–16	>90%	24	Weak	50% M, R
Glimepiride	Oral	5–9	>99%	24	Weak	99% M, R
Meglitinides						
Repaglinide	Oral	1–2	>98%	2–3	None	99% M, F
Nateglinide	Oral	1.5–2	>98%	2–3	Weak	85% M, R
Dipeptidyl Peptidase IV Inhibitors						
Sitagliptin	Oral	12–14	38%	24	None	R, M (minor)
Saxagliptin	Oral	2–3	<5%	24	Moderate	65% R, 35% M
Linagliptin	Oral	12	60–70%	24	None	F, M (minor)
Alogliptin	Oral	12–21	20%	24	Minor	75% R, M (minor)
Incretin Analogues						
Exenatide	SC[a]	1–2.4	–	24	None	90% R
Exenatide, extended release	SC[a]	1–2.4	–	168	None	90% R
Lixisenatide	SC[a]	3–5	–	24	None	R
Liraglutide	SC[a]	13	>98%	24	None	M
Dulaglutide	SC[a]	120	–	168	None	M
Albiglutide	SC[a]	120	–	168	None	M

[a]Subcutaneous.
F, Feces; *M*, metabolized; *R*, renal excretion.

bonds. Dimeric insulin is absorbed less rapidly than monomeric insulin and can self-aggregate into hexameric complexes or other large low-mobility clusters, when the insulin is at high concentrations and in the presence of Zn^{++}. Monomeric insulin diffuses faster from subcutaneous tissue to the blood, providing a rapid onset and shorter duration of action. In all rapid-acting insulins, the C terminal region of the B peptide has been modified (see Fig. 53.2). For some preparations, the pharmacokinetics is affected by the dose. The pharmacokinetics of unmodified human recombinant insulin (Humulin) is dose dependent, with the half-life increasing as the dose increases.

Intermediate- and long-acting insulins provide a steady basal level of insulin during fasting periods and have been modified to decrease their rate of diffusion from the SC injection site to the blood and to prevent degradation. Neutral protamine Hagedorn (NPH) insulin, a suspension at a neutral (N) pH of the complex of insulin and the arginine-rich cationic peptide protamine (P), developed by Christian Hagedorn (H), forms insoluble complexes, delaying the absorption and onset to extend action. Current analogous preparations contain protamine and insulin aspart or lispro in various mixtures. Insulin glargine contains two additional arginines, which decrease the overall charge of the molecule to near zero at neutral pH, greatly decreasing its solubility. In addition, insulin glargine precipitates at the site of injection, creating a depot that dissolves slowly and produces a stable baseline level of circulating drug. Insulin detemir contains modifications that allow it to associate with albumin both locally and in the blood, slowing diffusion and preventing degradation by proteases. Insulin degludec self-associates into a multihexameric state and slowly disassembles into monomers, allowing for steady release of insulin into the blood for more than 24 hours. Insulin degludec can bind albumin, which further extends the duration of action.

Insulin Secretagogues

The pharmacokinetics of the insulin secretagogues are summarized in Table 53.2.

Sulfonylureas and Meglitinides

The sulfonylureas are rapidly and completely absorbed from the GI tract and circulate highly bound to plasma proteins by ionic interactions, which can be competitively displaced by other drugs. Second-generation sulfonylureas interact through nonionic bonds with albumin, preventing competition with other molecules and increasing overall duration of action, allowing once-a-day dosage. Most sulfonylureas are metabolized in the liver, with inactive and weak metabolites excreted by the kidney.

The meglitinides, repaglinide and nateglinide, have more rapid onsets and shorter durations of action than the sulfonylureas. Hypoglycemic actions with the meglitinides may occur as early as 20 minutes after an oral dose. Consequently, these drugs are generally taken immediately before meals to ensure that the effect on enhancing insulin release coincides with the increase in blood glucose. The meglitinides are highly bound to plasma proteins but not readily displaced by other drugs. Repaglinide is metabolized by oxidation and conjugation with glucuronic acid to products eliminated in the feces. Nateglinide is metabolized in the liver to products excreted in the urine.

Gliptins and Incretin Analogues

All DPP-IV inhibitors are rapidly absorbed after oral administration, with peak plasma levels achieved in 1–3 hours. The drugs have differences in albumin binding and duration of action, reflected in their variability in volume of distribution in tissues. However, none of these drugs is extensively metabolized. Three of the agents, sitagliptin, saxagliptin, and alogliptin, are mainly eliminated by renal filtration, whereas lina-gliptin is mainly eliminated in the bile, which renders it especially valuable for patients with renal failure.

Exenatide, like all incretin peptide derivatives, is administered SC. Exenatide has a half-life of 2–3 hours in plasma, while lixisenatide is an extended-release formulation modified to increase its affinity for the GLP-1 receptor and bind for longer a period of time, leading to a greater delaying effect on gastric emptying. Exenatide and lixisenatide are predominantly eliminated by glomerular filtration and renal tubular proteolysis. All three human GLP-1 analogues have posttranslational modifications that prevent DPP-IV proteolysis and further modifications that increase their half-life in plasma. Liraglutide has increased resistance to DPP-IV degradation, a decreased rate of absorption from SC tissue, and the ability to bind albumin to prevent glomerular filtration, all of which increase its half-life to 11 hours. Liraglutide is eliminated by general metabolic pathways without a specific organ as a major route of elimination. Dulaglutide and albiglutide are also DPP-IV resistant modified GLP-1 analogues, which have been linked to human immu-noglobulin or albumin, respectively. These two fusion proteins have negligible glomerular filtration and are slowly metabolized by the liver and in other organs, like large endogenous plasma proteins, reaching a half-life of about a week.

Drugs That Decrease Insulin Resistance

Pharmacokinetic properties of drugs that decrease insulin resistance and other antihyperglycemic agents are summarized in Table 53.3.

Biguanides

Metformin, which is orally administered, is absorbed primarily in the duodenum, with a large volume of distribution. It does not bind to plasma proteins, has a half-life of about 6 hours, and is eliminated unchanged by the kidneys, mainly by tubular secretion; clearance of metformin is 3–4 times greater than creatinine clearance.

Thiazolidinediones

Rosiglitazone and pioglitazone are absorbed after oral administration rapidly and completely, reaching peak plasma concentrations within 2–4 hours. The drugs are highly bound to serum proteins. Rosiglitazone is inactivated by the liver, followed by glucuronidation and sulfation. Pioglitazone is extensively metabolized to several active metabolites, which accumulate in the blood to higher levels than the unmodified drug, thus increasing the duration of action. Pioglitazone and its metabolites are conjugated with glucuronic acid or sulfate and are excreted in the bile.

Amylin Analogues

Pramlintide is administered SC, with peak serum levels reached within 20 minutes. Pramlintide is metabolized primarily to the biologically active des-lys derivative by the kidneys.

Other Antihyperglycemic Agents

The pharmacokinetics of bromocriptine are discussed in Chapter 15, and those of the bile acid sequestrants are discussed in Chapter 42.

Gliflozins

The gliflozins are orally active and rapidly absorbed. They bind signifi-cantly to plasma proteins and are metabolized by the liver and eliminated primarily in the urine. The gliflozins have been categorized as intermedi-ate or long acting, reflecting differences in both pharmacokinetic and pharmacodynamic profiles.

TABLE 53.3 Pharmacokinetic Properties of Drugs Used to Decrease Insulin Resistance and Other Antihyperglycemic Agents

Drug	Administration	$t_{1/2}$ (hrs)	Plasma Protein Binding	Metabolite Activity	Elimination
Biguanides					
Metformin	Oral	3–7	Negligible	None	R
Thiazolidinediones					
Rosiglitazone	Oral	3–4	>99%	Weak	M, R
Pioglitazone	Oral	4–8	>99%	Moderate	>90% M, F, R
Amylin Analogues					
Pramlintide	SC[a]	0.84	60%	Moderate	M
D2 Dopaminergic Agonists					
Bromocriptine	Oral	5–7	90–96%	Moderate	M, F
Bile Acid Sequestrants					
Colesevelam	Oral	NA	–	–	F
Gliflozins					
Canagliflozin	Oral	10–13	99%	None	M, 60% R, F
Dapagliflozin	Oral	13	91%	None	M, 75% R, G
Empagliflozin	Oral	12	86%	None	M (minor), 55% R, F
α-Glucosidase Inhibitors					
Acarbose	Oral	NA	–	None	M, F 55%, R
Miglitol	Oral	2	–	None	R

[a]Subcutaneous.

F, Feces; M, metabolized; NA, not absorbed; R, renal excretion.

α-Glucosidase Inhibitors

Acarbose and miglitol are designed to have their action in the lumen of the small intestine. The amount of acarbose absorbed systemically is negligible. Miglitol is absorbed, although there is no evidence that the systemic absorption of the drug contributes to its therapeutic action. The half-life of circulating miglitol is 2 hours, and almost all the drug is eliminated unchanged in the urine.

PHARMACOVIGILANCE: ADVERSE EFFECTS AND DRUG INTERACTIONS

Controlling Blood Glucose

A major problem in treating DM is that blood glucose control cannot be achieved with a fixed concentration of insulin. Insulin release is subject to complex regulation by many factors (Box 53.1), and circulating concentrations can change dramatically with complex temporal patterns. Too little insulin results in hyperglycemia, whereas too much causes hypoglycemia and potentially insulin shock. Correlating insulin concentrations with the glucose load is a major challenge in insulin therapy, particularly because insulin sensitivity may vary greatly among individuals. Exercise or ethanol intake can greatly enhance insulin sensitivity, decreasing the hormonal requirement. Stress, pregnancy, or drugs, including thiazide diuretics and β-adrenergic receptor antagonists, decrease insulin sensitivity and exacerbate signs and symptoms of DM. As mentioned, the general strategy is to inject a short-acting insulin preparation to produce an insulin peak that coincides with the rise in blood glucose following a meal and to use an extended-action preparation to establish a baseline concentration to prevent hyperglycemia between meals and during the overnight period. Administering insulin with variable-rate infusion pumps provides a more flexible means to control circulating insulin. Tighter control of the blood glucose concentration to near-normal levels is always desired, but our current therapeutic strategies associate with a high incidence of severe hypoglycemic episodes. Careful monitoring of blood glucose levels is essential.

Insulin

Hypoglycemia, the most serious complication of insulin therapy, usually occurs because of errors in calculating doses or the timing of injections, changes in eating patterns, increased energy expenditure, or an increase in sensitivity. Severe hypoglycemia can cause unconsciousness, convulsions, brain damage, and death. Symptoms of hypoglycemia are often attributed to increases in epinephrine secretion, abnormal functioning of the central nervous system, or both. Compensatory epinephrine release will cause rapid heart rate, headache, cold sweat, weakness, and trembling with considerable variability, depending on the individual and the rate of fall of the blood glucose concentration, with impaired neural function often causing blurred vision, an incoherent speech pattern, and mental confusion also possible. The unconscious hypoglycemic state induced by an insulin overdose, insulin coma, is sometimes confused with diabetic coma, but the two have opposite causes and different therapeutic interventions. Diabetic coma results from an insulin deficit and involves ketoacidosis, electrolyte imbalance, and dehydration that usually develops over hours or days. In contrast, the onset of an insulin coma is typically very rapid. Management of an insulin coma requires rapid restoration of blood glucose by intravenous administration of concentrated dextrose solutions using large central veins and careful management.

Insulin has relatively few other adverse effects. General weight gain is associated with insulin therapy. Temporary visual disturbances may result from changes in the refractile properties of the lens brought about by decreasing osmolarity as glucose is brought under control.

Localized fat accumulation can occur if insulin is repeatedly administered at the same site due to stimulation of triglyceride accumulation in adipocytes surrounding the injection site. Curiously, lipoatrophy may also occur at the injection site. Both of these problems are typically remedied by rotating injection sites, a practice highly encouraged. Injected insulin preparations can cause localized allergic reactions leading to pain and itching. These reactions are usually not severe and may disappear with time. Systemic allergic reactions, which may trigger anaphylaxis, occur much less frequently.

Insulin Secretagogues
Sulfonylureas and Meglitinides

Multiple clinical trial evidence strongly indicates that the sulfonylureas have a higher risk of mild, moderate, or severe hypoglycemia than any other class of agents that promote insulin release, as well as drugs that decrease insulin resistance. Hypoglycemia could result from an overdose, increased insulin sensitivity, change in dietary pattern, or increased energy expenditure. If the response is mild, it can be corrected by decreasing the dose of drug. However, severe cases may persist for days and require glucose infusions. Weight gain is also commonly observed with sulfonylureas and is related to the excessive insulin triggering of triglyceride synthesis. In general, GI disturbances, allergic reactions, dermatological problems, mild anemia, and transient leukopenia can be expected in a small percentage of patients taking these agents. A disulfiram type of response (i.e., flushing, nausea, headache) caused by inhibition of aldehyde dehydrogenase is sometimes a problem if sulfonylureas are taken with alcohol, particularly with chlorpropamide.

Failure of evidence to establish correlations between the use of sulfonylureas and the risk of adverse cardiovascular effects suggests that these drugs do not produce a significant decrease in cardiovascular events. Sulfonylureas are mainly metabolized by CYP2C9, and inhibiting this enzyme increases plasma levels of these drugs. However, pharmacogenomic studies have shown that allelic variants of CYP2C9 with decreased metabolic activity do not have any clinical implications, although data are equivocal.

Repaglinide and nateglinide are usually taken prior to a meal to increase the clearance of postprandial glucose. Because of their short action, the meglitinides are associated with less hypoglycemia and weight gain compared with the sulfonylureas. Other common adverse effects are headache and upper respiratory infections. GI effects are uncommon, and meglitinides do not associate with increased cardiovascular risk, albeit large studies are lacking. The meglitinides are metabolized primarily by CYP3A4, and thus plasma levels will be affected by drugs that induce this enzyme, such as rifampin, barbiturates, and carbamazepine, as well as drugs that inhibit CYP3A4 such as erythromycin, ketoconazole, and miconazole. In addition, the antihyperlipidemic agent gemfibrozil interferes with the metabolism of repaglinide, and these drugs should not be coadministered.

Sulfonylureas and meglitinides are contraindicated in patients who do not have a proven pancreatic reserve of insulin. Consideration of metabolism and excretion must occur when considering drug therapy.

Gliptins and Incretin Analogues

The use of DPP-IV inhibitors is associated with a low risk of hypoglycemia and GI effects. These agents are weight neutral and do not increase the risk of pancreatitis or cardiovascular events. Compared to placebo, there is an increase in upper respiratory tract infections, urinary tract infections, and headache. Arthralgia and allergic and hypersensitivity reactions to gliptins have also been reported ranging from rashes, hives, facial, and neck swelling to anaphylaxis, angioedema, and exfoliative conditions, including Stevens-Johnson syndrome.

The incretins do not cause weight gain and rarely produce severe hypoglycemia in monotherapy or in combination with metformin and thiazolidinediones. These agents are commonly added to therapy with insulin, sulfonylureas, or meglitinides, where some patients may require a reduction in these agents to prevent hypoglycemia. The most common side effects include mild to moderate nausea, vomiting, diarrhea, and reactions at the injection site. Severe GI symptoms could result in volume contraction, which increases the risk of acute renal injury that could lead to renal failure in sensitive patients. These adverse effects associated with incretins are generally dose related and decrease over time, which make it advisable to start therapy with a low dose. Earlier warnings of pancreatitis and thyroid cell carcinomas have been lessened because more recent studies and metaanalysis of previous observational studies failed to show a significant increase in cases of pancreatitis or an increase in risk of pancreatic or cancer thyroid cell carcinomas, but these are quite rare cancers in humans, and further studies are needed. Incretins are synthetic peptides and, when injected subcutaneously, could be recognized as antigens for antibody formation. The incidence of antibody formation with exenatide is high (30%). The immunogenicity of human recombinant GLP peptides is lower but differs among the drugs, ranging from 9% with liraglutide to 1.8% with dulaglutide. Incretins do not produce significant drug-drug interactions directly, but because they delay gastric emptying, the rate of absorption of orally administered drugs may be affected. Exenatide should not be administered to patients with renal impairment or end-stage renal disease, and it is not recommended for patients with severe GI disorders.

Drugs That Decrease Insulin Resistance
Biguanides
Some form of GI distress occurs in more than half of individuals receiving metformin, at least partly due to inhibition of nutrient absorption, and may include diarrhea, nausea, vomiting, and flatulence. The severity usually diminishes with time, and only approximately 6% of individuals are ultimately unable to tolerate metformin. GI symptoms are less frequent with an extended-release preparation. Dose-dependent increased plasma lactate levels may occur due to inhibited hepatic mitochondrial respiration, causing a metformin-associated lactic acidosis. The incidence is very low and may include individuals with exacerbated mitochondrial sensitivity to biguanides. Those at highest risk appear to be elderly diabetic patients where metformin could accumulate at high levels, as occurs in patients who have significant renal or liver insufficiency. Excessive consumption of ethanol is contraindicated because ethanol potentiates effects of metformin on lactate metabolism.

Thiazolidinediones
Rosiglitazone and pioglitazone lead to weight gain in most patients, with increased adipocyte proliferation and insulin sensitivity and increased LDL and HDL cholesterol; rosiglitazone increases triglycerides, whereas pioglitazone slightly decreases triglycerides. Thiazolidinedione use is associated with fluid retention, complicating therapy with antihypertensives and diuretics. No evidence of hepatotoxicity has been obtained with rosiglitazone and pioglitazone, but troglitazone, a structurally related compound, has been associated with idiosyncratic hepatotoxicity. Therefore liver enzymes should be monitored before treatment and periodically during therapy.

Amylin Analogues
Adverse effects associated with pramlintide involve headache, nausea, vomiting, and other GI effects. Although pramlintide alone does not decrease blood glucose levels, when added to insulin therapy, the combination increases the incidence of hypoglycemic episodes, requiring a reduction of the insulin dose. Because pramlintide delays gastric emptying, the drug should not be used for patients who have gastroparesis or are taking other drugs that alter GI motility (i.e., anticholinergics).

Other Antihyperglycemic Agents
D₂ Dopamine Receptor Agonists
Bromocriptine is an oral medication that primarily affects the CNS. Common symptoms of the drug include hypotension, nausea, fatigue, dizziness, vomiting, and headache. Higher doses of bromocriptine, as used for other indications, could induce long-term psychotic disorders, including decreased cognition and delirium. Bromocriptine, as well as other ergot alkaloids, is associated with heart valvular complications, including fibrosis. Other adverse effects are discussed in Chapter 15.

Bile Acid Sequestrants
Colesevelam leads to adverse GI effects—that is, dyspepsia, constipation, and hemorrhoids—with a moderate increase of serum triglycerides producing contraindications in patients with hypertriglyceridemia. Colesevelam is not absorbed to the systemic circulation and can be used in pregnancy and lactation. However, it does interfere with the intestinal absorption of vitamins, folate, ascorbic acid, and other drugs (statins, diuretics, beta blockers, and warfarin), as discussed in Chapter 42.

Gliflozins
The gliflozins are associated with increased frequency of urinary tract and genital infections, especially in women, prompting an FDA warning indicating that the gliflozins can cause life-threatening urosepsis and pyelonephritis. SGLT2 inhibitors also produce episodes of hypoglycemia in 1%–4% of patients. Glucose in the renal tubules also induces osmotic diuresis, which could deplete plasma volume and cause hypotension, predisposing sensitive patients to acute kidney injury. As the drug decreases glucose under low insulin conditions, ketoacidosis could ensue due to an increased glucagon/insulin ratio that promotes lipolysis in adipocytes. There are no studies of gliflozins taken during pregnancy, but studies in animals suggest that some of these agents may affect renal development and maturation.

α-Glucosidase Inhibitors
Acarbose and miglitol disrupt the normal metabolism of complex carbohydrates in the GI tract, and side effects relating to carbohydrate malabsorption may be as high as 70%. The incidence and severity of side effects, which include abdominal pain, diarrhea, and flatulence, generally diminish with continued treatment. Nevertheless, α-glucosidase inhibitors are contraindicated in patients with inflammatory bowel disease, colonic ulceration, partial intestinal obstruction, or any other intestinal disease or condition that could be exacerbated by the increased formation of gas in the intestine.

Clinical problems associated with the use of these agents are summarized in the Clinical Problems Box.

NEW DEVELOPMENTS
Advances in the management of DM have been remarkable, and all evidence suggests that treatment will continue to improve in the future. Refinement of the combined use of modified forms of human insulin having a rapid onset and short duration of action or possessing a delayed onset and long duration of action with a flat insulin activity peak have proven very effective in sustaining low basal levels of insulin and more closely mimic endogenous insulin release in response to a carbohydrate challenge. Newer long-acting analogues and further improvement and development of "smart" insulin delivery systems are being developed along with new DPP-IV inhibitors, GLP-1 agonists, and SGLT2 inhibitors.

Pharmacogenomics is clarifying the basis for individual differences observed in the sensitivity to antidiabetic drugs. Studies have discovered several genetic polymorphisms in the genes coding for transporters,

CLINICAL PROBLEMS

Drug	Adverse Effects
Insulin	Symptoms of hypoglycemia, visual disturbances, peripheral edema, local or systemic allergic reactions
Sulfonylureas	Symptoms of hypoglycemia, gastrointestinal disturbances, hematological disturbances, ethanol intolerance
Meglitinides	Symptoms of hypoglycemia, headache, upper respiratory infections, blood levels affected by drugs altering CYP3A4
Incretin analogues	Gastrointestinal effects (nausea, vomiting, diarrhea), headache, hypoglycemia, development of antiincretin antibodies
Dipeptidyl peptidase-IV inhibitors	Nausea, hypoglycemia, urinary and respiratory infections, hypersensitivity reactions, including anaphylaxis and Stevens-Johnson syndrome
Metformin	Gastrointestinal effects (discomfort, diarrhea, pain), cough, lactic acidosis (in patients with impaired renal function)
Thiazolidinediones	Edema, mild dyslipidemia, weight gain, abdominal fat
Pramlintide	Nausea, vomiting, headache, hypoglycemia (when coadministered with insulin)
Bromocriptine	Hypotension, fatigue, nausea, psychosis
Colesevelam	Frequent gastrointestinal effects (constipation, diarrhea, hemorrhoids), hypertriglyceridemia, interferes with the absorption of drugs and vitamins
SGLT2-Inhibitors	Urinary and genital infections, hypoglycemia, hypotension, ketoacidosis
α-Glucosidase inhibitors	Abdominal pain, diarrhea, flatulence, malabsorption of carbohydrate, Ca^{++}, iron, thyroid hormones, and some hydrophobic drugs and vitamins

metabolizing enzymes, and other targets involved in the mechanism of action of metformin, sulfonylureas, incretins, and SGLT2 inhibitors. It is expected that studies in the near future, including clinical trials, will provide evidence for individualized treatments that maximize efficacy while minimizing side effects and costs.

The International Diabetes Federation Task Force on Epidemiology and Prevention of Diabetes has indicated that bariatric surgery can significantly improve glycemic control in severely obese patients with type 2 DM. The mechanisms underlying the relationship between obesity and insulin resistance (metabolic syndrome) are complex. Obesity, increased appetite, and changes in insulin sensitivity appear to be involved. The recently developed class of GLP-1 agonists has helped to better understand that several hormones and gut peptides, including ghrelin and leptin, interact with GLP-1 to modulate appetite. Many newer GLP-1 and DPP-IV agonists are in clinical trials (phase II and III). The pipeline and future of drug development includes multimolecular combinations based on GLP-1 plus other antiobesity or antidiabetic factors (amylin, gastrin, GIP, estrogens), as well as agents that prevent β-cell inflammation and dysfunction.

CLINICAL RELEVANCE FOR HEALTHCARE PROFESSIONALS

All healthcare professionals need to be aware of the fact that many of the agents used to treat DM produce altered blood glucose levels that may alter cognition and levels of consciousness and lead to other problems. In addition, the effect of these drugs on blood glucose levels may alter patient response to certain therapies and/or alter clinical protocols or interventions planned by various healthcare professionals. Knowledge of the adverse effects and interactions of antidiabetic agents with other drugs is crucial to understand the basis of altered patient response to therapy.

Additionally, knowledge that a patient is being treated with these agents will provide healthcare providers with a heightened sense of patient awareness to be able to recognize acute or chronic altered blood glucose manifestations and allow appropriate actions to be taken if hyper- or hypoglycemia should occur, particularly as an adverse effect of therapy.

TRADE NAMES

In addition to generic and fixed-combination preparations, the following trade-named materials are many of the important compounds available in the United States.

Recombinant Human Insulins
Rapid Acting
Lispro (Humalog)
Aspart (NovoLog)
Glulisine (Apidra)

Rapid-Acting Inhaled
Regular insulin (Afrezza)

Long Acting
Glargine (Lantus)
Detemir (Levemir)
Degludec (Tresiba)

Combinations
Mixture of 50% insulin lispro protamine suspension and 50% insulin lispro (Humalog Mix 50/50)
Mixture of 70% insulin aspart protamine suspension and 30% insulin aspart (Novolog 70/30)
Mixture of 70% insulin aspart and 30% insulin degludec (Tresiba)

Sulfonylureas
Chlorpropamide (Diabinese)
Glimepiride (Amaryl)
Glipizide (Glucotrol)
Glyburide (Micronase, DiaBeta)

Meglitinides
Repaglinide (Prandin)
Nateglinide (Starlix)

TRADE NAMES—cont'd

Gliptins
Sitagliptin (Januvia)
Linagliptin (Tradjenta)
Alogliptin (Nesina)
Saxagliptin (Onglyza)

Incretin Analogues
Exenatide (Byetta)
Exenatide, extended release (Bydureon)
Lixisenatide (Adlyxin)
Liraglutide (Saxenda, Victoza)
Dulaglutide (Trulicity)
Albiglutide (Tanzeum)

Biguanides
Metformin (Glucophage)
Metformin extended-release (Glucophage XR)

Thiazolidinediones
Rosiglitazone (Avandia)
Pioglitazone (Actos)

Modified Amylin Peptide
Pramlintide (Symlin)

Sodium-Glucose Cotransport 2 Inhibitors
Canagliflozin (Invokana)
Dapagliflozin (Farxiga)
Empagliflozin (Jardiance)

α-Glucosidase Inhibitors
Acarbose (Precose)
Miglitol (Glyset)

Bile Acid Sequestrants
Colesevelam (Welchol)

D_2 Dopamine Receptor Agonists
Bromocriptine (Cycloset)

Drug Combinations Containing Metformin
Glyburide plus metformin (Glucovance)
Pioglitazone plus metformin (Actoplus Met)
Glipizide plus metformin (Metaglip)
Alogliptin plus metformin (Kazano)
Canagliflozin plus metformin (Invokamet)

SELF-ASSESSMENT QUESTIONS

1. A 65-year-old man with type 2 diabetes mellitus is taking a drug that improves the tissue sensitivity of insulin by acting on the peroxisome proliferator–activated receptor. Which of the following is the patient taking?
   A. Acarbose.
   B. Metformin.
   C. Repaglinide.
   D. Sitagliptin.
   E. Pioglitazone.

2. A 44-year-old woman with type 1 diabetes mellitus takes glulisine insulin at mealtimes and glargine insulin at 8 a.m. However, during her physical therapy session at 10 a.m., she experiences dizziness, blurred vision, and loss of consciousness. Which of the following would best prevent the patient's side effects?
   A. Increase the glulisine insulin dose at breakfast.
   B. Reduce the glulisine insulin dose at breakfast.
   C. Increase the glargine insulin at breakfast.
   D. Omit the glargine insulin at breakfast.
   E. Omit the glulisine insulin at breakfast.

3. A 39-year-old obese man with type 2 diabetes mellitus is taking a drug that increases insulin secretion by blocking ATP-sensitive potassium channels on pancreatic β cells. This drug is:
   A. Sitagliptin.
   B. Pioglitazone.
   C. Metformin.
   D. Repaglinide.
   E. Acarbose.

4. A 55-year-old menopausal woman was recently diagnosed with type 2 diabetes based on her fasting blood glucose values. Her HbA1c was <7%, indicating that diet, exercise, and a single drug (monotherapy) may be sufficient to regulate her fasting glucose levels. Which of the following drugs should be prescribed for this patient?
   A. Acarbose.
   B. Colesevelam.
   C. Glyburide.
   D. Insulin aspart (with meals).
   E. Metformin.

5. Which of the following medications, when taken prior to eating, is especially effective for correcting postprandial hyperglycemia after a high-carbohydrate meal but also for the management of reactive hypoglycemia?
   A. Canagliflozin.
   B. Miglitol.
   C. Nateglinide.
   D. Pioglitazone.
   E. Tolbutamide.

6. A 62-year-old male became unconscious at his work late in the afternoon and was taken to the nearest emergency department. Laboratory results indicated a blood glucose of 55 mg/dL. Soon after, his wife arrived and told the doctor that her husband started a new medication 3 weeks ago that he takes once a day with breakfast to treat his diabetes mellitus type 2. She showed the pills to the doctor, who stated, "No wonder; this is a drug that commonly causes hypoglycemia." The drug belongs to which of the following classes?
   A. Biguanide.
   B. Bile acid sequestrant.
   C. Gliptin.
   D. Meglitinide.
   E. Sulfonylurea.

FURTHER READING

American Diabetes Association. Standards of medical care in diabetes-2016 abridged for primary care providers. *Clin Diabetes*. 2016;34:3–21.

De Meyts P. The insulin receptor and its signal transduction network. [Updated 2016 Apr 27]. In: De Groot LJ, Chrousos G, Dungan K, et al, eds. *Endotext [Internet]*. South Dartmouth (MA): MDText.com, Inc.; 2000. Available from: http://www.ncbi.nlm.nih.gov/books/NBK378978/.

Lyssenko V, Bianchi C, Del Prato S. Personalized therapy by phenotype and genotype. *Diabetes Care*. 2016;39:S127–S136.

Powers AC. Diabetes mellitus: diagnosis, classification, and pathophysiology. In: Kasper D, Fauci A, Hauser S, et al, eds. *Harrison's Principles of Internal Medicine*, 19e. New York, NY: McGraw-Hill; 2015.

Riehle C, Abel ED. Insulin signaling and heart failure. *Circ Res*. 2016;118:1151–1169.

Sterrett JJ, Bragg S, Weart CW. Type 2 diabetes medication review. *Am J Med Sci*. 2016;351:342–355.

Tancredi M, et al. Excess mortality among persons with type 2 diabetes. *N Engl J Med*. 2015;373:1720–1732.

WEBSITES

https://www.niddk.nih.gov/health-information/diabetes

This site is maintained by the National Institute of Diabetes and Digestive and Kidney Diseases of the National Institutes of Health and is a valuable resource for both patients and healthcare professionals on all aspects of diabetes, including the National Diabetes Education Program.

https://www.fda.gov/forpatients/illness/diabetes/default.htm

This site is maintained by the United States Food and Drug Administration and has numerous links to diabetes resources.

https://www.cdc.gov/diabetes/home/index.html

This site is maintained by the United States Centers for Disease Control and Prevention and has much information on diabetes and maintaining a healthy lifestyle.

54

Drug Therapy for the Management of Thyroid Disorders

Shelley Tischkau

MAJOR DRUG CLASSES

Thyroid hormones
Antithyroid drugs
- Thioureylenes
- Iodide

ABBREVIATIONS

D1	Iodothyronine deiodinase type 1
D2	Iodothyronine deiodinase type 2
D3	Iodothyronine deiodinase type 3
DIT	Diiodotyrosine
MIT	Monoiodotyrosine
PTU	Propylthiouracil
rT_3	Reverse T_3
T_3	Triiodothyronine
T_4	Thyroxine, tetraiodothyronine
TBG	Thyroxine-binding globulin
Tg	Thyroglobulin
TR	Thyroid hormone receptor
TRH	Thyrotropin-releasing hormone
TSH	Thyroid-stimulating hormone, thyrotropin

THERAPEUTIC OVERVIEW

Thyroid gland hormones, L-tetraiodothyronine (T_4, also known as thyroxine) or L-triiodothyronine (T_3), are potent effectors of energy metabolism. Levels of these hormones correlate directly with whole body O_2 consumption, heart rate and force of contraction, glucose and fatty acid use by muscle, lipolysis by adipose tissue, hepatic glycogenolysis, and gluconeogenesis. Moreover, thyroid hormones are essential for neonatal growth and development, especially of the brain. Levels of thyroid hormones are tightly regulated to maintain homeostatic function. Hyperthyroidism or hypothyroidism are abnormal states of thyroid gland function involving excess or reduced levels of thyroid hormones, respectively.

Pathophysiology

Graves disease is the most common form of hyperthyroidism. In Graves disease, the immune system synthesizes autoantibodies called thyroid-stimulating immunoglobulins (TSIs) or thyroid-stimulating hormone (TSH) receptor antibodies that bind to TSH receptors on thyroid cells and stimulate the production of thyroid hormone. Thus TSIs lead to effects similar to those of TSH. The second most common form of hyperthyroidism in the Western world is toxic nodular goiter, also known as Plummer disease, which consists of autonomously functioning thyroid nodules.

The most common cause of hypothyroidism is also autoimmune and is typically attributed to Hashimoto disease, also known as chronic lymphocytic thyroiditis, in which the immune system attacks the thyroid gland. This primary hypothyroidism is often associated with a firm goiter, progressing to a shrunken fibrotic gland, and results in a decreased production of thyroid hormones. Hypothyroidism may also result from insufficient stimulation of the gland by TSH as a consequence of a deficit either at the pituitary gland (secondary hypothyroidism) or in the hypothalamic production of thyroid-releasing hormone (TRH, tertiary hypothyroidism). Rarely, hypothyroidism may result from thyroid hormone resistance, in which mutations of either the thyroid hormone receptor prevent activation by thyroid hormones or downstream target genes prevent the physiological actions associated with thyroid hormones. In these cases, patients develop hypothyroid symptoms despite elevated levels of thyroid hormone as the body attempts to overcome the resistance by producing more hormone. Hypothyroidism in children in underdeveloped countries may result from iodine deficiency, but in developed countries, it is more commonly associated with thyroid dysgenesis.

Current options for the treatment of hyperthyroidism include pharmacological management, radioactive iodine glandular ablation, or surgical resection of the gland. Drug treatments are directed at inhibiting the synthesis of thyroid hormones with antithyroid drugs or reducing the effects of excessive thyroid hormone levels through the use of β-adrenergic receptor antagonists. Hypothyroidism is treated by thyroid hormone replacement with either T_4 or T_3.

Treatments are summarized in the Therapeutic Overview Box.

THERAPEUTIC OVERVIEW

Hyperthyroidism
Thioureylene drugs
Radioactive iodine
β-adrenergic receptor antagonists
Surgery

Hypothyroidism
Replacement therapy with synthetic thyroxine (T_4) or triiodothyronine (T_3)

MECHANISMS OF ACTION

Thyroid Hormones

Thyroid Hormone Biosynthesis

The follicular cells (thyrocytes) of the thyroid synthesize thyroglobulin, which serves as the substrate for the production of the two major thyroid

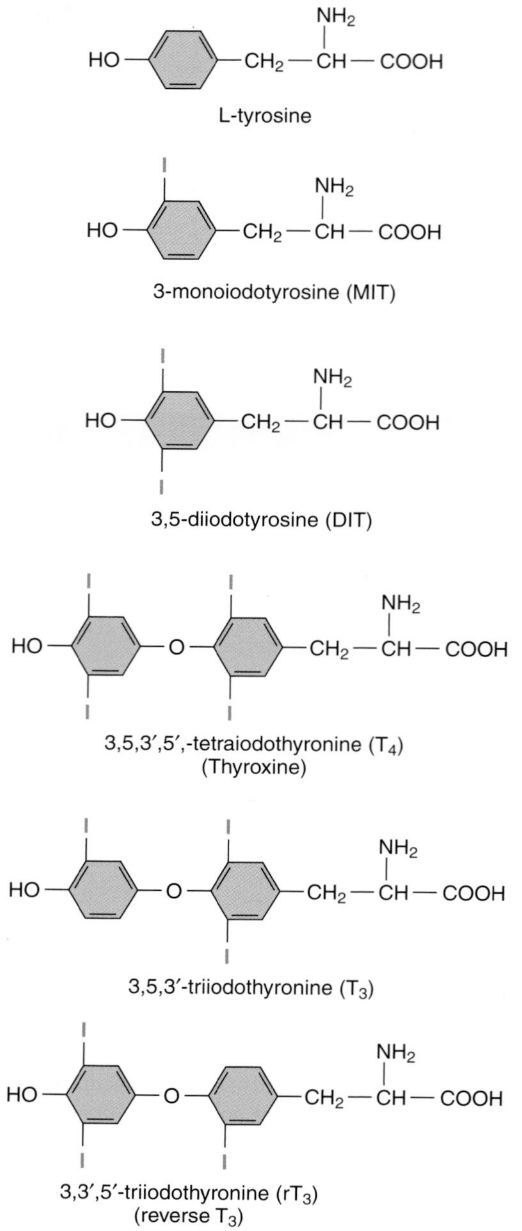

L-tyrosine

3-monoiodotyrosine (MIT)

3,5-diiodotyrosine (DIT)

3,5,3',5',-tetraiodothyronine (T_4)
(Thyroxine)

3,5,3'-triiodothyronine (T_3)

3,3',5'-triiodothyronine (rT_3)
(reverse T_3)

FIG. 54.1 Structures of Tyrosine and its Iodinated Derivatives.

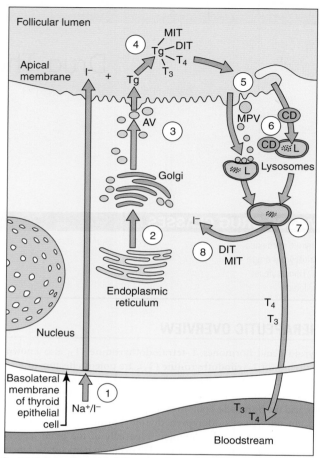

FIG. 54.2 Intrathyroidal Synthesis and Processing of Thyroid Hormones. *(1)* Iodide is taken up at the basolateral cell membrane and transported to the apical membrane. *(2)* Polypeptide chains of Tg are synthesized in the rough endoplasmic reticulum, and posttranslational modifications take place in the Golgi. *(3)* Newly formed Tg is transported to the cell surface in small apical vesicles (AV). *(4)* Within the follicular lumen, iodide is activated and iodinates tyrosyl residues on Tg, producing fully iodinated Tg containing MIT, DIT, T_4, and a small amount of T_3 (organification and coupling), which is stored as colloid in the follicular lumen. *(5)* Upon TSH stimulation, villi at the apical membrane engulf the colloid and endocytose the iodinated Tg as either colloid droplets (CD) or small vesicles (MPV). *(6)* Lysosomal proteolysis of the droplets or vesicles hydrolyzes Tg to release its iodinated amino acids and carbohydrates. *(7)* T_4 and T_3 are released into the circulation. *(8)* DIT and MIT are deiodinated, and the iodide and tyrosine are recycled.

hormones, T_4 and T_3, via enzymatic condensation of iodinated tyrosyl residues (Fig. 54.1). All circulating T_4, which is the predominant hormone produced by the gland, derives from the thyroid gland. In contrast, most T_3, the biologically active form, is produced by peripheral tissues via the action of 5'-deiodinase, which removes an iodide from the outer ring of T_4; only a small fraction of T_3 is produced and released from the thyroid.

The synthesis and release of T_3 and T_4 are shown in Fig. 54.2. Thyrocytes concentrate iodide from the circulation via a Na^+/I^- symporter on their basolateral membrane that transports Na^+ down its electrochemical gradient. This symporter is also present in salivary glands, breast, and stomach and can transport other anions such as pertechnetate and perchlorate, which can competitively inhibit iodide transport. Iodide is transported across the apical membrane to the follicular lumen by

the anion transporter, **pendrin**, where it is oxidized by thyroid peroxidase and hydrogen peroxide to its active form. Activated iodide forms covalent links with specific tyrosyl residues on thyroglobulin (Tg) to produce the thyroid hormone precursors **monoiodotyrosine (MIT)** and **diiodotyrosine (DIT)**. This process is referred to as **organification** of iodide. MIT or DIT donate their iodinated phenolic rings to acceptor iodotyrosyl residues on DIT in the Tg backbone and form an ether linkage with the acceptor phenolic ring to form T_4 and T_3 covalently bound to Tg. This process is called **oxidative coupling**. Iodinated Tg is stored as a colloid, and upon TSH stimulation when hormone is required, the colloid is endocytosed at the apical membrane, followed by proteolysis, releasing T_4 and T_3, which enter the circulation. MIT and DIT are deiodinated and reused.

T_4 is the predominant circulating form of thyroid hormone and is the most frequently used form of thyroid hormone in replacement therapies. In the periphery, deiodinase enzymes act on T_4 to remove an iodide from its outer ring to produce T_3, the more biologically active form of thyroid hormone. However, removing an iodide from the inner ring of T_4 (see Fig. 54.1) produces reverse T_3 (rT_3), which is biologically inactive. Similarly, removing an iodide from either ring inactivates T_3.

Thyrocytes use several mechanisms to maintain iodide homeostasis to prevent hormone overproduction. High levels of iodide lead to decreases in the activity of the Na^+/I^- symporter, preventing overproduction of thyroid hormone. In addition, high iodide levels also cause thyrocytes to shut down organification and coupling, an inhibitory response referred to as the Wolff-Chaikoff effect, a response that diminishes over time with persistently high levels of iodide. In some patients with thyroiditis or in the fetus, the thyroid does not escape from the Wolff-Chaikoff effect, and persistently high iodine levels can cause hypothyroidism, leading to goiter formation.

Regulation of thyroid hormone synthesis by thyrocytes also occurs at the level of the pituitary gland, which releases TSH (Chapter 49). When circulating levels of thyroid hormone are abnormally elevated, the sensitivity of the pituitary to TRH is reduced, causing decreased production of TSH. Further, the pituitary portal blood also carries counterregulatory compounds that inhibit TSH release (i.e., dopamine and somatostatin). In contrast, when levels of circulating thyroid hormone are abnormally decreased, the sensitivity of the pituitary to TRH increases, which stimulates TSH secretion and ultimately increases the release thyroid hormone.

Thyroid Hormone Receptors

Thyroid hormones exert their major effects by binding to thyroid hormone receptors (TRs), members of the nuclear receptor superfamily (Chapter 2). Two genes encode TRs, and each can be transcribed into alternatively spliced products. The relative proportions of each isoform expressed are developmentally dependent and tissue specific. TRs can homodimerize but are generally present as heterodimers, most commonly with the receptor for 9-cis-retinoic acid but also with other nuclear hormone receptors. TRs associate with DNA as part of a complex of transcription factors, even in the absence of thyroid hormone. When T_3 binds to its receptor, the interactions of the receptor with transcription corepressors and coactivators change, and local chromatin structure is modified by changes in histone acetylation. Binding of T_3 increases transcription of some genes and decreases the transcription of others. Thyroid hormones also regulate the processing of ribonucleic acid transcripts and the stability of specific messenger ribonucleic acids and have other nonnuclear actions. Another potential regulatory process is the expression of the TR splice variant (TRα2), which interacts with thyroid hormone response elements but is not activated by T_3. Consequently, expression of TRα2 can reduce sensitivity to thyroid hormone.

Antithyroid Drugs

As shown in Table 54.1, antithyroid drugs inhibit the synthesis, release, or metabolism of thyroid hormone. As depicted in Fig. 54.2, thyroid hormone synthesis involves uptake, organification, and coupling of iodide. Each of these steps provides a target to inhibit hormone production. Perchlorate decreases thyroid hormone production by competing with iodide for the Na^+/I^- symporter. Although perchlorate can be used briefly as a clinical antithyroid agent, cases of aplastic anemia have limited its usefulness. A single dose of perchlorate may be used as a diagnostic agent after administration of a tracer dose of radioactive iodine to determine whether a defect exists in a patient's ability to organify iodide.

TABLE 54.1 Antithyroid Drugs

Compound	Mechanism of Action
Perchlorate	Inhibition of iodide transport
Thioureylenes	Inhibition of organification and coupling
Iodide, lithium	Inhibition of deiodination of T_4 to T_3 Inhibition of hormone release
β-Adrenergic receptor blockers	Antagonize hypersensitivity for circulating catecholamines
Iopanoate (radiographic contrast agent)	Causes rapid decrease in serum T_4 and T_3

The thioureylene drugs propylthiouracil (PTU) and methimazole act as substrates for thyroid peroxidase to inhibit the organification of iodide and its coupling to thyroglobulin. Unlike methimazole, PTU also inhibits peripheral deiodination of T_4 to T_3, contributing to its antithyroid activity. The thioureylenes do not alter the action of existing thyroid hormones.

Administration of pharmacological doses of iodide transiently inhibits iodide uptake, synthesis, and release of thyroid hormone—namely, the Wolff-Chaikoff effect. Iodide is used for the treatment of a thyroid storm, which is a life-threatening untreated hyperthyroidism in which heart rate and blood pressure can increase to dangerously high levels. Lithium, an element used for the treatment of bipolar (manic depressive) disorder (Chapter 16), suppresses the release of thyroid hormone, but its chronic adverse effects limit its use for thyroid disorders.

In addition to drugs that inhibit hyperthyroidism by directly affecting the synthesis, release, or metabolism of thyroid hormone, other agents such as the β-adrenergic receptor antagonists inhibit the downstream symptoms of thyroid hormones. Hyperthyroidism is associated with tachycardia and other sympathomimetic effects as a consequence of thyroid hormone–induced increased density of β-adrenergic receptors, which facilitates the conversion of T_4 to T_3, increased expression of G-protein subunits, and cyclic adenosine monophosphate (cAMP) levels. In addition, thyroid hormones increase the expression of proteins that are both T_3- and cAMP-responsive, such as mitochondrial uncoupling protein 1, which is involved in thermogenesis. Consequently, β-adrenergic receptor blockers can be used to reduce the clinical symptoms of hyperthyroidism and are used as adjunct therapy.

Glucocorticoids are often included in acute therapy of severe hyperthyroidism such as occurs in thyroid storm. High doses are necessary, which decreases the conversion of T_4 to T_3, and may reduce pituitary TSH synthesis. Glucocorticoids may also have an antipyretic effect.

Several iodine-rich oral agents developed for radiological visualization of the gallbladder (cholecystography) are potent inhibitors of deiodinases. Iopanoic acid has been used as adjunct treatment of severe hyperthyroidism. However, because these compounds can provide iodide, they could exacerbate hyperthyroidism unless the patient has been pretreated with a thioureylene drug to inhibit organification. Further, the effects of the thioureylenes can be decreased by concurrent use of iopanate.

RELATIONSHIP OF MECHANISMS OF ACTION TO CLINICAL RESPONSE

Hyperthyroidism

Thioureylene drugs are commonly used for the initial treatment of hyperthyroidism. The American Thyroid Association and the American Association of Clinical Endocrinologists recommend methimazole for the treatment of Graves disease except in the first trimester of pregnancy

TABLE 54.2	**Pharmacokinetic Parameters of Thyroid Hormones and Antithyroid Drugs**				
Compound	Route of Administration	Oral Absorption	$t_{1/2}$ (Euthyroid State)	Disposition	Plasma Protein Binding
Thyroxine (T_4)	Oral, IV	Fair (50%–80%)	7 days	Metabolism, enterohepatic circulation	>99%
Triiodothyronine (T_3)	Oral	Good	24 hours	Metabolism, enterohepatic circulation	>99%
Propylthiouracil	Oral	Good	2 hours	Metabolism	82%
Methimazole	Oral	Good	8–12 hours	Metabolism	8%

or in patients who experience adverse reactions to this drug. Methimazole has better efficacy, a longer half-life ($t_{1/2}$) and duration of action, and fewer side effects relative to PTU. To establish return of the patient to the euthyroid state, thyroid hormone and TSH should be monitored. Once euthyroid status has been confirmed, the drug dose is typically reduced due to slower metabolism in euthyroid subjects. To avoid the risk of hypothyroidism once hormone levels return to normal, a small dose of T_4 can be administered and increased as required.

Long-term therapy for hyperthyroidism includes radioiodine, surgery, or continued treatment with thioureylene drugs. In the United States, the therapy used most commonly for the definitive treatment of hyperthyroidism is radioactive iodine. Antithyroid drugs are commonly used prior to surgery or radioactive iodine treatment in patients with toxic nodular goiter. Eventually, patients treated with radioactive iodine almost always become hypothyroid. Therefore it is common to intentionally ablate thyroid function with radioactive iodine rather than try to tailor the dose to attempt to achieve euthyroidism.

In selected patients, a partial thyroidectomy can offer definitive therapy, and thyroid hormone supplementation may not be required. If hyperthyroidism is due to Graves disease, which has an immune etiology, remission may occur. After maintaining euthyroidism with a thioureylene drug for 1–2 years, drug can be discontinued and the patient monitored for recurrence. Patients who have had the disease for a short time, or who have relatively small goiters, are more likely to experience remission. The percentage of patients likely to exhibit permanent remission varies but is less common (~20%) in areas where iodine intake is relatively high, such as in North America. If hyperthyroidism is due to autonomous thyroid nodules, spontaneous remission is unlikely.

Hypothyroidism

Maintenance of a hypothyroid patient is most commonly accomplished with T_4, which has a duration of action that allows daily administration. It is typically prescribed as the sodium salt to promote maximal absorption throughout the small intestine. Other commercially available forms include T_3, T_4 plus T_3, desiccated thyroglobulin, and thyroid extract. T_3 is not recommended for long-term management of hypothyroidism. Rather, it is primarily used in myxedema coma or for short-term management of postsurgical thyroid tumor patients during the process of diagnosis and treatment of residual tumor tissue. To treat most hypothyroid patients, the thyroid hormone dose is increased gradually while the patient's symptoms and serum levels of TSH are monitored. Several months may be required to establish the appropriate replacement dose because of the long $t_{1/2}$ of T_4 in euthyroid individuals, which is prolonged in hypothyroidism. If a patient has a functioning remnant of thyroid tissue initially, that remnant can either hypertrophy or atrophy, affecting the replacement dose. In addition, the dose will change if drugs that alter thyroid hormone absorption or metabolism are prescribed or discontinued. Thus symptoms and TSH levels should be monitored periodically in hypothyroid patients.

To reduce the risk of precipitating or worsening angina, particularly in aged patients, the dose of thyroid hormone should be increased gradually. However, more aggressive replacement is required occasionally in myxedema stupor/coma, despite the increased risk of precipitating acute cardiac disease.

PHARMACOKINETICS

The pharmacokinetic parameters for thyroid hormones and representative antithyroid drugs are listed in Table 54.2.

Thyroid Hormones

T_3 absorption is virtually complete, with a $t_{1/2}$ of 24 hours, reaching peak serum levels in 2–4 hours after oral administration in euthyroid subjects; thus blood levels rise and fall appreciably after each dose. In contrast, T_4 has a $t_{1/2}$ of approximately 7 days in euthyroid subjects, and thus blood levels do not display substantial variations after a daily dose. The oral absorption of T_4 varies depending on feeding state, with increased absorption in fasted patients. In addition, absorption can be impeded by several compounds, including dietary constituents such as ferrous sulfate, calcium, and soy flour. The sodium salt form of L-thyroxine enhances absorption.

T_4 and T_3 are almost completely protein-bound in the blood, with the highest affinity for thyroxine-binding globulin (TBG) plasma proteins, which bind approximately 70% of circulating hormones. Transthyretin (thyroxine-binding prealbumin, or TBPA) binds 15% of circulating hormones, whereas albumin, which has a lower affinity but massive binding capacity, accounts for 10% to 15%. Several drugs alter binding of thyroid hormones to plasma proteins: glucocorticoids, androgens, salsalate, salicylate, and phenytoin decrease binding, whereas estrogens, methadone, heroin, clofibrate, and 5-fluorouracil increase binding. When levels of binding proteins change, the total level of thyroid hormones measured in the blood also changes. Acute illness can decrease the levels of TBG and TBPA, thus reducing total blood levels of thyroid hormone. Sex hormone levels also influence expression of TBG; a rise in estrogen increases hepatic production of TBG, whereas a rise in androgen decreases TBG production. The effective level of binding proteins can be determined by measuring the amount of tracer-labeled T_3 that binds to a resin or by measuring free hormone level by dialysis. Given the effects of binding proteins on hormone levels, serum TSH levels provide a better measure for assessing a patient's thyroid status.

Three intrinsic membrane selenoproteins act as iodothyronine deiodinases to remove iodide from thyroid hormones. Deiodinase type 1 (D1) removes iodide from both rings, type 2 (D2) selectively deiodinates the outer ring, whereas type 3 (D3) selectively deiodinates the inner ring of iodothyronines, inactivating both T_4 and T_3. D1 is the major deiodinase present in liver, kidney, and thyroid and is regulated by thyroid hormone levels in some tissues. D1 acts primarily on the inner ring of T_3, with lesser activity on T_4 and the outer ring of T_3. D2 selectively deiodinates the outer ring of T_4, converting it to T_3, thereby forming the more active hormone in target tissues. D2 is the major enzyme in brown fat, heart, skeletal muscle, pituitary, and pineal gland. Thyroid hormone levels and adrenergic agents regulate D2 in some tissues. D3 is the major isoform in brain, fetal liver, and placenta.

The metabolism and excretion of the iodothyronines are increased by sulfation or glucuronidation. Because rT_3 is more susceptible to sulfate conjugation than either T_3 or T_4, it is metabolized faster. The alanine side chain of the amino acids on T_3 and T_4 can also be metabolized to form the thyroacetic acids, TRIAC and TETRAC, which have very short half-lives. Conjugated thyroid hormone metabolites are secreted in the bile, and there is substantial enterohepatic recirculation, which can be blocked by ingestion of drugs such as cholestyramine.

In hyperthyroidism, transcription of D1 and D3 increases in some tissues, whereas transcription of D2 is reduced and its degradation is increased, thereby decreasing T_4 conversion to T_3. In contrast, in hypothyroidism, D2 activity increases in some tissues, increasing conversion of T_4 to T_3.

Many factors influence the metabolism of thyroid hormones. Prolonged fasting reduces peripheral conversion of T_4 to T_3 by half while doubling the amount of T_4 converted to rT_3. Diet composition or nonthyroidal illness can also influence metabolism of thyroid hormones. Turnover of thyroid hormones is increased in hyperthyroidism and is slowed in hypothyroidism. Of the drugs that affect thyroid hormone metabolism, the iodine-rich antiarrhythmic agent amiodarone is the most egregious (Chapter 45). Amiodarone inhibits 5′-deiodinase activity, thus increasing serum T_4 and rT_3 levels while decreasing the level of T_3. However, amiodarone has direct effects on the thyroid, promoting thyroiditis, and can cause hyperthyroidism or hypothyroidism as it releases iodide.

Iodide

Daily intake of approximately 150 µg iodide is considered normal, and doses up to 500 µg do not affect thyroid function appreciably. Depending upon underlying pathophysiology, large doses of iodine can exacerbate hyperthyroidism, induce hypothyroidism, or cause goiter formation. Two solutions of iodine are used therapeutically: Lugol solution (which contains 5% KI and 5% elemental iodine, or approximately 6 mg per drop) and saturated solution of potassium iodide, which contains 1 g/mL KI, or approximately 40 mg per drop. Surgeons often administer 30 mg iodine twice a day for a few days or weeks before surgery to inhibit hormone release and reduce thyroid vascularity in patients with Graves disease who are undergoing a partial thyroidectomy. In general, iodine preparations should be administered only after blocking organification to prevent iodide from being incorporated into thyroid hormones.

Thioureylenes

Gastrointestinal absorption of thioureylenes is nearly complete. Because PTU has a relatively short serum $t_{1/2}$, it must be administered every 8 hours to maintain effective circulating levels. In contrast, methimazole is not bound appreciably to plasma proteins, has a longer serum $t_{1/2}$, and is concentrated substantially by the thyroid, with a slow turnover; thus it is effectively administered once a day. Because the thioureylenes act primarily by inhibiting thyroid hormone synthesis, long periods of administration are required before euthyroidism is achieved. Both agents are metabolized by oxidation and conjugation.

PHARMACOVIGILANCE: ADVERSE EFFECTS AND DRUG INTERACTIONS

Common adverse effects of thioureylene drugs include pruritus, rash, and fever. Some patients complain of a bitter or metallic taste following PTU administration. Rare side effects include agranulocytosis (0.1% to 0.3%), which appears within the first 90 days of therapy, and hepatic dysfunction (1%). A complete blood count should be obtained from patients prior to the initiation of therapy. It is important to warn the patient that if a persistent fever or other symptoms of infection develop, the drug must be stopped until it has been established that the white blood count is normal. The most common problem is hepatitis, although acute liver failure is also possible. Reports of liver damage have led to discouraging the use of PTU as first-line treatment. A serum liver profile is recommended before the initiation of therapy. PTU and methimazole both cross the placenta and are secreted in breast milk. Thus caution must be used for pregnant and nursing women.

Adverse effects of a large oral dose of iodine include gastrointestinal upset and rash. Longer exposure can cause swelling of the lacrimal or salivary glands with persistent tearing, salivation, and sore gums and teeth (iodism).

There are few side effects associated with the administration of T_4 when TSH is maintained within the normal range. Doses of T_4 leading to long-term suppression of TSH below the normal range increases the risk of ischemic heart disease and may cause left ventricular hypertrophy. Furthermore, TSH-suppressive doses may decrease bone mineral density in postmenopausal women. Numerous drugs have been reported to decrease the action of T_4, including central nervous system depressants, antihypertensive agents, antacids, and antibiotics. When prescribing thyroxine, it is critical to be aware of these important drug-drug interactions.

Potential problems associated with some of the important drugs for thyroid disorders are summarized in the Clinical Problems Box.

NEW DEVELOPMENTS

Up to 15% of patients who undergo replacement therapy with T_4 continue to experience symptoms despite having normal T_4 and TSH levels. Evidence suggests that this subset of patients may differentially express a certain polymorphism of the D2 enzyme responsible for the local conversion of T_4 to T_3. Animal studies indicate that supplementation of the T_4 regimen with T_3 may be beneficial, especially if a long-acting version of T_3 is used. A pharmacogenomics approach, identifying expression of specific polymorphisms in the gene that encodes D2 enzyme, may lead to the development of personalized treatment regimens that address this population. Additionally, studies on the unique nature of thyroid hormone receptor isoforms are providing information that may lead to the development of specific receptor agonists and antagonists that may selectively treat disturbances of homeostasis regulated by thyroid function.

CLINICAL RELEVANCE FOR HEALTHCARE PROFESSIONALS

The importance of understanding the role of thyroid hormones in the body is critical for the proper care of patients with thyroid dysfunction, either hyper- or hypofunction. Disruptions of thyroid hormone synthesis and release can alter many other organs and systems. For example, hyperthyroidism may predispose patients to arrhythmias, whereas hypothyroidism may alter lipid metabolism. Hyperthyroidism can be manifested as nervousness, irritability, sleep disturbances, and altered bowel habits, while patients with hypothyroid function can present with symptoms of fatigue, listlessness, altered mental status, irritability, and depression. All astute healthcare providers must consider altered thyroid function if individuals manifest any symptoms for which an etiology is not readily apparent. Simple blood tests measuring thyroid hormone levels, and levels of TSH, can reveal possible altered thyroid status.

CLINICAL PROBLEMS

Thyroid hormones	Acute overdose: angina, arrhythmias, or myocardial infarction
	Chronic overdose: accelerate osteoporosis or alter metabolism of other drugs
	Chronic low dose: bradycardia, sleepiness, hypercholesterolemia, and coronary artery disease
Thioureylene drugs	Pruritus and skin rash, granulocytopenia, serum sickness, hepatic toxicity, fever
Iodide	Goiter, hyperthyroidism, hypothyroidism, iodism (swollen salivary and lachrimal glands)

TRADE NAMES

In addition to generic and fixed-combination preparations, the following trade-named materials are some of the important compounds available in the United States.

Thyroid Hormones
Levothyroxine, T_4 (Levothroid, Levoxyl, Synthroid, Unithroid)
Liothyronine, T_3 (Cytomel, Triostat)
Liotrix, T_4:T_3 [4:1] (Euthyroid, Thyrolar)
Recombinant human TSH (Thyrogen)

Antithyroid Drugs
Methimazole (Tapazole, Thiamazole)
Propylthiouracil (generic)

SELF-ASSESSMENT QUESTIONS

1. A 40-year-old woman had a physical examination that revealed a slightly elevated heart rate and blood pressure, and palpation of her neck indicated an enlarged thyroid and elicited a complaint of tenderness. Laboratory tests revealed elevated TSH, decreased thyroid hormone levels, and elevated thyroglobulin antibodies. Which of the following is the most likely diagnosis?
   A. Graves disease.
   B. Hashimoto disease.
   C. Nontoxic goiter.
   D. Pituitary adenoma.
   E. Thyroid cancer.

2. Which of the following would be the most likely diagnosis if the patient who is described in Question 1 had laboratory results of low TSH, elevated thyroid hormones, and elevated thyroglobulin antibodies?
   A. Graves disease.
   B. Hashimoto disease.
   C. Pituitary adenoma.
   D. Thyroid cancer.
   E. Toxic goiter.

3. A patient with a history of hypertension was diagnosed with thyroid cancer requiring thyroid ablation. The patient rapidly developed hypothyroidism and required hormone replacement. Which of the following should be considered?

   A. Circulating levels of thyroxine should be restored rapidly because this patient's physiology has adapted to hypertension.
   B. Patient's hypertension will require a slower than normal rate of restoration of thyroid hormone levels.
   C. There are gender differences in the levels of thyroid hormone that must be considered.
   D. This patient is an ideal candidate for combination therapy with triiodothyronine and tetraiodothyronine.
   E. To prevent the growth-promoting properties of TSH, thyroid hormone levels must be adequate to suppress its formation by the anterior pituitary.

4. Which of the following potential problems can affect the pharmacological management of hypothyroidism and will most likely have the greatest influence on long-term management of thyroiditis?
   A. Effective immunosuppression by oral prednisone.
   B. Extent of thyroid gland function.
   C. Recovery of TSH levels.
   D. Regeneration of the thyroid gland.
   E. Responsiveness to levothyroxine replacement therapy.

FURTHER READING

Anonymous. Drugs for hypothyroidism. *Med Lett Drugs Ther.* 2015;57: 147–150.

Chakera AJ, Pearce SHS, Vaidya B. Treatment for primary hypothyroidism: current approaches and future possibilities. *Drug Des Devel Ther.* 2012;6:1–11.

De Leo S, Lee SY, Braverman LE. Hyperthyroidism. *Lancet.* 2016;388:906–916.

McAninch EA, Jo S, Preite NZ, et al. Prevalent polymorphism in thyroid hormone-activating enzyme leaves a genetic fingerprint that underlies associated clinical syndromes. *J Clin Endocrinol Metab.* 2015;100:920–933.

Werneck de Castro JP, Fonseca TL, Ueta CB, et al. Differences in hypothalamic type 2 deiodinase ubiquitination explain localized sensitivity to thyroxine. *J Clin Invest.* 2015;125:769–781.

WEBSITES

http://www.thyroid.org/guidelines-hyperthyroidism-thyrotoxicosis/
This website is maintained by the American Thyroid Association and contains guidelines for managing hyperthyroidism.

Calcium Regulating Hormones and Other Agents Affecting Bone

Jack W. Strandhoy

THERAPEUTIC OVERVIEW

Plasma Ca^{++} concentrations are normally maintained within narrow limits between 8.5 and 10.4 mg/dL (approximately 2.3 mM) in adults. Approximately 45% of plasma Ca^{++} (~2 mM) is bound to proteins and fatty acid anionic groups, and approximately 10% is complexed with inorganic anions. Intracellular Ca^{++} (100 nM–1 μM) is maintained by low membrane permeability to passive transport, and intracellular Ca^{++} exists unbound or stored in the mitochondria and endoplasmic reticulum. When ionized Ca^{++} levels fall outside the normal physiological range, compensatory mechanisms occur. Failure to restore normal levels adversely affects cellular and whole-body physiology. Calcium levels less than 8.5 mg/dL are indicative of **hypocalcemia**, which can lead to increased neuromuscular excitability and tetany and impairment of skeletal mineralization. Calcium levels exceeding 10.4 mg/dL are indicative of **hypercalcemia** and can precipitate life-threatening cardiac dysrhythmias, soft tissue calcification, kidney stones, and central nervous system abnormalities.

The primary sites of Ca^{++} regulation by the gastrointestinal (GI) tract, kidneys, and bone are depicted in Fig. 55.1. The GI tract normally absorbs 10%–20% of dietary Ca^{++}, with absorption dependent directly on **vitamin D** levels. **Renal tubular reabsorption** is highly efficient (99%) and recovers 10–20 g of calcium filtered per day. **Bone** is the major site of Ca^{++} storage, containing approximately 1 kg in a 70-kg human. Of this, more than 99% is normally in a bound and stable state, and 1% is an exchangeable pool that turns over at a rate of about 20 g/day.

Pathophysiology

Hypocalcemia often results from hypoparathyroidism or low levels of parathyroid hormone (PTH) or pseudohypoparathyroidism (resistance to PTH). Resulting imbalances of Ca^{++} metabolism include increased renal excretion of Ca^{++}, decreased formation of calcitriol (1,25-dihydroxyvitamin D, the hormonally active form of vitamin D), decreased bone resorption, and decreased intestinal absorption of Ca^{++}. Depending upon the severity of the disorder, therapeutic strategies include supplementation with oral or infused calcium salts and vitamin D.

Hypercalcemia can result from increases in PTH, with primary hyperparathyroidism common in the outpatient setting. Secondary (or unregulated tertiary) hyperparathyroidism often develops in response to chronic renal disease, bronchogenic carcinoma, or other related malignancies that secrete PTH-related peptide (PTHrP). Some lymphomas and granulomatous diseases, such as sarcoidosis, can also produce hypercalcemia by autonomous calcitriol production. Again, depending upon the severity of the disorder, therapeutic strategies may include the administration of the bisphosphonate zoledronic acid and calcitonin.

Disorders of bone turnover that are not usually associated with abnormal serum ion concentrations are also amenable to therapy. **Rickets** (inadequate bone mineralization during development) or **osteomalacia** (inadequate mineralization in adults) results in "soft" bones that may bow out of the normal straight position. These disorders typically result from the inadequate dietary intake or formation of active calcitriol from vitamin D. Treatment involves supplementation with Ca^{++}, vitamin D, and often phosphate, with the form of vitamin D administered depending on the patient's ability to produce calcitriol.

Osteopenia and **osteoporosis** are skeletal disorders in which decreased bone strength predisposes patients to an increased fracture risk. Risks include decreased estrogen levels in women and men, low initial bone thickness, small stature, family or personal history, chronic hyperparathyroidism, immunosuppression with corticosteroids, or periods of immobility. The diagnosis of milder osteopenia or more severe osteoporosis is made by measuring bone mineral density in multiple skeletal regions. Therapeutic interventions when appropriate include weight-bearing and muscle-strengthening exercises and reduction of falling risks. Pharmacological management involves replenishing Ca^{++} in bone with antiresorptive agents, such as the bisphosphonates or the selective estrogen receptor modulators (SERMs). If these approaches are insufficient, calcitonin, the PTH analogue teriparatide, or the monoclonal antibody denosumab is often indicated.

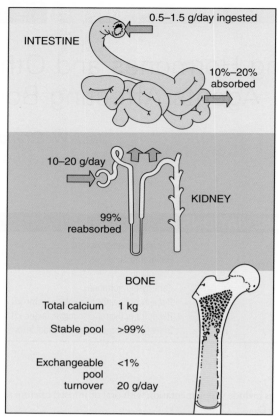

FIG. 55.1 Sites of Ca^{++} Regulation. Bone is the primary storage site, containing approximately 1 kg of Ca^{++}.

THERAPEUTIC OVERVIEW

Hypocalcemia

Disorders: Hypoparathyroidism; pseudohypoparathyroidism; renal failure; inadequate calcium intake or absorption; abnormal vitamin D ingestion, absorption, or metabolism

Management: Calcium salts and/or vitamin D or its analogues, parathyroidectomy if appropriate

Hypercalcemia

Disorders: Hyperparathyroidism, hypervitaminosis D, chronic kidney disease, neoplasia, sarcoidosis, hyperthyroidism

Management:

Mild hypercalcemia: dietary Ca^{++} restriction and adequate hydration, avoid thiazides and lithium

Moderate hypercalcemia: saline volume expansion, cinacalcet to suppress PTH if needed

Severe hypercalcemia: saline volume expansion, calcitonin, bisphosphonate (zoledronic acid), and calcitonin

Abnormal Bone Remodeling

Disorders: Paget disease, rickets, osteomalacia, osteoporosis

Management: zoledronic acid for Paget disease, adequate Ca^{++} and vitamin D, bisphosphonates, an SERM, denosumab

Paget disease of bone (osteitis deformans) is a chronic benign disorder with overactivity of both osteoclasts and osteoblasts, leading to high bone turnover with a less organized, weaker bone. Familial history, and potentially a chronic viral infection, may be involved. Skeletal deformity and bone pain may accompany the weakened bone, and cochlear damage may cause hearing loss. Besides ensuring that Ca^{++} and vitamin D intake are appropriate, infusion of the bisphosphonate zoledronic acid is recommended.

The loss of normal bone structure and integrity can also result from some drugs, disease, or nutritional deprivation, with resulting fractures often associated with increased morbidity and mortality. The treatments of Ca^{++} and bone metabolism depend on the cause and severity of the diseases and are summarized in the Therapeutic Overview Box.

MECHANISMS OF ACTION

Vitamin D, Metabolites, and Analogues

The structure and metabolism of vitamin D is shown in Fig. 55.2. Vitamin D is a secosteroid—that is, a steroid in which the B ring is cleaved and the A ring rotated. Vitamin D$_3$, cholecalciferol, is the natural form of vitamin D in humans and is synthesized from cholesterol in the skin in response to solar ultraviolet light. Vitamin D$_2$, ergocalciferol, is the plant-derived form. Both vitamins D$_2$ and D$_3$ are present in the diet and equally effective in adults. The primary circulating form of vitamin D is the metabolite 25-hydroxyvitamin D (calcifediol), which is formed in the endoplasmic reticulum and mitochondria of the liver. Calcifediol is further metabolized in the kidneys to 1,25-dihydroxyvitamin D (calcitriol), a reaction catalyzed by mitochondrial P450 27B1

(CYP27B1, also known as 1α-hydroxylase), and whose activity is stimulated by PTH and low plasma phosphate levels.

Calcitriol and active synthetic vitamin D analogues bind primarily to vitamin D receptors (VDRs) in the nucleus of target cells and act as ligand-activated transcription factors by modulating the synthesis of specific proteins. Among the protein products resulting from actions of vitamin D on the intestine are high-affinity Ca^{++}-binding proteins, the calbindins, which play a role in stimulation of intestinal Ca^{++} transport. Vitamin D metabolites increase the absorption of dietary Ca^{++} and PO$_4^{-3}$ by stimulating uptake across the GI mucosa, increasing serum Ca^{++} levels (Fig. 55.3). As a result of increased Ca^{++} and PO$_4^{-3}$ absorption, osteoblast mineralization is increased, responsible for the antirachitic effect of vitamin D.

In addition to the effects of vitamin D on bone, secondary to its effects on GI mineral absorption, vitamin D may also have a direct effect on bone, possibly through both VDR-independent and VDR-dependent mechanisms. Studies suggest that if mineral supply is sufficient, vitamin D promotes osteoblast formation and maturation. However, if Ca^{++} is limited, vitamin D acts in concert with PTH to maintain serum homeostasis at the expense of bone, promoting osteoclast maturation and recruitment of osteoclast precursors to resorptive sites in bone. Thus the functional roles of vitamin D may differ depending on age, stress, status of mineral homeostasis, and differentiation and maturity of osteoblasts.

Parathyroid Hormone and Analogues

PTH is an 84–amino acid polypeptide formed from the cleavage of larger precursors in the parathyroid gland. The first 34 amino acids of PTH (PTH 1–34) possess the full effects of the peptide on bone and Ca^{++} metabolism. PTH has multiple effects that influence Ca^{++} and PO$_4^{-3}$ metabolism and bone (Fig. 55.4). PTH acts directly at renal tubules to decrease PO$_4^{-3}$ and increase Ca^{++} reabsorption, resulting in decreased serum PO$_4^{-3}$ and increased serum Ca^{++} levels.

PTH also enhances Ca^{++} absorption indirectly by stimulating the formation of 1,25-dihydroxyvitamin D (see Fig. 55.2). PTH secretion is regulated by Ca^{++} through the extracellular Ca^{++}-sensing receptor (CaSR) that is highly expressed in the parathyroid gland and in renal

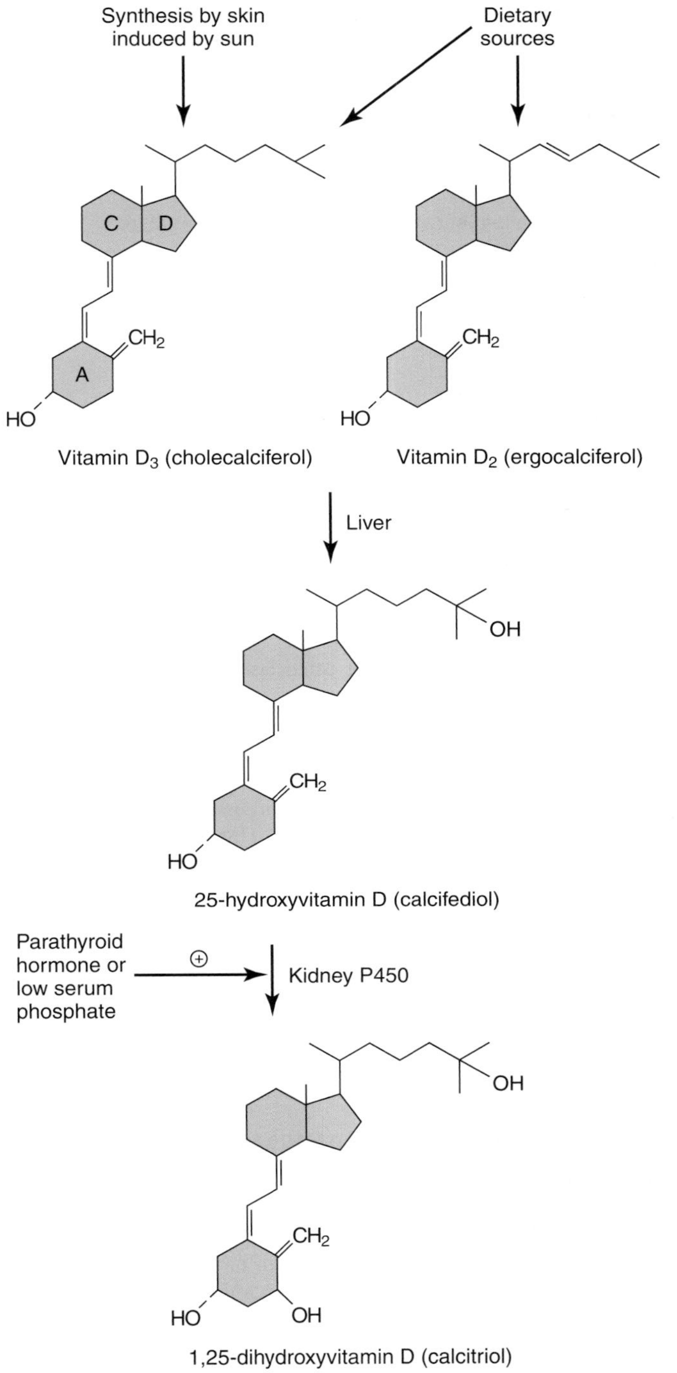

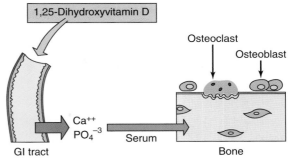

Vitamin D₃ (cholecalciferol)   Vitamin D₂ (ergocalciferol)

Liver

25-hydroxyvitamin D (calcifediol)

Parathyroid hormone or low serum phosphate → ⊕ → Kidney P450

1,25-dihydroxyvitamin D (calcitriol)

FIG. 55.2 Sources, Structure, and Metabolism of Vitamin D.

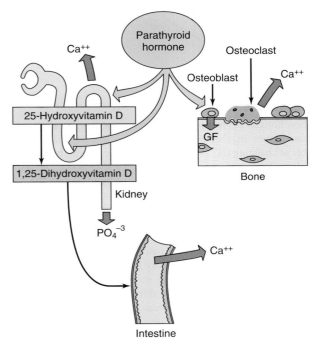

FIG. 55.3 Mechanism of the Antirachitic Effect of 1,25-Dihydroxyvitamin D. 1,25-dihydroxyvitamin D increases Ca^{++} and PO_4^{-3} absorption from the intestine, increasing serum concentrations. The ions deposit in bone, increasing bone mineralization.

FIG. 55.4 Direct and Indirect Effects of PTH on Ca^{++} Metabolism. Renal tubular reabsorption of PO_4^{-3} decreases, and that of Ca^{++} increases. Hormone-stimulated osteoblast activates osteoclast to release Ca^{++} into extracellular fluid. Intermittent stimulation of osteoblasts by PTH has anabolic effects mediated by growth factors (GF).

tubules. The CaSR is a membrane-associated G-protein–coupled receptor (GPCR) belonging to family C and, when activated, stimulates both cAMP-dependent protein kinase A and protein kinase C isozymes to inhibit the tonic secretion of PTH and the proliferation of parathyroid cells.

PTH also interacts with PTH receptors highly expressed in bone and the kidneys. The effects of PTH are dependent on whether it is administered intermittently or continuously. Intermittent administration to attain subphysiological levels leads to anabolic effects to promote bone formation, whereas continuous administration leads to bone loss.

The anabolic effect on bone may involve the induction of growth factors such as insulin-like growth factor-1 that promotes interaction with osteoblasts. Teriparatide is the active 1 to 34–amino acid portion of the PTH peptide.

Calcimimetics

Cinacalcet is the first drug in a category referred to as calcimimetics, drugs that mimic the effects of Ca^{++}. Cinacalcet is a positive allosteric modulator of CaSRs on the surface of the chief cells of the parathyroid gland. By increasing the sensitivity of CaSRs to activation by extracellular Ca^{++}, cinacalcet decreases the concentration of Ca^{++} required to suppress PTH secretion. Etelcalcetide is a newly developed calcimimetic with the same mechanism of action as cinacalcet that was approved for use in the United States in 2017.

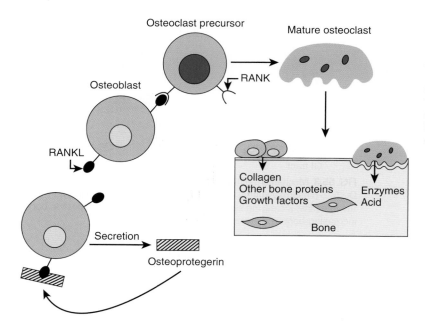

FIG. 55.5 Bone Remodeling and the Roles of Osteoblast and Osteoclast Proteins. Osteoclast precursors express receptors (RANK) that interact with the osteoblast membrane-associated cytokine, RANKL. This interaction leads to osteoclast maturation and the formation of a ruffled membrane, promoting binding to the bony surface and accompanied by protein secretion, acidification, and bone resorption. Osteoblasts also express osteoprotegerin that acts as a decoy receptor to block the interaction between RANK and RANKL, thereby inhibiting osteoclastogenesis.

Bisphosphonates

Bisphosphonates are pyrophosphate analogues that contain two phosphonate groups attached to a central carbon. Their spatial structure is capable of chelating Ca^{++}, so they strongly interact with hydroxyapatite crystals on bony surfaces undergoing active resorption. The bisphosphonates also promote osteoclast apoptosis by inhibiting the isoprenylation of small G proteins such as Rab, Rac, and Rho that are critical for osteoclast membrane ruffling, adherence to the bony surface, production of an acidic environment, and survival.

The first-generation bisphosphonates (etidronate, clodronate, and tiludronate) effectively inhibited osteoclast activity, decreased bone resorption, and reduced the incidence of fractures at high doses. However, they did not promote new bone growth and often led to bone demineralization. The second- and third-generation bisphosphonates (alendronate, risedronate, ibandronate, pamidronate, and zoledronic acid) also inhibit osteoclast activity but do not cause demineralization. Further, the third-generation drugs contain a heterocyclic N ring and are up to 10,000 times more potent than the first-generation drugs. Bisphosphonates are used to treat hypercalcemia, osteoporosis, and Paget disease of bone.

Selective Estrogen Receptor Modulators

Estrogens (Chapter 51) inhibit bone resorption and prevent fractures through the decreased production of interleukins that activate and promote the survival of osteoclasts. The selective estrogen receptor modulators (SERMs) such as raloxifene have tissue-selective activities at estrogen receptors. Raloxifene is an estrogen receptor agonist in liver and bone, is inactive in the uterus, and is an estrogen receptor antagonist in the breast. It inhibits bone resorption and stabilizes bone density, reducing the risk of vertebral compression fractures.

Calcitonin

Calcitonin is a 32–amino acid polypeptide secreted by the parafollicular cells of the thyroid. Calcitonin and a neuronal calcitonin gene-related peptide arise from differential splicing in parafollicular cells and neural tissue, and overproduction of calcitonin may be a marker for medullary thyroid carcinoma. Calcitonin decreases postprandial absorption of Ca^{++} and increases excretion of Ca^{++}, Na^+, Mg^{++}, Cl^-, and PO_4^{-3}—that is, its actions are generally opposite those of PTH. At the cellular level,

calcitonin inhibits the activity of osteoclasts, decreasing serum Ca^{++} and PO_4^{-3}.

Receptor Activator of Nuclear Factor-κB Inhibitors

Bone remodeling involves an interaction between the receptor activator of nuclear factor-κB (RANK) expressed on osteoclast precursors and its ligand, RANKL, expressed on osteoblasts. This interaction is necessary for osteoclast differentiation, survival, and activity, resulting in Ca^{++} release, and is a process affected by many factors such as PTH, prostaglandins, and inflammatory cytokines to stimulate bone resorption (Fig. 55.5). Osteoblasts also express and secrete osteoprotegerin (OPG, also known as osteoclastogenesis inhibitory factor), a protein that functions as a decoy receptor and binds to RANKL, preventing its binding to RANK, thereby inhibiting osteoclastogenesis. Denosumab is a monoclonal antibody directed against RANKL and represents the first in its class to inhibit osteoclast activity and bone resorption.

RELATIONSHIP OF MECHANISMS OF ACTION TO CLINICAL RESPONSE

Vitamin D, Metabolites, and Analogues

Adequate intake of vitamin D and calcium in food and supplements is essential for bone health. Increasingly, vitamin D is recognized to be an important component of the immune system, and its deficiency is linked to diseases beyond the skeletal system. Vitamin D, its metabolites, and synthetic analogues are all used in the treatment of rickets, osteomalacia, osteoporosis, and hypocalcemia. Drugs, doses, and regimens chosen depend on the disease treated and whether the patient can effectively synthesize endogenous calcitriol, which is dependent upon adequate PTH.

Hypocalcemia may be an incidental hallmark of disease severity and may normalize with disease treatment. Over half of patients admitted to intensive care units have hypocalcemia, and studies have shown that calcium supplements to these critically ill adults increase their 28-day survival. Mild hypocalcemia is not life threatening and can usually be remedied by oral calcium and an appropriate form of vitamin D. More severe hypocalcemia can present with cerebral and cardiac irregularities. Intravenous calcium gluconate or chloride can be cautiously administered into a central vein, along with replacement of oral calcium and vitamin D. Prevention of cardiac dysrhythmias is especially important to patients taking digoxin or other cardiac drugs. Hypocalcemia can be anticipated and prevented in patients undergoing a parathyroidectomy and often presents in hemodialysis patients. These complex patients often require frequent monitoring and supplementation of calcium, vitamin D analogues, and binding of phosphate.

Patients with 1α-hydroxylase deficiency benefit from calcitriol, 1α-hydroxyvitamin D$_2$, and dihydrotachysterol. Paricalcitol (19-nor-1α, 25-hydroxyvitamin D$_2$) and calcipotriene have a lesser effect on Ca^{++} metabolism than other analogues and therefore can be used with a reduced risk of hypercalcemia. Paricalcitol is used to suppress elevated PTH secretion in chronic kidney disease, and calcipotriene is used to promote normal skin cell differentiation in psoriasis.

Supraphysiological doses of vitamin D are used to treat hypoparathyroidism or vitamin D–resistant rickets.

Parathyroid Hormone and Analogues

Teriparatide is approved to treat severe osteoporosis for patients in whom antiresorptive agents have failed to prevent recurrent fractures. Teriparatide requires daily injection and has an anabolic effect on bone to increase density and reduce fractures. It is also approved for hypogonadal osteoporosis in men.

Calcimimetics

Cinacalcet is approved for primary and secondary hyperparathyroidism, which can result from parathyroid tumors and chronic renal failure. Further, preclinical and clinical studies suggest the possibility of using compounds like cinacalcet for the treatment of various forms of hypercalcemic hyperparathyroidism, such as lithium-induced hyperparathyroidism and that occurring after renal transplantation. Cinacalcet helps normalize serum Ca^{++} without altering bone mineral density but is less effective on a long-term basis at controlling PTH oversecretion than is parathyroidectomy. Nevertheless, cinacalcet represents a new approach to controlling blood Ca^{++} and bone health.

Etelcalcetide represents the first new treatment in many years for adult patients on hemodialysis to reduce secondary hyperparathyroidism. It is administered intravenously three times a week at the end of dialysis sessions. Studies to date support strong efficacy, but the drug has been on the market for only 1 year.

Bisphosphonates

Bisphosphonates constitute an increasingly useful group of agents used to treat osteoporosis, Paget disease of bone, and hypercalcemia, with newer agents in this class supplanting some of the early congers.

Although mild hypercalcemia (10.5–11.4 mg/dL) may be handled by dietary restriction and adequate hydration, moderate hypercalcemia (11.5–14 mg/dL) may require treatment with zoledronic acid administered intravenously. Severe hypercalcemia (>14 mg/dL) is a life-threatening condition often caused by advanced bone or renal pathology and requires immediate intensive treatment. The intravenous administration of a bisphosphonate such as zoledronic acid, calcitonin, or saline for volume expansion will reduce Ca^{++} rapidly. If renal or heart failure is involved, the addition of furosemide will increase Ca^{++} excretion.

Selective Estrogen Receptor Modulators

SERMs such as raloxifene and bazedoxifene play a major role in the prevention and treatment of osteoporosis. Decreased estrogen production commonly occurs as a result of ovarian failure, ovariectomy, chronic suppression with long-acting gonadotropin-releasing hormone agonists, and menopause, all of which lead to osteopenia and eventually osteoporosis. Estrogen supplementation or replacement is effective in delaying osteopenia and osteoporosis but is associated with an increased risk of cancer and cardiovascular diseases. The SERMs have become a mainstay of treatment for these disorders. Bazedoxifene is used alone in countries other than the United States; it is available in the United States only combined with conjugated estrogens.

Calcitonin

Injected calcitonin can be used to reduce acute hypercalcemia and in the secondary treatment of Paget disease. It inhibits osteoclast activity, decreases postprandial calcium absorption, and increases its renal excretion. However, the ability of calcitonin to decrease hypercalcemia diminishes with continued use. In addition, because it is a peptide with a short half-life, it must be injected frequently, rendering it less useful as a chronic medication. The usual source of pharmaceutical calcitonin is from salmon that cross-reacts with human receptors.

Receptor Activator of Nuclear Factor-κB Inhibitors

Denosumab is the prototype of an antibody targeted against RANKL that prevents osteoclast proliferation and bone dissolution. Because it lowers Ca^{++} release from bone, patients should not be hypocalcemic when beginning this drug. Denosumab is administered twice yearly by subcutaneous injection, and the American Association of Clinical Endocrinologists and National Osteoporosis Guideline Group suggest that denosumab should be considered with the bisphosphonates as first-line treatment for osteoporosis.

PHARMACOKINETICS

The pharmacokinetic parameters of selected agents are presented in Table 55.1.

Vitamin D, Metabolites, and Analogues

Calcifediol (25-OH vitamin D) and calcitriol (1,25-dihydroxyvitamin D) are absorbed rapidly after oral administration. Because they are members of the fat-soluble vitamin family (A, D, E, K), they require bile salts for adequate absorption. Patients with biliary cirrhosis or steatorrhea may have poorer absorption. Vitamin D binds to a glycoprotein, is metabolized to inactive glucuronides, and is stored in liver, fat, and muscle.

Parathyroid Hormone and Analogues

Teriparatide is administered by daily subcutaneous injections (20 μg). It is mandatory to achieve low, intermittent circulating levels to promote new bone growth because higher constant levels lead to resorption. Peak plasma concentrations are attained rapidly in normal individuals, and the drug is cleared with a mean half-life of 60 minutes. Because new bone is lost after cessation of teriparatide administration, termination of treatment is followed by administration of an antiresorptive agent such as a bisphosphonate or calcitonin.

Calcimimetics

Cinacalcet is administered orally and is best absorbed with food. Only about 20% of the drug is absorbed, and it is highly bound to plasma proteins. Cinacalcet is metabolized by several common hepatic cytochromes, but it is not excreted by the kidneys; thus it may be a logical choice in patients with compromised renal function.

Etelcalcetide is administered intravenously and has a longer elimination half-life (3–4 days) than cinacalcet. It is biotransformed in the blood and cleared by renal excretion in patients with normal kidney function or hemodiaylsis in patients with renal disease.

Bisphosphonates

The bisphosphonates are available orally for use at weekly or monthly intervals and by injection quarterly or once per year. Because of poor oral absorption (1%–6%), the bisphosphonates must be taken in the morning on an empty stomach with no food or other medication. In

TABLE 55.1	**Selected Pharmacokinetic Parameters**		
Agent	**Route of Administration**	**$t_{1/2}$**	**Disposition**
Vitamin D (calcifediol)	Oral	14 days	Bile for absorption, M
Calcitriol	Oral	1–3 days	Bile for absorption, M
Teriparatide	SC	5 min IV	M, R
		1 hour SC	
Cinacalcet	Oral	34 hours	M
Bisphosphonates	Oral, IV	Vary, some bound to bone for years	R
Raloxifene	Oral	28 hours	M
Calcitonin	SC, IM, nasal	20 min SC	M, R
Denosumab	SC	25 days	M

Abbreviations: *IM*, Intramuscular; *IV*, intravenous; *M*, metabolism; *R*, renal excretion; *SC*, subcutaneous.

addition, individuals must remain in a standing or sitting position for at least 30 minutes to minimize esophageal irritation. Bisphosphonates are not significantly metabolized, and after oral administration, approximately half the drug is excreted by the kidneys within 72 hours. The remainder of the absorbed drug is bound to hydroxyapatite in bone and can remain bound for years until resorption occurs at the sites where it is bound. Highly effective inhibition of osteoclast activity by drug incorporation directly into bone provides a long duration of action that can last up to a year.

Selective Estrogen Receptor Modulators

The pharmacokinetics of raloxifene, bazedoxifene, and other SERMs are discussed in Chapter 51.

Calcitonin

Calcitonin is weakly bound to plasma proteins, has a short plasma half-life, and is metabolized rapidly by both liver and kidney.

Receptor Activator of Nuclear Factor-κB Inhibitors

Denosumab is administered by subcutaneous injection twice a year. Its mean half-life is 25–28 days.

PHARMACOVIGILANCE: ADVERSE EFFECTS AND DRUG INTERACTIONS

Vitamin D, Metabolites, and Analogues

Excess vitamin D and its metabolites can lead to hypercalcemia. The adverse effects of hypercalcemia are dose dependent and include abdominal pain, constipation, nausea, increased risk of kidney stones, and soft tissue calcification. Although the immediate risk would seem greatest for 1,25-dihydroxyvitamine D, this compound has the shortest half-life; thus, cumulative effects and the risk of hypercalcemia are less frequent than with the other metabolites.

There is an increased risk of toxicity in patients with impaired renal function. Patients receiving vitamin D alone or with Ca^{++} must have serum Ca^{++} concentrations monitored, and treatment must be discontinued as Ca^{++} levels are restored or if hypercalcemia occurs. Benzothiadiazide diuretics, which decrease Ca^{++} excretion, can increase the risk of hypercalcemia from vitamin D. Drug interactions can occur with phenobarbital, phenytoin, and glucocorticoids, all of which interfere with vitamin D activation, as well as actions of metabolites on target tissues.

Parathyroid Hormone and Analogues

Teriparatide can lead to hypercalcemia because bone resorption can be stimulated if levels become elevated beyond those that produce an anabolic effect. This risk is lessened if the drug is administered intermittently, as for the treatment of osteoporosis. Adverse effects include nausea, headache, dizziness, and cramps; the safety of long-term use is unknown.

Calcimimetics

Common adverse effects of cinacalcet include GI disturbances, dizziness, decreased plasma testosterone, and muscle and chest pain. More serious side effects include hypocalcemia, muscle spasms, QT interval prolongation, GI bleeding, and seizures. Rash and hypersensitivity reactions have also been reported, as well as hypotension, heart failure and arrhythmias. A rare but serious adverse effect reported for cinacalcet is a **dynamic bone disease**, a renal osteodystrophy characterized by low bone turnover and decreased numbers of osteoclasts and osteoblasts, resulting from low levels of PTH.

Bisphosphonates

The major side effects of the bisphosphonates are GI problems including heartburn, abdominal pain, gastroesophageal reflux disease, diarrhea, and esophageal irritation and ulceration. All these effects can be minimized with parenteral administration. An association has been reported between bisphosphonate use and pathological conditions, including low bone turnover states with resultant pathological fractures, osteonecrosis of the jaw, and an increased incidence of atrial fibrillation.

Selective Estrogen Receptor Modulators

SERMs have been reported to exacerbate vasomotor symptoms associated with decreased estrogen. Some SERMs, such as bazedoxifene, are combined with conjugated estrogens that address this concern.

Calcitonin

Local hypersensitivity reactions including rashes, other allergic reactions, and nausea have been noted in patients receiving calcitonin. Although calcitonin could elicit hypocalcemia, this is not common. A potential problem with calcitonin is a loss of effectiveness with prolonged use.

Receptor Activator of Nuclear Factor-κB Inhibitors

The administration of denosumab for the treatment of osteoporosis in postmenopausal women commonly leads to back and musculoskeletal pain, hypercholesterolemia, and cystitis. Men also experience back pain as well as arthralgia. Constipation is also common.

The clinical problems associated with the use of compounds that alter Ca^{++} metabolism and bone formation are summarized in the Clinical Problems Box.

CLINICAL PROBLEMS

Drug Category	Adverse Effects
Vitamin D, metabolites, and analogues	Hypercalcemia, kidney stones
Teriparatide	Hypercalcemia
Cinacalcet	Nausea and vomiting, muscle spasms, QT interval prolongation, decreased testosterone, hypoparathyroidism, hypocalcemia
Bisphosphonates	Esophageal and GI irritation, ulcers, atypical femur fractures, osteonecrosis of the jaw
SERMs	Hot flashes, thromboembolism
Calcitonin	Local hypersensitivity reactions, loss of effectiveness with continued use
Denosumab	Back pain, hypercholesterolemia, constipation

NEW DEVELOPMENTS

Although many new approaches have been developed during the past several years, including the introduction of calcimimetics and RANKL inhibitor monoclonal antibodies, the need for better anabolic agents exists. Antiresorptive agents can only reduce nonvertebral fractures by 20%, necessitating the development of new therapies. Most compounds currently available target either bone resorption or formation, with limited information on combination approaches. Cinacalcet has been successful as a calcimimetic to decrease PTH and blood calcium, and similar compounds are being developed. Antibodies to proteins and receptors important to bone development or diseases are being explored as potential drugs. Some compounds currently in clinical testing include odanacatib, a reversible inhibitor of cathepsin K, a protease activated in an acidic environment that degrades several proteins in bone; romosozumab, a monoclonal antibody with anabolic properties that stimulates bone formation and inhibits resorption through blocking sclerostin, which inhibits bone formation; and abaloparatide, a parathyroid hormone-related peptide that induces bone formation without stimulating resorption and causing hypercalcemia. Undoubtedly, several new drugs will become available in the coming years.

CLINICAL RELEVANCE FOR HEALTHCARE PROFESSIONALS

All healthcare professionals should be aware of and should educate their patients on the numerous risk factors for bone health including age, sex, postmenopausal status, diet, medication and alcohol history, family history, concomitant disease, exercise, fall risks, and other environmental factors. Physical and occupational therapists should be especially aware of concerns of bone fragility. In addition, it is imperative that all dental professionals ask their patients about the prior use of the bisphosphonates or denosumab, as these drugs may lead to osteonecrosis of the jaw with potential complications from dental procedures. These individuals should also educate their patients on the value of fluoride for dental and bone health and on the association between osteoporosis and dental health.

TRADE NAMES

In addition to generic and fixed-combination preparations, the following trade-named materials are many of the important compounds available in the United States.

Vitamin D, Metabolites, and Analogues
Calcifediol (Calderol)
Calcipotriene (Dovonex)
Calcitriol (Rocaltrol)
Dihydrotachysterol (DHT, Hytakerol)
Doxercalciferol (Hectorol)
Ergocalciferol (Calciferol, Drisdol)
Paricalcitol (Zemplar)

Parathyroid Hormone and Analogues
Teriparatide (Forteo)

Calcimimetics
Cinacalcet (Sensipar)
Etelcalcetide (Parsabiv)

Bisphosphonates
Alendronate (Fosamax)
Etidronate (Didronel)
Ibandronate (Boniva)
Pamidronate (Aredia)
Risedronate (Actonel)
Zoledronic acid (Zometa, Reclast)

Selective Estrogen Receptor Modulators
Bazedoxifene + conjugated estrogens (DUAVEE)
Raloxifene (Evista)

Others
Calcitonin (Calcimar, Cibacalcin, Miacalcin)
Denosumab (Prolia)

SELF-ASSESSMENT QUESTIONS

1. A 62-year-old woman is concerned about ongoing gastric distress with mild esophagitis and dull pain around her lumbar vertebrae. Repeat bone density measurements by central dual-energy x-ray absorptiometry (DXA or DEXA) show moderate, progressive osteoporosis (T = −2.6). Her current medications include omeprazole, hydrochlorothiazide, losartan, multivitamins, calcium citrate, and vitamin D. Which of the following should be added to her treatment regimen?
   A. Alendronate.
   B. Calcipotriene.
   C. Calcitonin.
   D. Cinacalcet.
   E. Zoledronic acid.

2. A 45-year-old man with chronic kidney disease is on outpatient renal dialysis. He has secondary hyperparathyroidism and is on the list for a kidney transplant. As an alternative to parathyroid surgery at this time, which drug would be the best choice to regulate his elevated PTH secretion and hypercalcemia?
   A. Calcitonin.
   B. Etelcalcetide.
   C. Furosemide.
   D. Raloxifene.
   E. Teriparatide.

3. Which agent is a selective estrogen receptor modulator used to reduce bone loss associated with postmenopausal osteoporosis?
   A. Calcitonin.
   B. Clomiphene.
   C. Medroxyprogesterone acetate.
   D. Raloxifene.
   E. Teriparatide.
4. Which agent promotes bone deposition at low intermittent doses and bone resorption at higher chronic doses?
   A. Calcitonin.
   B. Calcitriol.
   C. Calcium salts.
   D. Teriparatide.
   E. Second-generation bisphosphonates.
5. Which agent increases bone density by antagonizing actions of osteoclasts and does not inhibit actions of osteoblasts?
   A. Calcium salts and DHT.
   B. Estrogen analogues.
   C. Inorganic phosphate (P_i).
   D. Raloxifene.
   E. Second-generation bisphosphonates.

FURTHER READING

Pazianas M, Miller P, Blumentals WA, et al. A review of the literature on osteonecrosis of the jaw in patients with osteoporosis treated with oral bisphosphonates: prevalence, risk factors, and clinical characteristics. *Clin Ther.* 2007;29(8):1548–1558.

Bernabei R, Martone AM, Ortolani E, et al. Screening, diagnosis and treatment of osteoporosis: a brief review. *Clin Cases Miner Bone Metab.* 2014;11(3):201–207.

McClung M, Harris ST, Miller PD, et al. Bisphosphonate therapy for osteoporosis: benefits, risks, and drug holiday. *Am J Med.* 2013;126(1):13–20.

Cruzado JM, Moreno P, Torregrosa JV, et al. A randomized study comparing parathyroidectomy with cinacalcet for treating hypercalcemia in kidney allograft recipients with hyperparathyroidism. *J Am Soc Nephrol.* 2016;27(8):2487–2494.

WEBSITES

https://www.aace.com/publications/guidelines

This website is maintained by the American Association of Clinical Endocrinologists and contains clinical practice guidelines for the diagnosis and treatment of osteoporosis.

https://www.iofbonehealth.org/content-type-semantic-meta-tags/guidelines

This is the International Osteoporosis Foundation website with links to treatment guidelines for osteoporosis throughout the world.

http://www2.kidney.org/professionals/KDOQI/guidelines_bone/

This is the National Kidney Foundation website that contains Clinical Practice Guidelines for Bone Metabolism and Disease in Chronic Kidney Disease from the Kidney Disease Outcomes Quality Initiative.

SECTION 8

Chemotherapy

56

Principles of Antimicrobial Use

Rukiyah Van Dross-Anderson and Eman Soliman

INTRODUCTION

Viruses, bacteria, and other unicellular and multicellular organisms in the environment can live in the human body and can produce desirable or undesirable responses within the host. In a healthy person, normal bacteria in the gastrointestinal tract have beneficial effects, assisting in the production of vitamins and food digestion. However, when nonbeneficial, pathogenic organisms enter the body and multiply, they can lead to an infection, which typically generates an inflammatory response.

The types of organisms that invade the human body and cause unwanted biological responses include acellular, unicellular, and multicellular organisms. The only acellular organisms known to induce infectious diseases in humans are viruses. Prions, which are proteinaceous particles lacking nucleic acids, can also lead to infections. The smallest known pathogens, known as viroids, are circular, single-stranded RNA molecules that typically lead to infections in plants and do not contribute to human disease. Bacteria are unicellular, nonnuclear organisms. Higher orders of size and complexity are found in unicellular, nucleated fungi (including yeast and filamentous forms) and protozoa. Major differences include the addition of a membrane-enclosed nucleus and mitochondria within the cell. More complex fungi are found in the multicellular, nucleated molds. Still higher orders of parasitic organisms are helminths (worms), which are a medical problem in both industrialized and developing countries.

Invading organisms can be destroyed using antimicrobial agents, provided they have not developed resistance. The availability of antimicrobial drugs for the successful eradication of invading organisms varies considerably with the type and location of the organisms within the human host. Selective antimicrobials interact with specific components in a microorganism to affect its growth or survival. These agents are used to eradicate pathogenic organisms such as bacteria (antibiotics), protozoa (antiprotozoals), fungi (antifungals), viruses (antivirals), and worms (anthelmintics). In contrast, nonselective antimicrobials do not target a specific microbe but decrease the spread of infectious organisms and include disinfectants, preservatives, and antiseptics. Disinfectants (such as bleach and ammonia) are used to decontaminate surfaces on inanimate objects; preservatives (such as formaldehyde and thimerosal) are additives used to prevent biodeterioration in food, pharmaceutical products, and biological specimens by bacterial action; and antiseptics (such as alcohol and soaps) are topically applied to decontaminate skin, thereby containing and preventing the spread of infections, particularly in clinical settings.

Traditionally, the term antibiotic was used to refer to substances produced by microorganisms that suppress the growth of other microorganisms, while antibacterial was more encompassing and used to describe not only natural antibiotics produced by microorganisms but also drugs synthesized in the laboratory. The distinction between these compounds is somewhat blurred today, and both terms are often used interchangeably to refer to any synthetic, semisynthetic, or natural compound used in medicine to eradicate or injure bacteria.

The selection of an appropriate antibiotic must consider the interrelationships among the host, the pathogenic organism, and the antimicrobial, often referred to as the "triangle" or "triad" of interactions among these factors, as depicted in Fig. 56.1. The pharmacodynamic effects of the antimicrobial agent on the invading organism cannot be appreciated without consideration of the development of resistance by the organism in response to the drug. Similarly, the adverse effects of the drug on the host must consider drug pharmacokinetics by the host. Further, the immune response of the host as a consequence of the pathogenicity or virulence of the invading organism must also be taken into consideration. An understanding of all of the interrelationships among these factors is critical for the selection of an appropriate agent (Box 56.1).

This chapter presents an overview of the principles governing the selection of antibiotic agents, with many principles also applicable to antiparasitic, antiviral, and chemotherapeutic agents.

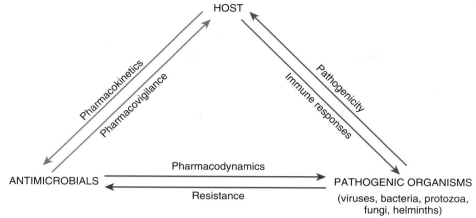

FIG. 56.1 Triad of Interactions Among the Host, Antimicrobial, and Pathogenic Organism.

BOX 56.1	Factors to Consider When Selecting Antimicrobial Agents for Therapy in Patients
Drug-Bacteria	Antibacterial spectrum, mechanism of action, selective toxicity, susceptibility of infecting microorganism, time-dependent and concentration-dependent killing effects, postantibiotic effect, need for bactericidal versus bacteriostatic agent, bacterial resistance
Host-Bacteria	Necessity for an antimicrobial agent, identification of the pathogen, host defense system, empiric, definitive and prophylactic therapy, combination therapy
Drug-Host	Pharmacokinetic factors (absorption, distribution, metabolism, elimination), age, adverse effects, allergy history, genetic or metabolic abnormalities

DRUG-BACTERIA INTERACTIONS

The primary consideration when selecting an antibacterial agent is often the nature of interactions between the drug and the bacteria. These interactions include pharmacodynamic considerations of the effect of the drug on the bacteria, including its spectrum of antibacterial activity and mechanism(s) of action, as well as the effect of the bacteria on the drug—that is, the development of resistance.

Antibacterial Spectrum

The antibacterial spectrum of a particular agent includes the pathogenic organisms effectively targeted by that drug. For example, the spectrum of penicillin includes various species of *Streptococcus*, other gram-positive bacteria, spirochetes, anaerobes, and *Neisseria meningitidis*. Because organisms have different levels of responsiveness to each antimicrobial agent, the antibacterial spectrum can be classified further into **drugs of choice** and **alternative drugs**. Drugs of choice are the first agents to consider when an infection by a particular organism is suspected or has been verified. These agents have the best activity against the organism and often have favorable adverse effect profiles. Alternative drugs, on the other hand, have activity against a specific organism but display properties that do not favor their use as a first choice, such as reduced efficacy, increased adverse effects, or use only for resistant organisms. In most cases, multiple choices are available for each organism. Although it is preferential to use a drug of choice, some situations favor the use of alternatives. For example, if a patient is pregnant and the drug of choice for the particular organism is unsafe during pregnancy, an alternative should be selected.

The activity of an agent against bacteria can also be described as **broad**, **narrow**, or **extended spectrum**. Broad-spectrum antibiotics are active against a wide range of pathogens and are often administered when the causative organism has not been identified. Tetracyclines, some cephalosporins, fluoroquinolones, and carbapenems are examples of broad-spectrum agents. Narrow-spectrum antibiotics are effective against a single or limited group of pathogens and are administered when the pathogen has been identified and its susceptibility is known. Natural penicillins, penicillinase-resistant penicillins, and monobactams are examples of narrow-spectrum agents. Extended-spectrum antibiotics possess an intermediate range of activity and include the aminopenicillins, antipseudomonal penicillins, and some cephalosporins.

Mechanisms and Sites of Action

The major antibacterial agents may be classified into three primary groups according to their mechanism(s) and sites of action—namely, agents affecting cell walls and membranes, agents inhibiting protein synthesis, and agents inhibiting DNA. The general structure of bacteria, illustrating the targets of antibacterial agents, is shown in Fig. 56.2. Further details about gram-negative and gram-positive cell walls are shown in Chapter 57, Fig. 57.1.

Cell wall synthesis inhibitors include the β-lactam drugs (penicillins, cephalosporins, carbapenems, monobactams) and the **non–β lactam drugs** (vancomycin, telavancin, bacitracin, fosfomycin, and cycloserine), while **agents that disrupt cell membranes** include the **polymyxins** (colistin and polymyxin B) and **daptomycin**. Inhibiting proteins involved in cell wall synthesis results in weakened cell walls, leading to cell death. Similarly, altering the integrity of bacterial cytoplasmic membranes causes cell lysis. These agents are discussed in detail in Chapter 57. The **protein synthesis inhibitors** include the **aminoglycosides** such as **streptomycin**, the **tetracyclines** and glycylcyclines, the **macrolides**, such as **erythromycin** and **azithromycin**, and others including **chloramphenicol** and **clindamycin**. These agents bind to and inhibit the function of bacterial ribosomes to prevent bacterial growth or survival and are discussed in detail in Chapter 58. **Drugs that affect DNA** include the **sulfonamides** and **trimethoprim**, the **quinolones** such as **ciprofloxacin**, the **nitrofurans** such as **nitrofurantoin**, and the **nitroimidazoles** such as **metronidazole**. These drugs target bacterial proteins involved in DNA synthesis and maintenance, thereby interfering with survival and propagation of the organism. These agents are discussed in detail in Chapter 59.

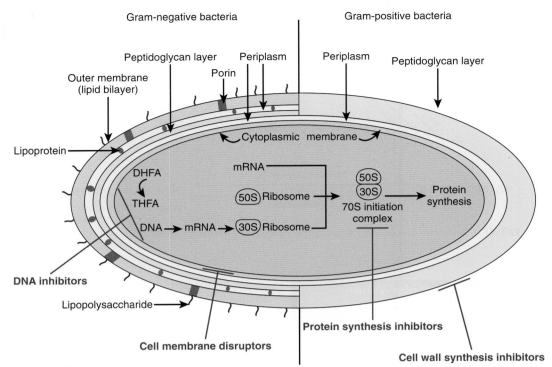

FIG. 56.2 Antimicrobial Sites and Mechanisms of Action. The cell walls of gram-negative and gram-positive bacteria are shown along with major sites and mechanisms of antibacterial drugs. *DHFA*, Dihydrofolic acid; *THFA*, tetrahydrofolic acid.

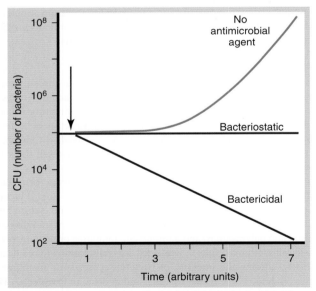

FIG. 56.3 Bactericidal Versus Bacteriostatic Antimicrobial Agents. A typical culture is started at 105 colony-forming units (CFU) and incubated at 37°C for various times. In the absence of an antimicrobial agent, there is cell growth. With a bacteriostatic agent added, no growth occurs, but neither are the existing cells killed. If the added agent is bactericidal, 99.9% of the cells are killed during the standardized test time.

Antimicrobial agents can also be classified as bactericidal (i.e., the organisms are killed) or bacteriostatic (i.e., the organisms are prevented from growing) as illustrated in Fig. 56.3. The major differences between bactericidal and bacteriostatic agents are summarized in Table 56.1. A given agent may demonstrate bactericidal actions under certain conditions and bacteriostatic actions under others, depending on the concentration of drug and the target bacteria. A bacteriostatic agent often is adequate in uncomplicated infections because the host defenses will help eradicate the microorganism. For example, in pneumococcal pneumonia, bacteriostatic agents suppress the multiplication of the pneumococci, and the pneumococci are destroyed by alveolar macrophages and polymorphonuclear leukocytes. For a neutropenic individual, such a bacteriostatic agent might prove ineffective, and a bactericidal agent may be necessary. Thus the status of the host may influence the selection of a bactericidal or bacteriostatic agent.

In addition, because the site of infection influences the ability of certain host defenses to contend effectively with microbes, bactericidal agents are required for the management of infections in areas "protected" from host immune responses, such as endocarditic vegetations and cerebrospinal fluid (CSF). In endocarditis, treatment with bacteriostatic antibiotics such as tetracyclines or erythromycin is associated with an unacceptably high failure rate; in contrast, treatment with bactericidal agents such as penicillin is associated with cure rates in excess of 95%.

Selective Toxicity

When an agent causes more harm to the bacteria than to the host by exploiting the differences between the host and the invading organism, it is referred to as selective toxicity. Because eukaryotic cells do not possess a cell wall, cell wall synthesis inhibitors are preferentially toxic to the organism. Similarly, protein synthesis inhibitors target prokaryotic ribosomes (50S and 30S) rather than eukaryotic ribosomes (60S and 40S), thereby exhibiting selective toxicity. Drugs that affect DNA achieve selective toxicity by targeting bacterial proteins needed for DNA replication and maintenance. In general, agents that are selectively toxic produce fewer adverse effects in the host because of the preferential activity toward the microbial target.

	Bactericidal	**Bacteriostatic**
Effect	Kills bacteria	Inhibits the growth of bacteria
Number of bacteria	Falls rapidly after drug exposure	Remains relatively constant
Activation of host immune system	NOT required (can be used in immunocompromised host)	Required (used only in immunocompetent host)
Uses	Life-threatening and deep-seated infections (e.g., endocarditis, meningitis)	Non–life-threatening infections
Examples	Cell wall synthesis inhibitors, aminoglycosides, fluoroquinolones, sulfonamide + trimethoprim	Tetracyclines, chloramphenicol, macrolides, clindamycin, sulfonamides, trimethoprim

TABLE 56.1 Comparison Between Bactericidal and Bacteriostatic Antimicrobial Agents

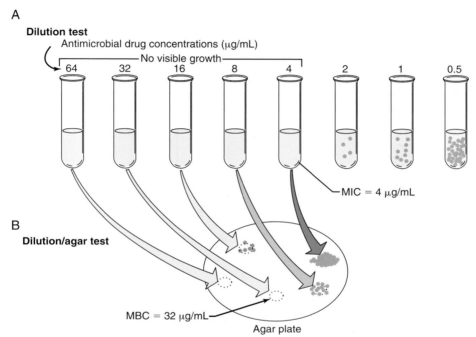

FIG. 56.4 Dilution/Agar Tests for Determination of MIC and MBC for a Given Drug and Microorganism. (A) Dilution test: each tube contains 5×10^5 colony-forming units of bacteria, plus antibiotic at the concentration indicated. The MIC is the minimal drug concentration at which no visible growth of bacteria is observed (4 µg/mL in this example). This method has been adapted to automated systems by using a microtiter plate instead of test tubes. (B) Dilution/agar test: each tube in A that shows no visible growth is cultured on a section of the new agar plate (no additional antibiotic is added to the agar plate). The MBC is the lowest concentration at which no growth occurs on the agar (32 µg/mL in this example).

Microorganism Susceptibility

The susceptibility of bacteria to specific antimicrobial agents can be determined in cell culture. The results of these tests are not generally available until 18–48 hours after an initial culture sample has been obtained. Susceptibility testing is often performed by automated systems based on the broth dilution method in which antibiotics are tested in serial dilutions that encompass the concentrations normally achieved in humans. This method detects the lowest concentration of antimicrobial agent that prevents visible growth after incubation for 18–24 hours, referred to as the minimal inhibitory concentration (MIC). The technique is shown in Fig. 56.4. This same test procedure can be extended to determine the minimal bactericidal concentration (MBC), or minimal concentration that kills 99.9% of cells. MBC determinations are no longer used regularly in most clinical laboratories.

Another method for determining bacterial susceptibility to antibiotics is the disk diffusion method, in which disks impregnated with the drugs to be tested are placed on an agar plate freshly inoculated with the bacterial strain in question (Fig. 56.5). After the plates have been

incubated for 18–24 hours, bacterial growth is apparent everywhere except near the disks, where a "zone of inhibition" may be present, indicating that the bacterial strain is susceptible to the antibiotic in the disk. This test is simple to perform, but only semiquantitative, and not useful for determining the susceptibility of many slow-growing or fastidious organisms; it has been replaced by automated broth dilution systems in many laboratories. A newer and related method is the E-test, which uses a strip containing the antibiotic in a concentration gradient along with a numerical scale instead of a disk. The point where the zone of inhibition touches the strip indicates the MIC (Fig. 56.6). Because of the many antimicrobial agents available, it is difficult to test all agents against an isolate. Thus laboratories often use one compound as representative of a class. It is important to recognize that susceptibility tests require interpretation, are not error proof, and may fail to identify a resistant population.

Drug Properties That Affect Dosing

Antibiotics may exhibit concentration- or time-dependent killing effects depending on their properties. Certain antibiotics, including the

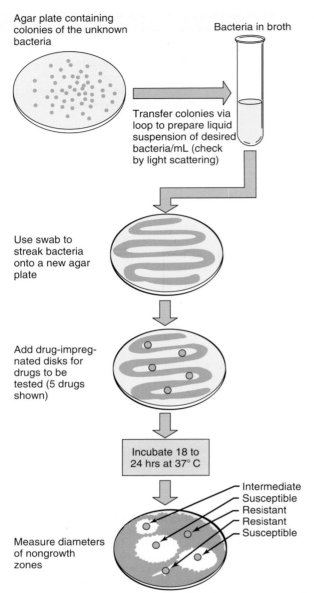

FIG. 56.5 Disk Diffusion Method for Testing Bacteria for Susceptibility to Specific Antimicrobial Agents.

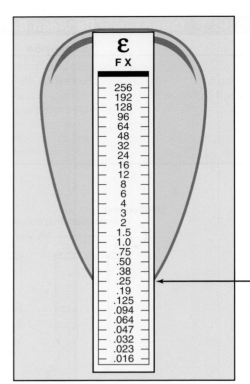

FIG. 56.6 E-Test Method for Susceptibility Testing. A labeled strip impregnated with a gradient of antibiotic is placed on a freshly inoculated agar plate. The point where the border of the zone of inhibition touches the strip defines the MIC *(arrow)*.

fluoroquinolones and aminoglycosides, exhibit **concentration-dependent killing** for which the rate and extent of effects increase with increasing plasma levels above the MIC. The clinical goal for administering this type of agent is to maximize the drug dosage and minimize the duration of exposure. Conversely, other agents, such as the β-lactam antibiotics and vancomycin, exhibit **time-dependent killing** for which the rate and extent of effects increase with time as long as the plasma concentration is above the MIC. The clinical goal for agents that kill bacteria in a time-dependent manner is to maximize the duration and minimize the concentration of drug exposure.

The **postantibiotic effect** is the period of time in which the serum concentration of the drug is below the MIC and bacterial growth is suppressed. Most bactericidal agents exhibit a postantibiotic effect, including the β-lactams, fluoroquinolones, aminoglycosides, rifampin, and vancomycin. In addition, some bacteriostatic agents, including tetracycline, clindamycin, and the macrolides, exhibit a postantibiotic effect. The mechanisms mediating this effect are unclear but may be due to the persistence of antibiotic at the target site, slow recovery after reversible nonlethal damage caused by the antibiotic, or the lag time required by bacteria to synthesize new enzymes and cellular components. The postantibiotic effect allows for less frequent drug dosing.

Bacterial Resistance

Drug resistance can be defined as the ability of bacteria to withstand the effects of an antibacterial agent. **Susceptible** (sensitive) bacteria have MIC values that can be achieved in the blood or other appropriate body fluid using the recommended doses. In contrast, **resistant bacteria** have MIC values that exceed recommended levels. Some bacteria have MIC values in between the susceptible and resistant levels. The importance of antibiotic resistance cannot be overstated, as the ability of bacteria to develop resistance to multiple drugs threatens many of the chemotherapeutic advances of the antimicrobial era. There are several consequences of antibiotic resistance; the most obvious is that treating a patient with an ineffective drug will lead to therapeutic failure or relapse. The development of resistance also forces physicians to use newer, more costly, and sometimes more toxic agents. Resistant bacteria have a competitive advantage over other flora and, under the pressure of heavy antibiotic use, can spread in the hospital environment. Because of resistance, the number of untreatable infections has increased dramatically in the past several decades. **Multidrug-resistant (MDR)** bacteria are increasing and spreading worldwide. Examples of MDR gram-positive bacteria include penicillin-resistant *Streptococcus pneumoniae* (PRSP), methicillin-resistant *Staphylococcus aureus* (MRSA), vancomycin-resistant *S. aureus* (VRSA), vancomycin-resistant enterococci (VRE), and *Clostridium difficile*. Examples of MDR gram-negative bacteria include carbapenem-resistant Enterobacteriaceae (CRE), *Neisseria gonorrhoeae*, *Pseudomonas aeruginosa*, and *Acinetobacter* species. Additionally, MDR tuberculosis (MDR-TB) and extensively drug-resistant TB (XDR-TB) are of major concern because limited therapeutic options are available, leading to extensive morbidity and mortality (Chapter 60). Knowledge of the resistance patterns of organisms in the community and hospital

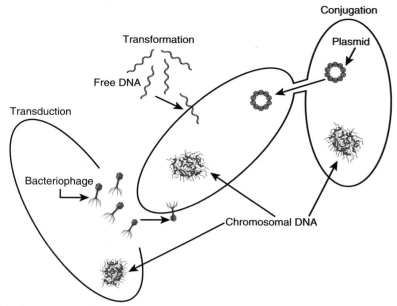

FIG. 56.7 Mechanisms of Genetic Exchange. Transformation is the ability of bacteria to take up free DNA from the environment. Transduction is the transfer of DNA from a bacteriophage to bacteria. Conjugation is the transfer of plasmid DNA from one bacterium to another and requires physical contact between cells.

setting helps direct therapy when the infecting organism and its drug susceptibility are unknown. In addition, recognizing that some bacteria have the propensity to develop resistance to certain antibiotics during a course of treatment should influence antibiotic selection even after the susceptibility profile is known.

Antibiotic resistance can be innate or acquired. **Innate resistance** is a result of natural structural or functional characteristics. For example, gram-negative bacteria are innately insensitive to many classes of antibiotics that are effective against gram-positive bacteria. This MDR phenotype is due to the presence of the gram-negative outer membrane (see Fig. 56.2), which is impermeable to many molecules, and to the expression of MDR efflux pumps that reduce the intracellular concentration of many drugs. **Acquired resistance** occurs via mutations in the genes associated with the antibiotic mechanism of action, such as mutations leading to alterations in the antibiotic target or in proteins enabling access of the antibiotic to the target, such as the porin proteins.

Acquired resistance can be due to the acquisition of foreign DNA coding for resistance determinants through **horizontal gene transfer**. Bacteria can acquire external genetic material through three main strategies: (1) **transformation**, (2) **transduction**, and (3) **conjugation** (Fig. 56.7). Transformation is the incorporation of naked DNA from the environment into bacteria, while transduction is the process in which viral bacteriophages inject genetic material into bacteria. Both transformation and transduction are not commonly associated with the development of clinically significant antibiotic resistance. However, conjugation is a very efficient method for spreading resistance genes that involves cell-to-cell contact. Conjugation uses mobile genetic elements such as plasmids and transposons, which play a crucial role in the development and dissemination of antimicrobial resistance among clinically relevant organisms. The transfer of plasmids by conjugation is the most important mechanism of acquisition of new resistance genes. Resistance plasmids (R plasmids) can carry resistance genes for one or several antimicrobial agents. The conjugative transfer of the plasmid requires that it contains the genes mediating conjugation and depends on its host range. Some plasmids can be transferred only to closely related strains; others can be transferred to a broad range of species;

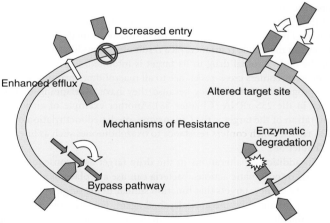

FIG. 56.8 The Major Mechanisms of Bacterial Resistance to Antibiotics. These mechanisms include altered receptors or targets to which the drug cannot bind, enhanced destruction or inactivation of drug, synthesis of resistant metabolic pathways, and decreases in the concentration of drug reaching the receptors by decreased entry or enhanced efflux.

thus they have great potential to spread resistance genes. **Transposons** are mobile genetic elements, which contain resistance genes. They can move from plasmid to plasmid or between plasmid and chromosome. They can be carried along with the plasmid genome to another strain by conjugation. Once transferred, the transposon either remains in the original plasmid, is inserted into a new plasmid, or is inserted into the chromosome. Transposons often have a broader host range than plasmids, and both are very effective means for spreading resistance genes.

The basic mechanisms of resistance to antimicrobial agents include:
- Modification of the drug target site
- Decreased drug access or accumulation
- Enzymatic inactivation of the drug
- Alteration of metabolic pathways

These mechanisms are depicted in Fig. 56.8. Microorganisms can utilize one or more of these mechanisms simultaneously.

Modification of the Drug Target Site

Modification of the drug target is one of the most common mechanisms of antibiotic resistance in bacteria. Changes to the drug target lead to resistance because the affinity of the drug for the modified drug target is reduced. Alterations in the drug target can result from gene-mediated mutations in the drug target, enzyme-mediated alterations of the drug target, and/or replacement of the original drug target.

A classic example of gene-mediated mutational resistance develops with rifampin. High-level rifampin resistance occurs by single-step point mutations in the *rpoB* gene encoding the β subunit of RNA polymerase, which is the target of rifampin (Chapter 60). Another well-characterized example of mutational resistance is the development of chromosomal mutations in the genes encoding the enzymes, DNA gyrase, and topoisomerase IV, the most frequent mechanism of acquired resistance to the fluoroquinolones (Chapter 59). Antibiotic resistance due to mutational changes is also responsible for resistance to the oxazolidinones such as linezolid, which involves the development of mutations in the genes encoding domain V of the 23S rRNA subunit, and/or the ribosomal proteins L3 and L4 (Chapter 58). Another example is resistance to trimethoprim-sulfamethoxazole (TMP/SMX), which can be attributed to mutations in the promoter region of the DNA-encoding dihydropteroic acid synthase and dihydrofolate reductase, leading to the production of increased quantities of the enzymes and overwhelming the ability of TMP-SMX to inhibit folate production (Chapter 59).

One of the best characterized examples of resistance through enzyme-mediated alterations of the drug target is the methylation of the 23S rRNA of the 50S ribosomal subunit catalyzed by an enzyme encoded by the *erm* genes (erythromycin ribosomal methylation), which results in macrolide resistance. As a result of this modification, binding of the antimicrobial drug to its target is inhibited. Expression of the *erm* genes confers cross-resistance to all macrolides, lincosamides, and streptogramin B antibiotics because they have overlapping binding sites in the 23S rRNA (Chapter 58). Another example of enzymatic alteration of the target is the Cfr enzyme–mediated methylation of the 23S rRNA, which confers resistance to oxazolidinones such as linezolid (Chapter 58).

In addition to alterations in the drug target as a consequence of genetic or enzymatic actions, bacteria can use a replacement strategy and develop new targets that function similar to the original target but are not inhibited by the antimicrobial agent. For example, resistance to methicillin in *S. aureus* results from the acquisition of the *mecA* gene, which encodes PBP2a, a PBP that has a low affinity for the β-lactams, including the penicillins, and all of the cephalosporins except the fifth-generation (Chapter 57). Another important example of resistance due to replacement is vancomycin resistance in enterococci, which involves the acquisition of *van* gene clusters. These gene clusters code for biochemical machinery that remodels the synthesis of the peptidoglycan by changing the normal D-alanine-D-alanine terminal peptide to D-alanine-D-lactate, which decreases the affinity of the antibiotic for its target by about 1000-fold (Chapter 61).

Decreased Drug Access or Accumulation

The access of the antibiotic to, or accumulation at, its sites(s) of action can be altered by bacteria by either decreasing drug influx or increasing drug efflux. Down regulation or mutations of the genes encoding the outer membrane channels known as porins confer resistance to antibiotics such as the β-lactams, tetracyclines, and some fluoroquinolones, all of which use these channels to enter the bacteria. Reductions in porin expression significantly contribute to the resistance of Enterobacteriaceae, and both *Pseudomonas* and *Acinetobacter* species, to the carbapenems and cephalosporins.

Bacteria can also overexpress efflux pumps, which actively transport many antibiotics out of the cell and contribute to the innate resistance of gram-negative bacteria to many drugs. Many classes of efflux pumps have been characterized in both gram-negative and gram-positive pathogens, several of which transport a wide range of structurally dissimilar substrates and confer resistance to several antimicrobial classes, including the tetracyclines, macrolides, fluoroquinolones, β-lactams, carbapenems, and polymyxins. For example, one family of MDR efflux pumps, the resistance-nodulation division in gram-negative bacteria (e.g., AcrB in *Escherichia coli* and MexB in *P. aeruginosa*), transport a wide array of substrates, conferring resistance to the tetracyclines, chloramphenicol, some β-lactams, novobiocin, fusidic acid, and the fluoroquinolones. Other resistance efflux pumps are the Tet and Mef systems, which contribute to the resistance to both the tetracyclines and macrolides, respectively.

Enzymatic Inactivation of the Drug

Enzyme-catalyzed inactivation of antibiotics is a major mechanism of resistance. Many enzymes have been identified that can degrade and modify antibiotics of different classes, including the β-lactams, aminoglycosides, and macrolides. For example, the main mechanism of resistance to the β-lactam antibiotics, such as the penicillins, cephalosporins, carbapenems, and monobactams, relies on destruction of these compounds by a diverse range of β-lactamase enzymes. Moreover, the enzyme-catalyzed addition of chemical groups to antibiotics causes resistance by preventing the drug from binding to its target due to steric hindrance. Modifying enzymes that acetylate, phosphorylate, and adenylate drugs are noted for producing this type of drug inactivation. For example, aminoglycoside-modifying enzymes (AMEs) that covalently modify the hydroxyl or amino groups of the aminoglycoside molecule have become the predominant mechanism of aminoglycoside resistance worldwide. Another classic example of enzymatic drug inactivation involves the modification of chloramphenicol by the expression of acetyltransferases known as CATs (chloramphenicol acetyltransferases).

Alteration of Metabolic Pathways

Another resistance strategy employed by bacteria is altering the metabolic pathways targeted by the antibacterial agent. For example, although most bacteria must synthesize folic acid for DNA synthesis, some bacterial strains have altered pathways that enable them to obtain folic acid from the environment. Because the sulfonamides exert their antibacterial action by inhibiting an enzyme needed for folic acid synthesis (Chapter 59), resistant bacteria acquire folic acid from an alternative source, thereby eliminating the need for folic acid synthesis and obviating the drug target.

Preventing Antibacterial Resistance

The persistence and spread of resistance are usually favored by human factors, such as the inappropriate use of antimicrobial agents. Prescribing antibacterial agents for viral infections, using broad-spectrum agents when narrow- or extended-spectrum agents are appropriate and using an agent at an improper dose or exposure duration all contribute to the development of resistance. In addition, many countries allow self-prescription of antibiotics, which may contribute to resistance. The addition of antimicrobials to livestock feed (for their growth-promoting effects) is also a major source of bacterial resistance. Animals fed antimicrobials can rapidly develop resistant enteric flora, which can be transferred to humans who handle or consume these animal products. Therefore many countries have banned the addition of antimicrobial agents (used in humans) to animal feeds. Eventually, bacteria will develop resistance to antibiotics in response to selective pressure, which has the potential to occur more rapidly than new antibiotics can be developed. Therefore coordinated and sustained efforts are required to minimize the spread of antimicrobial resistance. This coordinated response to antibiotic resistance is called "antimicrobial stewardship." Many hospitals now have formal stewardship programs as a part of their infection prevention efforts.

HOST-BACTERIA INTERACTIONS

The nature of interactions between the host and the bacteria influences the selection of an appropriate antimicrobial agent. These interactions include how the bacteria affect the host through the manifestation of disease, as well as how the host responds to the bacteria, primarily through immune responses.

Pathogen Identification and Disease Manifestation

Bacteria are capable of colonizing in virtually every location of the body, resulting in the development of a variety of infections. For many infections, samples of the possible pathogen or pathogens should be obtained and identified before initiating therapy because drug therapy can decrease the yield of a culture. Gram staining is the fastest, simplest, and most inexpensive method to identify bacteria and fungi, and results can be used to guide the initial antimicrobial choice. Normally sterile body fluids, as well as wound exudates, sputum, and fecal material, should be Gram stained to yield information about the infecting microorganisms.

Host Defenses

Considerations must be given to host defenses against the bacteria. An absence of white blood cells predisposes a patient to serious bacterial infections, and bacteriostatic agents are often ineffective in treating serious infections in neutropenic hosts. The critical white blood cell count is between 500 and 1000 mature polymorphonuclear cells/mm^3. Bactericidal agents are also required in the setting of other host defects, such as agammaglobulinemia or asplenia, the latter predisposing patients to pneumococcal or *Haemophilus* infection. The absence of complement components C7 to C9 predisposes patients to serious infection with *Neisseria* species. Knowledge of the organisms most frequently causing infections in patients with defects of white blood cells, complement, T cells, or immunoglobulin production aids in the selection of bactericidal agents when fever develops.

DRUG-HOST INTERACTIONS

The interactions between the host and the drug must also be considered carefully when selecting antibacterial agents. These interactions include how the host processes the drug (pharmacokinetics) and how the drug affects the host (adverse effects).

Pharmacokinetic Factors

Pharmacokinetic principles determine the amount of antimicrobial that is needed to obtain the appropriate drug concentration at the site of infection (Chapter 3). Considering the variation in absorption, distribution, metabolism, and elimination of the antimicrobial agents in concert with the effects of hepatic and renal function, as well as age, on pharmacokinetic parameters, it is no surprise that drug pharmacokinetics are critical in selecting the proper drug.

Absorption

Antimicrobial agents are usually administered by oral (PO), intramuscular (IM), or intravenous (IV) routes. Most oral antimicrobial agents reach peak serum concentrations within 1–2 hours. However, drug absorption may be less following oral administration than after other routes if the agent is unstable in the presence of stomach acids. Furthermore, the absorption of some drugs is delayed or inhibited when ingested with food or polyvalent cations or if patients have delayed intestinal transit time, such as occurs with diabetes. Consistent with this, antimicrobial agents vary widely in their oral bioavailability. For example, agents such as TMP/SMX, the fluoroquinolones, rifampin, and metronidazole are almost completely absorbed after oral administration and can often be used orally even when a severe infection is present. In contrast, the aminoglycosides, vancomycin, and some sulfonamides have poor bioavailability, necessitating administration through alternative routes. Parenteral therapy ensures adequate serum levels, and for many agents, higher drug levels can be achieved when administered IV. As such, most life-threatening infections are treated, at least initially, with IV agents.

Distribution

Antimicrobial agents must reach the anatomical site of infection in adequate concentrations to eliminate the infection. However, in some cases, the site of infection is not easily penetrated. Thus the dose, route, and duration of administration are critical determinants of antibacterial efficacy. The desired peak concentration of drug at the site of infection should be at least four times the MIC. However, if host defenses are adequate, peak concentrations may be much lower and even equal to the MIC and still be effective. When host defenses are absent or inoperative, peak concentrations 8- to 16-fold greater than the MIC may be required.

Most antimicrobial agents readily enter body tissues and compartments, except for the CSF, brain, prostate, and bone. Meningitis is a difficult infection to treat because many antimicrobial agents do not cross the blood-brain or blood-CSF barriers very well (Box 56.2). Therefore infections of the central nervous system (CNS) often require the use of lipid-soluble agents, which easily enter the CSF, such as chloramphenicol, metronidazole, minocycline, cefepime, and some fluoroquinolones. Aminoglycosides are ineffective against CNS infections because they do not enter the CSF, even in the presence of inflammation. The penicillins, aztreonam, the cephalosporins, and the carbapenems enter the CSF to variable degrees in the presence of inflamed meninges. The quinolones such as ciprofloxacin also enter the CSF at concentrations adequate to kill some microorganisms. Vancomycin is active against all pneumococci, and because of possible resistance to other agents, it is used routinely as part of empiric therapy for pneumococcal meningitis, yet microbiologic failures of vancomycin have been reported because this agent does not penetrate into the CSF sufficiently to guarantee acceptable bactericidal levels.

BOX 56.2 Ability of Antibiotics to Enter the Cerebrospinal Fluid in Effective Concentrations	
Readily enter CSF	Chloramphenicol, sulfonamides, trimethoprim, rifampin, metronidazole, cefepime, minocycline
Enter CSF only when inflammation is present	Penicillin G, ampicillin, piperacillin, oxacillin, nafcillin, cefuroxime, cefotaxime, ceftriaxone, ceftazidime, aztreonam, ciprofloxacin, vancomycin, meropenem, imipenem
Do not enter CSF adequately to treat infection	Cefazolin, cefoxitin, erythromycin, clindamycin, tetracycline, gentamicin, tobramycin, amikacin, streptomycin, doxycycline, clarithromycin, azithromycin

Similarly, the prostate epithelium is difficult to penetrate. Inflammation of the prostate reduces the intracellular pH, and thus antibiotics that are weak bases, such as trimethoprim, the sulfonamides, tetracyclines, fluoroquinolones, and metronidazole, are useful in prostatitis because they become trapped in the prostate.

Osteomyelitis is a bone infection that requires prolonged therapy. Drug administration for less than 4 weeks is usually associated with high rates of failure because the concentration of antibiotic in bone is often low, and the anatomy of bone is such that bacteria can avoid contact with the antibiotic.

Endocarditis is also difficult to treat because bacteria trapped in a fibrin matrix divide slowly, and many antibiotics are effective only on rapidly growing microorganisms. Therefore antibiotics used in endocarditis must be bactericidal, administered at high concentrations, and administered for prolonged periods to enable the antibiotic to diffuse into the matrix to kill all bacteria.

Frequently, antimicrobial drug therapy is ineffective in the presence of a foreign surface such as an artificial joint or a prosthetic heart valve. Many microorganisms grow at a slow rate in a sessile form that accumulates on the foreign surface and becomes covered with a glycocalyx. The coating protects the bacteria from attack by leukocytes and, most important, from destruction by antimicrobial agents.

Microorganisms also persist in abscesses because circulation is impaired, reducing delivery of antibody, complement, and leukocytes. Moreover, complement is destroyed in abscesses and cannot potentiate the destruction of bacteria by leukocytes. In addition, leukocytes function less effectively in an abscess because of the absence of adequate oxygen and the acidic environment. Bacteria in an abscess frequently grow slowly compared with other infection sites and are not as easily killed by antimicrobial agents that are effective when bacteria are rapidly dividing. In some situations, the antimicrobial agent is destroyed by enzymes induced by the microorganisms or by enzymes released when the microorganisms are killed by the antibiotic. Antibiotic therapy can rarely cure established abscesses, lesions containing foreign bodies, or infections associated with excretory duct obstruction unless these sites are drained surgically.

Some infections are the result of microorganisms that survive inside of polymorphonuclear phagocytes or macrophages following their ingestion. *Mycobacterium, Legionella,* and *Salmonella* species survive within phagocytic cells, and antimicrobial agents that fail to penetrate these cells are not successful in eradicating infection caused by these organisms. Compounds such as isoniazid and rifampin are successful in the treatment of *Mycobacterium tuberculosis* because these agents enter mononuclear cells in which tubercle bacilli survive, and the antimicrobial agents kill the bacilli within these phagocytic cells (Chapter 60).

Bacterial infections associated with obstructions of the urinary, biliary, or respiratory tracts tend to persist despite antibiotic therapy because antimicrobial agents penetrate these areas very poorly. In addition, bacteria present in the obstructed regions are in a quiescent state from which they emerge after antimicrobial therapy is discontinued, and most agents do not kill resting bacteria.

Placental distribution during pregnancy. Almost all antimicrobial agents cross the placenta to some degree and may affect the fetus. With most agents, the greatest risk of teratogenic and toxic effects on the fetus is in the first trimester. Metronidazole is teratogenic in lower animals, but it is not clear if this drug poses a risk to human fetuses. Other agents such as rifampin and trimethoprim may have a teratogenic potential and should be used only when alternative agents are unavailable. Quinolones cause cartilage abnormalities in animal models, but as with some other agents, it is not clear if these effects translate to significant human health risks.

The use of the tetracyclines in pregnancy should be avoided because they alter fetal dentition and bone growth. Tetracyclines have also been

BOX 56.3 Antimicrobial Agents to Be Used With Caution or Avoided During Pregnancy

Agent	Potential Toxicity
Aminoglycosides	Damage to cranial nerve VIII
Chloramphenicol	Gray baby syndrome
Clarithromycin	Possible increased spontaneous abortion risk
Erythromycin estolate	Cholestatic hepatitis in mother
Imipenem	Unclear
Linezolid	Various fetal toxicities
Sulfonamides	Hemolysis in newborn with glucose-6-phosphate dehydrogenase deficiency; increased risk of kernicterus
Tetracyclines	Limb abnormalities, dental staining, inhibition of bone growth
Trimethoprim	Altered folate metabolism
Quinolones	Abnormalities of cartilage
Vancomycin	Possible auditory toxicity

associated with hepatic, pancreatic, and renal damage in pregnant women. Streptomycin has been associated with auditory toxicity in children of mothers treated for tuberculosis, and the sulfonamides should not be used in the third trimester of pregnancy because they may displace bilirubin from albumin-binding sites and cause CNS toxicity in the fetus. Antimicrobial agents that should be used with caution or avoided during pregnancy are summarized in Box 56.3.

Many antibiotics are excreted in breast milk and can cause direct adverse effects, alter the microflora in the newborn, or act as sensitizing agents to cause future allergy. Therefore antibiotics also should be used cautiously in women who are breastfeeding.

Metabolism

Both host and bacteria can express enzymes that inactivate antibacterial agents before these drugs have a chance to interact with their cellular targets. For example, the β-lactam antibiotics are inactivated by β-lactamases produced by bacteria. To overcome this effect, innovative drug design has been employed to develop inhibitors of the β-lactamases and β-lactamase antibiotics that are more resistant to destruction by these enzymes, such as ceftriaxone (Chapter 57). Similarly, host enzymes can also destroy antibacterial agents. The host enzyme, renal dehydropeptidase, metabolizes imipenem to an inactive compound. To prevent drug inactivation, imipenem is available in a fixed-drug combination with cilastatin, an inhibitor of renal dehydropeptidase.

Elimination

Hepatic and renal excretion are the primary routes of elimination for drugs. In patients with compromised liver or kidney function, drug accumulation can occur and increase the risk of adverse effects. Therefore it is important to consider liver and kidney function when prescribing antimicrobial and other agents.

Hepatic function. Antimicrobials metabolized by the liver include chloramphenicol, erythromycin, clarithromycin, rifampin, metronidazole, and some of the quinolones. It may be necessary to reduce the doses of these agents to avert toxic reactions in patients with impaired hepatic function. Chloramphenicol toxicity in newborns stems from the inability of underdeveloped livers to convert the drug to an inactive, nontoxic glucuronide. The resulting toxicity is acutely life-threatening and is classically known as "gray baby syndrome."

Renal function. The presence of reduced renal function may influence the choice of an antibiotic and the dosage used. Many antimicrobial agents are eliminated from the body by renal filtration or secretion, and some of these agents can accumulate in the body and cause serious toxic reactions unless there is dose adjustment for reduced renal function. Antimicrobial agents that require dose adjustment include the aminoglycosides, vancomycin, certain penicillins, most cephalosporins, the carbapenems, and the quinolones. Failure to adjust dosage can lead to ototoxicity from aminoglycosides and neurotoxicity from the penicillins, imipenem, or the quinolones. The aminoglycosides can cause renal toxicity and should be used with caution in patients with preexisting renal insufficiency. Dose adjustments for agents eliminated by glomerular filtration usually can be estimated on the basis of the patient's age and body size and on serum creatinine concentration.

Age

Because pharmacokinetic properties change with age, it is important to consider this variable when selecting antimicrobial agents. Renal function decreases with age; therefore the dosage or administration interval of agents cleared by the renal route should be adjusted when used in elderly patients. The pH of gastric secretions is also affected by age, and this factor may influence selection of a drug. In addition, certain antibiotics such as the tetracyclines should not be given to children because they bind to developing teeth and bone. Similarly, sulfonamides should not be given to newborns because they displace bilirubin from serum albumin and can produce kernicterus, a CNS disorder.

Adverse Effects

Most commonly used antimicrobial agents have favorable safety profiles because of their selective toxicity. Although the potential for toxicity is always a concern, it is generally not the pivotal factor driving the selection process. Because of nephrotoxicity and ototoxicity, aminoglycoside use has decreased with the development of the β-lactams and fluoroquinolones with broad gram-negative activity. Unfortunately, the development of antibiotic resistance is beginning to force clinicians to return to antimicrobial agents that were once discarded for less toxic alternatives. For example, some strains of *P. aeruginosa* and *Acinetobacter* species have developed resistance to all commonly used agents, which has led to the recycling of parenteral polymyxin B, an agent with considerable toxicity that had not been used by a generation of physicians.

Allergy History

Obtaining a history of an adverse reaction to an antibiotic is valuable because a similar reaction to other members of the same drug class may occur. It is important to characterize the reaction to distinguish intolerance, such as gastrointestinal upset from a true allergy, and to recognize potentially life-threatening allergic reactions, such as anaphylaxis or exfoliative dermatitis. When these serious reactions occur, administration of chemically related compounds should be avoided. Significant allergy appears to be more common with the β-lactams, particularly the penicillins and sulfonamides. In anaphylactic reactions to penicillins, the immunoglobulin E antibody is usually directed at the penicillin nucleus, so the potential for allergic reactions to other penicillins is high. For many other allergic reactions, the potential for cross-allergy to related compounds is not known.

Genetic and Metabolic Abnormalities

Genetic abnormalities of host enzyme function may alter the toxicity of certain agents. For example, hemolysis in glucose-6-phosphate dehydrogenase–deficient individuals can be provoked by the sulfonamides, nitrofurantoin, pyrimethamine, the sulfones, and chloramphenicol. In addition, isoniazid may not be inactivated adequately in people who do not acetylate drugs well (50% of the United States population are slow acetylators), and peripheral neuropathy can develop in such patients unless they are treated with pyridoxine (vitamin B6). Thus pyridoxine is usually prescribed with isoniazid.

ANTIMICROBIAL THERAPY

Types of Antimicrobial Therapies

The three common types of antimicrobial therapies are definitive, empiric, and prophylactic therapy. Definitive drug therapy means that the selection of an antimicrobial agent is based upon the identification of the organism and its susceptibility to antibiotics. This type of therapy is not the initial therapeutic approach because 24–72 hours are needed to identify the pathogen(s) and determine drug susceptibility. Definitive drug therapy should be carried out with narrow- or extended-spectrum agents. Empiric therapy is the initial approach to treat bacterial infections and is guided by the clinical presentation and knowledge of the most common causative agents. This type of therapy utilizes broad-spectrum agents to cover multiple possible pathogens commonly associated with the specific clinical syndrome. In empiric therapy, other factors are important to consider, including where infection was acquired (hospital or community infection) and whether mechanical predisposing factors, such as indwelling catheters and respirators, were present. Also, common pathogens for certain infections, such as bacterial meningitis, are age dependent, and the age of the patient must be considered when utilizing empiric therapy. The use of agents with broad activity usually disturbs normal bacterial flora to a greater degree than narrow-spectrum therapy and may promote the development of antibiotic-resistant pathogens. Although empiric therapy is often used early in the course of therapy, the specter of antibiotic resistance and the added costs associated with broad therapy emphasize the importance of narrowing coverage when susceptibility testing results become available.

Prophylactic drug therapy is the use of an antimicrobial agent to prevent infection. Prophylaxis is often administered immediately after exposure to a virulent pathogen or before a procedure associated with an increased risk of infection. Chronic prophylaxis is sometimes administered to persons with underlying conditions that predispose to recurrent or severe infection. Several concepts are important in determining whether prophylaxis is appropriate for a particular situation. In general, prophylaxis is recommended when the risk of infection is high or the consequences of infection are significant. The nature of the pathogen, type of exposure, and immune competence of the host are important determinants of the need for prophylaxis. The antimicrobial agent should be able to eliminate or reduce the probability of infection, or, if infection occurs, reduce the associated morbidity. The ideal agent should be inexpensive, orally administered in most circumstances, have few adverse effects, have a minimal effect on the normal microbial flora, and have limited potential to select for antimicrobial resistance. Consequently, the choice of agents is critical, and the duration of prophylaxis should be as brief as possible; often a single dose is sufficient. The emerging crisis of antibiotic-resistant bacteria underscores the importance of rational, not indiscriminate use of antimicrobial agents.

The efficacy of prophylaxis is well established in situations such as perioperative antibiotic administration before certain surgical procedures, exposure to invasive meningococcal disease, and prevention of recurrent rheumatic fever. To prevent postoperative wound infections, the antimicrobial agent must be present at the surgical site when the area is exposed to the bacteria. The antibiotic should be given immediately preoperatively and should inhibit the most common and important bacteria likely to produce infection. Prophylaxis can be effective without eradication of all bacteria, so it is not essential to administer a broad-spectrum drug.

Prophylaxis is accepted in other situations without supporting data. When the risk of infection is low, such as the occurrence of bacterial endocarditis after dental procedures, randomized clinical trials of prophylaxis are not feasible. However, the consequences of infection may be catastrophic, providing a compelling argument for prophylaxis, despite the low risk of infection. People with valvular or structural lesions of the heart, in whom endocarditis is common, should receive antibiotic prophylaxis at the time of surgical, dental, or other procedures that may produce a transient bacteremia. Prophylaxis reduces the number of organisms that could lodge on the valvular tissue and alters the surface properties of the microorganism to reduce their affinity for cardiac tissue. The prophylactic antibiotic should be administered just before the procedure because limiting exposure minimizes the selection of resistant bacteria. Because viridans group streptococci from the mouth or intestine and enterococci from the intestine or genitourinary tract have a propensity to cause endocarditis, prophylaxis should be directed against these organisms.

Antimicrobial prophylaxis has been advocated after other exposures, including some bite wounds, *Haemophilus* meningitis, exposure to sexually transmitted diseases, and following sexual assault, influenza, and some potential agents of bioterrorism, including anthrax. Prophylaxis can prevent opportunistic infections in persons with AIDS and is sometimes used to prevent postsplenectomy infections, cellulitis complicating lymphedema, and recurrent lower urinary tract infections. Tuberculosis "prophylaxis" should be considered preemptive therapy because it is typically given to persons already infected with *M. tuberculosis* (by virtue of having a positive skin test) in an attempt to prevent clinical disease.

There are many other situations, some controversial, for which antimicrobial prophylaxis is used. When prophylaxis is advocated without data confirming efficacy, there should be a scientific rationale to support the use of a particular antimicrobial agent.

Drug Combination Therapy

The reasons for using antibiotic combinations are listed in Box 56.4. Although combination therapy is necessary, sometimes it tends to be overused. Some of the reliance on antibiotic combinations is due to an inability to identify the etiologic agent, forcing continuation of this type of therapy.

The consequences of using antimicrobial combinations directed at a single organism are shown in Fig. 56.9. **Synergism** is present if the activity of the combined antimicrobial agents is greater than the sum of the independent activities. **Indifferent** effects are present

---

BOX 56.4 Reasons for Concurrent Use of More Than One Antimicrobial Agent in a Patient

To treat a life-threatening or polymicrobial infection and provide coverage of multiple causative organisms

To provide coverage of potential causative agents during empiric therapy

To prevent the development of resistance in some but not all organisms (bacteria must develop resistance to multiple drug targets)

To achieve synergy (obtain enhanced antibacterial activity)

To permit the use of lower drug doses

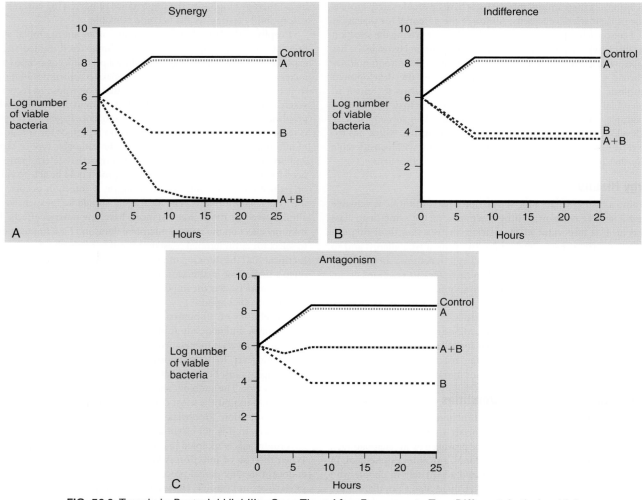

FIG. 56.9 Trends in Bacterial Viability Over Time After Exposure to Two Different Antimicrobial Agents (A and B) Demonstrating Synergy (A), Indifference (B), and Antagonism (C).

if the combined activity of the antimicrobial agents is similar to the greatest effect produced by an individual drug alone. Antagonism is present when the activity of the combination is less than what could have been achieved by using the agents separately.

When antimicrobial agents are used in combination, the desired effect is synergism. This effect has been documented for the following:

- The combination of an inhibitor of cell wall synthesis (such as penicillin or ampicillin) with an aminoglycoside antibiotic
- The combination of agents in which one compound (such as clavulanate, an inhibitor of β-lactamases) inhibits an enzyme that inactivates the other compound (such as amoxicillin)
- The combination of agents acting on sequential steps in a metabolic pathway (such as sulfonamide + trimethoprim)

A classic example of synergy is the use of penicillin or ampicillin plus an aminoglycoside to treat enterococcal endocarditis. Although penicillins are usually bactericidal, they affect enterococci in a bacteriostatic fashion, with a large difference between the inhibitory and bactericidal concentrations. Aminoglycosides alone are inactive against enterococci because they cannot get inside the cell to reach their ribosomal target site. The penicillins alter the cell wall of enterococci, allowing the aminoglycoside to enter the bacterial cell when both drugs are administered (Fig. 56.10). The combination is bactericidal, and this synergistic effect is critically important in the treatment of enterococcal endocarditis in humans.

The evidence that combination antimicrobial therapy is of value in life-threatening infections has been shown, albeit not consistently, in neutropenic patients. For example, the combination of an anti-pseudomonal penicillin and an aminoglycoside yielded better survival rates in some studies of patients with *Pseudomonas* sepsis. The major disadvantages of combination therapy for serious infections are the added cost and the risk of toxicity.

Combination therapy is sometimes used for polymicrobial infections, including those occurring at intraperitoneal and pelvic sites. Combination therapy is currently recommended for the empiric treatment of many patients with community-acquired pneumonia to treat both *S. pneumoniae* and atypical pathogens including *Mycoplasma*, *Chlamydia*, and *Legionella* species.

Combination therapy is essential for the treatment of tuberculosis because subpopulations of organisms intrinsically resistant to all first-line agents are present in patients with cavitary disease and a high organism burden (Chapter 60). In this setting, the use of multiple drugs prevents the resistant organisms from surviving. The ability of combination therapy to prevent the development of resistance by other bacteria is less well established.

Monitoring Antimicrobial Therapy

Because of the favorable safety profile of most antimicrobial agents, predictable pharmacokinetics, and the ability to achieve serum levels well above MICs, it is usually not necessary to monitor serum antibiotic concentrations. Agents for which serum levels are routinely obtained are those that have serious toxicity or narrow margins of safety, such as the aminoglycosides and vancomycin. Measuring serum concentrations of these agents can help ensure that therapeutic and not toxic levels are attained. This is particularly important in patients with diminished renal function, as these agents undergo renal elimination and have nephrotoxic potential.

Selection of an Antimicrobial Agent

The extensive variety of pathogenic bacteria, the numerous antibiotics available, and the significant list of factors to be considered in selecting antibiotic therapy on a rational basis can be confusing for students, as well as nonspecialists in infectious diseases. The relative activities of some representative antibiotics against individual microbial species are detailed in Table 56.2. Because the development of antibiotic resistance occurs at variable rates, the relative activities are approximate and subject to change.

In general, clinical personnel should resist prescribing antimicrobial therapy unless there is a reasonable probability that a bacterial infection is present. When the downside risk of withholding therapy is great, such as with bacterial meningitis or in clinically unstable patients, therapy should be started without delay, even when the presence of a bacterial infection is uncertain.

Bacteria and Anatomical Location

It is estimated that antimicrobial therapy is initiated in 75% of cases of bacterial infections before the pathogenic microorganisms have been identified and that the specific pathogenic organism is never identified in approximately 50% of treated infections. As discussed, because empiric therapy is often used in making treatment choices, it is important to be aware of the bacterial strains that may be present at selected anatomical sites. Many times, this may be the only meaningful way of guiding the selection of an antibiotic. Table 56.3 lists the common organisms that infect specific anatomical sites, and Table 56.4 lists organisms with the anatomical locations of the infection and the drugs often used for treatment. Most infections can be treated successfully with different antibiotics, and there may be more than one drug that results in successful therapy. When choosing a drug regimen, it is always important to consider the rates of local antibiotic resistance.

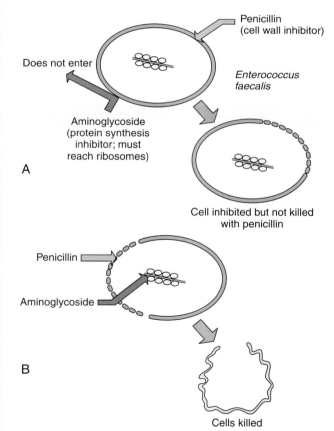

FIG. 56.10 An Example of Synergy Between Two Antibiotics. (A) Either penicillin or an aminoglycoside is administered; the cells are inhibited but not killed. (B) When penicillin and an aminoglycoside are administered concurrently, the penicillin compromises the cell wall, enabling the aminoglycoside to enter the cell and reach the ribosomes to prevent protein synthesis; therefore the cells are killed.

TABLE 56.2   Susceptibility of Common Bacteria to Antibiotics[a]

Organisms	Pen G	Ampicillin	Piperacillin	Piperacillin/ Tazobactam	Cefazolin (1st Gen)	Cefuroxime (2nd Gen)	Cefotaxime, Ceftriaxone, Ceftizoxime (3rd Gen)	Ceftazidime	Imipenem	Gentamicin	Amikacin	Doxycycline	Erythromycin	Clindamycin	Vancomycin	Ciprofloxacin	Levofloxacin
Gram Positive																	
Streptococcus pyogenes	4	4	4	4	4	4	4	3	4	0	0	3	3	4	4	2	4
Streptococcus pneumoniae	3	3	3	3	3	3	3	2	3	0	0	3	2	3	4	2	4
Staphylococcus aureus	0	0	0	2	2	2	2	1	2	1	2	2	2	2	4	1	2
Enterococcus faecalis	2	3	3	3	0	0	0	0	2	0[b]	0	0	1	0	3	1	1
Gram Negative																	
Escherichia coli	0	2	2	4	3	3	4	4	4	3	4	2	0	0	0	3	3
Klebsiella species	0	0	2	3	3	3	3	3	4	3	4	2	0	0	0	3	3
Enterobacter species	0	0	2	2	0	1	2	2	4	3	4	2	0	0	0	4	4
Pseudomonas aeruginosa	0	0	3	3	0	0	0	3	3	2	3	0	0	0	0	2	2
Haemophilus influenza	1	2	2	4	2	4	4	4	4	3	3	2	1	0	0	4	4
Anaerobes																	
Clostridium species	4	4	4	4	2	3	3	1	4	0	0	3	2	3	4	0	1
Bacteroides species	1	1	2	4	0	0	1	0	4	0	0	1	1	3	0	1	2

[a]Ratings based on tissue or plasma concentration expected for normal dosing schedule; 4, resistance uncommon; 3, clinically useful but not predictably active; 2, variably active; 1, limited activity or resistance widespread; 0, inactive.
[b]Has activity when combined with a cell wall active drug such as ampicillin.

TABLE 56.3   Common Microorganisms Causing Infections

Otitis Media
Streptococcus pneumoniae
Haemophilus influenzae
Moraxella catarrhalis
Viral

Sinusitis
Streptococcus pneumoniae
Haemophilus influenzae
Streptococcus species
Staphylococcus aureus
Anaerobes (chronic sinusitis)
Viral

Pneumonia
Streptococcus pneumoniae
Haemophilus influenzae
Moraxella catarrhalis
Chlamydia pneumoniae
Legionella pneumophila
Klebsiella pneumoniae
Staphylococcus aureus
Other gram-negative bacilli
Mixed anaerobes
Mycobacterium tuberculosis
Viral

Intraabdominal Sepsis
Escherichia coli
Klebsiella species
Enterobacter species
Proteus species
Enterococcus species
Bacteroides species
Anaerobic streptococci
Clostridium species

Gynecologic
Neisseria gonorrhoeae
Chlamydia species
Escherichia coli
Klebsiella species
Streptococcus species
Bacteroides species

Urinary Tract Infection
Escherichia coli
Klebsiella species
Proteus species
Enterococcus species
Staphylococcus saprophyticus
Pseudomonas species

Meningitis
Cryptococcus neoformans
Group B streptococci
Listeria monocytogenes
Haemophilus influenzae
Neisseria meningitidis
Streptococcus pneumoniae

Diarrhea
Salmonella species
Shigella species
Campylobacter species
Escherichia coli
Vibrio species
Yersinia species
Clostridium difficile
Viral

Skin
Group A streptococci
Staphylococcus aureus
Other streptococci
Gram-negative rods (rarer)

Endocarditis
Streptococcus viridans
Staphylococcus aureus
Enterococcus species
Coagulase-negative staphylococci
Gram-negative bacilli
Bartonella species

TABLE 56.4 Organisms With Common Infection Sites and Drugs of Choice for Treatment

Bacteria	Infection	First Choice	Alternatives
Gram Positive			
Staphylococcus aureus	Abscess, cellulitis, bacteremia, pneumonia, endocarditis	*Methicillin Susceptible* Cloxacillin, dicloxacillin (PO), nafcillin, oxacillin (parenteral) *Methicillin Resistant* Vancomycin + gentamicin + rifampin	1-Cephalosporin, vancomycin, clindamycin, imipenem, TMP-SMX, linezolid, daptomycin, tigecycline, fluoroquinolone
Streptococcus pyogenes (group A)	Pharyngitis Cellulitis	Penicillin V	1-Cephalosporin Clindamycin, macrolide
Streptococcus (group B) species	Meningitis Cellulitis, sepsis	Penicillin G Penicillin G or ampicillin	Cefotaxime, vancomycin 1-Cephalosporin
Enterococcus species	Bacteremia	Ampicillin	Vancomycin Linezolid if vancomycin resistant
	Endocarditis	Ampicillin/gentamicin	Vancomycin/gentamicin
	Urinary tract	Ampicillin	Fluoroquinolone, nitrofurantoin
Streptococcus viridans	Endocarditis	Penicillin/gentamicin	Cephalosporin, vancomycin
Streptococcus pneumoniae	Pneumonia	Penicillin G, ceftriaxone	Fluoroquinolone, vancomycin
	Otitis, sinusitis	Amoxicillin	Erythromycin
	Meningitis	Penicillin G (or, for penicillin-resistant strains, vancomycin)	Cefotaxime, ceftriaxone
Listeria monocytogenes	Bacteremia, meningitis, endocarditis	Ampicillin	TMP-SMX
Gram Negative			
Escherichia coli	Urinary tract	TMP-SMX, fluoroquinolone	Cephalosporin
	Bacteremia	3-Cephalosporin	TMP-SMX, fluoroquinolone
Klebsiella pneumoniae	Urinary tract	Fluoroquinolone	Cephalosporin, TMP-SMX
	Pneumonia, bacteremia	3-Cephalosporin	Imipenem, aztreonam, fluoroquinolone
Proteus mirabilis	Urinary tract	Ampicillin	TMP-SMX
Haemophilus influenzae	Otitis, sinusitis, bronchitis	Amoxicillin-clavulanate	2-3-Cephalosporin, TMP-SMX, azithromycin
	Epiglottitis	Cefotaxime, ceftriaxone	Cefuroxime
Pseudomonas aeruginosa	Urinary tract	Fluoroquinolone	Antipseudomonal penicillin, ceftazidime, aminoglycoside
	Pneumonia, bacteremia	Antipseudomonal penicillin, ceftazidime	Aztreonam, aminoglycoside, quinolones, carbapenem
Moraxella catarrhalis	Otitis, sinusitis	Amoxicillin-clavulanate	TMP-SMX, macrolide
Neisseria gonorrhoeae	Genital	Ceftriaxone	
Anaerobes			
Bacteroides species	Abdominal infections, abscesses	Metronidazole	Penicillin/β-lactamase inhibitor combinations, carbapenems, clindamycin
Clostridium perfringens	Abscesses, gangrene	Penicillin G	Metronidazole
Clostridium difficile	Diarrhea	Metronidazole	Vancomycin
Other			
Legionella species	Pulmonary	Azithromycin, fluoroquinolone	Erythromycin, doxycycline (± rifampin)
Mycoplasma pneumoniae	Pulmonary	Azithromycin, doxycycline	Ciprofloxacin, levofloxacin, clarithromycin
Chlamydia pneumoniae	Pulmonary	Doxycycline, azithromycin	Clarithromycin, fluoroquinolone
Chlamydia trachomatis	Genital	Azithromycin, doxycycline	Levofloxacin
Rickettsia species	Rocky Mountain spotted fever	Doxycycline	Chloramphenicol
Ehrlichia species	Ehrlichiosis	Doxycycline	Chloramphenicol

1-Cephalosporin, First-generation cephalosporin; *2-Cephalosporin*, second-generation cephalosporin; *3-Cephalosporin*, third-generation cephalosporin; *TMP-SMX*, trimethoprim-sulfamethoxazole.

SELF-ASSESSMENT QUESTIONS

1. Methicillin-resistant *Staphylococcus aureus* (MRSA) is a common nosocomial pathogen that is increasing in frequency in community settings. Which of the following statements best describes the most common mechanism of resistance by *S. aureus*?
   A. Acquisition of the novel protein PBP2a.
   B. Increased cell wall repair.
   C. Increased efflux of β-lactams.
   D. Increased synthesis of metabolic factors.
   E. Reduced permeability to β-lactams.

2. Antibiotics are commonly administered before surgical procedures. Which of the following statements best describes the guidelines for perioperative antimicrobial prophylaxis?
   A. Administer the antibiotic just prior to the procedure.
   B. Begin antibiotic prophylaxis at least 24 hours before surgery.
   C. Include an antifungal in the regimen.
   D. Select the broadest spectrum antibiotic for complete coverage.
   E. Use antibiotic combinations as opposed to monotherapy.

3. Individuals who are deficient in glucose-6-phosphate dehydrogenase are at a greater risk of developing hemolytic anemia in response to various drugs. Which one of the following classes of antibiotics has the greatest potential to result in this adverse effect in these patients?
   A. Cephalosporins.
   B. Macrolides.
   C. Quinolones.
   D. Sulfonamides.
   E. Tetracyclines.

4. When using combination antibiotic therapy, it is important to administer drugs that work synergistically if possible. Which one of the following represents a combination with known synergism?
   A. A β-lactam and an aminoglycoside.
   B. A penicillin and a cephalosporin.
   C. Two drugs in which the second drug will displace the first from plasma protein–binding sites.
   D. Two drugs that are eliminated by different routes.
   E. Two drugs that work on the same step in a metabolic pathway.

5. Bacteria develop resistance to tetracyclines by which primary mechanism?
   A. Altered ribosomal target.
   B. Bypass pathway in folic acid metabolism.
   C. Enzymatic inactivation.
   D. Increased drug efflux.
   E. Mutations of DNA gyrase gene.

FURTHER READING

Blanco P, Hernando-Amado S, Reales-Calderon JA, et al. Bacterial multidrug efflux pumps: much more than antibiotic resistance determinants. *Microorganisms*. 2016;4:14–32.

Bratzler DW, Houck PM. Antimicrobial prophylaxis for surgery: an advisory statement from the National Surgical Infection Prevention Project. *Clin Inf Dis*. 2004;38:1706–1715.

Leeka S, Terrell CL, Edson RS. General principles of antimicrobial therapy. *Med Lett Drugs Ther*. 2011;86(2):156–167.

Moellering RC, Graybill JR, McGowan JE, Corey L. Antimicrobial resistance prevention initiative—an update: proceedings of an expert panel on resistance. *Am J Med*. 2007;120:S4–S25.

WEBSITES

http://www.idsociety.org/Antimicrobial_Agents/

This website is maintained by the Infectious Diseases Society of America and is an excellent resource that contains guidelines on the uses of antimicrobial agents as well as information and guidelines regarding infectious diseases.

https://www.cdc.gov/getsmart/community/for-hcp/outpatient-hcp/adult-treatment-rec.html

This page is maintained by the Centers for Disease Control and Prevention and provides guidelines for the use of antimicrobial agents in both pediatric and adult patients.

Drugs Targeting Bacterial Cell Walls and Membranes

Rukiyah Van Dross-Anderson and Daniel A. Ladin

MAJOR DRUG CLASSES

β-Lactam cell wall synthesis inhibitors
  Penicillins
  Cephalosporins
  Carbapenems
  Monobactams
Non-β-lactam cell wall synthesis inhibitors
  Peptides
  Others
Cell membrane disrupters
  Lipopeptides

ABBREVIATIONS

CSF	Cerebrospinal fluid
ESBLs	Extended-spectrum β-lactamases
GI	Gastrointestinal
GlcNAc	*N*-Acetylglucosamine
IM	Intramuscular
IV	Intravenous
MRSA	Methicillin-resistant *Staphylococcus aureus*
MSSA	Methicillin-sensitive *Staphylococcus aureus*
MurNAc	*N*-Acetylmuramic acid
PBPs	Penicillin-binding proteins
VISA	Vancomycin-intermediate *Staphylococcus aureus*
VRE	Vancomycin-resistant *Enterococcus*
VRSA	Vancomycin-resistant *Staphylococcus aureus*

THERAPEUTIC OVERVIEW

Maintenance of the bacterial cell envelope, which consists of membranes, proteins, and other structures surrounding the cytoplasm, is critical for bacterial cell viability. The structures within the envelope not only protect the cell and serve as a barrier to the environment, but also carry out numerous functions that are conducted by intracellular organelles in mammalian cells.

The envelopes of gram-positive and gram-negative bacteria contain cell walls, as well as membranes, both of which serve as targets for antibiotic agents. Drugs affecting bacterial cell walls and membranes may be classified as the β-lactam cell wall synthesis inhibitors including the penicillins, cephalosporins, carbapenems, and monobactams; the non-β-lactam cell wall synthesis inhibitors, including the peptides vancomycin, telavancin, and bacitracin, and others such as fosfomycin and cycloserine, and the cell membrane disrupters that include the lipopeptides colistin, polymyxin B, and daptomycin. The organisms susceptible to and therapeutic applications of these groups of compounds are summarized in the Therapeutic Overview Box.

MECHANISMS OF ACTION

Bacterial Envelopes

The composition of gram-positive and gram-negative bacterial envelopes is shown in Fig. 57.1. Both gram-positive and gram-negative bacteria contain rigid cell walls composed of a highly cross-linked peptidoglycan matrix, but the relative thickness of the cell wall and presence and composition of membranes differ. Gram-positive bacteria contain a thicker (up to 100 nm), highly cross-linked peptidoglycan matrix with many more (15 to 30) layers than gram-negative bacteria, which have a peptidoglycan layer about 2–3 nm thick. In addition, gram-negative bacteria contain an outer membrane composed of phospholipids and lipopolysaccharides, that contain porin channels and other proteins, whereas gram-positive bacteria lack the outer membrane.

Both gram-positive and gram-negative bacteria have phospholipid cytoplasmic membranes that contain penicillin-binding proteins (PBPs), named because they covalently bind radiolabeled penicillin G. The PBPs are enzymes composed of two domains, the transglycosylase domain and the transpeptidase domain, both of which play a major role in the formation of the peptidoglycan layer.

The cell wall is assembled in a series of steps beginning within the cytoplasm and terminating on the outer side of the cytoplasmic membrane (Fig. 57.2). The glycan chain of the peptidoglycan is composed of repeating disaccharide units of *N*-acetylmuramic acid (MurNAc) attached to a pentapeptide and *N*-acetylglucosamine (GlcNAc), connected through β-1,4-linkages. The initial stage of peptidoglycan synthesis is known as the assembly stage during which MurNAc and GlcNAc are formed and the former attached to the pentapeptide. The GlcNAc-MurNAc-pentapeptide (a peptidoglycan unit) is transported by bactoprenol (undecaprenyl phosphate), which is a phospholipid carrier within the cytoplasmic membrane. Bactoprenol binds to and transports the peptidoglycan unit from the inner side to the outer side of the cytoplasmic membrane, after which it is monodephosphorylated to enable it to transport another peptidoglycan unit—that is, a recycling mechanism. The peptidoglycan units are linked in sequence to form long chains of alternating disaccharides, catalyzed by the transglycosylase subunit of PBP, followed by a polymerization stage that involves cross-linking to form continuous two-dimensional sheets, catalyzed by the transpeptidase subunit of PBP. During the cross-linking reaction, the transpeptidase displaces the final D-alanine (D-ala) from the D-ala-D-ala terminus of the pentapeptide, forming an acyl enzyme intermediate that readily couples to the free amino group of the third residue (L-lysine) of the pentapeptide of an adjacent chain. When cross-linking is complete, the enzyme is regenerated. Both bacterial cell walls and membranes are targets for several classes of pharmacological agents.

479

THERAPEUTIC OVERVIEW

β-Lactam Cell Wall Synthesis Inhibitors
Penicillins
Primarily aerobic and anaerobic gram-positive bacteria including *Clostridium*, *Listeria monocytogenes*, *Staphylococcus*, and *Streptococcus* species; some aerobic gram-negative bacteria including *Neisseria meningitidis* and *Pasteurella multocida*

Streptococcal skin and soft tissue infections, pneumococcal upper respiratory tract infections, oropharynx infections, scarlet fever, syphilis, bite wounds, sepsis (neutropenic patients)

Cephalosporins
Aerobic and anaerobic gram-positive and gram-negative bacteria (dependent on generation of cephalosporin) including *Staphylococcus aureus*, *Escherichia coli*, *Haemophilus influenzae*, *Moraxella catarrhalis*, *Pseudomonas aeruginosa*, *Proteus mirabilis*, *Neisseria gonorrhoeae*, *Streptococcus pneumoniae*, *N. meningitidis*, and Enterobacteriaceae, *Klebsiella*, *Proteus*, and *Streptococcus* species
Infections of the throat, lungs, ears, kidneys, bone and skin/soft tissue, urinary tract; gonorrhea; bacterial meningitis; Lyme disease

Carbapenems
Aerobic and anaerobic gram-positive and gram-negative bacteria including *P. aeruginosa*, *E. coli*, *Klebsiella pneumonia*, *Enterobacter cloacae*, *Citrobacter freundii*, *P. mirabilis*, *Serratia marcescens*, and *Acinetobacter*, *Staphylococcus*, and *Streptococcus* species
Abdominal and complicated urinary tract infections, sepsis, hospital-acquired pneumonia

Monobactams
Aerobic gram-negative bacteria including *P. aeruginosa* and Enterobacteriaceae
Bronchitis, pneumonia, sepsis, peritonitis, infections of the skin and urinary tract

Non-β-Lactam Cell Wall Synthesis Inhibitors
Vancomycin
Aerobic and anaerobic gram-positive bacteria including *Corynebacterium jeikeium* and *Bacillus anthracis* and *Clostridium*, *Enterococcus*, *Staphylococcus*, and *Streptococcus* species
Clostridium difficile infection, sepsis, pneumococcal meningitis, endocarditis

Telavancin
Aerobic gram-positive bacteria including MSSA, MRSA, VISA, *C. difficile*, and *Enterococcus* and *Streptococcus* species
Complicated skin and soft tissue infections, hospital-acquired pneumonia

Bacitracin
Aerobic and anaerobic gram-positive and gram-negative bacteria including *S. aureus*, *Staphylococcus epidermidis*, *Streptococcus pyogenes*, and *Clostridium* and *Neisseria* species
Uncomplicated skin and soft tissue wounds

Fosfomycin
Aerobic and anaerobic gram-positive and gram-negative bacteria including *E. coli*, *Enterococcus faecalis*, and Enterobacteriaceae
Uncomplicated urinary tract infections

Cycloserine
Aerobic gram-positive and gram negative bacteria including *E. coli*, *S. aureus*, *Nocardia*, and other *Enterococcus* species. Also includes *Mycobacterium tuberculosis* and *Chlamydia* species
Urinary tract infections, multidrug-resistant tuberculosis

Cell Membrane Disrupters
Colistin
Aerobic gram-negative bacteria including *E. coli*, *P. aeruginosa*, *Acinetobacter*, and *Enterobacter* and *Klebsiella* species
Eye infections; swimmer's ear (otitis externa); multidrug resistant gram negative infections

Daptomycin
Aerobic and anaerobic gram-positive bacteria including *C. difficile*, *Clostridium perfringens*, *E. faecalis* (vancomycin-susceptible only), *Streptococcus agalactiae*, *S. aureus* (including MSSA, MRSA, VISA, and VRSA), and *Enterococcus* and *Streptococcus* species
S. aureus bacteremia, complicated skin and skin structure infections, multidrug-resistant infections, endocarditis

β-Lactam Cell Wall Synthesis Inhibitors

The β-lactam antibiotics include the widely used **penicillins** and **cephalosporins**, as well as the **carbapenems** and **monobactams**. The general structures of agents in these classes are shown in Fig. 57.3. All β-lactam antibiotics have a four-membered ring containing a cyclic amide (the lactam) with the β denoting that the amine is located on the second carbon relative to the carbonyl group. This small ring is structurally strained with **low inherent stability** and is hydrolyzed in an acidic environment like the stomach, as well as by β-lactamases (also known as penicillinases), which represent a major mechanism of resistance to these compounds. Thus some penicillins (and some cephalosporins) that are susceptible to hydrolysis are administered in combination with an irreversible **β-lactamase inhibitor** such as **clavulanate**, **sulbactam**, and **tazobactam**.

The β-lactams are **bactericidal** under most conditions. These agents inhibit cell wall synthesis at the final cross-linking step and thus have maximal activity against rapidly dividing bacteria. Molecular modeling has demonstrated that the penicillins and cephalosporins can assume a conformation very similar to that of the D-ala-D-ala peptide. Thus the β-lactams serve as substrates for the enzyme, preventing peptidoglycan cross-linking and leading to weakened cell walls susceptible to lysis.

The effects of exposure to β-lactams depend on the bacterial species and the PBPs to which the drug binds. Some bacteria swell rapidly and burst; some develop into long filamentous structures that do not divide but eventually fragment, resulting in disruption of the organism, whereas others show no morphological change but cease to be viable. Lysis of gram-positive bacteria by β-lactams is ultimately dependent on **autolysins**, enzymes that normally hydrolyze the peptidoglycan matrix during cell division, hence promoting bacterial multiplication. There are "tolerant" bacteria that lack these autolysins, and in these organisms, the β-lactams are bacteriostatic rather than bactericidal.

Penicillins

The penicillins may be classified several different ways, typically according to either susceptible organisms (antistaphylococcal or broad or extended spectrum) or susceptibility to hydrolysis by β-lactamases. The natural penicillins, **penicillin G** and **penicillin V**, are the drugs of choice for many gram-positive organisms. The aminopenicillins,

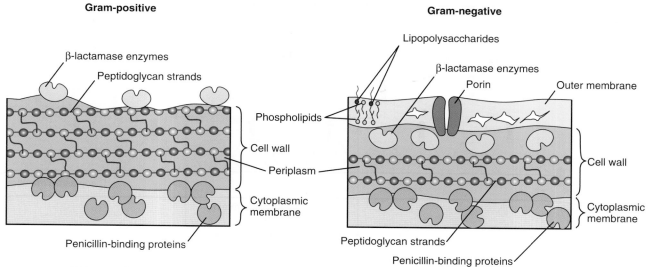

FIG. 57.1 Composition of Gram-Positive and Gram-Negative Bacterial Envelopes. Gram-positive bacteria contain a thicker cell wall composed of many (15–30) layers of rigid peptidoglycan strands, whereas gram-negative bacteria have a thinner wall (3–5 layers). Gram-negative bacteria also have an added outer membrane composed of phospholipids and polysaccharides that contains porin channels and other proteins. The inner or cytoplasmic phospholipid membrane present in both gram-positive and gram-negative cells contains penicillin-binding proteins that play a major role in the formation of the peptidoglycan layer.

amoxicillin and ampicillin, have a positively charged amino group that enhances transport through porin channels and are also inactivated by β-lactamases and therefore are most often combined with a β-lactamase inhibitor. The penicillinase-resistant penicillins (also known as the β-lactamase-resistant penicillins or antistaphylococcal penicillins) include oxacillin, cloxacillin, nafcillin, and dicloxacillin, and as their name implies, these compounds are resistant to destruction by most β-lactamases and are used principally to treat staphylococcal infections. The antipseudomonal penicillins include ticarcillin and piperacillin, are also subject to β-lactamase cleavage, and have an extended spectrum of activity.

Cephalosporins

The cephalosporins are structurally very similar to the penicillins; they contain a dihydrothiazine ring in place of the thiazolidine ring (see Fig. 57.3). Compounds that possess a methoxy group at position 7 are often called cephamycins, but for practical purposes, these agents can be considered cephalosporins. Similarly, agents in which the sulfur at position 5 has been replaced by an O_2 are oxycephems, and agents in which the sulfur is replaced with a carbon are called carbacephems. These agents are considered cephalosporins from both microbiological and pharmacological perspectives.

The cephalosporins have a broad spectrum of activity and encompass five generations of agents, with cefazolin and cephalexin representing the first generation, cefaclor and cefprozil representing the second generation, and ceftriaxone and cefixime representing the third generation; cefepime is the only fourth-generation compound and ceftaroline the only fifth-generation compound that is available in the US. The cephamycins include cefoxitin and cefotetan.

Carbapenems and Monobactams

The carbapenems contain a five-membered ring attached to the β-lactam ring like the penicillins, but the sulfur is external to the ring (see Fig. 57.3). These agents also have a broad spectrum of activity and include ertapenem, imipenem, and meropenem.

Aztreonam is the only available monobactam. This agent contains a single β-lactam ring (see Fig. 57.3) and is effective against aerobic gram-positive bacteria.

Non-β-Lactam Cell Wall Synthesis Inhibitors

Cell wall synthesis inhibitors lacking a β-lactam ring include the peptides vancomycin, telavancin, and bacitracin and other nonpeptides including fosfomycin and cycloserine.

Peptides

Vancomycin is a glycopeptide that was isolated originally from an actinomycete in soil and is active only against gram-positive bacteria. It inhibits cell wall synthesis by binding with high affinity to the D-ala-D-ala terminus of the nascent peptidoglycan pentapeptide, preventing subsequent cross-linking (see Fig. 57.2). Consequently, the peptidoglycans become weakened, and the cell becomes susceptible to lysis.

Telavancin is a semisynthetic lipoglycopeptide derivative of vancomycin. Like vancomycin, telavancin binds to the D-ala-D-ala terminus of the nascent peptidoglycan chain to inhibit polymerization. In addition, as a consequence of its lipophilic side chain like the polymyxins and daptomycin, telavancin disrupts bacterial cell membrane potential and increases membrane permeability. Thus it has a unique dual mechanism of action to affect both bacterial cell walls and membranes.

Bacitracin is a mixture of polypeptides isolated from the *Bacillus subtilis* that inhibits bacterial cell wall synthesis by binding to the bactoprenol phospholipid carrier and inhibiting its dephosphorylation. Thus bacitracin inhibits the recycling of the phospholipid carrier, preventing its ability to transport additional peptidoglycan units, blocking further chain elongation and causing bacteria to osmotically lyse.

Others

Fosfomycin is a small molecule isolated from a *Streptomyces* species that inhibits cell wall synthesis by blocking peptidoglycan precursor availability. Fosfomycin is a phosphoenolpyruvate analogue that irreversibly inhibits enolpyruvate transferase (MurA), a key enzyme involved

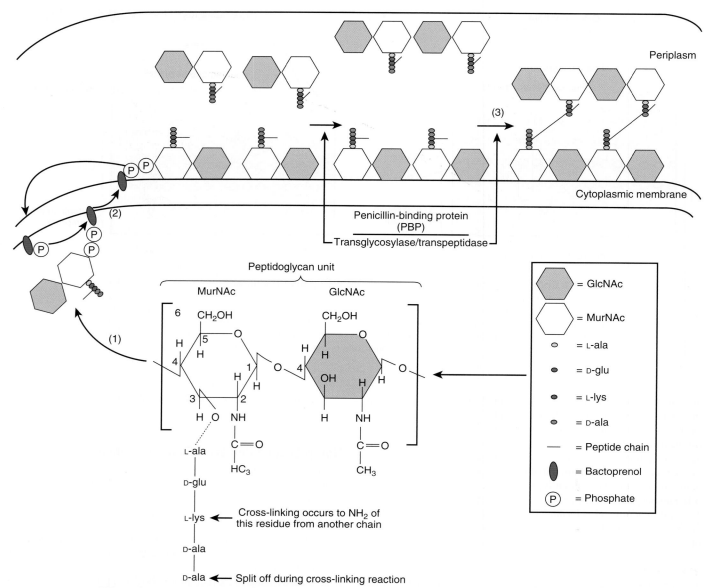

FIG. 57.2 Synthesis of the Peptidoglycan Cell Wall. The synthesis of the peptidoglycan layer occurs in a series of steps as follows: (1) the peptidoglycan repeat unit is synthesized by adding a pentapeptide chain with two terminal D-alanines to N-acetylmuramic acid (Mur NAc), which combines with N-acetylglucosamine (GlcNAc); (2) the repeat unit attaches to the bactoprenol pyrophosphate carrier, which transports the unit from the inner surface of the cytoplasmic membrane to the outer surface; and (3) the repeat unit is attached to the end of the peptidoglycan chain by the action of penicillin-binding proteins, which contain both a transglycosylase domain that attaches the units and a transpeptidase domain, which leads to cross-linking.

in the synthesis of MurNAc. Without MurNAc, bacteria cannot synthesize peptidoglycan units. Fosfomycin has a bactericidal effect and is effective against a broad range of organisms.

Cycloserine is another small molecule isolated from a *Streptomyces* species and is an analogue of D-alanine. Cycloserine also interferes with early steps in the synthesis of the cell wall by competitively inhibiting both L-alanine racemase, which converts L-alanine to D-alanine and D-alanylalanine synthetase, which incorporates the amino acid into the pentapeptide for peptidoglycan biosynthesis. Cycloserine has a broad spectrum of activity and can be bactericidal or bacteriostatic.

Cell Membrane Disrupters
Lipopeptides

The lipopeptide antibiotics include the polymyxins that were introduced in the 1960s and daptomycin, which was approved for use in 2003. The structures of colistin (polymyxin E) and daptomycin are shown in Fig. 57.4.

The polymyxins are bactericidal and include colistin and polymyxin B, the former the most widely used of the two. Although colistin was seldom used because of neurotoxicity and nephrotoxicity, its use has

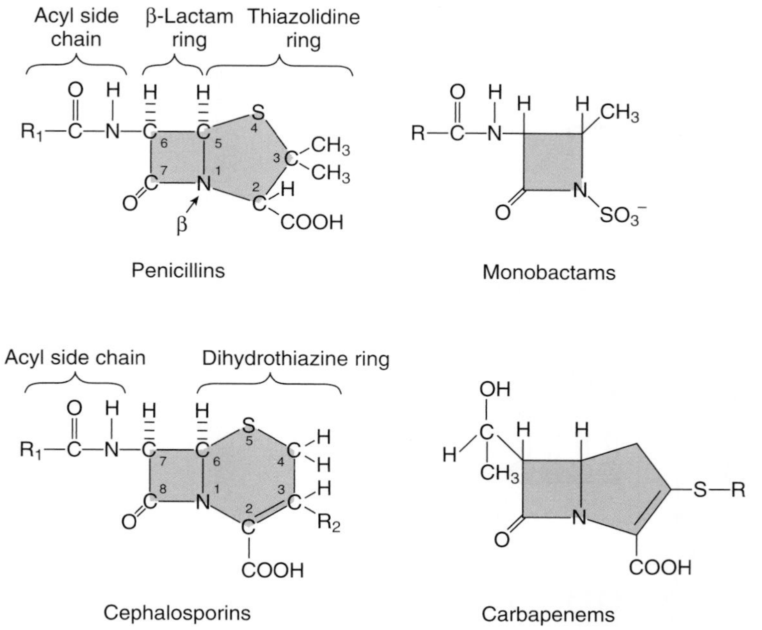

FIG. 57.3 General Structures of the β-Lactam Antibiotics. Shown are the four-membered β-lactam rings that are subject to hydrolysis by β-lactamases. All of the β-lactam antibiotics, except the monobactams, have a second ring fused to the β-lactam ring. For penicillins, the second ring is a thiazolidine, whereas for cephalosporins, it is a dihydrothiazine. Carbapenems have an unsaturated ring with an external sulfur. Different structural groups positioned at the side chains (R) give rise to compounds with differing antibiotic properties. Structures have been numbered according to the United States Pharmacopoeia (USP) system, with the nitrogen atom given the first position. Note that this numbering system may differ from others that assign the sulfur in penicillin as number one.

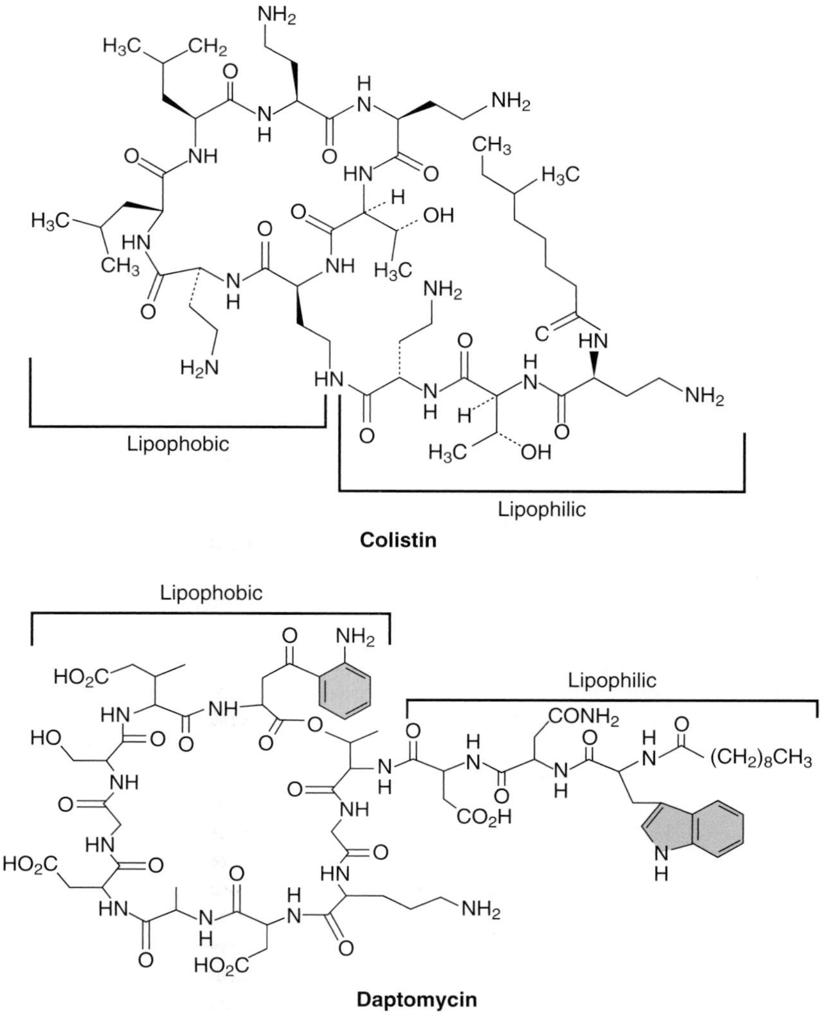

FIG. 57.4 Structures of Lipopeptides. The structures of colistin and daptomycin are shown, illustrating the hydrophilic and hydrophobic portions of the molecules.

Colistin

Daptomycin

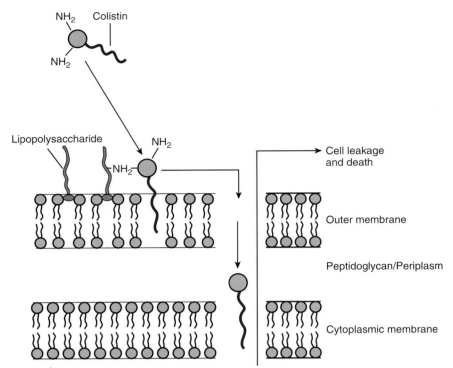

FIG. 57.5 Mechanism of Action of Colistin. The amino groups of the lipophobic peptide portion of the molecule interact with lipopolysaccharide cationic sites on the outer membrane of gram-negative bacteria, with the fatty acid (lipophilic) portion of the molecule penetrating the membrane, causing pore formation. The drug can enter through the pores and penetrate the cytoplasmic membrane, leading to the release of intracellular components and cell lysis.

increased due to the rise of multidrug-resistant organisms. Polymyxins are cyclic detergents with both lipophilic and lipophobic groups that interact with the lipopolysaccharides in the outer membrane of gram-negative bacteria. The amino groups of the peptide interact with divalent cationic sites on the lipopolysaccharides, while the fatty acid portion of the drug penetrates the hydrophobic areas to produce holes in the membranes, through which intracellular constituents leak out of the bacteria (Fig. 57.5). Thus the polymyxins are surface-active amphipathic agents.

Daptomycin is a lipopeptide derived from *Streptomyces roseosporus* that has a fatty acid moiety covalently attached to the cyclic peptide at its *N*-terminus and exerts rapid bactericidal activity. Several actions have been proposed to explain the unique mechanism of action of this compound. Studies support a calcium-dependent conformational rearrangement to an active micellar form, increasing the amphiphilicity of the compound, although it is unclear whether the compound oligomerizes prior to or after insertion into the membrane (Fig. 57.6). Once in the membrane, the daptomycin oligomers form pore-like structures that lead to depolarization, loss of membrane integrity, and leakage of ions (e.g., potassium) from the cytoplasm, followed by bacterial cell death. Daptomycin has specific activity against gram-positive organisms.

MECHANISMS OF RESISTANCE

β-Lactam Cell Wall Synthesis Inhibitors

Resistance to the β-lactam cell wall synthesis inhibitors became evident shortly after the introduction of penicillin. Three primary mechanisms are involved: (1) the overexpression of β-lactamases and expression of extended spectrum β-lactamases (ESBLs); (2) decreased affinity of bacterial PBPs; and (3) deletions or mutations in the expression of the porin protein channel in the outer lipid membrane of gram-negative bacteria through which the antibiotics gain access to the cell, thereby limiting drug permeability.

Penicillins

Resistance to penicillin by the induction of β-lactamases led to the development of both semisynthetic penicillins resistant to hydrolysis by these enzymes and compounds with greater activity against staphylococcal and gram-negative organisms, the latter producing a greater variety of β-lactamases than gram-positive bacteria. Currently, more than 95% of staphylococci are resistant to penicillin G due to the presence of PBPs that **bind poorly** to β-lactams. An important clinical example is methicillin-resistant *Staphylococcus aureus* (MRSA), which poses a serious hospital, and increasingly, community problem because these staphylococci have acquired a high-molecular-weight PBP-2a with a poor affinity for all β-lactams (except for the fifth-generation cephalosporin ceftaroline).

Cephalosporins

The first-generation cephalosporins are more stable in the presence of bacterial β-lactamases than the penicillins and thus are not combined with β-lactamase inhibitors. However, the introduction of these new β-lactams led to mutations in preexisting β-lactamases, producing the ESBLs that confer high-level resistance. Further, resistance of gram-negative bacteria has also been attributed to porin mutations leading to decreased drug entry, as well as to decreased affinity of and poor binding to PBPs.

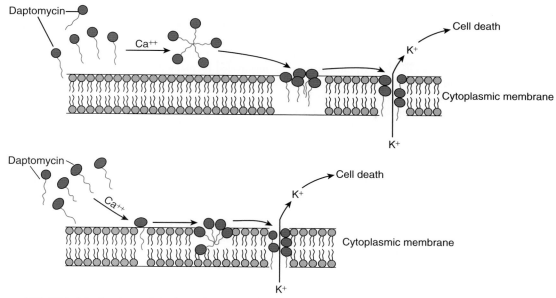

FIG. 57.6 Mechanism of Action of Daptomycin. Daptomycin interacts with gram-positive bacterial cell membranes in a Ca^{++}-dependent manner to cause pore formation and leakage of K^+ from the cytoplasm, leading to cell death. Two proposed mechanisms are depicted. The top scheme shows the Ca^{++}-mediated oligomerization and possible micelle formation, followed by insertion into the membrane and pore formation, while the bottom scheme depicts the Ca^{++}-mediated insertion of daptomycin into the membrane, followed by aggregation and pore formation.

Carbapenems

Decreased drug accumulation constitutes a major mechanism of resistance to the carbapenems. Organisms such as *Pseudomonas aeruginosa* develop resistance by deleting the porin protein through which imipenem gains entry to the cell. Similar to other classes of β-lactams, PBP mutations and ESBLs also provide bacteria with significant drug resistance to the carbapenems.

Monobactams

Resistance of gram-positive and anaerobic species of bacteria to aztreonam has been attributed to the decreased binding to PBPs, as well as the expression of ESBLs that degrade the compound.

Non–β-Lactam Cell Wall Synthesis Inhibitors

Resistance of *S. aureus* to vancomycin was first reported in the United States in 2002, characterized as vancomycin-intermediate *S. aureus* (VISA), and shortly thereafter, vancomycin-resistant *S. aureus* (VRSA) was described with a minimum inhibitory concentration more than double that for the intermediate resistant strain. The mechanism mediating vancomycin resistance in VISA strains involves an increased production of D-ala-D-ala residues that reside at the site of bacterial cell division (septum) close to the site of cell wall synthesis. Vancomycin binds to these residues, limiting access of the drug to its site of action to inhibit peptidoglycan cross-linking. Several studies have identified mutations in selected genes, including *vraR*, *graRS*, and *walRK*, that contribute to the development of resistance.

Vancomycin resistance in VRSA strains is similar to that in vancomycin-resistant enterococci (VRE) and involves alterations in the terminal D-ala-D-ala peptide. For both VRSA strains and VRE strains, bacteria acquire a set of *van* genes coding for enzymes that catalyze the synthesis of a D-ala-D-lactate terminal peptide instead of the normal D-ala-D-ala. Vancomycin binds D-ala-D-lactate with a much lower affinity (1000-fold for *Enterococcus faecium* and *Enterococcus faecalis*) than the

normal peptide. In addition, for some VRE strains, the D-ala-D-ala is replaced by D-ala-D-serine, to which vancomycin exhibits a sixfold lower affinity than for D-ala-D-ala.

Although resistance to topically applied antibiotics is not as common as that to systemically administered compounds, resistance may develop. The most common mechanism of resistance to bacitracin is an increased expression of several ABC transporters, leading to enhanced drug efflux.

Fosfomycin enters bacterial cells through the glycerophosphate transporter, and mutations in the transporter can render bacteria resistant. Fosfomycin can also be inactivated by bacterial enzymes of the glyoxalase family.

Resistance to cycloserine occurs by several mechanisms, including increased expression of alanine racemase raising the amount of D-ala available, and inhibition of alanine uptake.

Cell Membrane Disrupters

Resistance of gram-negative bacteria to the polymyxins typically involves modifications of the lipopolysaccharides in the outer membrane, decreasing the binding of the polymyxins.

Resistance to daptomycin has been reported to emerge during treatment of deep-seated infections such as osteomyelitis and endocarditis. Although the mechanisms involved have not been elucidated, evidence suggests that resistance may develop as a consequence of mutations in the *mprF* gene, which regulates the charge on the cell membrane, thereby affecting the ability of the drug to bind to and insert into the membrane bilayer.

RELATIONSHIP OF MECHANISMS OF ACTION TO CLINICAL RESPONSE

β-Lactam Cell Wall Synthesis Inhibitors
Penicillins

Although antibiotic resistance to penicillin G and penicillin V is widespread in many bacterial species, natural penicillins remain the drugs of choice for a variety of gram-positive infections caused by *Streptococcus* (streptococcal pharyngitis, other infections caused by β-hemolytic streptococci, and viridans streptococcal infections, including endocarditis), *Enterococcus*, *Listeria*, and *Corynebacterium*. Natural penicillins are also the drugs of choice for all forms of syphilis, meningococcal infections, actinomycosis, and several less common infections. Recent increases in resistance among *Streptococcus pneumoniae* reduce support for utilizing penicillin in meningeal infections unless the isolate is confirmed to be susceptible. Even moderately resistant extrameningeal pneumococcal infections (pneumonia), however, still respond to penicillin. Although *Neisseria meningitidis* remains highly susceptible, most strains of *Neisseria gonorrhoeae* are resistant through plasmid-mediated β-lactamase production. Many anaerobic species, including *Clostridium perfringens* and *Actinomyces* species, are susceptible to penicillin G, but organisms such as *Bacteroides fragilis* and *Clostridium difficile* are not. Aerobic gram-negative *Enterobacteriaceae* and *Pseudomonas* species are also resistant.

The penicillinase-resistant penicillins are still used principally to treat staphylococcal infections, although strains of *S. aureus* that contain altered PBPs conferring resistance to most β-lactams (MRSA) are increasing in frequency. The penicillinase-resistant penicillins retain sufficient activity against most streptococci to be clinically useful in treating soft tissue infections. This is important because streptococci and *S. aureus* are the major causes of cellulitis. These agents are less active against oral cavity anaerobic species than penicillin G and show no activity against gram-negative bacilli.

β-Lactamase Inhibitors

Clavulanate, sulbactam, and tazobactam are β-lactamase inhibitors, which inactivate the β-lactamases of *S. aureus* and many gram-negative bacteria, including plasmid-mediated common β-lactamases in *Escherichia coli*, *Haemophilus*, *Neisseria*, *Salmonella*, and *Shigella* species and chromosomal β-lactamases in *Klebsiella*, *Moraxella*, and *Bacteroides* species. None of the β-lactamase inhibitors bind to the chromosomal ampC β-lactamases in *Pseudomonas*, *Enterobacter*, *Citrobacter*, or *Serratia* species. These inhibitors differ in relative potency, reflected in the ratio of inhibitor to the paired penicillin. Sulbactam, the weakest inhibitor, is available in a 1:2 ratio of sulbactam to ampicillin; the ratio of tazobactam to piperacillin is 1:8.

Clavulanate has a β-lactam ring but only minimal antibacterial activity because it binds poorly to most PBPs. It irreversibly inhibits β-lactamases. Sulbactam is a penicillanic acid derivative with extremely weak antibacterial activity against gram-positive cocci and *Enterobacteriaceae* but inhibits several other organisms at higher concentrations. It also irreversibly inhibits the β-lactamases inhibited by clavulanate, although it is less potent. Tazobactam is another penicillanic acid derivative similar in structure to sulbactam but with a higher potency.

Ampicillin and amoxicillin have similar antibacterial activity that is 2–4 times greater than penicillin G against enterococci and *Listeria monocytogenes*. Ampicillin and amoxicillin are useful for treating some upper respiratory tract infections, provided the infection is not caused by β-lactamase–producing *Haemophilus* organisms. All aminopenicillin/β-lactamase inhibitor combinations have excellent activity against anaerobes. Combinations of amoxicillin with clavulanate are used to treat otitis media in children and sinusitis, bacterial exacerbations of bronchitis, and lower respiratory tract infections in adults. This combination is also effective in skin infections, particularly when anaerobic and aerobic organisms are present. It is also the drug of choice for human and animal bite wounds. Ampicillin is used in combination with sulbactam to treat mixed aerobic/anaerobic skin and soft tissue infections, including diabetic foot infections, mixed aerobic/anaerobic pulmonary and odontogenic infections, and intraabdominal infections.

Ticarcillin and piperacillin are active against *Pseudomonas* and certain species of *Proteus* that are resistant to ampicillin. Piperacillin is also useful for the treatment of *Klebsiella* infections. Both drugs inhibit streptococcal and enterococcal species to varying degrees and are inactivated by many β-lactamases of both gram-positive and gram-negative bacteria. Piperacillin has moderate activity against anaerobes and is similar to ticarcillin in activity against *Enterobacter*, *Serratia*, and *Providencia* species. These drugs are often combined with aminoglycoside antibiotics; both ticarcillin and piperacillin act synergistically with aminoglycosides to inhibit *Pseudomonas aeruginosa*. Because of their β-lactamase susceptibility, they are also combined with β-lactamase inhibitors. Piperacillin in combination with tazobactam is more effective than ticarcillin/clavulanate against pseudomonal and enterococcal activity due to superior antipseudomonal activity of piperacillin, likely the reason why the manufacture of ticarcillin/clavulanate terminated in 2015. Piperacillin/tazobactam has been used extensively to treat nosocomial infections and is the recommended drug of choice for serious blood infections in neutropenic patients.

Cephalosporins

The spectra of activity for the first-generation cephalosporins are similar, inhibiting most gram-positive cocci (except for enterococci and Listeria), many *E. coli*, *Klebsiella* species, and *Proteus mirabilis* (indole negative). Most other Enterobacteriaceae are resistant, as are *Pseudomonas*, *Bacteroides*, and *Haemophilus* species. First-generation cephalosporins are used to treat respiratory, skin, and urinary tract infections and as prophylaxis before cardiac surgery or orthopedic prosthesis procedures. Cefazolin has a similar antimicrobial spectrum as the oral agents but has slightly enhanced activity against *E. coli* and *Klebsiella* species.

Among the second-generation cephalosporins and the cephamycins, cefuroxime has greater activity against *S. pneumonia* and *Streptococcus pyogenes* than first-generation cephalosporins but less activity against *S. aureus*. Cefuroxime also possesses activity against *Borrelia burgdorferi* and *Moraxella*. Cefaclor, an oral cephalosporin, has similar activity to cephalexin, with somewhat greater activity against *Haemophilus influenzae*, *Moraxella catarrhalis*, *E. coli*, and *P. mirabilis*, and is used to treat upper respiratory tract infections in children. Loracarbef is a carbacephem that inhibits β-lactamase–producing *H. influenzae* and respiratory tract pathogens.

Cefoxitin is less active against gram-positive organisms than the first-generation agents but is more stable against β-lactamase degradation by Enterobacteriaceae (but not *Enterobacter* or *Citrobacter* species) and anaerobic bacteria. Also, it is not hydrolyzed by the plasmid-mediated ESBLs that destroy cefotaxime, ceftriaxone, and ceftazidime and has been used to treat aspiration pneumonia and intraabdominal and pelvic infections. Cefotetan inhibits many β-lactamase-producing Enterobacteriaceae and most *Bacteroides* species. It is also used to treat intraabdominal and pelvic infections. However, these two agents are not as active against *B. fragilis* as the penicillin-β-lactamase inhibitor combinations. Consequently, the use of second-generation cephalosporins has declined, although they are still used for perioperative prophylaxis.

Among the third-generation cephalosporins, cefotaxime has excellent activity against gram-positive streptococcal species, including *S. pneumoniae*, and gram-negative *Haemophilus* and *Neisseria* species. A metabolite of cefotaxime acts synergistically with cefotaxime, and the two compounds have better activity against *Bacteroides* species than the parent compound. The activity of ceftizoxime and ceftriaxone is similar to that of cefotaxime. These agents are used to treat lower respiratory tract infections, urinary tract infections, skin infections, osteomyelitis, and meningitis. Ceftriaxone also is used to treat gonorrhea and Lyme disease. Because of favorable pharmacokinetics allowing once-daily dosing, ceftriaxone is more widely used than the other two agents. Ceftazidime inhibits *P. aeruginosa*, most streptococci, *Haemophilus*, *Neisseria*, and most Enterobacteriaceae. It does not inhibit *Bacteroides* species and is inactivated by ESBL-producing organisms. It is less active against gram-positive and anaerobic organisms than other parenteral third-generation cephalosporins. Cefpodoxime inhibits streptococci, *Haemophilus*, *Moraxella*, *Neisseria*, and many Enterobacteriaceae.

Cefepime, which is the only **fourth-generation cephalosporin**, has an extended spectrum of activity against some gram-positive cocci and Enterobacteriaceae. Structurally related to third-generation cephalosporins, cefepime contains a quaternary nitrogen along with the negatively charged carboxyl, rendering it a zwitterion. Zwitterions have a net neutral charge but are capable of penetrating the outer membrane of gram-negative bacteria at higher rates than third-generation drugs. In addition, cefepime has a low affinity for class I ampC β-lactamases. Cefepime is active against most pathogenic gram-positive cocci (except *Enterococcus* and MRSA), Enterobacteriaceae, *P. aeruginosa*, *H. influenzae*, and *N. meningitidis*.

Ceftaroline is the only **fifth-generation cephalosporin** available and has activity against staphylococcal infections caused by *Enterococcus*, MRSA, and VRSA. This activity is thought to be due to the presence of a 1,3-thiazole ring, which increases the affinity of ceftaroline for PBP2a and PBP2x. Ceftaroline is widely used for treating community-acquired pneumonia and for eliminating skin and soft tissue infections caused by *Staphylococcus*, *Proteus*, *Klebsiella*, *Moraxella*, *E. coli*, and other species of Enterobacteriaceae. Ceftaroline does not exhibit appreciable activity toward *P. aeruginosa* or *Acinetobacter* species.

Carbapenems

Imipenem, meropenem, and ertapenem have high affinity for PBPs expressed by a wide variety of organisms, excellent stability against most β-lactamases, and good permeability, leading to very broad antibacterial activity. They inhibit most gram-positive organisms such as the hemolytic streptococci, *S. pneumoniae*, viridans group streptococci, and *S. aureus* (although not MRSA). Imipenem and meropenem have some activity against *E. faecalis* but not *E. faecium*. Most Enterobacteriaceae, *Haemophilus* species, *Moraxella* species, *Neisseria* species, and *P. aeruginosa* are also inhibited by these compounds. Ertapenem has a similar spectrum of activity but is not active against *P. aeruginosa*, *Enterococcus* species, or *Acinetobacter*. The carbapenems have extensive activity against anaerobic organisms, inhibiting most *Bacteroides* species, but not *Clostridium difficile*. They also inhibit *Nocardia* species and some mycobacteria.

The carbapenems can be used to treat bacteremias and lower respiratory tract, intraabdominal, gynecological, bone and joint, central nervous system, and complicated urinary tract infections caused by resistant bacteria. They may also be used in febrile neutropenic patients. Because of their broad spectrum of activity, these agents are useful as single-agent therapy in mixed aerobic/anaerobic bacterial infections. However, resistance in gram-negative nosocomial pathogens such as *Pseudomonas* and *Acinetobacter* is increasingly a problem.

Monobactams

Aztreonam is the only monocyclic β-lactam with a high affinity for the PBPs of certain aerobic gram-negative bacteria. It binds to PBP-3 of Enterobacteriaceae and *P. aeruginosa*, producing long filamentous bacteria that ultimately lyse and die. It does not bind to PBPs of gram-positive or anaerobic species. It is not hydrolyzed by most β-lactamases except for those expressed by *Klebsiella oxytoca* and *Stenotrophomonas maltophilia*, or by plasmid-encoded ESBLs. Aztreonam is effective for the treatment of bacteremia, respiratory and urinary tract infections, osteomyelitis, and skin infections. Like other β-lactams, it exhibits synergy when used in combination with aminoglycosides.

Non-β-Lactam Cell Wall Synthesis Inhibitors

Vancomycin is active against gram-positive bacteria such as staphylococci (including MRSA and coagulase-negative staphylococci), streptococci (such as hemolytic and viridans group streptococci and *S. pneumoniae*, including penicillin-resistant strains), and enterococci (such as *E. faecalis* and *E. faecium*). In addition, vancomycin displays activity against *Bacillus* species, *Corynebacterium jeikeium*, *L. monocytogenes*, and gram-positive anaerobes such as *Clostridium* and *Propionibacterium* species. Vancomycin is the first-line treatment for MRSA infections such as complicated skin infections, bloodstream infections, lower respiratory tract infections, and endocarditis. It is also useful for treating infections of prosthetic valves and catheters caused by coagulase-negative staphylococci and *Corynebacterium*. It is effective alone or in combination with an aminoglycoside for endocarditis caused by *Streptococcus viridans* or *Streptococcus bovis*, especially in patients allergic to β-lactam antibiotics. It is also used in combination with gentamicin for the treatment of enterococcal endocarditis in patients allergic to penicillins. Vancomycin in combination with cefotaxime, ceftriaxone, or rifampin is also recommended for the treatment of meningitis caused by penicillin-resistant pneumococci.

Oral vancomycin is used to treat colitis caused by *C. difficile*, an obligate anaerobic, gram-positive, spore-forming bacillus, particularly in severe cases or for mild to moderate cases that fail to respond to metronidazole (Chapter 59). *C. difficile* infection (CDI), also known as pseudomembranous colitis, is most often associated with antimicrobial use and disruption of the normal gastrointestinal (GI) microflora. CDI has become a major nosocomial problem, affecting three million hospitalized patients annually in the United States. Antibiotics that can lead to CDI include clindamycin (Chapter 58), ampicillin, second- and third-generation cephalosporins (particularly cefotaxime, ceftriaxone, cefuroxime, and ceftazidime), and the fluoroquinolones (Chapter 59).

Telavancin is active against methicillin-sensitive *S. aureus* (MSSA), MRSA, VISA, heteroresistant VISA, vancomycin-susceptible enterococci, some vancomycin-resistant enterococci, streptococci (including penicillin-resistant and multidrug-resistant strains), and several anaerobic bacteria including *C. difficile*. The drug is approved for the treatment of complicated skin and soft tissue infections and hospital-acquired pneumonia.

Bacitracin inhibits gram-positive cocci including *Streptococcus*, *Staphylococcus*, and *Enterococcus*, including vancomycin-resistant enterococci. Gram-negative species inhibited by bacitracin include bacilli, *Clostridium* (including *C. difficile*), and some *Neisseria* species and *Haemophilus* organisms. Enterobacteriaceae and *Pseudomonas* species are resistant. Bacitracin is typically applied topically but has no proven value for the treatment of furunculosis, pyoderma, carbuncles, or cutaneous abscesses. Topically administered bacitracin zinc has been shown to reduce the risk of infections in patients with uncomplicated soft tissue wounds.

Fosfomycin possesses broad-spectrum antibacterial activity that targets gram-positive and gram-negative organisms, including *E. faecalis*, *E. coli*, and other Enterobacteriaceae. Because fosfomycin is predominantly excreted in the urine and possesses increased activity in low pH environments, it is widely used for the treatment and prophylaxis of urinary tract infections.

Cycloserine is a broad-spectrum antibiotic with activity against *E. coli*, *S. aureus*, *Chlamydia*, *Enterococcus*, *Nocardia* species, and other Enterobacteriaceae and is used for urinary tract infections. It is also second-line treatment for tuberculosis (Chapter 60). The action of cycloserine may be bactericidal or bacteriostatic, depending on its concentration and the organism.

Cell Membrane Disrupters

The antimicrobial activities of colistin and polymyxin B are restricted to gram-negative bacteria, including *E. coli, Klebsiella, Salmonella, Enterobacter, Pasteurella, Bordetella, Shigella, P. aeruginosa,* and *Acinetobacter; Proteus* and *Serratia* species are intrinsically resistant. Colistin is available as otic drops in combination with other drugs. It is also available as colistin sulfate for oral use and as colistimethate sodium for parenteral administration. Polymyxin B sulfate is available for ophthalmic, otic, and topical use (in combination with other compounds) for the treatment of infections of the skin, mucous membranes, eye, and ear caused by sensitive microorganisms such as external otitis, which is frequently caused by *Pseudomonas.* The polymyxins are used as salvage therapy for the treatment of infections caused by multidrug-resistant gram-negative organisms, especially *Acinetobacter* species, *P. aeruginosa,* and *Klebsiella* species.

Daptomycin is selectively active against gram-positive bacteria including MSSA, MRSA, VISA, and VRSA, *Streptococcus* species, including penicillin-susceptible and penicillin-resistant strains of *S. pneumoniae,* and *Enterococcus species,* including vancomycin-susceptible and vancomycin-resistant strains of *E. faecium* and *E. faecalis.* Daptomycin is indicated for the treatment of complicated skin and soft tissue infections, complicated bacteremia, and endocarditis. It should not be used for the treatment of community-acquired pneumonia due to its inactivation by pulmonary surfactants.

PHARMACOKINETICS

β-Lactam Cell Wall Synthesis Inhibitors

Penicillins

Pharmacokinetic characteristics of the penicillins and the β-lactamase inhibitors are provided in Table 57.1.

Penicillin G is hydrolyzed rapidly in the stomach at low pH. Decreased gastric acid production improves absorption, whereas food intake impairs it. Absorption is rapid and occurs primarily in the duodenum.

Unabsorbed penicillin is destroyed by bacteria in the colon. Penicillin V is more acid stable and better absorbed than penicillin G, even when ingested with food. A peak plasma concentration of penicillin G is achieved in 15–30 minutes after intramuscular (IM) injection but declines quickly because of rapid removal by the kidneys. Repository forms are available as procaine or benzathine salts. Procaine penicillin is an equimolar mixture of procaine and penicillin and results in concentrations of penicillin G that last for 12 hours to several days after doses of 300,000 to 2.4 million units. Benzathine penicillin is a 1:2 combination of penicillin and the ammonium base and is slowly absorbed, with plasma concentrations detectable for up to 15–30 days.

Penicillin G is eliminated primarily by tubular secretion, and renal clearance is equivalent to renal plasma flow. Excretion can be blocked by probenecid (although the coadministration of probenecid with penicillin has declined in clinical practice). Renal elimination is also considerably less in newborns because of poorly developed tubular function; the half-life of penicillin G is 3 hours in newborns compared with 30 minutes in 1-year-old children. Excretion declines with age, but adjustments in dose are not necessary until renal clearance decreases to less than 30 mL/min. Hemodialysis removes penicillin G from the body; peritoneal dialysis is less efficient. A small amount is excreted in breast milk and saliva, but it is not present in tears or sweat. The natural penicillins enter the CSF in the presence of meningeal inflammation.

The penicillinase-resistant penicillins oxacillin, cloxacillin, nafcillin, and dicloxacillin are acid stable and orally absorbed, with absorption decreased in the presence of food. Peak plasma concentrations are achieved approximately 1 hour after ingestion, and they are all highly protein bound. Elimination is primarily via the kidneys, with some biliary excretion and hepatic metabolism. These drugs are minimally removed from the body by hemodialysis. Oxacillin is less effective orally; however, adequate plasma and cerebrospinal fluid (CSF) concentrations are achieved when it is administered by the intravenous (IV) route. Nafcillin is absorbed erratically following oral administration, and thus the preferred route is IV. Elimination of nafcillin is primarily by biliary excretion. In the presence of meningeal inflammation, the

TABLE 57.1	Pharmacokinetic Parameters of Penicillins and β-Lactamase Inhibitors			
Antimicrobial Agent	**Route(s) of Administration**	**$t_{1/2}$ (hrs)**	**Protein Binding (%)**	**Elimination**
Penicillin				
Penicillin G[a]	Oral[a]/IV	0.5	55	M, R (main)
Benzathine penicillin	IM	14 days	55	R (main)
Penicillin V	Oral	1.0	60	R (main
Oxacillin	Oral/IV	0.4	92	M, R (main), B
Dicloxacillin	Oral	0.6	97	M, R (main), B
Nafcillin	IV	0.5	90	R (some), mainly B
Ampicillin	IV	1.0	15	R (some), some B
Amoxicillin	Oral	1.0	15	R (main)
Ticarcillin	IV	1.2	50	M, R (main)
Piperacillin	IV	1.3	50	M, R
β-Lactamase Inhibitors				
Clavulanate				
(with amoxicillin)	Oral	1.0	30	M, R (main)
(with ticarcillin)	IV			
Sulbactam (with ampicillin)	IV	1.0	15	R (main)
Tazobactam (with piperacillin)	IV	1.0	20	M, R (main)

[a]Poor acid stability.
B, Biliary; *IM,* intramuscular; *IV,* intravenous; *M,* metabolized; *R,* renal.

penicillinase-resistant penicillins enter the CSF in concentrations adequate to treat staphylococcal meningitis or brain abscesses.

Ampicillin is moderately well absorbed after oral administration, with absorption decreased in the presence of food. Ampicillin is well distributed to most body compartments, and therapeutic concentrations are achieved in pleural, synovial, peritoneal, and cerebrospinal fluids. It is eliminated primarily by renal excretion with some biliary contribution. Amoxicillin is better absorbed than ampicillin after oral ingestion and absorption is delayed, but not decreased, by food. Its distribution is similar to that of ampicillin. Therapeutic concentrations of the aminopenicillins are achieved in the presence of meningeal inflammation.

Ticarcillin is administered parenterally, as it is not absorbed from the GI tract. It is distributed extensively throughout the body but does not reach sufficient concentrations in the CSF for the treatment of *Pseudomonas* meningitis. Ticarcillin is excreted primarily by the kidneys. Piperacillin is administered IV or IM and has nonlinear pharmacokinetics, with plasma concentrations not proportional to dose. Piperacillin reaches therapeutic levels in the CSF in the presence of inflammation.

β-Lactamase Inhibitors

The β-lactamase inhibitors are marketed only with a penicillin derivative. In general, the paired penicillin/β-lactamase inhibitors have similar half-lives. However, clearance of the two compounds may diverge in renal insufficiency. Clavulanate enters most body compartments, with therapeutic concentrations reached in middle ear fluid, tonsils, sinus secretions, bile, and the urinary tract. Sulbactam is widely distributed in the body, including the CSF in the presence of meningitis. It is excreted in the urine, and its half-life is increased to 6 hours in adults with renal failure and in newborns. The half-life of tazobactam is prolonged in the presence of piperacillin, and it is excreted primarily by the kidneys.

Cephalosporins

Pharmacokinetic properties of the cephalosporins are provided in Table 57.2. The first- and second-generation cephalosporins are generally well distributed but do not enter the CSF in sufficient concentrations

TABLE 57.2 Pharmacokinetic Parameters of Other β-Lactam Cell Wall Synthesis Inhibitors

	Route of Administration	$t_{1/2}$ (hrs)	Protein Binding (%)	Route of Elimination	CSF Penetration[a]
Cephalosporins					
First Generation					
Cefazolin	IV/IM	2.0	85	R	
Cephalexin	Oral	1.0	15	R	
Cefadroxil	Oral	1.5	20	R	
Second Generation					
Cefaclor	Oral	1.0	25	M, R	
Cefprozil	Oral	1	20	R	
Loracarbef	Oral	1	25	R	
Cefuroxime	IV/IM/Oral	1.7	35	R	Yes
Cefoxitin	IV/IM	0.8	70	R	
Cefotetan	IV/IM	3.5	85	R	
Cefprozil	Oral	1.3	45	R	
Third Generation					
Cefotaxime	IV/IM	1.0	50	R	Yes
Ceftizoxime	IV/IM	1.8	30	R	Yes
Ceftriaxone	IV/IM	6–8	90	R (50%), B (60%)	Yes
Cefixime	Oral	3.7	75	R (50%), (other)	Yes
Ceftazidime	IV/IM	1.8	15	R	Yes
Cefpodoxime	Oral	1.2	25	R	
Fourth/Fifth Generation					
Cefepime	IV/IM	2.1	20	R	Yes
Ceftaroline	IV	2.6	20	R	Yes
Carbapenems					
Imipenem	IV	1.0	20	M, R	Yes
Meropenem	IV	1	2	M, R	Yes
Ertapenem	IV	4	95	M, R	Yes
Monobactams					
Aztreonam	IV	1.5–2.0	45–60	R	Yes

[a]Adequate for therapeutic use.
B, Biliary; *IM*, intramuscular; *IV*, intravenous; *M*, metabolized; *R*, renal.

for the treatment of meningitis, with the exception of cefuroxime. These compounds are eliminated by the kidneys but achieve sufficient concentrations to treat urinary tract infections.

The third-generation cephalosporins are generally administered parenterally except for cefdinir, cefixime, and cefpodoxime, which can be administered orally. These agents are well distributed, and many of them penetrate the CSF in the presence of meningeal inflammation. The majority of these agents are excreted via the kidneys, although ceftriaxone undergoes biliary excretion.

Cefepime is administered parenterally and is widely distributed, readily entering the CSF with or without meningeal inflammation. Cefepime is excreted primarily unchanged in the urine.

Ceftaroline is administered parenterally and is rapidly converted in the plasma to its active form by phosphatases. It is widely distributed and penetrates the CSF in the presence of meningeal inflammation. Ceftaroline is eliminated in the urine unchanged.

Carbapenems

Pharmacokinetic parameters of the carbapenem antibiotics are also presented in Table 57.2. Imipenem enters the CSF only during inflammation and has high affinity for brain tissue. It is eliminated by glomerular filtration and tubular secretion and is inactivated by a dehydropeptidase in the renal tubules. To overcome inactivation, imipenem is combined with a renal dehydropeptidase inhibitor, cilastatin, which has no antibacterial activity itself and does not affect the properties of imipenem except to prevent its hydrolysis. The serum half-life of imipenem increases as creatinine clearance falls and is increased in patients with renal insufficiency, requiring dose adjustments. Meropenem also penetrates well into most fluids and tissues, including the CSF after IV administration. Meropenem is not hydrolyzed by renal dehydropeptidase and is excreted unchanged in the urine, requiring dose adjustment in patients with renal insufficiency. Ertapenem has a longer half-life than imipenem and meropenem, enabling once-daily dosing. It is highly protein bound and excreted primarily via the kidneys, requiring dose changes with severe renal impairment. It is also less susceptible to hydrolysis by renal dehydropeptidase.

Monobactams

Aztreonam is administered parenterally, with widespread distribution to all body sites and compartments, including the CSF (Table 57.3). It is eliminated by glomerular filtration and tubular secretion, requiring dose reductions for individuals with renal insufficiency.

Non–β-Lactam Cell Wall Synthesis Inhibitors

Pharmacokinetic properties of these agents are provided in Table 57.3.

Vancomycin is poorly absorbed from the GI tract and thus is administered IV. It is used orally only for the treatment of colitis caused by *C. difficile*. Vancomycin administered IV enters many body fluids, including bile, pleural, pericardial, peritoneal, and synovial. Bactericidal CSF concentrations of vancomycin are reached with high IV doses in patients with inflamed meninges. The half-life of vancomycin is 4–11 hours (5–9 days in anuric patients). Vancomycin is not metabolized and is eliminated by glomerular filtration; thus dosage should be adjusted on the basis of renal function. Vancomycin is not removed efficiently by hemodialysis or peritoneal dialysis. Monitoring plasma concentrations is necessary to ensure therapeutic concentrations are achieved and toxicity averted in patients with depressed renal function.

Fosfomycin is administered orally and is rapidly absorbed and well distributed to the kidneys, bladder, prostate, and seminal vesicles. Oral bioavailability may be decreased slightly by food. It is not bound to plasma proteins, has a half-life of 3–8 hours, and is excreted unchanged in the urine and feces.

Cycloserine is well absorbed following oral administration, with a half-life of approximately 10 hours. It is metabolized in the liver and eliminated via the kidneys. Thus accumulation may occur in individuals with impaired renal function.

Cell Membrane Disrupters

The pharmacokinetic properties of colistin and daptomycin are presented in Table 57.3. Both of these agents are poorly absorbed orally and are typically administered IV. Colistin is typically administered as colistimethate sodium, which is a prodrug that is hydrolyzed following IV administration to the active form. It is poorly distributed throughout the body and is tightly bound to membranes in liver, lungs, kidneys, brain, heart, and muscles. It has a half-life less than 5 hours and is excreted primarily via the kidneys.

Daptomycin is highly bound to plasma proteins, with a half-life following IV administration of 8–9 hours. Daptomycin has a very small volume of distribution and is eliminated primarily by renal excretion, with a small (<10%) biliary contribution.

PHARMACOVIGILANCE: ADVERSE EFFECTS AND DRUG INTERACTIONS

β-Lactam Cell Wall Synthesis Inhibitors
Penicillins

Although the penicillins can cause a wide variety of adverse effects, serious adverse reactions are fortunately rare. Adverse effects vary for each of the penicillins, with the most frequent effect being diarrhea that occurs in about 25% of patients, followed by delayed-type hypersensitivity and contact dermatitis in about 4%–8% of individuals.

TABLE 57.3 Pharmacokinetic Parameters of Non-β-Lactam Cell Wall Synthesis Inhibitors and Cell Membrane Disruptors

	Route of Administration	$t_{1/2}$ (hrs)	Protein Binding (%)	Route of Elimination	CSF Penetration[a]
Vancomycin	IV	4–11	55%	R	Yes
Fosfomycin	Oral	3–8	<1	R, B	Yes
Cycloserine	Oral	10	<1	M, R	Yes
Colistin	IV	5		R	Yes
Daptomycin	IV	8–9	>90%	R	No

[a]Adequate for therapeutic use.
B, Biliary; *IV*, intravenous; *M*, metabolized; *R*, renal.

Immediate hypersensitivity, which can be life-threatening, is the most important adverse effect and includes anaphylaxis, wheezing, angioedema, and urticaria. It occurs through immunoglobulin E–mediated antibody reactions, usually directed at the penicillin nucleus, which is common to all drugs of this class. Therefore a patient who develops anaphylaxis to a specific penicillin should be considered allergic to all of them. Penicillins can be partially degraded to compounds with varying allergenicity, with penicilloyl acid derivatives representing the major determinants and benzylpenicillin and benzylpenicilloate minor determinants contributing to penicillin allergy. Anaphylactic reactions to penicillins are uncommon, occurring in 1–5 of 10,000 cases. In contrast, a morbilliform skin eruption type of allergy occurs in 3%–5% of patients receiving penicillin. Any of the β-lactams can cause Stevens-Johnson syndrome, a rare, life-threatening immune complex–mediated hypersensitivity disorder of the skin and mucous membranes. Seizures can occur in patients possessing epileptogenic foci who receive large doses of penicillin G or other penicillins or who receive average doses but have impaired renal function.

Skin testing with benzylpenicilloyl polylysine, benzylpenicillin G, and Na$^+$ benzylpenicilloate is 95% successful in identifying people likely to have an anaphylactic reaction. However, a negative skin test does not exclude later development of a rash. Anaphylactic reactions to penicillins should be treated with epinephrine (Chapter 11). There is no evidence that antihistamines or corticosteroids are beneficial. Whenever there is a history of an allergic reaction to penicillin or any other β-lactam antibiotic, the most practical approach is to use a different class of antibiotics.

The penicillinase–resistant penicillins can also cause hypersensitivity reactions as well as interstitial nephritis. This is uncommon but produces fever, macular rash, eosinophilia, proteinuria, eosinophiluria, hematuria, and eventually anuria. Discontinuation of penicillin results in the return of normal renal function. Hepatic function abnormalities such as elevation of aspartate aminotransferase or alkaline phosphatase concentrations often follow the use of high doses of β-lactamase–resistant agents. In general, hepatic function rapidly returns to normal when agents are discontinued.

There are no unusual reactions noted for the penicillin/β-lactamase inhibitor combinations, although the incidence of diarrhea with oral amoxicillin/clavulanate is relatively high. This is not observed with the parenteral inhibitor combinations. Incidences of rash and other GI reactions are similar to those of a penicillin-class drug used alone.

Like most penicillins, aminopenicillins can cause hypersensitivity and nonallergic skin rashes, particularly in individuals with preexisting mononucleosis. Diarrhea is more common after oral ampicillin than amoxicillin, the reason why the latter is generally preferred. The aminopenicillins can cause enterocolitis due to superinfection of *C. difficile*. This organism can overgrow when the normal bowel flora is disrupted by antibiotic therapy, producing a cytotoxin and an enterotoxin that cause diarrhea and pseudomembrane formation (pseudomembranous colitis). Distortion of normal intestinal flora by penicillins can also cause bowel function to be altered and cause colonization with resistant gram-negative bacilli or fungi such as *Candida*.

Penicillin-induced neutropenia is rare but can occur as a result of the suppression of granulocyte colony–stimulating factor. All penicillins, particularly high concentrations of ticarcillin, alter platelet aggregation by binding to adenosine diphosphate receptors on the platelets. However, significant bleeding disorders are infrequent. High doses of antipseudomonal penicillins are also known to induce hepatic function abnormalities, including elevated aspartate aminotransferase or alkaline phosphatase levels. These values usually return to normal when agents are discontinued.

Cephalosporins

The cephalosporins are less likely to cause allergic reactions than the penicillins. Cephalosporins can produce anaphylaxis, but the incidence is extremely low. Anaphylaxis to cephalosporins in patients with known penicillin hypersensitivity appears to be <5%. If other therapeutic options exist, cephalosporins should be avoided in patients who have had a severe immediate hypersensitivity reaction to a penicillin. Patients who have exhibited a rash in response to penicillins are at low risk for a similar reaction to cephalosporins. However, maculopapular and morbilliform eruptions may occur in patients receiving cephalosporins. Interstitial nephritis is uncommon but may occur in patients receiving any of the cephalosporins, particularly when aminoglycoside antibiotics are coadministered. Generally, third-generation cephalosporins are well tolerated but are known to cause hypersensitivity in patients with penicillin allergy.

Some cephalosporins have unique adverse effects that are not shared by other members of this class. Cefaclor may lead to fever, joint pain, and local edema in addition to hypersensitivity, while cefotetan possesses a methylthiotetrazole (MTT) side chain that antagonizes vitamin K epoxide reductase and can cause bleeding and thrombocytopenia; it should be avoided in patients taking anticoagulants. The MTT side chain of cefotetan also blocks activity of aldehyde dehydrogenase, which causes a disulfiram-like reaction; thus alcohol consumption should be avoided. Ceftriaxone use has been associated with the formation of gallbladder precipitate, which is usually resolved promptly after discontinuation. In rare cases, hematological disorders such as neutropenia and granulocytopenia are seen.

Cefepime can cause hypersensitivity and anaphylaxis, especially in patients allergic to the penicillins, and can also lead to superinfection due to *C. difficile* overgrowth. Ceftaroline can also precipitate *C. difficile* overgrowth and subsequent formation of pseudomembranous colitis in rare cases.

Carbapenems

Imipenem, meropenem, and ertapenem can cause allergic reactions similar to those produced by the penicillins and should not be administered to patients who have had anaphylactic reactions to penicillins or cephalosporins. Diarrhea and superinfection due to *C. difficile* overgrowth can also occur. Rapid infusion of imipenem with cilastatin can produce nausea and emesis. Imipenem binds to brain tissue more avidly than penicillin G and can cause seizures, which constitute its most serious toxic reaction. Seizures have occurred in patients with decreased renal function and an underlying seizure focus; therefore, imipenem should not be used to treat meningitis. In contrast, meropenem is unlikely to cause seizures and can be used safely to treat bacterial meningitis caused by susceptible organisms.

Monobactams

Unlike other β-lactams, aztreonam does not cross-react with antibodies against penicillin and its derivatives. Consequently, it can be used in patients with a known hypersensitivity to penicillins and most cephalosporins. Because antibodies to cephalosporins can be directed at the side chain, however, aztreonam should be used with caution in patients with anaphylaxis to ceftazidime, a drug with the same side chain on the β-lactam ring as aztreonam.

Non-β-Lactam Cell Wall Synthesis Inhibitors

Most reactions to vancomycin are relatively minor and reversible. However, vancomycin is irritating to tissue, resulting in phlebitis at the site of injection. In addition, chills and fever may occur. Ototoxicity and nephrotoxicity are uncommon with current preparations. However, the risk of these toxicities increases with coadministration of another ototoxic or nephrotoxic drug, such as an aminoglycoside. The most common adverse reaction to vancomycin is the so-called red man syndrome, or infusion-related flushing caused by the release of histamine from basophils and mast cells. It presents as a rapid-onset erythematous rash or pruritus on the head, face, neck, and upper trunk. This reaction can be prevented by prolonging the infusion period to 2 hours or pretreating with an antihistamine such as diphenhydramine. Adverse reactions to telavancin are similar to those of vancomycin, including nephrotoxicity and infusion-related reactions.

Hypersensitivity rarely occurs after the topical use of bacitracin. If given parenterally, bacitracin can cause severe nephrotoxicity.

Fosfomycin is well tolerated but is associated with diarrhea.

Cycloserine may lead to central nervous system effects ranging from mild reactions, such as headache or restlessness, to severe reactions, including depression, psychosis, and seizures; it may exacerbate underlying seizure disorders or mental illness. Pyridoxine administration may help prevent or alleviate these effects. Cycloserine may cause peripheral neuropathy.

Cell Membrane Disrupters

Polymyxins are nephrotoxic, and therefore their administration with other nephrotoxic drugs like aminoglycosides should be avoided. The nephrotoxicity appears to result from drug binding to renal tubule cell membranes, producing proteinuria, casts, and a loss of brush border enzymes, which can progress to renal failure. Renal function usually returns when the drug is discontinued. Polymyxins also cause neurotoxicity manifested as neuromuscular block, paresthesias, ataxia, visual disturbances, and dizziness.

Daptomycin may cause damage to the musculoskeletal system. Myopathy in conjunction with increases in creatine phosphokinase have been reported; rhabdomyolysis has been reported to occur rarely. In addition, daptomycin can cause eosinophilic pneumonia and peripheral neuropathy. Caution is recommended when daptomycin is coadministered with aminoglycosides or statins because of potential risks of nephrotoxicity and myopathy, respectively.

The most commonly observed side effects of representative antibiotics affecting bacterial cell walls and membranes are summarized in the Clinical Problems Box.

NEW DEVELOPMENTS

The widespread use of antibiotics has resulted in increasing resistance through a variety of mechanisms. Inventive approaches to preventing resistance include the use of specific metabolic inhibitors, the development of newer structures that are less susceptible to degradation, and the development of new classes of compounds. The main approaches used currently are to restrict the use of the antibiotics unless absolutely necessary and to use the minimal durations of therapy needed. However, it is clear that new classes of compounds will be needed because most organisms eventually become resistant to these and other antibiotics. Fortunately, many new targets for antibiotic development are being identified by sequencing the genomes of specific bacterial species, which may shed new light on essential processes that can be targeted. Such new targets are likely to include both metabolic and structural proteins, including those involved in the synthesis and maintenance of bacterial cell walls.

CLINICAL RELEVANCE FOR HEALTHCARE PROFESSIONALS

All healthcare professionals are likely to come in contact with individuals taking a bacterial cell wall synthesis inhibitor at some point in their lives and need to be aware of the limitations and adverse effects associated with these agents.

CLINICAL PROBLEMS

β-Lactam Cell Wall

Penicillin G	Immunoglobulin E antibody allergic reaction (anaphylaxis or early urticaria), neutropenia
Ampicillin/Amoxicillin	Delayed hypersensitivity and contact dermatitis, skin rash and fever, diarrhea, enterocolitis
Oxacillin	Elevated aspartate aminotransferase activity, neutropenia
Nafcillin	Elevated aspartate aminotransferase activity
Cephalosporins	Skin rash and fever, diarrhea
Cefotetan	Disulfiram-like effects
Cefoxitin	Enterocolitis
Ceftriaxone	Precipitation in gallbladder, diarrhea
Cefepime	Enterocolitis
Imipenem	Seizures

Non-β-Lactam Cell Wall Synthesis Inhibitors

Vancomycin	Phlebitis, flushing
Bacitracin	Nephrotoxic if enters systemic circulation (limited to topical use)
Fosfomycin	Diarrhea, nausea, vaginitis
Cycloserine	Headache, drowsiness, tremor, central nervous system effects

Cell Membrane Disrupters

Colistin	Nephrotoxicity, neurotoxicity
Daptomycin	Musculoskeletal damage including myopathy and peripheral neuropathy, eosinophilic pneumonia

TRADE NAMES

In addition to generic and fixed-combination preparations, the following trade-named materials are some of the important compounds available in the United States.

Penicillins
Amoxicillin (Amoxil, Amoxicot, Trimox)
Ampicillin (Principen)
Benzathine penicillin (Bicillin L-A)
Carbenicillin (Geocillin)
Cloxacillin (Cloxapen)
Dicloxacillin (Dynapen)
Nafcillin (Nallpen)
Oxacillin (Bactocill)
Penicillin G (Pentids, Pfizerpen)
Penicillin V (PC Pen-VK, Veetids, V-Cillin)
Piperacillin (Pipracil)
Ticarcillin (Ticar)

Penicillin/β-Lactamase Inhibitor Combinations
Amoxicillin-clavulanate (Augmentin)
Ampicillin-sulbactam (Unasyn)
Piperacillin-tazobactam (Zosyn)

Cephalosporins
First generation
    Cefadroxil (Duricef, Ultracef)
    Cefazolin (Ancef, Kefzol)
    Cephalexin (Keflex)
    Cephapirin (Cefadyl)
    Cephradine (Velosef)
Second generation
    Cefaclor (Ceclor)
    Cefoxitin (Mefoxin)
    Cefprozil (Cefzil)
    Cefuroxime (Kefurox, Zinacef)

Cefuroxime axetil (Ceftin)
    Loracarbef (Lorabid)
Third generation
    Cefdinir (Omnicef)
    Cefixime (Suprax)
    Cefotaxime (Claforan)
    Cefpodoxime (Vantin)
    Ceftazidime (Fortaz, Tazicef, Tazidime)
    Ceftizoxime (Cefizox)
    Ceftriaxone (Rocephin)
Fourth generation
    Cefepime (Maxipime)
Fifth generation
    Ceftaroline (Teflaro)

Carbapenems
Ertapenem (Invanz)
Imipenem-cilastatin (Primaxin)
Meropenem (Merrem)

Monobactams
Aztreonam (Azactam)

Polypeptides and Non-β-Lactams
Vancomycin (Vancocin)
Telavancin (Vibativ)
Bacitracin (Baciguent, AK-Tracin)
Fosfomycin (Monurol)
Cycloserine (Seromycin)

Cell Membrane Disrupters
Polymyxin B
Colistin/Polymyxin E
Daptomycin (Cubicin)

SELF-ASSESSMENT QUESTIONS

1. An asthmatic patient is hospitalized for the treatment of a severe respiratory infection due to *S. pneumoniae*. The patient reports a prior allergic reaction to ampicillin. Which of the following would be the best choice for this patient?
   A. Amoxicillin.
   B. Aztreonam.
   C. Cefepime.
   D. Imipenem.
   E. Vancomycin.

2. A patient is administered an intravenous antibiotic for the treatment of bacterial meningitis, but a short time later, the patient experiences a seizure. Which of the following drugs was most likely administered?
   A. Ampicillin.
   B. Ceftriaxone.
   C. Imipenem.
   D. Nafcillin.
   E. Vancomycin.

3. Resistance to vancomycin is becoming increasingly more common in *S. aureus* species. Which of the following is the most common mechanism by which this occurs?
   A. Decreased affinity of PBPs for vancomycin.
   B. Increased efflux of vancomycin.

   C. Increased number of binding sites for vancomycin.
   D. Production of β-lactamases.

4. Although β-lactam antibiotics are considered primarily to be bactericidal, in some bacteria, they are only bacteriostatic. Which of the following statements best explains this phenomenon?
   A. The absence of autolysins.
   B. The absence of porin proteins.
   C. The formation of filamentous structures.
   D. Increased layers of peptidoglycan in the cell wall.
   E. Increased numbers of penicillin-binding proteins.

5. Some antibiotics exhibit a "postantibiotic effect" after plasma levels fall below the minimum inhibitory concentration (MIC). Which one of the following drugs exhibits a postantibiotic effect that causes inhibition of cell growth up to 4 hours after plasma levels are under the MIC?
   A. Aztreonam.
   B. Cefaclor.
   C. Meropenem.
   D. Oxacillin.
   E. Vancomycin.

FURTHER READING

Gardete S, Tomasz A. Mechanisms of vancomycin resistance in *Staphylococcus aureus*. *J Clin Invest*. 2014;124(7):2836–2840.

Nordmann P, Laurent D, Laurent P. Carbapenem resistance in *Enterobacteriaceae*: here is the storm! *Trends Mol Med*. 2012;18:263–272.

Paterson DL, Bonomo RA. Extended spectrum beta-lactamases: a clinical update. *Clin Microbiol Rev*. 2005;18:657–686.

Ofosu A. *Clostridium difficile* infection: a review of current and emerging therapies. *Ann Gastroenterology*. 2016;29:147–154.

Zhanel GG, Wiebe R, Dilay L, et al. Comparative review of the carbapenems. *Drugs*. 2007;67:1027–1052.

WEBSITES

https://medlineplus.gov/antibiotics.html

This website is maintained by the United States National Library of Medicine and has numerous links to many valuable resources on antibiotics.

http://www.idsociety.org/Antimicrobial_Agents/

This website is maintained by the Infectious Disease Society of America and contains guidelines for the use of antimicrobial agents as well as links to numerous excellent resources for healthcare professionals and patients.

https://www.cdc.gov/hai/organisms/visa_vrsa/visa_vrsa.html

This site is maintained by the United States Centers for Disease Control and Prevention and contains very useful information on VISA and VRSA in healthcare settings.

Drugs Targeting Bacterial Protein Synthesis

Rukiyah Van Dross-Anderson and Daniel A. Ladin

MAJOR DRUG CLASSES

Aminoglycosides and related compounds
Tetracyclines and glycylcyclines
Macrolides
Ketolides
Lincosamides
Oxazolidinones
Streptogramins
Others

ABBREVIATIONS

AIDS	Acquired immunodeficiency syndrome
CSF	Cerebrospinal fluid
GI	Gastrointestinal
IM	Intramuscular
IV	Intravenous
MLS_B	Macrolide-lincosamide-streptogramin B
mRNA	Messenger ribonucleic acid
tRNA	Transfer ribonucleic acid

THERAPEUTIC OVERVIEW

Bacterial ribosomes, which are composed of approximately 60% ribosomal RNA and 40% protein (by weight), represent a primary target for a diverse group of antibiotic agents that inhibit bacterial protein synthesis. Prokaryotic ribosomes are comprised of a small 30S and a large 50S subunit (where S is a Svedberg unit for sedimentation rate) that complex to form the 70S ribosome. The 30S subunit contains the 16S ribosomal RNA and guides messenger RNA (mRNA) into place by binding to three initiation factors to ensure that translation begins at the correct location. The larger 50S subunit, which contains two RNA species, the 5S and the 23S, functions as a catalyst for peptide bond formation. Because eukaryotic ribosomes consist of a 40S and 60S subunit, antibiotics that target the bacterial ribosome lead to selective inhibition of bacterial protein synthesis.

The drugs that target the bacterial ribosome fall into numerous chemical categories and include aminoglycosides, tetracyclines and glycylcyclines, macrolides, ketolides, lincosamides, oxazolidinones, and streptogramins. The organisms susceptible to and therapeutic applications of these agents are summarized in the Therapeutic Overview Box.

MECHANISMS OF ACTION

The steps involved in bacterial protein synthesis and sites of action of the protein synthesis inhibitors are shown in Fig. 58.1. The aminoglycosides, tetracyclines, and glycylcyclines bind to the 30S ribosomal subunit; all others bind to sites on the 50S subunit. Further, depending on the drug class and the bacteria, these agents may result in either bactericidal or bacteriostatic effects. In general, the aminoglycosides are bactericidal, while the others are bacteriostatic with a few exceptions for several specific bacteria.

Aminoglycosides

The aminoglycosides, including streptomycin, gentamicin, tobramycin, kanamycin, neomycin, and others, consist of amino sugars linked through glycosidic bonds to an aminocyclitol. The structures of streptomycin, gentamicin, kanamycin, and neomycin are shown in Fig. 58.2. The particular amino sugars and specific locations of the amino groups distinguish the compounds and are important for their antimicrobial effects and toxicity. The aminoglycosides exert a concentration-dependent bactericidal action and are effective primarily against aerobic gram-negative bacteria.

The aminoglycosides diffuse through the porin channels in the outer membrane of gram-negative bacteria, followed by active transport across the inner cytoplasmic membrane (Chapter 56, Fig. 56.1). This latter process is an energy-requiring, rate-limiting step driven by the membrane potential, which is compromised in an anaerobic environment or at low pH, and is inhibited by divalent cations such as Ca^{++} and Mg^{++}. After crossing the cytoplasmic membrane, the aminoglycosides bind to the 30S ribosomal subunit, maintaining a low concentration of intracellular free drug, which facilitates continued drug transfer.

Streptomycin, the most thoroughly studied aminoglycoside, binds to at least three proteins and the 16S ribosomal RNA in the 30S subunit. Thus mutations in any of these moieties can affect drug binding and effectiveness. As a consequence of binding, streptomycin inhibits protein synthesis by: (1) interfering with initiation, leading to abnormal initiation complexes; (2) misreading the mRNA template, leading to the synthesis of nonfunctional or toxic proteins; and (3) cleaving polyribosomes (mRNA ribosome complexes) into nonfunctional monosomes. Aminoglycosides also have a prolonged postantibiotic effect to suppress bacterial growth after serum concentrations fall below the minimal inhibitory concentration (MIC), which is attributed to the irreversible binding of the drug to the 30S ribosome, with intracellular drug accumulation that persists after plasma levels decline. Higher aminoglycoside concentrations are associated with a longer postantibiotic effect.

Tetracyclines and Glycylcyclines

The tetracyclines include tetracycline, chlortetracycline, doxycycline, minocycline, and others, while the only currently approved glycylcycline

THERAPEUTIC OVERVIEW

Aminoglycosides

Aerobic gram-negative bacteria including *Pseudomonas*, *Acinetobacter*, and *Enterobacter* species; some mycobacteria including *M. tuberculosis*

Peritonitis associated with peritoneal dialysis; bacterial endocarditis; sepsis; severe abdominal and urinary tract infections; skin and mucous membrane infections

Tetracyclines and Glycylcyclines

Aerobic and anaerobic gram-positive and gram-negative bacteria including *Chlamydia*, *Legionella*, and *Rickettsia* species; *M. pneumoniae*

Infections of the respiratory tract, skin and soft tissue, intraabdominal organs, gastrointestinal and urinary tract; sexually transmitted diseases; Rocky Mountain spotted fever; anthrax exposure

Macrolides

Aerobic gram-positive bacteria including *Streptococci*, *Pneumococci*, *Staphylococci*, and *Enterococci* species; *L. pneumophila*; some *Rickettsia*, *Chlamydia*, *Mycoplasma*, and *Mycobacteria* species

Respiratory tract infections (pneumonia, chronic bronchitis, acute otitis media, acute streptococcal pharyngitis, and acute bacterial sinusitis); skin and soft-tissue infections; diphtheria; pertussis (prophylaxis and treatment); peptic ulcer disease caused by *H. pylori*

Ketolides

Aerobic gram-positive bacteria including *S. aureus* and *S. pneumoniae*; *H. influenzae*, *M. catarrhalis*, *C. pneumoniae*, and *M. pneumoniae*

Community-acquired pneumonia

Lincosamides

Aerobic and anaerobic gram-positive and anaerobic gram-negative bacteria including *Streptococcus* species, *Fusobacterium* species, *B. fragilis*, *A. israelii*, and *N. asteroides*; some *Mycoplasma* species

Skin and soft-tissue infections, lung abscess and anaerobic lung and pleural space infections, acne vulgaris (topical use), bacterial vaginosis (topical use)

Oxazolidinones

Aerobic and anaerobic gram-positive organisms including *E. faecium* and *S. aureus*; *Chlamydia*, *Legionella*, and *Mycoplasma* species

Infections caused by vancomycin-resistant *E. faecium*; uncomplicated skin and skin-structure infections; community-acquired pneumonia; use reserved for treatment of infections caused by multiple-drug–resistant bacteria

Streptogramins

Aerobic and anaerobic gram-positive organisms including *E. faecium*, *Staphylococci*, and *Streptococci* species; *M. catarrhalis*, *C. pneumoniae*; *M. pneumoniae*; *Neisseria* and *Legionella* species

Infections caused by vancomycin-resistant *E. faecium* and complicated skin and skin-structure infections caused by methicillin-susceptible strains of *S. aureus* or *S. pyogenes*

Chloramphenicol

Aerobic and anaerobic gram-positive and gram-negative bacteria including *Rickettsia*, *Chlamydia*, *Chlamydophila*, *Clostridium*, *Streptococci*, and *Gemella* species

Only used clinically in life-threatening infections and if no other equally effective and potentially less toxic antimicrobials are available

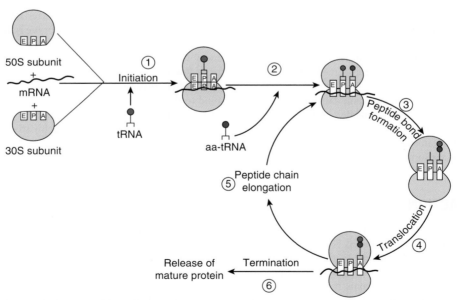

FIG. 58.1 Bacterial Protein Synthesis. Protein synthesis involves the formation of the 70S ribosome from the 50S and the 30S ribosomes. The 70S ribosome contains 3 sites. The P (peptidyl) site is the site where the first amino acid attaches to the ribosome, the A (aminoacyl or acceptor) site is the site where subsequent amino acids are added, and the E (exit) site is the site where the tRNAs are released. Protein synthesis inhibitors act at one or several steps in the cycle, which is composed of the following processes: (1) initiation; (2) attachment of amino acids to the A site; (3) peptide bond formation; (4) translocation; (5) peptide chain elongation; and (6) termination.

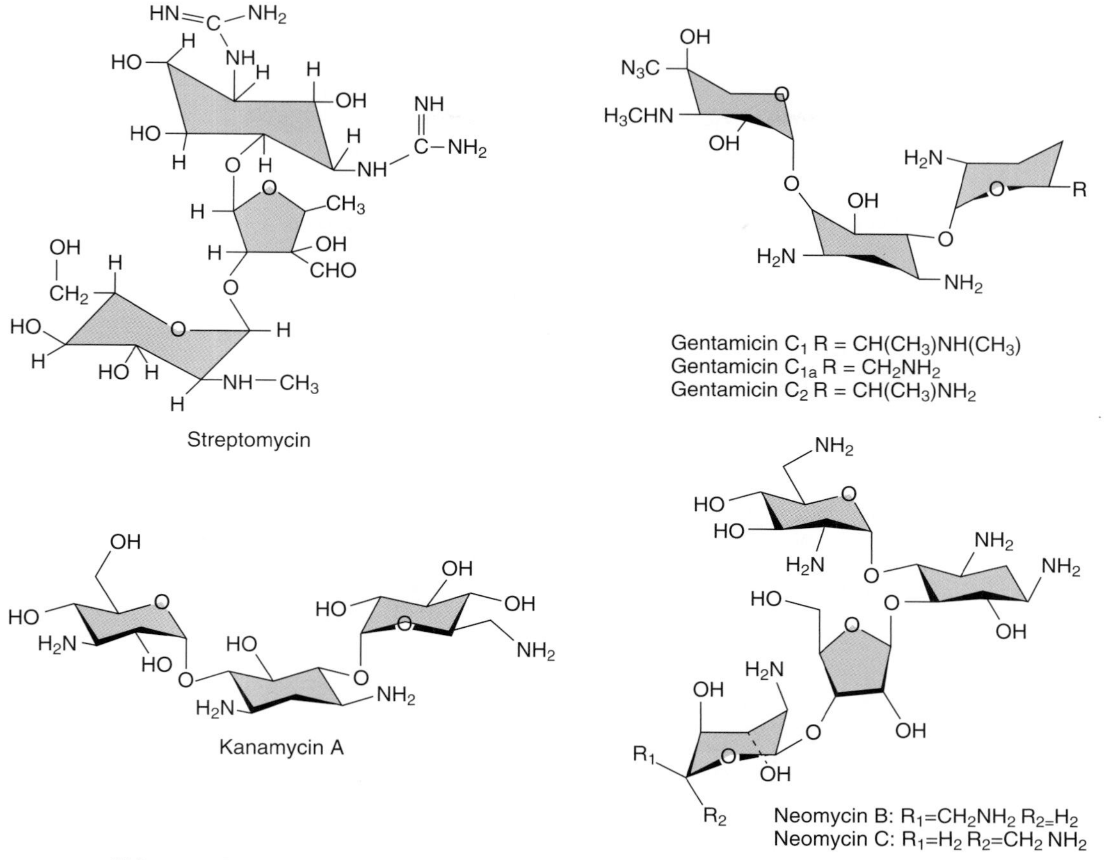

FIG. 58.2 Structures of Streptomycin, Gentamicin, Kanamycin A, and Neomycin.

antibiotic is tigecycline. The structures of tetracycline and tigecycline are shown in Fig. 58.3. These agents are bacteriostatic and are effective against a broad spectrum of aerobic and anaerobic gram-negative and gram-positive organisms.

These drugs diffuse through porin channels in the outer membrane of gram-negative bacteria, followed by active transport across the inner cytoplasmic membrane via a carrier system. The drugs enter the cytoplasm of gram-positive bacteria by an undefined active process. Differences in the activities of individual tetracyclines are related to their solubility in lipid membranes of the bacteria, with minocycline and doxycycline more lipophilic. Once inside the cell, the tetracyclines and tigecycline bind reversibly to the A site on the 30S ribosomal subunit, thereby inhibiting attachment of the aminoacyl-transfer RNA (tRNA) to its acceptor site and preventing the beginning of the elongation cycle.

Macrolides

The macrolides include erythromycin, clarithromycin, azithromycin, and dirithromycin; the structure of erythromycin, the prototype, is shown in Fig. 58.3. These agents contain large (12–16 membered) lactone rings with attached sugar molecules. In general, these agents are bacteriostatic, but may be bactericidal at higher concentrations for some organisms such as *Streptococcus pneumoniae* and *Streptococcus pyogenes*. They are effective primarily against aerobic gram-positive bacteria.

The macrolides penetrate the bacterial cytoplasmic membrane and bind reversibly to a single domain on the 23S RNA on the 50S ribosomal subunit, causing dissociation of peptidyl-tRNA from the ribosome and interfering with peptide chain elongation.

Ketolides

Telithromycin is a semisynthetic derivative of erythromycin, with keto and carbamate substitutions, rendering it less susceptible to resistance development. Telithromycin is currently the only ketolide available in the United States. It has a mechanism of action similar to the macrolides, viz., it also binds to the 50S ribosomal subunit and prevents protein and peptide elongation. However, unlike the macrolides, telithromycin binds to two domains of the 23S RNA.

Lincosamides

The lincosamides include lincomycin, clindamycin, and pirlimycin, with clindamycin the main lincosamide in clinical use. These agents are thiogalactosides, with the structure of clindamycin shown in Fig. 58.3. The lincosamides have a somewhat unique spectrum of activity and are effective against both aerobic and anaerobic gram-positive but only anaerobic gram-negative bacteria. The site of action of clindamycin is similar to that of erythromycin and telithromycin and involves binding on the 23S RNA on the 50S ribosomal subunit, and although the binding site for clindamycin overlaps that for erythromycin, it does not appear to be identical. Clindamycin blocks peptide bond formation between the A and P site tRNAs, thereby inhibiting the elongation cycle.

Oxazolidinones

The oxazolidinones include linezolid and tedizolid. These agents represent a newer class of antibiotics that are active against aerobic and anaerobic gram-positive organisms and may be bactericidal or bacteriostatic, depending on the bacteria. The mechanisms of action of the

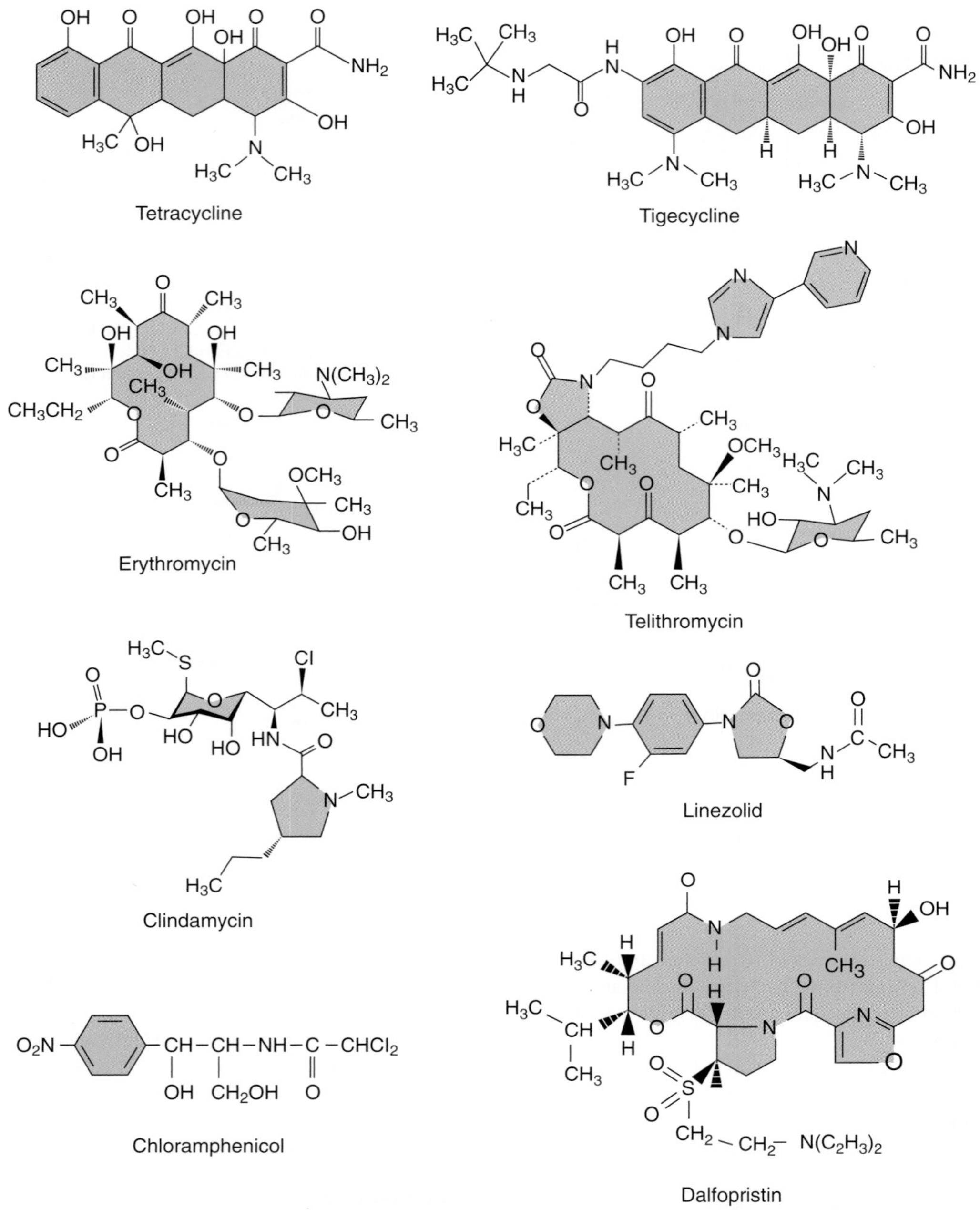

FIG. 58.3 Structures of Representative Bacterial Protein Synthesis Inhibitors Representing Major Drug Classes.

oxazolidinones is not fully understood. Studies have shown that these agents bind to the P site on the 50S ribosomal subunit to prevent formation of the 70S initiation complex, inhibit peptide bond formation like the lincosamides, and block peptidyl transferase like chloramphenicol, leading to inhibition of termination.

Streptogramins

The streptogramins include **quinupristin**, which is a streptogramin B, and **dalfopristin**, which is a streptogramin A, and represent semisynthetic derivatives of naturally occurring pristinamycins produced by *Streptomyces pristinaespiralis*. These agents are combined in a 30:70 ratio of quinupristin/dalfopristin. They are effective against aerobic and anaerobic gram-positive bacteria and can be bacteriostatic or bactericidal, depending on the specific bacteria. These agents bind to the 50S ribosomal subunit, with quinupristin binding to the same site as the macrolides to dissociate

peptidyl-tRNA from the ribosome, causing early termination of chain elongation, and dalfopristin leading to a conformational change in the ribosome, enhancing the binding of quinupristin 100-fold. Dalfopristin also inhibits peptidyl transferase to inhibit peptide bond formation.

Others

Chloramphenicol, which was isolated and has been used for more than 70 years, is a unique compound containing a nitrobenzene ring (see Fig. 58.3). Chloramphenicol is primarily bacteriostatic but is bactericidal for selected pathogens, including *S. pneumoniae, Neisseria meningitidis,* and *Haemophilus influenzae*. It is active against aerobic and anaerobic gram-positive and gram-negative bacteria. **Chloramphenicol** readily enters bacterial cells and binds reversibly to the 50S ribosomal subunit close to the site where erythromycin and clindamycin bind. Interestingly, erythromycin inhibits the binding of chloramphenicol to 50S ribosomes, but chloramphenicol does not inhibit erythromycin binding. Evidence suggests that chloramphenicol inhibits peptidyl transferase, inhibiting termination of the elongation cycle and preventing the release of the polypeptide chain.

Mupirocin (pseudomonic acid) is a monoxycarbolic acid derived from a fermentation product of *Pseudomonas fluorescens*. It binds reversibly to isoleucyl transfer-RNA synthetase, thus preventing the incorporation of isoleucine into nascent peptides during protein synthesis. Mupirocin is active against many gram-positive bacteria including *S. pyogenes* and methicillin-susceptible and methicillin-resistant strains of *Staphylococcus aureus*.

MECHANISMS OF RESISTANCE

Aminoglycosides

Bacterial resistance to the aminoglycosides results from: (1) enzymatic modification of the drug, (2) altered ribosomes, or (3) inadequate transport within the cell. The most common and clinically important form of resistance stems from modification of the aminoglycoside, which occurs through enzyme-catalyzed phosphorylation, adenylation, or acetylation. The genes for these enzymes are located on plasmids or transposons, which can be spread to many different bacterial species. Many such enzymes have been identified, some of which can inactivate only one or two compounds, whereas others can inactivate multiple compounds. For example, an enzyme that acetylates the amino group at position 6 of the amino hexose can inactivate kanamycin, neomycin, tobramycin, and amikacin but not gentamicin or streptomycin. The altered aminoglycosides do not bind as well to ribosomes. Amikacin is the most resistant of the aminoglycosides to inactivation by resistant organisms, and netilmicin is the second most resistant.

Resistance resulting from altered ribosomes occurs in enterococci but is relatively uncommon and rarely occurs with gram-negative bacteria. In addition, resistance as a consequence of the inadequate transport of drug across the cytoplasmic membrane is uncommon in aerobic or facultative species but does occur in strict anaerobes. Mutants with alterations in the electron transfer chain and in adenosine triphosphatase activity have been identified but are very rare. The resistance of some *Pseudomonas* species to aminoglycosides may be related to failure of the drug to distort the lipopolysaccharide of the outer membrane, thus not allowing drug to enter the bacterial cell.

Tetracyclines and Glycylcyclines

Resistance to the tetracyclines is primarily plasmid mediated, but can also be transposon mediated, and involves mainly decreased bacterial cell accumulation of the drug, as a consequence of decreased influx or increased efflux. Drug influx may be compromised by outer membrane protein alterations resulting from mutations in chromosomal genes. Drug efflux may be enhanced by the drug-induced induction of a new protein that promotes active efflux. A second resistance mechanism involves the plasmid-mediated generation of a protein that competes with the drug for binding to the ribosome, referred to as ribosomal protection. Lastly, resistance can arise through the induction of enzymes that inactivate the drug. Resistance to one tetracycline usually implies resistance to all tetracyclines. However, some staphylococci and some *Bacteroides* species are resistant to tetracycline but susceptible to minocycline and doxycycline because of the lipophilicity of these latter agents.

Macrolides

Bacterial resistance to macrolides occurs by several mechanisms, some of which also confer resistance to clindamycin and quinupristin (a streptogramin B). Efflux systems represent a prominent mechanism of macrolide resistance and is associated with macrolide efflux genes *(mef)*. This mechanism, which confers cross-resistance, exists among

erythromycin, clarithromycin, and azithromycin but does not confer resistance to clindamycin or streptogramin B. In addition, gram-negative bacteria may also possess esterases that hydrolyze erythromycin.

Another resistance mechanism involves alterations of ribosomal binding sites that occur via a plasmid-encoded enzyme that methylates the 50S ribosomal subunit. Methylation likely causes a conformational change of the ribosomal target and decreased binding. This type of resistance is associated with the erythromycin ribosome methylation gene *(erm)* and is referred to as the macrolide-lincosamide-streptogramin B (MLS$_B$) phenotype because it confers resistance to macrolides, clindamycin, and streptogramin B.

Ketolides

In contrast to the macrolides, telithromycin retains activity against most organisms whose ribosomal binding sites have been modified via methylation (MLS$_B$ phenotypes). In addition, ketolides do not appear to induce MLS$_B$ resistance in streptococci but may promote constitutive expression of *erm* genes in staphylococci with an inducible MLS$_B$ phenotype. Telithromycin-resistant strains of *S. pneumoniae* have been described in which both ribosomal modification and mutations in ribosomal proteins were present. Telithromycin has retained activity against streptococci, demonstrating *mef*-mediated efflux pumps.

Lincosamides

Resistance to clindamycin may arise from alterations in ribosomal binding sites, with a resultant MLS$_B$ phenotype conferring resistance to both clindamycin and macrolides. This form of resistance is often plasmid mediated and has been observed in clindamycin-resistant strains of *Bacteroides fragilis*. Innate resistance to clindamycin in *Enterobacteriaceae* and *Pseudomonas* results from poor permeability of the cell envelope to clindamycin.

Oxazolidinones

Resistance to linezolid typically arises as a consequence of alterations in the binding site on the 50S ribosomal subunit. Because linezolid binds to a site that is in a deep cleft surrounded by 23S RNA, any point mutations in nucleotides will lead to structural alterations that alter binding and thus efficacy. Because bacteria contain multiple copies of 23S ribosomal RNA genes, resistance generally requires mutations in more than one copy. Cross-resistance with other ribosomal inhibitors has not been demonstrated. Gram-negative organisms become resistant to linezolid via drug efflux.

Streptogramins

Resistance to quinupristin involves altered ribosomal binding as a consequence of a plasmid-encoded methylase, i.e., the MLS$_B$ phenotype. Resistance to dalfopristin involves two plasmid-mediated mechanisms, viz., enzymatic modification of the drug and enhanced efflux. The expression of an acetyltransferase inactivates dalfopristin, while the expression of ATP-dependent efflux proteins promotes drug efflux. Resistance to quinupristin is mediated by genes that encode lactonases, which inactivate the antibiotic. Innate resistance to quinupristin/dalfopristin occurs in Enterobacteriaceae and *Pseudomonas aeruginosa* related to cell membrane impermeability.

Others

Most resistance to chloramphenicol is attributed to the plasmid-encoded expression of chloramphenicol acetyltransferase, which catalyzes the acetylation of the hydroxy groups of chloramphenicol and inhibits drug binding to the 50S subunit. Less common mechanisms of resistance arise from alterations in cell wall permeability or ribosomal proteins.

Because mupirocin has a unique mechanism of action that is not shared with any other antibiotic, cross-resistance with other classes of antibiotics is not a problem. Mutations of the gene-encoding isoleucyl transfer-RNA synthetase or the presence of an extra copy of the gene may lead to a low-level resistance. In addition, expression of the *mupA* gene, which encodes a "bypass" synthetase that binds mupirocin with much lower affinity, can lead to a high-level resistance. Strains with high-level resistance have caused hospital-associated outbreaks of staphylococcal infection.

RELATIONSHIP OF MECHANISMS OF ACTION TO CLINICAL RESPONSE

Aminoglycosides

The aminoglycosides are effective primarily against aerobic gram-negative organisms, and in combination with other classes of antibiotics, are most often used in the treatment of bacteremia and sepsis. They are ineffective against anaerobic organisms. Because the therapeutic index of the aminoglycosides is narrow and toxicity can be serious, close attention must be paid to the pharmacokinetics of these drugs in individual patients. Renal function must be assessed, and monitoring of plasma concentrations is recommended.

Synergistic killing has been demonstrated when aminoglycosides are combined with cell wall synthesis inhibitors (e.g., β-lactams, glycopeptides), related partly to increased uptake of the aminoglycosides in the presence of cell wall active agents. Clinically, aminoglycosides and cell wall active agents are combined to achieve synergistic killing against enterococci, *S. aureus*, *P. aeruginosa*, and other Enterobacteriaceae.

Aminoglycosides should be reserved for the treatment of serious infections for which other agents, such as penicillins or cephalosporins, are not suitable. Aminoglycosides have no role in the initial therapy of gram-positive infections. They must be given in combination with penicillins or glycopeptides to treat endocarditis resulting from enterococci, viridans streptococci, or coagulase-negative staphylococci. Gentamicin is the preferred agent because streptomycin resistance is common.

The initial treatment of suspected sepsis has consisted of an aminoglycoside, such as gentamicin or tobramycin, in combination with a penicillin or cephalosporin, but newer cephalosporins and other β-lactams, such as aztreonam or imipenem, have lower toxicity and are being used with increased frequency in this setting (Chapter 57). Local antimicrobial resistance patterns should be used to help define empiric therapies for sepsis.

Aminoglycosides are used in combination with an antipseudomonal β-lactam to treat suspected sepsis in febrile neutropenic patients. Choice of the particular agent depends on local susceptibility patterns. In general, gentamicin is the first agent used, with tobramycin reserved for *Pseudomonas* infections or amikacin used in the event of resistance. Alternatives should be used for the treatment of neutropenic fever when patients have received previous nephrotoxic chemotherapy.

Nosocomial (hospital-acquired) pneumonia has been treated with aminoglycosides, and an aminoglycoside in combination with an antipseudomonal penicillin, cephalosporin, or monobactam is usually selected for the treatment of serious respiratory tract infections resulting from *P. aeruginosa*. In addition, aminoglycosides may be indicated in combination treatment regimens for nosocomial intraabdominal infections, where the potential for serious *Pseudomonas* and *Enterobacter* infections exists. In addition, the combination of an aminoglycoside with clindamycin can be used to treat gynecological infections, including pelvic inflammatory disease.

Streptomycin is used primarily to treat uncommon infections such as those caused by *Francisella tularensis*, *Brucella* species, *Yersinia pestis*, and resistant tuberculosis strains or infections in patients allergic to

BOX 58.1 **Therapeutic Uses of Tetracyclines**	
Drug of Choice	Rickettsial diseases: Rocky Mountain spotted fever, typhus, scrub typhus, Q fever; ehrlichiosis; *M. pneumoniae*; *C. pneumoniae*; *C. trachomatis*; *C. psittaci*; Lyme disease *(Borrelia burgdorferi)*; relapsing fever caused by *Borrelia* organisms; brucellosis
Alternative Agent As Treatment of Syndromes	Plague; pelvic inflammatory disease
	Acne, low-dose oral or topical; bacterial exacerbations of bronchitis; malabsorption syndrome resulting from bowel bacterial overgrowth

the usual antituberculosis drugs (Chapter 60). Amikacin is also used to treat multidrug-resistant tuberculosis.

Tetracyclines and Glycylcyclines

Tetracyclines are broad-spectrum agents that inhibit a wide variety of aerobic and anaerobic gram-positive and gram-negative bacteria and other microorganisms such as *Ehrlichia* species, *Mycoplasma* species, *Chlamydia* species, *Rickettsia* species, Spirochaetaceae, which includes *Borrelia* and *Treponema* species, and some mycobacterial species. The tetracyclines have many clinical uses, but because of increasing bacterial resistance and development of other drugs, they are no longer as widely used. For example, some *S. pneumoniae*, *S. pyogenes*, and staphylococci are now resistant to most tetracyclines, as are many *Escherichia coli* and *Shigella* species and virtually all *P. aeruginosa*. Doxycycline inhibits *B. fragilis*, but most *Bacteroides* species are resistant to the other tetracyclines. Other species susceptible to the tetracyclines include *Fusobacterium* and *Actinomyces*, *Borrelia burgdorferi* (the cause of Lyme disease), *Mycobacterium marinum* and *leprae*, and some *Plasmodium* species.

Tetracyclines are the preferred agents for the treatment of rickettsial diseases such as Rocky Mountain spotted fever, typhus, scrub typhus, rickettsial pox, and Q fever (Box 58.1), with doxycycline being the preferred agent from this class. Doxycycline is also the drug of choice for the treatment of ehrlichiosis and is used to treat Lyme disease and relapsing fever caused by *Borrelia* species. Atypical respiratory pathogens, including *Mycoplasma pneumoniae*, *Chlamydophila pneumoniae*, and *Chlamydophila psittaci*, respond to tetracyclines, which may be better tolerated by adults than erythromycin. Systemic *Vibrio* infections and peptic ulcer disease associated with *Helicobacter pylori* may also be treated with tetracyclines. Chlamydial infections of a sexual origin, such as nongonococcal urethritis, salpingitis, cervicitis, and lymphogranuloma venereum, are effectively treated with doxycycline. Tetracyclines are also effective for the treatment of inclusion conjunctivitis and trachoma caused by Chlamydiae. For penicillin-allergic patients, tetracycline or doxycycline represents an important alternative treatment for some forms of syphilis. In addition, doxycycline is a recommended treatment for granuloma inguinale.

Minocycline and doxycycline inhibit some methicillin-resistant staphylococci and has been used to treat these infections, but vancomycin remains the drug of choice. Doxycycline also is an important option for prophylaxis against *Plasmodium falciparum* for travelers to regions where malaria is endemic, particularly those with mefloquine-resistant species.

Macrolides

The macrolides are active primarily against gram-positive species such as staphylococci and streptococci but also inhibit some gram-positive bacilli (Box 58.2). Most aerobic gram-negative bacilli are resistant, although azithromycin inhibits *Salmonella*.

BOX 58.2 **Therapeutic Uses of Erythromycin**

Drug of Choice	*M. pneumoniae*; Group A streptococcal upper respiratory tract infection (penicillin-allergic patient); *Legionella* infection; *B. pertussis*; *C. jejuni*; *U. urealyticum*; *B. henselae*; *C. diphtheriae*
Alternative Agent	Lyme disease; *Chlamydia* infection
As Treatment of Syndromes	Bacterial bronchitis; otitis media (with sulfonamide); acne, topical
Prophylaxis	Endocarditis (penicillin-allergic patient); large bowel surgery; oral surgery

---

Erythromycin is relatively safe and widely used, especially for the treatment of infections in children. Erythromycin and other macrolides are used as an alternative to penicillin, particularly in children with streptococcal pharyngitis, erysipelas, scarlet fever, cutaneous streptococcal infections, and pneumococcal pneumonia. Because of the success of macrolides in the treatment of pulmonary infections, these drugs continue to be used in the treatment of respiratory tract infections in adults. The primary differences among **erythromycin**, **clarithromycin**, and **azithromycin** are related to relative activities against certain bacterial species such as *Mycobacterium*, gastrointestinal (GI) tolerability, and pharmacokinetics.

Both azithromycin and clarithromycin inhibit *H. influenzae*, but of all the macrolides, azithromycin is the most effective. Azithromycin and clarithromycin both have activity against *Mycobacterum avium* complex and *Mycobacterium chelonae*, although clarithromycin is more active against the latter. Both agents also have important activity against *H. pylori*. Dirithromycin is generally similar to erythromycin in its spectrum of antibacterial activity.

Although macrolide resistance in *S. pneumoniae* and *S. pyogenes* continues to increase, these agents continue to be used widely in combination with β-lactams for the treatment of community-acquired pneumonia because of their excellent activity against atypical respiratory pathogens. Although macrolides can cure *S. aureus* infections, they are not an initial choice for therapy because of the high frequency of resistance. Azithromycin is useful for treating sexually transmitted diseases, including those caused by Chlamydiae, and erythromycin can be used to treat chlamydial pneumonia of the newborn. Trachoma can be treated effectively with a single dose of azithromycin. Recent data also support the use of azithromycin for the treatment of traveler's diarrhea. Erythromycin is also useful for eradicating the carrier state of diphtheria and may shorten the course of pertussis if administered early. Clarithromycin and azithromycin are useful in both preventing and treating *M. avium* complex infections in patients with acquired immunodeficiency syndrome (AIDS). Bacillary angiomatosis in patients with AIDS has also been successfully treated with erythromycin. Erythromycin can be used to prevent bacterial endocarditis in penicillin-allergic patients with rheumatic fever.

Ketolides

Telithromycin displays excellent activity against most of the pathogens causing community-acquired pneumonia, acute exacerbations of chronic bronchitis, and acute sinusitis, including atypical intracellular pathogens. Potent in vitro activity against *S. pneumoniae*, *H. influenzae*, *Moraxella catarrhalis*, *M. pneumoniae*, *C. pneumoniae*, and *L. pneumophila* has been demonstrated. Telithromycin retains activity against most penicillin-resistant and macrolide-resistant *S. pneumoniae*, regardless of macrolide resistance phenotype. Given its activity against drug-resistant

pneumococci, telithromycin may prove to be especially useful in the treatment of community-acquired pneumonia in areas with high levels of penicillin and macrolide resistance.

Lincosamides

Clindamycin inhibits many anaerobes and most gram-positive cocci but not enterococci, aerobic gram-negative bacteria, or atypical bacteria. Clindamycin is useful for anaerobic pleuropulmonary and odontogenic infections and is appropriate therapy for intraabdominal or gynecological infections in which *Bacteroides* organisms are likely pathogens, although resistance in these species is increasingly common. Clindamycin should not be used for brain abscesses if anaerobic species are anticipated.

Clindamycin is an alternative to penicillin and may be preferable in certain situations in which β-lactamase–producing *Bacteroides* organisms are present. Clindamycin is also an alternative to penicillinase-resistant penicillins in the treatment of staphylococcal infections but is usually not preferred to a cephalosporin or vancomycin and should not be used for the treatment of endocarditis. Clindamycin may be useful for some methicillin-resistant *S. aureus* (MRSA) infections, but inducible clindamycin resistance may occur in isolates resistant to erythromycin. For severe group A streptococcal infections or toxic shock syndrome, clindamycin is often used in combination with penicillin to limit bacterial growth and reduce toxin production.

In AIDS patients with sulfonamide allergy or intolerance, clindamycin represents an important component of alternative combination treatments for central nervous system toxoplasmosis or *Pneumocystis jiroveci* (previously named *Pneumocystis carinii*) pneumonia.

Oxazolidinones

Linezolid displays activity directed primarily against gram-positive organisms such as staphylococci (including methicillin- and vancomycin-resistant strains), streptococci (including penicillin-resistant strains of *S. pneumoniae*), enterococci (including vancomycin-resistant strains), gram-positive anaerobic cocci, and gram-positive rods such as *Corynebacterium* species and *Listeria monocytogenes*. It has a moderate activity against mycobacteria, including *Mycobacterium tuberculosis* and *M. avium* complex, and a poor activity against most gram-negative bacteria. Linezolid is approved for vancomycin-resistant infections caused by *Enterococcus faecium*, complicated or uncomplicated skin and soft-tissue infections caused by *S. aureus*, and hospital- or community-acquired pneumonia caused by *S. aureus* or *S. pneumoniae*. Linezolid is also used off-label for the treatment of multidrug-resistant tuberculosis and *Nocardia* infections.

Streptogramins

The combination quinupristin/dalfopristin is active against gram-positive cocci, including all staphylococci, multidrug-resistant streptococci, penicillin-resistant *S. pneumoniae*, and *E. faecium* but not *Enterococcus faecalis*. The combination is also active against atypical pneumonia-causing organisms including *M. pneumoniae*, *Legionella* species, and *C. pneumoniae* but inactive against gram-negative organisms such as Enterobacteriaceae, *P. aeruginosa*, and *Acinetobacter* species.

Quinupristin/dalfopristin is used for the treatment of infections caused by vancomycin-resistant enterococci and complicated skin and skin-structure infections caused by methicillin-sensitive *S. aureus* or *S. pyogenes*. It is also used for the treatment of nosocomial pneumonia and infections caused by methicillin-resistant *S. aureus*.

Others

Chloramphenicol has an extremely broad spectrum of antimicrobial activity, inhibiting aerobic and anaerobic gram-positive and gram-negative bacteria, *Chlamydia*, *Rickettsia*, and *Mycoplasma* species. It is

TABLE 58.1   Selected Pharmacokinetic Parameters

Drug	Administration	Absorption	Plasma Protein Binding (%)	Normal Plasma $t_{1/2}$ (hrs)	Anuric Plasma $t_{1/2}$ (hrs)	Elimination
Aminoglycosides[*]						
Gentamicin	IV, IM	Poor	<10	2	35–50	R (100)
Streptomycin	IM	Poor	35	2–2.5	35–50	R (100)
Kanamycin	IV, IM	Poor	<10	2–2.5	35–50	R (100)
Tobramycin	IV, IM	Poor	<10	2	35–50	R (100)
Amikacin	IV, IM	Poor	<10	2–2.5	35–50	R (100)
Netilmicin	IV, IM	Poor	<10	2	35–50	R (100)
Tetracyclines						
Tetracycline	Oral, IV, IM, topical	75%	55	8	>50	M, R
Doxycycline	Oral, IV	93%	85	16	20–30	M, R, B
Oxytetracycline	Oral, IM	Good	30	9	Long	M, R (20–35%)
Minocycline	Oral, IV	95%	75	16	20–30	M, R (5%)
Chlortetracycline	Oral	30%	50	6	>50	M, R
Tigecycline	IV	Poor		27	Unchanged	B (59%), R (22%)
Other Drugs						
Chloramphenicol	Oral, IV	Good	50	3	–	M (90%), R
Erythromycin	Oral, IV	Good but variable	<70	1.5	4	M (90%), R
Azithromycin	Oral, IV	Good[a]	7–50	10–50	–	B
Clarithromycin	Oral	Good	–	4	–	B, R
Dirithromycin	Oral	Good[b]	20	30–44	–	M
Clindamycin	Oral, IV, IM	90%	90	2.4	6	M (90%), R
Spectinomycin	IM	Poor	<10	2.5	–	R (100%)
Telithromycin	Oral	57%[c]	70	13	–	M (70%)
Quinupristin/dalfopristin	IV	–	90	1–3	–	M, R (15%)
Linezolid	Oral, IV	100%	31	4.5–5.5	7	M, R

B, Biliary; M, metabolized; R, renal.
[*]Aminoglycosides have long half-lives in tissue (25 to 500 hours).
[a]Decreased by food.
[b]Slightly enhanced by food.
[c]Oral absorption is 90%, with 57% bioavailable after first-pass metabolism.

particularly active against *B. fragilis*. Although it is bacteriostatic for Enterobacteriaceae, staphylococci, and streptococci, it is bactericidal for *H. influenzae*, *N. meningitidis*, and *S. pneumoniae*. Because of the serious adverse side effects associated with its use, chloramphenicol should be used only when no other drug is suitable. In the United States, chloramphenicol is used mainly as an alternative therapy for patients with bacterial meningitis who have a severe penicillin allergy that precludes treatment with a β-lactam. However, clinical failures have been observed with chloramphenicol when used to treat meningitis caused by penicillin-resistant *S. pneumoniae*. Chloramphenicol also represents an alternative therapy for patients with rickettsial diseases who cannot be treated with a tetracycline. In certain parts of the world, chloramphenicol continues to be widely used to treat typhoid fever, given its low cost and availability. Unfortunately, chloramphenicol-resistant *Salmonella typhi* are becoming increasingly problematic. The activity of chloramphenicol is antagonized by the macrolides and clindamycin and thus should not be used concurrently.

Clinical evidence indicates that patients who potentially benefit from mupirocin prophylaxis are those who have *S. aureus* nasal colonization and also have risk factors for distant infection or a history of skin or soft-tissue infections.

PHARMACOKINETICS

Selected pharmacokinetic parameters for commonly used inhibitors of protein synthesis are presented in Table 58.1.

Aminoglycosides

The aminoglycosides are not absorbed to a significant extent after oral or rectal administration and thus are administered by the intramuscular (IM) or intravenous (IV) routes. The exception to this is in newborns with necrotizing enterocolitis, when significant oral absorption can occur. However, if renal impairment is present, even the small amount of drug absorbed by the oral route may accumulate and cause toxicity, even in adults. Peak plasma concentrations occur 30–60 minutes after IM injection, with plasma concentrations comparable to those achieved after a 30-minute infusion. Absorption from the IM site of injection is decreased in patients in shock, and thus the IM route is rarely used to treat life-threatening septic infections.

Topical application of aminoglycosides results in minimal absorption, except in patients with extensive cutaneous damage, such as burns or epidermolysis. Intraperitoneal and intrapleural instillations result in such rapid absorption that toxicity may develop; however, irrigation (of bladder), intratracheal, and aerosol delivery do not result in significant absorption. New techniques of aerosolization with correct particle size can produce concentrations of more than 100 μg/mL in the lung but only 4 μg/mL in plasma.

Because of their high polarity, aminoglycosides do not enter phagocytic or other cells, the brain, or the eye. They are distributed into interstitial fluid, with a volume of distribution essentially equal to that of the extracellular fluid. The highest concentrations of aminoglycosides occur in the kidney, where they concentrate in proximal tubular cells. Urine concentrations are generally 20–100 times greater than those in plasma and remain so for 24 hours after a single dose. These drugs enter peritoneal, pleural, and synovial fluids relatively slowly, but eventually achieve concentrations that are only slightly less than those in plasma.

Concentrations of aminoglycosides in cerebrospinal fluid (CSF) after IM, IV, or intrathecal administration into the lumbar space are inadequate for the treatment of gram-negative meningitis, requiring intraventricular instillation, which yields high concentrations in both areas. Subconjunctival injection produces high aqueous fluid concentrations but inadequate intravitreal concentrations.

Elimination of aminoglycosides occurs almost completely through glomerular filtration by the kidneys; a small amount of drug is reabsorbed into proximal renal tubular cells. Renal clearance is approximately two-thirds that of creatinine. However, these drugs can become trapped in tissue compartments, yielding tissue half-lives of 25–500 hours. Dosing schedules must be adjusted in patients who have reduced renal capacity. Because the clearance of aminoglycosides is linearly related to creatinine clearance, the latter can be used to calculate dosing. Aminoglycosides can be removed from the body by hemodialysis but not very well by peritoneal dialysis.

Tetracyclines and Glycylcyclines

Some tetracyclines are incompletely absorbed, whereas others are well absorbed when administered orally, but all attain adequate plasma and tissue concentrations. Minocycline and doxycycline are the most completely absorbed and chlortetracycline the least. Absorption is favored during fasting because tetracyclines form complexes with divalent metals, including Ca^{++}, Mg^{++}, Al^{++}, and Fe^{++}. Absorption of some tetracyclines is decreased when ingested with milk products, antacids, or Fe^{++} preparations. However, food does not interfere with the absorption of minocycline or doxycycline.

The tetracyclines are widely distributed in body compartments, with high concentrations in liver, kidney, bile, bronchial epithelium, and breast milk. These drugs can also enter pleural, peritoneal, synovial, and sinus fluids, cross the placenta, and enter phagocytic cells. Penetration into the CSF is poor and increases only minimally in the setting of meningeal inflammation; however, minocycline does achieve therapeutic concentrations in brain tissue.

Tetracyclines do not bind to formed bone but are incorporated into calcifying tissue and the dentin and enamel of unerupted teeth. Thus the deposition of tetracyclines in teeth and bones is more problematic in children than adults.

The tetracyclines are eliminated by renal and biliary routes and by metabolism. Although most of the biliary-eliminated drug is reabsorbed by active transport, some is chelated and excreted in feces. This occurs even when these drugs are administered parenterally. Renal clearance of the tetracyclines occurs by glomerular filtration. All tetracyclines, except doxycycline, accumulate in patients with decreased renal function, making doxycycline, which is eliminated by biliary excretion, the drug of choice for individuals with renal impairment. Similarly, chlortetracycline undergoes hepatic metabolism (75%) and is excreted by biliary and renal excretion.

Metabolism of doxycycline is increased in patients receiving barbiturates, phenytoin, or carbamazepine because these agents induce the formation of hepatic drug-metabolizing enzymes. The half-life of doxycycline decreases from 16 to 7 hours in such patients. In contrast, decreased hepatic function or common bile duct obstruction will prolong the half-life of the tetracyclines because of the reduction in biliary excretion.

Macrolides

In its free base form, erythromycin is inactivated by acid, and thus it is administered orally with an enteric coating that dissolves in the duodenum. Even in the absence of food, which delays absorption, peak plasma concentrations are difficult to predict. Ester forms of erythromycin are available to help overcome this problem. Lactobionate and gluceptate, water soluble forms of the drug, are available for IV administration.

Erythromycin is well distributed and produces therapeutic concentrations in tonsillar tissue, middle ear fluid, and lung. It enters prostatic fluid, where it reaches concentrations approximately one-third those in plasma. It does not diffuse well into brain or CSF. Erythromycin crosses the placenta and is found in breast milk, with high concentrations also observed in liver and bile, as well as in alveolar macrophages and neutrophils.

The main route of elimination of erythromycin is via metabolic demethylation by the liver and biliary excretion. Inactive metabolites are responsible for gastric intolerance. Only a small percentage is excreted unchanged. Erythromycin metabolites inhibit cytochrome P450 enzymes and can lead to increased plasma levels of drugs, including theophylline, oral anticoagulants, and digoxin. Care must be taken to monitor patients on other medications if erythromycin is added to their regimen.

In contrast to erythromycin, azithromycin is acid stable. Approximately 37% of a dose is absorbed but greatly reduced in the presence of food. Serum concentrations are low because of rapid distribution to tissues. Therapeutic concentrations are reached in lung, genitalia, and liver. Azithromycin is highly concentrated in phagocytic cells, macrophages, and fibroblasts, from which it is slowly released. Tissue concentrations of azithromycin may be 10–100 times greater than plasma concentrations. Release from the tissues is slow and may take from 2–4 days; however, the presence of bacteria causes the drug to be released from neutrophils. The prolonged tissue half-life of azithromycin allows for once-daily dosing and shorter durations of therapy.

Azithromycin is eliminated unchanged in feces and to a lesser extent in urine. Concentrations in the elderly and patients with decreased renal function are increased but are not significantly affected by hepatic disease. In contrast to erythromycin and clarithromycin, azithromycin does not inhibit hepatic cytochrome P450 enzymes.

Clarithromycin is approximately 55% absorbed by the oral route and is widely distributed to lung, liver, and soft tissues. Concentrations in phagocytic cells are approximately ninefold greater than those in serum. The drug is metabolized to a 14-hydroxy derivative, which has antibacterial activity greater than that of the parent compound. Approximately 30% of the drug is excreted in the urine and the remainder in feces. Currently, an intravenous preparation of clarithromycin is not available. As with erythromycin, clarithromycin is a hepatic cytochrome P450 inhibitor.

Ketolides

Telithromycin is well absorbed after oral administration, but 33% of an administered dose undergoes first-pass metabolism in the liver, with 57% reaching the systemic circulation. Absorption is not affected by food. Telithromycin achieves high intracellular concentrations, particularly within neutrophils and alveolar macrophages, and has extensive penetration into respiratory and tonsillar tissues. Metabolism occurs in the liver, with elimination primarily in feces and a smaller portion in urine. Telithromycin inhibits cytochrome P450 activity, which can lead to drug interactions. Dosing does not require modification in patients with hepatic or renal impairment.

Lincosamides

Clindamycin is well absorbed from the GI tract. Although absorption is delayed in the presence of food, overall bioavailability is not decreased. Mean peak plasma concentrations occur within 1 hour. Clindamycin is available as a palmitate ester, which is rapidly hydrolyzed to free drug, and is also available as a phosphate ester, with the latter used for IM administration. Distribution is widespread, with clindamycin entering most body compartments and achieving adequate concentrations in lung, liver, bone, and abscesses. It enters the CSF and brain tissue, but the concentrations are inadequate to treat meningitis and should not be relied on to treat brain infections except toxoplasmosis. This drug enters polymorphonuclear leukocytes and alveolar macrophages and crosses the placenta. Clindamycin is metabolized to the bacteriologically active *N*-dimethyl and sulfoxide derivatives, which are excreted in urine and bile. The half-life is prolonged in patients with severe liver disease.

Oxazolidinones

Linezolid is well absorbed after oral administration, with oral bioavailability approaching 100%. Therefore linezolid may be given orally or IV without dose adjustment. The half-life of linezolid is approximately 4–6 hours, and the drug distributes widely to well-perfused tissues. Linezolid is mainly metabolized by nonenzymatic oxidation to aminoethoxyacetic acid and hydroxyethyl glycine derivatives. Approximately 80% of the administered dose is eliminated by renal excretion (30% as active compound and 50% as the two oxidation products). Dosage adjustment is not required for either mild or moderate hepatic impairment or for renal insufficiency.

Streptogramins

The combination of quinupristin/dalfopristin is administered only by IV infusion. After IV administration, quinupristin/dalfopristin rapidly achieves a wide tissue distribution but does not have significant CSF penetration and does not cross the placenta. Both compounds are primarily metabolized by hepatic conjugation. About 80% of an administered dose is eliminated by biliary excretion, and the remainder is excreted unchanged by the kidneys. Dose adjustment is not required for either hepatic or renal impairment.

Others

Chloramphenicol is administered parenterally (IV or IM) as a prodrug that is activated in the plasma by cholinesterases. It is widely distributed throughout the body, achieving concentrations in CSF that are 60% of those in plasma. It is also present in breast milk and placental fluid. The major route of elimination of chloramphenicol is via hepatic metabolism, with both parent drug and glucuronidated metabolites excreted in the urine.

Mupirocin is available as a 2% cream and a 2% ointment for treatment of skin lesions and impetigo secondarily infected with *S. aureus* or *S. pyogenes*, and as a 2% intranasal ointment. Systemic absorption through intact skin or skin lesions is minimal. Mupirocin is only administered topically.

PHARMACOVIGILANCE: ADVERSE EFFECTS AND DRUG INTERACTIONS

Aminoglycosides

The aminoglycosides are used less commonly than other agents for many gram-negative infections because they have a low therapeutic index and toxicity can be serious. Thus plasma concentrations should be monitored, close attention must be given to the pharmacokinetics of these drugs in individual patients, and renal function must be assessed. The most important and most common serious adverse effects include those on the renal, cochlear, and vestibular systems.

Reversible renal impairment that can progress to severe renal insufficiency develops in 5%–25% of patients receiving an aminoglycoside for more than 3 days. These agents lead to an initial decrease in glomerular filtration that may result from inhibition of vasodilatory prostaglandins. The aminoglycosides are transported across the luminal brush border membrane and accumulate in proximal tubular cells, where they inhibit several enzymes and alter mitochondria and ribosomes. Of clinical significance is the decrease in renal concentrating ability, proteinuria, and the appearance of casts in the urine, followed by a reduction in the glomerular filtration rate and a rise in the serum creatinine concentration. Because tubules can regenerate, renal function usually returns to normal after the drug is cleared. A few patients whose renal function does not return to pretreatment values require dialysis.

Toxicity correlates with the amount of drug and duration of administration, and there is an increased risk associated with aged individuals, females, concomitant liver disease, and concomitant hypotension. Coadministration of aminoglycosides with loop diuretics, vancomycin, cisplatin, cyclosporin, or amphotericin B can potentiate renal toxicity and volume depletion. In addition, the risk of nephrotoxicity is higher when aminoglycosides are administered in two or three divided doses compared with a single daily dose. Specific aminoglycosides differ in their nephrotoxic potential, with neomycin the most nephrotoxic and streptomycin the least.

Aminoglycosides can damage either or both the cochlear and vestibular systems. As compared with renal toxicity, aminoglycoside-induced ototoxicity is usually irreversible. Although the exact frequency is unknown, some damage probably occurs in 5%–25% of patients, depending on the underlying auditory status and duration of therapy. Cochlear toxicity is a result of the destruction of hair cells of the organ of Corti, particularly the outer hair cells in the basal turn, accompanied by subsequent retrograde degeneration of the auditory nerves. Aminoglycosides also damage hair cells of the crista ampullaris, leading to vestibular dysfunction and vertigo. In addition, aminoglycosides accumulate in perilymph and endolymph and inhibit ionic transport, which is the cause of cochlear cell damage. The drugs accumulate when plasma concentrations are high for prolonged periods, and ototoxicity is probably enhanced by persistently elevated plasma concentrations. Single daily high-dose therapy produces less ototoxicity.

The amount of auditory or vestibular function loss correlates with the amount of hair cell damage. Repeated courses of therapy continue to cause damage to more hair cells. Concomitant use of loop diuretics, such as furosemide, is thought to increase the risk of ototoxicity. The incidence of vestibular toxicity is highest for patients who receive 4 weeks of therapy or longer.

Clinical signs of auditory problems, such as tinnitus or a sensation of fullness in the ears, are not reliable predictors of this toxicity. The initial hearing loss is of high frequencies outside the voice range; thus toxicity will not be recognized unless hearing tests are performed. Eventually the loss of hearing may progress into the auditory range. For patients receiving prolonged courses of aminoglycosides, serial high-frequency audiometric testing should be undertaken.

Vestibular toxicity is usually preceded by headache, nausea, emesis, and vertigo, so patients who are ill often have difficulty identifying the onset of vestibular toxicity. These patients may go through a series of stages from acute to chronic symptoms that are apparent only on standing, or the patients may achieve a compensatory state in which they use visual cues to adjust for the loss of vestibular function.

Neuromuscular paralysis is rare, but results from inhibition of the presynaptic release of acetylcholine and postsynaptic receptor blockade. Aminoglycosides inhibit the influx of Ca^{++} at the presynaptic nerve terminal, thus blocking acetylcholine release. Presynaptic blockade is more readily caused by neomycin and tobramycin than by streptomycin, whereas the opposite is true for the postsynaptic effects. Neuromuscular paralysis is most likely to occur during surgery when anesthesia and neuromuscular blockers such as succinylcholine are used but can also occur in patients with myasthenia gravis.

Aminoglycosides are contraindicated in pregnant women. Although controlled human studies have not been conducted, investigations in animals demonstrate that aminoglycosides cause ototoxicity and nephrotoxicity after in utero exposure.

Tetracyclines and Glycylcyclines

Although usually well tolerated, the tetracyclines may produce adverse effects ranging from minor to life-threatening. Allergy to a tetracycline precludes its further use. Photosensitization with a rash is a toxic rather than an allergic effect and is most often seen in patients receiving demeclocycline or doxycycline.

Effects on bone and teeth preclude the use of tetracycline in children less than 8 years of age because a permanent brown-yellow discoloration of teeth will develop in 80% of individuals. The effect is permanent, and the enamel becomes hypoplastic. The effects on bone and teeth may also result from maternal use of tetracyclines during pregnancy. Thus tetracyclines are contraindicated in this population.

Tetracyclines cause dose-dependent GI disturbances, including epigastric burning, nausea, and vomiting. Esophageal ulcers have also been reported. Pancreatitis is rarely observed. Hepatic toxicity is encountered most often in conjunction with parenteral use but can also occur with oral administration. Tetracyclines also aggravate existing renal dysfunction.

Demeclocycline can cause nephrogenic diabetes insipidus, and minocycline may produce vertigo, particularly in women. Superinfection caused by an overgrowth of other bacteria, particularly oral and vaginal candidiasis, frequently occurs after use of tetracyclines. Indeed, the effect of tetracyclines on normal GI flora is also suggested to interrupt enterohepatic cycling of oral contraceptives, leading to decreased effectiveness. As such, women taking tetracyclines should be advised to seek secondary means of birth control.

Macrolides

Erythromycin is one of the safest antibiotics, with epigastric pain, abdominal cramps, nausea, and emesis representing the most common side effects. Administration by the IV route may be associated with thrombophlebitis. Cholestatic hepatitis may occur in patients receiving estolate preparations of erythromycin, usually beginning 10–20 days into treatment and characterized by jaundice, fever, leukocytosis, and eosinophilia. The problem abates rapidly once drug administration is stopped. Erythromycin at high doses can cause reversible transient deafness. Rarely, erythromycin use has been associated with polymorphic ventricular tachycardia (torsades de pointes) due to prolongation of the QT interval. Erythromycin stimulates GI motility by acting as a motilin receptor agonist, leading to enhanced gastric emptying. Thus erythromycin can be used to improve gastric motility in patients with gastroparesis.

Erythromycin also inhibits the cytochrome P450 system, which can lead to significant drug-drug interactions. Erythromycin prolongs the half-life of theophylline and can lead to theophylline toxicity. It also inhibits the metabolism of carbamazepine, cyclosporine, corticosteroids, warfarin, and digoxin.

Azithromycin is generally well tolerated and has fewer GI side effects than erythromycin. Because it does not interfere with cytochrome P450 enzymes, it does not have the same drug-drug interactions.

Clarithromycin is similarly well tolerated. It is intermediate between erythromycin and azithromycin relative to the incidence of intolerance caused by GI side effects. Clarithromycin also inhibits cytochrome P450s, as does erythromycin, and may cause increased serum concentrations of other drugs.

Dirithromycin, like erythromycin, can also cause GI side effects. However, it does not interfere with cytochrome P450 metabolism.

Ketolides

The most serious effects with telithromycin involve hepatic damage. Multiple cases of liver failure have resulted in liver transplant or death. As such, the use of telithromycin has decreased considerably. Other adverse effects include diarrhea, nausea, and abdominal pain. More recently, telithromycin has been shown to cause visual disturbances and exacerbations of myasthenia gravis.

Lincosamides

Diarrhea may occur in up to 20% of patients treated with clindamycin. The most important adverse effect of clindamycin is pseudomembranous enterocolitis produced by *Clostridium difficile*, estimated to occur in 3%–5% of patients. This syndrome is characterized by diarrhea, abdominal pain, and fever, with diarrhea beginning either during or after drug therapy. Orally administered vancomycin or metronidazole may be needed for this secondary superinfection, if it occurs.

Oxazolidinones

The principal toxicity of linezolid is hematologic. Myelosuppression, including anemia, leukopenia, and thrombocytopenia, has been reported with linezolid use, often occurring with therapy duration greater than 2 weeks. Platelet counts should be monitored closely in patients with a history of thrombocytopenia, bleeding risk, or disorders of platelet function and in patients receiving treatment for longer than 2 weeks. Long-term (>8 weeks) linezolid use is also associated with the development of lactic acidosis, peripheral neuropathy, and optic neuritis and may be attributed to the actions of the drug on mitochondria. Other common side effects of linezolid include diarrhea, nausea, vomiting, headache, insomnia, constipation, and an alteration in taste perception.

Linezolid is a weak nonspecific inhibitor of monoamine oxidase. A boxed warning has been issued regarding the concomitant use of the drug with adrenergic or serotonergic agents, including selective serotonin reuptake inhibitors, due to the risk of serotonin syndrome, characterized by palpitations, headache, or hypertensive crisis. Therefore coadministration of these agents should be avoided. In addition, patients taking linezolid should avoid eating large quantities of food with high tyramine content.

Streptogramins

Local inflammation, pain, edema, and thrombophlebitis at the infusion site may occur with quinupristin/dalfopristin administration, particularly when infused via a peripheral vein. Therefore administration usually requires central venous access. In addition, arthralgias and myalgias have been reported in some patients and can be controlled by reducing the infusion frequency to every 12 hours. Hyperbilirubinemia can occur in some patients.

Quinupristin/dalfopristin inhibits CYP3A4. Therefore concomitant administration of this combination and drugs mainly metabolized by CYP3A4 may result in increased plasma drug concentrations that could increase both therapeutic effects and adverse reactions. Examples of CYP3A4-metabolized drugs affected by quinupristin/dalfopristin include antihistamines (e.g., azelastine and clemastine), anticonvulsants (e.g., fosphenytoin and felbamate), antibiotics (macrolides, fluoroquinolones, and ketoconazole), antidepressants (e.g., fluoxetine, imipramine, and venlafaxine); antipsychotics (e.g., haloperidol, risperidone, and quetiapine), and calcium-channel blockers (e.g., nifedipine, verapamil, and diltiazem).

Others

Chloramphenicol produces serious side effects attributed to its action on mitochondrial membrane enzymes, cytochrome oxidases, and adenosine triphosphatases. Because of these adverse effects, chloramphenicol has limited clinical uses, primarily used when no alternative treatment is suitable. Its hematological effects are the most important, and regular monitoring of complete blood count should be performed. Aplastic anemia occurs in 1 : 25,000 to 1 : 40,000 patients, with a high death rate in those in whom an aplastic state develops or who progress to acute leukemia. Aplastic anemia is usually not dose dependent and most often occurs weeks to months after therapy is completed, but it can occur concurrently with therapy.

A second important hematological side effect is reversible bone marrow suppression. This form of toxicity usually develops during therapy, is dose dependent, and is reversible. It is manifest by anemia, thrombocytopenia, or leukopenia, alone or in combination.

A complication known as gray baby syndrome may be encountered in infants receiving chloramphenicol. This syndrome of pallor, cyanosis, abdominal distention, vomiting, and circulatory collapse, resulting in approximately a 50% mortality rate, develops in neonates with excessively high plasma concentrations of drug. High concentrations result from inadequate glucuronidation and failure to excrete the drug by the kidneys. Children less than 1 month of age should receive only low doses of chloramphenicol, though in overdose situations, excess drug can be removed by hemoperfusion over a bed of charcoal. Chloramphenicol also can produce optic neuritis in children and GI side effects including nausea, vomiting, diarrhea, and hypersensitivity rashes. Chloramphenicol inhibits hepatic cytochrome P450 enzymes, thereby prolonging the half-life of phenytoin, tolbutamide, and other drugs; barbiturates, on the other hand, decrease the half-life of chloramphenicol.

Mupirocin may cause irritation at the site of application. Contact with the eyes should be avoided because mupirocin causes burning and irritation that may take several days to resolve. Systemic reactions to mupirocin rarely occur. Polyethylene glycol present in the ointment can be absorbed from open wounds and damaged skin and is excreted by the kidneys. Application of the ointment to large surface areas should be avoided in patients with renal failure to avoid accumulation of polyethylene glycol.

The most commonly observed side effects and drug interactions for representative agents are listed in the Clinical Problems Box.

NEW DEVELOPMENTS

Emerging antimicrobial resistance continues to be problematic, and the need for agents active against drug-resistant organisms is expanding. Development of new inhibitors of bacterial ribosomes may provide additional options. Currently, the glycylcyclines represent a promising new group of agents within the tetracycline class. With the approval of tigecycline offering treatment for tetracycline- and macrolide-resistant organisms, the glycylcyclines have an expanded spectrum of activity, with in vitro activity against methicillin-resistant *S. aureus*, vancomycin-resistant enterococci, and penicillin-resistant *S. pneumoniae*, and may be active against some resistant gram-negative organisms.

CLINICAL RELEVANCE FOR HEALTHCARE PROFESSIONALS

All healthcare professionals will come in contact with individuals taking a bacterial protein synthesis inhibitor at some point in their lives and need to be aware of the limitations and adverse effects associated with these agents.

CLINICAL PROBLEMS

Aminoglycosides
Nephrotoxicity
Ototoxicity; vestibular (associated with intense headaches) and cochlear (associated with high-pitched tinnitus) sensory cells are highly sensitive to aminoglycosides; may be due to genetic predisposition
Acute neuromuscular blockade and apnea (infrequent but myasthenia gravis patients are particularly susceptible)
Drug interactions with other agents that increase the risk of renal toxicity such as diuretics, angiotensin-converting-enzyme inhibitors, nonsteroidal antiinflammatory drugs, cisplatin, amphotericin, and other nephrotoxic compounds.

Tetracyclines and Glycylcyclines
Gastrointestinal tract upsets
Alteration of enteric flora leading to vaginal candidiasis
Photosensitivity
Hepatic toxicity, particularly in patients who are pregnant or have renal failure
Renal dysfunction in patients with renal disease
Discoloration of teeth of children exposed to tetracyclines during gestation through to 8 years of age
Increased intracranial pressure in young infants
Vertigo (minocycline)
Drug interactions with products containing magnesium such as antacids, calcium supplements and laxatives and products containing iron. Do not administer with food.

Macrolides and Ketolides
GI tract disturbances
Hepatotoxicity (particularly erythromycin estolate and telithromycin)
Prolongation of QT interval

Auditory impairment with high doses
Drug interactions with other agents that are metabolized by or induce cytochrome P450 enzymes.

Lincosamides
Gastrointestinal effects
Pseudomembranous colitis caused by toxin from *C. difficile*
Serious rash (uncommon, seen in HIV infected patients)
Stevens-Johnson syndrome (uncommon)

Oxazolidinones
Hematological toxicity including anemia, leukopenia, pancytopenia, and thrombocytopenia. Reduction in platelets is related to duration of treatment.
Drug interactions in patients receiving concomitant treatment with an adrenergic or serotonergic agent due to oxazolidinone inhibition of monoamine oxidase

Streptogramins
Pain and phlebitis at infusion site
Joint and muscle pain
Drug interactions with other agents that are cytochrome P450 3A4 substrates can raise blood pressure and result in significant toxicity.

Chloramphenicol
Hematological toxicity; bone marrow suppression leading to life-threatening pancytopenia; increased incidence of acute leukemia in patients who recover from chloramphenicol-induced bone marrow aplasia
Gray baby syndrome in neonates, particularly if premature
Drug interactions with other agents that are metabolized by or induce cytochrome P450 enzymes

TRADE NAMES

In addition to generic and fixed-combination preparations, the following trade-named materials are some of the important compounds available in the United States.

Aminoglycosides

  Amikacin sulfate (Amikin)
  Gentamicin sulfate (Cidomycin, Garamycin, G-Myticin)
  Kanamycin sulfate (Kantrex)
  Netilmicin sulfate (Netromycin)
  Tobramycin sulfate (Bethkis, Nebcin)

Tetracyclines

  Demeclocycline (Declomycin)
  Doxycycline (Doryx)
  Doxycycline Ca^{++} (Vibramycin calcium)
  Minocycline HCl (Dynacin, Minocin)
  Oxytetracycline (Terramycin)
  Tetracycline (Achromycin, Sumycin)

Macrolides

  Azithromycin (Zithromax)
  Clarithromycin (Biaxin)
  Dirithromycin (Dynabac)
  Erythromycin (EryDerm, Erygel, Ilotycin)
  Erythromycin ethylsuccinate (contains sulfisoxazole) (Pediamycin, Eryzole, Wyamycin)
  Erythromycin estolate (Ilosone)

Others

  Chloramphenicol (Chloromycetin)
  Clindamycin (Cleocin)
  Telithromycin (Ketek)
  Quinupristin/dalfopristin (Synercid)
  Linezolid (Zyvox)
  Mupirocin (Bactroban)

SELF-ASSESSMENT QUESTIONS

1. A 45-year-old man with a history of a severe penicillin allergy is undergoing treatment for bacterial meningitis. Several days into therapy, he reports a severe headache, general malaise, and visual disturbances. Blood tests reveal that he is severely anemic. Which of the following drugs is most likely responsible for these adverse effects?
   A. Azithromycin.
   B. Chloramphenicol.
   C. Doxycycline.
   D. Penicillin.
   E. Tigecycline.

2. Which of the following classes of drugs acts by binding reversibly to the 50S ribosomal unit, blocks peptidyl transferase, and results in preventing translocation from the aminoacyl site to the peptidyl site?
   A. Aminoglycosides.
   B. Glycylcyclines.
   C. Ketolides.
   D. Streptogramins.
   E. Tetracyclines.

3. An antibiotic is administered once daily in the intensive care unit to treat sepsis caused by an abdominal wound. Serum and urine concentrations of the drug are monitored during the course of therapy. Ten days after therapy is discontinued, the drug is still detectable in the urine. Which of the following antibiotics was administered?
   A. Azithromycin.
   B. Chloramphenicol.
   C. Doxycycline.
   D. Gentamicin.
   E. Amoxicillin.

4. A macrolide antibiotic is required to treat a streptococcal infection in a 71-year-old penicillin-sensitive man who is also receiving digoxin and warfarin therapy. Which of the following drugs would be best for this patient?
   A. Azithromycin.
   B. Clarithromycin.
   C. Erythromycin.
   D. Telithromycin.

FURTHER READING

Ackermann G, Rodloff AC. Drugs of the 21st century: Telithromycin (HMR 3647)—the first ketolide. *J Antimicrob Chemother*. 2003;51:497–511.

Hancock RE. Mechanisms of action of newer antibiotics for gram-positive pathogens. *Lancet Infect Dis*. 2005;5:209–218.

Noskin GA. Tigecycline: A new glycylcycline for treatment of serious infections. *Clin Infect Dis*. 2005;41(suppl):S303–S314.

Orelle C, Carlson S, Kaushal B, et al. Tools for characterizing bacterial protein synthesis inhibitors. *Antimicrob Agents Chemother*. 2013;57:5994–6004.

Wilson DN. Ribosome-targeting antibiotics and mechanisms of bacterial resistance. *Nat Rev Microbiol*. 2014;12:35–48.

WEBSITES

https://www.cdc.gov/ncird/dbd.html

This website is maintained by the United States Centers for Disease Control and Prevention and provides an excellent overview of bacterial diseases.

Drugs Targeting Bacterial DNA

Rukiyah Van Dross-Anderson and Ahmed E.M. Elhassanny

MAJOR DRUG CLASSES

Sulfonamides and trimethoprim
Fluoroquinolones
Nitrofurans
Nitroimidazoles

ABBREVIATIONS

AIDS	Acquired immunodeficiency syndrome
CNS	Central nervous system
CSF	Cerebrospinal fluid
GI	Gastrointestinal
IV	Intravenous
MSSA	Methicillin-susceptible *Staphylococcus aureus*
MRSA	Methicillin-resistant *Staphylococcus aureus*
PABA	*p*-Aminobenzoic acid
TMP-SMX	Trimethoprim-sulfamethoxazole

THERAPEUTIC OVERVIEW

The discovery of the antibacterial action of the sulfa drugs in the first half of the past century preceded our knowledge of DNA and the mechanisms regulating nucleic acid and protein synthesis. Many drugs have been developed since that time that target diverse processes involved in bacterial DNA replication, ranging from those that target the simplest mechanism limiting precursors for DNA synthesis to those that target more complex mechanisms, such as inhibition of DNA uncoiling. Many agents have a broad spectrum of antibacterial activity and are useful for their bacteriostatic or bactericidal effects against organisms that have not developed resistance. In addition, several of these agents are also effective against protozoal infections (Chapter 63).

The drugs that target DNA include the sulfonamides and trimethoprim, the quinolones, the nitrofurans, and the nitroimidazoles. The therapeutic applications of these agents are summarized in the Therapeutic Overview Box.

MECHANISMS OF ACTION

Structures of representative agents from each class are shown in Fig. 59.1.

Sulfonamides and Trimethoprim

Sulfonamides are structural analogues of *p*-aminobenzoic acid (PABA) and include sulfanilamide, sulfamethoxazole, sulfadiazine, sulfisoxazole, and sulfacetamide. These agents competitively inhibit dihydropteroate synthase, the first step in the synthesis of tetrahydrofolate from PABA (Fig. 59.2). Tetrahydrofolate is the physiologically active form of folic acid and is required as a cofactor for the synthesis of thymidine, purines, and bacterial DNA. Although humans rely on dietary sources of folate, most bacteria must synthesize folic acid, rendering inhibition of folate synthesis a selective target. Thus inhibition of folate synthesis inhibits bacterial cell growth. Only bacteria that synthesize their own folic acid are sensitive to sulfonamides; those that lack the enzymes required for folate synthesis from PABA, like mammals, depend on exogenous sources of folate, and, as such, are not susceptible to sulfonamides.

THERAPEUTIC OVERVIEW

Sulfonamides
Treatment of nocardiosis and toxoplasmosis
Topical agents for burn wounds

Trimethoprim-Sulfamethoxazole Combination
Urinary tract infections
Treatment and prevention of *Pneumocystis jirovici (carinii)* infections and *Toxoplasma gondii* encephalitis in AIDS patients (significant side effects)
Prevention of spontaneous bacterial peritonitis in patients with cirrhosis
Resistant bacteria

Fluoroquinolones
Urinary tract infections
Prostatitis
Sexually transmitted diseases (resistance in *Neisseria gonorrhoeae*)
Bacterial diarrheal infections
Community-acquired pneumonia (third-generation agents only)
Osteomyelitis
Agents of biowarfare
Mycobacterial infections

Nitrofurans
Urinary tract infections

Nitroimidazoles
Trichomoniasis, amebiasis, and giardiasis
Infections caused by obligate anaerobic bacteria such as *Bacteroides* and *Clostridium*

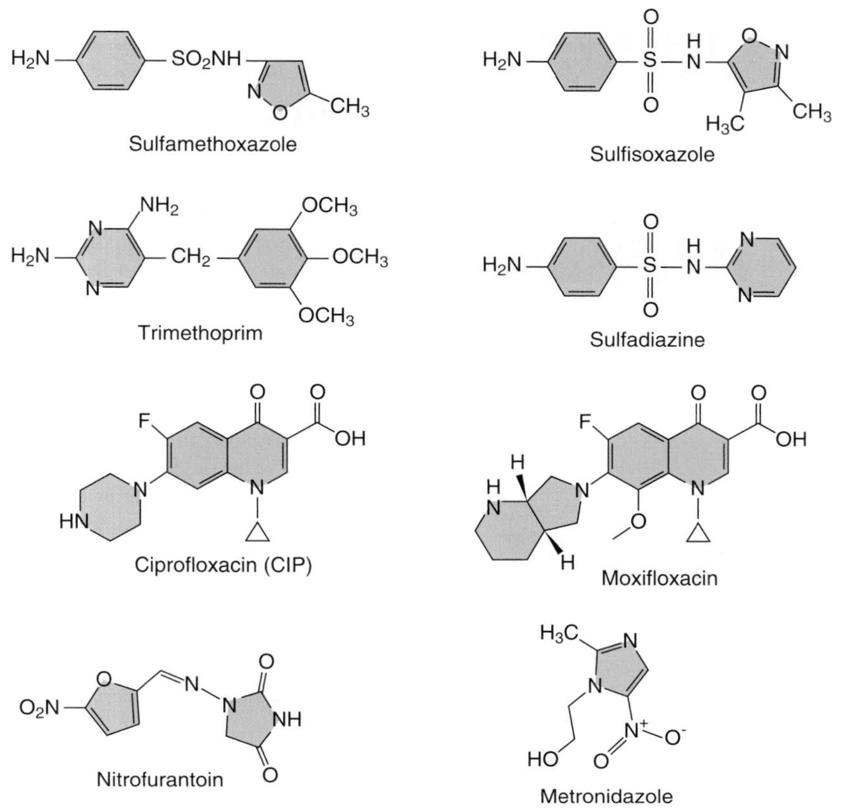

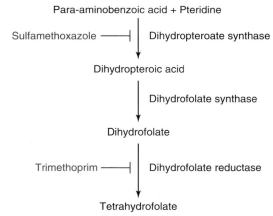

FIG. 59.1 Structures of Representative Agents.

FIG. 59.2 Folate Synthesis Pathway and Sites of Action of Trimethoprim and Sulfamethoxazole.

Trimethoprim was used initially as an antimalarial drug but was replaced by pyrimethamine, which acts by a similar mechanism. The antibacterial actions of trimethoprim stem from its high affinity for bacterial dihydrofolate reductase. Trimethoprim binds competitively and inhibits this enzyme in both bacterial and mammalian cells, but inhibition of the human enzyme requires approximately 100,000 times higher concentrations of drug relative to the bacterial enzyme. Thus trimethoprim prevents conversion of dihydrofolate to tetrahydrofolate and blocks formation of thymidine, some purines, methionine, and glycine in bacteria, leading to rapid death of the microorganisms.

Trimethoprim and sulfamethoxazole (TMP-SMX) are used effectively in combination to achieve synergistic effects by blocking sequential steps in folic acid synthesis. The combination of the two drugs is bactericidal.

Quinolones

The quinolones, which were first developed in the 1960s and represent one of the most commonly prescribed classes of antibiotics, are synthetic fluorinated analogues of nalidixic acid, and include norfloxacin, ciprofloxacin, ofloxacin, levofloxacin, moxifloxacin, and gemifloxacin. These compounds all have a fluorine at position six in the two-ring structure (see Fig. 59.1) and directly inhibit bacterial DNA synthesis by inhibiting bacterial type II topoisomerases, (DNA gyrase) and topoisomerase IV. DNA gyrase catalyzes the introduction of negative supercoils into DNA, while topoisomerase IV separates interlinked replicated chromosomal DNA during cell division. Both processes are required for normal bacterial DNA transcription and duplication. The fluoroquinolones bind to and trap the enzyme-DNA complexes, blocking gyrase-mediated supercoiling and topoisomerase IV-mediated separation of catenated DNA, resulting in inhibition of DNA synthesis and cell growth, with a lethal effect on the cell (Fig. 59.3).

Nitrofurans

Nitrofurantoin is a member of a group of synthetic nitrofuran compounds that also includes nitrofurazone. These compounds are converted to short-lived intermediates by a bacterial nitroreductase and interact with DNA to cause strand breakage and deleterious macromolecular alterations that have a lethal effect on the cells.

Nitroimidazoles

Metronidazole and related compounds are nitroimidazole prodrugs with a broad spectrum of activity against both protozoa and anaerobic bacteria. Metronidazole is reduced by ferredoxins or their equivalents

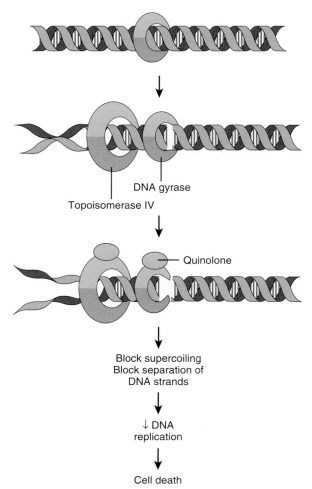

DNA gyrase

Topoisomerase IV

Quinolone

Block supercoiling
Block separation of
DNA strands

↓ DNA
replication

Cell death

FIG. 59.3 Mechanism of Action of the Quinolones. Normal bacterial DNA transcription and duplication requires the sequential actions of type II topoisomerases. DNA gyrase catalyzes the introduction of negative supercoils into DNA, and topoisomerase IV separates interlinked replicated DNA during cell division. The quinolones bind to the topoisomerase-DNA complexes, blocking both the supercoiling and separation of DNA strands, resulting in DNA synthesis inhibition and cell death.

present only in anaerobic and microaerophilic pathogens but not in human cells or aerobic organisms. The reduced products and free radicals generated bind covalently to DNA, causing damage and death (Chapter 63).

MECHANISMS OF RESISTANCE

Sulfonamides and Trimethoprim

Resistance to sulfonamides is widespread, and its incidence continues to increase among all major bacterial pathogens. Several mechanisms mediate the development of resistance, including: (1) reduced cellular uptake of the drug, which can be chromosomal or plasmid in origin; (2) decreased affinity of dihydropteroate synthase for sulfonamides by a point mutation replacing a single amino acid; and (3) increased synthesis of PABA, which is not common, but exhibited by some staphylococci.

Resistance to trimethoprim can stem from: (1) reduced cell permeability, (2) overproduction of dihydrofolate reductase, or (3) production of an altered reductase with reduced affinity for the drug. Resistance can develop by a chromosomal mutation or more commonly from

plasmid-encoded trimethoprim-resistant dihydrofolate reductases. Resistance can develop when the drug is used alone. *Pseudomonas aeruginosa*, *Bacteroides fragilis*, and enterococci are usually resistant.

Quinolones

Bacterial resistance is the most common and serious problem confronting the clinical use of the fluoroquinolones. Mechanisms of resistance include: (1) decreased intracellular drug accumulation via the production of efflux pumps or changes in porin structure (in gram-negative bacteria) and (2) mutations in *gyrA* and *gyrB*, which encode the α- and β-subunits of DNA gyrase, and mutations in *parC* and *parE*, which encode the α- and β-subunits of topoisomerase IV. These mutations account for most bacterial resistance to the fluoroquinolones, as stepwise increases in resistance are associated with sequential mutations in these genes. Recently, two types of plasmid-mediated resistance to fluoroquinolones have been described, the first mediated by Qnr proteins, which protect DNA gyrase from the fluoroquinolones, and the second mediated by an acetyltransferase, which is capable of modifying ciprofloxacin. Although both mechanisms confer low-level resistance, they may facilitate the point mutations that confer high-level resistance. Resistance to one fluoroquinolone generally leads to cross-resistance to all other members of this class. Fluoroquinolone resistance of clinical significance occurs in *Staphylococcus aureus*, *Pseudomonas aeruginosa*, *Campylobacter* species, *Escherichia coli* and other Enterobacteriaceae, *Neisseria gonorrhoeae*, and, more recently, *Streptococcus pneumoniae*.

Nitrofurans

Resistance to the nitrofurans is infrequent and not plasmid mediated. Rather when resistance develops, it is the result of a mutation associated with a loss of bacterial nitroreductase activity.

Nitroimidazoles

Clinical resistance to metronidazole has been reported for a variety of anaerobic and microaerophilic bacteria, with mechanisms involved differing according to the organism. Metronidazole resistance in *Trichomonas vaginalis* can be attributed to two mechanisms. The first is impaired oxygen scavenging, leading to high intracellular O_2 concentrations and decreased activation of metronidazole, while the second is due to low levels of ferredoxin as a consequence of reduced gene transcription. Resistance of anaerobic bacteria to metronidazole is increasing, with important clinical consequences. For *Bacteroides* species, metronidazole resistance has been linked to a family of nitroimidazole (*nim*) resistance genes (on the chromosome or plasmids). Although the exact mechanisms of resistance are unknown, these genes appear to encode a nitroimidazole reductase, which converts a 5-nitroimidazole to a 5-aminoimidazole, thus inhibiting the formation of the reactive nitroso group. Despite the fact that metronidazole has been used widely for the treatment of the microaerophilic organism *Helicobacter pylori*, this bacterium can develop resistance to this drug rapidly via a mechanism that is not yet fully understood.

RELATIONSHIP OF MECHANISMS OF ACTION TO CLINICAL RESPONSE

Sulfonamides and Trimethoprim

Sulfonamides have activity against a broad range of gram-positive and gram-negative bacteria, *Nocardia* species, *Chlamydia trachomatis*, as well as parasites (*Plasmodia* and *Toxoplasma*). However, there are few indications for the use of sulfonamides because of the many other agents available with fewer side effects or better therapeutic profiles. Most sulfonamide use is in the form of TMP-SMX.

Oral **sulfisoxazole** acetyl is used in combination with erythromycin ethylsuccinate for the treatment of otitis media in children due to its activity against *S. pneumoniae, Moraxella catarrhalis,* and *Haemophilus influenzae.* Sulfisoxazole or **sulfamethoxazole** are used to treat urinary tract infections caused by *E. coli* and other *Enterobacteriaceae,* while sulfisoxazole or **sulfadiazine** are drugs of choice for the treatment of nocardiosis, but clinicians usually prefer the TMP-SMX combination for this indication. Sulfadiazine is commonly prescribed in combination with pyrimethamine to treat central nervous system (CNS) toxoplasmosis, an opportunistic infection common in acquired immunodeficiency syndrome (AIDS), because it achieves the highest concentrations in the cerebrospinal fluid (CSF) and brain. **Sulfadoxine** is also available in combination with pyrimethamine to treat malaria (Chapter 63).

Of the poorly absorbed sulfonamides, **sulfasalazine** is used to treat rheumatoid arthritis, ulcerative colitis, regional enteritis, and inflammatory bowel disease; it has little effect on intestinal flora.

Sulfacetamide, a topical agent, is used in ophthalmic preparations because it penetrates into ocular tissues and fluids. Both **silver sulfadiazine** and **mafenide** are active against many bacterial species, including *P. aeruginosa,* and are used topically in burn patients to reduce the bacterial population in the burn eschar to concentrations low enough to prevent wound sepsis and hasten healing. The activity of silver sulfadiazine also results from the slow release of silver into the surrounding medium, which inhibits the growth in vitro of nearly all pathogenic bacteria and fungi, including some species resistant to sulfonamides. However, the toxicity of silver limits it use to topical application.

Trimethoprim has an antibacterial spectrum similar to that of sulfamethoxazole but is 20–100 times more potent. It inhibits many gram-negative and gram-positive microorganisms. Although trimethoprim is rarely used alone to treat infections because of increasing resistance and the availability of alternative agents, it can be given alone for the definitive therapy of acute urinary tract infections and prostate infections.

TMP-SMX inhibits many gram-positive bacteria including: *S. aureus* (most methicillin-susceptible *S. aureus* [MSSA] and some methicillin-resistant *S. aureus* [MRSA]), especially community-acquired strains, coagulase-negative staphylococci (e.g., *Staphylococcus saprophyticus*), and some *S. pneumoniae* and *Listeria monocytogenes.* The combination is also active against gram-negative bacteria including *H. influenzae, Neisseria meningitidis, E. coli, Klebsiella, Enterobacter, Citrobacter, Serratia, Salmonella, Shigella, Yersinia pseudotuberculosis,* and *Yersinia enterocolitica. Nocardia asteroides* may be susceptible, but enterococci and *Campylobacter* species are resistant.

TMP-SMX has been the drug of choice in the United States for the treatment of uncomplicated urinary tract infections, but the prevalence of resistance in *E. coli* now threatens its empiric use. Recent guidelines recommend that once the local prevalence of *E. coli* resistant to TMP-SMX exceeds 20%, quinolones should be used for the empiric treatment of urinary tract infections. TMP-SMX is considered an alternative to quinolones for prostatitis resulting from Enterobacteriaceae.

TMP-SMX has also been used for the treatment of upper and lower respiratory tract infections because of its activity against *H. influenzae, Moraxella* species, and *S. pneumoniae.* It is effective for acute exacerbations of chronic bronchitis, acute otitis media in children, and acute maxillary sinusitis in adults. However, emerging resistance among *S. pneumoniae, H. influenzae,* and *Moraxella* in the United States, Canada, and Europe has changed recommendations for use. TMP-SMX is also no longer recommended as empiric therapy for community-acquired pneumonia, for the treatment of traveler's diarrhea, or for most identified bacterial diarrhea because of the high prevalence of resistance in *Shigella* and enterotoxigenic *E. coli.* TMP-SMX is now considered an alternative to

high-dose amoxicillin in patients allergic to β-lactam antibiotics (adults and children) for the treatment of mild acute bacterial sinusitis.

TMP-SMX provides effective treatment and prophylaxis against *Pneumocystis jirovici (carinii)* pneumonia in patients with cell-mediated immune defects, such as in patients with AIDS and in some solid organ transplant recipients. An oral regimen of trimethoprim in combination with dapsone, which is a sulfone with properties similar to the sulfonamides (Chapter 60), is one of several alternatives to oral high-dose TMP-SMX in mild to moderate *P. jiroveci* pneumonia. TMP-SMX is also used for the treatment of Whipple disease caused by *Tropheryma whippleii* and is useful in preventing bacterial peritonitis in patients with underlying cirrhosis.

TMP-SMX has been used successfully to treat *Nocardia* infections, but failures have been reported. TMP-SMX may be an effective substitute for the doxycycline combination (doxycycline and streptomycin or gentamicin) in the treatment of brucellosis.

Quinolones

Quinolones can be classified into three generations based on antimicrobial activity. The **first generation** includes **norfloxacin,** which has activity against the common pathogens that cause urinary tract infections. However, it is the least active of the fluoroquinolones against both gram-negative and gram-positive organisms. The **second-generation** fluoroquinolones (e.g., **ciprofloxacin** and **ofloxacin**) have greater activity than first-generation compounds against gram-negative bacteria including *Enterobacter* species, *P. aeruginosa, Neisseria meningitidis, Haemophilus* species, and *Campylobacter jejuni* and moderate to good activity against many gram-positive cocci (MSSA, streptococci, and enterococci). Ciprofloxacin is also effective against diarrhea, prostatitis, and osteomyelitis and has the highest activity against *P. aeruginosa.* The **third-generation** fluoroquinolones such as **levofloxacin** (the L-isomer of ofloxacin), **gemifloxacin,** and **moxifloxacin** are slightly less active than the second-generation drugs against gram-negative bacteria, but have greater activity against gram-positive cocci, including *S. pneumoniae,* enterococci, and MRSA. Gemifloxacin and moxifloxacin have enhanced activity against anaerobes. Fluoroquinolones also are active against agents of atypical pneumonia (e.g., mycoplasmas and *Chlamydiae*), intracellular pathogens such as *Legionella,* and some mycobacteria, including *Mycobacterium tuberculosis* and *Mycobacterium avium* complex (Chapter 60).

Fluoroquinolones (other than moxifloxacin, which achieves relatively low urinary tract levels) are effective for the treatment of uncomplicated and complicated urinary tract infections caused by Enterobacteriaceae and have become drugs of choice in areas where the prevalence of TMP-SMX resistance is over 20% (Table 59.1). Because of activity against *Chlamydia trachomatis* and Enterobacteriaceae, fluoroquinolones (e.g., norfloxacin, ciprofloxacin, and ofloxacin) are drugs of choice for both acute and chronic prostatitis.

For sexually transmitted diseases such as chlamydia, fluoroquinolones such as ofloxacin or levofloxacin are considered possible alternatives to azithromycin or doxycycline. Fluoroquinolones are used in combination with other agents for the treatment of pelvic inflammatory disease. Fluoroquinolone-resistant *N. gonorrhoeae* limits the efficacy of these drugs in Asia, the Pacific (including Hawaii), and more recently, in regions of the United States. Resistance of *N. gonorrhoeae* to fluoroquinolones has spread, and gonorrhea is typically treated with third generation cephalosporins. Chancroid (infection by *Haemophilus ducreyi*) can be treated with ciprofloxacin. Fluoroquinolones (e.g., norfloxacin, ciprofloxacin, and ofloxacin) are efficacious for treating diarrhea caused by *Shigella* organisms, toxigenic *E. coli, Campylobacter, Salmonella,* and typhoid and are drugs of choice in the empiric treatment of traveler's diarrhea.

TABLE 59.1 Clinical Uses of Fluoroquinolones

Disease	Recommendations
Respiratory Tract Infections	
Pseudomonas infection of the lung in cystic fibrosis patients	Ciprofloxacin and levofloxacin
Necrotizing otitis	Ciprofloxacin for *Pseudomonas aeruginosa*
Community-acquired pneumonia	Third-generation fluoroquinolone
Hospital-acquired pneumonia	Ciprofloxacin, for susceptible gram-negative pathogens
Urinary Tract Infections	
Cystitis, uncomplicated	All effective except moxifloxacin (second generation most appropriate)
Pyelonephritis	All effective except moxifloxacin (second generation most appropriate)
Prostatitis	All effective
Osteomyelitis	
Gram-negative bacterial infections	Ciprofloxacin
Bacterial Diarrheal Diseases	
	Ciprofloxacin used most commonly; all considered likely to be effective
Sexually Transmitted Diseases	
Gonorrhea	Resistance testing required
Chlamydia	Ofloxacin, levofloxacin
Chancroid	All likely to be effective
Mycobacterial Diseases	
Disseminated *M. avium* complex	Ciprofloxacin, levofloxacin as fourth agent if needed
M. tuberculosis	Ofloxacin, levofloxacin for drug resistance or intolerance to first-line agents

Because of their enhanced activity against gram-positive organisms, including pneumococci (both penicillin-susceptible and penicillin-resistant *S. pneumoniae*), levofloxacin and moxifloxacin are drugs of choice for treating community-acquired pneumonia. They, like other fluoroquinolones, are also active against atypical causes of pneumonia, such as *Chlamydia* species, *Mycoplasma pneumoniae*, and *Legionella pneumophila*. Ciprofloxacin is effective in the treatment of susceptible *Pseudomonas* infection of the lung in cystic fibrosis patients.

Fluoroquinolones are also useful for the treatment of osteomyelitis, and, in particular, ciprofloxacin is an effective therapy for susceptible *Pseudomonas* osteomyelitis. The potential for rapid development of quinolone resistance in staphylococci during quinolone therapy limits the role of fluoroquinolones in the treatment of skin and soft tissue infections, especially if *S. aureus* is suspected. In combination with a gram-positive agent such as clindamycin, fluoroquinolones may be used for the treatment of complicated diabetic foot infections. In addition, a single dose of ciprofloxacin constitutes an alternative to rifampin for eradication of *N. meningitidis* in asymptomatic carriers.

Fluoroquinolones are also drugs of choice for the treatment of and postexposure prophylaxis against several agents that could be used in biowarfare, including anthrax, cholera, plague, brucellosis, and tularemia. Fluoroquinolones are also useful in the treatment of mycobacterial infections. Multidrug treatment of *M. avium* complex infections may include a fluoroquinolone as a third or fourth agent (Chapter 60). Ofloxacin and levofloxacin are commonly used in the treatment of multidrug-resistant tuberculosis and for tuberculosis patients intolerant to first-line therapies. Moxifloxacin pharmacokinetics and potency predict that it may be useful as an additional first-line therapy for tuberculosis.

Nitrofurans

Nitrofurans inhibit a variety of gram-positive and gram-negative bacteria, including most *E. coli*, staphylococci, many *Klebsiella* species, enterococci, *Neisseria*, *Salmonella*, *Shigella* organisms, and *Proteus* species, and are used to treat urinary tract infections. Nitrofurazone is used only for topical applications.

Nitroimidazoles

Metronidazole is used clinically to treat trichomoniasis, amebiasis, and giardiasis (Chapter 63). It is also effective against a variety of infections caused by obligate anaerobic bacteria, including *Bacteroides*, *Clostridium*, and microaerophilic bacteria, such as *Helicobacter* and *Campylobacter* species. It is also used in combination with other antimicrobial agents to treat microbial infections with mixed aerobic and anaerobic bacteria. Metronidazole is used as primary therapy for mild to moderate *Clostridium difficile* infection, the major cause of pseudomembranous colitis. However, with increasing reports of treatment failures and higher rates of recurrence with metronidazole, oral vancomycin is used (Chapter 61). It is used as a single agent to treat bacterial vaginosis and in combination with other antibiotics (e.g., clarithromycin) and a proton pump inhibitor to treat infection with *H. pylori*. Metronidazole is extremely effective against anaerobic bacterial infections and is used to treat Crohn's disease, antibiotic-associated diarrhea, and rosacea.

PHARMACOKINETICS

The pharmacokinetic properties of the antimicrobial drugs that target DNA are shown in Table 59.2.

Sulfonamides and Trimethoprim

Sulfonamides differ markedly in absorption, plasma protein binding, and half-lives. For highly absorbed sulfonamides, absorption occurs primarily from the small intestine. There is minimal absorption from topical application. Plasma protein binding ranges from a low of 45% for sulfadiazine to >90% for sulfisoxazole, sulfadoxine, and sulfasalazine, and half-lives range from 6 hours for sulfisoxazole (short-acting) to more than 100 hours for sulfadoxine (long-acting). The sulfonamides enter most body compartments, including ocular, pleural, peritoneal, synovial, and the cerebrospinal fluid (CSF). The highest concentrations in the CSF are achieved with sulfadiazine, reaching 30%–80% of plasma concentrations. Sulfonamides cross the placenta and enter the fetal circulation. Hepatic acetylation and glucuronidation represent major mechanisms of inactivation, with metabolites excreted in the urine. Some sulfonamides, such as sulfadiazine and sulfisoxazole, are poorly soluble and precipitate in the acidic urine forming crystalline deposits (crystalluria) that can cause urinary obstruction.

Sulfasalazine is poorly absorbed from the gastrointestinal (GI) tract, making it ideal for use in the therapy of ulcerative colitis and regional enteritis. The poor absorption properties allow high levels of the drug to be achieved in the GI tract. Sulfasalazine is metabolized by intestinal bacteria to sulfapyridine and 5-aminosalicylate (5-ASA, mesalamine). Sulfapyridine is responsible for most of the antibacterial activity and is absorbed from the intestine and excreted in the urine. On the other hand, 5-ASA is an antiinflammatory agent that is useful in treatment of inflammatory bowel disease.

Trimethoprim is usually administered orally, alone, or in combination with sulfamethoxazole. Trimethoprim is well absorbed from the GI

TABLE 59.2	Pharmacokinetic Properties			
Drug	**Route of Administration**	**Plasma Protein Binding (%)**	**$t_{1/2}$ (hrs)**	**Elimination**
Sulfonamides				
Sulfacetamide	Topical	-	-	-
Sulfisoxazole	Oral	90	6	M, R
Sulfamethoxazole	Oral, IV	70	11	M, R
Sulfadiazine	Oral, IV	45	17	M, R
Sulfadoxine	Oral	98	120–200	M, R
Sulfasalazine	Oral	99	6–10	M, R
Trimethoprim	Oral	70	11	R (60%)
Quinolones				
Norfloxacin	Oral	10–15	4 (8 in anuria)	M (20%), R (27%)
Ciprofloxacin	Oral, IV	20–40	4 (10 in anuria)	M, R (50%)
Levofloxacin	Oral, IV	24–38	7	R (80%)
Moxifloxacin	Oral, IV	50	10–14	M (25%), R (20%), F (25%)
Nitrofurans				
Nitrofurantoin	Oral	20–60	0.6–1.2	M, R
Nitroimidazoles				
Metronidazole	Oral, IV, topical	<20	8	M, R (20%)

F, Fecal; *M*, metabolized; *R*, renal excretion.

tract, with peak plasma concentrations reached in approximately 2 hours. Absorption is not influenced by sulfamethoxazole. Trimethoprim has a larger volume of distribution than sulfamethoxazole because it is more lipid soluble. Therefore the ratio of trimethoprim:sulfamethoxazole in TMP:SMX is 1:5, which results in peak plasma concentrations 1:2; that is optimal for the combined effects of these drugs in vitro. Trimethoprim is rapidly and widely distributed to body tissues and compartments, entering pleural, peritoneal, and synovial fluids, as well as the aqueous fluid of the eye, the CSF, and brain. Because of its high lipid solubility, trimethoprim crosses biological membranes and enters bronchial secretions, prostate and vaginal fluids, and bile. In addition, because trimethoprim is a weak base, it concentrates in prostatic and vaginal fluids, which are more acidic than plasma. Both trimethoprim and sulfamethoxazole cross the placenta.

Only 10%–20% of trimethoprim is metabolized by oxidation and conjugation to inactive oxide and hydroxyl derivatives. It is excreted in the urine, with 60% of the dose excreted within 24 hours in patients with normal renal function. There is a linear relationship between the serum creatinine concentration and the half-life of trimethoprim. The half-life of 11 hours in normal adults and children is shortened to approximately 6 hours in young children. Urinary concentrations of trimethoprim are high, even in the presence of decreased renal function, and a small amount of trimethoprim is excreted in the bile.

Quinolones

Most fluoroquinolones are available in both oral and intravenous (IV) formulations. The fluoroquinolones are well absorbed from the upper GI tract (bioavailability of 80%–95%), but absorption is decreased in the presence of divalent and trivalent cations, including those in antacids such Ca^{++} and Al^{+++}, as well as Zn^{++} and Fe^{++}. Therefore oral fluoroquinolones should be taken 2 hours before or 4 hours after products containing these cations. The fluoroquinolones have good tissue penetration, with levels that exceed serum concentrations in prostate, stool, bile, lung, and neutrophils. Urine and kidney tissue concentrations are usually high when renal elimination is high. Concentrations of fluoroquinolones in bone are usually lower than in serum, but are still adequate for treatment of osteomyelitis. CSF penetration is not usually sufficient for treatment of meningitis.

The half-lives of norfloxacin and ciprofloxacin require twice-a-day dosing, but levofloxacin, moxifloxacin, and ofloxacin can be given once daily. The principal route of elimination for most of these agents is via the kidneys, and dose adjustments are required for patients with compromised renal function. Moxifloxacin is eliminated by hepatic excretion and is contraindicated in patients with hepatic failure.

Nitrofurans

Nitrofurantoin is well absorbed from the GI tract, and food increases its bioavailability. It has a short half-life in healthy individuals as a result of rapid excretion and metabolism in tissues. The drug is excreted into bile, after which it is reabsorbed and eliminated through glomerular filtration and tubular secretion to yield brown urine. Less drug enters the urine in patients with declining renal function, making this drug ineffective in the treatment of urinary tract infections in patients with creatinine clearances <40 mL/min.

Nitroimidazoles

Metronidazole is available for oral, IV, intravaginal, and topical administration. It is well absorbed after oral administration and is widely distributed in tissues. The drug penetrates well into body tissues and fluids, including vaginal secretions, seminal fluid, breast milk, and CSF. The half-life of metronidazole in plasma is approximately 8 hours, and less than 20% of the drug is bound to plasma proteins. Metronidazole is metabolized in the liver to a hydroxy derivative, an acid, and glucuronides, and the metabolites are eliminated in the urine.

PHARMACOVIGILANCE: ADVERSE EFFECTS AND DRUG INTERACTIONS

Sulfonamides and Trimethoprim

The most common adverse effects associated with the sulfonamides are skin rashes, photosensitivity, exfoliative dermatitis, urticaria, fever, nausea, vomiting, and diarrhea. Although allergic rashes occur in only 2%–3% of patients, these drugs should not be used in patients with a known sulfonamide allergy. Most rashes occur after 1 week of therapy, but can occur earlier in previously sensitized individuals. Stevens-Johnson syndrome (a potentially fatal condition) can also occur but is relatively uncommon (<1%). A serum sickness–like illness also is seen, with fever, joint pains, and rash, which can be of the erythema nodosum type.

Other adverse effects include hematological, urinary, and hepatic toxicities. The hematological toxicities include agranulocytosis, megaloblastic, aplastic, and hemolytic anemias, and thrombocytopenia. Hemolytic anemia can occur in patients deficient in glucose-6-phosphate dehydrogenase, in which the sulfonamide serves as an oxidant. However, hemolysis can also occur in patients who have normal glucose-6-phosphate dehydrogenase concentrations. Some sulfonamides, including sulfadiazine and sulfisoxazole, may precipitate in urine, especially at neutral or acidic pH, producing crystalluria, hematuria, or even urinary obstruction. Crystalluria can be treated by administration of sodium bicarbonate to alkalinize the urine and fluids to increase urine flow. Hepatotoxicity occurs in less than 0.1% of patients receiving sulfonamides and manifests as headache, nausea, vomiting, fever, hepatomegaly, and jaundice, which usually appear 3–5 days after sulfonamide administration is started.

Drug interactions include potentiation of the action of sulfonylurea hypoglycemic agents, orally administered anticoagulants, phenytoin, and methotrexate. Mechanisms of these interactions include displacement of albumin-bound drug and competition for drug-metabolizing enzymes. Sulfonamides cross the placenta and are secreted in breast milk. When they are taken near the end of pregnancy, they may displace bilirubin from plasma proteins in the newborn (especially premature infants). Free bilirubin can be deposited in the basal ganglia of the brain, causing an encephalopathy called kernicterus. Therefore sulfonamides should not be used in the third trimester of pregnancy.

Trimethoprim alone can cause nausea, vomiting, and diarrhea but rarely causes a rash. It can increase creatinine concentrations because it competes with creatinine for the same renal clearance pathways. Trimethoprim can lead to hyperkalemia as a consequence of decreased K$^+$ secretion in the distal tubule.

Side effects encountered with TMP-SMX include all those associated with both agents. Hematological toxicity in the form of megaloblastic anemia, thrombocytopenia, and leukopenia occurs more often in patients receiving the combination than in those receiving single agents and can be dose related. Other toxicity-related conditions include glossitis, stomatitis, and occasional pseudomembranous enterocolitis. CNS effects include headache, depression, and hallucinations.

The incidence of rash and neutropenia is greater in patients with AIDS than in other patients. The importance of TMP-SMX in the prevention of *P. jirovici (carinii)* pneumonia has prompted an investigation of ways to manage allergic reactions to TMP-SMX in these patients. Both symptomatic treatment (using antihistamines or steroids) of the allergy and oral desensitization have been effective.

Fluoroquinolones

Fluoroquinolones can cause GI reactions such as nausea, vomiting, and abdominal pain. Outbreaks of pseudomembranous colitis have been reported in hospitals following the inclusion of a third-generation fluoroquinolone on the formulary. Although CNS effects such as dizziness, headache, restlessness, depression, and insomnia are infrequent, they tend to be more common in the aged and may be potentiated by the concomitant use of nonsteroidal antiinflammatory drugs. Seizures are rare. Common dermatologic reactions include rash, photosensitivity reactions, and pruritus. In addition, hepatotoxicity occasionally occurs in association with these agents, and prolongation of the QTc interval

has been reported with ciprofloxacin, levofloxacin, gemifloxacin, and moxifloxacin. Therefore these drugs should be used with caution in patients receiving other agents known to increase the QTc interval, such as antiarrhythmic agents, erythromycin, and tricyclic antidepressants. High rates of these adverse events observed in postmarketing surveillance have caused several fluoroquinolones to be removed from the market.

Fluoroquinolones are not recommended for patients under 18 years of age or for athletes, as therapy has been associated with multiple reports of tendon rupture (usually the Achilles tendon). Because this effect is reversible, fluoroquinolones may be used in children for the treatment of pseudomonal infections associated with cystic fibrosis. Fluoroquinolones have also been associated with peripheral neuropathy, which may persist for months to years after the drug is stopped or may become permanent. Ciprofloxacin inhibits CYP1A2 and prevents the metabolism of drugs that are substrates for this cytochrome P450.

Nitrofurans

The most common adverse reactions to the nitrofurans are GI, with anorexia, nausea, and vomiting being most prevalent. Hypersensitivity reactions involving the skin, lungs, liver, or blood have been observed and appear to be associated with fever and chills. Cutaneous effects include maculopapular, erythematous, urticarial, and pruritic reactions.

Two major types of pulmonary reactions occur in patients receiving nitrofuran. An acute immunologically mediated reaction, characterized by fever, cough, and dyspnea, begins approximately 10 days into treatment. A second form occurs in patients receiving long-term therapy, which develops insidiously, with patients exhibiting cough, shortness of breath, and radiological signs of interstitial fibrosis. Patients' conditions improve when the drug is stopped, but many have residual effects believed to be caused by peroxidative destruction of pulmonary membrane lipids as a consequence of the reactive oxygen species produced by the action of reductase on the nitrofurans. The nitrofurans also cause cholestatic and hepatocellular liver disease and granulomatous hepatitis and can lead to nephrotoxicity, particularly in patients with severely depressed renal function.

Hematological reactions related to the nitrofurans include granulocytopenia, leukopenia, and megaloblastic anemia, with acute hemolytic anemia occurring in patients deficient in glucose-6-phosphate dehydrogenase. Several neurological reactions have been reported, including headache, drowsiness, dizziness, nystagmus, and peripheral neuropathy of an ascending sensorimotor type.

Nitroimidazoles

Common side effects of **metronidazole** include headache, nausea, dry mouth, metallic taste, diarrhea, and stomatitis. Development of neurotoxic effects, such as dizziness, vertigo, encephalopathy, convulsions, numbness of the extremities, and ataxia, requires drug discontinuation. Because of its potential neurotoxicity, metronidazole should be used with caution in patients with CNS disease. Drug sensitivity is manifest as urticaria, flushing, and pruritus and requires withdrawal of metronidazole. Dysuria and cystitis have been reported as well. Metronidazole has a disulfiram-like effect, and patients should be cautioned to avoid alcohol during treatment.

The most commonly observed side effects for representative agents are listed in the Clinical Problems Box.

NEW DEVELOPMENTS

Due to the development of multidrug resistance, new drug targets are constantly being sought to fight bacterial pathogens. An increased understanding of the bacterial DNA replication machinery and specific proteins involved has led to pursuit of new antimicrobials targeting DNA. A particular focus has been on essential proteins that are conserved among pathogens but differ from humans. Novel bacterial nonquinolone topoisomerase inhibitors are being developed to target fluoroquinolone-resistant pathogens as are DNA ligase inhibitors, DNA polymerase III inhibitors, and inhibitors of other replication-related proteins. In addition, drugs that target protein-protein interactions essential for bacterial DNA replication are also being sought. As our knowledge of the macromolecules and processes involved in bacterial DNA replication increases, so will the development of drugs that target these specific proteins. A diverse group of agents are currently in preclinical development that will undoubtedly yield newer effective agents.

CLINICAL RELEVANCE FOR HEALTHCARE PROFESSIONALS

All healthcare professionals will employ these antimicrobial agents frequently in many patients. It is important for these healthcare providers to have knowledge of the most common adverse effects to monitor individuals for increased susceptibility to infection and alterations in cardiac and kidney function. It is important to recognize that many patients are allergic to sulfur-containing agents, such as the sulfonamides, while hypersensitivity and photosensitivity may also be an issue for some patients.

CLINICAL PROBLEMS

Trimethoprim-Sulfamethoxazole
Hypersensitivity: rashes, fever
Stevens-Johnson syndrome
Hematological reactions
Urinary toxicity (crystalluria)
Hepatotoxicity
Increased serum creatinine concentration (trimethoprim)
Hyperkalemia (trimethoprim)
Drug interactions due to protein binding displacement and competition for metabolizing enzymes

Fluoroquinolones
Gastrointestinal effects
CNS agitation (rarely seizures)
Dermatologic reactions
Hepatotoxicity
Damage to growing cartilage (not recommended for use in children)
Peripheral neuropathy
Prolongation of the QTc interval
Theophylline metabolism inhibition (ciprofloxacin)

Nitrofurans
Gastrointestinal effects
Cutaneous reactions
Pulmonary reactions
Hematological reactions
Hepatotoxicity
Neurological reactions

Metronidazole
Gastrointestinal effects
Neurotoxic effects (requires discontinuation)
Dysuria and cystitis
Disulfiram-like effect (avoid alcohol during treatment)

TRADE NAMES

In addition to generic and fixed-combination preparations, the following trade-named materials are some of the important compounds available in the United States.

Sulfonamides and Trimethoprim
Mafenide (Sulfamylon)
Sulfacetamide (Sulamyd, Cetamide, Bleph-10)
Sulfadiazine
Silver sulfadiazine (Silvadene, Thermazene)
Sulfadoxine (Fansidar)
Sulfamethizole (Thiosulfil Forte)
Sulfamethoxazole (Gantanol)
Sulfanilamide (AVC)
Sulfisoxazole (Gantrisin, Truxazole)
Trimethoprim (Proloprim, Trimpex)
Trimethoprim-sulfamethoxazole (Bactrim, Septra)
Pyrimethamine-sulfadoxine (Fansidar)

Fluoroquinolones
Ciprofloxacin (Cipro)
Enoxacin (Penetrex)
Gemifloxacin (Factive)
Levofloxacin (Levaquin)
Lomefloxacin (Maxaquin)
Norfloxacin (Noroxin)
Ofloxacin (Floxin)
Moxifloxacin (Avelox)

Nitrofurans
Nitrofurantoin (Macrobid, Macrodantin, Furadantin)
Nitrofurazone (Furacin)

Nitroimidazole
Metronidazole (Flagyl)

SELF-ASSESSMENT QUESTIONS

1. A 27-year-old woman develops an exfoliative rash along with painful joints, anemia, and nephritis while being treated for a first episode of a urinary tract infection. Which of the following drugs is responsible for these effects?
   A. Ciprofloxacin.
   B. Nitrofurantoin
   C. Norfloxacin.
   D. Polymyxin b.
   E. Trimethoprim-sulfamethoxazole.

2. A 20-year-old woman presents to the University Student Health Care center with a 2-day history of painful urination, dysuria, frequency, and urgency. She had been in good health before the abrupt onset of these symptoms. Physical examination reveals moderate suprapubic tenderness and a normal vaginal exam. Which of the following is the best empiric therapy while awaiting culture results?
   A. Metronidazole.
   B. Sulfisoxazole.
   C. Levofloxacin.

D. Trimethoprim-sulfamethoxazole.

E. Nitrofurantoin.

3. Which one of the following agents exerts a bactericidal action by inhibiting topoisomerases and DNA gyrase of microorganisms?

A. Ciprofloxacin.

B. Nitrofurantoin.

C. Polymyxin B.

D. Sulfamethoxazole.

E. Azithromycin.

4. A chromosomal mutation in dihydrofolate reductase may lead to resistance to which antibacterial agent?

A. Ciprofloxacin.

B. Nitrofurantoin.

C. Sulfamethoxazole.

D. Trimethoprim.

E. Polymyxin B.

FURTHER READING

Aldred KJ, Kerns RJ, Osheroff N. Mechanism of quinolone action and resistance. *Biochemistry*. 2014;53(10):1565–1574.

Price JR, Guran LA, Gregory WT, McDonagh MS. Nitrofurantoin vs other prophylactic agents in reducing recurrent urinary tract infections in adult women: a systematic review and meta-analysis. *Am J Obstet Gynecol*. 2016;215(5):548–560.

Robinson A, Causer RJ, Dixon NE. Architecture and conservation of the bacterial DNA replication machinery, an underexploited drug target. *Curr Drug Targets*. 2012;13(3):352–372.

van Eijk E, Wittekoek B, Kuijper EJ, Smits WK. DNA replication proteins as potential targets for antimicrobials in drug-resistant bacterial pathogens. *J Antimicrob Chermother*. 2017;72:1275–1284.

WEBSITES

https://aidsinfo.nih.gov/drugs/401/sulfamethoxazole---trimethoprim/0/patient

This site is maintained by the United States Department of Health and Human Services. It contains information on the use of sulfonamides and trimethoprim, especially in the prevention and treatment of opportunistic infections in HIV-infected teenagers and adults.

http://www.merckmanuals.com/professional/infectious-diseases/bacteria-and-antibacterial-drugs/fluoroquinolones

This site is the Merck Manual, Professional Version, and is an excellent source of information regarding the use of fluoroquinolones and metronidazole.

Antimycobacterial Agents

Rukiyah Van Dross-Anderson and Ahmed E.M. Elhassanny

MAJOR DRUG CLASSES

First-line drugs for tuberculosis
   Isoniazid, rifamycins, pyrazinamide, ethambutol
Second-line drugs for tuberculosis
   Antibacterial agents targeting DNA, protein, and cell wall synthesis
Drugs for leprosy
   Dapsone, rifampin, clofazimine
Drugs for *Mycobacterium avium* complex
   Macrolides, ethambutol

ABBREVIATIONS

CDC	Centers for Disease Control and Prevention
CNS	Central nervous system
CSF	Cerebrospinal fluid
GI	Gastrointestinal
HIV	Human immunodeficiency virus
IM	Intramuscular
INH	Isoniazid (isonicotinic acid hydrazide)
IV	Intravenous
LTBI	Latent TB infection
MAC	*Mycobacterium avium* complex
MDR-TB	Multidrug-resistant TB
PAS	*p*-Aminosalicylic acid
POA	Pyrazinoic acid
PZA	Pyrazinamide
PZase	Nicotinamidase/pyrazinamidase
TB	Tuberculosis
WHO	World Health Organization
XDR-TB	Extensive drug-resistant TB

THERAPEUTIC OVERVIEW

Mycobacteria are relatively slow-growing, obligate gram-positive aerobic bacilli with a unique cell wall that contains mycolic acids, which are long-chain fatty acids that render the cell wall relatively impermeable. Mycobacteria are stained by basic dyes and resist decolorization with acid-alcohol; thus they are termed acid-fast organisms. The major human mycobacterial pathogens are the virulent *Mycobacterium tuberculosis* complex and *Mycobacterium leprae*. Most other types of mycobacteria, classified as nontuberculous mycobacteria, occasionally cause human disease. For example, *Mycobacterium avium* complex (MAC) causes infections among highly immunocompromised patients with human immunodeficiency virus (HIV) infection or in persons with prior pulmonary disorders. More rapidly growing nontuberculous mycobacteria can cause skin and soft tissue infection after trauma or surgery (e.g., *Mycobacterium chelonae* or *Mycobacterium fortuitum*) or after exposure to salt water *(Mycobacterium marinum)*.

Tuberculosis

Tuberculosis (TB) is an airborne disease transmitted by droplet nuclei (small particles 1 to 5 μm in diameter) and caused by *M. tuberculosis* species. The World Health Organization (WHO) estimated that in 2015, 10.4 million individuals developed active disease, and more than 1.8 million deaths occurred, with TB in the top 10 causes of death worldwide. Further, according to the United States Centers for Disease Control and Prevention (CDC), one-third of the world's population is infected with TB, and TB represents a leading killer of individuals infected with HIV.

In most cases, mycobacterial proliferation occurs in the lung, but it can also occur in the spine, hips, and gastrointestinal (GI) tract. Symptoms of pulmonary TB include chronic cough, night sweats, blood-tinged sputum, weight loss, shortness of breath, fever, and chest pain. About 90% of people infected with *M. tuberculosis* complex are asymptomatic and do not transmit the disease to others, reflecting the dormant stage, referred to as a latent tuberculosis infection (LTBI). The risk of progression from latent infection to active disease ranges from a 5%–10% lifetime risk in immunocompetent individuals to a 10% lifetime risk in immunocompromised individuals, including those with HIV, intravenous drug users, and patients with other illnesses such as silicosis, diabetes mellitus, and certain malignancies. Others at increased risk include recent immigrants from areas with a high incidence of TB and racial/ethnic minorities.

Leprosy

Leprosy (also known as Hansen disease) is caused by *M. leprae*. Although this disease is rare in the United States and Canada, it is not uncommon in developing countries. According to the WHO, 200,000 new cases of leprosy were reported in 2015, with 19,000 children diagnosed. It is estimated that 23 million people are living with leprosy-related disabilities throughout the world.

The route of transmission of leprosy remains uncertain and may involve nasal droplet infection, contact with infected soil, and even insect vectors. *M. leprae* multiplies very slowly, with a generation time of 14 days and an incubation period that can vary between 1 and 20 years. The clinical manifestations are largely confined to the skin, peripheral nervous system, upper respiratory tract, eyes, and testes and depend highly on the immune response of the infected person to *M. leprae*. Two distinct forms of leprosy exist—namely, paucibacillary (also known as tuberculoid) and multibacillary (also known as lepromatous). Paucibacillary leprosy is characterized by a small number of hypopigmented, well-bordered, anesthetic skin lesions with few acid-fast bacilli and is limited by cell-mediated immune responses. In contrast, multibacillary leprosy is characterized by numerous infiltrated skin lesions containing large numbers of acid-fast bacilli, and there is a poor cell-mediated response to the organism.

Mycobacterium avium Complex Disease

MAC consists of *Mycobacterium intracellulare* and *M. avium*, the former a pulmonary pathogen affecting immunocompetent individuals with abnormal lung anatomy or physiology and the latter leading to disseminated disease in immunocompromised individuals (patients with HIV infection and CD4+ T lymphocyte counts of <75/μL). MAC is a common organism found in both fresh- and salt water, soil, and farm animals. MAC is transmitted via ingestion or inhalation, and unlike TB, it is not transmitted from person to person.

MAC may cause both asymptomatic infection and symptomatic disease in humans. It crosses the mucosal epithelium to infect macrophages, spreads to submucosal tissue, and is transported by the lymphatic system to the lymph nodes. The most common manifestation of MAC is pulmonary disease; it can also cause lymphadenitis in children.

Treatment of Mycobacteria

The treatment of mycobacteria is more difficult than the treatment of other bacterial diseases for several reasons, including their slow growth and ability to become dormant for extended periods of time. Multidrug therapy is the standard for disorders resulting from mycobacterial infections, with the goals of killing the bacilli rapidly, minimizing or preventing the development of drug resistance, and eliminating persistent organisms from the host to prevent relapse. Treatment regimens for *M. tuberculosis* complex, *M. leprae*, and *M. avian* complex are presented in the Therapeutic Overview Box.

THERAPEUTIC OVERVIEW

Infection	Goal
Tuberculosis	Latent disease: prophylaxis with isoniazid or rifampin for high-risk patients to prevent active disease
	Active disease
	If susceptible, multidrug (4) therapy with first-line agents: isoniazid, rifampin, pyrazinamide, and ethambutol
	If resistant, multidrug (4–6) therapy with second-line agents
Leprosy	Paucibacillary: rifampin and dapsone
	Multibacillary: rifampin, dapsone. and clofazimine
Mycobacterium avium complex	Pulmonary disease
	Newly diagnosed: rifampin, ethambutol, and a macrolide antibiotic, such as clarithromycin or azithromycin
	Advanced disease or recurrence: rifabutin
	Disseminated disease
	Prophylaxis with clarithromycin or azithromycin
	Active disease: clarithromycin or azithromycin and ethambutol

---

MECHANISMS OF ACTION

First-Line Drugs for Tuberculosis

Four drugs are used as first-line treatment for TB, including isoniazid, a rifamycin such as rifampin, pyrazinamide, and ethambutol. The structures of these agents are shown in Fig. 60.1.

Isoniazid

Isoniazid (INH) is a bactericidal agent that inhibits the synthesis of mycolic acid, a major constituent of mycobacterial cell walls (Fig. 60.2). INH is a prodrug that enters the cytoplasm of bacilli by passive diffusion and is activated by the *M. tuberculosis* catalase-peroxidase enzyme KatG, leading to the formation of an isonicotinoyl radical. This activated form of INH inhibits two enzymes, enoyl acyl carrier protein (ACP) reductase (InhA) and a β-ketoacyl ACP synthase (KasA), decreasing the synthesis of mycolic acid and leading to cell death. The isonicotinoyl radical also leads to the generation of peroxides and superoxides that may also contribute to mycobacterial cell death. Deletions or mutations in the *katG* gene is the major cause of resistance to INH. Mutations in the regulatory regions of a gene encoding for alkyl hydroperoxide reductase C (the *ahp*C gene) has also been associated with some INH-resistant strains.

Rifamycins

The rifamycins are also bactericidal and include rifampin, rifabutin, and rifapentine. These agents enter *M. tuberculosis* in a concentration-dependent manner and inhibit DNA-dependent RNA polymerase of mycobacteria and many gram-positive and gram-negative bacteria but not the mammalian enzyme. The rifamycins bind to the β subunit of the enzyme, blocking the growing RNA chain. Resistance is conferred by single mutations that tend to occur (>95%) in an 81–base pair region of the *rpoB* gene that codes for the β subunit. Because of the broad spectrum of activity of these agents, they are also used against *M. leprae* and *M. avian* complex.

Pyrazinamide

Pyrazinamide (PZA) is a bactericidal prodrug that enters *M. tuberculosis* by passive diffusion followed by deamination to the active metabolite pyrazinoic acid (POA) by the enzyme nicotinamidase/pyrazinamidase (PZase) encoded by the *pncA* gene (Fig. 60.3). POA exits the cell through passive diffusion, and in an acidic environment, a portion of it becomes protonated to HPOA, which diffuses readily back into the cell. Once inside the cell, the active HPOA inhibits fatty acid synthase I, interfering with the synthesis of mycolic acid (see Fig. 60.2). It also decreases the intracellular pH and disrupts mycobacterial plasma membrane transport, all of which contribute to its bactericidal activity. Selected mutations in *pncA* are associated with PZA resistance in *M. tuberculosis*. Unlike other agents, PZA targets nongrowing bacilli; it has little to no effect against growing cells.

Ethambutol

Ethambutol interferes with the synthesis of mycobacterial cell walls by inhibiting arabinosyl transferase III, preventing the polymerization of arabinose into arabinogalactan (see Fig. 60.2). The target is encoded by a three-gene operon (*embC*, *emb*A, *emb*B), particularly *emb*B, with resistance to ethambutol likely due to mutations in *emb*B.

Second-Line Drugs for Tuberculosis

Second-line drugs for TB are used for individuals who have drug-resistant TB or fail to respond to conventional therapy. Most second-line drugs are less active against *M. tuberculosis* than the first-line agents and have significantly greater toxicity.

The second-line agents for TB include ethionamide, which is chemically related to INH and has a similar mechanism of action to block the synthesis of mycolic acids. Also included is cycloserine, which is an analogue of the amino acid D-alanine and inhibits peptidoglycan biosynthesis. The pharmacology of cycloserine is discussed in Chapter 57.

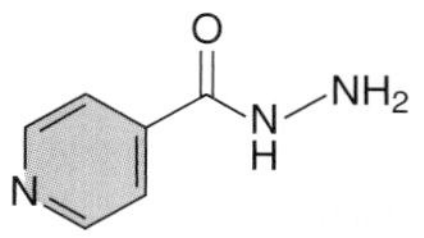

Isoniazid

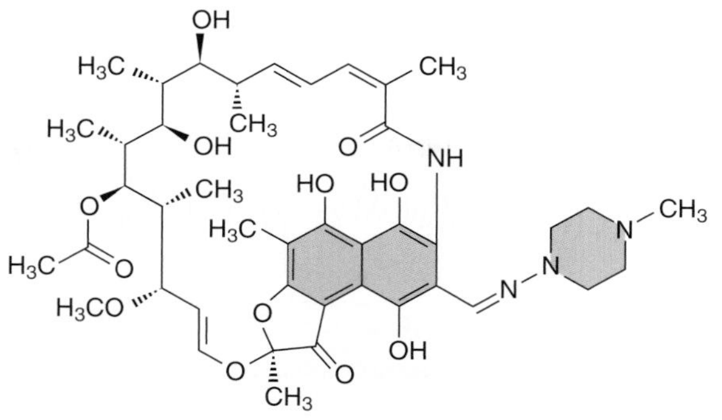

Rifampin

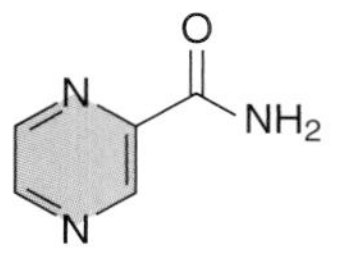

Pyrazinamide

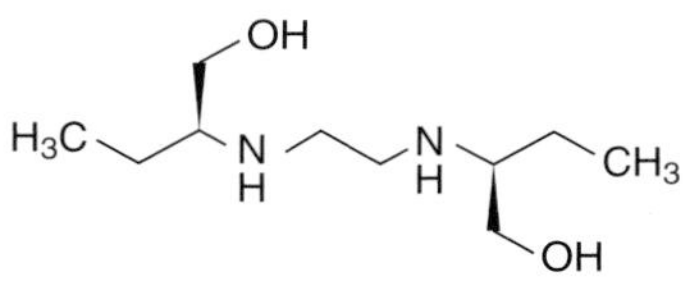

Ethambutol

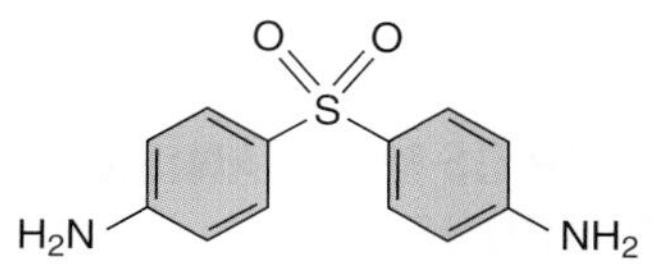

Dapsone

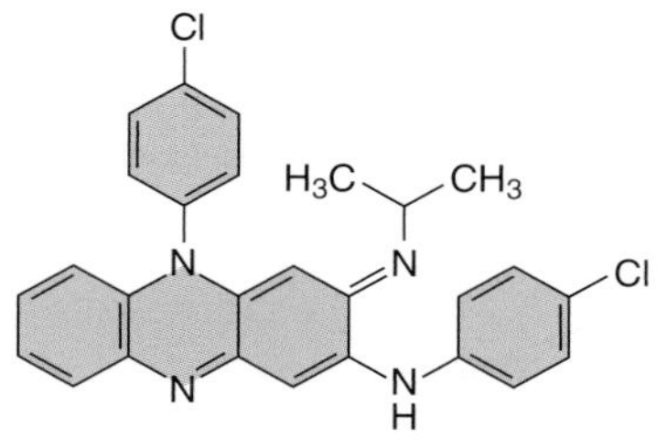

Clofazimine

FIG. 60.1 Chemical Structures of Selected Antimycobacterial Drugs.

Among the protein synthesis inhibitors used as second-line drugs for TB are **streptomycin**, **capreomycin**, and other aminoglycosides, including **amikacin** and **kanamycin**. Streptomycin is recommended as first-line therapy in some settings. However, it should be used only when an injectable drug is needed or desirable and for the treatment of infections resistant to other drugs. Capreomycin is an effective protein synthesis inhibitor but exhibits only bacteriostatic activity. The pharmacology of streptomycin and other aminoglycosides is discussed in Chapter 58.

Other agents used for drug-resistant TB include **para-aminosalicylic acid (PAS)** and the **fluoroquinolones**, both of which target DNA. PAS is a structural analogue of para-amino benzoic acid (PABA) and competes with PABA for incorporation into the folate pathway in the reaction catalyzed by dihydropteroate synthase. The product of this reaction is further processed by dihydrofolate synthase to generate a hydroxyl dihydrofolate antimetabolite, which inhibits dihydrofolate reductase enzymatic activity, thereby blocking the folate pathway (Chapter 59, Fig. 59.2).

The pharmacology of the fluoroquinolones levofloxacin, moxifloxacin, ciprofloxacin, and gatifloxacin is discussed in Chapter 59.

Drugs for Leprosy

The standard treatment of leprosy also involves multidrug therapy with **dapsone** and **rifampin**, with or without **clofazimine**. The structures of these compounds are shown in Fig. 60.1.

Dapsone is a structural analogue of PABA with properties similar to those of the sulfonamides (Chapter 59). It is an inhibitor of dihydropteroate synthase in the folate pathway to produce a bacteriostatic effect (Chapter 59, Fig. 59.2). It has a very broad spectrum of activity against bacteria, protozoa, and fungi. It also exhibits antiinflammatory activity by inhibiting several enzymes expressed by neutrophils, and it inhibits neutrophil migration.

Clofazimine is also bactericidal with antiinflammatory activity. The antibacterial effects of clofazimine are mediated by binding to mycobacterial DNA, but it also may be a prodrug that releases reactive oxygen species to interfere with the mycobacterial electron transport chain. Its antiinflammatory activity is due to inhibition of macrophage, T cell, and neutrophil function.

Drugs for *Mycobacterium avium* Complex

MAC infection also often requires multidrug therapy, mainly including a macrolide (clarithromycin or azithromycin), ethambutol, and a

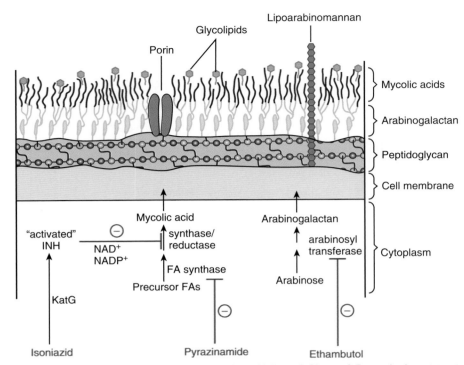

FIG. 60.2 Composition of the Mycobacterial Cell Wall and Sites of Drug Action. Mycobacteria contain an inner cell membrane, a thin peptidoglycan layer, and the highly branched arabinogalactan that connects the peptidoglycan with the thick outer layer of mycolic acids. Porin channels penetrate arabinogalactan and mycolic acid layers, with glycolipids and other proteins present. The glycolipid lipoarabinomannan, which contains a mannose polymer, extends from the cell membrane to the cell surface, and is a major virulence factor for *Mycobacterium tuberculosis*. Isoniazid (INH), pyrazinamide, and ethambutol all inhibit the synthesis of the *M. tuberculosis* cell wall.

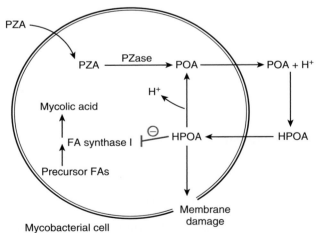

FIG. 60.3 Proposed Mechanism of Action of Pyrazinamide (PZA). PZA is a prodrug that diffuses into the cell and is converted to pyrazinoic acid (POA) by the enzyme pyrazinamidase (PZase) encoded by the *pncA* gene. POA exits the cell, where it is protonated in an acidic environment to HPOA, which diffuses back into the cell. HPOA inhibits mycobacterial fatty acid synthase I, acidifies the cytoplasm, and disrupts mycobacterial membranes.

rifamycin (rifampin or rifabutin). The use of rifamycins for disseminated nontuberculous mycobacterial disease in HIV-infected patients may cause special problems because of their interactions with protease inhibitors. Other drugs with activity against MAC organisms include the aminoglycosides, fluoroquinolones, and clofazimine.

RELATIONSHIP OF MECHANISMS OF ACTION TO CLINICAL RESPONSE

Drug Treatment of Tuberculosis

The goals of TB therapy are to kill tubercle bacilli rapidly, to minimize or prevent the development of drug resistance, and to eliminate persistent organisms from the host's tissues to prevent relapse. **Multidrug therapy** is required for prolonged periods (at least 6 to 9 months for susceptible disease). There are two phases for the treatment of patients with TB disease: the **initiation phase** (bactericidal or intensive phase) and the **continuation phase** (subsequent sterilizing phase). Patients with TB, or a high clinical suspicion for TB, should be started on a **four-drug regimen** consisting of **INH**, **rifampin**, **PZA**, and **ethambutol** for 2 months. Once a definitive diagnosis for *M. tuberculosis* is obtained through an acid-fast bacilli smear and culture, isolates should undergo susceptibility testing. If studies demonstrate susceptibility to first-line drugs, INH and rifampin should be continued for 4 more months (the continuation phase), and PZA and ethambutol can be discontinued. Patients at high risk for relapse (those with cavitary pulmonary disease at initial presentation and who remain culture positive after 2 months of therapy) should extend the continuation phase for 3 more months, for 9 months of total therapy. Specific schedules for the treatment of active TB disease have been developed.

INH is the most active drug for the treatment of TB and is indicated for both latent and active TB. Similarly, **rifampin** is indicated for the treatment of both latent and active TB, as well as a single drug for patients with latent TB who are unable to take INH or who have been exposed to a case of active TB caused by an INH-resistant rifampin-susceptible strain. The antimicrobial effects of rifabutin and rifapentine are similar to those of rifampin. In addition, rifabutin can be substituted for rifampin for HIV+ patients with TB because it has fewer drug interactions. PZA is used in conjunction with INH and rifampin in short-course (6-month) regimens.

Drug Treatment of Multidrug-Resistant and Extensively Drug-Resistant Tuberculosis

There are two types of drug-resistant tuberculosis, multidrug-resistant TB (MDR-TB) and extensively drug-resistant TB (XDR-TB). MDR-TB is defined as TB resistant to at least INH and rifampin, while XDR-TB, which has emerged recently, is resistant to INH and rifampin, as well as the fluoroquinolones, and at least one of the injectable drugs such as amikacin, kanamycin, or capreomycin. Drug-resistant strains of *Mycobacterium* are associated with higher morbidity and mortality than nonresistant strains.

Drug resistance is an important factor in determining the appropriate therapeutic regimen and requires a directly observed therapy plan under the supervision of an experienced clinician. Treatment regimens are based on the patient's health status and the results of susceptibility testing and require 18–24 months of treatment with second-line drugs. About 3.3% of newly diagnosed and 20% of patients previously treated for TB worldwide have MDR-TB, with 9.7% of these exhibiting XDR-TB. In 2014, approximately 480,000 people worldwide were diagnosed with MDR-TB.

The second-line agents include ethionamide, cycloserine, streptomycin, capreomycin, other aminoglycosides, and PAS, as well as drugs currently under clinical investigation.

Drug Treatment of Leprosy

Recommended therapy for leprosy is based on the classification of disease and includes multidrug therapy with dapsone and rifampin, with or without clofazimine.

The WHO recommends that patients with paucibacillary (or tuberculoid) disease receive rifampin once monthly and dapsone on a daily basis for 6 months. Furthermore, patients with single-lesion paucibacillary disease can be treated with single-dose multidrug therapy (rifampin, ofloxacin, and minocycline). Patients with multibacillary disease require a minimum of 12 months of triple-drug therapy (rifampin and dapsone monthly plus clofazimine either daily or monthly), although they are frequently treated for 24 months. Unfortunately, chemoprophylaxis with rifampin or dapsone for high-risk contacts of leprosy patients has proven unsuccessful.

Immune Reactions in Leprosy

Patients with leprosy can experience episodic, immunologically mediated acute inflammatory responses, termed *reactions*, that can cause nerve damage. These reactions can be characterized by swelling and edema in preexisting skin lesions or peripheral neuropathy/neuritis, which can cause pain, tenderness, and loss of function. They occur in up to one-third of patients with leprosy and, if not recognized and treated aggressively, can lead to irreversible nerve damage and limb deformity. They can occur before, during, or after treatment for leprosy. The two common types of reactions are type 1, or reversal reactions, characterized by cellular hypersensitivity and manifest with skin lesions and inflammation of the nerve trunk, and type 2, or erythema nodosum leprosum (ENL), characterized by a systemic inflammatory response to immune complex deposition and manifest with skin lesions, fever, arthralgia, neuritis, vasculitis, adenopathy, iridocyclitis, orchitis, and dactylitis. Type 1 reactions are best treated with glucocorticoids such as prednisone, while type 2 reactions are treated with prednisone and thalidomide, with clofazimine reserved as a second-line agent.

Treatment of *Mycobacterium avium* Complex Disease

Treatment of MAC disease requires at least 12 months of multidrug therapy with macrolide antibiotics (clarithromycin or azithromycin), ethambutol, and rifampin, or single-drug therapy with rifabutin, depending on the status of the disease. Among immunocompetent patients with pulmonary MAC, treatment is often recommended for 12 months after sputum conversion. If HIV-infected individuals have a CD4+ T lymphocyte count of <50 cells/μL, they should receive prophylaxis against disseminated MAC disease throughout their life, unless immune reconstitution occurs as a consequence of highly active antiretroviral therapy. Patients with an increase in CD4+ T lymphocyte counts to >100 cells/μL for more than 3 months can safely discontinue prophylaxis.

PHARMACOKINETICS

Pharmacokinetic properties of agents used for the treatment of TB are provided in Table 60.1.

First-Line Drugs for Tuberculosis
Isoniazid

INH is well absorbed orally and is widely distributed, with peak concentrations achieved in pleural, peritoneal, and synovial fluids. Cerebrospinal

TABLE 60.1	Selected Pharmacokinetic Properties			
Drug	**Administered**	**$t_{1/2}$ (hrs)**	**Average C_{max} (μg/mL)**	**Elimination**
Isoniazid	Oral, IV, IM	<2–4	2–8	M, R
Rifampin	Oral, IV	2–4	4–12	M, R
Rifabutin	Oral	32–67	0.2–0.6	M, R, F
Rifapentine	Oral	14–18	10–20	M, F
Pyrazinamide	Oral	2–10	30–60	M, R
Ethambutol	Oral	2–4	1–4	R
Capreomycin	IV, IM	4–6	20–45	R
p-aminosalicylic acid	Oral	1	20	M, R
Ethionamide	Oral	3	1.5	M, R
Dapsone	Oral	25	11–23	M, R
Clofazimine	Oral	10–14 days	0.5–2	F

C_{max}, Peak plasma levels; *F*, fecal; *IM*, intramuscular; *IV*, intravenous; *M*, metabolized; *R*, renal excretion.

fluid (CSF) concentrations are approximately 20% of plasma levels but can increase to 100% with meningeal inflammation. INH is metabolized by a liver *N*-acetyltransferase, and the rate of acetylation determines its concentration in plasma and its half-life. However, there is little evidence that differences in rates of acetylation are therapeutically important if INH is administered once daily because plasma levels are well above minimum inhibitory concentrations.

Rifamycins (Rifampin, Rifabutin, Rifapentine)

Rifampin is well absorbed orally and widely distributed, achieving therapeutic concentrations in lung, liver, bile, bone, and urine, and entering pleural, peritoneal, synovial fluids, CSF, tears, and saliva. Its high lipid solubility enhances its entrance into phagocytic cells, where it kills intracellular bacteria. Rifampin is metabolized in the liver to a desacetyl derivative that is also biologically active. Unmetabolized drug is excreted in bile and reabsorbed from the GI tract through entero-hepatic circulation; the deacetylated metabolite is poorly reabsorbed with eventual elimination in urine. Rifampin induces the expression of cytochrome P450s, which increases its own metabolism, resulting in increased biliary excretion with continuation therapy. Induction of metabolism results in reduction of the plasma half-life by 20%–40% after 7–10 days of therapy. Patients with severe liver disease may require dose reduction.

The oral bioavailability of rifabutin is less than that of rifampin, but the plasma half-life of rifabutin is approximately 10 times greater than rifampin. Rifabutin is more lipid soluble than rifampin and is extensively distributed. Rifabutin also induces its own metabolism through the cytochrome P450 system but to a lesser extent than rifampin. It is metabolized in a similar manner but does not significantly induce its own metabolism.

Pyrazinamide

PZA is well absorbed orally and widely distributed, readily penetrating cells and cavities. It enters the CSF if the meninges are inflamed. PZA is metabolized by the liver, and its metabolic products are excreted mainly by the kidneys. Dose modifications are necessary in renal failure.

Ethambutol

Approximately 75%–80% of ethambutol is orally absorbed and widely distributed. Ethambutol crosses the placenta and, under normal circumstances, does not penetrate into the CSF. However, with meningeal inflammation, CSF concentrations can reach 10%–50% of plasma values. Ethambutol is mainly excreted unchanged by the kidneys, and dose adjustments are necessary in renal failure. It can be removed from the body by peritoneal dialysis or hemodialysis.

Second-Line Drugs for Tuberculosis

Capreomycin is administered by intramuscular (IM) or intravenous (IV) routes and is eliminated by the kidneys. It enters the CSF poorly and accumulates during renal dysfunction.

PAS is available as granules and as a solution for IV administration. PAS is well absorbed orally and enters lung tissue and pleural fluid. It is metabolized in the liver by an acetylase different from the one that metabolizes INH. Most of the absorbed dose is excreted in the urine as metabolites.

Ethionamide is well absorbed orally and widely distributed, entering the CSF and reaching concentrations equal to those in plasma. It is metabolized in the liver, with metabolites excreted through the kidney. Ethionamide interferes with INH acetylation. Ethionamide should be taken with food to reduce gastrointestinal effects and with pyridoxine to limit neuropathic side effects.

The pharmacokinetics of cycloserine are discussed in Chapter 57, those of the aminoglycosides in Chapter 58, and those of the fluoroquinolones in Chapter 59.

Drugs for Leprosy

Dapsone is well absorbed from the upper GI tract, is distributed to all body tissues, and achieves therapeutic concentrations in skin. It is approximately 70% bound to plasma proteins, excreted in bile, and reabsorbed via the enterohepatic circulation. It is acetylated in liver by the same enzyme that acetylates INH, and acetylation phenotype does not affect its half-life. Dapsone is excreted as glucuronide and sulfate conjugates in urine. It has a plasma half-life of 25 hours, which is reduced in patients receiving rifampin. The dosage should be reduced in renal failure.

Clofazimine is variably absorbed from the GI tract and distributed in a complex pattern, with high concentrations reached in subcutaneous fat and the reticuloendothelial system. It is not metabolized but is excreted slowly by the biliary route. It is estimated to have a half-life of 70 days.

PHARMACOVIGILANCE: ADVERSE EFFECTS AND DRUG INTERACTIONS

First-Line Drugs for Tuberculosis

Isoniazid

Although adverse reactions to INH are uncommon, a few are serious. Hepatotoxicity is the most potentially serious side effect, although recent data suggest the incidence is lower than previously thought (0.1%–0.15%). The risk of hepatotoxicity is age related and is rare in persons <20 years old; however, the incidence in people 50–64 years old is approximately 2%. The risk of hepatitis is higher when INH is administered with other potentially hepatotoxic drugs such as PZA or rifampin. The risk may also increase with underlying liver disease, a history of heavy alcohol consumption, or in the postpartum period. Asymptomatic elevation of aminotransferases, which are generally transient, can occur in 10%–20% of those taking INH for LTBI. Although the incidence of clinical hepatitis is low (approximately 1%), it can be fatal when it occurs. The drug should be discontinued when aminotransferases are increased by more than five times normal levels in asymptomatic patients or more than threefold in symptomatic patients. Patients should be advised to discontinue INH at the onset of symptoms consistent with hepatitis, such as nausea, loss of appetite, and dull midabdominal pain. Routine laboratory monitoring is recommended for persons at increased risk of toxicity. Liver function tests should be obtained on any patient who develops symptoms that could suggest hepatitis.

Other side effects of INH include peripheral neuropathy, which occurs more commonly in slow acetylators, those with a nutritional deficiency, diabetes, HIV infection, renal failure, and alcoholism, and in pregnant and breastfeeding women. The neuropathy is due to pyridoxine (vitamin B6) deficiency because INH increases pyridoxine excretion. Thus pyridoxine is recommended for all patients with risk factors to help prevent neuropathy and may be administered to reverse a neuropathy, should it occur. INH-induced central nervous system (CNS) toxicity is less common than peripheral neuropathy and includes dysarthria, irritability, psychosis, seizures, dysphoria, and inability to concentrate, but the prevalence is not well quantified. CNS toxicity can also be treated with pyridoxine. Other side effects include rare hypersensitivity reactions such as fever, rash, hemolytic anemia, and vasculitis. Also, a lupus-like syndrome is rare (<1%), although approximately 20% of patients develop antinuclear antibodies.

Rifamycins (Rifampin, Rifabutin, Rifapentine)

Rifampin is generally well tolerated. Patients should be advised that rifampin results in an orange discoloration of sputum, urine, sweat, and tears, and soft contact lenses may become stained. Rifampin causes nausea and vomiting in 1%–2% of patients but is rarely severe enough to warrant discontinuation. The major toxicity of rifampin is hepatitis. Transient, asymptomatic hyperbilirubinemia may occur in up to 0.6% of patients. More severe hepatitis that has a cholestatic pattern may also occur. It is more common when the drug is given in combination with INH (2.7%) than when given alone or in combination with other drugs (1.1%). Severe hepatic toxicity has been reported when rifampin is used in combination with PZA for short-course (2-month) therapy for treatment of LTBI, and the risk of death has been estimated to be as high as 0.09%. This combination is no longer recommended for LTBI, but both drugs remain important components of multidrug regimens described previously. Hypersensitivity reactions are uncommon but include thrombocytopenia, hemolysis, transient leukopenia, and renal failure caused by interstitial nephritis. A flu-like syndrome with fever, chills, muscle aches, headache, and dizziness may occur when patients take the drug on a biweekly regimen, but it does not occur with a daily regimen.

There are many drug interactions between rifamycins and other drugs, including antiretroviral agents. Paradoxical or immune reconstitution reactions are more common among HIV-infected patients with TB who are started on antiretroviral therapy early in the course of TB treatment. Therefore a delay of initiation of antiretroviral therapy in HIV-infected patients may be recommended, if possible, until after 1–2 months of TB disease therapy. Recommendations on the use of antiretroviral therapies in HIV-infected patients with TB continue to evolve.

Rifamycins (especially rifampin) are among the most potent inducers of hepatic cytochrome P450 oxidative enzymes and the P-glycoprotein transport system and have a large number of drug interactions (Box 60.1). Rifampin usually results in increased metabolism and enhanced clearance of other drugs. Rifampin cannot be used with protease inhibitors, although it can be used with nucleoside and some nonnucleoside reverse transcriptase inhibitors (Chapter 66). Rifabutin has less of an effect on cytochrome P450s than rifampin and can be used with several protease inhibitors. It is substituted for rifampin when treating HIV-infected patients taking protease inhibitors. Women of childbearing age should be advised to use alternative contraceptive methods while on rifampin because oral contraceptives will not be effective.

Adverse effects of rifabutin are similar to those of rifampin. In addition, neutropenia has been described, especially among persons with advanced HIV/acquired immunodeficiency syndrome. Rifabutin can also cause uveitis, and the risk is increased with higher doses or when used in combination with macrolide antibiotics that reduce its clearance. It may also occur with other drugs that reduce clearance, such as protease inhibitors and azole antifungal drugs. Although drug interactions are less problematic with rifabutin than with rifampin,

they still occur, and close monitoring is required. Adverse effects of rifapentine are similar to those of rifampin.

Pyrazinamide

Hepatotoxicity is the most serious adverse effect of PZA, with elevation of liver aminotransferase concentration the first indication. The effect is less frequent in patients who receive the more current lower dose regimens compared to the higher doses used in earlier trials. Mild anorexia and nausea are common, but severe nausea and vomiting are rare. PZA causes hyperuricemia by inhibiting the renal excretion of urate. Clinical gout caused by PZA is rare, although nongouty polyarthralgia can occur in up to 40% of patients. As mentioned earlier, severe hepatotoxicity has been reported among patients taking rifampin and PZA for short-course therapy for LTBI, and liver function should be carefully monitored.

Ethambutol

The most important toxicity of ethambutol is a dose-related optic neuritis. This is manifest as decreased visual acuity or decreased red-green color discrimination. Patients should have baseline visual acuity and color discrimination monitored and be questioned about possible visual disturbances. Monthly testing is recommended for patients taking doses greater than 15 mg/kg/day, receiving the drug for longer than 2 months, or with renal insufficiency. Other reported side effects include elevated serum uric acid levels, precipitation of acute gout, and liver toxicities.

Second-Line Drugs for Tuberculosis

Ethionamide frequently causes significant GI reactions, and many patients cannot tolerate elevated doses. Nausea, vomiting, abdominal pain, diarrhea, a metallic taste in the mouth, and many CNS complaints are typical including depression, headache, and feelings of restlessness. Endocrine disturbances including gynecomastia, alopecia, hypothyroidism, and impotence have also been described. Diabetes may be more difficult to manage. Ethionamide is similar in structure to INH and may cause similar side effects, including hepatitis (approximately 2%). Liver function tests should be monitored if there is underlying liver disease and if symptoms develop. Thyroid hormone levels should also be monitored.

The adverse effects of capreomycin and the other aminoglycosides are similar and include nephrotoxicity and ototoxicity (Chapter 58). Close monitoring of renal function is required.

The most common side effects of PAS include nausea, vomiting, abdominal pain, and diarrhea. The incidence of GI side effects is lower with the granular formulation, which is the only formulation available in the United States. A malabsorption syndrome has been described, and hypothyroidism is common, especially among those taking PAS and ethionamide. Hepatitis is uncommon. With prolonged therapy, thyroid function should be monitored. In addition, it may cause crystalluria.

Drugs for Leprosy

The most common adverse effects of dapsone are hemolytic anemia and methemoglobinemia. Hemolysis is greatly enhanced in patients with glucose-6-phosphate dehydrogenase deficiency. Methemoglobinemia is caused by a dapsone *N*-oxidation product and is usually asymptomatic but may become important if the patient develops hypoxemia from lung disease. Although bone marrow suppression is rare, agranulocytosis and aplastic anemia may occur. GI intolerance, including anorexia, nausea, and vomiting, can occur, as well as hematuria, fever, pruritus, and rash.

The most common adverse effects of clofazimine are GI intolerance, including anorexia, diarrhea, and abdominal pain. Skin pigmentation resulting from drug accumulation and producing red-brown to black discoloration is common, especially in dark-skinned persons.

BOX 60.1   Examples of Drugs With Reduced Half-Lives Caused by Concomitant Administration of Rifampin

Barbiturates, chloramphenicol, cimetidine, clarithromycin, clofibrate, contraceptives (oral), cyclosporin, dapsone, digitoxin, digoxin, efavirenz, estrogens, fluconazole, itraconazole, ketoconazole, metoprolol, methadone, phenytoin, prednisone, propranolol, quinidine, protease inhibitors, ritonavir, sulfonylureas, tacrolimus, theophylline, thyroxine, verapamil, warfarin

The adverse effects of prednisone, used for the treatment of leprosy-associated immune reactions, are discussed in Chapter 50. Thalidomide, which is used for type 2 reactions, is teratogenic, cannot be taken by women who are pregnant or may become pregnant during therapy, and should not be given to women of childbearing age without reliable forms of birth control. Because thalidomide passes into semen, males taking thalidomide must use a latex or synthetic condom during sexual contact with women who are pregnant or could become pregnant and for up to 4 weeks following discontinuation of therapy. Other adverse effects of thalidomide include peripheral neuropathy, constipation, hypothyroidism, and increased risk of deep vein thrombosis.

Drugs for *Mycobacterium avium*

Rifabutin is generally well tolerated at the lower doses used for prophylaxis against MAC infections, although serious side effects such as uveitis have been reported.

Adverse effects associated with the use of drugs for the treatment mycobacterial diseases are summarized in the Clinical Problems Box.

NEW DEVELOPMENTS

Human TB is a major global health problem. In 2014, the WHO set a goal of reducing mortality by 95% of active TB by 2035. However, current TB control strategies will not be sufficient to reach this goal without the development of novel vaccines that can prevent TB infection and progression to TB disease. The only available vaccine is *Mycobacterium bovis* bacillus Calmette-Guerin (BCG) vaccine, which is a live attenuated strain of *M. bovis*. Although this vaccine provides some protection against severe TB in children when administered at birth, its efficacy for protection against pulmonary TB in adults is variable (0%–80%). Thus the development of new vaccine strategies against human TB remains a global health priority. There are some TB vaccine candidates (e.g., *Mycobacterium vaccae*), which have completed phase III clinical trials, and several candidates in the clinical development pipeline. Further research is needed to understand the nature of the immune response required for protection against infection with TB and progression to disease.

In addition to developing new vaccines, there is a critical need for new anti-TB drugs to shorten the length of therapy for drug-susceptible disease; improve treatment options and outcomes for patients with MDR-TB, which is a serious global problem; and provide more effective and shorter regimens for the treatment of LTBI. There are several promising drugs against TB in both preclinical and clinical trials, including bedaquiline that inhibits ATP synthase, new inhibitors of mycolic acid such as delamanid, and small, cationic, amphipathic antimicrobial peptides that are part of the innate immune system.

Leprosy remains one of the leading causes of physical disability from an infectious disease, and despite almost 30 years of effective multidrug treatment, the prevalence and incidence of leprosy have not changed significantly since 2005. Effective chemoprophylaxis would be welcome for high-risk contacts, but the use of rifampin and dapsone has unfortunately been unsuccessful. The only prophylactic measure with any degree of success has been vaccination with BCG, with one dose conferring approximately 50% protection. An effective vaccine would be highly desirable.

A clear understanding of the pathogenesis and physiology of *M. leprae* is still lacking. Further research is needed in the areas of diagnosis, as well as treatment and prevention. New drug discovery is needed due to the threat of drug resistance. The sequencing of the genome of *M. leprae* was one of the most exciting scientific achievements that can help to better understand transmission and enhance the development of vaccines and potentially eliminate leprosy in the future.

CLINICAL RELEVANCE FOR HEALTHCARE PROFESSIONALS

A major concern for all healthcare providers dealing with patients with a mycobacterial infection is protection of the provider from the infection. Thorough handwashing and sterilization of any instruments used are essential. Furthermore, since these diseases are treated using a multidrug therapeutic approach, it will be important for healthcare providers to know the scope of therapeutic agents that the patient is taking to reduce the potential for drug-drug interactions. In addition, mycobacterial infections are often present in patients with reduced immunity, which may involve the use of several other types of medications.

SELF-ASSESSMENT QUESTIONS

1. A 24-year-old patient receiving combination therapy for the treatment of tuberculosis becomes pregnant, although she has been using oral contraceptives. Which of one the following drugs is responsible for interfering with the action of the oral contraceptives, resulting in medication failure?
   A. Ethambutol.
   B. Isoniazid.
   C. Pyrazinamide.
   D. Rifampin.
   E. Streptomycin.
2. A patient is newly diagnosed with active tuberculosis. Which one of the following drug combinations should be initiated in this patient?
   A. Amikacin, isoniazid, pyrazinamide, streptomycin.
   B. Ciprofloxacin, cycloserine, isoniazid, ethionamide.
   C. Ethambutol, isoniazid, rifabutin, moxifloxacin.
   D. Ethambutol, pyrazinamide, rifampin, streptomycin.
   E. Isoniazid, rifampin, pyrazinamide, ethambutol.
3. A 58-year-old woman is being treated for leprosy. She becomes severely anemic during treatment, and her drug regimen is changed. Which one of the following drugs was she initially taking that led to her anemia?
   A. Ciprofloxacin.
   B. Clofazimine.
   C. Dapsone.
   D. Ethionamide.
   E. Rifampin.
4. Mycolic acids are major components of mycobacterial cell walls. Which of the following drugs inhibits the synthesis of mycolic acids?
   A. Clofazimine.
   B. Ethambutol.
   C. Ethionamide.
   D. Isoniazid.
   E. Rifampin.

FURTHER READING

Fogel N. Tuberculosis: a disease without boundaries. *Tuberculosis*. 2015;95(5): 527–531.

Johnson MM, Odell JA. Nontuberculous mycobacterial pulmonary infections. *J Thorac Dis*. 2014;6:210–220.

Neurmberger E, Grassert J. Pharmacokinetics and pharmacodynamic issues in the treatment of mycobacterial infections. *Eur J Clin Microbiol Infect Dis*. 2004;23:243–255.

Rodrigues LC, Lockwood DNJ. Leprosy now: epidemiology, progress, challenges, and research gaps. *Lancet Infect Dis*. 2011;11:464–470.

WEBSITES

http://www.cdc.gov/tb/pubs/mmwr/maj_guide.htm
This website is maintained by the United States Centers for Disease Control and Prevention and is an excellent source for tuberculosis information, including guidelines.

https://www.cdc.gov/tb/publications/guidelines/tb_hiv_drugs/default.htm
This page is maintained by the United States Centers for Disease Control and Prevention and contains information on managing drug interactions in the treatment of HIV-related tuberculosis.

http://apps.who.int/medicinedocs/en/d/Jh2988e/5.html
This site is maintained by the World Health Organization and provides information on drug treatment for leprosy.

http://www.who.int/tb/publications/global_report/en/
This site is maintained by the World Health Organization and provides information on tuberculosis.

Drugs Targeting Resistant Organisms

Rukiyah Van Dross-Anderson and Ahmed E.M. Elhassanny

MAJOR DRUG CLASSES

Drugs for multidrug-resistant gram-positive bacteria
Drugs for multidrug-resistant gram-negative bacteria

ABBREVIATIONS

CA-MRSA	Community-acquired methicillin-resistant *Staphylococcus aureus*
CDC	Centers for Disease Control and Prevention
CRA	Carbapenem-resistant *Acinetobacter*
CRE	Carbapenem-resistant *Enterobacteriaceae*
HA-MRSA	Hospital-acquired methicillin-resistant *Staphylococcus aureus*
LPS	Lipopolysaccharide
MDR	Multidrug resistant
MIC	Minimum inhibitory concentration
MRSA	Methicillin-resistant *Staphylococcus aureus*
PBPs	Penicillin-binding proteins
VISA	Vancomycin-intermediate *Staphylococcus aureus*
VRSA	Vancomycin-resistant *Staphylococcus aureus*
VRE	Vancomycin-resistant enterococci

THERAPEUTIC OVERVIEW

Antibiotic resistance is one of the biggest threats to global health today. Infections caused by multidrug-resistant (MDR) organisms lead to higher medical costs, prolonged hospital stays, and increased morbidity and mortality. In the United States, at least 2 million people become infected annually with bacteria that are resistant to antibiotics, which causes at least 23,000 deaths and costs over $20 billion every year. Moreover, it is estimated that by 2050, antibiotic resistance will cause approximately 10 million deaths per year unless alternative treatments are identified. Clinically important MDR gram-positive and gram-negative bacteria and the antimicrobial agents commonly used to treat infections caused by these bacteria are presented in the Therapeutic Overview Box.

THERAPEUTIC OVERVIEW

Gram-Positive Bacteria

Methicillin-resistant *S. aureus* (MRSA) is a major concern. Approved treatments include clindamycin, trimethoprim/sulfamethoxazole, doxycycline, minocycline, vancomycin, linezolid, daptomycin, telavancin, and tigecycline.

Vancomycin intermediate and resistant *S. aureus* (VISA and VRSA) are increasing in presence. Treatment includes daptomycin, quinupristin/dalfopristin, linezolid, telavancin, tigecycline, or ceftaroline.

Vancomycin-resistant enterococci (VRE) are developing worldwide. Treatment includes daptomycin, linezolid, quinupristin/dalfopristin, and tigecycline.

Gram-Negative Bacteria

Neisseria gonorrhoeae has developed resistance to almost all agents used to treat the infection, which is the second leading sexually transmitted bacterial infection. Treatment includes ceftriaxone with or without azithromycin or doxycycline.

Carbapenem-resistant *Enterobacteriaceae* has increased significantly and poses substantial clinical challenges, as there is no defined treatment.

Pseudomonas aeruginosa–resistant organisms are found in patients with cystic fibrosis and in immunocompromised patients. Treatments utilize a wide variety of antimicrobial drugs from nearly all classes.

Acinetobacter species that are resistant to the carbapenems pose a concern for patients who are critically ill and maintained on a ventilator. Treatment includes colistin, polymyxin B, tigecycline, or minocycline. Long-term treatment is needed, usually with multidrug therapy.

MULTIDRUG-RESISTANT GRAM-POSITIVE BACTERIA

The common gram-positive organisms that develop drug resistance, resistance mechanisms, and drug treatment options are listed in Box 61.1.

Methicillin-Resistant *Staphylococcus aureus* (MRSA)

S. aureus, a gram-positive coccus, is one of the most common pathogens that cause nosocomial infections. This bacterium has developed resistance to different classes of antibiotics using a variety of mechanisms. Although methicillin is no longer used in clinical practice, methicillin resistance is still used as a marker of staphylococcal resistance to β-lactams. Many strains of *S. aureus* are now resistant to methicillin, as well as agents belonging to the methicillin subclass (oxacillin, cloxacillin, dicloxacillin, and nafcillin), cefazolin, and all other β-lactams except for fifth-generation cephalosporins (Chapter 57).

Hospital-acquired MRSA (HA-MRSA) causes invasive disease, especially in immunocompromised individuals, including pneumonia, endocarditis, deep wound infections, and/or osteomyelitis. Although the incidence of HA-MRSA is geographically diverse, most hospitals in the United States report MRSA rates of 5% to 25%, but outbreaks are increasing, and resistance rates over 50% have been reported in other countries. MRSA has also become an established community-based pathogen. Since the late 1990s, community-acquired MRSA (CA-MRSA) has spread across the United States and Europe. Numerous outbreaks of CA-MRSA infections have been reported throughout the world. CA-MRSA most commonly causes pyogenic skin and soft tissue infections, necrotizing fasciitis, necrotizing pneumonia, and bacteremia.

BOX 61.1 Common Multidrug-Resistant Gram-Positive Bacteria

Methicillin-Resistant *Staphylococcus aureus* (MRSA)

Resistance to methicillin in *S. aureus* results from the altered peptidoglycan transpeptidase (also known as penicillin-binding protein 2a) that has low affinity for all β-lactams, including penicillins, cephalosporins (except for fifth-generation compounds), and carbapenems.

Hospital-associated MRSA (HA-MRSA) causes invasive disease in immuno-compromised individuals.

Community-acquired MRSA (CA-MRSA) strains have spread across the United States and Europe.

Antibiotic options for treating MRSA infections include clindamycin, trimethoprim/sulfamethoxazole, tetracyclines (doxycycline or minocycline), vancomycin, linezolid, daptomycin, telavancin, and tigecycline. Mupirocin is used for nasal decolonization in patients with recurrent infections.

Vancomycin-Intermediate *S. aureus* (VISA)

Vancomycin-intermediate *S. aureus* (VISA) strains show reduced vancomycin susceptibility (MIC = 4–8 mcg/mL) due to a thickened cell wall with increased production of D-alanine-D-alanine residues, which are capable of binding and sequestering vancomycin.

Vancomycin-Resistant *S. aureus* (VRSA)

Vancomycin resistance in vancomycin-resistant *S. aureus* (VRSA) (MIC ≥16 mcg/mL) is due to the synthesis of altered target D-alanine-D-lactate instead of the normal target D-alanine-D-alanine.

Antimicrobial regimen for *S. aureus* strains that show reduced susceptibility or resistance to vancomycin includes daptomycin, quinupristin/dalfopristin, linezolid, telavancin, tigecycline, or ceftaroline.

Vancomycin-Resistant Enterococci (VRE)

Vancomycin resistance in VRE is due to altered drug target (the production of D-alanine-D-lactate instead of the normal D-alanine-D-alanine).

Treatment options for VRE include daptomycin, linezolid, quinupristin/dalfopristin, and tigecycline.

Mechanism of Resistance

Resistance to methicillin in *S. aureus* results from the acquisition of the *mecA* gene, often located in a large DNA fragment designated staphylococcal chromosomal cassette *mec (SCCmec)*. The *mecA* gene encodes an altered peptidoglycan transpeptidase (also known as penicillin-binding protein 2a [PBP2a]) that has low affinity for all β-lactams, including penicillins, cephalosporins (except for fifth-generation compounds), and carbapenems.

Treatment

The Centers for Disease Control and Prevention (CDC) supports the guidelines published by the Infectious Diseases Society of America (IDSA) in 2011, which recommended treatment with clindamycin, trimethoprim/sulfamethoxazole (TMP/SMX), tetracyclines (doxycycline or minocycline), vancomycin, linezolid, daptomycin, telavancin, or tigecycline. Mupirocin is used for nasal decolonization in patients with recurrent infections.

Vancomycin-Intermediate *Staphylococcus aureus* (VISA) and Vancomycin-Resistant *Staphylococcus aureus* (VRSA)

Vancomycin-intermediate *S. aureus* (VISA) strains show reduced vancomycin susceptibility (minimum inhibitory concentration [MIC] = 4–8 mcg/mL). Several VISA strains associated with clinical infection have been described. The first reported case was observed in Japan in 1997. Subsequently, clinical infections with similar strains have been reported in the United States and worldwide.

VRSA strains (MIC ≥16 mcg/mL) have also emerged worldwide. In the United States, a small number of cases have been identified. Sporadic cases have been reported elsewhere.

Mechanism of Resistance

The reduced vancomycin susceptibility in VISA strains is due to altered cell wall metabolism that results in a thickened cell wall with increased production of D-alanine-D-alanine residues, which are capable of binding vancomycin. Thus vancomycin is sequestered within the cell wall by these targets and cannot reach its site of action. The genetic basis for these cell wall alterations is not fully understood, but studies have identified mutations in several genes, including *vraR*, *graRS*, and *walRK*, that seem to contribute to the development of resistance.

Heteroresistant (hVISA) refers to VISA strains that contain subpopulations of bacteria with vancomycin MICs in the intermediate range, but the vancomycin MIC for the entire population remains within the susceptible range. Similar to VISA, hVISA strains resist vancomycin due to an unusually thickened cell wall. There are several reports of vancomycin failure and persistent infection due to hVISA. The basis of such clinical vancomycin failure is still not fully understood.

Resistance in VRSA is conferred by acquisition of a plasmid carrying the *vanA* gene cluster from vancomycin-resistant enterococci (via transposon Tn1546). The *vanA* gene cluster encodes enzymes, which catalyze the synthesis of the D-alanine-D-lactate terminal peptide instead of the normal D-alanine-D-alanine. Vancomycin binds D-alanine-D-lactate with a much lower affinity than the normal peptide.

Treatment

Antimicrobial regimens for *S. aureus* strains with reduced susceptibility or resistance to vancomycin include daptomycin, quinupristin/dalfopristin, linezolid, telavancin, tigecycline, or ceftaroline. These may be given as a single agent or in combination with other antibiotics.

Vancomycin-Resistant Enterococci (VRE)

Enterococci are gram-positive cocci, which are part of the resident intestinal flora. They are the second most common cause of nosocomial infection (after staphylococci). Enterococci cause urinary tract infections, bacteremia related to intravascular catheters, bacterial endocarditis, meningitis, and soft tissue infections. *Enterococcus faecalis* and *Enterococcus faecium* are two predominant enterococci causing nosocomial infections. *Enterococci* are inherently resistant to a variety of commonly used antibiotics. VRE were first described in Europe in the late 1980s and, subsequently, rapidly spread worldwide, including to the United States, where more than 80% of *E. faecium* isolates are VRE, while only 7% of *E. faecalis* isolates are resistant to vancomycin.

Mechanism of Resistance

Resistance to vancomycin by enterococci is due to the acquisition of a set of *van* genes, which code for a biochemical machinery that remodels the synthesis of peptidoglycan through the production of D-alanine-D-lactate instead of the normal D-alanine-D-alanine at the end of the pentapeptide moiety of the nascent peptidoglycan precursors, and the destruction of the normal D-alanine-D-alanine precursors to prevent vancomycin from binding to the cell wall precursors. Vancomycin binds D-alanine-D-lactate with a much lower affinity (about 1000-fold) than D-alanine-D-alanine.

Treatment

Treatment options for VRE include daptomycin, linezolid, quinupristin/dalfopristin, and tigecycline.

MULTIDRUG-RESISTANT GRAM-NEGATIVE BACTERIA

The common gram-negative organisms that develop drug resistance, resistance mechanisms, and drug treatment options are listed in Box 61.2.

Resistance of *Neisseria gonorrhoeae*

N. gonorrhoeae (also known as gonococci) is a gram-negative diplococci bacterium that causes the second most commonly reported sexually transmitted bacterial infection in the United States after *Chlamydia trachomatis*. In 2013, about 100 cases of *N. gonorrhoeae* per 100,000 persons were reported in the United States, representing approximately an 8% increase in incidence from 2009. *N. gonorrhoeae* has a remarkable capacity to alter its antigenic structures and adapt to changes in the microenvironment. The major surface structures that undergo antigenic variations include pili, opacity-associated proteins (Opa), and lipooligosaccharides.

BOX 61.2   Common Multidrug-Resistant Gram-Negative Bacteria

Neisseria gonorrhoeae

Gram-negative cocci that has a remarkable capacity to alter its antigenic structures and adapt to changes in the microenvironment.

Mechanisms of antibiotic resistance include enzymatic inactivation of the antibiotics, alteration of antimicrobial targets, increase in drug export (through efflux pumps), and decreased uptake (through porin modifications) of the antibiotics.

A single dose of the third-generation cephalosporin ceftriaxone is the first-line therapy for uncomplicated gonococcal infections.

Initial treatment regimens must also incorporate azithromycin or doxycycline that are effective against coinfection with *C. trachomatis*.

Alternative treatment for gonococcal infections include cefixime, ceftizoxime, cefotaxime, spectinomycin.

Carbapenem-Resistant Enterobacteriaceae (CRE)

CRE are resistant to most β-lactam antibiotics, including "last-line" carbapenems.

They are responsible for serious infections (such as intraabdominal infections, pneumonia, urinary tract infections, and device-associated infections).

Carbapenem resistance is mediated by carbapenemase enzymes or a decrease in the uptake of antibiotics by modifications of porins in association with overexpression of β-lactamases.

CRE treatment options include polymyxins (colistin and polymyxin B), tigecycline, fosfomycin, and aminoglycosides (amikacin, gentamicin, and tobramycin).

Pseudomonas aeruginosa

Strains resistant to all classes of antipseudomonal agents except polymyxins are increasing worldwide.

Multidrug resistance is mediated by diverse mechanisms such as decreased influx due to porin alterations, enzyme-catalyzed degradation or modification of antibiotics, target site alterations, and efflux systems.

P. aeruginosa resistant to all other treatment options can be treated with polymyxins.

Carbapenem-Resistant Acinetobacter (CRA)

Acinetobacter baumannii possess a diversity of resistance mechanisms that may lead to multidrug resistance.

The most significant mechanism of carbapenem resistance in *A. baumannii* is the production of carbapenemases.

Treatment of CRE includes colistin, polymyxin B, tigecycline, and minocycline.

Mechanisms of Resistance

N. gonorrhoeae has developed resistance to almost all antimicrobial agents introduced for gonorrhea treatment. This bacterium has utilized all known mechanisms of antibiotic resistance, including enzymatic inactivation, alteration of antimicrobial targets, increased export (through efflux pumps), and decreased uptake (through porin modifications) of the antibiotics.

The most common mechanism of resistance to the penicillins is chromosomally mediated mutations of the *penA* and *ponA* genes that encode for PBP2 and PBP1, respectively, which decrease the affinity of these proteins for penicillin. The plasmid-located bla_{TEM-1} gene coding for a TEM-1-type β-lactamase that hydrolyzes the β-lactam ring is another mechanism of penicillin resistance that is disseminated worldwide. Furthermore, penicillin resistance can arise from specific mutations, resulting in overexpression of the MtrCDE efflux pump system, which exports the penicillin out of the cell and, less commonly, from mutations of the outer membrane channel porin PorB1b, resulting in a decreased influx of penicillin.

Resistance to the macrolides by *N. gonorrhoeae* is conferred by mutations in the 23S ribosomal subunit and by modification of this subunit by RNA methylase encoded by *erm* genes, which block macrolide binding to the 23S subunit. Resistance to fluoroquinolones is mediated through plasmid-mediated mutations of *gyrA* and/or *parC*, which reduce binding affinity to DNA gyrase and topoisomerase IV. Tetracycline resistance is mediated by the plasmid-borne *tetM* gene, whose product binds to bacterial ribosomes and subsequently causes release of the tetracycline molecule. Additionally, alterations in target structures, overexpression of efflux pumps, and decreased influx can contribute to the tetracycline resistance in gonococci. Resistance to the cephalosporins, ceftriaxone and cefixime, occurs as a result of mutations in *penA* gene encoding PBP2, which decreases the affinity to PBPs. In addition, increased efflux and decreased influx of these antibiotics also play a role in the development of resistance.

Treatment

Currently, a single dose of the cephalosporin ceftriaxone (Chapter 57) is the first-line therapy for uncomplicated gonococcal infections. Coinfection with *C. trachomatis* occurs frequently with gonococcal infections, and thus initial treatment regimens must also incorporate azithromycin or doxycycline, which are effective against chlamydial infection. Alternative treatments include cefixime, ceftizoxime, cefotaxime, and spectinomycin. Although third-generation cephalosporins have remained highly effective against gonococcal infections, the recent isolation of strains highly resistant to ceftriaxone in Japan and some European countries is a major concern.

Carbapenem-Resistant Enterobacteriaceae (CRE)

Enterobacteriaceae are gram-negative bacilli that are normal inhabitants of the intestinal tract. They are the most common cause of both community- and hospital-acquired infections of the urinary tract, bloodstream, and/or lower respiratory tract infections. *Escherichia coli* and *Klebsiella* species are members of Enterobacteriaceae and represent the most important pathogens for humans. Enterobacteriaceae have a natural tendency to acquire genetic material through horizontal gene transfer mediated by plasmids and transposons. The recent emergence of CRE is a major concern for clinical therapy. CRE are resistant to most β-lactam antibiotics, including "last-line" carbapenems. The prevalence of CRE infections has increased significantly over the past decade, especially in healthcare settings. They are responsible for serious infections, such as intra-abdominal infections, pneumonia, urinary tract infections, and device-associated infections. According to the CDC, more than 9000 healthcare-associated infections are caused by carbapenem-resistant *Klebsiella* and *Escherichia* species. Infections caused by CRE are of major concern because they are associated with high mortality rates, which range from 18% to 48%.

Mechanisms of Resistance

Carbapenem resistance develops from acquisition of genes encoding for carbapenemases, enzymes capable of degrading carbapenems. The most important carbapenemases are the KPC-type enzymes first reported in the United States, but now found worldwide; the metallo-β-lactamases (VIM, IMP, and NDM); and the OXA-48–type enzymes. Additionally, resistance to carbapenems in Enterobacteriaceae can arise from a decrease in the uptake of antibiotics by modifications of porins in association with overexpression of β-lactamases that possess very weak affinity for carbapenems. For example, a combination of plasmid-encoded AmpC (a cephalosporinase) expression together with decreased cell membrane permeability due to modifications of porins contributes to carbapenem resistance in *Klebsiella pneumoniae*, *E. coli*, and *Salmonella typhimurium*. Similarly, production of extended-spectrum β-lactamases (ESBLs) (e.g., plasmid-located bla_{TEM}, bla_{SHV}, and bla_{CTX-M}), in combination with outer membrane permeability defects, is responsible for carbapenem resistance in some members of the Enterobacteriaceae.

Treatment

Despite being a major health concern, the optimal treatment for CRE infections is still unknown because there are no published data from randomized controlled trials assessing antimicrobial treatment options. Therefore much of the existing evidence is limited to reviews of case reports and small retrospective studies. Potential CRE treatment options include the polymyxins (colistin and polymyxin B), tigecycline, fosfomycin, and aminoglycosides (amikacin, gentamicin, and tobramycin). In addition, case reports have shown that dual-carbapenem combination treatment may be an effective option for infections caused by CRE.

Resistance of *Pseudomonas aeruginosa*

P. aeruginosa is a rod-shaped, gram-negative bacterium found in many environments including soil, plants, vegetables, tap water, and countertops. The ubiquity of *P. aeruginosa* is due to its simple nutritional needs. Importantly, it causes significant bloodstream, urinary tract, pulmonary, and device-related infections in hospitalized patients and in patients with cystic fibrosis. It is frequently isolated from immunocompromised hospitalized patients in the intensive care unit.

Mechanisms of Resistance

P. aeruginosa was one of the first pathogens to develop resistance to multiple antibiotics. Strains resistant to all classes of antipseudomonal agents except polymyxins have emerged and are increasing worldwide. *P. aeruginosa* utilize a diversity of resistance mechanisms that lead to multidrug resistance. *P. aeruginosa* can develop carbapenem resistance by several mechanisms, which include porin alterations, PBP modifications, enzyme production, and efflux pumps, with porin changes the most common cause of resistance. Mutation of the *oprD* gene and subsequent loss of its encoded porin is the most common cause of imipenem resistance in *P. aeruginosa*. Resistance to meropenem or doripenem requires this porin change combined with overexpression of AmpC, β-lactamase, or efflux pump overexpression. Up regulation of the MexAB-OprM efflux system may confer resistance to meropenem in addition to fluoroquinolones, penicillins, and cephalosporins. Carbapenem resistance in *P. aeruginosa* can also be mediated by metallo-β-lactamases (e.g., the IMP, VIM, and NDM-1 types), which are the predominant group of carbapenemases found in *P. aeruginosa*. The genes encoding these enzymes are normally encoded in class 1 integrons,

which are usually associated with a plasmid or a transposon, thus allowing transfer between bacteria.

P. aeruginosa developed a high level of resistance to aminoglycosides (such as amikacin, gentamicin, and tobramycin), which is mediated by the 16S rRNA methylases that interfere with the binding of these antibiotics to their site of action. The genes encoding these enzymes are usually associated with mobile genetic elements (transposons and plasmids) that enhance their horizontal spread. High-level resistance to fluoroquinolones in *P. aeruginosa* is conferred by mutational changes in the fluoroquinolone targets DNA gyrase (*gyrA* and *gyrB*) and/or topoisomerase IV (*parC* and *parE*). Overexpression of multidrug efflux pumps (e.g., MexAB-OprM RND-type system) is another common mechanism of resistance to fluoroquinolones (in addition to chloramphenicol, tetracyclines, and β-lactams) in *P. aeruginosa*. The emergence of colistin-resistant *P. aeruginosa* isolates has been reported worldwide, which is associated with modifications of the lipid A component of lipopolysaccharides.

Treatment

Antibiotic options for the treatment of resistant *P. aeruginosa* infections include piperacillin/tazobactam, cefepime or ceftazidime, aztreonam, carbapenems (e.g., imipenem, doripenem, meropenem), fluoroquinolones (ciprofloxacin, levofloxacin), and/or aminoglycosides (gentamicin, tobramycin, amikacin). When *P. aeruginosa* develops resistance to all other treatment options, the polymyxins (e.g., colistin and polymyxin B) have been used. Despite their high rate of associated nephrotoxicity and neurotoxicity, the lack of a well-defined optimal dosing regimen for colistin, and a paucity of clinical experience with polymyxin B, this class of antibiotics is considered the last resort to treat MDR gram-negative bacteria, including *P. aeruginosa*, because they have a good activity against these resistant bacteria.

Resistance of *Acinetobacter*

Acinetobacter species are gram-negative bacilli. *Acinetobacter baumannii* is a particularly major concern because of its tendency to acquire antibiotic resistance genes. Carbapenem-resistant *Acinetobacter* (CRA) strains, which are usually resistant to all the available anti-*Acinetobacter* agents except polymyxins, are an important cause of hospital-acquired infection in several countries, especially in Europe and Latin America. According to a 2013 CDC report, *Acinetobacter* was the cause of 2% of nosocomial infections, and it was responsible for about 7% of the infections in critically ill patients on mechanical ventilators. Additionally, 7300 out of 12,000 annual *Acinetobacter* infections were multidrug resistant, which led to about 500 annual deaths.

Mechanisms of Resistance

A. baumannii employ diverse mechanisms to produce multidrug resistance. Carbapenem resistance can develop via several molecular mechanisms, of which the most significant one is the production of intrinsic or acquired OXA-type carbapenemases. *A. baumannii* naturally produces basal levels of chromosomally encoded OXA-51–group carbapenemase. However, acquisition of a stronger promoter by transposition of an insertion sequence, upstream of the *OXA-51* group gene, results in overexpression of this gene and consequently high-level carbapenem resistance. Recently, resistance to carbapenem in *A. baumannii* has been shown to be mediated by certain acquired metallo-β-lactamases (e.g., NDM-1), which have carbapenem-hydrolyzing activity. The majority of *A. baumannii* clinical isolates are also resistant to cephalosporins, including third- and fourth-generation agents, which is mediated by the production of AmpC β-lactamase and ESBLs.

A. baumannii develops resistance to aminoglycosides through the production of various aminoglycoside-modifying enzymes and the production of 16S ribosomal RNA methyltransferase. The *Acinetobacter* ArmA enzyme methylates the aminoglycoside-binding site (A-site) of 16S rRNA, protecting it from aminoglycosides, leading to high-level resistance to gentamicin, tobramycin, and amikacin. The primary mechanism of high-level resistance to fluoroquinolones is mutation of genes encoding DNA gyrase and topoisomerase IV, which are the targets of these antibiotics. Moderate levels of fluoroquinolone resistance in *A. baumannii* are mediated by the overexpression of active efflux pumps, such as the RND efflux system encoded by the *adeABC* operon.

Acinetobacter has also developed resistance to polymyxins by two mechanisms—namely, mutations causing alterations in lipid A (a component of lipopolysaccharide polymyxin target) by addition of phosphoethanolamine and mutations in the genes encoding the enzymes that catalyze the first steps in lipopolysaccharide biosynthesis. These mutations are associated with decreased fitness and impaired virulence, which is why the resistance to polymyxins among CRA has remained uncommon. Finally, resistance of *A. baumannii* to tigecycline has been reported by several groups and might be due to up regulation of the multidrug efflux pumps AdeABC and AdeIJK.

Treatment

Treatment of MDR *A. baumannii* includes colistin, polymyxin B, tigecycline, and minocycline. The role of combination therapy in the treatment of highly drug-resistant *A. baumannii* remains unclear.

NEW DEVELOPMENTS

The development of agents that can be used to manage carbapenem-resistant infections is a high priority, according to the WHO. The development of resistance to vancomycin by enterococci and staphylococci is also considered a high priority because vancomycin was the drug of choice for MRSA and is now finding resistant strains. Teixobactin is a novel antibiotic isolated from soil that is effective against a large number of resistant microorganisms, including *S. aureus* and *M. tuberculosis*. The drug binds to lipid II (the molecular target for vancomycin) and lipid III, which are important precursors for the synthesis of the cell wall. Teixobactin could change the landscape for the treatment of resistant microorganisms from a variety of standpoints. First, because of the unique mechanism of teixobactin, it may take 30 years for the development of resistant organisms. Second, the isolation and identification of teixobactin was made possible through the development of methods to grow organisms that were previously uncultured. Soil contains a plethora of bacteria that until now were not successfully cultured; thus there is anticipation that many novel antimicrobial agents may be developed in the future using this technology.

CLINICAL RELEVANCE FOR HEALTHCARE PROFESSIONALS

The treatment of infections produced by resistant organisms provides a significant challenge to healthcare professionals. Many of the issues described for healthcare professionals with respect to other types of antimicrobial agents applies to those agents used for resistant organisms. Healthcare providers need to be aware of the serious adverse effects of antimicrobial agents in addition to being extremely cautious regarding their own personal hygiene to prevent contracting the infection. Since many of these infections develop in soft tissues, it will be especially important for providers to monitor contact very closely and be certain to wear protective gear to reduce the possibility of inadvertent contact. It is also important to understand the other drugs patients may be taking to reduce the potential for drug-drug interactions.

SELF-ASSESSMENT QUESTIONS

1. Antibiotic options for treating MRSA infections include all of the following except:
   A. Vancomycin.
   B. Clindamycin.
   C. Daptomycin.
   D. Polymyxins.
   E. Trimethoprim/sulfamethoxazole.
2. Initial treatment regimens for uncomplicated gonococcal infections include:
   A. Vancomycin.
   B. Azithromycin or doxycycline.
   C. Cefotaxime.
   D. Ceftriaxone.
   E. B and D.
3. The resistance of VRSA and VRE strains to antimicrobials is due to:
   A. Thickening of the peptidoglycan layer.
   B. Alterations in the D-alanine-D-alanine drug target.
   C. Plasmid-encoded β-lactamases.
   D. Enzyme-catalyzed phosphorylation, adenylation, or acetylation.
   E. Alterations in the penicillin-binding protein.

4. Infections caused by CRE are of major concern because:
   A. They are resistant to most β-lactam antibiotics.
   B. The optimal treatment is unknown.
   C. They are associated with high mortality rates.
   D. Their prevalence has increased significantly over the past decade.
   E. All of the above
5. A last resort treatment for *P. aeruginosa* resistant to all other treatment options is the:
   A. Penicillins.
   B. Carbapenems.
   C. Polymyxins.
   D. Monobactams.
   E. Amphenicols.

FURTHER READING

Doi Yohei, Murray Gerald L., Peleg Anton Y. *"Acinetobacter baumannii: Evolution of Antimicrobial Resistance—Treatment Options."* Seminars in respiratory and critical care medicine. Vol. 36. No. 01. Thieme Medical Publishers; 2015.

Iredell Jon, Brown Jeremy, Tagg Kaitlin. Antibiotic resistance in *Enterobacteriaceae*: mechanisms and clinical implications. *BMJ.* 2016;352:h6420.

Karaiskos Ilias, Giamarellou Helen. Multidrug-resistant and extensively drug-resistant Gram-negative pathogens: current and emerging therapeutic approaches. *Expert Opin Pharmacother.* 2014;15(10): 1351–1370.

Lin Ming-Feng, Lan Chung-Yu. Antimicrobial Resistance in *Acinetobacter Baumannii*: From Bench to Bedside. *World J Clin Cases. WJCC2.12,* 2014;787–814. *PMC.* Web. 13 Sept. 2016.

Liu Catherine, et al. Clinical practice guidelines by the Infectious Diseases Society of America for the treatment of methicillin-resistant *Staphylococcus aureus* infections in adults and children. *Clin Infect Dis.* 2011;52(3):e18–e55.

Miller William R., et al. Vancomycin-Resistant Enterococci: Therapeutic Challenges in the 21st Century. *Infect Dis Clin North Am.* 2016;30(2): 415–439.

Nagel Jerod L., et al. Antimicrobial Stewardship for the Infection Control Practitioner. *Infect Dis Clin North Am.* 2016;30(3):771–784.

Oliver Antonio, et al. The increasing threat of *Pseudomonas aeruginosa* high-risk clones. *Drug Resist Updat.* 2015;21:41–59.

Potron Anaïs, Laurent Poirel, Patrice Nordmann. Emerging broad-spectrum resistance in Pseudomonas aeruginosa and *Acinetobacter baumannii*: mechanisms and epidemiology. *Int J Antimicrob Agents.* 2015;45(6): 568–585.

Rossolini Gian Maria, et al. Update on the antibiotic resistance crisis. *Curr Opin Pharmacol.* 2014;18:56–60.

Unemo Magnus, Shafer William M. Antimicrobial resistance in *Neisseria gonorrhoeae* in the 21st century: past, evolution, and future. *Clin Microbiol Rev.* 2014;27(3):587–613.

WEBSITES

https://www.cdc.gov/drugresistance/

This website is maintained by the Centers for Disease Control and Prevention and provides information for both clinicians and consumers about resistant microbes.

http://www.who.int/mediacentre/news/releases/2017/bacteria-antibiotics-needed/en/

This website, maintained by the World Health Organization, provides a list of bacteria for which new antibiotics are urgently needed, as well as additional links to information regarding antibiotic/antimicrobial resistance.

62

Antifungal Agents

Mona M. McConnaughey and J. Scott McConnaughey

THERAPEUTIC OVERVIEW

Fungi that cause cutaneous and subcutaneous mycoses: Treat with dermatological preparations, occasionally systemic agents
  Epidermophyton species
  Microspora species
  Sporothrix species
  Trichophyton species
Fungi that cause systemic mycoses: Difficult to treat; available drugs often cause deleterious side effects; often need long-term therapy
  Aspergillus species
  Candida species
  Blastomyces dermatitidis
  Cryptococcus neoformans
  Coccidioides immitis
  Fusarium species
  Histoplasma capsulatum
  Paracoccidioides brasiliensis
  Rhizopus and *Mucor* species

THERAPEUTIC OVERVIEW

Fungal infections are not uncommon, and evidence suggests that their incidence is increasing, affecting more than 1 billion people worldwide. These infections can manifest in a specific tissue or organ such as the skin, nails, respiratory, or urogenital or alimentary tracts or can be systemic. Anyone can acquire a fungal infection, but the aged, critically ill, and immunocompromised individuals are most susceptible to opportunistic infections, as are individuals with burns or intravascular catheters, enabling fungi to easily enter the body and bloodstream.

Fungal infections can be mild, such as skin rashes or those affecting the nails, or can be life-threatening, such as fungal pneumonia. Life-threatening infections are becoming increasingly common in the hospital setting (nosocomial), with the two predominant nosocomial infections caused by species of *Candida* and *Aspergillus*.

Major types of fungal infections and examples of prevalent causative species are summarized in the Therapeutic Overview Box.

MECHANISMS OF ACTION

Fungi are more complex than bacteria or viruses. They can be uni- or multicellular with rigid cell walls containing complex polysaccharides (glucans and chitin) and cell membranes containing the steroid ergosterol rather than cholesterol present in animal cell membranes.

The typical structure of a fungal cell and sites of action of antifungal drugs are shown in Fig. 62.1. The principal classes of antifungal drugs include the allylamines, azoles, polyenes, echinocandins, and others, and structures of representative agents from each class are shown in Fig. 62.2.

Allylamines

The allylamines, such as terbinafine and naftifine, decrease the synthesis of ergosterol by fungal cells through selective inhibition of the enzyme squalene epoxidase (also called squalene monooxygenase), which catalyzes the conversion of squalene to squalene epoxide. Inhibition of squalene epoxide synthesis has a twofold effect. It increases the intracellular accumulation of squalene, which is toxic to the cells, and it decreases membrane ergosterol, which leads to increased membrane permeability, with leakage of cellular components. Both of these actions underlie the fungicidal activity of these compounds. Although butenafine is not a true allylamine, it has the same mechanism of action as the allylamines.

Azoles

The azoles comprise the imidazoles, such as miconazole and ketoconazole, and the triazoles, such as voriconazole and fluconazole. The azoles inhibit the synthesis of ergosterol in actively growing fungi by

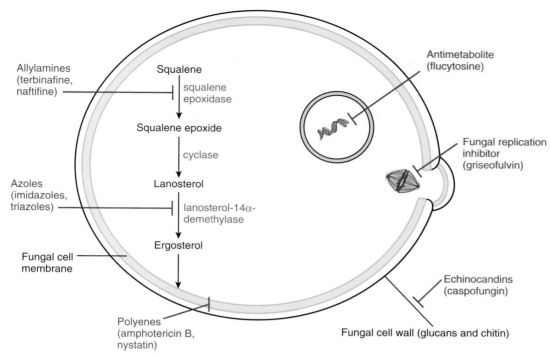

FIG. 62.1 A Fungal Cell Depicting Sites of Action of Antifungal Agents.

inhibiting the enzyme lanosterol-14α-demethylase (CYP51) that converts lanosterol to ergosterol. At high concentrations, azoles cause K^+ and other components to leak from the cell, an action that may involve inhibition of plasma membrane Na^+, K^+-ATPase. Thus the azoles are generally fungistatic but can be fungicidal, depending on concentration and fungal species. Resistance to azoles can develop as a consequence of increased azole efflux or increased production of lanosterol-14α-demethylase. A point mutation in the gene encoding for lanosterol-14α-demethylase, *ERG11*, can lead to cross-resistance to all azoles.

Polyenes

Polyenes are macrocyclic lactones containing a hydrophilic hydroxylated portion and a hydrophobic conjugated double-bond portion. The prototype polyenes are amphotericin B and nystatin. Polyenes bind to ergosterol in fungal cell membranes and form channels or pores, enabling K^+ and Mg^{++} to leak out of the cell, thus reducing viability (Fig. 62.3). Emergence of resistance to polyenes is rare but can occur with long-term use and is usually a result of the organism producing reduced amounts of membrane ergosterol. Fungi that lack ergosterol, which are rare but do exist, are not susceptible to these agents.

Amphotericin B is available as a conventional formulation complexed with deoxycholate and as three lipid-based formulations. It has been postulated that by incorporating amphotericin B into the lipid moieties, the active drug can be transferred selectively to ergosterol-containing fungal membranes without interfering with the cholesterol-containing human membranes, thereby decreasing toxicity. Amphotericin B and nystatin may be either fungistatic or fungicidal, depending on the concentration of drug that reaches the target and the fungal species.

Echinocandins

Echinocandins, such as caspofungin, micafungin, and anidulafungin, consist of large cyclic peptides linked to a long-chain fatty acid. These agents have a unique mechanism of action and disrupt the fungal cell wall rather than the cell membrane. The echinocandins inhibit β-(1,3)-D-glucan synthase, blocking the production of β-(1,3)-D-glucan, the major structural component of the fungal cell wall. These agents may be either fungistatic or fungicidal, depending on drug concentration and the fungal species. Resistance to these agents is increasing and has been shown to develop through mutations in various subunits of the target enzyme.

Others

Flucytosine is an antimetabolite with a dual mechanism of action. The drug is transported into susceptible fungi by a permease system for purines, competitively inhibiting purine and pyrimidine uptake and mediating a direct effect of the drug on the fungus. In addition, following uptake, flucytosine is deaminated by cytosine deaminase to the active form, 5-fluorouracil, which is converted by uridine monophosphate pyrophosphorylase and other enzymes to 5-fluoro-2′-deoxyuridine 5′-monophosphate, which inhibits thymidylate synthase and interferes with DNA synthesis (Chapter 68). Flucytosine can be either fungistatic or fungicidal, depending on drug concentration and fungal species. Fungi can be resistant to flucytosine if they lack a permease, have a defective cytosine deaminase, or express low levels of the uridine monophosphate pyrophosphorylase enzyme.

Griseofulvin binds to α and β tubulin comprising the fungal microtubules that form the mitotic spindles, thereby blocking polymerization and interfering with fungal mitosis. Griseofulvin is deposited in the keratin precursor cells of the skin, hair, and nails, rendering the newly formed keratin resistant to fungal invasion. As the infected keratin is shed, it is replaced by fungal-free tissue. Thus this agent is fungistatic.

Ciclopirox is a synthetic compound thought to exert its activity through chelation of trivalent metal cations including Fe^{3+} and Al^{3+}, leading to alterations in enzymatic activities that disrupt cellular metabolism, fungal membranes, DNA repair mechanisms, and mitosis, all of which contribute to its fungicidal activity. It also has antiinflammatory activity.

Tolnaftate is a topical fungicide that appears to act like the allylamines and can be either fungistatic or fungicidal.

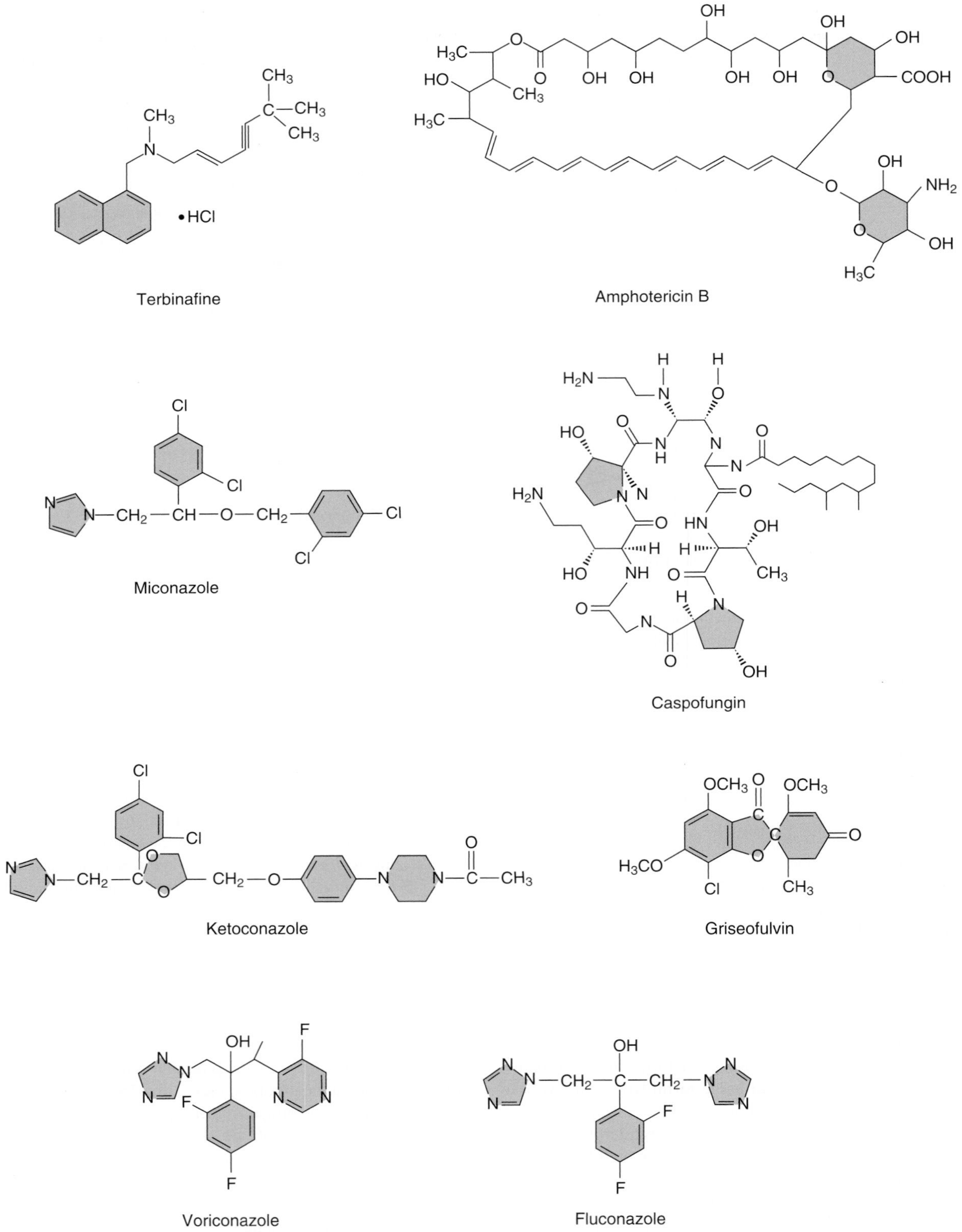

Terbinafine

Amphotericin B

Miconazole

Caspofungin

Ketoconazole

Griseofulvin

Voriconazole

Fluconazole

FIG. 62.2 Structures of Representative Antifungal Agents.

Undecylenic acid is another topical agent that is thought to interact nonspecifically with fungal cell membranes for its fungistatic action.

RELATIONSHIP OF MECHANISMS OF ACTION TO CLINICAL RESPONSE

The activity of representative antifungal agents against specific causative organisms is presented in Table 62.1.

Allylamines

The allylamines are mainly used for dermatophyte infections. Terbinafine is used both orally and topically to treat onychomycosis, a fungal infection of the nail, and "ringworm" infections, including tinea corporis, tinea cruris, tinea pedis, and tinea capitis. Treatment can last up to 6 months, depending on the type of infection. Naftifine and butenafine are also used topically for the treatment of dermatophyte infections. The potential to develop resistance to the allylamines is attributed to multidrug resistance efflux mechanisms.

Azoles

The azoles are active against a broad spectrum of fungi, including many dermatophytes, yeasts, dimorphic fungi, and some *Phycomycetes.* Ketoconazole, the oldest of the azoles, inhibits most of the common dermatophytes as well as many of the fungi that cause the systemic mycoses. Ketoconazole is effective for the treatment of cutaneous mycoses as well as oral and esophageal candidiasis in immunocompromised patients. It is less effective than fluconazole for *Candida* and has no activity against *Aspergillus* organisms or *Phycomycetes.*

Itraconazole is an effective treatment for histoplasmosis, paracoccidioidomycosis, blastomycosis, coccidioidomycosis, and sporotrichosis. It has some activity against *Cryptococcus, Pseudallescheria boydii,* and *Candida,* although other agents may be preferable for candidiasis. This agent is also frequently taken by oral administration for a prolonged period for the treatment of fungal nail infections and other dermatophytes.

Fluconazole is an effective treatment for candidiasis, blastomycosis, coccidioidomycosis, pseudallescheriasis, histoplasmosis, as well as meningitis caused by *Coccidioides immitis* or *Cryptococcus neoformans.* Fluconazole is effective for preventing serious fungal infections in select hosts, including liver transplant recipients and other immunocompromised patients. Fluconazole is a popular treatment for vaginal candidiasis and frequently is effective after one oral dose.

Voriconazole may have a higher affinity for lanosterol-14α-demethylase than other azoles, which improves activity against *Candida, Aspergillus* species, *P. boydii,* and *Fusarium.* Because data suggest synergy with other antifungal agents, voriconazole can also be used in combination with caspofungin for the treatment of severe infections with *Aspergillus fumigatus.* Voriconazole is also likely to be effective against most *Candida* isolates that are resistant to fluconazole. Its primary use is to treat invasive aspergillosis.

Posaconazole is useful for the treatment of serious fungal infections, including aspergillosis, candidiasis, and zygomycosis. This agent is also effective for infections caused by *Scedosporium apiospermum* or *Fusarium* species in patients who do not respond to other treatments.

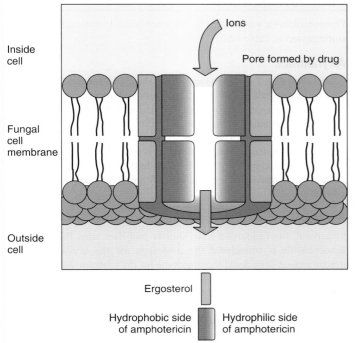

FIG. 62.3 Action of Polyenes to Form Pores in the Fungal Cell Membrane Through Which K$^+$ and Mg^{++} Can Leak Out of the Cell.

TABLE 62.1	Activity of Various Antifungal Agents											
Agent	*Aspergillus* species	*Blastomyces dermatitidis*	*Candida albicans*	*Candida,* other species	*Fonsecaea* species, *Phialophora verrucosa, Cladosporium carrionii*	*Cryptococcus neoformans*	*Coccidioides immitis*	*Fusarium* species	*Histoplasma capsulatum*	*Rhizopus* species, *mucor* species, and others	*Paracoccidioides brasiliensis*	*Pseudallescheria* species	*Sporothrix* species
Ketoconazole	−	+	+	±	−	+	+	±	+	−	+	−	+
Itraconazole	+	+	+	±	+	+	+	±	+	−	+	−	+
Fluconazole	−	+	+	±	−	+	+	±	+	−	+	−	+
Voriconazole	+	+	+	+	−	+	+	+	+	−	+	+	±
Amphotericin B	+	+	+	+	−	+	+	±	+	+	+	−	+
Caspofungin	+	±	+	+	−	−	−	−	±	−	±	−	−
Flucytosine	±	−	+	+	+	+	−	−	−	−	−	−	−

Isavuconazonium is used primarily to treat aspergillosis and invasive mucormycosis. Patients who benefit the most are those who are immunocompromised and those at high risk for developing aspergillosis.

Miconazole and the other topical azoles have activity similar to that of ketoconazole, but miconazole also inhibits *P. boydii*, the only systemic infection for which intravenous (IV) miconazole may be appropriate. Miconazole is used topically primarily for vulvovaginal candidiasis. It is comparable to the other azoles in the management of cutaneous candidiasis, ringworm, and tinea versicolor.

Polyenes

The polyenes are broad-spectrum antifungal agents. **Amphotericin B** is important for most life-threatening mycoses, although newer, less toxic antifungals are frequently preferred. For serious systemic fungal infections, amphotericin B is still a drug of choice for induction therapy, with a systemic azole given for chronic therapy or prevention of relapse. Prolonged treatment of systemic fungal infections with amphotericin B may last up to 3 or 4 months. A variety of organisms are susceptible to amphotericin B. In addition to those listed in Table 62.1, these include *Rhodotorula*, *Leishmania braziliensis*, *Leishmania mexicana*, and *Pneumocystis jirovecii*. Resistance is rare but has been seen in *P. boydii*, *Trichosporon*, *Aspergillus terreus*, *Fusarium*, and *Candida lusitaniae*.

Disseminated cryptococcal infections, including meningitis, can be treated with either amphotericin B alone or in combination with flucytosine. Amphotericin B acts synergistically with flucytosine against *Candida* organisms and *C. neoformans*. Synergy of amphotericin B with other agents, such as rifampin and tetracyclines, can be demonstrated in vitro, but clinical studies to support this observation are lacking. Severe cases involving *Histoplasma capsulatum*, *Blastomyces dermatitidis*, and *C. immitis* can be treated with amphotericin B. This agent is also a drug of choice for *Zygomycetes* infections.

It is unclear whether lipid formulations of amphotericin B result in improved activity against fungal pathogens as compared to deoxycholate amphotericin B. Limited clinical data suggest that lipid formulations may show improved efficacy for select fungi, including *H. capsulatum*, *C. neoformans,* and *A. fumigatus*. In addition, the lipid formulations may be superior in certain clinical scenarios, including fungal infections of the central nervous system and those occurring in patients with a low neutrophil count.

Nystatin has a spectrum of activity similar to that of amphotericin B but is too toxic for parenteral administration and is only used topically to treat *Candida* infections of the skin and mucous membranes. It is effective for oral and vaginal candidiasis and *Candida* esophagitis.

Echinocandins

The echinocandins have a narrow antifungal spectrum. **Caspofungin** inhibits *Candida* and *Aspergillus* species and exhibits dose-dependent fungicidal activity, although the drug is fungistatic for *Aspergillus* species. Caspofungin is indicated for the treatment of serious *Candida* infections, particularly those involving azole-resistant *Candida*. It can be used for patients with invasive aspergillosis who are unresponsive to other agents. Caspofungin has also been used in combination with voriconazole or amphotericin B for the treatment of severe *Aspergillus* infections.

Micafungin and **anidulafungin** are used primarily for serious *Candida* infections, resistant esophageal candidiasis, and prevention of *Candida* infections in patients undergoing bone marrow transplantation.

Others

Flucytosine is administered orally and has a narrow antifungal spectrum. Fungicidal activity is greatest against *C. neoformans* and *Candida* species. Activity may also include *Cladosporium* and *Phialophora* species. Resistance of *Candida* species to this drug is extremely variable. Flucytosine

acts synergistically with amphotericin B and will enhance activity as well as reduce the emergence of resistant fungi. Human cells do not contain cytosine deaminase and hence cannot activate the drug.

Griseofulvin is administered orally to treat superficial mycoses of the skin, nails, or hair. It primarily inhibits dermatophytes of *Microsporum*, *Trichophyton*, and *Epidermophyton* species and has no effect on filamentous fungi such as *Aspergillus*, yeasts such as *Candida* organisms, or dimorphic species such as *Histoplasma*. Treatment lasts for weeks to months until the new fungal-free keratin has replaced the infected tissue.

Ciclopirox is a broad-spectrum topical nail lacquer used for onychomycosis and is active against the dermatophyte *Trichophyton rubrum*. Tolnaftate and undecylenic acid are available in several topical preparations to treat dermatophyte infections.

PHARMACOKINETICS

Pharmacokinetic parameters for commonly used antifungal drugs are summarized in Table 62.2.

Allylamines

Terbinafine is well absorbed orally from the gastrointestinal (GI) tract, with a plasma half-life of about 16 hours and a prolonged terminal half-life of approximately 16 days. Terbinafine is highly lipophilic and keratophilic, resulting in high concentrations in the stratum corneum, sebum, hair, and nails. The drug may be detected in nails for up to 90 days after treatment is discontinued. It is metabolized extensively by the liver and excreted in the urine and feces as inactive metabolites. **Naftifine** and **butenafine** are used topically and exhibit minimal systemic absorption.

Azoles

In general, the imidazoles have shorter half-lives than the triazoles. Ketoconazole is considered the prototype for the imidazoles, and itraconazole is considered the prototype for the triazoles. All azoles can be used topically, although some are exclusively topical, including clotrimazole, econazole, oxiconazole, sulconazole, butoconazole, terconazole, tioconazole, efinaconazole, and sertaconazole. Azoles that can be used systemically include ketoconazole, miconazole, itraconazole, fluconazole, voriconazole, posaconazole, and isavuconazonium. The agents are all metabolized extensively by the hepatic cytochrome P450 system, and many of them inhibit these enzymes, leading to drug-drug interactions.

Ketoconazole, when given orally, requires an acidic environment for absorption. Therefore coadministration of antacids, histamine (H_2) receptor antagonists, or proton pump inhibitors will reduce absorption. Ketoconazole is distributed in saliva, skin, bone, aqueous humor, and pleural, peritoneal, and synovial fluids. The drug crosses the blood-brain barrier poorly. Ketoconazole is metabolized extensively by hepatic hydroxylation and oxidative *N*-dealkylation.

Itraconazole is frequently considered the prototype for the azole family. Like ketoconazole, its oral absorption is favored in an acidic pH, and therefore coadministration of drugs that decrease stomach acid will reduce absorption. Food increases absorption of capsules but decreases absorption of suspensions. An IV formulation is also available but rarely used. Itraconazole is distributed mainly to lipophilic tissues and does not cross the blood-brain barrier well. Very little is found in saliva or the cerebrospinal fluid (CSF). The drug undergoes extensive hepatic metabolism.

Fluconazole is water soluble and rapidly absorbed after oral administration. Fluconazole does not require an acidic environment for absorption. Approximately 70%–80% is eliminated unchanged through the kidneys, with small amounts of metabolites present in urine and

TABLE 62.2 Pharmacokinetic Parameters for Antifungal Drugs

Drug	Administration	Absorption	t$_{1/2}$ (hrs)	Urine Concentration	Elimination	Plasma Protein Bound (%)
Terbinafine	Oral, topical	>70%	16 (16 days)[a]	Poor	M (main)	99
Ketoconazole	Oral, topical	75%[b]	8	Poor	M (95%), R (3%)	99
Miconazole	Topical, IV	Poor	0.5	–	M (95%)	90
Econazole	Topical	<1%	–	–	M (95%)	–
Clotrimazole	Topical	<1%	–	–	M (95%)	–
Fluconazole	Oral, IV	85%	25–30	Good	R (main), M	12
Itraconazole	Oral	9% (40%[c])	17–60	Poor	M	99
Voriconazole	Oral, IV	>90% (fasting)	6–24	Poor	M	58
Posaconazole	Oral	10–40%[c]	20–35	Poor	M	98
Amphotericin B	Topical, oral, IV	No	24 (15 days)[a]	Good	B (some) (main)	>90
Lipid-based amphotericin B	IV	No	24 (15 days)[a]	Poor	–	–
Nystatin	Topical	No	–	–	–	>90
Caspofungin	IV	Poor	9–11	Poor	M (>98%)	>97
Anidulafungin	IV	Poor	43–50	Poor	B	84
Micafungin	IV	Poor	1417	Poor	M (>98%)	>99
Flucytosine	Oral	Good	3–6	Good	R (85%)	<10
Griseofulvin	Oral, topical	Poor[d]	20	–	M (main)	–

[a]Terminal elimination phase.
[b]Needs acidic pH to be absorbed.
[c]Less well absorbed during fasting.
[d]Particles taken up by unknown process.
B, Biliary; M, metabolism; R, renal.

feces. Fluconazole is widely distributed to tissues and body fluids and crosses the blood-brain barrier, with therapeutic concentrations attained in the CSF. Fluconazole has been reported to produce less inhibition of hepatic P450 enzymes than either ketoconazole or itraconazole.

Voriconazole is rapidly absorbed orally, with greater than 90% bioavailability that decreases when the drug is taken with food. More than 95% of this drug is metabolized by hepatic cytochrome P450s to inactive compounds, with only a small amount excreted unchanged in the urine. The half-life of the drug is dose dependent, and the dosage should be adjusted in patients with liver disease.

Posaconazole is rapidly absorbed following oral administration with food, greatly enhancing absorption. Posaconazole is extensively glucuronidated with very limited hepatic metabolism. The glucuronide conjugates are eliminated in the urine and feces.

Isavuconazonium is rapidly absorbed after oral administration and is distributed extensively throughout the body, with a half-life as long as 5–6 days. It is metabolized primarily by the hepatic cytochrome P450 system.

Polyenes

Amphotericin B is insoluble in water, has a large lipophilic domain, and is not absorbed from the GI tract. It is administered orally only to treat fungal infections of the GI tract, which sometimes develop after depletion of bacterial microflora from broad-spectrum antibacterial drugs. For IV administration, amphotericin B is either complexed with deoxycholate to form a colloidal suspension or given as a lipid-based formulation. Amphotericin B enters pleural, peritoneal, and synovial fluids and aqueous humor, where it reaches a concentration approximately half that in serum. The agent does not readily penetrate into the CSF. It has been speculated that amphotericin B is bound to cholesterol-containing membranes in tissues in the body.

The principal pathway for amphotericin B elimination is not known. Some drug is excreted by the biliary route, and about 3% is eliminated unchanged in urine. Complete elimination of amphotericin B may take

months. Patients with renal dysfunction may require a dose or frequency reduction. Amphotericin B is not removed by hemodialysis. Lipid-based formulations of amphotericin B achieve higher serum levels and improved penetration of the central nervous system, as well as more rapid plasma clearance than deoxycholate preparations.

Echinocandins

Caspofungin is not absorbed from the GI tract and must be administered by IV infusion. It is rapidly distributed to tissues and exhibits extensive (97%) binding to plasma albumin. The plasma half-life for caspofungin is about 10 hours, and it is redistributed to tissues where it gradually undergoes metabolism by hydrolysis and N-acetylation to inactive metabolites that are excreted in both bile and urine. Micafungin and anidulafungin have similar pharmacokinetics, although anidulafungin is excreted primarily in the feces.

Others

Flucytosine is well absorbed from the GI tract and is distributed in the body, with CSF concentrations about 80% of those in plasma. It enters the peritoneum, synovial fluid, bronchial secretions, saliva, and bone. The majority of the drug is excreted unchanged by glomerular filtration, with a half-life of approximately 4 hours, which increases greatly as creatinine clearance diminishes. For patients with renal insufficiency, the half-life is greatly prolonged, and the dosage must be reduced. If necessary, the drug can be removed by hemodialysis and peritoneal dialysis. A small fraction of the dose can be converted by intestinal bacteria to 5-fluorouracil and can lead to potential hematological toxicity.

Griseofulvin is relatively insoluble, with approximately half of an oral dose entering the circulation after GI absorption. Absorption can be significantly enhanced by taking the drug with a fatty meal. Griseofulvin is widely distributed and is taken up in fat, liver, and muscle. It concentrates in keratin precursor cells in the stratum corneum of the skin, nails, and hair. Griseofulvin is metabolized in the liver by dealkylation and excreted in the urine as a glucuronide. Griseofulvin induces hepatic cytochrome P450s, leading to drug-drug interactions.

PHARMACOVIGILANCE: ADVERSE EFFECTS AND DRUG INTERACTIONS

Allylamines

Terbinafine can lead to headache, diarrhea, dyspepsia, and abdominal pain. Some patients experience disturbances in taste. Rarely, rashes, including toxic epidermal necrolysis, have been reported. Increases in liver transaminase levels occur in less than 5% of patients, but rare cases of severe hepatotoxicity and death have been reported. It is generally advised to avoid terbinafine in patients with preexisting liver disease. Terbinafine inhibits CYP2D6, which increases plasma levels of tricyclic antidepressants, selective serotonin reuptake inhibitors, and other drugs metabolized by this enzyme. Depressive symptoms have been reported during postmarketing surveillance of terbinafine.

Naftifine and butenafine are used topically and may lead to local reactions include burning, stinging, and itching.

Azoles

All azoles can inhibit hepatic cytochrome P450s, particularly CYP3A4. As a consequence, significant drug-drug interactions can occur. Some examples of drugs that may have interactions with various azoles include warfarin, cyclosporine, digoxin, sulfonylureas, quinidine, dofetilide, phenytoin, and simvastatin.

Ketoconazole can lead to nausea and vomiting that can be reduced if the drug is taken with food. The most serious adverse effect is hepatic toxicity in 5%–10% of patients, manifest as transient elevations of serum aminotransferase and alkaline phosphatase levels. However, fulminant hepatic damage is rare, with an incidence of 1 in 12,000, although jaundice, fever, liver failure, and even death have been reported in a few patients. Ketoconazole is rarely used for systemic mycoses because the newer azoles are less toxic.

Ketoconazole is a potent inhibitor of CYP3A4 and significantly inhibits steroid synthesis. It can cause transient gynecomastia and breast tenderness by blocking testosterone synthesis. High doses can lead to azoospermia and impotence and may block cortisol secretion and suppress adrenal responses to adrenocorticotropic hormone. Some animal studies have demonstrated teratogenic effects.

Drugs that decrease stomach acid will decrease absorption because ketoconazole needs an acidic environment for absorption. Because ketoconazole interferes with the synthesis of ergosterol, it may decrease the effectiveness of amphotericin B, which binds to ergosterol to form pores.

Itraconazole is generally well tolerated, but some mild GI side effects are common, such as nausea and diarrhea. Other side effects may include rash, headache, and edema. More serious side effects include cardiac suppression and liver damage. Rare cases of liver failure have been reported. Since itraconazole can decrease ejection fraction due to negative inotropic effects, it should be used with caution in patients with heart failure or ventricular dysfunction. Some animal studies have demonstrated teratogenic effects in the first trimester. Like ketoconazole, any drug that decreases stomach acid will result in decreased absorption, and inhibition of CYP3A4 and other cytochrome P450s can lead to drug-drug interactions.

Fluconazole is generally well tolerated, with the most common side effects being nausea, headache, rash, abdominal pain, and diarrhea. Rare reports have included hepatic necrosis and Stevens-Johnson syndrome. High doses of fluconazole during the first trimester have been shown to cause birth defects in humans, and a single dose may increase the risk of miscarriage. Like other azoles, fluconazole can inhibit CYP3A4 and increase levels of other drugs metabolized by this enzyme.

Voriconazole causes transient reversible visual disturbances in approximately 40% of patients. These changes include blurriness and alterations in color vision and usually occur immediately after a dose, resolve within 30 minutes, and reverse with discontinuation of the drug. It is recommended that patients not drive at night due to possible visual impairment. Although rare, voriconazole can cause hepatitis and hepatic failure. There have been reports of rash and Stevens-Johnson syndrome, as well as anaphylactic reactions. Voriconazole is teratogenic and contraindicated during pregnancy. Voriconazole is both a substrate for and inhibitor of hepatic cytochrome P450s, leading to drug-drug interactions.

Isavuconazonium is relatively new and has been shown to cause nausea and headaches as well as dyspnea, cough, and peripheral edema. Increased liver enzymes and decreased potassium levels have been noted, along with shortened QT interval and hypersensitivity reactions, including Stevens-Johnson syndrome. Isavuconazonium causes fetal abnormalities in laboratory animals and is both a substrate for and inhibitor of hepatic cytochrome P450s.

Miconazole is rarely used systemically. Intravenous infusion of miconazole produces nausea and vomiting in 25% of patients. It may also cause chills, malaise, tremors, confusion, dizziness, or seizures.

Polyenes

Amphotericin B, administered IV, causes many adverse effects. The initial reactions usually include chills, fever, headache, vomiting, pain, and occasionally hypotension or hypertension. These symptoms, caused by release of proinflammatory cytokines, are related to the infusion rate and can be controlled with antipyretics, antihistamines, antiemetics, narcotics, and glucocorticoids. Dantrolene can be administered if rigors occur.

Some degree of renal toxicity develops in most patients treated with amphotericin B. This adverse effect presents as an early decrease in glomerular filtration rate resulting from vasoconstrictive actions on glomerular afferent arterioles. The drug may also have an effect on the distal renal tubule, leading to K^+ loss, hypomagnesemia caused by failure to reabsorb Mg^{++}, or tubular acidosis. Potassium supplements may be needed. The extent of renal damage is related to the total dose of drug, and although most renal function recovers even if therapy is continued, some residual damage occurs. Loading with normal saline before infusion of amphotericin B may reduce the degree of renal toxicity. Lipid formulations of amphotericin B are better tolerated, with fewer infusion-related effects and considerably less nephrotoxicity than deoxycholate-complexed amphotericin B. Increased kidney damage can occur when amphotericin B is used with other nephrotoxic agents such as cyclosporine, aminoglycosides, or nonsteroidal antiinflammatory drugs (NSAIDs); these combinations should be avoided if possible.

Amphotericin B can cause bone marrow suppression as a consequence of inhibition of erythropoietin production, resulting in normochromic, normocytic anemia. This effect generally returns to normal after therapy is stopped. Other adverse effects include neurotoxicity (rare), cardiac dysrhythmias, pulmonary infiltrates, rash, and anaphylaxis. Hepatotoxicity and diabetes insipidus have also been reported.

Nystatin has minimal side effects because it is not absorbed systemically. Some nausea or GI side effects can occur if the drug is swallowed. When used as an oral rinse, an unpleasant taste has been reported.

Echinocandins

Caspofungin is usually well tolerated, with adverse effects including fever, phlebitis, headache, nausea, and rash. Studies suggest that caspofungin may release histamine, which can cause flushing and pruritus. Teratogenic effects have been reported in laboratory animals. Drugs that induce hepatic cytochrome P450s may decrease serum levels of caspofungin, and combining cyclosporine with caspofungin may increase the risk of liver damage.

Micafungin and anidulafungin have side effects similar to caspofungin but have less interaction with the hepatic cytochrome P450 system.

Others

Flucytosine can cause serious hematological side effects, including anemia, leukopenia, and thrombocytopenia. Rarely, fatal agranulocytosis can develop. Toxicity is primarily attributable to the metabolite 5-fluorouracil. Mild liver dysfunction occurs frequently, but is usually reversible, and severe hepatic injury is rare. Since this drug is usually coadministered with amphotericin B, there may be reduced renal clearance because amphotericin B is nephrotoxic. This renal damage can inhibit flucytosine excretion, leading to increased blood levels.

Flucytosine can inhibit hepatic drug-metabolizing enzymes and raise levels of drugs metabolized by the cytochrome P450 system. Combining flucytosine with cisapride, pimozide, dofetilide, or quinidine has been shown to increase the risk of fatal arrhythmias. Animal studies have demonstrated some teratogenic effects.

Griseofulvin may cause headaches, rash, insomnia, and nausea upon initial exposure. Occasionally leukopenia, neutropenia, hepatotoxicity, or photosensitivity may occur. Although renal function is not decreased, albuminuria can develop. Since griseofulvin induces hepatic drug-metabolizing enzymes and increases the metabolism of other drugs metabolized by the same system, it should not be administered to patients with porphyria. Due to reports of teratogenic effects in animals, griseofulvin is not recommended for use during pregnancy.

Clinical problems and major side effects encountered with the antifungal agents are summarized in the Clinical Problems Box.

NEW DEVELOPMENTS

As fungi and yeast continue to develop resistance to current drugs, the need exists for antifungals with novel mechanisms of action. One of the major mechanisms contributing to multidrug resistance in *Candida albicans* is the plasma membrane drug efflux system. Therefore, inhibiting this efflux pump may be a potential strategy to increase the susceptibility of *C. albicans* to antifungals. New mechanisms of action selectively targeting the fungal cell wall or cell membrane are always being investigated. Two recent topical drugs for onychomycosis include tavaborole that inhibits fungal protein synthesis by inhibition of an aminoacyl-transfer ribonucleic acid synthetase and efinaconazole that has increased penetration into the infected cells. A novel mechanism for a drug to treat invasive aspergillosis involves a decrease in levels of the fungal cell wall component galactomannan. Other novel antifungal compounds that are being investigated include myriocin and fulvic acid, which target fungal biofilm formation and host inflammatory responses. The newly developed orotomide class of antifungal agents, which is active against *Aspergillus* and other resistant organisms, inhibits dihydroorotate dehydrogenase (DHODH), which is involved in pyrimidine biosynthesis.

CLINICAL RELEVANCE FOR HEALTHCARE PROFESSIONALS

All healthcare professionals need to be aware of the side effects associated with the use of antifungal agents because many individuals are using these compounds. It is especially critical for physicians, physician assistants, and nurse practitioners to be aware of possible drug-drug interactions because many patients take over-the-counter medications and herbal supplements, which can interact with antifungal medications. Because all the azoles inhibit cytochrome P450s to some extent, healthcare professionals should be watchful for drug-drug interactions and the potential for increased adverse events.

Physical therapists, occupational therapists, and other healthcare professionals working with patients being treated with antifungal drugs should be aware of the major side effects associated with these agents. In particular, the infusion-related effects of amphotericin B can limit a patient's ability to participate in rehabilitation, while flucytosine can result in a decreased capacity to exercise and lead to increased bleeding after injury, and voriconazole can cause visual disturbances that can interfere with functional performance of patients participating in rehabilitation.

The dental use of antifungals frequently involves immunocompromised patients (including cancer chemotherapy or HIV-positive individuals) who are very susceptible to oral fungal infections. Diabetes, nutritional deficiencies, acid saliva, xerostomia, night use of prosthetic dentures, smoking, diets rich in sugars, as well as poor oral hygiene increase the risk for oral candidiasis. Drugs the dentist may prescribe for the frequent management of oral fungal infections are available as lozenges, gels, ointments, oral suspensions, and tablets. For oral candidiasis, dentists often prescribe a polyene (nystatin, hamycin, natamycin, or amphotericin B). Even though these agents are not absorbed by the GI tract, the dentist should remember that these agents can produce adverse effects such as mouth irritation and, if swallowed, stomach upset, rash, nausea, and diarrhea. Dentists should be aware that azoles work by a different mechanism from the polyenes (inhibiting the synthesis of ergosterol) and can be used topically or given orally. A variety of azoles are available for topical administration and come as rinses, creams, ointments, or

CLINICAL PROBLEMS

Drug	Adverse Effects
Terbinafine	Taste disturbance, liver toxicity, depression
Ketoconazole	GI disturbances, hepatotoxicity, inhibition of hepatic P450 enzymes, inhibition of steroid synthesis
Itraconazole	GI disturbances, rare hepatotoxicity, cardiac suppression
Fluconazole	GI disturbances, rare hepatotoxicity, rare Stevens-Johnson syndrome, teratogenic
Voriconazole	Reversible photopsia, mild rash, Stevens-Johnson syndrome, toxic epidermal necrolysis, hepatotoxicity, visual hallucinations
Isavuconazonium	Headache, nausea, cough, dyspnea, peripheral edema, allergic reactions, hypokalemia, increased liver enzymes
Miconazole	Headache, pruritus, thrombophlebitis, hepatotoxicity
Amphotericin B	Nephrotoxicity, fever, chills, phlebitis, hypokalemia, anemia, vomiting, pain
Caspofungin, micafungin, anidulafungin	Fever, headache, thrombophlebitis, rash, pruritus, rare hepatotoxicity
Flucytosine	Bone marrow suppression, hepatotoxicity, GI disturbance
Griseofulvin	Headache, rash, induction of hepatic P450 enzymes

suspensions. Oral ketoconazole, itraconazole, and fluconazole are sometimes prescribed for severe cases of oral candidiasis or prophylactically to prevent oral candidiasis in immunocompromised patients, so it is important to know the major side effects. The dentist needs to be aware that the oral absorption of ketoconazole and itraconazole is facilitated by gastric acidity because these drugs are more soluble at lower pH, so drug absorption will be reduced if these agents are taken at the same time as antacids, H_2 blockers, or proton pump inhibitors. Dentists should know that all oral azoles have the potential for drug interactions. A particularly important drug interaction involves azoles and warfarin because this combination can increase the levels of the anticoagulant and increase the risk of bleeding.

TRADE NAMES

In addition to generic and fixed-combination preparations, the following trade-named materials are some of the important compounds available in the United States.

Amphotericin B deoxycholate (Fungizone)
Amphotericin B lipid complex (Abelcet)
Amphotericin B cholesteryl sulfate complex (Amphotec)
Liposomal amphotericin B (AmBisome)
Anidulafungin (Eraxis)
Butenafine (Lotrimin Ultra, Mentax)
Caspofungin (Cancidas)
Clotrimazole (Lotrimin, Mycelex, Canesten)
Ciclopirox (Loprox, Penlac Nail Lacquer)
Econazole nitrate (Spectazole, Ecoza)
Fluconazole (Diflucan)

Flucytosine (Ancobon)
Griseofulvin (Grifulvin V, Gris-PEG)
Isavuconazonium (Cresemba)
Itraconazole (Sporanox, Onmel)
Ketoconazole (Nizoral)
Miconazole (Monistat, Micatin, Oravig)
Micafungin (Mycamine)
Naftifine (Naftin)
Nystatin (Mycostatin, Nystex, Nilstat)
Posaconazole (Noxafil)
Terbinafine (Lamisil, Terbinex)
Tolnaftate (Tinactin, Podactin, Tinamar)
Voriconazole (Vfend)

SELF-ASSESSMENT QUESTIONS

1. A 24-year-old man presents to the emergency department reporting chest pain and a nonproductive cough that began approximately 1 week ago. His symptoms are progressing, and he now has a low-grade fever, productive cough, hemoptysis, weakness, and anorexia. A chest x-ray reveals an infiltrate in the upper left lobe of the lungs, and culture and staining of deep sputum reveal fungal elements of *Blastomyces dermatitidis*. The patient was started on an intravenous antifungal. Two weeks later, the patient's serum creatinine was significantly elevated to 3.0 mg/dL. Which of the following antifungal agents was most likely prescribed for this patient?
   A. Caspofungin.
   B. Colloidal amphotericin B.
   C. Flucytosine.
   D. Itraconazole.
   E. Voriconazole.

2. An HIV-infected patient develops rapidly progressing cryptococcal meningitis, for which he was hospitalized and administered amphotericin B and flucytosine. Which of the following drugs would be best for this patient as prophylactic therapy when he is released from the hospital?
   A. Clotrimazole.
   B. Fluconazole.
   C. Nystatin.
   D. Metronidazole.
   E. Voriconazole.

3. A 48-year-old woman has an obvious case of onychomycosis of the toes. Which of the following agents would be the most appropriate oral drug for this fungus?
   A. Caspofungin.
   B. Fluconazole.

   C. Miconazole.
   D. Nystatin.
   E. Terbinafine.

4. A 19-year-old student presents to the emergency department reporting that while driving to work, he suddenly experienced blurred vision and a loss of ability to distinguish color. His history reveals that he is currently taking an antifungal medication. Which of the following drugs would result in these effects?
   A. Flucytosine.
   B. Griseofulvin.
   C. Nystatin.
   D. Terbinafine.
   E. Voriconazole.

5. A patient is prescribed an oral drug for a fungal infection, but a week later, there was no improvement. He sought his physician who learned that the patient was having gastric reflux issues and began taking an over-the-counter proton pump inhibitor. It is likely that the antifungal drug he was taking was:
   A. Amphotericin B.
   B. Caspofungin.
   C. Fluconazole.
   D. Itraconazole.
   E. Griseofulvin.

FURTHER READING

Ashbee HR, Barnes RA, Johnson EM, et al. Therapeutic drug monitoring (TDM) of antifungal agents: guidelines from the British Society for Medical Mycology. *J Antimicrob Chemother*. 2014;69(5):1162–1176.

WEBSITES

http://www.merckmanuals.com/professional/infectious-diseases/fungi/overview-of-fungal-infections

This is the Merck Manual professional version and provides an overview of fungal infections, as well as links to detailed information on many fungal species.

Antimalarial and Other Antiprotozoal Agents

Adonis McQueen

THERAPEUTIC OVERVIEW

Parasitic infections are an important cause of morbidity throughout the world. Parasites, which live in (endoparasites) or on (ectoparasites) host organisms, may affect specific internal organs or systems such as the gastrointestinal (GI) tract or the circulation. The manifestations of parasitic infections can range from mild disturbances, such as itching or diarrhea, to severe and fatal diseases, such as malaria. A variety of conditions that promote parasitic infections include poor sanitation and public health measures, increased population density, and increased world travel. Enteric parasites are prevalent in developing areas and intermittently cause epidemics in industrialized countries when they gain access to water or food supplies. In industrialized countries, parasitic diseases most commonly affect refugees, immigrants, military personnel, returning international travelers, and occasionally residents who have not traveled. Several protozoa have also emerged as important opportunistic pathogens in patients with acquired immunodeficiency syndrome (AIDS).

The three major groups of parasites include the protozoa, helminths, and arthropods. Protozoa are composed of a single cell and can multiply in their human hosts. Theoretically, infection with only one cell can result in overwhelming disease. Protozoal species differ widely in their sensitivity to drugs. Common protozoal diseases, causative organisms, transmission vectors, and geographical distributions are shown in the Therapeutic Overview Box. Disorders associated with helminths and the pharmacological agents used to treat these parasites are presented in Chapter 64.

MECHANISMS OF ACTION

Malaria

Malaria poses a major health problem for residents of many tropical areas and for international travelers. More than 1 million deaths are attributed annually to malaria in sub-Saharan Africa alone. *Plasmodium* species, which cause malaria, are transmitted by *Anopheles* mosquitoes. Four species of *Plasmodium* infect humans, including *Plasmodium falciparum*, the predominant species worldwide; *Plasmodium vivax* and *Plasmodium ovale*, which have dormant liver stages; and *Plasmodium malariae*, which is least frequently associated with infections.

THERAPEUTIC OVERVIEW

Common Protozoal Diseases
Causative organism, transmission vector, and geographical distribution

Malaria
Plasmodium species, *Anopheles* mosquitoes, Africa, Asia, Middle East, Central and South America, western Pacific islands

Leishmaniasis
Leishmania species, sand flies, tropics, subtropics, and southern Europe

African Trypanosomiasis
Trypanosoma brucei gambiense and *Trypanosoma brucei rhodesiense*, tsetse flies, Africa

Chagas Disease (American Trypanosomiasis)
Trypanosoma cruzi, triatomine (reduviid) bugs, Americas

Amebiasis
Entamoeba histolytica, contaminated food and water, Africa, Mexico, South America, and India

Giardiasis
Giardia lamblia, contaminated food and water, worldwide

Toxoplasmosis
Toxoplasma gondii, cats and undercooked meats, worldwide

Trichomoniasis
Trichomonas vaginalis, sexually transmitted, worldwide

The malaria parasite life cycle in the host is shown in Fig. 63.1. Sporozoites are inoculated into the host when an infected female *Anopheles* mosquito takes a blood meal. The sporozoites travel through the circulation to the liver, where they invade hepatocytes. Within the liver, the sporozoites pass through several stages. For *P. falciparum*, the sporozoites develop into schizonts, eventually producing merozoites,

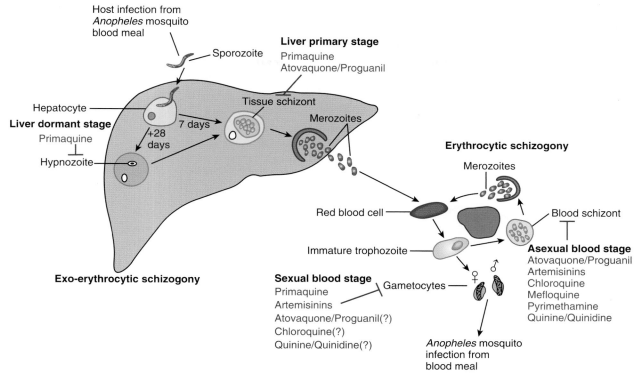

FIG. 63.1 The Malaria Parasite Life Cycle in the Human Host and Sites of Action of Antimalarial Drugs.

which are released into the circulation to invade red blood cells. The sporozoites from *P. vivax* and *P. ovale* also follow this pathway, but a portion of the sporozoites can produce hypnozoites, which can persist dormant in the liver for a prolonged period before completing development into schizonts. These hepatic stages represent exo-erythrocytic schizogony.

During erythrocytic schizogony, the merozoites in the red blood cells multiply asexually to form immature trophozoites. The trophozoites can mature to schizonts, which rupture to release merozoites, destroying the erythrocytes in the process. The immature trophozoites can also differentiate via the sexual erythrocytic stage into gametocytes, which can be ingested by another *Anopheles* mosquito during a blood meal. The erythrocytic stage is the only symptomatic stage.

The sites of action of antimalarial drugs are shown in Fig. 63.1, and structures of representative antimalarial and other antiprotozoal agents are shown in Fig. 63.2.

Blood Schizonticides

The site of action of most antimalarial drugs is on the asexual erythrocytic form of the parasite to prevent or treat malaria symptoms. These drugs include the artemisinins, chloroquine, mefloquine, pyrimethamine, and quinine/quinidine.

Artesunate is a water-soluble semisynthetic derivative of the artemisinin group of drugs. Artesunate and other artemisinin relatives, including **dihydroartemisinin** and **artemether**, are endoperoxide-containing compounds. These agents represent the most rapid-acting antimalarial agents and kill the malarial parasite at all erythrocytic stages, targeting both the asexual and sexual stages. The artemisinins bind to heme iron that is rich in the acidic digestive vacuole of the parasite as a consequence of hemoglobin digestion. By inhibiting hemoglobin metabolism, the artemisinins interfere with processes critical for the survival of both the schizonts and the developing gametocytes.

In addition, these agents produce free radicals that can alkylate critical parasitic proteins, such as Ca^{++}-ATPase and a glutathione S-transferase, and increase the clearance of infected erythrocytes through the spleen by reducing cell adherence.

Chloroquine is a 4-aminoquinoline that is also active against the erythrocytic forms of *Plasmodium*. Chloroquine is concentrated in the hemoglobin-containing digestive vesicles of *Plasmodium* species and inhibits the heme polymerase that incorporates heme into the insoluble, nontoxic crystalline material hemozoin, resulting in disruption of heme sequestration. Chloroquine-resistant strains of *P. falciparum* transport chloroquine out of the intraparasitic compartment more rapidly than susceptible strains. Although chloroquine clearly inhibits the asexual erythrocytic stage of the parasite, some evidence supports an effect on the sexual stage producing gametocytes as well.

Mefloquine is an analogue of quinine that appears to have several actions that kill the erythrocytic forms of *Plasmodium*. It may form complexes with heme iron that are toxic, and it leads to swelling in the digestive vacuoles. It may also associate with hemozoin.

Pyrimethamine binds to and irreversibly inhibits dihydrofolate reductase. It is approximately 1000-fold more active against *Plasmodium* dihydrofolate reductase-thymidylate synthetase than against human dihydrofolate reductase. Inhibition of this enzyme interferes with the synthesis of purines and pyrimidines required for DNA and cell replication. Pyrimethamine is often used with one of the sulfonamides to inhibit sequential steps in folate metabolism. Similarly, **trimethoprim** also inhibits dihydrofolate reductase of some protozoa, as well as many bacteria, and is frequently administered with sulfamethoxazole (Chapter 59).

Quinine has been used to treat malaria for centuries. It is concentrated in the acidic food vacuoles of *Plasmodium* and is thought to inhibit the activity of heme polymerase like chloroquine. **Quinidine**, the stereoisomer of quinine, presumably acts in the same manner. Both of

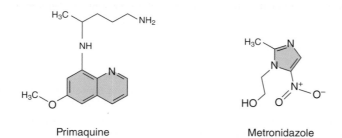

R = H Dihydroartemisinin
R = CH₃ Artemether
R = CH₂CH₃ Arteether
R = CO(CH₂)₂CO₂H Artesunate

Artemisinin

Chloroquine

Mefloquine

Pyrimethamine

Quinine

Atovaquone

Proguanil

Primaquine

Metronidazole

FIG. 63.2 Structures of Representative Antimalarial and Other Antiprotozoal Agents.

these agents interfere with the asexual, and may affect the sexual, erythrocytic stage.

Tissue and Blood Schizonticides

A limited number of agents are effective for both the hepatic and erythrocytic stages of the parasite. These agents include atovaquone, proguanil, and primaquine.

Atovaquone targets the primary liver stages of *Plasmodium* in addition to the asexual erythrocytic stage. It may also affect gametocytes. Atovaquone selectively inhibits mitochondrial electron transport, resulting in a loss of ubiquinone required as a cofactor for pyrimidine biosynthesis.

Proguanil is a prodrug that is activated to cycloguanil and is an inhibitor of dihydrofolate reductase-thymidylate synthetase, like pyrimethamine. As a consequence, DNA and cell replication are inhibited both in the liver and blood. Proguanil may also affect gametocytes.

Primaquine is an aminoquinoline that is unique in its ability to target both the primary (merozoite) and latent (hypnozoite) hepatic stages, as well as the gametocytes. Its mechanism of action is not well understood but may involve the generation of reactive oxygen species and interference with electron transport, both of which alter protozoal DNA.

Other Antiprotozoals

Many antiprotozoal drugs also have antibacterial activity and typically target DNA, RNA, or protein synthesis, intermediary metabolites, or membrane structure. Many of the antibiotics discussed in other chapters have activity against some protozoa, including tetracycline, doxycycline, and clindamycin that inhibit protein synthesis (Chapter 58) and the sulfonamides that inhibit dihydropteroate synthetase and para-aminobenzoic acid binding (Chapter 59). Amphotericin B is thought to affect leishmania the same way it affects susceptible fungi, by disrupting membranes (Chapter 62). In addition, liposomal and lipid-associated amphotericin B selectively target macrophages, the cells in which leishmania reside.

Eflornithine is an irreversible inhibitor of ornithine decarboxylase, the enzyme that catalyzes the rate-limiting step in polyamine synthesis. Although polyamines are essential for growth and differentiation of all cells, eflornithine has clinical activity only against *Trypanosoma brucei gambiense*.

Furazolidone is a nitrofuran derivative with both antiprotozoal and antibacterial activity. Furazolidone and its related free radical products interfere with several bacterial enzyme systems and bind to bacterial DNA. Its mechanism of action against *Giardia lamblia* is uncertain.

Iodoquinol, also known as diiodohydroxyquinoline and uidoquinol, is a quinolone derivative effective for amebiasis against *Entamoeba histolytica* cysts and, to a lesser extent, trophozoites. Although it has amoebicidal activity, its mechanism of action is unknown.

Melarsoprol is an arsenical and reacts with sulfhydryl groups on proteins to inhibit many enzymes, including trypanothione, which provides a reducing environment in parasites analogous to glutathione in mammalian cells. *Trypanosoma brucei rhodesiense* and *T. brucei gambiense* have an unusual purine transporter that concentrates melarsoprol in the organisms.

Metronidazole and **tinidazole** are nitroimidazole prodrugs with a broad spectrum of activity against both protozoa and anaerobic bacteria. These compounds are reduced by ferredoxins or their equivalents, and the reduced products and free radicals generated bind covalently to DNA, causing damage and death.

Nifurtimox has been proposed to lead to oxidative stress through the formation of superoxide anion, hydrogen peroxide, and hydroxyl radicals that damage cell membranes and DNA. Recent evidence suggests that nifurtimox may also be a prodrug reduced by a trypanosomal nitroreductase to a metabolite that inhibits parasitic cell growth.

Nitazoxanide is an antifolate and interferes with all folate-dependent enzymes. It also interferes with the pyruvate:ferredoxin oxidoreductase enzyme–dependent electron transfer reaction essential for anaerobic energy metabolism.

Paromomycin is a broad-spectrum aminoglycoside antibiotic whose action is similar to that of neomycin (Chapter 58). Paromomycin binds to the 16S ribosomal RNA, leading to defective polypeptide chains and cell death. It is thought to have its antiprotozoal action by inhibiting translation.

Pentamidine isethionate has an unknown mechanism of action but may interfere with polyamine biosynthesis and inhibit topoisomerase II.

Sodium stibogluconate and **meglumine antimoniate** affect bioenergetics in leishmania, inhibiting glycolysis and fatty acid β-oxidation.

RELATIONSHIP OF MECHANISMS OF ACTION TO CLINICAL RESPONSE

Malaria Prophylaxis

Efforts to prevent malaria focus on minimizing mosquito contact and using chemoprophylaxis. Persons traveling to areas where *Plasmodium* species remain sensitive to chloroquine should take **chloroquine** weekly, and people with intense or prolonged exposure to *P. vivax* or *P. ovale* should receive a course of **primaquine** after leaving the endemic area. For travelers to chloroquine-resistant areas, there are three choices of comparable efficacy: **doxycycline, atovaquone/proguanil,** and **mefloquine**. Doxycycline is administered daily starting 2 days before travel and continued for 4 weeks after exposure to kill parasites released into the blood after completing their incubation in the liver. The combination of atovaquone/proguanil is the best tolerated and is also administered 2 days before travel and for 1 week after leaving the endemic area. **Mefloquine** has the advantage of being used weekly but has neuropsychiatric effects in some individuals. It is started 1–2 weeks before departure and is continued for 4 weeks after leaving the endemic area. Recent data suggest that **primaquine** taken daily can also be used for prophylaxis. However, recipients must be screened to ensure that they are not glucose-6-phosphate dehydrogenase (G6PD) deficient because primaquine can lead to oxidative stress and hemolysis in these individuals. Doxycycline, atovaquone/proguanil, or primaquine cannot be used during pregnancy.

Malaria Treatment

Artesunate and other artemisinins have been used successfully for the treatment of severe *P. falciparum* malaria in areas where mefloquine- and quinine-resistant strains are endemic. In many instances, artemisinin derivatives are used concurrently with mefloquine or another antimalarial drug. Artemisinin combination therapy for the treatment of *P. falciparum* malaria is highly effective against gametocytes and thus can potentially decrease parasite transmission. Currently available artemisinin derivatives are not useful prophylactically because of their short half-lives and concern about neurotoxicity with long-term use. Other antimalarials are being studied in combinations to determine their additive or synergistic effects and whether they may be useful against drug-resistant isolates.

Chloroquine is recommended for treatment of acute infections with *P. ovale, P. malariae,* and chloroquine-sensitive strains of *P. vivax* and *P. falciparum*. Primaquine is administered to patients with *P. vivax* and *P. ovale* to prevent relapses. Oral **proguanil** or **quinine** plus **doxycycline** or **tetracycline** are used for the treatment of chloroquine-resistant *P. falciparum* malaria. Clindamycin is used in place of doxycycline with quinine in children or pregnant women. Mefloquine used at full treatment doses is effective but has frequent side effects.

Atovaquone/proguanil is formulated as a fixed dose for the prophylaxis and treatment of chloroquine-resistant *P. falciparum* malaria. Proguanil acts synergistically with atovaquone.

Treatment of Other Protozoal Diseases

Nifurtimox and **benznidazole** are currently approved for the treatment of Chagas disease. These drugs have a limited ability to effect cure in chronically infected patients and are used primarily to manage the lesions associated with the disease. The drugs are not effective in patients with chronic chagasic cardiomyopathy, megaesophagus, or megacolon.

Agents for the treatment of trypanosomiasis depend on the species and stage of the disease. **Pentamidine isethionate** is used for patients with the hemolymphatic stage of *T. brucei gambiense*, and **suramin** is used for *T. brucei rhodesiense*. **Melarsoprol** is used in patients with central nervous system (CNS) disease but is highly toxic. Eflornithine, also known as the "resurrection drug," is effective for the treatment of *T. brucei gambiense* in both the hemolymphatic and later CNS stages of infection, but supplies are very limited.

Liposomal amphotericin B is the only drug approved for the treatment of visceral leishmaniasis in the United States. The pentavalent antimonials sodium stibogluconate and meglumine antimoniate have been used historically for the treatment of visceral and cutaneous leishmaniasis around the world, but resistance is increasing. Miltefosine, an orally administered drug, is now considered the treatment of choice for visceral leishmaniasis in India. Amphotericin B deoxycholate and pentamidine isethionate are more toxic treatment alternatives.

The treatment of symptomatic toxoplasmosis consists of pyrimethamine and a short-acting sulfonamide, such as sulfadiazine. Leucovorin (folinic acid) is administered concurrently to prevent bone marrow suppression (Chapter 68). The combination of pyrimethamine and clindamycin is also effective and frequently used in patients with AIDS. The macrolide spiramycin has been used to treat women infected with *Toxoplasma gondii* during pregnancy.

PHARMACOKINETICS

Pharmacokinetic parameters for selected antiprotozoal drugs are listed in Table 63.1.

Antimalarials

Artesunate is administered by intravenous (IV) or intramuscular (IM) administration. After administration, artesunate is metabolized rapidly by plasma esterases to its active metabolite, dihydroartemisinin (DHA). A minor amount of the drug is metabolized by CYP2D6. DHA is glucuronidated and represents a major metabolite in the urine. Elimination is slower following IM than IV administration with a half-life after IV administration of less than 5 minutes for the parent and 21–64 minutes for DHA. The half-life after IM administration is approximately 40 minutes. DHA accumulates significantly in parasite-infected erythrocytes.

Chloroquine phosphate is well absorbed when taken orally, with peak serum concentrations reached in 3.5 hours. It is eliminated slowly

after treatment is terminated. Approximately 50% of the drug is excreted unchanged in the urine, and the rest is metabolized in the liver.

Mefloquine is slowly and incompletely absorbed after oral administration, with peak serum concentrations reached in 7–24 hours. The drug is highly protein bound with a long half-life.

Quinidine gluconate is administered by IV injection to patients with acute malaria who are unable to take oral medications.

Atovaquone is highly lipophilic, and administration with food enhances absorption twofold. Plasma concentrations do not correlate with dose, and the drug is highly protein bound, with a half-life exceeding 60 hours due to enterohepatic recycling with eventual fecal elimination. There is little excretion in urine.

Proguanil is well absorbed slowly after oral administration, with peak serum levels reached in 5 hours and an elimination half-life of 12–21 hours. The concentration in erythrocytes is approximately six times that in plasma.

Atovaquone/proguanil combinations have pharmacokinetics as described for the individual drugs.

Other Antiprotozoals

Eflornithine can be administered orally or IV. Peak plasma concentrations are reached approximately 4 hours after oral administration. The drug is widely distributed in the body, including the CNS, with the bulk of drug excreted in the urine.

Furazolidone is well absorbed after oral administration and extensively metabolized. More than 60% is excreted in the urine.

Melarsoprol is administered IV, and a small but therapeutically significant amount enters the CNS. It is rapidly excreted in the feces.

Metronidazole is rapidly and completely absorbed after oral administration and reaches peak plasma concentrations in 1 hour. More than half of the administered dose is metabolized in the liver, and the parent drug and metabolites are excreted in the urine.

Nifurtimox is well absorbed when taken orally, with a peak serum concentration reached in approximately 3.5 hours. It is rapidly metabolized.

Nitazoxanide is well absorbed orally and rapidly hydrolyzed to its active metabolite, tizoxanide, which undergoes conjugation to

TABLE 63.1	Pharmacokinetic Parameters of Selected Antiprotozoal Drugs				
Drug	**Administration**	**Absorption**	**$t_{1/2}$**		**Disposition**
Antimalarials					
Artesunate	IV, IM	Good	21–64 minutes (major metabolite)		M, R
Chloroquine	Oral	Good	4 days		M, R
Mefloquine	Oral	Good	6–23 days		M
Pyrimethamine	Oral	Good	3–4 days		R
Quinine	Oral, IV	Good	16–18 hrs		M, R
Atovaquone/proguanil	Oral	Adequate/good	12–60 hrs		F
Primaquine	Oral	Good	4 hrs		M
Other Antiprotozoals					
Eflornithine	Oral, IV	Good	3–4 hrs		R
Furazolidone	Oral (liquid)	Good	–		M, R
Metronidazole	Oral, IV	Good	8 hrs		M, R
Nitazoxanide	Oral (liquid)	Good	Active metabolite		M, R, F
Paromomycin	Oral	Poor			R
Pentamidine isethionate	IM or IV	–	IV 6 hrs, IM 9–13 hrs		R
Sodium stibogluconate	IM or IV	–	Variable		R

F, Fecal; *IM*, intramuscular; *IV*, intravenous; *M*, metabolized; *R*, renal excretion.

glucuronide. Tizoxanide is highly protein bound and is excreted in urine, bile, and feces, whereas the glucuronide is excreted in urine and bile.

Pentamidine isethionate is administered via IM or IV injection and has a plasma half-life of approximately 6 hours and a terminal elimination phase of approximately 12 days. It accumulates in tissue and is only slowly eliminated by the kidneys.

Sodium stibogluconate and meglumine antimoniate are administered IM or IV daily for a period of 3–4 weeks. These compounds have biphasic kinetics, with a short first-phase half-life of 2 hours and a second-phase half-life of 1–3 days. Excretion is via the kidneys.

Doxycycline, tetracycline, ciprofloxacin, and the sulfonamides are well absorbed when taken orally. Their pharmacokinetics are discussed in detail in Chapters 58 and 59. The pharmacokinetics of amphotericin B are discussed in Chapter 62.

PHARMACOVIGILANCE: ADVERSE EFFECTS AND DRUG INTERACTIONS

Antimalarials

The artemisinins are generally well tolerated but have been associated with mild to moderate increases in serum aminotransferase. In addition, idiosyncratic acute hepatic reactions have occurred, and there have been sporadic reports of ataxia. Because these compounds are metabolized extensively by CYP3A4, drug-drug interactions may occur with CYP3A4 inducers or inhibitors.

Chloroquine is relatively well tolerated when used for malaria treatment or prophylaxis. The side effects are dose related and reversible and include headache, nausea, vomiting, blurred vision, dizziness, and fatigue. When high doses are used, as in the treatment of rheumatologic diseases, serious and permanent retinal damage may occur. Chloroquine is contraindicated in persons with retinal disease, psoriasis, or porphyria. Children are especially sensitive to chloroquine, and cardiopulmonary arrest has occurred after accidental overdoses and in adults attempting suicide.

Mefloquine is relatively well tolerated when used for prophylaxis, but CNS side effects have limited its use. Side effects are more frequent and severe in patients receiving higher doses. Neuropsychiatric reactions such as seizures, acute psychosis, anxiety, and other disturbances occur in a small percentage of individuals but can be severe. Mefloquine should not be used in persons with a history of seizures or psychiatric disturbances.

Pyrimethamine is generally well tolerated. Blood dyscrasias, rash, vomiting, and seizures are rare. Bone marrow suppression may occur with high doses but can be prevented by concurrent administration of leucovorin (folinic acid).

Quinine has the poorest therapeutic index among antimalarial drugs. Common side effects include tinnitus, decreased hearing, headache, dysphoria, nausea, vomiting, and mild visual disturbances. Quinine therapy has been associated with severe hypoglycemia in persons with severe *P. falciparum* infections as a result of glucose utilization by the parasite and the quinine-mediated release of insulin from the pancreas. The hypoglycemia may be alleviated by the IV administration of glucose. Rare complications include allergic skin rashes, pruritus, agranulocytosis, hepatitis, and massive hemolysis in patients with *P. falciparum* malaria, which has been termed *blackwater fever*. Quinine causes respiratory paralysis in persons with myasthenia gravis, stimulates uterine contractions, and may induce abortion but has been used successfully to treat serious cases of malaria during pregnancy. Quinidine gluconate, the stereoisomer of quinine, is also a Class 1A antiarrhythmic drug (Chapter 45). It decreases ventricular ectopy, affects cardiac conduction, and prolongs the QT_c interval. Life-threatening dysrhythmias can occur,

but are rare. Hypotension may result if the drug is administered too rapidly.

Atovaquone is generally well tolerated but has been associated with GI side effects, including nausea, vomiting, and diarrhea. It has also been reported to cause skin rash and pruritus.

Proguanil can cause GI signs and symptoms with occasional nausea, diarrhea, urticaria, or oral ulceration when administered in low doses.

The combination atovaquone/proguanil is the best tolerated of all medications available for prophylaxis against chloroquine-resistant *P. falciparum*. Side effects include those of both drugs. Asymptomatic transient elevations in liver enzymes have also been reported.

Primaquine is also relatively well tolerated, although abdominal discomfort and nausea occur in some persons. The major toxicity is hemolysis in persons with G6PD deficiency. Primaquine is contraindicated during pregnancy because intrauterine hemolysis can occur in a G6PD-deficient fetus. Neutropenia, GI disturbances, and methemoglobinemia have been reported.

Other Antiprotozoals

Eflornithine is tolerated much better than other antitrypanosomal medications. Its side effects include flatulence, nausea, vomiting, diarrhea, anemia, leukopenia, and thrombocytopenia. On rare occasions, diplopia, dizziness, cutaneous hypersensitivity reactions, hearing loss, or seizures may occur.

Iodoquinol is contraindicated in persons sensitive to iodine. It occasionally causes rash, anal pruritus, acne, slight enlargement of the thyroid gland, nausea, and diarrhea.

Melarsoprol is extremely toxic, which limits its use to patients with CNS involvement by *T. brucei rhodesiense*. Myocardial toxicity, albuminuria, hypertension, abdominal pain, vomiting, and peripheral neuropathy have been reported. Approximately 10% of recipients develop allergic encephalitis, which may be fatal.

Metronidazole administration is commonly associated with GI complaints such as nausea, vomiting, diarrhea, and a metallic taste. Neurotoxicity including dizziness, vertigo, and numbness is rare but is a basis for discontinuation of treatment. Metronidazole has a disulfiram-like effect, and patients undergoing treatment should abstain from alcohol while taking this drug. Tinidazole has a similar spectrum of adverse effects but is generally better tolerated.

Nifurtimox is often toxic. Side effects include anorexia, vomiting, weight loss, memory loss, sleep disorders, tremor, paresthesias, weakness, and polyneuritis.

Nitazoxanide is very well tolerated. On rare occasions, the eyes may appear yellow, and the urine may be similarly discolored.

Paromomycin may lead to GI disturbances and diarrhea. Because paromomycin is an aminoglycoside antibiotic, it can produce ototoxicity and renal toxicity, the latter particularly in persons with preexisting renal disease.

Pentamidine isethionate toxicity is common, including GI complaints, dizziness, flushing, hypotension, renal damage, and blood dyscrasias. A major adverse reaction is hypoglycemia caused by acute damage to β cells of the pancreatic islets, resulting in insulin release and the long-term consequence of insulin-dependent diabetes mellitus.

Sodium stibogluconate and meglumine antimoniate have frequent side effects, but they usually do not prevent completion of therapy. Chemical pancreatitis is common, and recipients also frequently experience myalgias, arthralgias, fatigue, and nausea. Nonspecific S- and T-wave changes may be observed on the electrocardiogram. Untoward effects are more common in persons with renal failure.

An overview of the adverse effects associated with the antiprotozoal drugs is summarized in the Clinical Problems Box.

CLINICAL PROBLEMS

Metronidazole	GI side effects, metallic taste, neurotoxicity, alcohol intolerance
Paromomycin	GI side effects, ototoxicity, renal toxicity
Chloroquine	Headache, nausea, vomiting, blurred vision, retinal damage
Primaquine	GI side effects, hemolysis in people with glucose-6-phosphate deficiency
Quinine	Tinnitus, decreased hearing, headache, dysphoria, GI side effects, visual disturbances, hypoglycemia
Mefloquine	Neuropsychiatric reactions
Pyrimethamine	Rare blood dyscrasias, rash, vomiting, seizures
Artesunate	Idiosyncratic acute hepatic reactions, ataxia

TRADE NAMES

In addition to generic and fixed-combination preparations, the following trade-named materials are some of the other compounds used for parasitic diseases around the world.

Antimalarials
Artesunate (from the U.S. CDC)
Atovaquone and proguanil (Malarone)
Chloroquine (Aralen)
Mefloquine (Lariam)
Primaquine (generic)
Quinine (Qualaquin)
Quinidine (Quinora, Quin-G, Cardioquin)

Antiprotozoals
Eflornithine (Vaniqa)
Furazolidone (Furoxone)
Iodoquinol (Yodoxin, Diquinol)
Melarsoprol (Arsobal)
Metronidazole (Flagyl)
Nitazoxanide (Alinia)
Paromomycin (Humatin)
Pentamidine isethionate (Pentam 300, Nebupent)
Pyrimethamine (Daraprim)
Sodium stibogluconate (Pentostam)
Tinidazole (Tindamax)

NEW DEVELOPMENTS

Antimalarials

The emergence of multidrug-resistant *P. falciparum* has stimulated the search for new forms of treatment and prophylaxis for malaria. Among the newer compounds are the artemisinin derivatives, which include artesunate. These were identified in studies of qinghaosu, the Chinese herbal treatment for malaria derived from the wormwood plant *Artemisia annua*. Studies are ongoing in search of agents to treat drug-resistant strains.

Drugs used to treat Chagas disease are toxic and variably effective in eradicating *Trypanosoma cruzi*, and better and more tolerable drugs are needed. With respect to African sleeping sickness, eflornithine is effective and reasonably well tolerated for the treatment of *T. brucei gambiense*, but economic and logistical factors have restricted its production, and supplies are very limited. Drugs for the treatment of the hemolymphatic and CNS stages of *T. brucei rhodesiense* have substantial and, at times, life-threatening toxicity.

Pentavalent antimonials remain the treatment of choice for leishmaniasis in many areas, despite their toxicity and reports of clinical failures and resistance. Liposomal and lipid-associated amphotericin B preparations are effective and theoretically attractive because they target macrophages, the only cells infected by *Leishmania* species. Unfortunately, these preparations are expensive and must be administered parenterally. The most exciting recent advance in this area has been the development of miltefosine, a phosphocholine analogue administered orally. It is currently the drug of choice for treating visceral leishmaniasis in India, where resistance to sodium stibogluconate is common. Although it has adverse GI and hepatic effects, these are seldom severe enough to require discontinuation of therapy. In time, this drug may become more widely used.

Several potential drug targets have been identified recently for *Cryptosporidium* and *Toxoplasma*, and drug development is ongoing, with several lead candidates identified.

CLINICAL RELEVANCE FOR HEALTHCARE PROFESSIONALS

Healthcare providers are less likely to encounter individuals with parasitic diseases, as they are relatively uncommon. However, with a mobile society, many individuals may travel to areas where malaria is endemic and may contract the disease. Individuals receiving antiprotozoal drugs may experience skin rashes, varying degrees of GI distress, and neurological complications that could range from headaches and tremors to confusion, acute psychosis, and seizures. The severity of the infection will also impact the ability of a patient to actively engage in aerobic activities. It is important to know the medications an individual patient is taking to understand the potential for other drug interactions that may occur.

SELF-ASSESSMENT QUESTIONS

1. Why is chloroquine ineffective for treating recurrent episodes of fever and headache caused by infection with *Plasmodium ovale*?
   A. It does not cross the blood-brain barrier.
   B. It does not eradicate the dormant hepatic forms of the organism.
   C. It does not kill infected mosquitoes upon their next blood meal.
   D. It is an ineffective blood schizonticide.
   E. It is an ineffective gametocide.

2. Which of the following drugs leads to hemolysis in persons with glucose-6-phosphate dehydrogenase deficiency?
   A. Chloroquine.
   B. Doxycycline.
   C. Mefloquine.
   D. Primaquine.
   E. Pyrimethamine.

3. A 27-year-old woman has just returned from a trip to Southeast Asia. Over the past 24 hours, she has developed a fever of 104°F, shaking, and chills. A blood smear reveals *P. vivax*. Which one of the following drugs would you prescribe to eradicate the exoerythrocytic phase of the organism?
   A. Chloroguanide.
   B. Chloroquine.
   C. Primaquine.
   D. Pyrimethamine.
   E. Quinacrine.

4. Which of the following drugs or drug combinations would you prescribe to treat the erythrocytic stage of malaria?
   A. Primaquine.
   B. Chloroquine.
   C. Atovaquone/proguanil.
   D. A and B are both correct.
   E. B and C are both correct.

FURTHER READING

Griffith KS, Lewis LS, Mali S, Parise ME. Treatment of malaria in the United States. *JAMA*. 2007;297:2264–2277.

Krishna S, Bustamante L, Haynes RK, Staines HM. Artemisinins: their growing importance in medicine. *Trends Pharmacol Sci*. 2008;29(10):520–527.

WEBSITES

www.cdc.gov/travel
This website is maintained by the United States Centers for Disease Control and Prevention, and provides an interactive module on traveler health issues around the world for both clinicians and consumers.

http://apps.who.int/iris/bitstream/10665/162441/1/9789241549127_eng.pdf
This is a direct link to the World Health Organization Guidelines for the Treatment of Malaria, 3rd edition, 2015.

https://www.cdc.gov/malaria/index.html
This website is maintained by the United States Centers for Disease Control and Prevention and is a valuable source of information about malaria.

https://www.cdc.gov/parasites/about.html
This an also a link to the website maintained by the United States Centers for Disease Control and Prevention and is an excellent source for information about parasites and associated disorders.

Anthelmintics and Ectoparasiticides

Mona M. McConnaughey and J. Scott McConnaughey

MAJOR DRUG CLASSES

Anthelmintics
    Benzimidazoles (mebendazole and albendazole)
    Diethylcarbamazine
    Ivermectin
    Praziquantel
    Pyrantel pamoate
Ectoparasiticides

ABBREVIATIONS

GABA	γ-Aminobutyric acid
GI	Gastrointestinal

THERAPEUTIC OVERVIEW

Helminths, or parasitic worms, are large multicellular organisms that infect millions of people worldwide and lead to numerous diseases. The helminths include the nematodes (roundworms), the platyhelminths (flatworms) that include the trematodes (flukes) and cestodes (tapeworms), and the acanthocephalins (thorny-headed worms). According to the United States Centers for Disease Control and Prevention (CDC), roundworms affect more than 800 million people worldwide, and hookworm, which is a leading cause of iron-deficiency anemia in many areas, affects more than 550 million people worldwide.

Humans become exposed to mature helminths or larvae through soil, water, by ingesting raw or undercooked meat from an infected intermediate host, or transmission through a bite from an arthropod vector. The clinical manifestations of helminthic diseases are proportionate to both the worm burden and type of worm.

Soil-transmitted helminths, which are most prevalent, include roundworm, whipworm, and hookworm and are typically present in regions with warm, moist climates and poor sanitation. These worms reside in the intestines of the host, and if the individual defecates outdoors or if the feces is used as fertilizer, the eggs in the feces will be deposited in the soil. Roundworm and whipworm eggs mature in the soil to species that can infect humans if they consume unwashed or uncooked fruits or vegetables. In contrast, hookworm eggs hatch in soil and release larvae that mature to a form that can penetrate human skin, such as may occur if walking barefoot on contaminated soil. Pinworms, which are common in industrialized countries, are frequently spread among children after the mature female worm migrates from the rectum and deposits ova in the perianal area. Soil-transmitted infestations can lead to no symptoms or can result in gastrointestinal (GI) disturbances, blood and protein loss, and growth retardation in children.

Water-transmitted helminths include the blood flukes (trematode worms) of the genus *Schistosoma*, which are released from snails into freshwater and enter humans through direct penetration of the skin after contact with infested water. The larvae entering the body mature, and the adults live in blood vessels, where females release more eggs that can become sequestered in tissues leading to immune reactions and organ damage. Depending on the specific species, the resulting schistosomiasis can produce hematuria, fibrosis of the bladder and ureter predisposing to bladder cancer, renal damage, genital lesions, and possible irreversible alterations such as infertility.

Infection from the cestodes or tapeworms that live as adults in the GI tract of their definitive hosts and in cystic forms in organs of their intermediate hosts can be asymptomatic or lead to mild symptoms. In contrast, infections resulting from transmission through a bite from an arthropod vector lead to more serious consequences. Filarial helminths are transmitted by mosquitoes in a manner somewhat similar to that of *Plasmodium* (Chapter 63). Mosquitoes become infected through a blood meal from an infected host; the larvae mature within the mosquito, and when the mosquito takes another blood meal, the mature parasite larvae are deposited on the skin and enter lymphatic vessels. Although acute infections may be asymptomatic, they cause damage to the lymphatic and renal systems. Chronic lymphatic filariasis leads to lymphedema or elephantiasis. Infection with another filaria that has major consequences is transmitted by black flies and can result in river blindness and "lizard" skin.

In addition to the endoparasites, ectoparasites such as mites, fleas, ticks, and lice can attach to the skin, remain there for a prolonged period, and also lead to diverse consequences ranging from scabies-associated pruritis and pediculosis pubis to ulcers and paralysis.

Diseases caused by helminths, the causative organisms, and susceptibility to treatments are presented in the Therapeutic Overview Box.

MECHANISMS OF ACTION

Anthelmintics

The anthelmintics represent a diverse, albeit limited, group of compounds that have major importance for both human and veterinary medicine. Many of these agents may be considered "broad spectrum" because they are effective against several helminth species, whereas others are highly selective. Chemical structures of the anthelmintics are shown in Fig. 64.1.

The benzimidazoles include mebendazole and albendazole and are broad-spectrum anthelmintics. These agents are carbamates that bind to β-tubulin in susceptible nematodes, preventing microtubule polymerization necessary for many cell functions, including glucose uptake and mitosis (Fig. 64.2). These agents lead to cell death in rapidly

THERAPEUTIC OVERVIEW

Helminth-Associated Diseases and Treatments

Ascariasis (roundworm infection)
  Ascaris lumbricoides; susceptible to benzimidazoles and pyrantel pamoate
Ancylostomiasis (hookworm infection)
  Ancylostoma duodenale and *Necator americanus*; susceptible to albendazole, mebendazole and pyrantel pamoate
Enterobiasis (roundworm/pinworm infection)
  Enterobius vermicularis; susceptible to benzimidazoles and pyrantel pamoate
Lymphatic filariasis (roundworm infection; elephantiasis)
  Filarioidea family (*Wuchereria bancrofti, Brugia malayi*, and *Brugia timori*); susceptible to albendazole plus ivermectin or diethylcarbamazine
Onchocerciasis (river blindness)
  Onchocerca volvulus; susceptible to ivermectin
Schistosomiasis (flatworm/fluke infection)
  Schistosoma species; susceptible to praziquantel
Strongyloidiasis (roundworm infection)
  Strongyloides species; susceptible to ivermectin and albendazole
Taeniasis (tapeworm infection)
  Taenia saginata (from beef), *Taenia solium* (from pork), and *Taenia asiatica* (Asian); susceptible to praziquantel
Trichinosis (roundworm infection)
  Trichinella spiralis and others; susceptible to benzimidazoles
Trichuriasis (whipworm infection)
  Trichuris trichiura; susceptible to benzimidazoles

dividing cells and promote nematode expulsion in nondividing cells. The inhibition constant of these agents for nematode tubulin is 25–400 times greater than that for the mammalian protein, and serum glucose concentrations are not affected in the human host.

Diethylcarbamazine is used exclusively for filarial species. Although its mechanism of action is not well understood, it sensitizes microfilariae to phagocytosis, inhibits immune and inflammatory responses, perhaps as a consequence of cyclooxygenase inhibition, and inhibits nitric oxide synthase. Diethylcarbamazine also promotes organelle damage and filarial apoptosis.

Ivermectin activates glutamate- and possibly other ligand-gated Cl^- channels present only in invertebrates to hyperpolarize muscle membranes. This leads to tonic paralysis of the muscles and death of the parasite.

Praziquantel is rapidly taken up by tapeworms and flukes and increases membrane permeability to Ca^{++}, causing tetanic contractions and paralysis. It also generates reactive oxygen species and causes alterations in morphology, exposing parasitic surface antigens that can be destroyed in the intestines or passed into the feces.

Pyrantel pamoate is a tetrahydropyrimidine that is an alternative to the benzimidazoles with a similar spectrum of activity. The drug is a depolarizing neuromuscular blocker that causes a persistent activation of muscle nicotinic receptors, resulting in a spastic paralysis. The paralyzed helminths are expelled in the feces. Pyrantel also inhibits acetylcholinesterase, leading to increased spike discharge frequency, perhaps increasing susceptibility of the muscle receptors to depolarization blockade.

Ectoparasiticides

Most ectoparasiticides are used to kill organisms on livestock, horses, and pets but are also used superficially when these parasites live on the skin of humans. Adulticides kill the adult parasites, larvicides kill the larvae, and ovicides kill the eggs.

Benzyl alcohol kills lice by suffocation, while lindane blocks γ-aminobutyric acid $(GABA)_A$ channels and causes death of mites and lice by inducing convulsions.

Malathion is an organophosphate cholinesterase inhibitor insecticide (Chapter 7) that kills adult lice and ova by inhibiting the inactivation of acetylcholine. Permethrin is a pyrethroid insecticide that interferes with Na^+ channels and delays membrane repolarization, leading to parasite paralysis and death. Spinosad is a mixture of spinosyn A and D, two metabolites of a soil actinomycetes, that has insecticidal properties. The agent antagonizes both GABA and nicotinic receptors, leading to parasite paralysis and death.

RELATIONSHIP OF MECHANISMS OF ACTION TO CLINICAL RESPONSE

Anthelmintics

Treatment of helminthic infections is effective and generally well tolerated. Drug resistance has been reported but is infrequent.

Albendazole and mebendazole are active against common intestinal nematodes such as *Ascaris lumbricoides, Enterobius vermicularis*, and *Necator americanus* and may be effective for *Trichuris trichiura*. Albendazole may be superior to mebendazole for these infections, especially when used as a single dose, and is probably superior to mebendazole against most tissue-dwelling helminths. Albendazole is active against many cestode and nematode parasites and can be used to treat larval forms of pork and dog tapeworm infections.

Diethylcarbamazine is effective for the adjunctive treatment of lymphatic filariasis caused by all members of the *Filarioidea* family.

Ivermectin is widely used for veterinary parasitic diseases. Its major use in humans is in treatment of onchocerciasis and strongyloidiasis and as an adjunctive treatment for lymphatic filariasis. Ivermectin can also be used to treat cutaneous larva migrans, mites, and lice.

Praziquantel is active against all *Schistosoma* species as well as other flukes. It is a drug of choice for cestodes (tapeworms).

Pyrantel pamoate is effective for the treatment of intestinal nematodes such as *E. vermicularis* and *N. americanus*. It also may have activity against *Trichostrongylus* species.

Ectoparasiticides

These agents are all used topically to treat lice and mites. Lindane is considered a second-line agent because it can increase the risk of seizures in the patient.

PHARMACOKINETICS

Pharmacokinetic parameters for selected anthelmintic and ectoparasiticide drugs are listed in Table 64.1.

Anthelmintics

Albendazole is poorly absorbed from the GI tract, although absorption is enhanced when taken with a fatty meal. The drug is metabolized to the active form, albendazole sulfoxide. Albendazole sulfoxide reaches peak serum concentrations in 2–3 hours and has a half-life of 8–12 hours. Excretion is primarily in the bile.

Mebendazole is only slightly soluble in water and is poorly absorbed from the GI tract. Up to 10% of an orally administered dose is absorbed, metabolized, and excreted in the urine within 48 hours, while the remainder is excreted unchanged in the feces.

Diethylcarbamazine is readily absorbed following oral administration, with peak plasma levels reached in 1–2 hours. It is partially metabolized

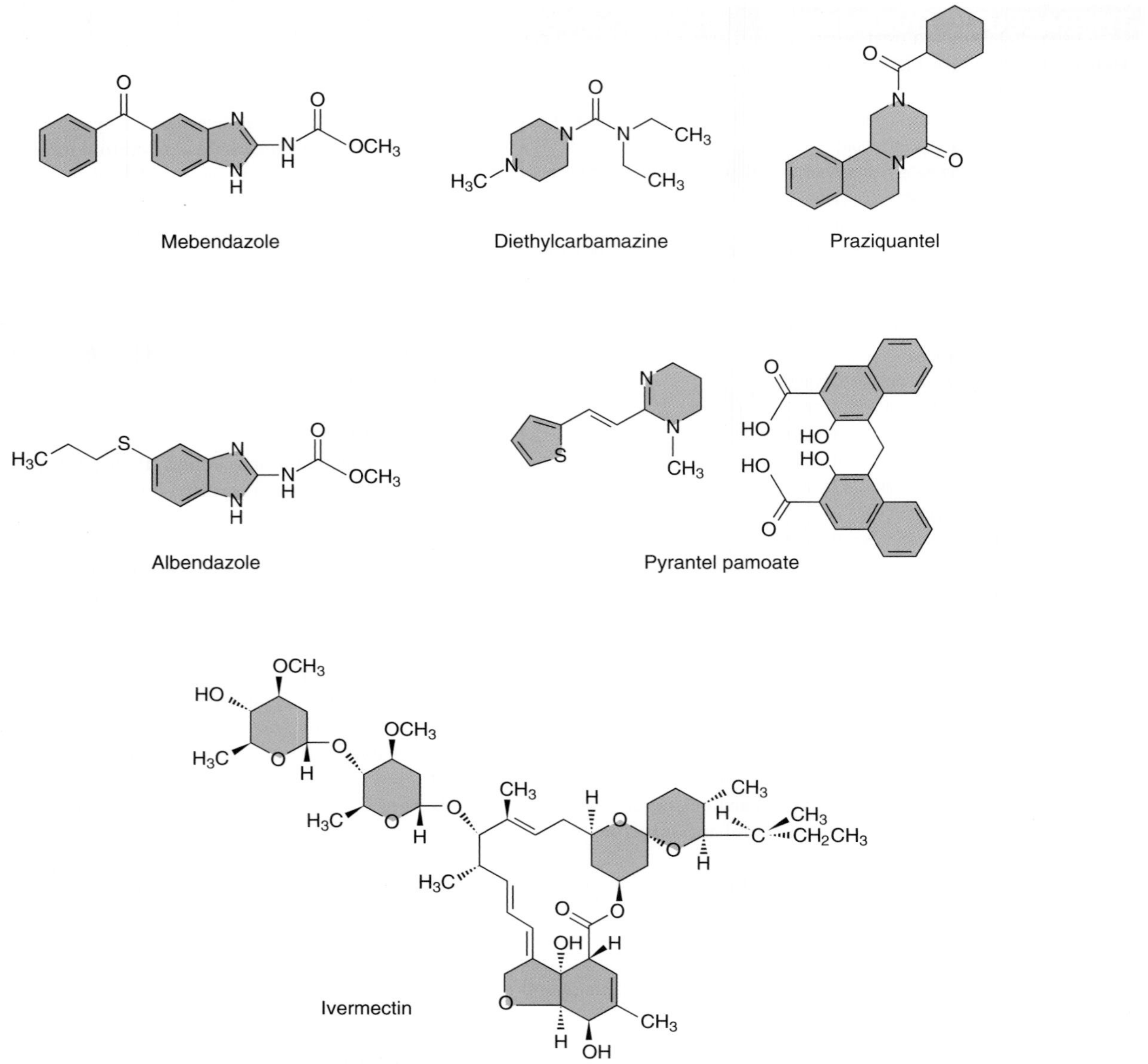

FIG. 64.1 Structures of Anthelmintic Drugs.

to an *N*-oxide, has a half-life of 8–12 hours, and is excreted via the kidneys.

Ivermectin is rapidly absorbed following oral administration and reaches peak serum levels in 4–5 hours. It is highly protein bound and has a half-life of about 12–16 hours. It tends to accumulate in adipose and hepatic tissues and is eliminated by biliary excretion with some enterohepatic circulation.

Praziquantel is well absorbed orally and reaches peak serum levels in 1–3 hours. Praziquantel undergoes extensive first-pass metabolism, generating inactive metabolites that are excreted primarily in the urine. Serum concentrations of praziquantel are increased in patients with moderate to severe hepatic impairment. Concentrations of praziquantel in cerebrospinal fluid are 15%–20% of that of the serum.

Pyrantel pamoate is poorly absorbed from the GI tract and therefore is mainly effective against susceptible helminths in the lumen of the GI tract. Most of the dose is excreted unchanged in the feces.

PHARMACOVIGILANCE: ADVERSE EFFECTS AND DRUG INTERACTIONS

Anthelmintics

Albendazole is usually well tolerated when given as a single dose for treatment of intestinal helminthic infections. Diarrhea and abdominal discomfort occur in some cases. Albendazole can cause some liver dysfunction and elevated transaminases. It rarely causes bone marrow suppression but has been shown to be teratogenic.

Mebendazole is well tolerated when used to treat intestinal nematodes. Some abdominal pain and diarrhea may occur. When administered at high doses for prolonged periods, it can produce alopecia, dizziness, transient bone marrow suppression with neutropenia, and hepatocellular injury.

Diethylcarbamazine may lead to itching and swelling of the face, particularly around the eyes. It can also lead to fever, skin rash, and painful and tender glands, although these adverse effects are uncommon. When used chronically to treat onchocerciasis (river blindness), it can cause inflammation and degeneration on the optic disc and retina.

Ivermectin is generally well tolerated with some mild GI effects, but when used to treat onchocerciasis (river blindness), it may trigger an allergic and inflammatory Mazzotti-type reaction resulting from the death of the microfilariae. Symptoms may include fever, pruritus, tender lymph nodes, headache, and arthralgias. Hypotension has been reported on rare occasions.

Praziquantel is frequently associated with mild side effects such as dizziness, headache, nausea, and abdominal pain. Allergic reactions can occur and are usually attributed to release of worm antigens.

Pyrantel pamoate has minimal toxicity at the recommended dose. Some nausea, diarrhea, and abdominal pain can occur. There have been some rare reports of dizziness, headache, and insomnia.

An overview of the adverse effects associated with various anthelmintic drugs is summarized in the Clinical Problems Box.

NEW DEVELOPMENTS

Anthelmintics

In the recent years, there has been a growing interest in novel approaches for the treatment of parasitic diseases. An increased understanding of helminthic neurotransmitters and receptors has led to the development of potential agents targeting the helminthic nervous system and its

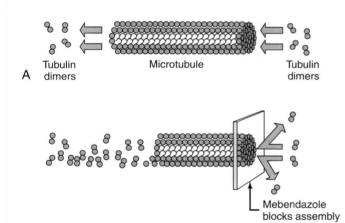

FIG. 64.2 Mechanism of Action of the Benzimidazoles. (A) Under normal conditions, tubulin dimers are continually being polymerized and depolymerized from the ends of the microtubule. (B) Albendazole and mebendazole can bind to β-tubulin and prevent polymerization, resulting in breakdown of microtubules.

components. Organometallic compounds have been found to be effective against various helminths, increasing interest in these compounds for new drug design. Essential antioxidant enzymes that are unique to helminths have recently been identified, making these appealing drug targets. Research is being done using solid lipid nanoparticles for the treatment of filariasis. Recent advances in schistosome genomics and transcriptomics have identified components that regulate an intrinsic apoptotic cell death pathway, raising the prospect of developing novel treatments for schistosomiasis that affect this pathway.

CLINICAL RELEVANCE FOR HEALTHCARE PROFESSIONALS

Healthcare providers treating patients with anthelmintic and ectoparasitic drugs should be aware of the major side effects and drug interactions associated with these agents. Nematode infestations such as pinworm or roundworm are common and will be dealt with frequently. Flukes and tapeworms are less commonly seen. It is important to understand how these infections are transmitted and which major drugs are effective. Lice and mites infest up to 12 million or more people annually in the United States, and it is important for the primary healthcare provider to understand transmission and treatment. Caution should be exercised when prescribing these agents to women who might be pregnant.

Patients with poor sanitation practices and poor dental hygiene have increased risk for gum disease and the risk of acquiring a parasitic infection, so dentists should be aware of the major symptoms. Parasites can contribute to malnutrition and anorexia, which predispose patients to malodor and coated tongue. It is also important for all healthcare professionals to remember that many anthelmintic agents cause dizziness, hypotension, and tachycardia that may interfere with positional change. These medications must be used with caution in women who are or might be pregnant without confirmation of nonpregnant status or consultation with the patient's obstetrician.

TABLE 64.1	Pharmacokinetic Parameters of Selected Anthelmintic Drugs			
Drug	**Administration**	**Absorption**	**$t_{1/2}$ (hours)**	**Disposition**
Albendazole	Oral	Good with fatty meal	Extensive first-pass metabolism, 8–9	M, R
Mebendazole	Oral	Poor (5%–10%)	2.5–5.5	F
Diethylcarbamazine	Oral	Good	8–12	M, R
Ivermectin	Oral	Good	12–16	F
Praziquantel	Oral	Good	0.8–1.5	M, R
Pyrantel pamoate	Oral	Very little	—	F

F, Fecal; *M*, metabolized; *R*, renal excretion.

TRADE NAMES

In addition to generic and fixed-combination preparations, the following trade-named materials are some of the other compounds used for anthelmintic and ectoparasitic diseases around the world. Some anthelmintics are obtained only abroad or through the United States Centers for Disease Control and Prevention (CDC).

Anthelmintics

Albendazole (Albenza)
Diethylcarbamazine (Hetrazan; obtained from the CDC)
Ivermectin (Stromectol)
Mebendazole (Vermox, Emverm)

Praziquantel (Biltricide)
Pyrantel pamoate (Antiminth, Pin-X)

Ectoparasiticides

Benzyl alcohol (Ulesfia)
Ivermectin (Sklice)
Lindane (generic only)
Malathion (Ovide)
Permethrin (Elimite, Nix, Lyclear, Acticin)
Spinosad (Natroba)

SELF-ASSESSMENT QUESTIONS

1. A 5-year-old boy developed localized erythema and severe itching on his feet. He appears malnourished and lethargic despite reportedly eating a well-balanced diet. His mother reports that he typically plays barefooted in the yard and sandbox. Fecal samples reveal evidence of *Necator americanus*. Which of the following is the best treatment for this patient?
   A. Diethylcarbamazine.
   B. Ivermectin.
   C. Mebendazole.
   D. Metronidazole.
   E. Praziquantel.

2. While traveling overseas, a 35-year-old man and his wife eat pork prepared by a street vendor, which appears slightly undercooked. Within the next few weeks, they experience vague abdominal discomfort and generalized weakness. They both notice strange things in their bowel movements and take a sample to the physician, who identifies them as proglottids (tapeworm). Which of the following is the best treatment for these patients?
   A. Albendazole.
   B. Mefloquine.
   C. Mebendazole.
   D. Metronidazole.
   E. Praziquantel.

3. A 9-year-old girl is brought to the clinic by her mother who states that when combing through her hair, she thinks she found head lice. The diagnosis is confirmed, and a topical drug is prescribed that interferes with sodium channels. This drug is most likely:
   A. Malathion.
   B. Tetracycline.
   C. Permethrin.
   D. Ivermectin.
   E. Spinosad.

4. A 7-year-old male patient presents complaining of pruritis in the anal area. He is diagnosed as having a pinworm infection (*Enterobius vermicularis*) and prescribed an agent that binds to β-tubulin, preventing polymerization, thus decreasing ATP level and killing the worm. This drug is most likely:
   A. Albendazole.
   B. Ivermectin.
   C. Diethylcarbamazine.
   D. Pyrantel pamoate.
   E. Praziquantel.

5. A 25-year-old male medical student presents with mild fever, arthralgia in multiple joints, and hepatomegally. CBC shows marked eosinophilia, and upon questioning, the patient reveals a recent volunteer aid trip to Egypt, where he waded in the Nile about 1 month before presentation. Stool examination and serum antibody testing are positive for *Schistosoma mansoni*. The recommended medication would be:
   A. Ivermectin.
   B. Chloramphenicol.
   C. Praziquantel.
   D. Pyrantel pamoate.
   E. Mebendazole.

FURTHER READING

Rana AK, Misra-Bhattacharya S. Current drug targets for helminthic diseases. *Parasitol Res.* 2013;112(5):1819–1831.

Tchuem Tchuente LA. Control of soil-transmitted helminthes in sub-Saharan Africa: diagnosis, drug efficacy concerns and challenges. *Acta Trop.* 2011;120(suppl 1):S4–S11.

WEBSITES

https://www.cdc.gov/parasites/about.html
This website is maintained by the United States Centers for Disease Control and Prevention and is an excellent source for general information on parasites both for clinicians and consumers.

https://www.neglecteddiseases.gov/usaid-target-diseases/soil-transmitted-helminths
This website is maintained by the United States Agency for International Development (USAID) and contains resources and additional links regarding soil-transmitted helminths.

https://www.cdc.gov/ticks/
This website is maintained by the United States Centers for Disease Control and Prevention and provides information on ticks, the health problems associated with ticks, and strategies/treatments to manage tickborne illnesses.

65

Antiviral Agents

LaToya M. Griffin and Margaret Nelson

THERAPEUTIC OVERVIEW

Viruses are responsible for significant morbidity and mortality in populations worldwide. These infectious agents consist of a core genome of nucleic acid (either DNA or RNA) contained in a protein shell (capsid), sometimes surrounded by a lipoprotein membrane known as an envelope (Fig. 65.1).

Although viruses can survive as viral particles (virions) outside of a host, they cannot replicate independently. Rather, they must enter cells and use the energy-generating, DNA- or RNA-replicating, and protein-synthesizing pathways of the host cell to replicate. In essence, viruses hijack the cellular machinery of its host to multiply. Thus viral infections cause a wide range of structural and biochemical effects on host cells and often lead to cell death. Some viruses can integrate a copy of their genetic material into host chromosomes, achieving viral latency, in which clinical illness can recur without reexposure to the virus.

Many antiviral agents inhibit single steps in the viral replication cycle and are considered virustatic—that is, they do not destroy a given virus but temporarily halt replication. Further, for an antiviral agent to be optimally effective, the patient must have a competent host immune system that can eliminate or effectively stop virus replication. Patients with immunosuppressive conditions are prone to frequent and often severe viral infections that may recur when antiviral drugs are discontinued. Thus prolonged suppressive therapy is often necessary. Further, there is no antiviral agent that eradicates latent viruses, and viral strains can develop that are resistant to specific drugs. Approaches to the treatment of viral infections are summarized in the Therapeutic Overview Box, and some virus families that infect humans and associated illnesses are listed in Table 65.1.

MECHANISMS OF ACTION

The Viral Replication Cycle

The mechanism of action of antiviral agents is not always well understood, but most currently available antiviral drugs interfere with various steps involved in the virus replication cycle (Fig. 65.2). The infection is initiated by the binding of the virus to an appropriate host cell, followed by endocytosis, uncoating of enveloped viruses, and the transfer of viral nucleic acids (either DNA or RNA) into the host cell nucleus. Within the nucleus, viral nucleic acids are replicated and transcribed into viral mRNA. The mRNA initiates protein synthesis followed by protein processing and assembly with the viral DNA/RNA to yield the

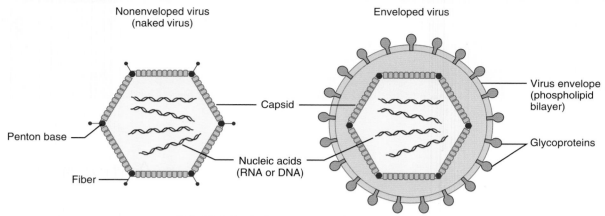

FIG. 65.1 Basic Components of Virus Particles.

TABLE 65.1	Virus Groups of Clinical Importance		
Virus Family	**Nucleic Acid**	**Associated Illnesses**	**Enveloped (E) or Nonenveloped (NE)**
Adenoviridae	DNA	Acute upper respiratory tract infections, common cold, conjunctivitis	NE
Hepadnaviridae	DNA	Hepatitis B, liver cancer	E
Herpesviridae	DNA	Genital and orolabial herpes, chickenpox and shingles, meningoencephalitis, mononucleosis, retinitis, roseola, Kaposi's sarcoma	E
Papillomaviridae	DNA	Papillomas (warts); cervical, vaginal, penal, anal, and oropharyngeal cancers	NE
Parvoviridae	DNA	Erythema infectiosum	NE
Arenaviridae	RNA	Aseptic meningitis, hemorrhagic fever, Lassa fever	E
Bunyaviridae	RNA	Encephalitis, four corners disease	E
Coronaviridae	RNA	Upper respiratory tract infections, severe acute respiratory syndrome (SARS)	E
Influenzaviridae	RNA	Influenza	E
Paramyxoviridae	RNA	Measles, mumps, respiratory tract infections in children	E
Picornaviridae	RNA	Poliomyelitis, diarrhea, respiratory tract infections, hepatitis A, aseptic meningitis	NE
Retroviridae	RNA	Leukemia, acquired immunodeficiency syndrome	E
Rhabdoviridae	RNA	Rabies	E
Togaviridae	RNA	Rubella, yellow fever	E

virion, which is released from the host cell to infect other host cells. The replication of retroviruses, such as human immunodeficiency virus (HIV), is described in Chapter 66.

The structures of representative antiviral agents are shown in Fig. 65.3.

Inhibitors of Cell Penetration

Docosanol is an aliphatic alcohol that inhibits the fusion of many enveloped viruses, such as herpes simplex virus (HSV), to the host cell membrane, thereby preventing virus entry; it does not act on the virus itself.

Palivizumab is a recombinant humanized monoclonal antibody that also inhibits viral entry into cells. It is directed against an epitope in the A antigenic site of the fusion (F) protein of the respiratory syncytial virus (RSV) envelope and prevents the entry of RSV into host cells.

Inhibitors of Viral Uncoating

Amantadine and rimantadine inhibit the replication of the enveloped influenza A virus by binding to the M_2 protein in the viral envelope, thereby preventing uncoating. The M_2 protein is a proton ion channel that facilitates acidification of the virus core at the onset of cell infection, which subsequently activates viral RNA transcriptase. Since influenza B lacks the M_2 protein, it is not susceptible to the action of amantadine and rimantadine. Further, a single amino acid change in the M_2 protein in the influenza A virus results in drug resistance. Although once extremely effective against influenza A, amantadine and rimantadine are no longer recommended for the treatment or prevention of influenza A due to the high resistance rates of the H1N1 and H3N2 viral subtypes.

Inhibitors of Viral Replication

Ribavirin is a synthetic guanosine nucleoside analogue mainly used in the treatment of hepatitis C virus (HCV), but it is also active against RSV, HIV, and influenza viruses. Ribavirin has several mechanisms that inhibit viral RNA and protein synthesis. Ribavirin may be considered a prodrug, as it is phosphorylated by adenosine kinase to the triphosphate, which binds to the nucleotide binding site on viral mRNA polymerase to decrease viral replication or produce defective virions.

Acyclovir is a synthetic deoxyguanosine analogue and is the prototypical agent used for the treatment of HSV-1, HSV-2, and varicella-zoster

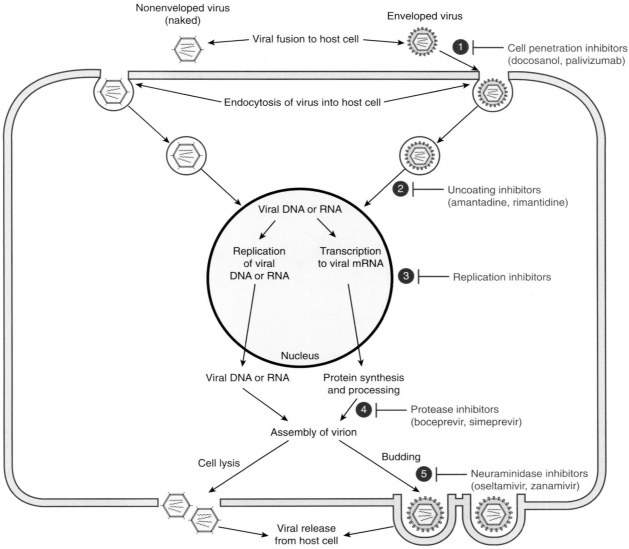

FIG. 65.2 Viral Replication. Shown are the processes involved in viral replication and the sites of drug action including (1) cell penetration, (2) uncoating, (3) replication, (4) protein processing by proteases, and (5) budding and release (via neuraminidase).

virus (VZV). Acyclovir may also be considered a prodrug, as it is metabolized to more active compounds. Acyclovir is activated by viral thymidine kinase, with selectivity due to its affinity for the HSV and VZV enzymes. Following thymidine kinase phosphorylation, acyclovir monophosphate is subsequently phosphorylated to the diphosphate by guanylate kinase and to the triphosphate by several other kinases. Acyclovir triphosphate inhibits DNA replication in two ways. It competes with deoxyguanosine triphosphate for incorporation into viral DNA, leading to viral DNA polymerase inhibition. Further, after incorporation into the DNA, acyclovir terminates viral DNA elongation. Acyclovir selectively accumulates in infected cells because the thymidine kinase required for initial phosphorylation is much more active in the virus than in host cells. Moreover, the subsequent active compound, acyclovir triphosphate, cannot cross cell membranes. The resulting concentration of acyclovir triphosphate is 50–100 times greater in infected cells compared to uninfected cells, resulting in minimal toxic effects on healthy host cells.

Several agents related to acyclovir with a similar spectrum of activity are available. Valacyclovir, an L-valyl ester of acyclovir, is a prodrug of acyclovir that is rapidly converted to acyclovir in the intestines and liver and leads to serum levels of acyclovir that are 3–5 times greater than those following oral acyclovir. Penciclovir is another guanosine analogue, and famciclovir is the oral prodrug of penciclovir. Like acyclovir, penciclovir activation requires phosphorylation by viral kinases. Importantly, penciclovir triphosphate exhibits a lower affinity for DNA polymerase compared to acyclovir triphosphate but accumulates in the cell to a much more appreciable extent than acyclovir.

Ganciclovir is another synthetic deoxyguanosine analogue and is used to inhibit replication of cytomegalovirus (CMV). Like acyclovir, ganciclovir is a prodrug that is phosphorylated by the CMV serine/threonine kinase phosphotransferase UL97. Triphosphorylated ganciclovir inhibits viral DNA polymerase and leads to early chain termination. Valganciclovir is a prodrug of ganciclovir and is rapidly converted to ganciclovir via first-pass metabolism.

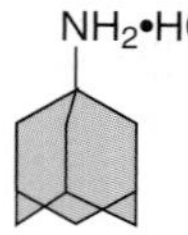

FIG. 65.3 Structures of Representative Antiviral Drugs.

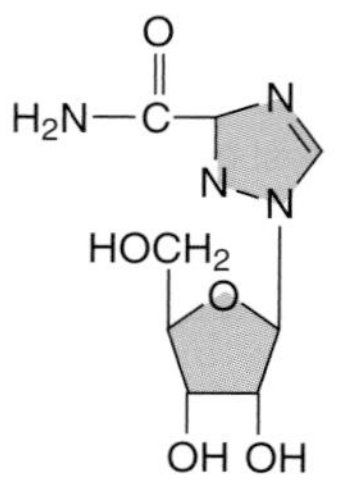

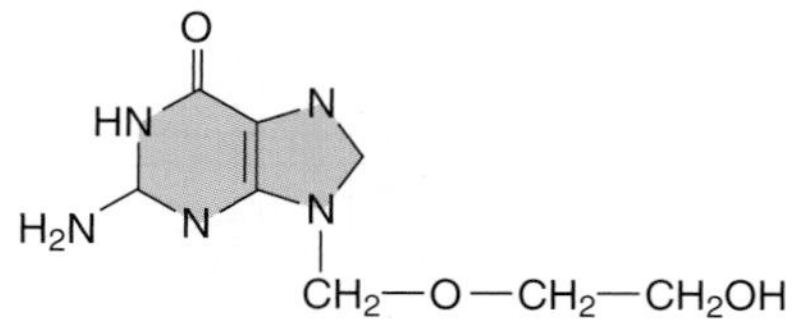

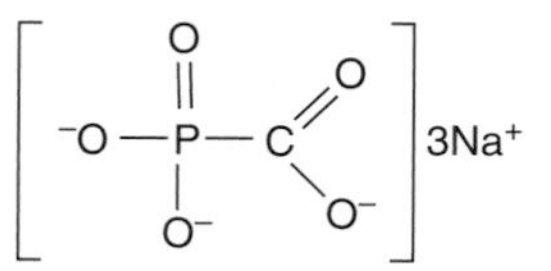

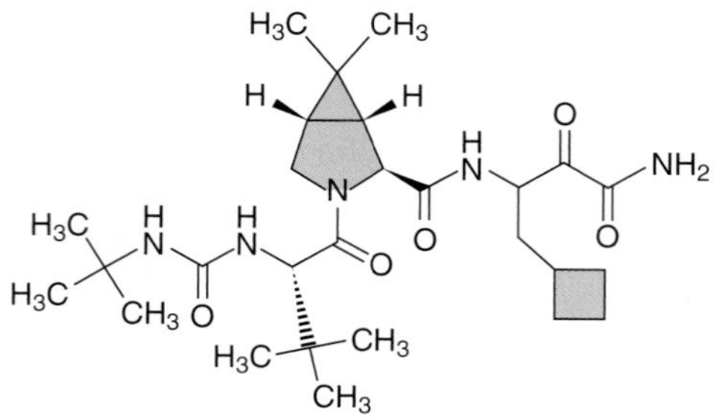

Trifluridine, or trifluorothymidine, is a fluorinated pyrimidine analogue that is incorporated into viral DNA during replication, thereby leading to the formation of mutant proteins and inhibition of viral DNA synthesis. It also inhibits thymidylate synthetase, inhibiting DNA synthesis. **Idoxuridine** is an iodinated deoxyuridine analogue that is also incorporated into viral DNA during replication in place of thymidine, leading to inhibition of thymidylate synthetase and viral DNA polymerases, thereby inhibiting further DNA chain elongation. The activation of trifluridine and idoxuridine is dependent upon host cell kinases, rather than viral thymidine kinases. Because viral thymidine kinase is not required for activation, trifluridine and idoxuridine have activity against HSVs that contain thymidine kinase–deficient mutants, which are resistant to acyclovir.

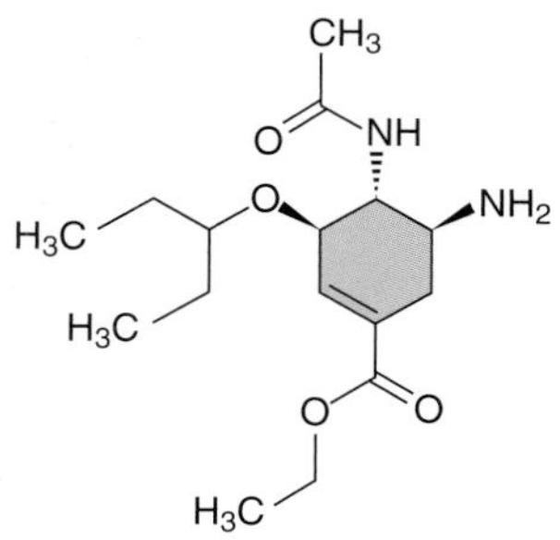

Cidofovir is a synthetic cytosine analogue used primarily to treat CMV retinitis. Unlike acyclovir, the conversion of cidofovir to its active form, cidofovir diphosphate, is independent of viral kinases. Upon activation by host cell kinases, cidofovir inhibits DNA replication via inhibition of viral DNA polymerase. Because it does not require viral enzyme activation, cidofovir shows activity against many acyclovir- and ganciclovir-resistant viral strains.

Foscarnet is an organic pyrophosphate analogue active against acyclovir-resistant herpes and varicella viruses. Foscarnet does not require activation by cellular enzymes, and it exerts it antiviral activity by attaching to the pyrophosphate site on replicative enzymes, thereby inhibiting the activity of DNA polymerases, RNA polymerases, and reverse transcriptases. Structural alterations in CMV DNA polymerase have led to resistance against foscarnet.

Adefovir dipivoxil is a diester prodrug of adefovir, an acyclic adenine nucleotide analogue of adenosine monophosphate that is phosphorylated by host cell kinases to the active diphosphate, which inhibits hepatitis B virus (HBV) DNA polymerase and causes chain termination after incorporation into viral DNA.

Telbivudine is a thymidine nucleoside analogue that also possesses antiviral activity against HBV. Following phosphorylation by host cell enzymes, telbivudine triphosphate inhibits HBV DNA polymerase and is incorporated into viral DNA, leading to chain termination. Although highly effective against HBV, the development of telbivudine resistance following prolonged (>1 year) drug exposure is common due to the development of mutations in the HBV gene *M204I*. **Lamivudine** is another thymidine nucleoside analogue active against HBV DNA polymerase, while **entecavir** is a guanosine nucleoside analogue also used to treat HBV. Entecavir competes with deoxyguanosine triphosphate to inhibit HBV DNA replication by inhibiting HBV DNA polymerase.

Sofosbuvir is a nucleotide analogue that inhibits HCV NS5B (nonstructural protein 5B) RNA-dependent RNA polymerase and is active for patients with the HCV genotypes 1, 2, 3, 4, 5, and 6. Sofosbuvir binds to the Mg^{++} ions in the active site motif of the polymerase to prevent replication of the HCV genetic material. Sofosbuvir is referred to as a direct-acting antiviral agent.

Approved as a chemotherapeutic agent, **5-fluorouracil (5-FU)** is an anticancer drug (Chapter 68) that irreversibly inhibits thymidylate synthase and interrupts normal cellular DNA and RNA synthesis. 5-FU is most effective on rapidly dividing cells.

Protease Inhibitors

Boceprevir and **simeprevir** are protease inhibitors approved for the treatment of HCV genotype 1 infection. All three agents inhibit HCV replication by attaching to the NS3/4A protease, which cleaves HCV-encoded polyproteins, thereby prohibiting viral maturation.

Neuraminidase Inhibitors

Influenza A and B express a unique neuraminidase enzyme that is highly conserved in both viruses. Neuraminidase catalyzes the removal of terminal sialic acid residues linked to glycoproteins and glycolipids that promote the release of progeny virions. Oseltamivir and zanamivir are analogues of sialic acid that inhibit neuraminidase, preventing virion budding and release.

Other Agents

Interferons (IFNs) are endogenous glycoproteins produced by lymphocytes, macrophages, fibroblasts, and other human cells in response to viral proliferation. IFNs inhibit the synthesis of viral proteins within a host cell. They bind to specific cell receptors, which activate signaling pathways that result in inhibition of viral penetration, uncoating, synthesis, or methylation of mRNA, translation of viral proteins, or assembly and release of virus. IFNs are used to suppress rather than treat HBV and to eradicate the virus in HCV and papillomavirus (HPV) infections.

Immunoglobulins are primarily used prophylactically, but some preparations possess antiviral activity against specific viruses, such as hepatitis A or B, and can be used for both treatment and prevention.

RELATIONSHIP OF MECHANISMS OF ACTION TO CLINICAL RESPONSE

All antiviral agents are virustatic and are active against replicating, not latent viruses. Viral infection genotype, severity, and location all determine the formulation, duration, and often, the number of drugs in a therapeutic regimen. Some infections require monotherapy for a short duration, such as acyclovir for the treatment of HSV, while others require continuous combination drug therapy (e.g., interferon alfa and ribavirin for the management of HCV). Many of the most effective antiviral agents target viral cycle pathways or undergo activation mediated by enzymes present only in viruses, processes that minimize toxicity to uninfected host cells. Due to the increasing specificity of drugs for viral targets, viruses are modifying the structures of their enzyme and protein targets and developing resistance. While useful for the prevention of infection or recurrent outbreak, antiviral drugs are often administered after infection has occurred and, as such, are most effective when administered early in treatment.

Generally, a drug is classified as active against a given virus if a greater than 50% reduction in plaque-forming units at an attainable serum concentration is achieved. In recent years, the polymerase chain reaction has provided the technology to allow detection of individual virus mutations, enabling physicians to predict viral susceptibility to many antiviral agents.

Inhibitors of Penetration

In the development of antivirals, certain agents that were used systemically were determined to be more toxic to host cells than infected cells. As such, the utility of these compounds is limited to localized topical administration. As an example, docosanol is available as an over-the-counter 10% topical cream to treat HSV. Docosanol reduces the healing time of HSV infection on the face or lips and decreases symptoms associated with HSV outbreak including itching, burning, and pain.

Palivizumab is recommended for the prevention of RSV in infants and children who are at high risk for infection, such as premature infants or pediatric patients with congenital heart defects.

Inhibitors of Viral Uncoating

Amantadine and rimantadine were used for many years for the treatment and prophylaxis of influenza A infections, with higher efficacy when given before exposure to the virus or within 48 hours of developing symptoms. These agents are no longer recommended for the treatment of influenza A due to the development of resistant influenza A virus strains (H1N1 and H3N2).

Inhibitors of Viral Replication

Ribavirin demonstrates antiviral activity against RSV, paramyxoviruses, and Lassa fever virus. Ribavirin is also approved for the treatment of HCV in combination with IFNs or sofosbuvir.

Oral acyclovir can be effective in suppressing recurrences of mucocutaneous HSV infections in immunosuppressed patients and can be used prophylactically in bone marrow and other transplant patients to prevent herpes recurrence in which it is most effective when started prior to and continuing after transplantation. Acyclovir is also effective in the management of moderate to severe varicella in specific groups, including patients with pulmonary or cutaneous disorders or those receiving long-term salicylate therapy or corticosteroids. Patients whose treatment is initiated within 72 hours of the onset of symptoms show decreased viral shedding and more rapid healing. Acyclovir is not effective in treating CMV pneumonia or visceral disease, Epstein-Barr virus, mononucleosis, or chronic fatigue syndrome.

For initial episodes of genital herpes, oral acyclovir decreases the duration of symptoms, time to lesion healing, and duration of viral shedding. Acyclovir also shortens recurrent episodes by several days. Recurrences are common after the termination of therapy as a consequence of latent virus because acyclovir only inhibits an actively replicating virus. To treat primary genital HSV, intravenous (IV) or oral acyclovir is recommended. To reduce the frequency of recurrences, shorten the duration of lesion, and prevent HSV-2 transmission to partners, oral suppressive therapy should be provided within the first day of lesion presence or during the prodrome that can occur prior to outbreaks. Suppressive acyclovir therapy decreases recurrences in patients by 70%–80% and improves quality of life. After discontinuation of acyclovir, recurrence rates generally return to near pretreatment levels.

Acyclovir administered IV is also used in the treatment of HSV encephalitis, neonatal HSV, and serious VZV infections. HSV encephalitis requires 14 to 21 days of IV therapy in which high-dose acyclovir is used to improve penetration across the blood-brain barrier. After HSV encephalitis is diagnosed, acyclovir should be administered as soon as possible to decrease patient morbidity and mortality.

Like acyclovir, valacyclovir has antiviral activity against HSV-1, HSV-2, and varicella infections and is often used for initial and recurrent genital herpes. Penciclovir is used to treat recurrent herpes labialis and is available as a topical cream. Famciclovir is used to treat new and recurrent HSV-1 and HSV-2 as well as acute zoster virus infection.

Ganciclovir and valganciclovir are used in the treatment of CMV retinitis, colitis, and pneumonitis, particularly in immunocompromised patients such as those with acquired immunodeficiency syndrome (AIDS) and transplant patients. In immunocompromised patients with CMV retinitis, ganciclovir administered IV delays disease progression, and combination therapy of ganciclovir and foscarnet is more effective than either drug alone. Genetic mutations in *UL97* confer viral resistance to ganciclovir. Valganciclovir is also used to treat CMV retinitis and to prevent CMV infection in transplant recipients.

HSVs that contain altered thymidine kinase have developed resistance to these guanosine analogues and are acyclovir-penciclovir–resistant strains. Resistance can also occur as a result of alterations in protein structures of viral DNA polymerase. Although these mutated viruses are resistant to acyclovir and related agents, they are susceptible to the antiviral drugs trifluridine, cidofovir, and foscarnet.

Initially developed as anticancer therapies, idoxuridine and trifluridine have been found to exert potent antiviral activity against HSV. Both agents can be used topically to treat herpes simplex keratitis. Trifluridine is formulated as an ophthalmic cream used for keratoconjunctivitis and recurrent epithelial keratitis caused by HSV-1 and HSV-2.

Cidofovir is used primarily to treat CMV retinitis. Because cidofovir does not require viral enzyme activation, it has activity against many acyclovir- and ganciclovir-resistant viral strains.

Foscarnet is also active against acyclovir-resistant herpes and varicella viruses and is used primarily to treat end-organ CMV diseases, such as retinitis. Foscarnet is only approved for IV administration in the treatment of end-organ CMV disease and is also effective against acyclovir-resistant HSV and VZV. To prevent toxicity, foscarnet should be titrated according to the calculated creatinine clearance of the patient prior to infusion. When used in combination, foscarnet and ganciclovir are more efficacious against CMV; however, toxicity is also increased when both agents are administered together. Structural alterations in CMV DNA polymerase have led to resistance against foscarnet.

Adefovir dipivoxil is approved for the treatment of hepatitis B.

Lamivudine rapidly decreases HBV replication with minimal toxic effects; however, its long-term utility is limited due to the increase in the emergence of lamivudine-resistant HBV when the drug is used alone. In addition, lamivudine has been effective in preventing mother-to-child HBV transmission if taken during the last 4 weeks of gestation.

Sofosbuvir is often used in combination with pegylated IFN alfa as well as ribavirin. Sofosbuvir is also available in a fixed-dose combination tablet with the HCV NS5A protein inhibitor ledipasvir for the treatment of HCV genotype 1a and 1b.

5-FU acts primarily as an ablative agent, destroying both infected and healthy cells and therefore should only be used externally over relatively small areas. 5-FU kills cells infected with papillomavirus (warts) and is formulated as a 5% topical cream for this purpose. It has also been used topically to treat condylomas caused by HPV.

Protease Inhibitors

Boceprevir and simeprevir are used for the treatment of HCV genotype 1 infection and are frequently combined with pegylated IFNs and ribavirin. Simeprevir, in combination with peginterferon and ribavirin, is a once-daily pill that can be used in patients with liver disease as well as HIV-coinfected patients with HCV genotype 1 infection.

Neuraminidase Inhibitors

Oseltamivir and zanamivir are approved for the prevention and treatment of influenza A and B. Zanamivir is administered via inhalation directly to the respiratory tract, where the concentration of drug is estimated to be greater than 1000 times that needed to cause 50% inhibition of neuraminidase. In recent screening, resistant strains have remained susceptible to oseltamivir and zanamivir.

Other Agents

IFNs have wide antiviral activity based on their mechanism of action. In addition to disrupting the replication of a large spectrum of viruses, IFNs also possess immunomodulatory and antiproliferative actions, further enhancing their antiviral activity. All three classes of human IFNs (α, β, γ) are nonspecific immune stimulators used to suppress, rather than treat, HBV and to eradicate the virus in HCV and papillomavirus infections. Various formulations of interferon alfa are available for the treatment of acute hepatitis C and chronic hepatitis B or C (often in combination with ribavirin).

Immunoglobulins are primarily used prophylactically but can be used for both treatment and prevention. Immunoglobulins have the ability to neutralize some viruses. The spectrum of immunoglobulin activity depends upon the presence of neutralizing antibody and the capacity of the virus to be neutralized by antibody. Hepatitis C is not neutralized by currently available immunoglobulin preparations, so administration is not recommended after exposure to these viruses. All agents are significantly less effective in immunosuppressed patients.

Standard human immunoglobulin contains antibodies that prevent and destroy hepatitis A infection; the vaccine is formulated as an intramuscular injection. Some human immunoglobulins have high titers against specific viruses such as hepatitis B and rabies and are more efficacious against these viruses than nonspecific immunoglobulins. Immunoglobulins are usually given intramuscularly as close as possible to the time of exposure to the virus. In some circumstances, an immunoglobulin should also be administered very close to the lesion (as in rabies) to provide high concentrations to lymphatic tissues. In most situations, intramuscular injection provides systemic immunoglobulin concentrations adequate to prevent the development of clinical infection. However, because immunoglobulins do not confer long-term immunity, they must often be given in a series of injections, together with vaccine therapy.

PHARMACOKINETICS

For most antiviral agents to be active, they must become concentrated within cells. Many compounds are nucleoside analogues and are rapidly metabolized to inactive compounds, which are then eliminated from the body. This necessitates frequent dosing to maintain adequate intracellular drug concentrations. The pharmacokinetic parameters for some antiviral drugs are listed in Table 65.2.

TABLE 65.2	**Pharmacokinetic Parameters of Some Commonly Used Drugs**			
Drug	**Routes of Administration**	**Peak Serum Concentrations (μg/mL)**	**$t_{1/2}$ (hrs)**	**Disposition**
Amantadine	Oral	0.3–0.7	12–18 (doubles in aged)	R (90%), M (9%)
Rimantadine	Oral	0.2–0.3	24–36	M (90%), R (10%)
Ribavirin	Aerosol, oral	0.8–3.5	9	M (60%), R (30%)
Acyclovir	Topical, oral, IV	0.6–10.0	3–4	R (80%), M (20%)
Valacyclovir	Oral	3.0 (ACV)	3–4	R (80%), M (20%)
Famciclovir	Oral	4.0 (PCV)	2–3 (PCV serum)	R (90%)
Ganciclovir	IV, oral	4–6	3–4	R (90%)
Foscarnet	IV	30	3	R (80%)
Lamivudine	Oral	2–3	5–7	R (70%), M (30%)

ACV, Acyclovir; *M*, metabolic; *PCV*, penciclovir; *R*, renal.

Inhibitors of Viral Uncoating

Amantadine is well absorbed and distributes throughout the body, where 65% of amantadine is protein bound. The plasma half-life of amantadine is 12–18 hours and doubles in the aged, necessitating dosage reductions. Drug concentrations in serum can vary widely based upon the age of the patient, although peak drug concentrations occur 2–4 hours after ingestion. Amantadine is eliminated by glomerular filtration and tubular secretion and is primarily excreted unchanged. Rimantadine is also well absorbed, and approximately 40% is protein bound. Rimantadine has a half-life of 24–30 hours in young adults and 32 hours in aged patients and those with compromised liver function and thus requires dosage adjustments in such patients. Rimantadine is extensively metabolized in the liver, undergoing hydroxylation, conjugation, and glucuronidation prior to urinary excretion.

Inhibitors of Viral Replication

Ribavirin is rapidly and extensively absorbed following oral administration, with a bioavailability of approximately 45%. Peak concentrations after IV administration are 10-fold greater than after oral administration. Ribavirin is administered via aerosol as a monotherapy for patients with severe respiratory RSV. Approximately 3% of the ribavirin absorbed accumulates in red blood cells in the form of ribavirin triphosphate, prolonging serum half-life to 40 days, during which time the compound is slowly metabolized and eliminated by the kidneys as the unchanged parent and metabolites.

Acyclovir is available as topical, oral, or IV formulations. The bioavailability of acyclovir is low (<20%), and the drug is modestly protein bound. Due to the short half-life, approximately 3 hours, oral administration of acyclovir requires frequent dosing. Poor absorption and the need for higher drug concentrations has led to different dosage formulations of acyclovir for the treatment of shingles. Percutaneous absorption of topical acyclovir is very low. Acyclovir is eliminated by glomerular filtration and tubular secretion and is mainly excreted unchanged. Other drugs that are also eliminated renally, such as methotrexate and probenecid, decrease the renal excretion of acyclovir by competing for elimination and can cause higher than desirable drug plasma levels.

Valacyclovir is only available in an oral form and has a higher oral bioavailability (54%–70%) than oral acyclovir. Valacyclovir quickly undergoes first-pass metabolism in the liver and intestines to acyclovir, resulting in serum concentrations of acyclovir that are 3–4 times higher than after oral acyclovir. Famciclovir is also only orally available and metabolized in the liver to its active compound, penciclovir. Bioavailability of famciclovir, once metabolized to penciclovir, is 70%. Penciclovir is also renally eliminated.

Due to its poor oral bioavailability, ganciclovir is administered IV and is readily bioavailable. Ganciclovir is eliminated primarily unchanged in urine, and therefore the plasma half-life can increase substantially in patients with severe renal insufficiency. Ganciclovir can also be administered intravitreally to treat CMV retinitis, in which it has a half-life of 50 hours. Valganciclovir is recommended to be taken with food and has a high oral bioavailability (60%). Valganciclovir is rapidly hydrolyzed in the intestines and liver to ganciclovir, with a half-life of 4 hours. Valganciclovir is eliminated through glomerular filtration and active tubular secretion.

Cidofovir is administered IV, and the half-life of its active metabolite, cidofovir diphosphate, is 17–65 hours, allowing for weekly dosing for 2 weeks followed by dosing every 2 weeks. Cidofovir undergoes renal elimination, with the dose based on renal clearance of the patient. To reduce the risk of drug-induced nephrotoxicity, cidofovir is administered with saline and probenecid.

Foscarnet is available only as an IV formulation with high bioavailability. Because foscarnet can bind calcium and other divalent cations,

up to 30% of the agent can accumulate in bone, with a half-life of several months. It is mainly excreted unchanged in the urine, and therefore dosage must be adjusted for impaired renal function.

Adefovir dipivoxil is quickly hydrolyzed by intestinal and serum enzymes into adefovir, which has a bioavailability of approximately 60%. Adefovir is eliminated through glomerular filtration and active tubular secretion. Dose modifications are recommended for patients with impaired renal function.

Telbivudine has a high volume of distribution, with approximately 3% of the drug plasma protein bound. Telbivudine has a half-life of 15 hours and is eliminated primarily by glomerular filtration. Lamivudine displays a high bioavailability, and absorption is slower when taken with food. Lamivudine undergoes minor metabolism; it is renally eliminated unchanged.

Entecavir has high bioavailability following oral administration (>99%), with a plasma half-life of 128–149 hours, thus requiring only intermittent dosing. Entecavir undergoes glomerular filtration and tubular secretion.

Sofosbuvir is approximately 60% plasma protein bound and reaches peak plasma concentrations within 2 hours after oral ingestion. Sofosbuvir undergoes hepatic metabolism to form the active nucleoside analogue and is eliminated primarily via the kidneys.

Protease Inhibitors

Simeprevir and boceprevir should be taken with food to maximize absorption. Simeprevir is highly bound to plasma proteins (>99%) with a half-life of 40 hours in HCV infected patients. Simeprevir and boceprevir undergo hepatic metabolism. Simeprevir is metabolized by CYP3A4, and boceprevir is metabolized primarily by aldo-keto reductases and to some extent via CYP3A4 and CYP3A5. Both drugs and metabolites are eliminated mainly through biliary excretion.

Neuraminidase Inhibitors

Oseltamivir is administered orally and is a prodrug of oseltamivir carboxylate. Once converted to its active form by hepatic esterases, oseltamivir is 75% bioavailable, with a half-life of 13 hours. Excretion of oseltamivir occurs mainly in the kidneys, and dosage adjustments are recommended for patients with renal insufficiency. Zanamivir is administered as an inhaled formulation and has a pulmonary half-life of 3 hours. Zanamivir undergoes minimal metabolism and is mainly excreted in urine unchanged.

Other Agents

IFN alfa-2a and alfa-2b are formulated as injectable (subcutaneous or intramuscular) preparations for the treatment of HBV and HCV, and absorption from injection sites is slow, with serum concentrations peaking within 8 hours and declining within the next several days. The biological activity of IFNs begins quickly after injection, reaches an apex at 24 hours, and decreases over 4–6 days. IFNs distribute throughout the body and can be detected in brain and cerebrospinal fluid, with trace amounts in urine. Elimination is complex, with liver, lung, kidney, heart, and skeletal muscle all contributing to inactivation. Approximately 30% of IFN undergoes renal elimination, and doses should be adjusted in patients with impaired renal function. Due to the short half-life of IFNs, formulations conjugated with polyethylene glycol (PEG) have been developed. These pegylated IFNs have slower subcutaneous rates of absorption and longer serum half-lives, and have more sustained antiviral activity. In the management of chronic hepatitis, IFNs are injected three times per week, whereas pegylated IFNs are injected once per week. IFNs are also effective when injected directly into condylomas or administered subcutaneously or intramuscularly for the management of papillomavirus infections.

As antiviral therapy, immunoglobulins are administered IV, subcutaneously, or intramuscularly. After intramuscular injection, immunoglobulin serum concentrations peak in 4–6 days and decline, with half-lives ranging from 20–30 days. After exposure to rabies, it is recommended that the wound be infiltrated with high-titer immunoglobulin to neutralize virus, with the remaining immunoglobulin administered intramuscularly. IV gamma globulin is administered every 3–4 weeks to agammaglobulinemic patients.

PHARMACOVIGILANCE: ADVERSE EFFECTS AND DRUG INTERACTIONS

Because many antiviral drugs are derivatives of nucleic acids, significant toxicities to uninfected cells can occur. Most toxicity involves bone marrow suppression with a loss of granulocytes, platelets, and erythrocytes. In many instances, systemic toxicities are so severe that the drug can only be administered topically. Further, because these compounds often interfere with human DNA or RNA synthesis, any antiviral agent should be used with the utmost caution in pregnancy and only when the potential benefits of treatment clearly outweigh the potential risks.

Inhibitors of Cell Penetration

Docosanol is generally well tolerated. Because it is provided as a topical cream, common side effects are burning, swelling, or redness at the site of application. Allergic reactions such as difficulty breathing, facial swelling, and delirium are rare but serious adverse effects.

Inhibitors of Viral Uncoating

Common side effects observed after administration of amantadine and rimantadine include nausea, anorexia, insomnia, nervousness, and light-headedness. More severe central nervous system effects, including delirium, hallucinations, and seizures that have been attributed to increased dopaminergic neurotransmission, are more often observed with the use of amantadine. These effects are often seen in aged patients or patients with impaired renal function or seizure disorders. In addition, these effects may increase while using antihistamines, anticholinergic agents, hydrochlorothiazide, and trimethoprim-sulfamethoxazole. Both agents are classified as pregnancy category C.

Inhibitors of Viral Replication

Ribavirin use often leads to flu-like symptoms. Approximately 10% of recipients exhibit hemolytic anemia and dyspnea in the initial weeks of therapy. Patients should have serial measurements of hemoglobin levels while on ribavirin. Aerosolized ribavirin is generally well tolerated, but bronchospasm may occur. Significant deterioration of pulmonary function has been reported in adults with chronic obstructive pulmonary disease and asthmatics receiving aerosol therapy. Ribavirin is contraindicated in pregnant women, as it is teratogenic and embryolethal in animal models. Patients exposed to ribavirin are advised not to conceive children for at least a 6-month period after exposure to the drug.

Acyclovir is generally well tolerated, with 1% of patients experiencing nausea, diarrhea, and vomiting. Due to the basic nature of acyclovir (pH 9–11), phlebitis is the most common side effect, occurring in 15% of patients. Acyclovir undergoes renal excretion, and although uncommon, crystalline nephropathy and transient elevated creatinine concentrations can occur. Such effects can be prevented by sufficient hydration and avoidance of rapid infusion rate. Probenecid and cimetidine decrease

the renal clearance of acyclovir and thus prolong its half-life. Acyclovir has not shown teratogenic effects in animal models, but at extremely high doses, chromosomal damage has been observed. Because its safety in pregnancy is unknown, acyclovir should be given only after its potential benefits and risks are carefully evaluated. To date, no congenital disorders have been identified in children of women who received acyclovir.

Although valacyclovir is well tolerated, nausea, headache, and diarrhea can occur. Confusion, hallucinations, and seizures have been reported at high doses. Famciclovir and penciclovir are also well tolerated, with minimal adverse effects. Most clinical experiences with ganciclovir involve its use in the treatment of CMV retinitis in HIV coinfected patients, with the most common side effects including myelosuppression (up to 40%), nausea, diarrhea, fever, and rash. The neutropenia and thrombocytopenia associated with bone marrow suppression are typically observed in the second week of therapy and are usually reversible. Concomitant use with nucleoside reverse transcriptase inhibitors increases bone marrow toxicity. To decrease significant side effects, some patients with CMV retinitis receive intraocular ganciclovir implants. Systemic toxicities associated with these implants include leukopenia, thrombocytopenia, hepatic dysfunction, seizures, and mucositis. When used in conjunction with zidovudine, azathioprine, or mycophenolate mofetil, ganciclovir can lead to enhanced myelosuppression. Ganciclovir is teratogenic, carcinogenic, and mutagenic.

Topical antivirals (idoxuridine, trifluorothymidine, trifluridine) are generally well tolerated. The most common side effects include mild local irritation, headaches, and nausea. Glucocorticoids are often used with these agents to lessen inflammation.

The major adverse effect associated with cidofovir exposure is a dose-dependent nephrotoxicity that is often avoided by adequate hydration. Cidofovir should not be used with other nephrotoxic drugs, including amphotericin B and aminoglycoside antibiotics. Importantly, cidofovir is contraindicated in patients with renal insufficiency. Cidofovir is embryotoxic and mutagenic.

Foscarnet is a strongly anionic compound that can chelate divalent cations, resulting in hypocalcemia, hypomagnesemia, and electrolyte imbalances in up to 20% of patients. The incidence of hypocalcemia increases with concurrent use of the antimicrobial agent pentamidine. Seizures, hallucinations, and headaches can occur, presumably as a result of hypocalcemia, and can be worsened with concurrent use of the antimicrobial drug imipenem. Foscarnet causes renal insufficiency, and doses must be adjusted in patients with decreased creatinine clearance. Up to 30% of HIV-infected patients receiving foscarnet therapy for CMV retinitis exhibit increases in serum creatinine. Foscarnet can cause anemia, which is exacerbated in the presence of zidovudine. Foscarnet has been shown to be mutagenic in animal models.

Adefovir dipivoxil is generally well tolerated but has been associated with renal damage. It is also embryotoxic and teratogenic at high doses. Oral adefovir is well tolerated with less serious side effects, but high doses of adefovir can lead to nephrotoxicity, lactic acidosis, and severe hepatomegaly with steatosis.

Telbivudine is associated with mild adverse effects, including fatigue, headache, and cough. Myopathy and peripheral neuropathy have also been reported. As in the case with nucleoside analogues, severe hepatomegaly with steatosis and lactic acidosis may occur both during and after therapy. In doses used for HBV therapy, minimal side effects are observed when taking lamivudine, as it has an excellent safety profile. Headache, nausea, malaise, and fever were reported in less than 15% of patients. When used as a monotherapy for HBV treatment, lamivudine is nontoxic, yet in patients coinfected with HIV, the use of lamivudine increases the risk of pancreatitis.

Most common side effects observed with entecavir include headache, dizziness, fatigue, and nausea. Patients discontinuing entecavir treatment

CLINICAL PROBLEMS

Amantadine	Dizziness, headache, insomnia
Rimantadine	Gastrointestinal upset, central nervous system effects
Ribavirin	Headache, gastrointestinal upset, dyspnea, teratogenic
Acyclovir	Central nervous system effects (nervousness)
Valacyclovir	Headache, dizziness, malaise
Famciclovir	Headache
Ganciclovir	Bone marrow suppression, central nervous system effects, rash, fever
Foscarnet	Bone marrow suppression, granulocytopenia, myositis
Adefovir Dipivoxil	Pancreatitis, neuropathy
Telbivudine	Dizziness, lactic acidosis
Entecavir	Myalgia, light-headedness
Sofosbuvir	Fatigue and headache
Oseltamivir	Vomiting, diarrhea, otitis media
Zanamivir	Headache, dizziness, fever, joint pain
Interferons	Neutropenia, fatigue, drowsiness

TRADE NAMES

In addition to generic and fixed-combination preparations, the following trade-named materials are some of the important compounds available in the United States.

Cell Penetration Inhibitors
Docosanol (Abreva)
Palivizumab (Synagis)

Viral Uncoating Inhibitors
Amantadine (Symmetrel)
Rimantadine (Flumadine)

Inhibitors of Viral Replication
Acyclovir (Zovirax, Sitavig buccal tablets)
Adefovir (Hepsera)
Cidofovir (Vistide)
Famciclovir (Famvir)
Foscarnet (Foscavir)
Ganciclovir (Cytovene)
Lamivudine (Epivir, Epivir-HBV)
Penciclovir (Denavir)
Ribavirin (Rebetol, Virazole, Copegus)
Ribavirin/interferon alfa-2b (Rebetron)
Telbivudine (Tyzeka)
Trifluridine (Viroptic)
Valacyclovir (Valtrex)
Valganciclovir (Valcyte)

Protease Inhibitors
Boceprevir (Victrelis)
Entecavir (Baraclude)
Sofosbuvir (Sovaldi)

Neuraminidase Inhibitors
Oseltamivir (Tamiflu)
Zanamivir (Relenza)

Immune Modulators
Immunoglobulins (H-Big, HyperHep, HyperRab, VariZIG)
Interferon alfa-2a (Roferon-A)
Interferon alfa-2b (Intron A)
Interferon alfa-n3 (Alferon N)
Interferon alfacon-1 (Infergen)

should be closely monitored, as severe acute exacerbation of HBV infection can occur. Patients who are also coinfected with HIV should not take entecavir unless the patient is also receiving highly active antiretroviral therapy due to the potential development of resistance against the latter.

Common side effects observed with sofosbuvir are fatigue, headache, nausea, and insomnia. Bradycardia has been reported in patients when sofosbuvir is coadministered with amiodarone and β-adrenergic receptor blockers. Additionally, patients with a history of cardiac disease are at an increased risk of experiencing heart dysrhythmia with sofosbuvir. As a substrate of P-glycoprotein, sofosbuvir is not advised when taking other agents that modify P-glycoprotein activity, including rifampin.

Protease Inhibitors

In patients receiving triple therapy for the treatment of HCV genotype 1 with simeprevir in conjunction with peginterferon alfa and ribavirin, the combination use of simeprevir leads to nausea, photosensitivity, and rash. A reduced efficacy has been observed with the *NS3 Q80K* polymorphism of HCV, and thus genotype screening is recommended prior to the initiation of therapy with simeprevir. Because simeprevir is metabolized primarily via cytochrome P450s, caution is advised during coadministration with other agents metabolized by such enzymes, as higher plasma concentrations of simeprevir have been reported. In addition, simeprevir contains a sulfur and is contraindicated in patients with a sulfonamide allergy.

Neuraminidase Inhibitors

Possible side effects of oseltamivir include nausea, vomiting, and headache. Adverse effects observed with zanamivir are cough, bronchospasm, transient decrease in pulmonary function, and nasal and throat discomfort. Administration of zanamivir is not recommended in persons with an underlying airway disease, including asthma or chronic obstructive pulmonary diseases.

Other Agents

Systemic IFN use is associated with significant and frequent side effects, and patients should be monitored closely for signs of toxicity. Common adverse effects in acute therapy include flu-like symptoms (e.g., severe malaise, fevers, and chills), myelosuppression, depression, leukopenia, and thyroid abnormalities. Adverse effects observed in chronic therapy include neutropenia, alopecia, reversible hearing loss, thyroid dysfunction, mental confusion, and severe depression. IFNs produce pain at the injection site, and in approximately 10%–20% of patients, the side effects experienced are too severe to warrant continuing therapy. Contraindications to IFN-alfa therapy are patients with autoimmune disease, history of cardiac arrhythmias, hepatic compensation, and pregnancy. In addition, caution is advised in patients with psychiatric pathologies, ischemic cardiac disease, thyroid disease, and epilepsy. Possible drug-drug interactions include theophylline, methadone, didanosine, and zidovudine, as concurrent use can worsen cytopenias.

Immunoglobulins are well tolerated, with pain at the injection site and brief low-grade fever the most commonly reported side effects.

True allergic reactions with urticaria or angioedema rarely occur, but IV gamma globulin can activate the alternative complement pathway, producing an anaphylactoid reaction.

Several of the clinical problems associated with the use of these agents are summarized in the Clinical Problems Box.

NEW DEVELOPMENTS

Antiviral agents are relatively selective toward specific viruses, and many viruses have developed resistant strains. Further, the discovery of emergent viruses, such as the Zika virus, necessitates new strategies for the continuous development of antiviral agents. Pathogenic viruses seem to be continuously emerging and reemerging, and major efforts are needed in many scientific arenas to combat unanticipated outbreaks. Although much progress has occurred in the past 20 years, more research is needed.

Recently, studies have reported that the G-protein–coupled receptor formyl-peptide receptor-2 (FPR2), which promotes viral replication, is activated following infection of a host cell with the influenza A virus and decreases the host immune response, leading to disease. Further, an antagonist of this receptor has been shown to protect animals from lethal infections. Thus further studies identifying new targets, such as this receptor, will undoubtedly lead to advances in drug development.

CLINICAL RELEVANCE FOR HEALTHCARE PROFESSIONALS

All healthcare professionals need to be vigilant, especially during the winter months when influenza may be rampant. Both professionals and their patients need to be aware of the early symptoms of viral infections and take all precautions not to spread disease.

SELF-ASSESSMENT QUESTIONS

1. A 78-year-old man presents for evaluation of a painful rash. He reports a sharp, burning pain radiating from his midback to his left side. He noticed a "rash" that spread "like a line" in the same area where he had pain. The rash has a dermatomal distribution from his spine around the left flank to the midline of the abdomen. It has erythematous patches with clusters of vesicles. He reports a history of chickenpox as a child. Among the following, which would be the most appropriate agent to prescribe?
   A. Abacavir.
   B. Entecavir.
   C. Famciclovir.
   D. Oseltamivir.
   E. Rimantadine.

2. A 25-year-old man was recently diagnosed with genital herpes and was prescribed acyclovir. Although acyclovir is well distributed into most cells throughout the body, it is more active in herpesvirus (HSV)–infected cells. Which of the following mechanisms best accounts for the selective action of acyclovir in HSV-infected cells as compared with uninfected cells?
   A. Competitive inhibition of viral thymidine kinase by acyclovir.
   B. Greater affinity of acyclovir triphosphate for cellular DNA polymerase.
   C. Greater inhibition of viral DNA repair enzymes.
   D. Inability to be converted to acyclovir triphosphate in virus-infected cells.
   E. Preferential conversion to acyclovir monophosphate in virus-infected cells.

3. Which of the following drugs is indicated for the treatment of either influenza A or influenza B?
   A. Amantadine.
   B. Foscarnet.
   C. Oseltamivir.
   D. Ribavirin.
   E. Rimantadine.

4. A patient is being treated for hepatitis C. Which drug combination would be the preferred treatment to eradicate the viral infection?
   A. Acyclovir and valganciclovir.
   B. Ribaviron and interferon alfa.
   C. Ledipasvir and sofosbuvir.
   D. Palivisumab and tenofovir.
   E. Cidofovir and valacyclovir.

5. Which nucleoside analogue that was used previously to treat HIV is now used to treat resistant forms of hepatitis B?
   A. Zanamivir.
   B. Valganciclovir.
   C. Lamivudine.
   D. Adefovir dipivoxil.
   E. Acyclovir.

FURTHER READING

Cento V, Chevaliez S, Perno CF. Resistance to direct-acting antiviral agents: clinical utility and significance. *Curr Opin HIV AIDS*. 2015;10(5):381–389.

Friborg J, et al. Combinations of lambda interferon with direct-acting antiviral agents are highly efficient in suppressing hepatitis C virus replication. *Antimicrob Agents Chemother*. 2013;57(3):1312–1322.

Herrick TM, Million RP. Tapping the potential of fixed dose combinations. *Nat Rev Drug Discov*. 2007;6:663–664.

Razonable RR. Antiviral drugs for viruses other than human immunodeficiency virus. *Mayo Clin Proc*. 2011;86(10):1009–1026.

Tcherniuk S, Cenac N, Comte M, et al. Formyl peptide receptor 2 plays a deleterious role during influenza A virus infections. *J Infect Dis*. 2016;214(2):237–247.

WEBSITES

https://www.cdc.gov/flu/professionals/antivirals/index.htm
This website, maintained by the United States Centers for Disease Control and Prevention, provides information to healthcare professionals on the use of antiviral agents in the treatment of influenza.

Antiretroviral Drugs for HIV

Amy Wecker

THERAPEUTIC OVERVIEW

The human immunodeficiency virus (HIV) is responsible for significant morbidity and mortality in populations worldwide. As per the Joint United Nations Programme on HIV/AIDS fact sheet (http://www.unaids.org), as of December 2016, 36.7 million people globally were living with HIV. Of those, 1.8 million people were newly infected with HIV in 2016, and 1.0 million people died from acquired immunodeficiency syndrome (AIDS)-related illnesses. Unfortunately, of the 36.7 million infected people, only about half were accessing antiretroviral therapy. Nearly 80 million people have become infected with HIV since the start of the epidemic in 1981, and more than 35 million people have died from AIDS-related illnesses. Fortunately, a remarkable amount of progress has been made in terms of understanding and treating the HIV virus given the relatively short time the epidemic has existed.

HIV belongs to a group of **retroviruses** called **lentiviruses**. The genome of retroviruses is made of RNA (ribonucleic acid), and each virus has two single chains of RNA. For replication, the virus needs a host cell, and the RNA must first be transcribed into DNA (deoxyribonucleic acid), which is accomplished with the enzyme **reverse transcriptase**. HIV infects mainly the **CD4+ lymphocytes** (T cells) but also infects monocytes, macrophages, and dendritic cells to a lesser degree, as these cells are also CD4+. Once infected, the cell is transformed into an HIV-replicating cell and loses its original function.

HIV is contracted through contact with infected bodily fluid, most commonly via sexual transmission or sharing needles. It is not generally contracted by contact with saliva. After transmission, the newly infected patient will "seroconvert," becoming HIV antibody positive in 2–12 weeks. This process is often accompanied by a flu-like illness, which will resolve on its own after a few weeks. The patient will then be asymptomatic for a variable period of time, usually 3–5 years. During this time, the CD4+ lymphocyte count will slowly decrease as the cells are killed by the virus, and the viral load (VL) will increase as the virus replicates. If the patient does not get tested and diagnosed at some point during this process, he or she will ultimately progress to AIDS.

A normal CD4+ lymphocyte count is roughly between 500–1500 cells/mm³ of blood. In an HIV-positive patient, when the CD4+ count drops below 200 cells/mm³, when the VL increases to over 100,000 copies/mL, or when an opportunistic infection develops, the patient is considered to have AIDS. When the CD4+ count drops below 200 cells/mm³, patients become susceptible to a variety of infections, including thrush and *Pneumocystis jirovecii* **pneumonia (PCP)**. When the CD4+ count drops below 50 cells/mm³, the list of opportunistic infections grows to include **mycobacterium avium complex (MAC)** infection, as well as **cytomegalovirus (CMV)** infection. Treatment can become very complicated. With early diagnosis and treatment of HIV infection, AIDS is completely preventable, and HIV becomes a chronic, manageable disease.

HIV Structure

An HIV virus particle is spherical, with a diameter of about 1/10,000 mm. Like other viruses, HIV lacks a cell wall and a nucleus. It has an outer coat, the viral envelope, which consists of two layers of lipids. Different proteins are embedded in the viral envelope, forming "spikes" consisting of the outer glycoprotein 120 (gp120) and the transmembrane gp41 (Fig. 66.1). HIV obtains this lipid membrane from its host cell during the budding process (Chapter 65). The gp120 is needed to attach to the host cell, and gp41 is critical for the cell fusion process. The HIV matrix proteins (including the p17 protein) lie between the envelope and core.

The viral core contains the viral capsule protein p24, which surrounds two single strands of HIV RNA and the enzymes needed for HIV replication: reverse transcriptase, protease, ribonuclease, and integrase. Of the nine virus genes, there are three—namely, *gag*, *pol*, and *env*—which contain the information needed to make structural proteins for new virus particles.

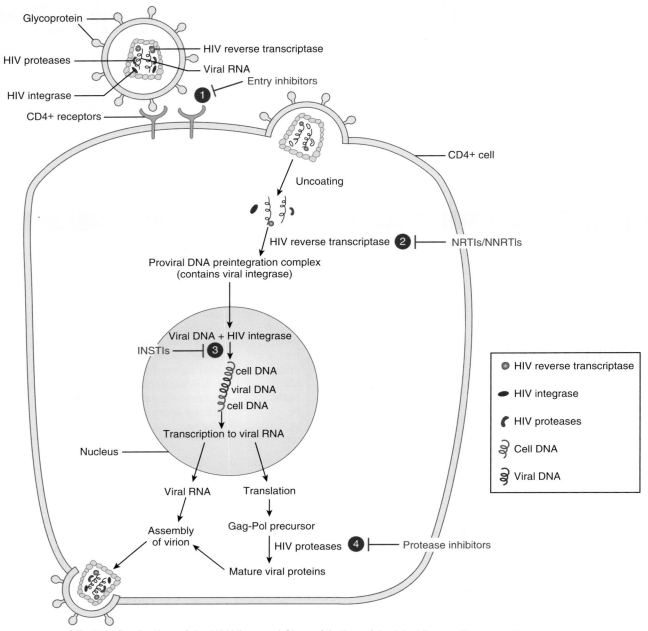

FIG. 66.1 Replication of the HIV Virus and Sites of Action of Antiviral Drugs. Shown are the processes involved in retroviral replication and the sites of drug action including (1) viral attachment and entry, (2) reverse transcription, (3) DNA integration, and (4) protein processing by proteases.

Currently available antiretroviral therapy (ART) consists of various combinations of antiretroviral agents, each of which inhibits a single step in the replication cycle. Because the optimal effectiveness of an antiviral agent depends on a competent host immune system that can help eliminate or effectively halt virus replication, immunosuppressed patients are prone to frequent and often severe infections that may recur when antiviral drugs are stopped.

For HIV, lifelong suppressive therapy with multiple active antiretroviral agents is necessary. Treatment usually consists of three active agents with or without a boosting agent. Currently, there is no antiviral agent that eliminates viral latency. Strains of HIV resistant to specific drugs can also develop. Several agents are converted in the body to active compounds (e.g., tenofovir prodrugs), and all antiretrovirals must

be present continuously to have a lasting antiviral effect. Approaches to the treatment of HIV with drugs are summarized in the Therapeutic Overview Box.

THERAPEUTIC OVERVIEW

Approaches to treatment of HIV include:
Block viral entry to CD4+ cells
Inhibit reverse transcriptase
Inhibit integration of the viral DNA into the host DNA
Inhibit protein processing

MECHANISMS OF ACTION

HIV Viral Replication Cycle

Understanding the steps involved in HIV infection and replication has led to the development of drugs that interfere with this process at various stages. This replication cycle and sites of drug action are shown in Fig. 66.1.

An HIV virion first binds to a receptor on the surface of its appropriate host cell, the CD4+ T-lymphocyte, to initiate an infection. This is usually the chemokine receptor 5 (CCR5) in a patient who has not been exposed previously to HIV therapy (CCR5-tropic virus), the chemokine receptor type 4 (CXCR4) in treatment-experienced patients (CXCR4-tropic virus), or both receptors (dual/mixed-tropic virus). Through a fusion process, the viral genome enters the cell, uncoats, and disassembles. An HIV-specific **reverse transcriptase** converts viral RNA into DNA, which enters the CD4+ cell nucleus. Within the host nucleus, the **HIV integrase** incorporates the HIV DNA into the cell's chromosomes. The host cell produces a copy of the HIV genome for packaging as new virions and viral messenger RNA, which is the template for protein synthesis. An HIV-specific **protease** hydrolyzes HIV polyproteins into smaller subunits, which assemble to form mature infectious virions.

Five classes of compounds have been used to interfere with the HIV reproductive cycle. These include **entry inhibitors, nucleoside reverse transcriptase inhibitors (NRTIs), nonnucleoside reverse transcriptase inhibitors (NNRTIs), integrase inhibitors (INSTIs), and protease inhibitors (PIs)**. Anti-HIV therapy with multiple agents has been very effective in limiting the progression to AIDS in persons carrying HIV. Chemical structures of representative drugs from each class are shown in Fig. 66.2.

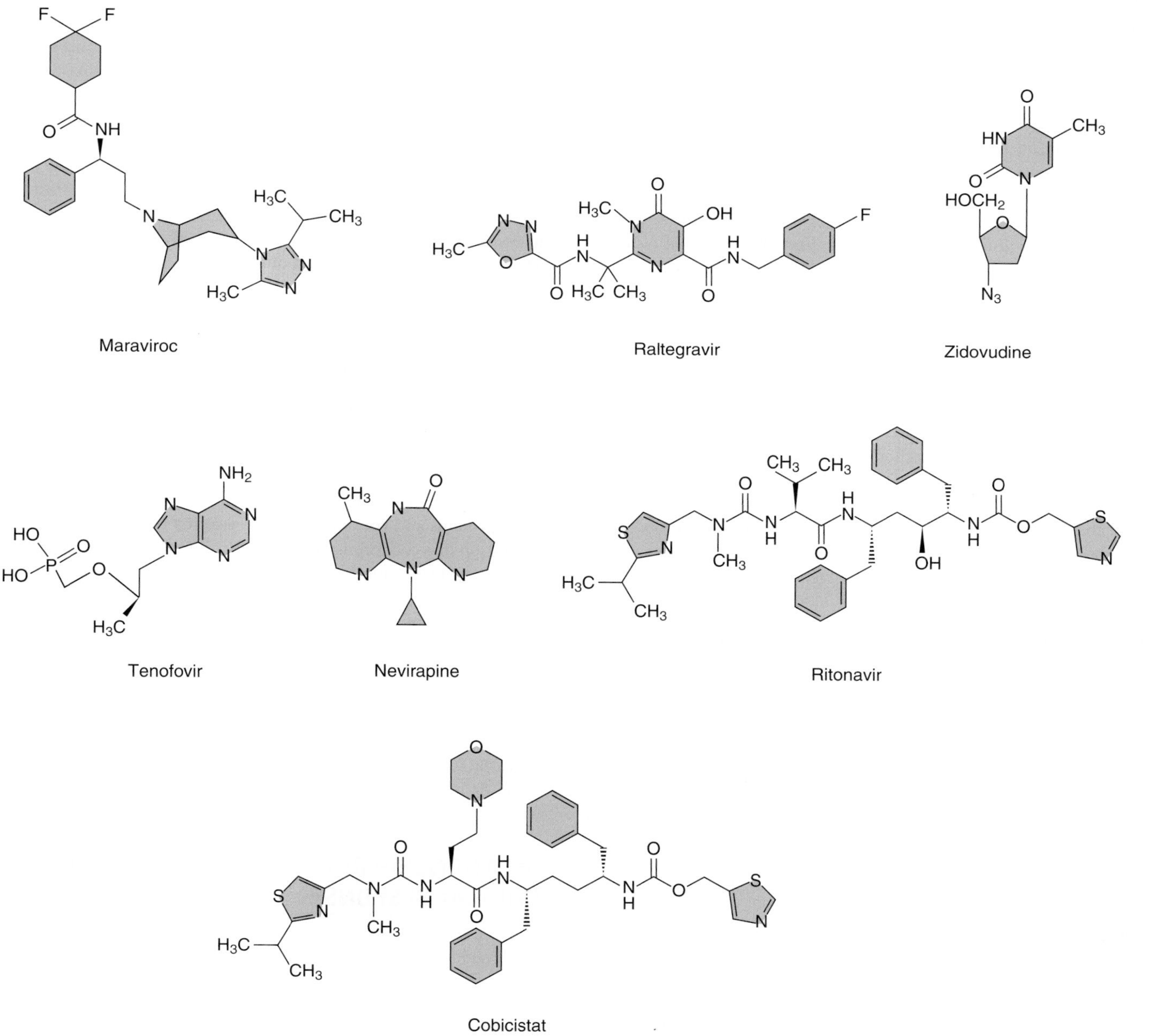

Maraviroc

Raltegravir

Zidovudine

Tenofovir

Nevirapine

Ritonavir

Cobicistat

FIG. 66.2 Structures of Representative Drugs Used for the Treatment of HIV.

Entry Inhibitors

HIV entry into cells is accomplished by a complex series of virus host interactions. Initially, virus approximates the CD4+ cell by interactions of HIV surface proteins and the host CD4+ receptor. After approximation, host receptors (either CCR5 or CXCR4) interact with HIV surface proteins, resulting in folding of the HIV protein gp41. This folding results in fusion of the HIV envelope with the host cell membrane and insertion of the HIV nucleoid into the cell. Maraviroc is a small molecule, a slowly reversible antagonist of CCR5 that inhibits the binding of gp120 on CCR5-tropic viruses, preventing entry of HIV into cells. Resistance occurs when CXCR4-tropic or dual/mixed-tropic HIV viruses are present. Enfuvirtide is a 36–amino acid synthetic peptide that prevents entry of HIV into cells by engaging the gp41 coils, causing steric hindrance of protein folding required for fusion. Resistance occurs when mutations of gp41 are induced that alter conformation and folding.

Nucleoside/Nucleotide Reverse Transcriptase Inhibitors

Zidovudine (AZT) is the prototype NRTI for use in HIV infection. It is a thymidine analogue that is phosphorylated to mono-, di-, and triphosphate forms by cellular kinases in both infected and uninfected cells. NRTIs have two primary mechanisms of action. First, the triphosphate form is a competitive inhibitor, binding to the active site of HIV reverse transcriptase. Second, after the nucleoside is incorporated into the elongating DNA chain, the forming sugar phosphate backbone of the DNA is blocked from further elongation by substitution at the 3 position. This results in chain termination. In the case of AZT, this substitution is an azido (N3) group. AZT inhibits HIV reverse transcriptase at much lower concentrations than those needed to inhibit cellular DNA polymerases, leading to a more targeted effect against HIV.

Tenofovir is an adenosine monophosphate analogue that also inhibits HIV reverse transcriptase and causes chain termination and is the only nucleotide currently available for use. After ingestion, tenofovir is phosphorylated by cellular enzymes to the diphosphate, which also inhibits mammalian and mitochondrial DNA polymerases, albeit weakly relative to inhibition of HIV reverse transcriptase.

Differences in NRTIs are based primarily on which nucleic acid is used and the type of substitution that causes chain termination. NRTIs have been produced for each of the four nucleic acids. The most commonly used NRTIs include emtricitabine, tenofovir, lamivudine, and abacavir.

Nonnucleoside Reverse Transcriptase Inhibitors

The NNRTIs include nevirapine, delavirdine, efavirenz, rilpivirine, and etravirine. As a class, the NNRTIs bind to HIV reverse transcriptase at a site distant from the catalytic site, the "NNRTI-binding pocket" that causes a conformational change in the enzyme, disrupting enzyme activity. Because NRTIs and NNRTIs do not bind at the same site, they can be used effectively as combination therapy with significant inhibition of HIV reverse transcriptase. Unlike NRTIs, NNRTIs do not require intracellular metabolism (i.e., phosphorylation) for activity. When resistance to NNRTIs occurs, multiple drugs within the class may be affected, and often only etravirine will remain available for therapy.

Integrase Strand Transfer Inhibitors

The INSTIs include raltegravir, dolutegravir, bictegravir, and elvitegravir. These agents block the integration of HIV-1 proviral DNA into the host cell genome, thus interrupting the HIV life cycle. Following reverse transcription of the viral RNA into a double-stranded DNA copy, the viral DNA remains associated with a "preintegration complex" that contains both viral and cellular proteins, including the viral integrase. The integration of the viral DNA into the host chromosome is subsequently achieved through a series of DNA cutting and joining reactions and occurs in three steps. First, two nucleotides are removed from each 3′-end of the viral DNA, a process termed 3′-end processing. Second, the processed viral DNA ends are inserted or joined into the host DNA, a process termed *DNA strand transfer*. The HIV-1 integrase catalyzes these first two steps of integration. Finally, cellular enzymes repair the single gaps in the DNA chain by removing the two unpaired nucleotides at the 5′-ends of the viral DNA.

Protease Inhibitors

The PIs, darunavir, atazanavir, ritonavir, and lopinavir, are very potent antiviral agents and inhibit HIV by blocking the HIV aspartyl protease, a viral enzyme that cleaves the HIV gag and gag-pol polyprotein backbone at nine specific cleavage sites to produce shorter, functional proteins, therefore inhibiting the production of infectious HIV virions. PIs also have a variety of nonretroviral activities, which can contribute to adverse effects via actions on the glucose transporter Glut4, bilirubin UDP-glucuronosyltransferase, apolipoprotein B degradation and secretion, and enzymes involved in adipocyte, osteoclast, or osteoblast function and differentiation.

PIs also have additional beneficial effects, as they inhibit inflammatory cytokine production and modulate antigen presentation and T-cell responses. This may increase the therapeutic efficacy of ART by directly reducing immune activation, inflammation, T-cell apoptosis, and opportunistic infections. These agents generally have a higher barrier to resistance than other agents and are usually given with a boosting agent to increase PI concentrations.

Boosting Agents

Ritonavir is itself a PI that is used in low doses (100–200 mg/day) to boost the efficacy of other PIs. It is an effective pharmacologic enhancer because it inhibits two key stages of metabolism. First, it inhibits first-pass metabolism, which occurs during absorption. Enterocytes that line the intestine contain both CYP3A4, one of the key cytochrome P450 isoenzymes associated with drug metabolism, and P-glycoprotein, an efflux transporter that can effectively pump drugs out of the gut wall and back into the intestinal lumen (Chapter 3). Ritonavir inhibits both of these proteins and consequently increases the maximum plasma concentration of a coadministered drug that interacts with these proteins. Second, ritonavir inhibits hepatic CYP3A4, thereby inhibiting the catabolism and increasing the plasma half-life of coadministered drugs that are metabolized by this pathway. Further, because ritonavir also inhibits P-glycoprotein in CD4+ cells, less drug is transported out of the cell, thereby increasing its intracellular accumulation.

Cobicistat is a pharmacokinetic enhancer that has no activity against HIV. It is a mechanism-based inhibitor of cytochrome P450 enzymes, including CYP3A4. Inhibition of CYP3A-mediated metabolism by cobicistat increases the systemic exposure of PIs and INSTIs; it is available alone or in combination with the PIs atazanavir and darunavir and with the INSTI elvitegravir.

RELATIONSHIP OF MECHANISMS OF ACTION TO CLINICAL RESPONSE

HIV is a relatively new disease, and therapy has changed rapidly since the development of the first antiretroviral drug. The relationship between the mechanisms of action of anti-HIV drugs and clinical response is best appreciated from a historical perspective. The historical account of the management of the disease also illustrates how an increased understanding of the life cycle of the virus and identification of new targets permitted the development of more highly efficacious agents based on their mechanisms of action.

The first cases of *Pneumocystis jirovecii* pneumonia (PCP) were reported in the *Morbidity and Mortality Weekly Report* (MMWR) published by the United States Centers for Disease Control and Prevention (CDC) on June 5, 1981. This marked the first official reporting of what would become known as the AIDS epidemic. At the time, the HIV virus had not been isolated, and not much was known. As rapidly increasing numbers of people, primarily gay men, but also intravenous drug users, began to get very sick and die, intensive research began.

On September 24, 1982, the CDC used the term *AIDS* for the first time and released the first case definition of AIDS as "a disease at least moderately predictive of a defect in cell-mediated immunity, occurring in a person with no known case for diminished resistance to that disease." In 1984, Dr. Robert Gallo and his colleagues at the National Cancer Institute identified the cause of AIDS, a retrovirus they initially called HTLV-III and later changed to HIV, and a diagnostic blood test was developed.

Three years later, in 1987, the first antiretroviral drug, AZT, was approved. Initial studies with AZT monotherapy seemed very promising, demonstrating that inhibition of HIV reverse transcriptase improved CD4+ counts and clinical outcomes in patients. Unfortunately, these effects were not sustained, as reverse transcriptase mutations developed rapidly, viral replication progressed, CD4+ counts fell, and clinical illnesses recurred. Other NRTIs were developed, initially used as salvage therapy and then used in combination, in an attempt to halt HIV replication. Because all of the NRTIs inhibit the reverse transcriptase the same way at the same active site, inhibitors of other stages of the HIV replication cycle were actively sought.

By 1992, AIDS had become the number one cause of death for men aged 25 to 44 in the United States. Intensive research was being conducted to develop new antiretroviral agents. The first rapid HIV test was also licensed in 1992, making it possible to receive a diagnosis in about 10 minutes.

In June 1995, the first PI, saquinavir, was approved, ushering in a new era of highly active antiretroviral therapy (HAART). Within 6 months, saquinavir was being used in combination with AZT and lamivudine (3TC). Multiple other PIs were rapidly developed. HAART became widely available to people living with HIV/AIDS in 1996, and AIDS morbidity and mortality fell almost immediately in the industrialized world. The way people thought about AIDS also changed forever. In 1997, the CDC reported the first substantial decline in AIDS deaths in the United States. Due largely to the use of HAART, AIDS-related deaths in the United States declined by 47% compared to the previous year.

However, HIV resistance developed rapidly when medications were used as single agents or irregularly, and it was apparent that strict adherence to therapy was crucial in achieving the best outcomes, which occur when viral replication is low. The initial HAART regimens were quite complex, involving large numbers of pills that had to be taken multiple times daily, which made adherence difficult. In 1997, two antiretroviral drugs, AZT and lamivudine, combined into one tablet was approved, making it easier for people living with HIV to take their medications.

Unfortunately, the lifesaving PIs were associated with many unpleasant gastrointestinal (GI) side effects, as well as other toxicities, leading to the search for alternative therapies. The NNRTIs were being developed at the time, and the first NNRTI, nevirapine, was approved in 1996. In the next 2 years, two other NNRTIs were approved, delavirdine in 1997 and efavirenz in 1998. These three drugs represent the first-generation NNRTIs. Because genetic barriers to the development of resistance were low, the need to develop NNRTIs with better resistance profiles led to the next generation of NNRTIs. The first drug in this class, etravirine,

was approved in 2008, and the second drug in this class, rilpivirine, was approved in 2011.

The first-single tablet regimen containing efavirenz, emtricitabine, and tenofovir was approved for use in 2006. The single-tablet regimen radically simplified treatment, improved adherence to therapy significantly, was also fairly well tolerated, and shifted the focus of HIV therapy from merely keeping people alive to keeping them alive with a good quality of life.

The newest class of antiretroviral agents, the INSTIs, were subsequently developed, with approval of raltegravir in 2007. Approval of dolutegravir and elvitegravir followed a few years later, and the newest INSTI, bictegravir, was approved in 2017. These agents are very well tolerated and have a fairly high genetic barrier to resistance.

Multiple new single-tablet regimens have been developed in the past few years, consisting of two NRTIs and either an NNRTI or an INSTI. The first PI-based single-tablet regimen is in development. There is also a new single-tablet drug on the market containing the two active compounds dolutegravir and rilpivirine that may avoid potential toxicities associated with the NRTIs. Currently, most HIV-positive individuals are able to take a single-tablet regimen with minimal adverse effects, and for those who cannot, due to resistance mutations, a once-daily or, at most, twice-daily regimen is generally available, making HIV a chronic disease, which, at this point in time, is fairly easy to manage.

PIs originally required very high dosing, and patients were taking multiple pills many times a day. The need to improve both the convenience and effectiveness of PIs led to research focusing on pharmacologic enhancement of their activity. To achieve higher concentrations of drug with fewer adverse effects, boosting agents are now commonly used.

PHARMACOKINETICS

The pharmacokinetic parameters for some anti-HIV drugs are listed in Table 66.1.

Entry Inhibitors

Maraviroc is rapidly absorbed after oral administration and reaches peak plasma concentrations at 0.5–4 hours after administration. Maraviroc has very poor bioavailability of only 23% and is dosed at 300 mg orally twice daily in the absence of potent CYP3A4 modulators. It is bound to plasma proteins (76%) and has a half-life of 14–18 hours. Maraviroc is metabolized mainly by CYP3A4 and is eliminated as both the unchanged parent (33%) and metabolites in the urine.

Enfuvirtide is available only for subcutaneous injection. Peak concentrations of 5 µg/mL occur 4–6 hours after injection. Enfuvirtide is poorly water soluble and is highly protein bound. Elimination is thought to be mainly through enzymatic catabolism of the polypeptide to constituent amino acids.

Nucleoside/Nucleotide Reverse Transcriptase Inhibitors

NRTIs and nucleotides are available for oral administration. AZT is the only drug in this class available for intravenous administration and can be helpful in managing pregnant women during labor. It is recommended for all HIV-positive women giving birth with a VL >1000 copies/mL. Peak serum concentrations for NRTIs and nucleotides generally occur within 30–90 minutes. Importantly, the intracellular half-lives of the phosphorylated compounds are many hours. This can allow once- or twice-daily dosing for many of these agents, improving compliance and decreasing toxicity.

Drug absorption is unique for each of the drugs in this class, and food or stomach pH can affect absorption for some of these agents. Didanosine and tenofovir are most affected in this regard. Didanosine

TABLE 66.1 Pharmacokinetic Parameters of Some Commonly Used Antiretroviral Drugs

Drug	Routes of Administration	Bioavailability and Protein Binding	Time (hrs) to Peak Serum Levels	Serum $t_{1/2}$ (hrs)	Elimination
Entry Inhibitors					
Enfuvirtide	SC	84% bioavailable, 92% protein bound	4–8	~4	M (peptidases)
Maraviroc	Oral	23%–33% bioavailable, 70% protein bound	0.5–4	14–18	M (CYP3A4); R (20%); F (76%)
Integrase Strand Transfer Inhibitors					
Raltegravir	Oral	83% protein bound	3	~9	M (UGT); R (32%); F (51%)
Dolutegravir	Oral	>98% protein bound; 50% bioavailable	2–3	14	M (UGT1A1); R (31%); F (53%)
Elvitegravir	Oral	98%–99% protein bound	4	~9 (boosted with ritonavir)	M (CYP3A4; UGT1A1/3); R (7%); F (95%)
Bictegravir	Oral	>99.7% protein bound	2–4	17.3	M (UGT1A1; CYP3A4); R (35%); F (60%)
Nucleoside/Nucleotide Reverse Transcriptase Inhibitors					
Abacavir	Oral	83% bioavailable; 50% protein bound	0.7–1.7	1.5	M (alcohol dehydrogenase; glucuronyl transferase); Exc, U (80%); F (16%)
Emtricitabine	Oral	93% bioavailable; <4% protein bound	1–2	10	M (oxidation); R (86%); F (14%)
Lamivudine	Oral	87% bioavailable; <36% protein bound	<0.5	5–7 (adults) 2 (children)	M (~6% sulfoxide metabolite); R (80%–90%)
Tenofovir disoproxil	Oral	25% fasting, 40% with high-fat meal, bioavailable, <7% protein bound	1–2	17	R (70%–80%)
Tenofovir alafenamide	Oral	80% protein bound	0.5	0.5	M (carboxylesterase; cathepsin A)
Zidovudine (AZT)	Oral; IV	25%–40% protein bound		1	M (CYP3A4)
Nonnucleoside Reverse Transcriptase Inhibitors					
Efavirenz	Oral	99% protein bound	2.5–4	41 ± 20	M (CYP3A4, 2B6); R (14%–34%); F (16%–61%)
Etravirine	Oral	99.9% protein bound	3–5	41 ± 20	M (CYP3A4, 2C9); F (94%)
Nevirapine	Oral	>90% bioavailable; 50%–60% protein bound	2–4	45 over first 2–4 weeks; 23 after due to autoinduction	M (CYP3A4); R (81%); F (10%)
Rilpivirine	Oral	99.7% protein bound	4–5	50	M (CYP3A4); R (6%)
Protease Inhibitors					
Atazanavir	Oral	86% protein bound	2–3	7–8 unboosted; 9–18 boosted	M (CYP3A4); R (13%); F (79%)
Darunavir	Oral	95% protein bound	2.5–4	15	M (CYP3A4); R (14%); (80%)
Lopinavir/Ritonavir	Oral	98%–99% protein bound	4	5–6 with ritonavir	M (CYP3A4); R (11%); F (86%)
Ritonavir	Oral	98%–99% protein bound	2	3–5	M (CYP3A4); R (11%); F (86%)

B, Biliary excretion; *F*, % excreted in feces; *IV*, intravenous; *M*, metabolic; *R*, % excreted in urine; *SC*, subcutaneous; *UGT*, uridine diphosphate glucuronosyltransferase.

is extremely acid labile and is formulated with a buffer to neutralize stomach acid and maximize absorption. Tenofovir is not well absorbed by itself and is available as the alafenamide salt, which is a relatively new preparation that is less toxic than the traditional disoproxil salt. The alafenamide salt is much more stable in plasma than the disoproxil salt, enabling the achievement of higher intracellular levels of tenofovir at lower doses, leading to a >90% reduction of free tenofovir in plasma, greatly reducing potential toxicities.

Penetration into the cerebrospinal fluid (CSF) varies widely among the drugs. NRTIs and nucleotides are eliminated by a combination of renal excretion and glucuronidation. Drugs that can interfere with hepatic glucuronidation (e.g., acetaminophen) or renal tubular transport (e.g., probenecid) may inhibit elimination of some agents and should be used with caution. Also, patients with renal insufficiency may need dosage adjustments. The improved dosing pattern of NRTIs and the need to use multiple NRTIs in the management of HIV disease have allowed the manufacture of fixed drug combinations, further improving patient compliance.

Nonnucleoside Reverse Transcriptase Inhibitors

The bioavailability of the NNRTIs is generally high. These agents are rapidly absorbed, with half-lives of 6–40 hours. Nevirapine is extensively metabolized by and induces CYP3A4 and CYP2B6, necessitating a modification in the doses of other drugs metabolized by this route. Efavirenz and rilpivirine possess the longest half-lives and can be given once daily. Efavirenz should be taken on an empty stomach, and rilpivirine should be taken with food to be most effective.

Integrase Strand Transfer Inhibitors

INSTIs generally have favorable pharmacokinetic profiles. Raltegravir is dosed twice a day, while dolutegravir, bictegravir, and elvitegravir (which is always administered with cobicistat, for boosting) can be given daily, although dolutegravir is dosed twice daily in people with some INSTI resistance and when taken with certain other antiretroviral agents. Raltegravir and dolutegravir have no food restrictions, but elvitegravir/cobicistat should be taken with food.

Raltegravir does not have the substantial drug-drug interaction potential of many other antiretrovirals because it is metabolized by glucuronidation, a low-affinity, high-capacity pathway. The primary enzyme is UGT1A1, and interactions can occur when concomitant medications induce or inhibit the activity of this enzyme. Elvitegravir undergoes extensive primary metabolism by hepatic and intestinal CYP3A4 and secondary metabolism by UGT1A1/3. Dolutegravir is primarily metabolized via UGT1A1 with a minor contribution by CYP3A and is a substrate for P-glycoprotein.

Protease Inhibitors

Several PIs are available for use. Because the absorption of these medications is usually improved with food, atazanavir and darunavir should both be taken with food. Peak serum concentrations of PIs are reached by 1–3 hours after ingestion, and the drugs are eliminated primarily via metabolism by CYP3A4. Inhibition of this enzyme can cause significant interactions with other medications. The elimination of PIs can be decreased preferentially by "boosting" with low-dose ritonavir or cobicistat. Patients with liver disease who need PI therapy must be monitored carefully.

PHARMACOVIGILANCE: ADVERSE EFFECTS AND DRUG INTERACTIONS

Because many antiretroviral drugs are derivatives of nucleic acids, significant toxicities to uninfected cells can occur.

Entry Inhibitors

Maraviroc is usually very well tolerated, though it can produce GI side effects like most HIV medications. Unfortunately, resistance significantly limits its use. Because maraviroc was never recommended for initial therapy, it is generally evaluated as an option for salvage therapy in treatment-experienced patients. However, many treatment-experienced patients have a CXCR4-tropic or dual/mixed tropic virus and are no longer good candidates for maraviroc therapy.

The main side effects associated with enfuvirtide are reactions at the injection site, which can be quite severe and involve possible hypersensitivity reactions. Patients need to rotate injection sites to allow resolution of the problem. Analgesics are sometimes necessary. This has significantly limited the utility of enfuvirtide, which is rarely used any more.

Nucleoside Reverse Transcriptase Inhibitors

Side effects of NRTIs and nucleotides vary with clinical stage of HIV disease. Persons with CD4+ counts above 200 cells/mm^3 generally tolerate these medications very well. The most common side effects in this group are GI upset, nausea, and headache. These effects occur in approximately 5% of patients and may decrease with time. Lamivudine and emtricitabine are among the better tolerated NRTIs. Patients with more advanced HIV disease often experience more frequent and more significant side effects to NRTIs. Megaloblastic erythrocyte changes occur within 2 weeks in most patients on AZT therapy. All NRTIs inhibit mitochondrial DNA formation to some extent. Severe lactic acidosis and hepatic steatosis occurred with some of the older NRTIs, which are no longer used, and while these are still concerns, the newer NRTIs are much less toxic. NRTIs have also been associated with lipodystrophy, but again, the newer ones not so much.

Abacavir can produce a sometimes-fatal hypersensitivity reaction characterized by fever, rash, and GI symptoms. Due to the potential severity of this reaction, it is recommended to screen patients for *HLA-B*5701* prior to initiating therapy. A positive test increases the chances of having a hypersensitivity reaction, so if the test is positive, alternative agents should be used. Abacavir may also increase the risk of acute cardiovascular events.

Tenofovir, as discussed, was formulated initially as the disoproxil salt, which causes proximal renal tubulopathy. Although this effect is generally subclinical, occasionally frank renal failure occurs, usually due to Fanconi syndrome. This preparation also leads to bone demineralization. The recent reformulation of tenofovir as the alafenamide salt almost completely eliminates these toxicities by decreasing the amount of tenofovir present in plasma by over 90%. The disoproxil salt should not be used in patients with a glomerular filtration rate (GFR) <70 mL/min, but the alafenamide salt can be used in patients with a GFR >30 mL/min.

Tenofovir is also effective for the treatment of hepatitis B; thus in coinfected patients, this must always be taken into consideration. If tenofovir is discontinued, patients may have a severe flare-up of their hepatitis B, and treatment with another agent should be initiated promptly.

Nonnucleoside Reverse Transcriptase Inhibitors

NNRTIs, although a single class of drugs, have widely varying side effects and treatment issues. One of the most significant side effects is rash. One-third of patients taking nevirapine can develop significant rash, with life-threatening hypersensitivity reactions. Patients who experience the rash should not be rechallenged. Rash is less common in patients taking the other NNRTIs but can certainly occur. Efavirenz use can be associated with severe depression and sleep disturbances, especially vivid dreams. It should be taken at bedtime, as it can cause drowsiness. A history of clinically significant depression is a relative contraindication for the use of efavirenz.

Rilpivirine is a good alternative to efavirenz. It is very well tolerated, rendering it an excellent choice for patients who are very sensitive to medication adverse effects. However, virologic failure (HIV-1 VL ≥50 copies/mL) was higher in subjects with baseline HIV-1 VL >100,000 copies/mL and in subjects with baseline CD4+ cell counts <200 cells/mm^3 (regardless of baseline HIV-1 VL levels). Compared to efavirenz, virologic failure in rilpivirine-treated subjects conferred a higher rate of overall resistance and cross-resistance to the NNRTIs, and more subjects developed tenofovir- and lamivudine/emtricitabine-associated resistance. Thus rilpivirine is only indicated for use in patients who have a CD4+ cell count of 200 cells/mm^3 or higher, with a VL of less than 100,000 copies/mL.

Etravirine is only indicated for treatment-experienced patients and can often be used even when there is resistance to other NNRTIs, but genotyping must be performed.

Protease Inhibitors

PIs are primarily metabolized by the cytochrome P450 system and thus have the potential to alter the metabolism of other drugs. Ritonavir has the greatest likelihood of drug-drug interactions, although this may occur with any PI. Patients on PI therapy must have their medications reviewed routinely to check for significant drug-drug reactions. Lipodystrophy was common with the older PIs. Glucose intolerance and dyslipidemia may also occur, and patients on PIs have an increased risk of myocardial infarctions. Indinavir may precipitate in renal tubules and create clinically significant kidney stones, and thus adequate hydration is required for patients receiving this agent. Other common side effects for PIs include GI upset and diarrhea.

The newer PIs, atazanavir and darunavir, are much safer and better tolerated than the older agents, are currently the most commonly used PIs, and are almost always given "boosted," in combination with either ritonavir, or now more commonly, cobicistat. Atazanavir is associated with unconjugated hyperbilirubinemia in nearly 50% of the patients as a result of inhibition of the UGT1A1 enzyme. However, the hyperbilirubinemia leads to jaundice or scleral icterus in only 5% of patients overall; less than 1% need to discontinue the drug due to this side effect. Several cases of cholelithiasis, with high levels of atazanavir found in the calculi, have been reported in patients who received atazanavir, and the use of atazanavir with or without ritonavir has also been associated with the development of nephrolithiasis. Atazanavir is unique among the PIs in that it requires an acidic gastric pH for absorption. Thus concomitant administration of proton pump inhibitors can reduce serum levels dramatically, and if needed, another PI should be used.

Darunavir is the newest PI, approved in 2006. It has activity against a broad range of drug-resistant clinical isolates. In vitro, darunavir has activity against viral isolates with resistance to five other PIs and demonstrates a high genetic barrier to the development of resistance.

Integrase Strand Transfer Inhibitors

INSTIs are generally very well tolerated. The most common adverse effects include diarrhea, nausea, headache, and insomnia. Raltegravir can cause elevations in amylase and in liver enzyme, but allergic reactions and drug interactions are infrequent.

Boosting Agents

Cobicistat, used to enhance the activity of both INSTIs and PIs, can increase serum creatinine by inhibiting its renal tubular secretion. This is not an actual toxicity but needs to be distinguished from renal toxicity induced by tenofovir disoproxil, which can be difficult, as these agents are often given together in a single tablet. This tablet should not be given to patients with a creatinine clearance <70 mL/min and should be discontinued if the creatinine clearance drops below 50 mL/min. Discontinuation should be considered if the serum creatinine increases by more than 0.4 mg/dL.

Several of the clinical problems associated with the use of these agents are summarized in the Clinical Problems Box.

NEW DEVELOPMENTS

Currently, most HIV-positive individuals are able to take a single-tablet regimen with minimal adverse effects and for those who cannot, due to resistance mutations, a once-daily or, at most, twice-daily regimen is generally available, making HIV a chronic disease, which, at this point, is fairly easy to manage. Multiple new single-tablet regimens

CLINICAL PROBLEMS	
Zidovudine	Bone marrow suppression, granulocytopenia, myositis
Abacavir	Hypersensitivity reactions
Tenofovir disoproxil	Proximal renal tubulopathy, bone mineralization defects
Efavirenz	Rash, sleep disturbances, vivid dreams
Ritonavir	Drug-drug interactions
Indinavir	Precipitation in renal tubules leading to kidney stones
Raltegravir	Increases liver amylase
Cobicistat	Inhibits renal tubular secretion of creatinine

have been developed in the past few years, consisting of two NRTIs and either an NNRTI or an INSTI. There is also a new single tablet on the market containing two active drugs, an NNRTI and an INSTI.

In addition to treating the disease once it develops, a major advance in this field has been to prevent HIV transmission. This approach is referred to as preexposure prophylaxis (PrEP) and uses a fixed-dose combination of tenofovir disoproxil and emtricitabine. This has been available since 2012, is now widely prescribed, and represents a cornerstone of public heath efforts to control the spread of HIV. Taking one dose daily has been shown to decrease the transmission of HIV by more than 90%. However, the efficacy of this strategy requires an ongoing commitment to adherence by patients. The risk of HIV acquisition should be determined by sexual risk behaviors of patients over the prior 6 months. Once on PrEP, patients should be monitored every 3 months, including an assessment of renal function due to the tenofovir disoproxil.

CLINICAL RELEVANCE FOR HEALTHCARE PROFESSIONALS

Healthcare providers treating HIV/AIDS patients receiving anti-HIV drugs should be aware of the major side effects and drug interactions associated with these agents. AIDS patients are at risk for various opportunistic infections and are likely receiving multiple drugs beyond the combination used to control the virus. Immune-compromised patients are at risk for developing fungal infections, especially of the oral cavity, as well as malnutrition and anorexia, which predispose patients to malodor and coated tongue. It is important to determine the other agents being taken by these individuals to ensure that drug-drug interactions do not have a negative impact. Assessment of over-the-counter medications is also essential because many of these agents pose additional interactions. Fortunately, most patients who adhere to therapy can now achieve full virologic suppression with an undetectable viral load, which reduces the risk of transmission to a neglibigle amount.

All healthcare providers should assess the relative risk of their patients contracting the virus to determine if PrEP is an appropriate therapy. If there is a risk for infection, PrEP should be prescribed and maintained as long as necessary. Caution should be exercised at all times to avoid inadvertent contact with bodily fluids, especially blood products.

TRADE NAMES

In addition to generic and fixed-combination preparations, the following trade-named materials are some of the important compounds available in the United States.

Entry Inhibitors
Enfuvirtide (Fuzeon)
Maraviroc (Selzentry)

NRTIs
Abacavir (Ziagen)
Emtricitabine (Emtriva)
Lamivudine (Epivir)
Tenofovir
   TDF (Viread)
   TAF
   FTC-TDF (Truvada)
   FTC-TAF (Descovy)
Zidovudine (AZT, Retrovir)

NNRTIs
Efavirenz (Sustiva)
Etravirine (Intelence)
Nevirapine (Viramune)
Rilpivirine (Edurant)

Protease Inhibitors
Atazanavir (Reyataz)
Darunavir (Prezista)
Lopinavir/Ritonavir (Kaletra)
Nelfinavir (Viracept)
Ritonavir (Norvir)

Integrase Strand Transfer Inhibitors
Raltegravir (Isentress)
Dolutegravir (Tivicay)
Elvitegravir (Vitekta)
Bictegravir

Single-Tablet Regimens
FTC-TAF, ELV, COBI (Genvoya)
FTC-TDF, ELV, COBI (Stribild)
Lamivudine, abacavir, dolutegravir (Triumeq)
FTC-TDF, efavirenz (Atripla)
FTC-TDF, rilpivirine (Complera)
FTC-TAF, rilpivirine (Odefsey)
Rilpivirine, dolutegravir (Juluca)
FTC-TAF, bictegravir (Biktarvy)

SELF-ASSESSMENT QUESTIONS

1. An HIV-positive patient has been treated with FTC-TDF and efavirenz for the past 3 years, and plasma HIV RNA levels have been undetectable. However, recent plasma RT-PCR reveals that her HIV RNA levels are greater than 20,000 copies/mL. A new regimen was proposed that included abacavir, lamivudine, and raltegravir. One year later, the patient's HIV RNA level is again found to be elevated with 50,000 copies/mL. Which of the following most likely describes the reason for the failure of this second regimen?
   A. The second regimen contained abacavir, which is not indicated for the treatment of HIV infections.
   B. The second regimen contained an NRTI that was cross-resistant with FTC.
   C. The second regimen contained all protease inhibitors.
   D. The second regimen did not contain ritonavir.
   E. The second regimen did not include a boosting agent.

2. A 25-year-old man was recently diagnosed with HIV infection and presents to you for treatment. He has also had diabetes mellitus since childhood and has renal insufficiency as a result, with a glomerular filtration rate of only 20 mL/min. Which drug should be avoided in this patient?
   A. Tenofovir disoproxil.
   B. Abacavir.
   C. Ritonavir.
   D. Efavirenz.
   E. Raltrgravir.

3. Which of the following drugs is indicated for the treatment of either HIV or hepatitis B?
   A. Tenofovir.
   B. Etravirine.
   C. Abacavir.
   D. Ritonavir.
   E. Entecavir.

4. Which of the following drugs does not need to be administered with a boosting agent?
   A. Darunavir.
   B. Dolutegravir.
   C. Atazanavir.
   D. Elvitegravir.
   E. Lopinavir.

5. Treatment of HIV typically involves the use of three active agents and a "boosting" agent such as cobicistat. The efficacy of the booster is due to its ability to inhibit:
   A. P-glycoprotein.
   B. Viral fusion.
   C. Virion assembly.
   D. Glucuronidation.
   E. CYP3A4.

FURTHER READING

Das M, Isaakidis P, Van den Bergh R, et al. HIV, multidrug-resistant TB and depressive symptoms: when three conditions collide. *Glob Health Action.* 2014;7(1):24912.

Stein R, Song W, Marano M, et al. HIV testing, linkage to HIV medical care, and interviews for partner services among youths – 61 health department jurisdictions, United States, Puerto Rico and the U.S. Virgin Islands, 2015. *MMWR Morb Mortal Wkly Rep.* 2017;66(24):629–635.

Van Wyhe KS, van de Water T, Boivin MJ, et al. Cross-cultural assessment of HIV-associated cognitive impairment using the Kaufman assessment battery for children: a systematic review. *J Int AIDS Soc.* 2017;20(1):1–11.

WEBSITES

http://aidsinfo.nih.gov/guidelines

This site is maintained by the United States National Institutes of Health and contains guidelines for the use of antiretroviral agents in HIV-1-infected adults and adolescents.

https://www.hiv.gov/hiv-basics

This site is maintained by the United States Department of Health and Human Services and is an excellent source for HIV-related information, including a historical account of the development of our understanding of HIV and its associated diseases.

www.aids.gov

This is the United States Government website that provides an excellent comprehensive timeline of our domestic epidemic.

Principles of Antineoplastic Drug Use

John S. Lazo

THERAPEUTIC OVERVIEW

In the past decade, remarkable advances in the treatments for human malignancies have been achieved in part because of the recognition that cancer is a disease with aberrant signaling pathways often caused by genetic changes. This does not mean that all cancers are inherited, rather that neoplastic cells generally have an altered genetic content. This was first recognized with the leukemias, which were found to be associated with an abnormal karyotype. Eventually it was noted that chromosomal rearrangements are common in malignant cells, and even cells with apparently normal karyotypes almost always have definable abnormalities, such as translocations, insertions, deletions, duplications, inversions, and/or single-nucleotide alterations.

A neoplasm, by definition, is an abnormal growth of a tissue, which can be either benign or malignant. The cells of a malignant neoplasm usually exhibit loss of cellular differentiation (anaplasia) along with abnormal or unregulated proliferation and invasive properties, allowing for the violation of the basement membrane of the tissue of origin, entrance into the blood or lymphatic system, and eventual dissemination to distant organs in a process called metastasis. Solid tumors arising from epithelial cells are termed carcinomas, whereas those originating from connective or mesenchymal tissue are classified as sarcomas. Malignancies that arise from the hematopoietic system include the leukemias and lymphomas. Within these general groups, there are more than 100 types of malignant human neoplasms defined primarily according to their anatomical location and the nature of the cell involved. The classification schemes are rapidly evolving, however, with the use of sophisticated molecular diagnostic methods, which will likely increase the number of recognized tumor types.

In the United States, malignant neoplasms are responsible for causing approximately 600,000 deaths per year, with approximately 1,700,000 new cases developing each year. The 5-year survival rate for all cancers diagnosed in the United States during 2005–2011 was 69%, which is a 40% increase from 1975–1977. This improvement in survival reflects both newer cancer treatments and earlier diagnoses. Lung, intestine, breast, pancreatic, and prostate neoplasms account for approximately half of the cancer deaths in the United States (Fig. 67.1).

The mechanisms by which human neoplasms originate are beginning to be understood. Malignant neoplastic cells result from the activation, or in some cases the acquisition, of specific dominant growth genes, called oncogenes, or a loss of functional negative growth effectors, called tumor-suppressor genes. It is now believed that genetic or epigenetic changes in both of these gene classes accompany the development of a full malignant phenotype. Proto-oncogenes, when activated, beget oncogenes, which encode modified proteins that cause cellular dedifferentiation and proliferation characteristics of the neoplastic state. Frequently, the resulting cells have attributes that resemble stem cells, with the ability to replicate indefinitely. Activation of proto-oncogenes can occur by several pathways that often involve exposure of cells to chemicals, radiation, or viruses. Activation can result from a single-point mutation or from gene duplication. The most common oncogenes found thus far in human tumors belong to the *RAS* gene family, which encodes guanosine triphosphate–binding proteins. Mutated *RAS* fails to dephosphorylate guanosine triphosphate and is constitutively active, leading to cells that are transformed to a neoplastic phenotype. Unfortunately, there currently are no drugs that specifically target *RAS*. More than 100 proto-oncogenes are known to exist. Most, if not all, products of these variously dominant-acting oncogenes are components of cellular signaling pathways. Other genes, known as tumor-suppressing genes, also are present in human cells and function to suppress excessive cellular growth. Retinoblastoma (tumor of the eye) is a prototype of a malignancy caused by a genetic loss of the tumor-suppressor gene *RB*. A second common tumor-suppressor gene is *tumor protein 53 gene (TP53)*, which possesses the important function of protecting genomic stability. Mutations in *TP53* are the single most prevalent lesion in human cancers, which is one cause for the instability of the cancer cell genome.

Tumor growth represents a balance between cancer cell division and death. Stromal cells, such as fibroblasts, endothelium, macrophages, and immune cells, create a tumor microenvironment and regulate this dynamic relationship. The relatively low oxygen, glucose, nutrients, and pH of the microenvironment also influence tumor growth. Cells die from necrosis and energy-dependent programmed cell processes, such as apoptosis, which is important for normal development (e.g., thymic involution). Many of our antineoplastic agents exert an apoptotic death mechanism (Chapter 68). Indeed, the apoptotic pathway is now being targeted in the development of drugs. Interestingly, some oncogenes—namely, *B cell lymphoma protein* gene *(BCL2)*—act by blocking apoptosis. There is also growing evidence that cellular senescence can limit tumor growth.

From the clinical standpoint, the successful control and treatment of malignant neoplasms are challenging because at the time of detection, the tumors are relatively large and genetically diverse. A single dose of an anticancer drug kills with first-order kinetics (Chapter 68), leaving a fraction of the tumor cells alive. Therefore multiple doses are always required. It is generally believed that reproductively proficient cancer

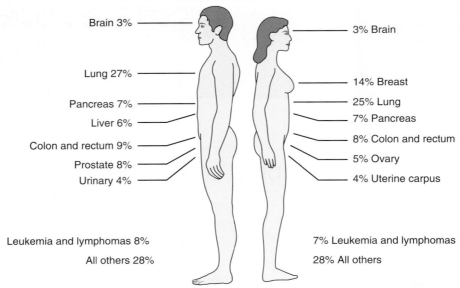

FIG. 67.1 Estimated Cancer Deaths in the United States in 2017. Percentage distribution of sites by sex (excludes basal and squamous cell skin cancers and carcinoma in situ, except bladder). (Data from American Cancer Society: Cancer Facts and Figures 2017.)

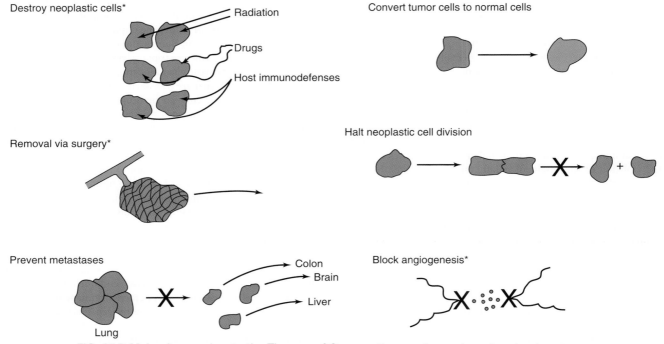

FIG. 67.2 Major Approaches to the Therapy of Cancers. Tumor cells are shown in red and nontumor cells in green. *In clinical use. Others are experimental.

stem cells are intrinsically resistant to anticancer drugs. In addition to the intrinsically **resistant** cell population, the surviving cells can develop drug resistance, reducing the overall response to subsequent treatment. Once a tumor has metastasized extensively (stage IV), local treatments, such as surgery and radiation, are much less efficacious. Unfortunately, drugs that selectively target tumor metastases, which is the primary cause of death, are lacking. Sadly, clinical trials in oncology have one of the highest failure rates, approximately 95%, compared to other therapeutic areas.

The generally accepted strategy for the clinical management of neoplastic diseases (Fig. 67.2) remains the removal or destruction of the

neoplastic cells while minimizing the toxic effects to nonneoplastic cells. Historically, individual drugs have been approved by regulatory agencies for use in specific types of tumors based on the tissue of origin—for example, breast, colon, brain, and lung. With the advent of affordable genetic testing, predictive biomarkers, and agents that block specific oncogenes, the classification and use of anticancer drugs are evolving to be more mechanistically oriented. Furthermore, as the understanding of cancer biology grows, there is considerable interest in discovering clinically useful agents that will prevent metastases formation and growth (antimetastatic agents), irreversibly convert tumor cells to more normal cells (differentiation agents), halt proliferation and cause senscence, or limit stromal cell support. Currently, drugs affecting these processes are either not available or highly experimental.

Chapters 68 and 69 address the principles using chemotherapy and the mechanisms of action and problems associated with the use of antineoplastic drugs in humans. There are now more than 180 anticancer drugs approved by the United States Food and Drug Administration (FDA), with almost half of the recently approved drugs for orphan disease indications—that is, for neoplastic diseases affecting fewer than 200,000 individuals in the United States. Mechanistic clustering of the drugs, therefore, provides a valuable method to organize this impressive array of pharmacological agents. Chapter 68 is dedicated to the cytotoxic drugs, which were the first agents to be identified and developed, while Chapter 69 discusses drugs that have been labeled targeted therapies along with hormones and biologics. It should be noted, however, that most of the cytotoxic agents have identified molecular targets and most of the target drugs, hormones, and biologics are cytotoxic to tumor cells.

There are now a growing number of tumor types responding to antineoplastic drug treatment. The Therapeutic Overview Box lists the response characteristics of patients to chemotherapy with advanced-stage tumors. Chemotherapy has been very effective in the management of leukemias and lymphomas, both in children and adults, such that most cases of leukemia in children are now curable. The success of treatment for adult leukemias is somewhat less, but complete remission in response to induction therapy is often achievable. On the other hand, advanced-stage solid tumors remain a challenge for complete response to chemotherapy. Choriocarcinoma, Ewing sarcoma, and testicular carcinoma are examples of solid tumors that can be cured with chemotherapy, even if they have metastasized.

DRUG SELECTION AND ISSUES

One of the difficulties in treating neoplastic diseases is that the tumor burden often is excessive at the time of diagnosis. This is illustrated in Fig. 67.3, which depicts the number of cells in a typical solid tumor over time, with 10^9 cells roughly equivalent to a volume of 1 cubic centimeter and representing the minimum size tumor that normally can be detected with current conventional methods. A single malignant cell requires approximately 30 doublings to reach 10^9 cells. On the other hand, it takes only 10 additional doublings for 10^9 cells to reach a population of 10^{12} cells, which is no longer compatible with life. Thus by the time a tumor is detected with the current methods, only a relatively small number of cell doublings are required before the tumor is fatal. Of course, not all tumor cells are cycling, so no meaningful predictions about longevity can be made purely on the basis of doubling times. Also, the doubling times of human tumors vary greatly. For acute lymphocytic leukemia, the doubling time during log-phase (first order) growth is 3 to 4 days, whereas the doubling time for lung squamous cell carcinoma is approximately 90 days. Thus in theory, in roughly 100 days, two lymphocytic leukemia cells could continue doubling and reach 10^9 cells. In addition, by the time a tumor is clinically detectable, it already has a well-developed vascular supply and most probably has already metastasized. If the tumor has outgrown the angiogenesis or vascularization process, areas of poor circulation will exist, which will limit exposure to drugs. Moreover, the intrinsic genetic instability of cancer cells enhances the likelihood of developing drug resistance.

Drug Therapy

The objective of chemotherapy in any given individual patient may be:
- curative, to obtain complete remission (e.g., Hodgkin disease);
- palliative, to alleviate symptoms but with little expectation of complete remission (e.g., carcinoma of the esophagus, with chemotherapy performed to ease the dysphagia);

THERAPEUTIC OVERVIEW

Cancers in Which Complete Remission to Chemotherapy Is Common and Cures Are Achieved, Even in Advanced Disease[a]
Acute lymphocytic leukemia (adults and children)
Acute myelogenous leukemia
Hodgkin disease (lymphoma)
Non-Hodgkin lymphoma
Choriocarcinoma
Testicular cancer
Burkitt lymphoma
Ewing sarcoma
Wilms tumor
Small cell lung cancer
Ovarian cancer
Hairy cell leukemia

Cancers in Which Objective Responses Are Achieved, but Chemotherapy Often Does Not Have Curative Potential in Advanced Disease
Multiple myeloma
Breast cancer
Head and neck cancer
Colorectal carcinomas
Chronic lymphocytic leukemia
Chronic myelogenous leukemia
Transitional cell carcinoma of bladder
Gastric adenocarcinomas
Cervical carcinomas
Melanoma
Neuroblastoma
Non–small cell lung cancer

Cancers in Which Only Occasional Objective Responses to Chemotherapy Are Achieved
Renal tumor
Pancreatic carcinomas
Hepatocellular carcinoma
Prostate carcinomas (hormone-unresponsive)

[a]Depending on tumor type, complete remission may result in cure.

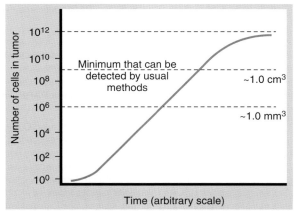

FIG. 67.3 Typical Tumor Growth Curve Showing That Roughly 10^9 Cells Are Needed For a Diagnosis.

- **adjuvant**, to improve the chances for a cure or prolong the period of disease-free survival when no detectable cancer is present but subclinical numbers of neoplastic cells are suspected (e.g., chemotherapy for breast cancer after surgical resection of all known tumor); or
- **debulking**, to reduce the tumor burden to allow for a more effective surgical removal of the tumor.

Targeted therapies are becoming increasingly important in the treatment of cancer (Chapter 69). Examples include bevacizumab, which targets vascular endothelial growth factor; I^{131} tositumomab, rituximab, and Y-90-ibritumomab tiuxetan, which target CD20 and are used for treatment of chemotherapy-refractory non-Hodgkin's lymphoma; and gefitinib and the antibody cetuximab, which target the epidermal growth factor receptor pathway. Immunotherapy includes biological response modifiers, which stimulate the human **immune** system to destroy tumor cells. The α and β human interferons are examples of efficacious agents for hairy cell leukemia and certain skin cancers. Other compounds include tumor necrosis factor, human growth factors, and monoclonal antibodies. Notably important immuno-oncology targets are the **programmed death ligand 1 (PD-L1)** and its cognate receptor, PD-1, which is found on activated T cells, B cells, and myeloid cells. PD-L1 up regulation allows melanoma, lung, renal, and gastric cancers to evade the host immune system. PD-1 checkpoint inhibitors, such as **nivolumab** and **pembrolizumab**, have been approved. Another example of effective immuno-oncology therapy is the blocking antibody against cytotoxic T-lymphocyte–associated protein 4 (CTLA-4), which down regulates cytotoxic T-lymphocytes and is used for the treatment of melanoma.

Drug Regimens

Although choriocarcinoma (gestational trophoblastic disease) and hairy cell leukemia are treated by using single drugs, nearly all other neoplasms are treated with drug **combinations**. The choice of drugs and dosing schedule for multiple-drug therapy emerged from empirical drug studies, especially for the cytotoxic agents. This has resulted in several guidelines, which continue to be the foundation for selecting most

drug combinations. Of noteworthy interest, many of these guidelines are similar to the guidelines for treating infectious organisms.

- Use drugs that show **activity** against the type of tumor being treated. The rationale is that seldom will a compound that shows no activity alone have an effect when used in combination.
- Use drugs that have different **mechanisms of resistance**. An example is the multidrug resistance protein (MRP) family, which includes cellular efflux pumps that transport anticancer drugs out of cells.
- Use drugs that have minimal or no **overlapping toxicities**. Although this may broaden the range of undesirable side effects of the drug combination, the goal is to reduce the possibility of life-threatening side effects that act in concert. For this reason, the side effects of the drugs selected should be diverse and not centered on the same organ system.
- Use drugs that have different **mechanisms of action** or that affect tumor cells at different stages of the **cell cycle**. Because tumor cells are in different stages of the cell cycle, a high proportion of the total tumor cell population can be targeted with each treatment.

The **dosing schedule** for each drug should be optimal to maximize the antitumor effect and minimize toxicity to the patient. In establishing the frequency of a dosing regimen, it is usual to allow sufficient time between dosage sequences to permit the most sensitive tissues (often bone marrow) to recover. As noted in Chapter 68, most drugs are more effective against tumor cells that are cycling rather than cells resting in the stationary (G_0) phase, but cells in a tumor may be present in any part of the cycle. Some drugs cause cell cycle arrest, which can limit the effectiveness of other drugs and thus should be avoided.

An increase in the number of drug combinations employed is a consequence of an improved understanding of the pathways shared by cancer drug targets and by discovery efforts using **synthetic lethal** approaches, which seek agents that alone have limited pharmacological actions but when combined together or used in tumors with a genetic defect, lead to selective tumor cell death. One example of this approach is the use of the poly-ADP ribose polymerase (PARP) inhibitor **olaparib** for the treatment of ovarian cancers, which have lost the brain cancer resistance protein 1 (BRCA1)-mediated homologous repair process for

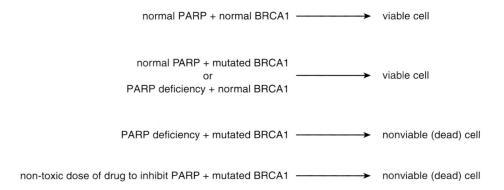

FIG. 67.4 Synthetic Lethal Strategy. Current approaches involve screening cells that exhibit death when the products from two different genes are lost but are viable when only one gene product is aberrant. Shown are the consequences of the interaction between poly-ADP ribose polymerase (PARP) and brain cancer resistance protein 1 (BRCA1). PARP repairs damage to single-strand breaks in DNA, whereas BRCA1 is critical for repairing double-strand DNA breaks by homologous recombination. Cells that do not express PARP and have BRCA1 mutations cannot repair DNA and die. Thus the use of a nontoxic dose of the PARP inhibitor olaparib to mimic the loss of PARP in patients with a BRCA1 mutation, such as may exist in ovarian and breast cancers, will lead to cell death due to a loss in the rescue pathway.

TABLE 67.1   Examples of Common Combination Drug Regimens

Terminology	Cancer	Drugs
MOPP	Hodgkin lymphoma	Mechlorethamine, vincristine, procarbazine, prednisone
ABVD	Hodgkin lymphoma	Doxorubicin, bleomycin, vinblastine, dacarbazine
BEP	Germ cell cancers	Bleomycin, etoposide, cisplatin
CMF	Breast cancer	Cyclophosphamide, methotrexate, 5-fluorouracil
CAF	Breast cancer	Cyclophosphamide, doxorubicin, 5-fluorouracil
CHOP	Non-Hodgkin lymphoma	Cyclophosphamide, doxorubicin, vincristine, prednisone
CHOP-R		Agents above + rituximab
Hyper-CVAD	Non-Hodgkin lymphoma	Hyperfractionated cyclophosphamide, vincristine, adriamycin, dexamethasone
FOLFIRI-Cetuximab	Colorectal cancer	Leucovorin, 5-fluorouracil, irinotecan, cetuximab
PVC	Anaplastic oligodendrogliomas	Procarbazine, vincristine, lomustine
R-EPOCH	B-cell non-Hodgkin lymphoma	Rituximab, etoposide, prednisone, vincristine, cyclophosphamide, doxorubicin
XELIRI	Colorectal, esophageal, gastric cancer	Capecitabine, irinotecan

double-strand DNA breaks, as shown in Fig. 67.4. Combinations of cytotoxic, hormone, biologic, and immunological agents are now accepted as valuable and improve patient response rates. Drugs are being used as an adjuvant therapy after surgical or radiation removal of the primary tumor. For example, adjuvant therapy is commonly employed in the management of completely resected breast cancer and colorectal cancer, with significant improvement in survival. Some examples of common combination drug regimens are given in Table 67.1.

SPECIAL CLINICAL PROBLEMS

Because chemotherapy is a systemic treatment, it is frequently challenging to deliver drug to the tumor without injuring normal tissue. In fact, normal tissue toxicity is the dose-limiting factor for almost all antineoplastic agents. Normal tissue toxicity can either be acute (with or shortly after chemotherapy) or delayed (months to years after chemotherapy). Most acute side effects (nausea, vomiting, alopecia, bone marrow suppression) are reversible or able to be reduced in severity. Agents that act like or stimulate the production of granulocyte colony–stimulating factor and granulocyte macrophage colony–stimulating factor can be used to reduce chemotherapy-induced neutropenia and infections (Chapter 70).

Delayed side effects of cytotoxic chemotherapy are quite diverse and include pulmonary fibrosis, sterility, neuropathy, and nephropathy, but the most important are leukemia and cardiotoxicity. Chemotherapy-induced leukemias are associated mainly with the alkylating agents. Cardiotoxicity is associated with the anthracyclines. Nausea and vomiting can be expected in a high fraction of patients receiving cytotoxic antineoplastic drugs. Some of the drugs most and least likely to trigger emesis and the current agents and guidelines for managing this adverse effect are listed in the Clinical Problems Box. Although the clinical management of nausea and vomiting can become a serious problem, as indicated, many drugs now exist that successfully control these symptoms.

Pediatric cancers represent a distinct challenge for the cytotoxic anticancer drugs because of their low therapeutic index and the lifetime risk of secondary malignancies being induced by the drugs. Drug toxicities align more closely with a child's body surface area than mass, and consequently drug dosage for children can be calculated as mg/m^2 rather than mg/kg. Because cancer occurs more frequently with aging (median age for cancer diagnosis is 66 years old in the United States), attention to other coadministered medications as well as kidney and liver function is important.

NEW DEVELOPMENTS

Fueled with an explosion in our understanding of the basic science of cancer, there have been significant advances in the treatment of the hematological neoplastic diseases and many solid tumors. For example, the past few decades have witnessed the description of RNA and DNA tumor viruses, oncogenes, and antioncogenes (tumor-suppressor genes) as well as dramatic advances in our understanding of cell cycle regulation, apoptosis, tumor immunology, and the signaling pathways in DNA damage responses. Many gene products involved in these pathways are new targets in the treatment of malignancies (Chapter 68). The development of cancer treatments, based on our increased understanding of these basic molecular mechanisms, will narrow the chasm between the molecular biology of cancer and clinical oncology. Moreover, new preclinical models of the disease, such as three-dimensional culturing systems, genetically modified mouse models and patient-derived xenografts, offer the possibility of providing better predictors of the ultimate efficacy of clinical trial candidates.

Pharmacogenomics is making significant advances in determining risks of recurrence, mortality, and response to adjuvant chemotherapy. Inexpensive genomic sequencing and methods to capture circulating tumor cells or DNA offer potential biomarkers that could enable the application of precision medicine strategies in which the drug treatment is tailored specifically to the molecular nature of the patient's disease (Chapter 4). In combination with new tumor imaging methods, diagnostic platforms, drug delivery systems, and clinical trial design, there is considerable hope that improved cancer treatments will emerge in the future.

CLINICAL PROBLEMS

Emetogenic Potential of Antineoplastic Agents

Level 1 (Minimal Risk, <10%)	Level 2 (Low Risk, 10%–30%)	Level 3 (Moderate Risk, 31%–89%)	Level 4 (High Risk, >90%)
Bevacizumab	Bortezomib	Carboplatin	Carmustine
Bleomycin	Cetuximab	Cyclophosphamide (<1.5 g/m² BSA)	Cisplatin
Busulfan	Cytarabine (<100 mg/m² BSA)	Cytarabine (>1 gm/m² BSA)	Cyclophosphamide (>1.5 g/m² BSA)
Vinblastine	Docetaxel	Daunorubicin	Dacarbazine
Vincristine	Etoposide	Doxorubicin	Dactinomycin
	5-Fluorouracil	Epirubicin	Lomustine
	Gemcitabine	Idarubicin	Mechlorethamine
	Ixabepilone	Ifosfamide	Pentostatin
	Lapatinib	Irinotecan	
	Methotrexate	Oxaliplatin	
	Mitomycin		
	Mitoxantrone		
	Paclitaxel		
	Pemetrexed		
	Topotecan		
	Trastuzumab		

Percentages in each level are estimates of the relative risk of emesis by the agent in the absence of any antiemetic treatment. Do not confuse risk level with severity of emesis.

Antiemetic treatment is based upon the emetogenic risk level of the antineoplastic agent.

Antiemetic Agents Used for Chemotherapy-Induced Nausea and Vomiting (CINV)

Serotonin (5-HT₃) Receptor Antagonists	Tachykinin Receptor Antagonists	Corticosteroids	Dopamine Receptor Antagonists	Cannabinoid Receptor Agonists
Dolasetron	Aprepitant	Dexamethasone	Metoclopramide	Nabilone
Granisetron	Fosaprepitant	Methylprednisolone	Phenothiazines	Dronabinol
Ondansetron	Casopitant			
Palonosetron	Netupitant			
Ramosetron	Rolapitant			
Tropisetron				

Recommended Antiemetic Regimens for CINV Prophylaxis

Emetic Risk Level	Acute Phase Treatment	Delayed Phase Treatment
High (Level 4)	Combination treatment with aprepitant, 5-HT₃ antagonist, and dexamethasone	Combination treatment with aprepitant and dexamethasone
Moderate (Level 3)	Combination treatment with 5-HT₃ antagonist and dexamethasone	Dexamethasone
Low (Level 2)	Dexamethasone	
Minimal (Level 1)	No routine prophylaxis needed	

SELF-ASSESSMENT QUESTIONS

1. Which of the following guidelines are applied to the design of combination chemotherapy?
   A. Use only orally active drugs together.
   B. Combine drugs with the same molecular target.
   C. Employ drugs that have minimal or no overlapping toxicities.
   D. Administer drugs with the same molecular mass.
   E. Apply drugs that are metabolized by the same route.

2. There are several goals for the administration of chemotherapeutic agents in the treatment of cancer. Which of the following terms describes chemotherapy administered after surgery, radiation, or both?
   A. Adjuvant.
   B. Curative.
   C. Elective.
   D. Palliative.

3. Drugs that selectively target tumor metastases:
   A. Do not exist.
   B. Typically inhibit angiogenesis.
   C. Are more effective than radiation therapy.
   D. Are more effective than surgery.

4. The primary objective of chemotherapy for a given patient may involve:
   A. Reducing tumor burden.
   B. Adjunctive therapy following surgery.
   C. Complete remission
   D. All of the above.

FURTHER READING

Begley CG, Ellis LM. Drug development: raise standards for preclinical cancer research. *Nature.* 2012;483:531–533.

Kinch MS. An analysis of FDA-approved drugs for oncology. *Drug Discov Today.* 2014;19:1831–1835.

Lazo JS, Sharlow ER. Drugging undruggable molecular cancer targets. *Annu Rev Pharmacol Toxicol.* 2016;56:23–40.s

WEBSITES

https://www.cancer.org/

The American Cancer Society website is useful for information regarding cancer and cancer chemotherapy.

https://www.cancer.gov/

This is the National Cancer Institute website and is a valuable resource for all cancer-related issues.

Cytotoxic Agents

Mary-Ann Bjornsti

THERAPEUTIC OVERVIEW

The goal of chemotherapy with antineoplastic agents is to kill tumor cells in solid or hematologic cancers while limiting the toxic effects of these drugs. Additional drugs and biologics have been developed that either enhance host immune response mechanisms or selectively target essential pathways in cancer cells (Chapter 69). Nevertheless, cytotoxic antineoplastic drugs remain the mainstay of effective chemotherapy. In clinical practice, most neoplastic diseases are treated using combinations of drugs; some of the common multimodality protocols are described in Chapter 67 (Table 67.1). This chapter will focus only on individual drugs that possess the ability to kill cells using a variety of mechanisms that form the basis for multiple-drug therapy.

The effectiveness of antineoplastic drugs varies with the type of cancer, the age and physiological condition of the patient, and the extent of tumor growth or spread (local versus metastatic disease). Other important factors include the specific endpoint used to evaluate effectiveness (e.g., a surrogate endpoint of tumor response rate versus clinical benefits, such as time to disease progression or patient survival) and adverse drug effects that limit patient dosing (dose-limiting toxicities). Most antineoplastic agents, particularly chemotherapeutic agents, are more effective in killing cells that are progressing through the cell cycle (Fig. 68.1) than in killing quiescent cells, which are resting in the G_0 phase. The growth fraction is the percentage of cells progressing through the cycle. In addition to proliferating tumor cells, there are also normal cells undergoing division, especially those of hair follicles, bone marrow, and the intestinal epithelium. These rapidly dividing cells are particularly sensitive to antineoplastic drugs and contribute to the dose-limiting adverse side effects and toxicities associated with select agents. It is widely held that most anticancer drugs kill cells primarily through an energy-dependent process of programmed cell death or apoptosis rather than through necrosis.

The action of cytotoxic chemotherapeutic agents typically follows first-order kinetics (Fig. 68.2), where the same fraction of cells is killed with each drug dose. Consequently, repeated cycles of chemotherapy are needed to reduce tumor size, and a functional host immune system is needed to kill all neoplastic cells and effect a cure. The frequency and duration of these treatments may be limited by patient toxicity.

Further evident in the "survival shoulder" in Fig. 68.2 is the fact that treatment with some agents requires a threshold of drug concentration to overcome endogenous repair or resistance pathways that suppress the cytotoxic activity of the drug.

Of the four major types of tumors, the faster-growing leukemias and lymphomas are generally more responsive to treatment than slower-growing carcinomas and sarcomas. Factors responsible for this difference include more rapid doubling times and the greater ease of drug distribution. Typically, the outer edges of solid tumors contain newly replicated cells, are well vascularized, and are readily accessible to drugs. This, in part, is attributed to the growth of new blood vessels by angiogenesis. However, the new tumor vasculature is typically less organized and "leakier" than normal vessels. In contrast, the central portions of many solid tumors are often hypoxic and necrotic, as angiogenesis is inadequate, making them poorly accessible to drugs. The inner cells may be dead or merely quiescent (noncycling), the latter still capable of returning to the cell cycle. Drug delivery to inner portions of solid tumors remains a major clinical challenge. In spite of the challenges, the endogenous factors that contribute to angiogenesis have become molecular targets for chemotherapeutic agents (Chapter 69).

Antineoplastic drugs must also enter the cell to produce cytotoxic effects. Some agents pass through the membrane by passive diffusion, with uptake driven by local concentration gradients. Other drugs must bind to carrier proteins for transport through the membrane and release into the cytoplasm, a mechanism particularly common with antimetabolites. Carrier-mediated transport is an active process and is not concentration driven, and the rate of transport is limited by the number of carrier molecules expressed on the cancer cells. Once in the cell, drugs diffuse into the nucleus or other cellular compartment and interact with target molecules to disrupt critical processes necessary for cell viability. Considerations for using antineoplastic agents are provided in the Therapeutic Overview Box.

THERAPEUTIC OVERVIEW

Goal
Kill tumor cells selectively with minimal side effects

Uses
Treatment of local or metastatic disease (curative or palliative)
Treatment of solid tumors (carcinomas, sarcomas, lymphomas) and hematological cancers (leukemias)
Decrease tumor burden

Effects
Some, but not all tumors, respond

Considerations
Issues of drug delivery to individual cancer cells
Cycling versus noncycling cell log-kill (same fraction of cells killed per dose)
Need for active immune system (host defenses) to eradicate residual cancer cells
Lack of vascularization, central hypoxic zone of tumors
Drug resistance (intrinsic or acquired)

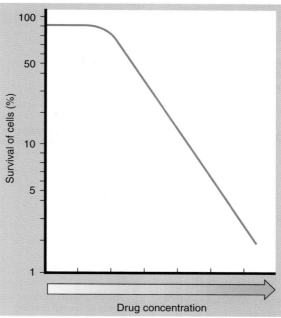

FIG. 68.2 Decline in the fraction of viable cells is first order with respect to drug concentration. Many antineoplastic agents and cultured cancer cells follow this log–cell kill principle of a fixed percentage of viable cells killed per dose of drug. This relationship also appears to apply in vivo, although the actual situation may be more complex. A threshold concentration of drug must often be achieved to cause a noticeable decrease in cell survival. This phenomenon, called "survival shoulder," may reflect endogenous repair and drug modification processes.

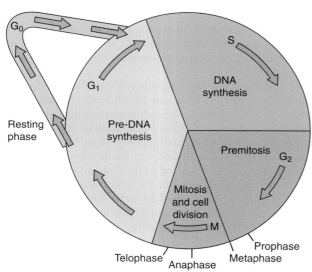

FIG. 68.1 Growth Cycle for Human Cells. The cells are quiescent or dormant in the G_0 (resting) phase. Growth stimulants promote the cycling of cells by inducing entry into the G_1 phase (pre-DNA synthesis), where the precursors needed for the replication of DNA are formed. DNA synthesis occurs in the S, or synthetic phase. This is followed by premitotic events and structural developments in the G_2 phase. Mitosis occurs in the M phase to produce two daughter cells, each of which has a full complement of replicated chromosomes and can either continue to cycle into G_1 or can enter the resting phase, G_0. Growth fraction is defined as the total cells in the growth cycle (G_1, S, G_2, M) divided by the total cells (G_1, S, G_2, M, G_0).

MECHANISMS OF ACTION

The basic mechanisms by which antineoplastic drugs and **antibody-drug conjugates (ADCs)** kill tumor cells are summarized in Fig. 68.3. Only drugs, conjugates, or biologics that exhibit some selectivity for neoplastic cells are used clinically. The difference in doses that elicit a therapeutic effect versus those that produce a toxic effect is termed the **therapeutic index** (Chapter 3). In general, **antimetabolites** inhibit DNA synthesis,

whereas **alkylating agents**, **ADCs**, and **antitumor antibiotics** typically damage or disrupt DNA, interfere with topoisomerase activity, or alter RNA transcription or structure. Representative structures of different classes of these agents are shown in Fig. 68.4. Several **plant alkaloids** used in cancer chemotherapy either disrupt microtubule dynamics or target topoisomerase. Other agents include **asparaginase**, a biologic that destroys essential amino acids needed for protein translation. Many clinically used antineoplastic agents are prodrugs, which must undergo either chemical or enzymatic modification to become actively cytotoxic.

Alkylating Agents

Alkylation involves the covalent attachment of an alkyl group to another molecule. The development of alkylating agents for the treatment of cancer was derived from early observations on the effects of mustard gases on cell growth. Although these compounds proved too toxic for clinical use, the first effective antineoplastic drugs, such as mechlorethamine, were developed from nitrogen mustard alkylating agents and are still in use today.

Alkylation is accomplished by the chemical formation of a positively charged carbonium ion, which reacts with an electron-rich group on DNA or RNA to covalently modify the nucleic acid. Most alkylating drugs in clinical use have two functional groups (i.e., **bifunctional agents**), allowing for the formation of **covalent links** between adjacent bases in a single strand of nucleic acid or between bases in different polynucleotide strands. Such crosslinks are more difficult to repair than monofunctional adducts. Interstrand crosslinks also prevent separation of the DNA strands during the S phase of the cell cycle. Although other nucleophilic constituents of cells are also alkylated, including RNA,

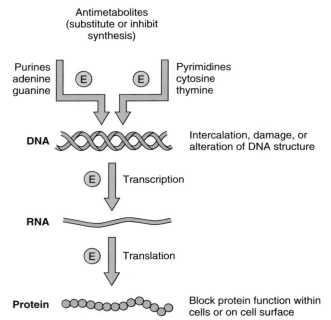

FIG. 68.3 Basic Mechanisms by Which Antineoplastic Drugs Selectively Kill Tumor Cells. *E* represents enzymes, some of which are inhibited by these drugs. Inhibition of DNA or RNA synthesis, production of miscoded nucleic acids, and formation of modified proteins are key mechanisms of action for many of these drugs.

proteins, and membrane components, the primary basis for cytotoxicity is alkylation of DNA, especially at the N-7 position of deoxyguanylates in either single- or double-stranded DNA. The mechanism of sequential alkylation of the N-7 position of guanine by mechlorethamine is illustrated in Fig. 68.5; other nitrogen mustards work through a similar mechanism. Cyclophosphamide undergoes sequential enzymatic and chemical activation to form the active phosphoramide mustard alkylating agent (Fig. 68.6), and ifosfamide, like cyclophosphamide, is also activated. Melphalan, a phenylalanine derivative of mechlorethamine, is actively transported into the cell by leucine and glutamine transport carriers. Busulfan is also thought to alkylate both the N-7 of guanine of DNA via the formation of carbonium ions, as well as the sulfhydryl groups (-SH) of glutathione and protein thiols.

Nitrosoureas are another group of antineoplastic alkylating agents in clinical use and include lomustine, carmustine, and semustine. The primary mechanism of activation of the nitrosoureas is DNA alkylation, as shown in Fig. 68.7. However, nitrosoureas can also carbamylate proteins, which may contribute to the cytotoxic activity of these agents.

The triazene alkylating agents include dacarbazine, procarbazine, and temozolomide. These drugs primarily methylate guanine at the O-6 and N-7 positions, resulting in the misincorporation of thymidine in newly synthesized DNA (across from the methylated guanine), which is not corrected by the mismatch repair system. However, increased expression of the 6-methylguanine-DNA methylase (MGMT) gene allows tumor cells to repair this form of DNA damage and acquire resistance to temozolomide. Unlike most alkylating agents, temozolomide is able to cross the blood-brain barrier.

Platinum antineoplastic agents, or platins, are coordinated complexes of platinum that are termed *alkylating-like* because they also modify DNA, mostly at the N-7 position of guanine. These drugs include cisplatin, carboplatin, nedaplatin, and oxaliplatin. Cisplatin is a planar platinum complex with two ammonia molecules and two chloride ions.

The reaction mechanism is complex and involves the replacement of chlorine with water, which is then replaced by N-heterocyclic bases in DNA (such as guanine). A second round of chloride displacement in the *cis* stereoisomer configuration forms intrastrand crosslinks, primarily at two adjacent deoxyguanylates in DNA. Less frequent interstrand crosslinks are formed by the *trans* isomer. Both contribute to the cytotoxic activity of cisplatin. Similar DNA crosslinks are formed with carboplatin and nedaplatin, although these analogues appear to be slightly less potent but less nephrotoxic than cisplatin. Oxaliplatin is a diaminocyclohexane platinum analogue that forms the same inter- and intrastrand crosslinks as cisplatin and carboplatin and inhibits DNA replication and transcription. However, the presence of the 1,2-diaminocyclohexane adduct reduces the development of some drug resistance attributed to specific repair pathways of platinum adducts formed by cis-/carboplatin.

Antimetabolites

Antimetabolites are compounds that mimic the structures of normal components required for DNA or RNA synthesis, including folic acid, pyrimidines, and/or purines. As a consequence, antimetabolites inhibit enzymes necessary for folic acid regeneration, pyrimidine or purine synthesis, or DNA or RNA synthesis in neoplastic cells. These agents frequently kill cells in the S phase (see Fig. 68.1). Examples of antimetabolites in clinical use for cancer therapy include methotrexate (MTX), pemetrexed, pralatrexate, 5-fluorouracil (5-FU), capecitabine, cytarabine (Ara-C), gemcitabine, 6-thioguanine (6-TG), 6-mercaptopurine (6-MP), and clofarabine. Structures of some of these agents are provided in Fig. 68.4.

Folic acid is essential for enzymatic reactions that transfer methyl groups during purine and pyrimidine biosynthesis. The antimetabolite MTX is a folate antagonist that competitively inhibits the enzyme dihydrofolate reductase (DHFR), which catalyzes the reduction of dihydrofolate to tetrahydrofolate (FH_4; Fig. 68.8). As a consequence, the regeneration of FH_4 is blocked, and the de novo synthesis of the thymidine nucleoside as well as the synthesis of purine and pyrimidine bases are prevented. MTX inhibits the synthesis of DNA, RNA, and proteins. MTX has about a 1000-fold higher affinity for DHFR than folate. Moreover, intracellular glutamylation of MTX greatly enhances its inhibitory activity and prevents efflux from the cell. Thus the selectivity of MTX for tumor cells derives, in part, from the higher levels of polyglutamylating enzyme activity in cancer cells, which traps higher concentrations of the more active glutamylated MTX.

Transport of MTX into cells is carrier mediated, and reduced MTX uptake is a prominent mechanism by which tumor cells develop resistance. When high-dose MTX is administered, it is typically followed within 24 hours by a "rescue process" that employs leucovorin (5-formyl-FH_4; folinic acid) to suppress MTX toxicity in normal tissue, such as bone marrow and gastrointestinal mucosa. Leucovorin is a reduced FH_4 analogue and at low doses enters nonmalignant cells by a carrier-mediated process, bypassing the requirement for DHFR activity, and enabling purine and pyrimidine synthesis to proceed in normal cells (see Fig. 68.8).

The MTX analogue pemetrexed inhibits three folate-dependent enzymes (i.e., thymidylate synthase, DHFR, and glycinamide ribonucleotide formyltransferase) involved in the synthesis of thymidine and purine nucleotides and inhibits DNA and RNA synthesis. Like MTX, pemetrexed is preferentially polyglutamylated in malignant cells, while another analogue, pralatrexate, selectively enters cancer cells expressing high levels of the reduced folate carrier type 1 (RFC-1). Although not an MTX analogue, pentostatin is a purine nucleotide analogue antibiotic that inhibits adenine deaminase, an essential enzyme for purine metabolism, especially in cells of the lymphoid system.

Alkylating Agents

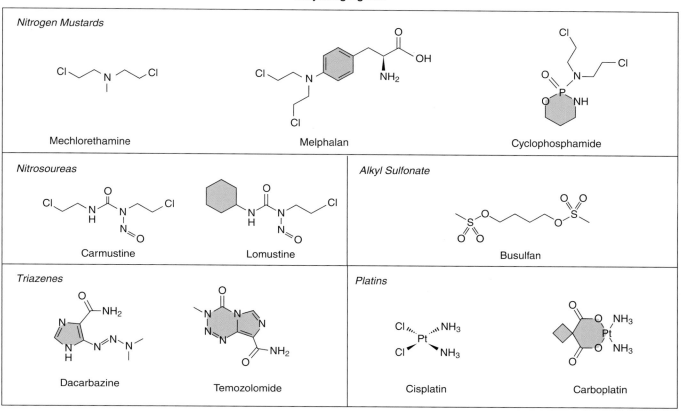

Antimetabolites

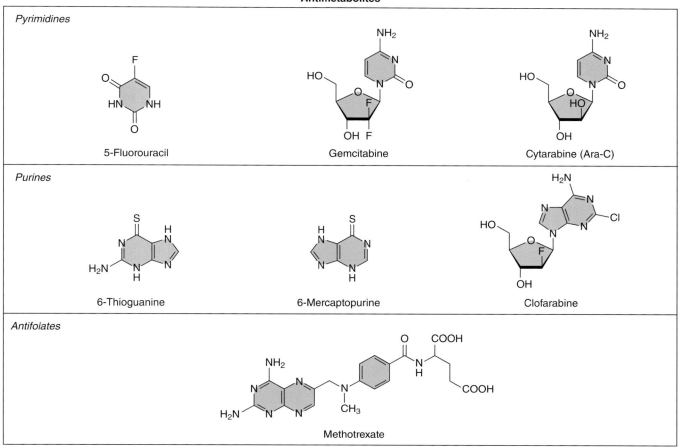

FIG. 68.4 Structures of Different Classes of Cytotoxic Anticancer Drugs. Shown are representative members of alkylating agents, antimetabolites, antitumor antibiotics, plant alkaloids, and others.

Continued

Antitumor Antibiotics

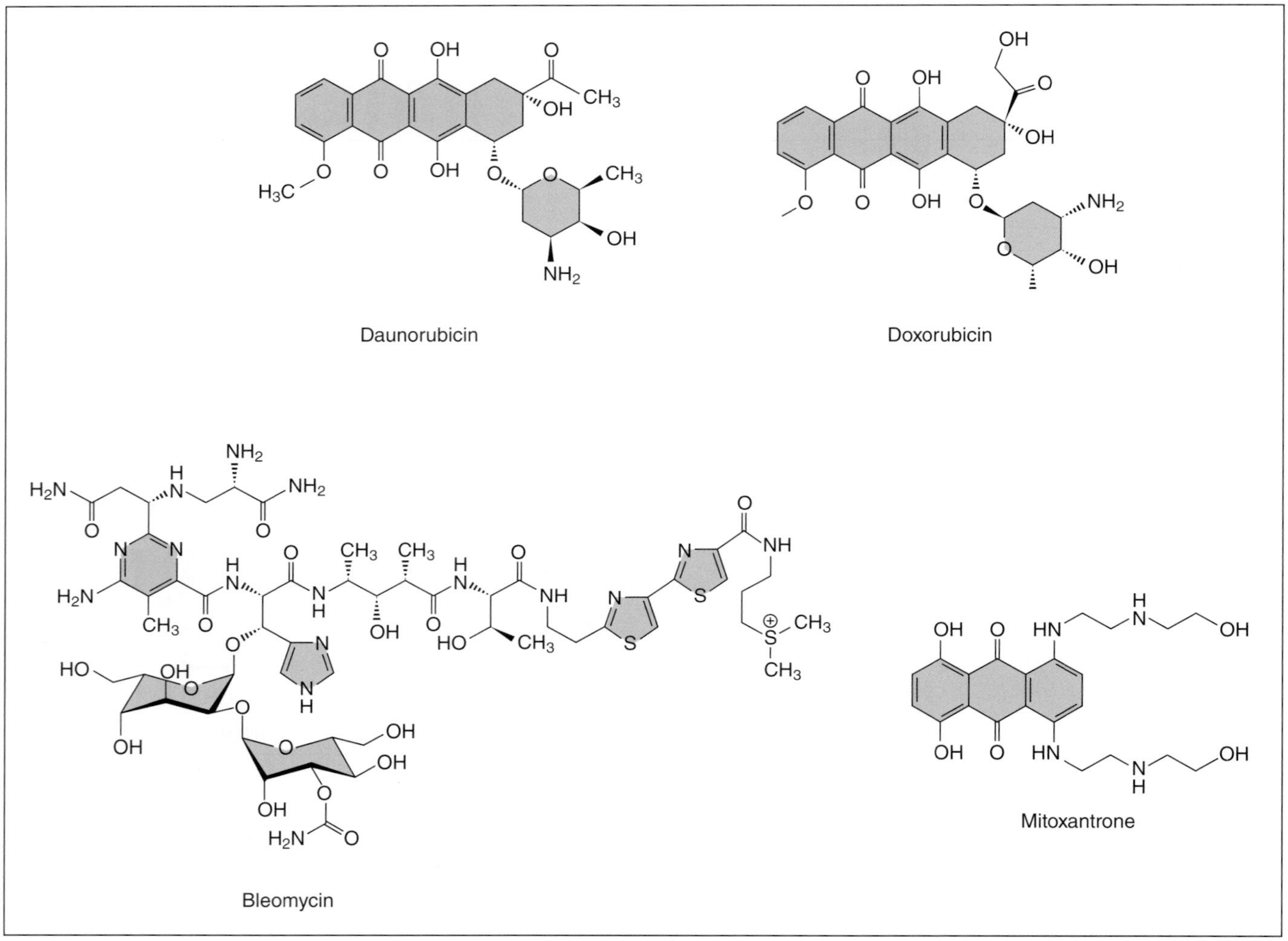

Daunorubicin

Doxorubicin

Bleomycin

Mitoxantrone

FIG. 68.4, cont'd

Plant Alkaloids

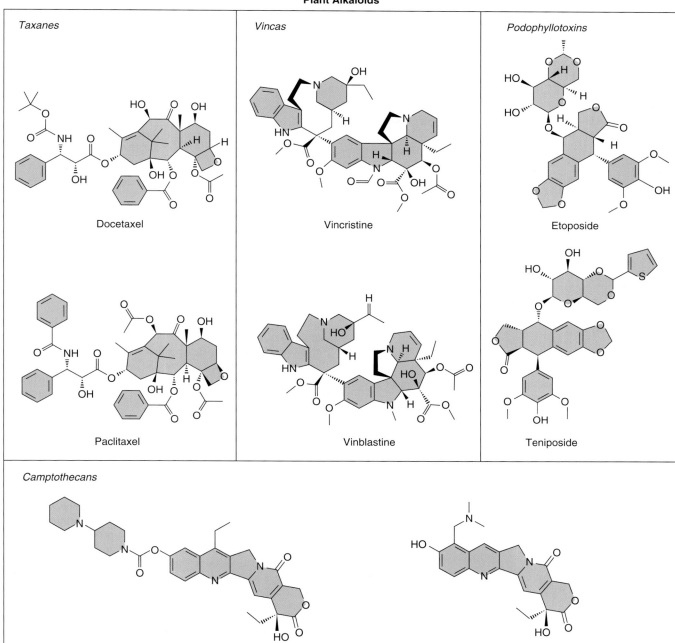

Taxanes

Docetaxel

Paclitaxel

Vincas

Vincristine

Vinblastine

Podophyllotoxins

Etoposide

Teniposide

Camptothecans

Irinotecan

Topotecan

Others

Ixabepilone

Eribulin

FIG. 68.4, cont'd

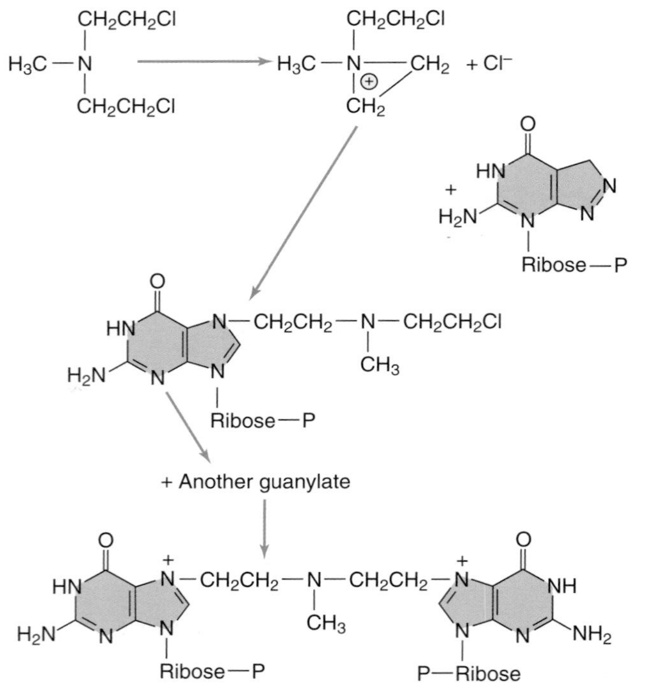

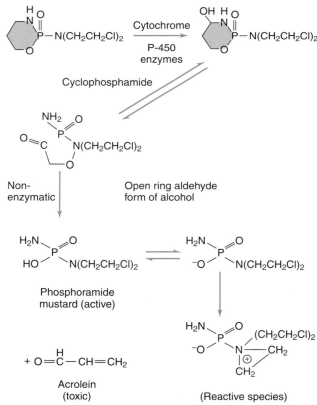

FIG. 68.5 DNA Alkylation by Mechlorethamine. Shown is the positively charged intermediate ion and its covalent attachment to the N-7 position of two deoxyguanylate nucleotides of DNA.

FIG. 68.6 Mechanism of Enzymatic and Chemical Activation of Cyclophosphamide to Form Active Phosphoramide Mustard. The acrolein formed has some antitumor activity but much less than that of the phosphoramide mustard.

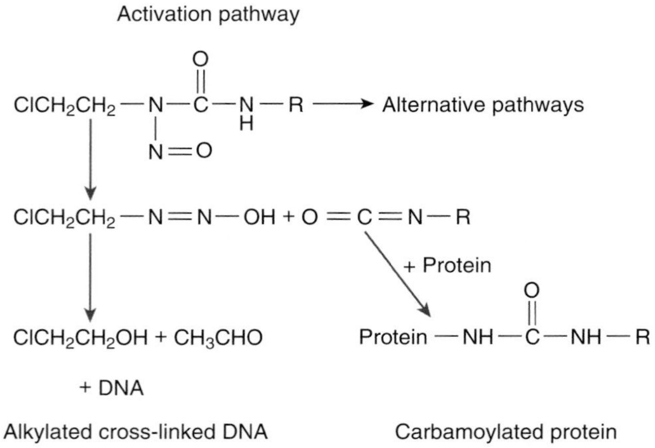

FIG. 68.7 Activation Pathways for Nitrosourea Alkylating Agents. Carbamylation of proteins also occurs but is believed to be a lesser cause of cell cytotoxicity than alkylation of DNA.

The pyrimidine antimetabolite, 5-FU, inhibits pyrimidine synthesis and thus DNA replication (Fig. 68.8). This agent is metabolized to the 5-fluoronated analogue of deoxyuridine monophosphate, which inhibits **thymidylate synthase** and prevents the conversion of deoxythymidine monophosphate (dTMP) from deoxyuridine monophosphate (dUMP). Capecitabine is an oral fluoropyrimidine and an inactive prodrug of 5-FU that is selectively converted to 5-FU in the liver and in tumors. Thymidine phosphorylase, an enzyme responsible for the final step in the conversion to 5-FU, may be endogenously overexpressed in neoplastic tissues. Floxuridine is rapidly converted into 5-FU.

Cytarabine, or Ara-C, is also a pyrimidine-based antimetabolite that combines a cytosine base and an arabinose (instead of deoxyribose) sugar. Ara-C is subject to inactivation or conversion to the active cytosine triphosphate by competing enzymatic activities (Fig. 68.9). Following activation, Ara-CTP is incorporated into DNA, terminating chain elongation. At high doses, Ara-C also is a competitive inhibitor of DNA polymerase. Some patients exhibit high cytidine deaminase activity and low deoxycytidylate kinase activity, resulting in considerable inactivation of the drug, a mechanism by which resistance develops.

Gemcitabine is a fluorine-substituted deoxycytidine antimetabolite. The sequential phosphorylation of this prodrug in cells, first by deoxycytidine kinase, then by other kinases, yields active forms of the drug that inhibit DNA synthesis. The diphosphate form inhibits ribonucleotide reductase to deplete deoxynucleotide triphosphate (dNTP) pools, while the triphosphate form inhibits DNA polymerase or acts to terminate chain elongation once incorporated into DNA.

The purine antimetabolites 6-mercaptopurine (6-MP) and 6-thioguanine (6-TG) are also activated by enzymes, including hypoxanthine-guanine phosphoribosyl transferase, to form nucleotides, which then inhibit several enzymes in purine synthesis pathways. The incorporation of the triphosphate nucleotides into DNA or RNA may also contribute to the cytotoxicity of these drugs.

Antitumor Antibiotics

Microbial antibiotics, isolated from a variety of microbes and representing several chemical classes, have proven to be very effective in the treatment of cancer and are collectively known as the antitumor antibiotics. These agents include the anthracyclines **doxorubicin** and **daunorubicin**, the analogues **idarubicin** and **epirubicin**, and the related anthracene **mitoxantrone**. Other antitumor antibiotics include **bleomycin**, **dactinomycin**, and **mitomycin**.

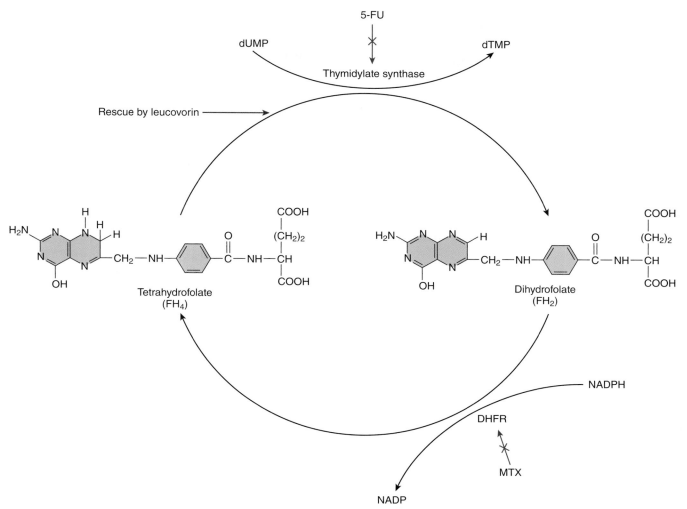

FIG. 68.8 Actions of Methotrexate (MTX) and 5-Fluorouracil (5-FU). Deoxythymidine monophosphate (dTMP) is synthesized from deoxyuridine monophosphate (dUMP) in a reaction catalyzed by the enzyme thymidylate synthase. This reaction requires tetrahydrofolate (FH_4) as a cofactor, which is concomitantly oxidized to dihydrofolate (FH_2). FH_4 is regenerated from FH_2 in a reduction reaction catalyzed by dihydrofolate reductase (DHFR). MTX reversibly inhibits DHFR, while 5-FU inhibits thymidylate synthase. Also shown is the rescue path by leucovorin, a reduced FH_4 analogue that bypasses DHFR, enabling purine and pyrimidine synthesis to proceed in normal cells. The synthesis of purine and pyrimidine bases is required for DNA, RNA, and protein synthesis.

The anthracycline antibiotics were isolated from *Streptomyces* and are widely used cytotoxic antineoplastic agents. The mechanism of action of doxorubicin, daunorubicin, and their analogues is complex and results from their ability to intercalate between bases in double-stranded DNA, poison DNA topoisomerase II, generate semiquinone and oxygen-free radicals, and possibly disrupt the fluidity of the cell membrane. As illustrated in Fig. 68.10, the poisoning of DNA topoisomerase II is thought to constitute the major cytotoxic activity of these drugs. Topoisomerase II is an enzyme that plays an important role in DNA replication and is essential for chromosome segregation. It catalyzes the uncoiling and unlinking of both strands of double-stranded DNA to modify DNA coiling and the intertwining of DNA duplexes. Doxorubicin and analogues poison the enzyme by stabilizing a covalent topoisomerase II-DNA reaction intermediate, which prevents the protein-linked DNA breaks from rejoining, ultimately leading to cell death.

Bleomycin is a mixture of several basic glycopeptides, with the structure of the A2 form used as representative. Among the most commonly used cytotoxic anticancer drugs, it has a unique mechanism of action. Bleomycin forms a tertiary complex with O_2 and Fe^{++} to induce sequence-specific single- and double-stranded DNA breaks. Double-stranded DNA cleavage is thought to cause cell lethality.

Dactinomycin (actinomycin D) is also a DNA intercalator, where the resulting blockade of transcription is a major source of its antitumor activity. Dactinomycin also induces single-stranded DNA breaks, possibly through the production of free radicals. Mitomycin-C undergoes reductive activation to form the active species, mitosene, which cross-links DNA by N-alkylation of DNA bases, typically guanine in the sequence 5'-CpG-3'.

Antibody-Drug Conjugates

Recent advances in the design of new cancer therapies involve the development of ADCs, in which a monoclonal antibody is covalently attached to a cytotoxic drug. The monoclonal antibody directs the conjugate to the surface of cancer cells, where it specifically interacts

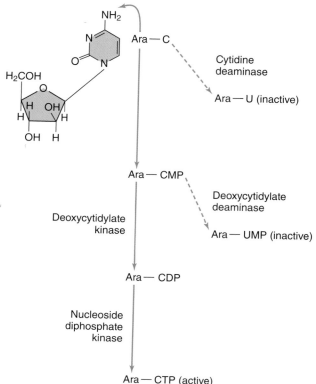

FIG. 68.9 Competing Activation and Deactivation Pathways for the Conversion of Cytarabine (Cytosine Arabinoside, Ara-C) to the Active Form That Inhibits DNA Polymerase.

with a surface-exposed protein that is only expressed on tumor cells. Binding of the conjugate to the surface protein triggers internalization of the conjugate, followed by cleavage of the linker between the drug and the antibody, leaving the cytotoxic molecule free to interact with its cellular target. The premise is that selective targeting of the cytotoxic payload to tumor cells will avoid, or at the very least, reduce substantially, the toxicities associated with drug exposure of normal cells and allow for local delivery of higher drug doses. Both cleavable and noncleavable linkers have been used to connect the cytotoxin to the antibody and have been shown to be stable and safe in preclinical and clinical trials. To date, three ADCs have received approval in the United States, and a fourth has been approved in Europe.

The first ADC approved in the United States in 2000, **gemtuzumab ozogamicin**, is comprised of an antibody to CD33 linked to an antitumor antibiotic, for the treatment of acute myelogenous leukemia. However, it was withdrawn from the market in 2010 due to toxicity and lack of efficacy. Two ADCs currently marketed in the United States are **brentuximab vedotin** and **trastuzumab emtansine**. Brentuximab vedotin is a CD30-targeted antibody, with a cathepsin-cleavable linker attached to a highly toxic antimicrotubule agent, monomethyl auristatin E (MMAE). MMAE blocks tubulin polymerization but is too toxic for use as a single agent. Trastuzumab emtansine combines the human epidermal growth factor 2 (HER2)-specific antibody with the microtubule inhibitor emtansine through a noncleavable linker.

Plant Alkaloids

Plants have served as a rich source for the development of active cytotoxic cancer drugs, including the vinca alkaloids (**vincristine** and **vinblastine**), taxanes (**paclitaxel**, **docetaxel**, and **cabazitaxel**), podophyllotoxins (**teniposide** and **etoposide**), and camptothecins (**topotecan** and irinotecan). Vinblastine and vincristine are close analogues derived from the periwinkle plant, with very different spectrums of clinical activity and dose-limiting toxicities, whereas the taxanes include **paclitaxel**, first isolated from yew trees, and other semisynthetic derivatives. The vincas and taxanes are both antimitotics. The vincas bind to **tubulin** to block microtubule polymerization, and the taxanes stabilize microtubules in the polymerized form (Fig. 68.11). In each case, the net effect is disruption of mitotic spindle function during the M phase of the cell cycle (see Fig. 68.1), resulting in an inability to properly segregate chromosomes and cell death.

Etoposide is a semisynthetic D-glucose derivative of podophyllotoxin, which is from the rhizobium of the mandrake plant. Etoposide and its close analogue **teniposide** poison topoisomerase II, as described for doxorubicin (see Fig. 68.10).

Camptothecins are natural products derived from a tree indigenous to China. Two approved analogues are **topotecan** and the prodrug **irinotecan**. Camptothecins target the enzyme DNA **topoisomerase I**, which is critical for unwinding DNA during replication and transcription. Thus the cytotoxic action of the camptothecins is highly S-phase dependent (see Fig. 68.1). Topoisomerase I makes transient single-stranded nicks in duplex DNA to allow for DNA unwinding or rewinding. Camptothecins stabilize a covalent enzyme-DNA reaction intermediate to prevent DNA relegation and inhibit DNA replication. Topotecan is a water-soluble derivative, while irinotecan is a prodrug that must be converted into the active metabolite, SN-38, predominantly by a liver carboxyl esterase.

Although not derived from plants, **ixabepilone** (an analogue of epothilone B from a myxobacterium) also acts to stabilize microtubules and is active in tumors with tubulin mutations. **Eribulin**, a macrocyclic ketone derived from a marine organism, has a unique mechanism of action by driving microtubule depolymerization.

Others

The enzyme L-**asparaginase**, isolated from either *Escherichia coli* or *Dickeya dadantii* (formerly known as *Erwinia chrysanthemi*), has antileukemic activity. The enzyme hydrolyzes the amino acid L-asparagine, which is present in low amounts in leukemia cells yet is essential for tumor cell growth. Depletion of L-asparagine terminates protein and eventually nucleic acid synthesis. This approach is selective for tumor cells that are devoid of asparagine synthetase and are unable to synthesize this essential amino acid.

Hydroxyurea inhibits the enzyme ribonucleotide reductase that catalyzes the rate-limiting step in the synthesis of deoxyribonucleotides required for DNA synthesis. Hydroxyurea is thought to complex with the non-heme Fe^{++}, which is required for enzyme activity and is an S phase–specific agent.

Arsenic trioxide is metabolized by arsenate reductase to trivalent arsenic, which then undergoes methylation predominantly in the liver. Arsenic accumulates mainly in liver, kidney, heart, lung, hair, and nails. Arsenic trioxide is thought to induce the degradation of the promyelocytic leukemia (PML) protein component of the onco-protein PML–retinoic acid receptor α complex, which then induces apoptosis of the leukemic promyelocytes. Arsenic trioxide also appears to have activity in multiple myeloma.

MECHANISMS OF RESISTANCE

In general, mechanisms of resistance to antineoplastic drugs can be distinguished as intrinsic or acquired. With intrinsic resistance, a specific drug protocol does not yield a positive response, even though the same therapeutic regimen has proved beneficial to other patients with the same disease. With acquired resistance, a patient initially has a positive response,

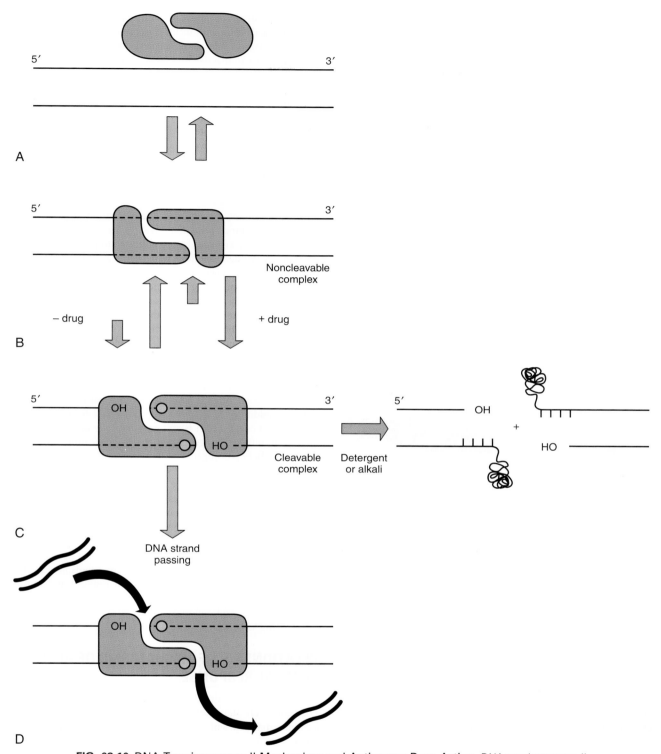

FIG. 68.10 DNA Topoisomerase II Mechanism and Anticancer Drug Action. DNA topoisomerase II binds to DNA (A) and forms two different types of protein-DNA complexes that are in rapid equilibrium: the noncleavable complex (B) and the cleavable complex (C). These complexes can be identified in vitro by the ability of detergent or alkali to separate DNA strands. The cleavable complex is transient but is stabilized by doxorubicin, daunorubicin, etoposide, or actinomycin (D). In the absence of drug, DNA strand passage occurs, whereas drugs block DNA strand passage and DNA relegation.

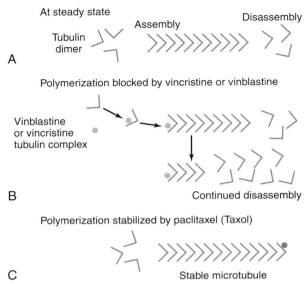

At steady state

Tubulin
dimer   Assembly   Disassembly

A

Polymerization blocked by vincristine or vinblastine

Vinblastine
or vincristine
tubulin complex

B   Continued disassembly

Polymerization stabilized by paclitaxel (Taxol)

C   Stable microtubule

FIG. 68.11 Microtubule Dynamics in the Presence of Vincristine, Vinblastine, or Paclitaxel. A dynamic steady state exists, with microtubule assembly occurring at one end and disassembly at the other (A). Vincristine and vinblastine (B) bind to tubulin dimers and block polymerization, allowing disassembly to predominate. In contrast, paclitaxel (C) blocks disassembly, causing stable microtubules to form even in the absence of normally essential cofactors. Cells treated with any of these agents are blocked in mitosis.

BOX 68.1   Possible Mechanisms of Resistance to Antineoplastic Agents

Antineoplastic Agent
Decreased uptake of active agent into cancer cell
Failure of agent to be metabolized to a chemical species capable of producing a cytotoxic effect
Enhanced conversion of agent to inactive metabolite
Increase in transport of agent from the cancer cell

Cancer Cell (DNA, Target Enzyme, or Other Macromolecule)
Repair of drug-induced DNA damage
Gene amplification or increased gene transcription leading to greater amount of target enzyme within the cancer cell
Reduced ability of target enzyme to bind agent
Increase in concentration of sulfhydryl scavengers
Altered concentrations of target protein
Increased expression of antiapoptotic genes, such as *BCL2*

---

but unfortunately, the tumor returns and is no longer responsive to subsequent treatments with the same drug or drug combination. In both cases, the reduced effectiveness in resistant patients can often be attributed to decreased intracellular concentration of the drug, alterations in drug metabolism, increased repair of drug-induced damage, or modification or mutation of drug targets. Increased expression of proteins that block the energy-dependent process of apoptosis, such as the oncogene *BCL2*, can also cause resistance to many agents. Mechanisms accounting for these differences in drug sensitivity are indicated in Box 68.1.

One mechanism of resistance is decreased drug uptake, such as in the case of MTX, which requires carrier proteins for transmembrane transport into the cell. Dactinomycin resistance also results from decreased uptake. A second mechanism of resistance involves a lack of

or decreased drug activation. For example, cyclophosphamide requires metabolic activation, and in the absence of this pathway, tumor cells will be resistant. A third mechanism is the enhanced conversion of an active agent to an inactive metabolite. For instance, an increase in the activity of aldehyde dehydrogenase promotes the catabolism of cyclophosphamide and the development of drug resistance.

Enhanced cellular efflux of a drug is another common mechanism of resistance. Human cells may express the transmembrane phospho-glycoprotein **P-glycoprotein**, which is an ATP-driven transport protein. This P-glycoprotein actively transports hydrophobic compounds with aromatic and basic properties out of the cell. Cells with an elevated expression of the *multidrug resistance (MDR1)* gene that encodes the multidrug-resistant P-glycoprotein manifest resistance to doxorubicin, daunorubicin, dactinomycin, etoposide, teniposide, vincristine, and vinblastine. Other structurally related drug transporters, such as multidrug resistance protein 1 (MRP1) and breast cancer resistance protein (BCRP), have also been implicated to play a role in multidrug resistance. Considerable efforts have been made to develop compounds that can block the action of the P-glycoprotein and related pumps and thus circumvent multidrug resistance. However, clinical trials with such agents have largely failed to overcome drug resistance due to toxicities associated with the inhibition of the normal physiological function of these membrane-bound transporters.

Another mechanism of resistance, exemplified by bleomycin resistance, involves the ability of cells to rapidly repair the DNA breaks caused by the drug. Gene amplification or gene mutation can also confer drug resistance. For example, cells with increased intracellular levels of DHFR as a consequence of gene amplification are resistant to the actions of MTX. In addition, MTX resistance may result from a mutation that produces an enzyme that is still enzymatically active but has a lower binding affinity for the drug. Alternatively, a gene mutation may prevent MTX from being conjugated with polyglutamates and would therefore not be retained in the tumor cell. In this case, higher unconjugated MTX concentrations would be required to inhibit DHFR.

Cells may also develop resistance to reactive drugs, particularly alkylating agents, by increasing intracellular concentrations of sulfhydryl compounds, such as glutathione and metallothioneins, which protect cells by scavenging highly reactive compounds. Last, resistance may be attributed to decreased expression of drug targets by tumor cells. For example, a decrease in topoisomerase II or topoisomerase I activity leads to resistance to etoposide or topotecan, respectively. Unfortunately, cancer cells often possess multiple pathways to effect drug resistance, which limits therapeutic efforts to block one or two pathways to effectively restore drug sensitivity.

RELATIONSHIP OF MECHANISMS OF ACTION TO CLINICAL RESPONSE

Most antineoplastic drugs are used as one component of a multiagent protocol where the cytotoxic effects of each drug may interact in a complex manner, with the preferred outcome being synergistic cell killing of malignant cells. The clinical use of combination chemotherapy is discussed in Chapter 67. All of the agents have specific cytotoxic properties, yet there are differences in the types of cancers for which the agents are approved.

Alkylating Agents

Cyclophosphamide is a component of multiple chemotherapy regimens used to treat leukemia, non-Hodgkin lymphoma, rhabdomyosarcoma, and breast and ovarian germ cell cancers. Temozolomide was approved in 2005 for the treatment of malignant gliomas, while a hydrochloride gel formulation of mechlorethamine was approved for second-line topical treatment of a subtype of cutaneous T cell lymphoma in 2014. In 2016, a more stable intravenous cyclodextrin formulation of melphalan was approved, which allows for high-dose conditioning of patients with multiple myeloma prior to hematopoietic progenitor (stem) cell transplantation. A regimen of busulfan and melphalan is also used for conditioning prior to stem cell transplantation. Chlorambucil, which is structurally similar to melphalan, is primarily used to treat chronic lymphocytic leukemia, while ifosfamide is active against several cancers, including small cell lung cancer, sarcomas, lymphomas, testicular carcinoma, and gynecological cancers. The nitrosoureas are lipophilic, readily cross the blood-brain barrier, and are often used to treat brain tumors, while the platins are widely used as frontline chemotherapeutic regimens to treat solid malignancies, including breast; ovarian; non–small cell lung, cervical, testicular, head, and neck cancers; and mesothelioma. Oxaliplatin is approved for treatment of metastatic colorectal carcinoma in combination with 5-FU and leucovorin (folinic acid) and has demonstrated activity in lung cancer.

Antimetabolites

MTX is widely used in the treatment of breast, head and neck, colorectal, and bladder cancers, as well as lymphomas and leukemia. Pemetrexed is approved for the treatment of malignant mesothelioma in combination with cisplatin and has demonstrable activity in cervical, breast, and non–small cell lung cancer. Pralatrexate is approved for recurrent peripheral T-cell lymphoma., while 5-FU is used to treat pancreatic, renal, and liver cancers and in frontline combination regimens with leucovorin for the treatment of colon cancer. Capecitabine is part of irinotecan- or oxaliplatin-containing regimens for the treatment of breast, colorectal, gastric, and esophageal cancers, while floxuridine is used to treat colon, kidney, and stomach cancers.

Ara-C is used in the treatment of leukemias and non-Hodgkin lymphoma. Gemcitabine was initially approved for the treatment of advanced pancreatic cancer but also has demonstrated activity in breast, ovarian, non–small cell lung, and bladder cancers. The purine antimetabolites, 6-MP and 6-TG, are used to treat acute lymphocytic leukemia and chronic myeloid leukemia, while 6-TG is also used in patients with acute myeloid leukemia. The purine nucleotide analogue **pentostatin** is active against hairy cell leukemia.

Antitumor Antibiotics

Doxorubicin is one of the most important therapeutic agents in the clinic, with activity in breast, ovarian, testicular, bladder, and liver cancers; lymphomas; hematologic malignancies; and childhood solid tumors, and is frequently used in combination with other agents. A pegylated liposomal formulation was developed to treat Kaposi sarcoma. Epirubicin is also used to treat breast cancer, while daunorubicin and idarubicin are frequently used to treat leukemias. Bleomycin is typically used in combination with other drugs to treat Hodgkin and non-Hodgkin lymphoma, and testicular, ovarian, and cervical cancers, among others. Mitomycin-C has activity in hypoxic tumor cells of upper gastrointestinal tract tumors, anal cancer, and breast cancer. It is also used to treat superficial bladder cancer.

Antibody-Drug Conjugates

Brentuximab vedotin is approved for relapsed Hodgkin lymphoma and acute lymphocytic leukemia. Trastuzumab emtansine and the antibody by itself are used for the treatment of HER2-positive metastatic breast cancer (Chapter 69).

Plant Alkaloids

Vinblastine is part of a chemotherapy regimen for the treatment of Hodgkin lymphoma and is also active in breast and testicular cancers.

In contrast, vincristine is used to treat acute lymphoblastic leukemia, both Hodgkin and non-Hodgkin lymphoma, and pediatric tumors (neuroblastoma and Wilm tumor). Paclitaxel is active against a wide range of solid tumors, including ovarian carcinomas, breast cancer, and small cell and non–small cell lung cancers. A nanoparticle, albumin-bound formulation of paclitaxel is approved for use with metastatic breast cancer, pancreatic cancer, and non–small cell lung cancer. Etoposide is a component of multidrug regimens for the treatment of non-Hodgkin lymphoma and has significant activity against small cell lung cancer, leukemias, and testicular cancer. Teniposide is active against acute leukemias in children, topotecan has activity in refractory ovarian and small cell lung cancers and in pediatric solid tumors, while irinotecan is approved for treatment of metastatic colorectal carcinoma, has activity in cervical and non–small cell lung and gastric cancers, and is active in pediatric solid malignancies.

Others

Ixabepilone and eribulin are approved for treatment of metastatic breast cancer, while eribulin was approved in 2016 for treating inoperable liposarcoma. Arsenic trioxide is an organic compound that has received approval as a single agent for the treatment of refractory acute promyelocytic leukemia.

PHARMACOKINETICS

Pharmacokinetic parameters can be calculated and used to describe the bodily distribution of a drug, based on measurements of drug plasma concentrations obtained at various times following administration of a single dose (Chapter 3). A graph of drug concentration over time can be described by the area under the curve (AUC), which provides a measure of drug exposure. A standard compartment model is often used to describe drug distribution and is useful in providing guidance to plan dosing schemes that maximize efficacy, yet minimize toxicity. For instance, with antitumor agents that disappear rapidly from the plasma, continuous intravenous infusion rather than bolus injection may be needed to obtain a high enough concentration to achieve a therapeutic effect. Cancer drugs typically have a narrow therapeutic index. Consequently, slight differences in metabolism, uptake, or elimination of drugs can have profound impacts on pharmacokinetic parameters and the clinical effects of therapy. For example, mutations that alter the activity of drug metabolizing enzymes, or differences in drug-drug interactions, can affect the steady-state levels of chemotherapeutic drugs. Another factor is the mode of action of the drug. Topotecan, for example, is highly S-phase dependent in its mode of action. In this case, a schedule of daily dosing is more efficacious than weekly administration of the same total dose. Another factor to consider is whether the drug is readily absorbed following oral administration. In cases where uptake is limited, intravenous administration of the drug is performed. The modes of administration and disposition of several antineoplastic agents are listed in Table 68.1.

PHARMACOVIGILANCE: ADVERSE EFFECTS AND DRUG INTERACTIONS

Typical side effects of many antitumor drugs, which may limit drug dosing, are listed in Table 68.2. Most of these effects reflect drug activity on rapidly proliferating normal cells. Myelosuppression (including anemia, thrombocytopenia, and neutropenia) results from drug-induced suppression of rapidly dividing bone marrow cells. Chemotherapy-induced nausea and vomiting (CINV) are quite common adverse events and can be attributed to effects on both cycling and nondividing cells. The potential for agents to produce CINV and therapeutic agents and

TABLE 68.1 Pharmacokinetic Parameters for Selected Drugs

Drug	Administration	Disposition	Notes
Nitrogen mustard	IV	M	—
Melphalan	Oral	M	—
Cyclophosphamide	IV, oral	M	—
Nitrosoureas	IV	M	Lipid soluble, crosses blood-brain barrier
Cisplatin	IV	R	90% Protein bound
Carboplatin	IV	R	2- to 3-hour $t_{1/2}$
Oxaliplatin	IV	R	Rapidly protein bound; ultrafilterable agent is active
Busulfan	IV, oral	M	Oral: 26-minute $t_{1/2}$; crosses blood-brain barrier
Paclitaxel	IV	M, B	Nonlinear pharmacokinetics, 88%–98% plasma protein bound
Methotrexate	IV, oral	R	50%–60% plasma protein bound
Pralatrexate	IV	R, B	Renal clearance 35%
5-Fluorouracil	IV	M	Crosses blood-brain barrier; 8- to 20-minute $t_{1/2}$
Cytarabine	IV	M, R	3-minute $t_{1/2}$
6-MP and 6-TG	Oral	M,[a] R	Large first-pass effect (10-minute $t_{1/2}$)
Doxorubicin	IV	M, B	50%–85% plasma protein bound
Daunorubicin	IV	R, B, M	—
Bleomycin	IV, IM	R (65%), M	—
Arsenic trioxide	IV	R, M	—
Asparaginase	IV, IM	—	—
Vincristine	IV	M, B	Minimal entry into the cerebrospinal fluid
Vinblastine	IV	B	—
Etoposide	IV, oral	R (main), M, B	97% plasma protein bound
Irinotecan	IV	M, B, R	6- to 12-hour $t_{1/2}$; active metabolite SN-38 is glucuronidated

[a]See text for drug interaction.

B, Biliary excretion; *IM*, intramuscular; *IV*, intraventricular; *M*, metabolized; *R*, renal excretion; $t_{1/2}$, half-life.

TABLE 68.2 Typical Undesirable Side Effects of Antineoplastic Drugs in Humans[a]

Tissue	Undesirable Effects
Bone marrow	Myelosuppression, including: Neutropenia and resulting infections Thrombocytopenia Anemia
Gastrointestinal tract	Oral or intestinal ulceration Nausea and vomiting Diarrhea
Nervous system	Neurotoxicity, neuropathies
Hair follicles	Alopecia
Gonads	Menstrual irregularities, including premature menarche; impaired spermatogenesis
Wounds	Impaired healing
Fetus	Teratogenesis (especially during first trimester)

[a]Many of these effects are caused by drug action on nontumor cells that usually are growing (i.e., cycling).

strategies for ameliorating these effects are described in Chapter 67. Regimens based on combinations of different drugs are generally designed to avoid overlapping dose-limiting toxicities, such as those listed in the Clinical Problems Box. These toxicities are generally unrelated to rapidly proliferating populations of normal cells.

Alkylating Agents

High-dose cyclophosphamide and ifosfamide are associated with a significant incidence of hemorrhagic cystitis that is not age or sex related and is associated with a 9–45 times greater risk of bladder cancer. The risk of this relatively rare event is greater following the intravenous administration of these agents and lower with oral administration and can be largely eliminated through vigorous hydration of the patient during treatment. In addition, the coadministration of mesna (sodium-2-mercaptoethane sulfonate) with cyclophosphamide or ifosfamide can prevent or reduce this urinary tract toxicity. The cystitis is apparently caused by acrolein, a toxic by-product of the metabolism of cyclophosphamide and ifosfamide. Mesna becomes a free thiol after glomerular filtration and reacts with acrolein and other urotoxic metabolites in the bladder to form nontoxic compounds.

As with most cytotoxic agents, it is important to administer the maximally tolerated dose to achieve maximal tumor cell kill. However, exposure of cells to cyclophosphamide and other alkylating agents can also lead to carcinogenesis. For example, leukemia is a well-known, long-term complication in patients with Hodgkin disease treated with a regimen including mechlorethamine. Melphalan treatment is also associated with induction of secondary leukemias and lymphomas. In addition to alkylating agents, high-dose regimens of topoisomerase II inhibitors and anthracyclines have also been associated with the occurrence of secondary malignancies, mostly leukemias.

With cisplatin, the major toxicities include nephrotoxicity, peripheral neuropathy, and ototoxicity. Damage is induced in renal tubules, which in turn decreases glomerular filtration rates and increases reabsorption. This nephrotoxicity develops 1–2 weeks after treatment has begun and is more common in patients who receive a bolus injection of cisplatin. Fractionating the dose over several days has been observed to reduce the intensity of this toxicity. The severity of renal toxicity can also be reduced by appropriate hydration of the patient and administration of mannitol (Chapter 38). Drug-induced neuropathy occurs mainly in large sensory fibers, resulting in numbness and tingling, followed by the loss of joint position sensation and a disabling sensory ataxia. Toxicity

CLINICAL PROBLEMS

Arsenic Trioxide

Cytopenia, nausea, vomiting, diarrhea, hepatotoxicity, prolongation of the QT interval, cardiac arrhythmias including *torsades de pointes* and complete heart block, acute promyelocytic leukemia differentiation syndrome, and sudden death

Bleomycin

Pulmonary fibrosis ("bleomycin lung")

Busulfan

Pulmonary fibrosis ("busulfan lung")

Doxorubicin

Cardiotoxicity

Pemetrexed, Pralatrexate

Stomatitis, nausea, vomiting, diarrhea, constipation, fatigue, pulmonary toxicity, and rash

Cisplatin

Nephrotoxicity and peripheral neuropathy

Oxaliplatin

Peripheral neuropathy, hypersensitivity, pulmonary fibrosis (rare), and abdominal pain

Cyclophosphamide, Ifosfamide

Hemorrhagic cystitis

Vincristine

Neurotoxicity

Irinotecan

Diarrhea (early and late), nausea and vomiting, cholinergic syndrome, myelosuppression

Cytarabine

Cerebral damage

Mitoxantrone

Cardiomyopathy

---

is generally reversed with discontinuation of drug treatment, but it may take a year or longer to resolve. Moreover, cisplatin neuropathy is a cumulative dose-limiting side effect. In contrast, carboplatin causes less neurotoxicity and nephrotoxicity but more pronounced myelosuppression than cisplatin.

Antimetabolites and Plant Alkaloids

The main toxicities associated with MTX, vinblastine, etoposide, and 5-FU is bone marrow suppression. Vinca alkaloids such as vincristine can cause peripheral neuropathy, but this is a less frequent problem with vinblastine.

Antitumor Antibiotics

Doxorubicin and daunorubicin are associated with long-term, dose-limiting myocardial toxicity. Although the acute cardiac effects of hypotension, tachycardia, and dysrhythmias are typically not clinically significant, long-term effects of congestive heart failure can be life-threatening and necessitate discontinuing drug therapy. Such long-term

effects have been proposed to be due to oxidative stress, appear weeks to months after therapy, and have been observed up to several years following therapy, especially in pediatric cancer patients. Thirty-five percent of patients receiving a cumulative dose of greater than 600 mg/m^2 experience congestive heart failure that is refractory to medical management. The potential for the development of congestive heart failure can be mitigated somewhat by the addition of dexrazoxane, a metal chelator, through a mechanism that may involve inhibition of free radical production. Bone marrow and gastrointestinal toxicity vary with plasma concentrations of doxorubicin.

Bleomycin and the alkylating agent busulfan both produce drug-induced pulmonary fibrosis, but this toxic effect is dose limited. Although more than 50% of unmodified bleomycin is excreted in the urine, bleomycin accumulates in the lungs and skin, which, in contrast to other tissues, have low levels of bleomycin hydrolase. Consequently, bleomycin is not metabolized, and continued elevated concentrations of the drug lead to the recruitment of lymphocytes and polymorphonuclear leukocytes in the bronchoalveolar fluids, although it is unclear how this leads to fibrosis. Hypersensitivity pneumonitis also is observed in patients who receive bleomycin, but it is less frequent in those who receive MTX, mitomycin-C, nitrosoureas, and other alkylating agents. The major side effects of Ara-C are myelosuppression and dose-limiting cerebellar damage. Ocular toxicity is occasionally associated with high doses.

Nearly all cytotoxic cancer drugs have adverse side effects that patients find objectionable.

NEW DEVELOPMENTS

Recent advances in understanding the molecular and cellular biology of cancer have identified novel targets for therapeutic development (Chapter 69), new biomarkers of response to stratify patients for specific therapeutic regimens, and improved formulations for drug delivery and stability. Several nanoparticle and liposomal formulations have improved the safety profile and stability of reactive cytotoxic therapeutics. The development of combination therapies that incorporate classic cytotoxics with molecularly targeted therapeutics are particularly exciting and hold promise. The advent of patient profiling and genomic medicine also provides opportunities for further stratification of patient populations to achieve even greater therapeutic benefit while minimizing the adverse events associated with dose-intensive cytotoxic regimens. Continued progress in the development of orally active compounds permits more patients to be treated outside of a hospital setting. The recent success of immune checkpoint inhibitors, in concert with cytotoxic therapies, is particularly exciting and will undoubtedly continue to advance the development of more effective clinical strategies to treat cancer patients.

CLINICAL RELEVANCE FOR HEALTHCARE PROFESSIONALS

The treatment of cancers involves many different modalities ranging from radiation therapy to pharmacotherapy using agents that have many different mechanisms of action. Nearly one-third of cancer patients receiving therapy will develop complications that affect the mouth. Therefore dentists should be aware of the potential for patients to develop dry mouth and the potential elevated risk for infection. Patients should be monitored prior to initiation of treatment if possible, and a plan for managing the patient during and after treatment should be developed to reduce the anxiety often associated with cancer treatment. Patients should be encouraged to maintain good oral hygiene, which should reduce the risk of complications and infection. Many of the cytotoxic

TRADE NAMES

In addition to generic and fixed-combination preparations, the following trade-named materials are available in the United States.

Alkylating Agents
Nitrogen Mustards
Chlorambucil (Leukeran)
Cyclophosphamide (Cytoxan, Neosar)
Ifosfamide (Ifex)
Mechlorethamine (Mexate)
Melphalan (Alkeran)

Alkyl Sulfonates
Busulfan (Myleran)

Nitrosoureas
Carmustine (BiCNU, Gliadel)
Lomustine (CeeNU, Gleostine)
Streptozocin (Zanosar)

Triazenes
Dacarbazine (DTIC-Dome)
Temozolomide (Temodar)
Procarbazine (Matulane)

Platinum Drugs
Carboplatin (Paraplatin)
Cisplatin (Platinol)
Oxaliplatin (Eloxatin)

Antimetabolites
Pyrimidines
Capecitabine (Xeloda)
Cytarabine, Ara-C (Cytosar-U)
Gemcitabine (Gemzar)
5-Fluorouracil (Efudex, Adrucil)
Floxuridine (FUDR)

Purines
Fludarabine (Fludara)
6-Mercaptopurine (Purinethol)
6-Thioguanine (Tabloid)
Clofarabine (Clolar)

Folates
Methotrexate (Trexall)
Pemetrexed (Alimta)
Pralatrexate (Folotyn)

Others
Pentostatin (Nipent)

Antitumor Antibiotics
Anthracyclines
Daunorubicin (Cerubidine)
Doxorubicin (Adriamycin, Doxil)
Epirubicin (Ellence)
Idarubicin (Idamycin)

Others
Bleomycin sulfate (Blenoxane)
Dactinomycin, actinomycin D (Cosmegen)
Mitomycin-C (Mitozytrex, Mutamycin)
Mitoxantrone (Novantrone)

Antibody-Drug Conjugates
Brentuximab vedotin (Adcetris)
Trastuzumab emtansine (Kadcyla)

Plant Alkaloids
Microtubule Targeting Agents
Vinblastine (Velban, Velsar)
Vincristine (Oncovin, Vincasar, Marqibo)
Paclitaxel (Taxol)
Paclitaxel albumin-bound formulation (Abraxane)
Cabazitaxel (Jevtana)

Topoisomerase Inhibitors
Etoposide (VePesid)
Teniposide (Vumon)
Irinotecan (Camptosar)
Topotecan (Hycamtin)

Others
Arsenic trioxide (Trisenox)
Asparaginase (Elspar, Erwinase)
Hydroxyurea (Hydrea)
Eribulin (Halaven)
Ixabepilone (Ixempra)

---

agents produce significant nausea and vomiting, which makes managing the patient challenging.

It is also important for all healthcare providers to maintain good communication with the patient undergoing chemotherapy and know where the patient is in the process of treatment because most treatment regimens are lengthy. Patients will experience fatigue and depression, which reduces their ability, as well as desire, to engage in rehabilitation programs. However, rehabilitation programs are an integral component of the treatment regimen in cancer patients. Programs should begin as early as possible and alternate between intensity levels, dependent upon where the patient is in the treatment protocol. It is important to include both aerobic and resistive exercise components; range of motion and stretching exercises are also important for those agents for which edema is a common side effect. It is well documented that physical rehabilitation programs have great benefit to cancer patients from both a physical and a mental standpoint.

SELF-ASSESSMENT QUESTIONS

1. A patient with Hodgkin lymphoma is determined to have a tumor burden of approximately 10^{28} cells. The standard chemotherapeutic regimen has a log-kill equal to 4. How many courses of therapy are necessary to reduce the tumor burden to 10^4 in this patient?
   A. 4.
   B. 6.
   C. 7.
   D. 20.
   E. 24.

2. Multidrug resistance commonly develops in response to the use of a single cancer chemotherapeutic agent. Which of the following is the most common mechanism by which this type of resistance occurs in cancer cells?
   A. Amplification of gene coding for enzymatic breakdown of specific drugs.
   B. Cytoplasmic drug-receptor complex travels to nucleus, binds to DNA, and results in expression of new messenger RNA.
   C. Inhibition of expression of genes specific for active drug uptake.
   D. Overexpression of the gene coding for surface glycoprotein (P-glycoprotein) involved in active drug efflux.
   E. Transfer of plasmids from one cancer cell to another.

3. Which of the following drugs binds to the toxic metabolite of cyclophosphamide and is administered to patients to protect them from cyclophosphamide-induced hemorrhagic cystitis?
   A. Allopurinol.
   B. Leucovorin.
   C. Leuprolide.
   D. Mercaptoethane sulfonate-Na$^+$ (Mesna).
   E. Mitotane.

4. Which of the following drugs is a prodrug?
   A. Cyclophosphamide.
   B. Methotrexate.
   C. 5-fluorouracil (5-FU).
   D. Vincristine (vinca alkaloid).
   E. Melphalan.

5. Which drug or drug group inhibits thymidylate synthetase?
   A. Antitumor antibiotics.
   B. Methotrexate.
   C. Vinca alkaloids.
   D. 5-fluorouracil (5-FU).
   E. Cytarabine (Ara-C).

6. Which of the following statements applies to bifunctional alkylating agents?
   A. Require activation by two CYPs in the liver.
   B. Can crosslink two guanines in DNA.
   C. Stabilize microtubules during mitosis.
   D. Act as antimetabolites.
   E. None of the above.

FURTHER READING

Bouwman P, Jonkers J. The effects of deregulated DNA damage signalling on cancer chemotherapy response and resistance. *Nat Rev Cancer*. 2012;12:587–598.

Holohan C, Van Schaeybroeck S, Longley DB, Johnston PG. Cancer drug resistance: an evolving paradigm. *Nat Rev Cancer*. 2013;13:714–726.

Lefrak EA, Pitha J, Rosenheim S, Gottlieb JA. A clinicopathologic analysis of adriamycin cardiotoxicity. *Cancer*. 1973;32(2):302–314.

WEBSITES

https://www.cancer.gov/publications/dictionaries/cancer-drug
This website is maintained by the National Cancer Institute and is a drug dictionary that contains definitions and additional information pertaining to drugs used for cancer and related conditions, including links to clinical trials.

https://www.fda.gov/Drugs/InformationOnDrugs/ApprovedDrugs/ucm279174.htm
This is the United States Food and Drug Administration website for Hematology/Oncology that contains approvals and safety notifications for drugs used to treat cancer.

69

Targeted Anticancer Agents

Jill Marie Siegfried

MAJOR DRUG CLASSES

Antihormonal agents
Receptor and nonreceptor tyrosine kinase inhibitors
Angiogenesis inhibitors
Proapoptotic agents
Immunomodulators

ABBREVIATIONS

ADCC	Antibody-dependent cell-mediated cytotoxicity
ALL	Acute lymphoblastic leukemia
ATP	Adenosine triphosphate
CLL	Chronic lymphocytic leukemia
CML	Chronic myelogenous leukemia
c-KIT	Proto-oncogene receptor tyrosine kinase
EGFR	Epidermal growth factor receptor
FDA	United States Food and Drug Administration
FGFR	Fibroblast growth factor receptor
GIST	Gastrointestinal stromal tumors
HER	Human epidermal growth factor receptor
HPV	Human papillomavirus
IFN-α	Interferon-α
IL-2	Interleukin-2
IV	Intravenous
LH-RH	Luteinizing hormone–releasing hormone
MDSC	Myeloid-derived suppressive cell
mRNA	Messenger ribonucleic acid
NK	Natural killer (cell)
NSCLC	Non–small cell lung cancer
PDGFR	Platelet-derived growth-factor receptor
RCC	Renal cell carcinoma
SERM	Selective estrogen receptor modulator
Treg	T regulatory cell
VEGFR	Vascular endothelial growth factor receptor

THERAPEUTIC OVERVIEW

Inhibitors that block specific oncogenic molecules belong to a relatively new class of cancer drugs called *targeted agents*, whose use is increasing as more information is gained about the pathways that drive cancer growth and survival. The properties of a malignant tumor have been categorized by Hanahan and Weinberg in a highly cited review (see Further Reading). These "hallmarks of cancer" include sustained proliferative signaling, induction of angiogenesis, resistance to cell death, and evasion of the immune system. All four of these hallmarks have been successfully targeted with agents that attack the pathways responsible for the relevant protumorigenic effects. Other hallmarks of cancer have been identified, such as aberrant energy generation, for which treatments are still in development.

Traditional chemotherapy, as discussed in the prior two chapters, involves the destruction of rapidly dividing tumor cells. However, newer approaches involve drugs that target specific cellular entities that are overactive or mutated in cancer cells, with reduced effects on normal cells. Targeted agents do not necessarily result in tumor cell death but may place the tumor cell in a nonproliferative state. Thus these agents typically have less severe side effects than traditional chemotherapeutic agents but require longer (sometimes continuous) therapy. In addition to being administered alone for the treatment of certain cancers, many of these targeted agents are also used in combination with traditional chemotherapeutic regimens to enhance their efficacy.

Cellular targets toward which agents are directed are listed in the Therapeutic Overview Box.

MECHANISMS OF ACTION

Antihormonal Agents

Steroid hormones such as estrogen or testosterone cross through the plasma membrane and bind to their cytoplasmic receptors, which dimerize and enter the nucleus, where they interact with hormone-responsive elements on chromatin to induce the synthesis of specific messenger ribonucleic acids (mRNAs). Translation of these mRNA species leads to the formation of new proteins that alter physiological or biochemical reactions, for example, to promote development and

THERAPEUTIC OVERVIEW

Targets
Hormones and their receptors
Growth factor receptors
Intracellular kinases
Angiogenesis
The apoptotic pathway
The immune system

Major Classes of Agents
Hormones and anti-hormones
Kinase inhibitors
Monoclonal antibodies
Small molecules
Cytokines

maintenance of the mammary gland or prostate. Tumors arising from these organs often express steroid hormone receptors and retain the same dependence on hormones for growth and survival as the tissue of origin.

Antihormonal drug treatment strategies for estrogen receptor–positive breast cancer include:

- Blockade of estrogen receptors with antiestrogen drugs (selective estrogen receptor modulators, or SERMs)
- Destruction of estrogen receptors
- Inhibition of estrogen production

Approximately 70% of all postmenopausal patients whose breast tumors are estrogen receptor positive respond favorably to SERM therapy, as opposed to less than 10% of those whose tumors are estrogen receptor negative. Tamoxifen is the main SERM used clinically and is an estrogen receptor partial agonist that binds to estrogen receptors and prevents estrogen-dependent gene transcription in most tissues (Chapter 51). By blocking the binding of estrogens, tamoxifen decreases estrogen-dependent increases in proteins needed for growth such as transforming growth factor-α, insulin-like growth factors, cyclin D1, and Myc. Because the partial agonist action of tamoxifen in the endometrium somewhat mimics estrogen, there is a small risk of uterine cancer development with prolonged tamoxifen use. Toremifene, closely related to tamoxifen, is a newer SERM that is an estrogen receptor antagonist and is also used to treat estrogen receptor–positive breast cancer, as well as breast cancers with unknown estrogen sensitivity. Toremifene does not require metabolic activation to be effective (unlike tamoxifen) and appears to have a better safety profile than tamoxifen. Fulvestrant is a SERM that also blocks the estrogen receptor, but unlike tamoxifen and toremifene, fulvestrant directs the receptor to the proteasome, where it is degraded.

Although postmenopausal women have very low levels of circulating estrogen after the ovaries cease estrogen production, estrogen can still be produced through the conversion of androstenedione to estrogen via the enzyme aromatase, which is located in the adrenal gland and several tissues, including fat cells (Chapters 48 and 51). Aromatase is also expressed in the normal mammary gland and even by some breast tumor cells. When estrogen is produced locally in the tumor microenvironment, it can directly stimulate estrogen-sensitive breast cancer. The aromatase inhibitors letrozole, anastrozole, and exemestane effectively block the production of estrogen and are alternatives to SERMs in postmenopausal women. Aromatase inhibitors are not used in the treatment of breast cancer in premenopausal women because they have a low ability to block the ovarian secretion of estrogen.

In metastatic prostate cancer, as in breast cancer, hormonal manipulations can produce objective responses. For prostate cancer, this involves either orchiectomy or pharmacological castration. Androgen concentrations can be reversibly reduced by suppression of the pituitary-gonadotropic axis. Leuprolide and goserelin are analogues of luteinizing hormone–releasing hormone (LH-RH) that inhibit the release of luteinizing hormone (LH) by the pituitary gland, which signals the testes and adrenal gland to produce testosterone (Chapter 49). The absence of LH results in a reduction in testosterone. Both agents are available in depot form and can be administered monthly. Leuprolide and goserelin are both agonists of LH-RH and produce an initial rise in LH, followed by a decline in 2–3 weeks due to reduced expression of the LH-RH receptor. The transient increase in LH leads to an initial rise in testosterone levels, after which hormone levels fall to castration levels. Degarelix is a newer drug that is an antagonist of LH-RH and causes an immediate reduction in LH followed by a reduction in testosterone. The advantage of degarelix is that there is no transient testosterone increase, which can cause an initial flare-up in prostate tumor growth before inhibition occurs.

Flutamide is an antiandrogen that inhibits androgen binding to its receptors in prostate cancer cells (Chapter 52). Unlike other agents, it increases levels of testosterone as a consequence of feedback signals to the pituitary to release more LH following the blockade of androgen receptors; however, the testosterone is ineffective because flutamide is a receptor antagonist and blocks its action. There has been recent interest in achieving total blockade of the androgen receptor through use of an antiandrogen combined with a drug to inhibit androgen synthesis. Enzalutamide is an androgen receptor antagonist that prevents both the binding of testosterone and the translocation of the androgen receptor to the nucleus, thereby preventing stimulation of gene transcription. Enzalutamide can be combined with abiraterone, an agent that inhibits CYP17A1, the cytochrome P450 enzyme responsible for synthesis of precursors of testosterone (Chapters 48 and 52). Lack of precursors for conversion to testosterone lowers testosterone levels.

Receptor and Nonreceptor Tyrosine Kinase Inhibitors

Since the introduction of imatinib in 2001 as the first in-class tyrosine kinase inhibitor, a remarkable increase in attention has been devoted to tyrosine kinases as targets for drug development. Many of these enzymes serve as receptors for various growth factors and cytokines, as well as intermediate participants in a variety of signaling pathways. Since 2001, 28 small-molecule tyrosine kinase inhibitors have been approved by the United States Food and Drug Administration (FDA) for use in the management of a variety of cancers, as well as rheumatoid arthritis, age-related macular degeneration, and promotion of wound healing. The agents that target tyrosine kinases and receptors and have been approved for use in the treatment of cancers are presented in Table 69.1 with their molecular targets, approved therapeutic use, and primary adverse effects. The number of agents currently in active clinical trials is also very large, as altered expression of specific tyrosine and other kinases and growth factors have been identified as specific for certain types of cancers. This area of research has produced the single largest number of new chemical entities in clinical practice in the past decade. There are also a number of growth factor receptors for which inhibitors have been developed as small-molecule tyrosine kinase inhibitors or antibodies.

Inhibitors of Epidermal Growth Factor Receptors

Many types of growth factor receptors exist that are overactive in cancer cells and can serve as targets for therapy. For example, the epidermal growth factor receptor (EGFR) is present on a variety of solid tumors, including non–small cell lung cancer (NSCLC), head and neck cancer, and malignant gliomas. EGFR expression correlates with poor clinical outcome and resistance to cytotoxic agents. The EGFR consists of an extracellular ligand-binding domain, a hydrophobic transmembrane domain, and an intracellular domain with tyrosine kinase activity. Upon stimulation by ligands such as epidermal growth factor, amphiregulin, or transforming growth factor α, the EGFR dimerizes, which initiates an intracellular prosurvival signaling cascade, resulting in increased cell proliferation, metastasis, and decreased apoptosis (Fig. 69.1). The EGFR pathway can be inhibited by either blocking the extracellular domain with monoclonal antibodies or using small-molecule tyrosine kinase inhibitors to block adenosine triphosphate (ATP) binding and inhibit kinase activity. The EGFR gene is sometimes mutated or amplified in several cancers, most commonly in NSCLC. When mutated in the tyrosine kinase domain, the receptor becomes constitutively active, and the signaling cascade propagates in the absence of ligands. In response to ligand, the signaling cascade can also be abnormally prolonged. When EGFR is amplified, sufficient receptor numbers are present to allow dimerization without ligand, also causing constitutive signaling.

TABLE 69.1 Agents Targeting Specific Cytokine Receptors and Tyrosine Kinases Used in the Treatment of Cancers

Drug (Trade Name)	Target	FDA-Approved Indications	Adverse Effects and Precautions
Afatinib	EGFR	NSCLC (PO)	Diarrhea, rash, stomatitis, paronychia
Axitinib	VEGFR	RCC	Diarrhea, hypertension, fatigue, nausea, "hand-foot" syndrome (HFS; palmar-plantar erythrodysesthesia), dysphonia
Bosutinib	BCR-ABL, Src family kinases	CML	Diarrhea, nausea and vomiting, thrombocytopenia, rash, abdominal pain, fatigue
Dasatinib	BCR-ABL, c-KIT, PDGFR, Src family kinases	CML, ALL Ph+	Rash, diarrhea, edema, pleural effusion including CHF, mucositis, myelosuppression, QT prolongation, fatigue, dyspnea
Erlotinib	EGFR	NSCLC, PC	Rash, diarrhea, loss of appetite, nausea and vomiting, fatigue, elevated LFTs
Gefitinib	EGFR	NSCLC	Rash, diarrhea, loss of appetite, elevated LFTs, patients cannot smoke while on treatment
Ibrutinib	Bruton tyrosine kinase	MCL, CLL	Increased serum creatinine; decreased platelets; diarrhea; hemorrhage, neutropenia; fatigue; peripheral edema; nausea, diarrhea; dyspnea; bruising
Idelalisib	Phosphoinositide 3-kinase	CLL, B-cell non-Hodgkin lymphoma, small lymphocytic lymphoma	Neutropenia (reduced ANC), pneumonia, diarrhea or colitis, hepatotoxicity
Imatinib	BCR-ABL, c-KIT, PDGFR	ALL, CML, GIST	Rash, weight gain, edema, pleural effusion, cardiac toxicity (depression of LVEF), nausea and vomiting, arthralgias and myalgias, myelosuppression
Lapatinib	HER2/neu, EGFR	BC HER2/neu+	Cardiac toxicity (LVEF depression, QT prolongation), rash, HFS, diarrhea, nausea, vomiting and dyspepsia, elevated LFTs
Nilotinib	BCR-ABL, c-KIT, PDGFR	Ph+ CML in patients resistant or intolerant to imatinib therapy	Rash; nausea and vomiting; myelosuppression; QT prolongation; sudden death; electrolyte abnormalities; hepatic dysfunction; avoid in patients with hypokalemia, hypomagnesemia, or long QT syndrome
Ponatinib	BCR-ABL, c-KIT, Src family kinases, FGFR, PDGFR	CML	Hypertension, neutropenia, leukopenia, anemia, thrombocytopenia, rash, constipation, fatigue, nausea, abdominal pain, oral mucositis, neutropenic fever
Regorafenib	c-KIT, ABL, VEGFR, PDGFR, FGFR	CC, GIST, HCC	Anemia, increased AST, asthenia, proteinuria, HFS, mucositis, thrombocytopenia, hypertension, diarrhea, altered LFT, increased INR
Sunitinib	VEGFR, PDGFR, c-KIT, FLT3	RCC, GIST	Nausea and vomiting, yellow discoloration of skin, hypothyroidism, depression of LVEF, adrenal function abnormalities, diarrhea, myelosuppression, mucositis, elevated LFTs, increased uric acid levels
Sorafenib	BRAF, VEGFR, EGFR, PDGFR	RCC	Hypertension, alopecia, HFS, myelosuppression, nausea and vomiting, bleeding

Targets: *BRAF*, Gene encoding B-Raf; *c-KIT*, proto-oncogene receptor tyrosine kinase; *EGFR*, epidermal growth factor receptor; *FGFR*, fibroblast growth factor receptor; *FLT3*, fms-like tyrosine kinase 3; *HER2/neu*, human epidermal growth factor 2/receptor tyrosine kinase erb-2; *PDGFR*, platelet-derived growth factor receptor; *Src*, family of non-receptor tyrosine kinases; *VEGFR*, vascular endothelial growth factor receptor.
Indications: *ALL*, Acute lymphoblastic leukemia; *BC*, breast cancer; *CC*, colorectal cancer; *CLL*, chronic lymphocytic leukemia; *CML*, chronic myelogenous leukemia; *GIST*, gastrointestinal stromal tumors; *MCL*, mantle cell lymphoma; *MTC*, medullary thyroid cancer; *NSCLC*, non–small cell lung carcinoma; *PC*, pancreatic cancer; *RCC*, renal cell carcinoma; *HCC*, hepatocellular carcinoma.

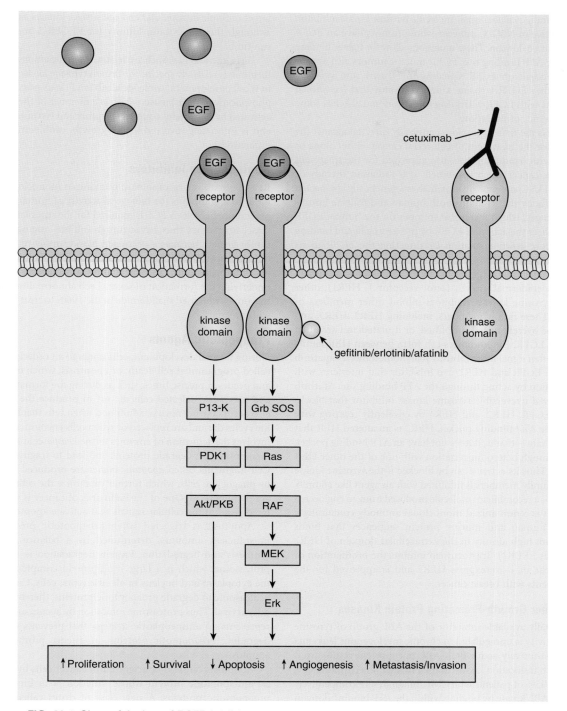

FIG. 69.1 Sites of Action of EGFR Inhibitors. The EGFR family is a group of structurally similar human growth factor receptors (HERs) with tyrosine kinase activity (kinase domain). These receptors play a critical role in regulating cell cycle progression and metastasis. Stimulation by ligands, including epidermal growth factor (EGF), transforming growth factor, and mitogenic signals, leads to receptor dimerization, activating the intracellular tyrosine kinase, which transmits progrowth signals to effector molecules. The EGFR can be inhibited either with the monoclonal antibody cetuximab that prevents ligand binding or with small molecules such as gefitinib, erlotinib, or afatinib that bind to the ATP binding site, inhibiting tyrosine kinase activity. Overexpression of EGFR is frequent in non–small cell lung cancers and in head and neck cancers.

Gefitinib, an orally available small-molecule tyrosine kinase inhibitor, is especially effective in NSCLC patients whose tumors have an *EGFR* mutation in the kinase domain. These mutations allow for tighter binding of gefitinib to the ATP binding site. EGFR mutant tumors also appear to be more dependent on EGFR signaling for growth and survival. **Erlotinib** is another EGFR tyrosine kinase inhibitor that has shown efficacy in patients with EGFR-activating mutations and also has some activity in the absence of mutations.

Cetuximab was the first monoclonal antibody directed against the EGFR approved for the treatment of colorectal cancer, either alone or in combination with irinotecan. It is also approved for the treatment of head and neck cancer when combined with radiation therapy or 5-fluorouracil (5-FU, Chapter 68). Cetuximab is a genetically engineered version of an antibody that contains both human and murine immunoglobulin sequences, which recognize epitopes on the human EGFR protein. It neutralizes the action of EGFR by preventing ligand binding and causes receptor down regulation by directing the EGFR to its degradation pathway.

In addition to selectively targeting the EGFR (also known as human EGFR or human epidermal growth factor receptor 1, HER1), other small-molecule tyrosine kinase inhibitors inhibit other members of the HER family. These family members, including HER2, HER3, and HER4, can also be overexpressed, amplified, or mutated and are often coexpressed with EGFR. Heterodimers can form between HER family receptors, which often signal more robustly than homodimers. **Lapatinib** is an orally active EGFR and HER2/neu inhibitor that interferes with self-phosphorylation by acting through the ATP binding site. **Afatinib** is a newly approved irreversible tyrosine kinase inhibitor that blocks ATP binding to EGFR, HER2, and HER4 by covalently reacting with amino acids in the ATP binding pocket. HER3 is an altered HER that lacks a kinase domain—that is, it does not have an ATP binding pocket. It only signals through heterodimerization with one of the other HER family members. Thus its activity can be blocked if the tyrosine kinase activity of other family members is inhibited with an agent like afatinib.

Trastuzumab is a recombinant molecule produced from an engineered DNA sequence. It is a humanized monoclonal antibody containing a combination of human and murine protein sequences that binds selectively and with high affinity to the extracellular domain of HER2 (also referred to as ERBB2). Trastuzumab inhibits the proliferation of human tumor cells that overexpress HER2 and is approved for the treatment of patients with breast cancer.

Inhibitors of Other Growth-Promoting Protein Kinases

Imatinib is an orally available inhibitor of the ABL group of tyrosine kinases whose activity is unregulated in chronic myelogenous leukemia (CML). The constitutively active BCR-ABL oncoprotein results from the chromosomal translocation known as the **Philadelphia chromosome,** which is found in 95% of patients with CML. Imatinib semicompetitively inhibits the BCR-ABL kinase by binding within the ATP binding domain of ABL in the closed, inactive conformation, preventing ABL from shifting to the active conformation that allows ATP binding. Imatinib is also able to bind within the ATP domain of the proto-oncogene receptor tyrosine kinase (c-KIT) and produce inhibition. **Nilotinib, bosutinib, ponatinib,** and **dasatinib** also target multiple tyrosine kinases, including BCR-ABL and platelet-derived growth factor receptor (PDGFR). Both bosutinib and dasatinib also target the Src family of kinases as well, while ponatinib targets those kinases as well as fibroblast growth factor receptor (FGFR) and c-KIT.

Sunitinib inhibits several transmembrane tyrosine kinases, including vascular endothelial growth factor receptors (VEGFR) types 1, 2, and 3 and PDGFR types α and β; these are important for cellular signaling in tumor proliferation and angiogenesis. **Sorafenib** and **regorafenib**

target multiple intracellular and cell surface kinases similar to sunitinib, although they have lower affinity for VEGFR-2 and PDGFR-β than sunitinib.

Ibrutinib and **idelalisib** are relatively unique among kinase inhibitors. Ibrutinib is relatively specific for Bruton tyrosine kinase, which is essential to B cell development, while idelalisib is a first in-class agent that targets phosphoinositide 3-kinase, which is a member of the family of kinases activated by G-protein–coupled receptors and tyrosine kinase receptors, and is intimately involved in cell growth, proliferation, survival, and differentiation.

Angiogenesis Inhibitors

Bevacizumab is a recombinant humanized monoclonal antibody that binds to and inhibits the biological activity of human VEGF expressed on endothelial cells. VEGF is required for the stimulation of new blood vessel formation; thus bevacizumab inhibits angiogenesis and slows tumor growth because a decreased blood supply reduces oxygen and other nutrients needed for growth. **Thalidomide** inhibits the proliferation of endothelial cells, also preventing angiogenesis, the mechanism underlying the formation of severe limb abnormalities in infants born to women who used thalidomide in the 1960s to treat nausea associated with pregnancy.

Proapoptotic Agents

During normal development, cells undergo an orderly process of dying called programmed cell death, or **apoptosis,** which is highly regulated and occurs at precise times, such as during the formation of the fingers and toes when selected cells die off to produce the digits. Apoptosis also occurs during normal adulthood when cells that have fulfilled their life cycles die and are replaced or when cells encounter stress. Apoptosis involves the activation of enzymes termed *caspases* at the mitochondrial membrane that degrade proteins and lead to fragmentation of DNA. Cell fragments called *apoptotic bodies* are produced that are engulfed by phagocytic cells, which further catabolize the cellular contents and are then recycled. One of the hallmarks of cancer is the failure of cells to respond to the cellular signals that activate apoptosis.

Apoptosis is triggered when proapoptotic proteins accumulate in sufficient amounts, determined by a balance between protein synthesis and degradation. Protein degradation is controlled by the proteasome, which is a large multiprotein complex present in both the cytoplasm and nucleus of all eukaryotic cells. Cancer cells use the proteasome to degrade proapoptotic proteins, thereby ensuring cancer cell survival. Thus proteasome inhibition by agents such as **bortezomib** represents an antineoplastic strategy that prevents cancer cells from degrading proapoptotic proteins, in essence promoting cancer cell apoptosis.

Apoptosis can also be triggered in cancer cells by blocking BCL-2, an antiapoptotic protein whose function is to bind and neutralize proapoptotic proteins. A new class of drugs called **BH3-mimetics,** such as **venetoclax,** bind to and inhibit members of the BCL-2 family. Normally, proteins that inactivate BCL-2 contain a BH3 domain, which inserts into a groove on BCL-2, causing BCL-2 to release proapoptotic proteins such as BAX, enabling apoptosis to proceed. BH3-mimetics bind to BCL-2 in this same groove, mimicking the proteins that neutralize BCL-2 and causing it to release BAX and other proapoptotic proteins.

Immunomodulators

"Biological therapy" attempts to use our native host defense system and its humoral and cellular components as weapons to fight cancer. Many of these weapons are intended to stimulate the immune system to destroy malignant cells. The immune system involves the action of many different cell types acting in concert, particularly lymphocytes, which include B cells, T cells, and natural killer (NK) cells (Chapters 34 and 35). Lymphocytes secrete antibodies, which possess unique affinities for their conjugate antigens and impart specificity to the immune system. They also secrete cytokines, which have wide-ranging cellular influences. Modulation of these systems may introduce remarkable therapeutic target specificity at the risk of induction of autoimmunity and unique toxicities such as fever and prolonged inflammation. Agents currently in use include cytokines, monoclonal antibodies, and vaccines.

Cytokines

Interleukin-2 (IL-2) is one of a family of cytokines, the interleukins, that are involved in direct communication between leukocytes. IL-2 is produced by activated T lymphocytes and is a growth factor for T cells. Interferon-α (IFN-α) belongs to another family of cytokines, the interferons, that are synthesized by macrophages and lymphocytes, and whose synthesis is stimulated by mitogens, antigens, RNA, or viruses. Interferons also express a wide variety of biological activities, often making it difficult to determine which ones might be operant in a particular context. The interferons modulate immune responses, augmenting T cell and NK cell–mediated cytotoxicity, participate in the regulation of cellular differentiation and antigenic expression, and possess antiviral activity.

Antibodies

Antibodies are products of B cells that are produced following exposure to specific protein sequences called *antigens*, which are determined to be foreign (nonself). The exact peptide to which a particular B cell reacts is called an *epitope*. Technological advances, including the development of murine hybridoma methodologies, have allowed the production of large quantities of pure antibodies specific for individual epitopes. Antibodies have been constructed to target and neutralize selected cancer-related proteins by blocking the ability of the proteins to carry out their functions. Recombinant DNA technology allows for replacement of some of the murine sequences with human sequences that are less likely to trigger rejection by the immune system. Cetuximab, the antibody directed against the EGFR, may also elicit B cell reactions that lead to tumor cell lysis when the antibody binds the tumor cell. This process is called antibody-dependent cell-mediated cytotoxicity (ADCC). Antibodies may also be used as the missile of biological "smart bombs" carrying a radiopharmaceutical or biological toxin warhead to a specific target. This type of approach is becoming more investigated as a potential mechanism to target specific cells.

Rituximab is a chimeric immunoglobulin G_1-κ monoclonal antibody raised against the CD20 antigen, constructed with a murine light- and heavy-chain variable region and a human constant region sequence. CD20 is a transmembrane protein expressed by most B cells at various stages of development and by malignant B lymphocytes. The protein is expressed on more than 90% of B cell non-Hodgkin lymphomas but importantly is not expressed by hematopoietic stem cells or other normal tissues. Rituximab binds to B lymphocytes after intravenous (IV) administration; therefore serum concentrations vary inversely with tumor burden. Complement-dependent cytotoxicity and ADCC are both mechanisms through which this agent may cause target cell lysis.

Vaccines

Vaccines for the prevention and treatment of cancer have been studied for many years, but advances in this area have been slow to develop. For the most part, vaccines are still primarily experimental treatments. The one notable exception is the approval of a recombinant quadrivalent human papillomavirus (HPV)-like particle vaccine (Gardasil) to prevent diseases related to HPV types 6, 11, 16, and 18, including precancerous cervical lesions, cervical cancer, vaginal or vulvar lesions, and genital warts. HPV is sexually transmitted, but initial infections typically go undetected. However, the presence of the virus can lead to abnormalities in the cervical epithelium that may progress to cancer.

Immune Checkpoint Inhibitors

A new form of therapy that has recently shown promise is the use of monoclonal antibodies that block immune checkpoints. The immune system is highly regulated, with specialized immune cell types that prevent an unchecked immune reaction that could lead to tissue damage or autoimmunity. Cells such as T regulatory cells (Tregs) and myeloid-derived suppressor cells (MDSCs) prevent cytotoxic T cells, dendritic cells, NK cells, and macrophages from working together to carry out prolonged cell lysis. Normally, only immunosuppressive cells such as Tregs and MDSCs express the protein PD-L1, which binds to its receptor PD-1 on cytotoxic T cells. This interaction suppresses T cells so they are "exhausted," or unable to carry out their cytolytic function, and prevents unchecked immune cell destruction of tissues. Tumor cells mimic the role of the normal immunosuppressive components of the immune system, placing the T cells into the "exhaustion" state by expressing PD-L1 on their cell surfaces. The discovery of the PD-L1 and PD-1 interaction helps explain why tumors are often not rejected by the host, even though ample cytotoxic T cells are present. Two antibodies are currently approved that inhibit this pathway; one is a humanized monoclonal antibody that neutralizes PD-L1 (nivolumab), and the other is a humanized monoclonal antibody that neutralizes PD-1 (pembrolizumab). Another immune checkpoint target is CTLA-4, a protein expressed by Tregs that suppresses cytotoxic T cell function. The monoclonal antibody ipilimumab has been developed to selectively target this protein.

RELATIONSHIP OF MECHANISMS OF ACTION TO CLINICAL RESPONSE

Prostatic and Breast Cancer

Enzalutamide and abiraterone are approved for use in metastatic prostate cancer refractory to castration or other antiandrogen treatments. Trastuzumab and lapatinib are indicated only for the treatment of breast cancer in patients whose tumors overexpress the HER2 protein (which is scored in tumor tissue sections using an approved immunohistochemistry test). For HER2-positive patients, approved indications in breast cancer include tumors that have spread locally to the lymph nodes, when trastuzumab is administered as an adjuvant treatment after chemotherapy, and in the metastatic setting, when patients have progressed after one or more chemotherapy regimens. It is also indicated for administration in combination with paclitaxel for the treatment of patients with metastatic breast cancer who are chemotherapy naive and whose tumors are HER2 positive. Lapatinib in combination with capecitabine has shown promise in patients for whom trastuzumab has lost efficacy and may be used in place of trastuzumab based upon a better adverse profile. Fulvestrant is also approved for the treatment of estrogen receptor–positive breast cancer in postmenopausal women. Toremifene is indicated in postmenopausal women whose cancer has metastasized.

Lung Cancer

For lung cancer, pembrolizumab is only used in patients whose tumors have been shown to be PD-L1 positive by an FDA-approved test. Both pembrolizumab and nivolumab are approved in metastatic lung cancer with progression after chemotherapy or with progression after a targeted agent specific for the patient's mutation in *EGFR* or the *ALK* fusion oncogene. Pembrolizumab is also used to treat some melanomas and cancers of the head and neck, while nivolumab has activity against renal cell cancers. Ipilimumab, the monoclonal antibody to CTLA-4, has been approved for melanoma treatment and also for NSCLC when combined with nivolumab. Although responses to these checkpoint inhibitors have been very encouraging in some patients, many are resistant to immune checkpoint inhibitors. Current research is determining if these drugs can be combined with other targeted agents.

Afatinib inhibits EGFR tyrosine kinase and HER2 and HER3 and is currently approved for treatment of NSCLC in the setting of EGFR-activating mutations. It is also being investigated in the management of breast cancer due to the similarity of action with lapatinib. Erlotinib is a small-molecule tyrosine kinase inhibitor of EGFR that is currently approved for treatment in NSCLC after failure of at least one prior chemotherapy regimen, with or without EGFR mutation, and in the EGFR mutant population, it is approved for first-line therapy. It can also be given as a maintenance regimen in lung cancer after successful treatment with chemotherapy. Erlotinib is also approved in metastatic pancreatic cancer, a tumor type that also shows dependency on EGFR signaling, in combination with the chemotherapy agent gemcitabine. Gefitinib is an orally active agent currently approved for first-line treatment of metastatic NSCLC patients whose tumors harbor an activating EGFR mutation.

Colorectal, Renal, and Gastrointestinal Cancers

Bevacizumab and cetuximab are approved for the treatment of metastatic colorectal cancer. Imatinib, originally introduced to treat disseminated cancers, is approved for use in the treatment of an unusual tumor known as gastrointestinal stromal cell tumor (GIST). This tumor is known to contain a c-KIT mutation that results in increased tyrosine kinase activity, which is inhibited by imatinib. Several other tyrosine kinase inhibitors are also approved for the treatment of patients with GIST who do not respond to imatinib, including sunitinib and regorafenib. Sunitinib, axitinib, and sorafenib are tyrosine kinase inhibitors that have been approved for treatment of advanced renal cell carcinoma (RCC). Recombinant IL-2 therapy as a single agent (aldesleukin) has activity in treatment of malignant melanoma and RCC, producing durable resolution of all disease in 6% to 7% of patients with metastatic disease. IL-2 is also being investigated as an adjunct with chemotherapy, monoclonal antibodies, and vaccines.

Blood-Borne Cancers

Imatinib has revolutionized the treatment of CML by producing complete remissions in the vast majority of patients with Philadelphia-positive chronic myelogenous leukemia (Ph+ CML). Despite the success of imatinib, mutations in the BCR-ABL kinase domain occur that lead to resistance. Bosutinib, dasatinib, nilotinib, and ponatinib are tyrosine kinase inhibitors approved for the treatment of a variety of leukemias and lymphomas, including CML, acute lymphoblastic leukemia (ALL), and Ph+ ALL. IFN-α has demonstrated clinical activity in the treatment of hairy cell leukemia, CML, indolent lymphoma, multiple myeloma, Kaposi sarcoma, superficial bladder carcinoma, RCC, and melanoma. Interferons are especially useful clinically for the treatment of viral hepatitis and as antitumor agents due to their antiangiogenic and antiproliferative effects. Venetoclax is a BH3-mimetic drug approved for treatment of chronic lymphocytic leukemia (CLL).

Rituximab is used in the treatment of indolent low-grade non-Hodgkin lymphoma, where it may be used as monotherapy and in combination with CHOP (cyclophosphamide, doxorubicin, vincristine,

and prednisone) or HyperCVAD part A (cyclophosphamide, vincristine, Adriamycin [doxorubicin], dexamethasone) chemotherapy as treatment for CD20-positive diffuse large B cell non-Hodgkin lymphoma. Rituximab is a component of a combination regimen using ibritumomab tiuxetan (another antibody raised against the CD20 protein to which a radio-isotope is conjugated) and is being evaluated in the treatment of CLL and other cancers. Other antibody-drug conjugation molecules are discussed in greater detail in Chapter 68. Ibrutinib and idelalisib are approved for use in CLL and other non-Hodgkin lymphomas. Ibrutinib has shown particular promise in the treatment of a relatively rare non-Hodgkin lymphoma called *mantle cell lymphoma*.

Bortezomib is a proteasome inhibitor that is indicated for the treatment of refractory multiple myeloma. Thalidomide is an angio-genesis inhibitor that is also approved for use in the treatment of multiple myeloma but only in patients where pregnancy has been ruled out.

Preventive Therapy

The most appropriate use of the HPV vaccine is to administer it to young girls before sexual activity; however, girls and women who are sexually active should also be vaccinated. Vaccination is indicated in all girls and women between 9 and 26 years of age. Since the vaccine can also protect against anal cancer, it is also indicated in boys and men in the same age group.

PHARMACOKINETICS

The pharmacokinetics of some of the drugs described in this chapter are summarized in Table 69.2. Of major consideration when administering these drugs is the fact that many of them are extensively metabolized by cytochrome P450 enzymes; thus the potential for serious drug interactions exists. Patients receiving these drugs typically receive other medications as well, including chemotherapeutic drugs, antimicrobials, antifungals, antiemetics, analgesics, and drugs to stimulate the bone marrow. In addition, many cancer patients are aged individuals who may be prescribed other drugs metabolized by the cytochrome P540 system for conditions such as heart disease or diabetes.

It is important to note that the pharmacokinetics of bevacizumab vary with age, gender, body weight, and tumor burden. Therefore the dosing of this agent must be individualized for each patient. Dosage adjustments may be required for any of these drugs in the presence of hepatic or renal failure, and therefore careful monitoring of the patient's status is required.

PHARMACOVIGILANCE: ADVERSE EFFECTS AND DRUG INTERACTIONS

Antihormonal Agents

The side effects of the antihormonal agents are related to the antagonism of the normal hormones. Hot flashes are the most common side effects reported for all of the hormone antagonists and aromatase inhibitors. These episodes can be intense and frequent but often abate with time. Other side effects common to these classes of drugs include the risk of blood clots, mood swings, and changes in libido. Tamoxifen can induce changes in the endometrium, leading to endometrial hyperplasia, endometriosis, or endometrial cancer. The incidence of these alterations is lower in premenopausal as compared with postmenopausal women; however, continued surveillance during therapy is required. Aromatase inhibitors, by virtue of blocking the production of even low levels of estrogen that are produced in postmenopausal women, lead to the development of osteoporosis. The use of bone density–supportive drugs such as the bisphosphonates (Chapter 55) is often required to diminish

TABLE 69.2   Pharmacokinetic Parameters for Selected Drugs

Drug	Administration	Disposition	Notes
Hormonal Agents			
Anastrozole	Oral	M	Metabolized by glucuronidation
Enzalutamide	Oral	M	Metabolized by CYP2C8 and CYP3A4; potential drug interactions
Exemestane	Oral	M	Metabolized by CYP3A4; potential drug interactions
Flutamide	Oral	M[a]	Contraindicated in hepatic failure
Fulvestrant	IM depot	M	Enterohepatic cycling
Letrozole	Oral	M	Metabolized by CYP3A4 and CYP2A6; potential drug interactions
Tamoxifen	Oral	M[a] (main)	Enterohepatic cycling
Cytokines			
Interferon-α	IV, SC	R	—
Interleukin-2	IV, SC	R	Rapid clearance by renal excretion and metabolism
Antibodies			
Bevacizumab	IV	M, R	Pharmacokinetics variable with gender, age, body weight, and tumor burden
Ipilimumab	IV	R	Severe and fatal immune-mediated adverse reactions
Nivolumab	IV	R	$t_{1/2}$ ~27 days
Pembrolizumab	IV	R	$t_{1/2}$ 26 days
Rituximab	IV	R	Fatal infusion reaction
Trastuzumab	IV	R	$t_{1/2}$ 6 days
Proteasome Inhibitors			
Bortezomib	IV	M	Metabolized by CYP1A2, 2C9, 2C19, 2D6, and 3A4; potential drug interactions
Tyrosine Kinase-Growth Factor Receptor Inhibitors			
Afatinib	Oral	M	95% protein bound; protein adducts primary metabolites
Axitinib	Oral	M	>99% protein bound; glucuronide and sulfoxide metabolites
Bosutinib	Oral	M[a]	Metabolized by CYP3A4
Dasatinib	Oral	M	Metabolized by CYP3A4 and also serves as an inhibitor of CYP3A4
Erlotinib	Oral	M[a]	Metabolized by CYP3A4 and CYP1A1; potential drug interactions
Gefitinib	Oral	M	Metabolized by CYP3A4; potential drug interactions
Ibrutinib	Oral	M[a]	>95% protein bound; metabolized by CYP3A4 and CYP2D6 (minor)
Idelalisib	Oral	M	Metabolized by aldehyde dehydrogenase and CYP3A4; minor glucuronidation
Imatinib	Oral	M[a]	Metabolized by CYP3A4 and CYP3A5; potential drug interactions
Lapatinib	Oral	M	Metabolized by CYP3A4 and CYP3A5 and inhibits CYP3A4 and CYP2C8
Nilotinib	Oral	M	Metabolized by CYP3A4; inhibits CYP3A4, 2C8, 2C9, 2D6, and UGT1A1; induces CYP2B6, 2C8, 2C9
Ponatinib	Oral	M	Metabolized mainly by CYP3A4 but also CYP2C8, 2D6 and 3A5 as well as esterases and amidases and P-gp
Regorafenib	Oral	M[a]	Metabolized by CYP3A4 and UGT1A9
Sorafenib	Oral	M[a]	Metabolized by CYP3A4; potential drug interactions
Sunitinib	Oral	M[a]	Metabolized by CYP3A4; potential drug interactions

[a]Active metabolites.

IM, Intramuscular; *IV*, intravenous; *M*, metabolized; *R*, renal excretion; *SC*, subcutaneous; $t_{1/2}$, half-life.

this effect. Additional adverse effects include bone and joint pain and elevated serum cholesterol levels.

Receptor and Nonreceptor Tyrosine Kinase Inhibitors

The tyrosine kinase inhibitors typically lead to diarrhea and formation of a rash. The adverse effects specific for some of these agents are listed in Table 69.1.

Angiogenesis Inhibitors

The most common toxicities of bevacizumab are hypertension, fatigue, blood clots, diarrhea, neutropenia, headache, appetite loss, and mouth sores. Less common but more serious side effects include gastrointestinal perforations that may require surgery, impaired wound healing, and bleeding from the lungs or other organs.

Proapoptotic Agents

Common adverse effects of bortezomib include gastrointestinal disturbances, headache and mild dizziness, muscle, bone or joint pain, and insomnia, while toxicities of bortezomib include peripheral neuropathy and myelosuppression. Common side effects associated with venetoclax include neutropenia, diarrhea and nausea, anemia, thrombocytopenia, and fatigue.

Immunomodulators

Toxicities of IL-2, although extensive and potentially severe, are manageable and include symptoms unlike those of chemotherapy. Patients routinely develop features of inflammatory disease including flu-like symptoms with fever, chills, and myalgias; capillary leak syndrome with attendant hypotension, acute kidney failure, adult respiratory distress syndrome, and rarely, respiratory failure requiring intubation; diarrhea, nausea, and emesis; anorexia; confusion and seizures; sepsis; and intensification or induction of autoimmune and inflammatory disorders.

IFN-α toxicities are multiple and include features of inflammatory disease like those of IL-2: flu-like symptoms such as fever, chills, fatigue, and myalgia; gastrointestinal toxicities such as anorexia, nausea, vomiting, and weight loss; depression; hepatotoxicity; neutropenia and thrombocytopenia; autoimmune diseases; renal toxicity; and thyroid abnormalities induced by autoimmunity.

Because rituximab is a protein, severe hypersensitivity reactions may occur. This is true of any of the antibody treatments discussed, which the body will detect as a foreign protein. Infusion reactions may include life-threatening cardiac arrhythmias and angina. A less severe infusion-related complex of symptoms often includes fever, chills, hypotension, nausea, urticaria, and bronchospasm. These symptoms may be attenuated by reducing the infusion rate, but patients need to be closely monitored, especially during the initial treatment when infusion reactions are most common. Tumor lysis syndrome, hemolytic anemia, and severe mucocutaneous reactions (i.e., Stevens-Johnson syndrome) have also been reported. The most significant toxicities of trastuzumab include cardiomyopathy, hypersensitivity reactions including anaphylaxis, infusion reactions, pulmonary events, and exacerbation of chemotherapy-induced neutropenia. The two most common side effects of gefitinib, erlotinib, and afatinib are skin rash and diarrhea.

The toxicities of the monoclonal antibodies, which are given as IV infusions, can be very severe. Immune checkpoint inhibitors need to be given with caution because life-threatening or even fatal inflammatory reactions have occurred as the immune system is activated throughout the body. Common organs affected include the lungs, intestines, and liver. These agents can also cause severe infusion reactions, fatigue, and cough.

The most commonly observed side effects for representative agents are listed in the Clinical Problems Box.

NEW DEVELOPMENTS

Research continues to discover specific tumor cell targets for therapeutic action that will reduce toxicity to normal tissues and improve efficacy in selected patients whose tumors are dependent on a particular target for growth and survival. This approach has been given the term *personalized medicine*. Many cancer targets are known, and the number of new agents under clinical development continues to grow. Promising new drugs include agents that inhibit the fibroblast growth factor receptor family (FGFRs), which can drive tumor growth when mutated or overexpressed; cyclin-dependent kinases (CDKs), which control the cell cycle; the hepatocyte growth factor (HGF), which is important in metastasis; and telomerase, which confers immortality on tumor cells. The "holy grail" of targeted cancer therapy is to use sequencing of the individual patient's tumor genome and/or analysis of gene expression as a way to determine which targets might be active so each patient is given the drug or drug combination most likely to be effective. New clinical trials focus on the molecular characteristics of the tumor to allow each patient to be assigned the drug most likely to be effective, rather than treating all patients with the same experimental agent or protocol. Drug combinations that improve overall activity are also under active study.

CLINICAL PROBLEMS

Anastrozole, Letrozole, and Exemestane
Hot flashes, ischemic heart disease, venous thromboembolic events, osteoporosis

Bevacizumab
Impaired wound healing (potentially fatal), hypertension, arterial thromboembolic events, neutropenia

Bortezomib
Sensory neuropathy, cardiomyopathy, hypotension, thrombocytopenia, neutropenia, infiltrative pneumonitis, reversible posterior leukoencephalopathy syndrome (RPLS)

Flutamide
Hot flashes, diarrhea, nausea, gynecomastia, impotence

Interferon-α
Flu-like symptoms, cytopenias, anorexia and weight loss, fatigue, depression, intensification or induction of autoimmune and inflammatory disorders

Interleukin-2
Flu-like symptoms, cytopenias, hypotension, capillary leak syndrome, acute kidney failure, adult respiratory distress syndrome, intensification or induction of autoimmune and inflammatory disorders

Tamoxifen
Thromboembolic events, endometrial hyperplasia, endometrial cancer, hot flashes

Trastuzumab
Cardiomyopathy, especially when coadministered with doxorubicin; infusion reactions; pulmonary toxicity; myelosuppression

Rituximab, Nivolumab, Pembrolizumab, and Ipilimumab
Severe infusion reactions; severe inflammation including pneumonitis, colitis, hepatitis, and nephritis; rash; cough; fatigue; diarrhea

CLINICAL RELEVANCE FOR HEALTHCARE PROFESSIONALS

The increasing prevalence of cancers suggests that patients undergoing chemotherapy will be seen by all healthcare professionals. The mechanisms of action of these agents modifies the immune system in a variety of ways that increase the risk for development of infections and reduces the ability of patients to heal. Dentists should be wary of the potential for bleeding because many of these drugs target blood-forming organs and blood cells, which impair the clotting cascade. It is also important to remember that patients will likely be receiving therapy for extended periods of time that are intermingled with treatment and nontreatment phases. During the nontreatment phases, some of the potential challenges may be reduced or absent, so it is essential to know whether the patients are actively being treated.

Many of these agents produce significant nausea and vomiting, which makes managing the patient challenging. The patients are also prone to low oxygen delivery to tissues, making them less able to engage in active exercise programs for extended periods of time. The goal of therapy programs should be to improve cardiovascular and pulmonary function so patients can complete the activities of daily living. The capacity of patients to perform these daily activities also provides a psychological benefit as patients begin to feel more engaged in social activities.

TRADE NAMES

In addition to generic and fixed-combination preparations, the following trade-named materials are available in the United States.

Hormonal Agents
Anastrozole (Arimidex)
Enzalutamide (Xtandi)
Exemestane (Aromasin)
Flutamide (Eulexin)
Goserelin (Zoladex)
Letrozole (Femara)
Leuprolide (Lupron, Eligard)
Tamoxifen (Nolvadex, Soltamox)

Antibodies
Bevacizumab (Avastin)
Cetuximab (Erbitux)
Ipilimumab (Yervoy)
Nivolumab (Opdivo)
Pembrolizumab (Keytruda)
Rituximab (Rituxan)
Trastuzumab (Herceptin)

Kinase Inhibitors
Afatinib (Gilotrif)
Axitinib (Inlyta)

Bosutinib (Bosulif)
Dasatinib (Sprycel)
Erlotinib (Tarceva)
Gefitinib (Iressa)
Ibrutinib (Imbruvica)
Idelalisib (Zydelig)
Imatinib (Gleevec)
Lapatinib (Tykerb)
Nilotinib (Tasigna)
Ponatinib (Iclusig)
Regorafenib (Stivarga)
Sorafenib (Nexavar)
Sunitinib (Sutent)

Cytokines
Interferon-α2b, recombinant (Intron A)
Interferon-α2a, recombinant (Roferon-A)
Interleukin-2, aldesleukin (Proleukin)

Proteasome Inhibitors
Bortezomib (Velcade)

Vaccine
Human papillomavirus vaccine (Gardasil)

SELF-ASSESSMENT QUESTIONS

1. Several drugs are administered as adjuvant agents in the treatment of estrogen receptor–positive breast cancer. Which of the following inhibits the conversion of androstenedione to estrogen?
   A. Anastrozole.
   B. Fulvestrant.
   C. Rituximab.
   D. Tamoxifen.
   E. Trastuzumab.

2. A 59-year-old patient is receiving a monoclonal antibody that inhibits vascular endothelial growth factor for the treatment of metastatic colorectal cancer. While receiving therapy, he cuts his foot on a piece of glass, requiring stitches. One month later, the wound has not healed and has become severely infected. Which of the following drugs is responsible for this effect?
   A. Bevacizumab.
   B. Bortezomib.
   C. Cetuximab.
   D. Gefitinib.
   E. Rituximab.

3. A 72-year-old woman with advanced renal carcinoma has not responded to traditional chemotherapeutic agents. Which of the following drugs can be added to her regimen to inhibit tyrosine kinase activity associated with vascular endothelial growth factor?
   A. Bevacizumab.
   B. Fulvestrant.

   C. Gefitinib.
   D. Interferon-α2b.
   E. Sunitinib.

4. A 64-year-old man is prescribed a drug for the treatment of his prostate cancer that blocks testosterone from binding to its intracellular receptor. Which of the following drugs has this mechanism of action?
   A. Flutamide.
   B. Fulvestrant.
   C. Goserelin.
   D. Leuprolide.
   E. Tamoxifen.

5. A 65-year-old man with lung cancer is prescribed an antibody that rescues cytotoxic T cells from suppression, resulting in higher ability of cytotoxic T cells to attack the tumor. Which agent was prescribed?
   A. Bevacizumab.
   B. Cetuximab.
   C. Rituximab.
   D. Interleukin-2.
   E. Nivolumab.

FURTHER READING

Hanahan D, Weinberg RA. Hallmarks of cancer: the next generation. *Cell.* 2011;144:646–674.

Margolin K. The promise of molecularly targeted and immunotherapy for advanced melanoma. *Curr Treat Options Oncol.* 2016;17:48. doi:10.1007/s11864-016-0421-5.

Nicolini A, Carpi A, Ferrari P, et al. Immunotherapy and hormone-therapy in metastatic breast cancer: a review and an update. *Curr Drug Targets.* 2016;17:1127–1139.

Rocco G, Morabito A, Leone A, et al. Management of non-small cell lung cancer in the era of personalized medicine. *Int J Biochem Cell Biol.* 2016;78:173–179.

Wu P, Nielson TE, Clausen MH. FDA-approved small-molecule kinase inhibitors. *Trends Pharmacol Sci.* 2015;36:422–439.

WEBSITES

https://www.cancer.gov/about-cancer/treatment/types/targeted-therapies/targeted-therapies-fact-sheet

This website is maintained by the National Cancer Institute of the National Institute of Health. It provides an overview of targeted cancer therapies with links to related resources.

http://oncologypro.esmo.org/Oncology-in-Practice/Drug-Drug-Interactions-with-Kinase-Inhibitors

This website is maintained by the European Society for Medical Oncology and provides information on the use of kinase inhibitors as well as links to other specific, targeted anticancer agents.

Special Considerations

Therapeutic Use of Hematopoietic Growth Factors

Pamela Potter

MAJOR DRUG CLASSES

Erythropoietin-stimulating agents
Colony-stimulating factors (G-CSF and GM-CSF)
Thrombopoietin analogues and activators

ABBREVIATIONS

EPO	Erythropoietin
ESA	Erythropoietin-stimulating agent
G-CSF	Granulocyte colony–stimulating factor
GI	Gastrointestinal
GM-CSF	Granulocyte macrophage colony–stimulating factor
IL	Interleukin
ITP	Idiopathic thrombocytopenic purpura
IV	Intravenous
JAK-STAT	Janus kinase/signal transducers and activators of transcription
SC	Subcutaneous
TPO	Thrombopoietin

THERAPEUTIC OVERVIEW

Hematopoiesis is the process of forming mature blood cells necessary for both ongoing cell replacement and enhancing formation during increased demand, such as occurs in response to infection requiring increased leukocyte (white blood cell) proliferation. Blood cells are formed in the bone marrow from hematopoietic stem cells, which are always being renewed and which can differentiate into both common myeloid and lymphocyte progenitor cells. The myeloid progenitor cells further divide and differentiate into cell lines that form thrombocytes (platelets), erythrocytes (red blood cells), mast cells, granulocytes (basophils, neutrophils, and eosinophils), and macrophages. The lymphoid progenitor cells give rise to natural killer cells, part of the innate immune response, T cells, and B cells involved in the adaptive immune response (Fig. 70.1).

Hematopoiesis is tightly controlled by several growth factors that regulate the proliferation and differentiation of the various cell types. Erythropoiesis, the differentiation of progenitor cells into red blood cells, is stimulated by erythropoietin (EPO), most of which is synthesized in the kidneys in response to low arterial oxygen tension. Thrombopoiesis, the formation of thrombocytes within the bone marrow, is stimulated by thrombopoietin (TPO), which is synthesized primarily in the liver and kidneys, and possibly by several cytokines, including interleukin-11 (IL-11), which promotes megakaryocyte maturation. The differentiation of myeloblasts is supported by granulocyte macrophage colony–stimulating factor (GM-CSF), which stimulates the formation of both granulocytes and macrophages, while granulopoiesis, forming neutrophils, basophils, and eosinophils, is stimulated selectively by granulocyte colony–stimulating factor (G-CSF). Lastly, the differentiation and maturation of lymphoid progenitor cells, or lymphopoiesis, are stimulated by several factors and cytokines that determine cell lineage.

In addition to growth factors, hematopoiesis also requires iron, vitamin B_{12}, and folic acid. The role of these factors and supplementation for deficiency anemias is discussed in Chapter 47.

Pathophysiology

Anemia is characterized by a decrease in the number of red blood cells, impairing the oxygen-carrying capacity of the blood and leading to fatigue, weakness, pallor, dizziness, exercise intolerance, shortness of breath, and tachycardia. The treatment of megaloblastic macrocytic anemia, which most often results from deficiencies of vitamin B_{12} or folate, and microcytic anemia, which is commonly due to iron deficiency, are discussed in Chapter 47.

Anemia may also occur in patients with chronic kidney failure due to decreased EPO production or may be drug induced following treatment for human immunodeficiency virus and other viral diseases, especially following the use of zidovudine and ribavirin, and from cancer chemotherapy. Drug-induced anemia and that associated with kidney disease are treated with EPO or erythropoietin-stimulating agents (ESAs).

Patients undergoing cancer chemotherapy or antiviral drug treatment may also exhibit neutropenia. Abnormally low levels of neutrophils render patients highly vulnerable to infection. GM-CSF and G-CSF can be used for treatment.

Thrombocytopenia, characterized by a deficiency of platelets, leads to tissue bleeding, easy bruising, and impaired blood clotting. Thrombocytopenia may result from autoimmune destruction of platelets, vitamin B_{12} or folic acid deficiencies, liver failure, or as a side effect of cancer chemotherapy. Treatment may involve transfusions, steroids, immunosuppressants, or, if drug induced, changing medications.

A summary of the therapeutic uses of agents that affect hematopoiesis is presented in the Therapeutic Overview Box.

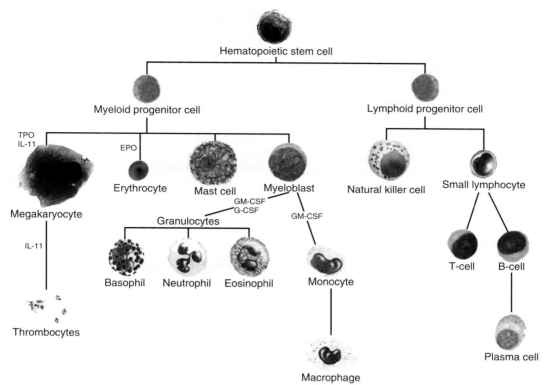

FIG. 70.1 Differentiation of Hematopoietic Stem Cells and Regulation By Growth Factors. *EPO*, Erythropoietin; *G-CSF*, granulocyte colony-stimulating factor; *GM-CSF*, granulocyte macrophage colony–stimulating factor; *IL-11*, interleukin-11; *TBO*, thrombopoietin.

THERAPEUTIC OVERVIEW

Erythropoietin-stimulating agents	Drug-induced anemias
Colony-stimulating factors	Neutropenia
Thrombopoietin analogues and	Idiopathic thrombocytopenic purpura
activators	Aplastic anemia
	Thrombocytopenia

MECHANISMS OF ACTION

Erythropoietin and Erythropoietin-Stimulating Agents

EPO was the first of the growth factors isolated and for which recombinant preparations became available. Epoetin alfa and darbepoetin alfa are erythropoietin-stimulating agents (ESAs) that mimic the effect of EPO on receptors located on progenitor cells and stimulate the formation and release of erythrocytes and reticulocytes from bone marrow. Stimulation of EPO receptors activates the Janus kinase–signal transducer and activator of transcription (JAK-STAT) pathway to increase gene transcription, a process requiring iron.

Colony-Stimulating Factors

GM-CSF and G-CSF are growth factors that promote progenitor cell differentiation. GM-CSF increases the production of many progenitor cells, whereas G-CSF acts more specifically to increase the proliferation of granulocytes, particularly the concentration and duration of activity of neutrophils in the bloodstream. G-CSF also mobilizes hematopoietic stem cells from the bone marrow into blood and reduces inflammation

by inhibiting IL-1 and tumor necrosis factor. These colony-stimulating factors increase the proliferation of myeloid cells through activation of JAK-STAT–associated receptors.

Recombinant DNA technology has been used to produce human G-CSF and GM-CSF. **Filgrastim** is recombinant nonpegylated human G-CSF, while **sargramostim** is recombinant nonpegylated human GM-CSF. The most commonly used preparation is **pegfilgrastim**, which is attached to polyethylene glycol, with a long half-life following injection.

Thrombopoietin Analogues and Activators

TPO increases platelet production by activating the Mp1 receptor, which is a member of the hematopoietic cytokine receptor family. Although recombinant forms of TPO are not yet available in the United States, analogues of TPO have been synthesized and are used to increase platelet production. **Romiplostim** is a fusion protein analogue of TPO with an immunoglobulin attached to increase its duration of action, and is approved by the United States Food and Drug Administration (FDA) for the treatment of chronic idiopathic thrombocytopenic purpura (ITP). **Eltrombopag** is a nonpeptide TPO receptor agonist also approved for the treatment of patients with ITP, as well as aplastic anemia or thrombocytopenia induced by interferon treatment of hepatitis C.

Oprelvekin is recombinant human IL-11, which also regulates the production of platelets. Oprelvekin binds to the IL-11 receptor and stimulates the maturation and differentiation of megakaryocytes. The actions of oprelvekin involve activation through the common receptor subunit glycoprotein 130 and activation of JAK-STAT–associated receptors. Oprelvekin also stimulates intestinal epithelial cells, inhibits adipogenesis, and increases the secretion of acute phase proteins.

RELATIONSHIP OF MECHANISMS OF ACTION TO CLINICAL RESPONSE

Erythropoietin and Erythropoietin-Stimulating Agents

EPO compounds are used to treat anemia associated with chronic renal disease in which there is a failure to produce sufficient EPO. The ESAs epoetin alfa or darbepoetin alfa increase erythrocyte production following administration, but their effectiveness may be limited by the amount of iron available for formation and function of red blood cells. Thus concomitant iron and folic acid supplementation are frequently recommended for these patients. Treatment is generally targeted to produce a maximum hemoglobin level of 10–12 g/dL, as higher amounts are associated with an increased risk of thromboembolism. Increases in hematocrit typically begin within 2 weeks after initiation of therapy.

ESAs are also used for other types of anemia that occur in patients with immunodeficiency disease, especially those treated with zidovudine, as well as for patients who develop anemia following treatment for hepatitis C and cancer, and the use of some antiviral medications.

Colony-Stimulating Factors

While G-CSF levels are normally low, its production in monocytes, macrophages, endothelial cells, fibroblasts, and bone marrow cells is induced by bacteria, endotoxins, and some cytokines, including tumor necrosis factor and IL-1. G-CSF is frequently used to reverse neutropenia induced by cancer chemotherapy, as well as that induced by some antiviral treatments. It is also used in patients with other forms of neutropenia, including congenital neutropenia and aplastic anemia. Use of G-CSF may reduce the likelihood of infection in patients with neutropenia. G-CSF is also used in transplantation of peripheral blood stem cells because it appears that pretreatment increases the number of cells available for transplantation.

Filgrastim increases total neutrophils due to increased production in the bone marrow. The response is similar to that induced by infection. Filgrastim is effective for the treatment of severe neutropenia resulting from autologous hematopoietic stem cell transplantation, as well as for neutropenia caused by cancer chemotherapy or treatment with antiviral drugs. By increasing the production and activation of neutrophils, filgrastim can decrease the likelihood of bacterial and fungal infections. It can also reduce the development of febrile neutropenia in patients undergoing cancer chemotherapy and allow for continuation of treatment if neutropenia develops in patients receiving antiviral and cancer therapy. The increase in neutrophils is also useful in patients undergoing peripheral blood stem cell transplantation. GM-CSF is used to decrease neutropenia primarily for patients having autologous bone marrow transplantation.

Thrombopoietin Analogues and Activators

Eltrombopag is approved for the treatment of thrombocytopenia and aplastic anemia. It is useful in patients with ITP who have not demonstrated sufficient improvement with other treatments. It allows patients on interferon treatment to continue therapy, as well as to increase platelets and decrease the risk of bleeding in patients with aplastic anemia. Eltrombopag may have mechanisms other than stimulation of TPO receptors, as TPO levels are already high in these patients, but eltrombopag is still effective at increasing platelet production. Romiplostim is also approved for the treatment of ITP and has been shown to increase platelet counts in more than 80% of patients. Both drugs increase platelet concentrations within about 2 weeks in most patients.

Oprelvekin is approved for the prevention of thrombocytopenia in patients undergoing chemotherapy for nonmyeloid cancers; it appears to decrease the number of transfusions required by these patients.

PHARMACOKINETICS

Erythropoietin and Erythropoietin-Stimulating Agents

Epoetin alfa is administered intravenously (IV) or subcutaneously (SC), with a half-life of about 4–8 hours. Because its effects are mediated by altering gene transcription, it is usually administered once a week. Darbepoetin alfa contains carbohydrate groups that increase its duration of action. It is also administered once a week by IV or SC injection, with a half-life of 20–40 hours, depending on the renal function status of the patient.

Colony-Stimulating Factors

Filgrastim is administered IV or SC and has a half-life of about 3.5 hours, requiring daily administration. Pegfilgrastim is a sustained duration form of filgrastim with a longer half-life and is typically administered 24 hours following each chemotherapy or radiation therapy cycle and may be continued once a week as needed.

Thrombopoietin Analogues and Activators

Romiplostim is administered SC once a week, as it has a half-life of approximately 3.5 days. Eltrombopag is administered orally once per day and has a half-life of 21–30 hours. Eltrombopag is extensively metabolized by CYP1A2 and CYP2C8, but the effects of inducers or inhibitors of these enzymes on plasma drug levels are unknown.

Oprelvekin is administered SC within 6–24 hours following each chemotherapy cycle and continued daily for 1–21 days until the platelet count exceeds 50,000/mm^3. The half-life is about 7 hours.

PHARMACOVIGILANCE: ADVERSE EFFECTS AND DRUG INTERACTIONS

Erythropoietin and Erythropoietin-Stimulating Agents

The most common side effects of ESAs are abdominal pain, cough, dyspnea, edema, and hypertension. ESAs should be avoided in people with uncontrolled hypertension. The most severe, but rare, adverse effect is venous thrombosis, the risk of which is generally reduced by ensuring that hemoglobin levels stay below 11 mg/dL. Iron deficiency may occur during treatment, and supplemental iron is frequently administered if serum ferritin levels fall below 100 ng/mL. In patients with some cancers, the risk of tumor progression or recurrence may increase, and thus use of these agents is contraindicated in patients receiving myelosuppressive therapy if the expected outcome is a cure. If these compounds are used, the lowest dose possible is recommended and only if anemia is present. Before physicians prescribe ESAs for cancer patients, they must complete specific training and enroll in the ESA APPRISE Oncology Program to enable continuous risk evaluation and mitigation by the United States Food and Drug Administration.

Colony-Stimulating Factors

Filgrastim (G-CSF) and pegfilgrastim are used more commonly than GM-CSF because they are better tolerated. The most common side effect of these agents is bone pain, occurring in about 30% of patients. Serious allergic reactions, acute respiratory distress, and spleen rupture may occur, but these are rare. GM-CSF can lead to arthralgias, myalgias, and capillary leak syndrome.

Thrombopoietin Analogues and Activators

The adverse effects of romiplostim are generally mild, with headache, dizziness, arthralgias, myalgias, and insomnia most common. While rare, thromboembolism can occur in patients in whom platelet levels are increased excessively (>50,000/mm^3). Eltrombopag may lead to headache, dizziness, myalgia, and GI side effects such as nausea, vomiting, and diarrhea. Elevations in hepatic enzymes, neutropenia, and anemia, as well as peripheral edema and dyspnea, have been reported. Hepatic function should be monitored, especially in patients being treated for thrombocytopenia secondary to treatment of hepatitis C. Thrombo-embolism is a potentially severe side effect if platelet levels become excessive.

Oprelvekin has many cardiovascular side effects, including atrial fibrillation and tachycardia, as well as dyspnea, which may result from edema and pleural effusion. It may also cause anemia due to increased plasma volume. Visual disturbances and ocular infections also occur.

A summary of the adverse effects of these agents is presented in the Clinical Problems Box.

NEW DEVELOPMENTS

Our knowledge of the regulation of hematopoiesis has increased dramatically during the past 50 years. Although research has led to an increased understanding of both extrinsic and intrinsic regulators of this process, the development of therapeutic approaches is still in its infancy as our knowledge base continues to expand. Controversies still exist at the most basic level regarding iron absorption and the effects of pharmacological agents on this fundamental process, as well as on the role of specific cytokines regulating thrombopoiesis. As research continues, the possibilities of differentiating and expanding hematopoietic stem cells in culture represents a new generation of cellular therapeutics with multiple clinical applications.

CLINICAL RELEVANCE FOR HEALTHCARE PROFESSIONALS

All healthcare professionals need to be aware of the use of hematopoietic agents, vitamins, and minerals by their patients. Use of these agents is indicative of compromised function with numerous implications. Restrictions and cautions may be required for any treatment that may induce abnormal bleeding or exposure to infections, such as may occur with dental procedures. The adverse effects of many of these agents, such as myalgias and arthralgias, may limit the ability of patients to participate in or respond to physical or occupational therapy. Further, all healthcare professionals must be aware of the adverse effects of these drugs that can become serious and life-threatening.

CLINICAL PROBLEMS

Erythropoietin-stimulating agents	Abdominal pain, cough and dyspnea, edema, hypertension, venous thrombosis
Colony-stimulating Factors	Bone pain, allergic reactions, acute respiratory distress, spleen rupture, capillary leak syndrome
Thrombopoietin analogues and activators	Atrial fibrillation, tachycardia, respiratory distress, anemia, visual problems, headache, dizziness, insomnia, myalgia, nausea, vomiting, diarrhea, liver dysfunction

---

TRADE NAMES

In addition to generic and fixed-combination preparations, the following trade-named materials are some of the important compounds available in the United States.

Erythrocyte-Stimulating Agents
Erythropoietin (EPO)
Epoetin alfa (Epogen, Procrit)
Darbepoetin (Aranesp)
Epoetin beta (Mircera)

Colony-Stimulating Factors
Filgrastim (G-CSF, Neupogen)
Pegfilgrastim (G-CSF, Neulasta)
Sargramostim (GM-CSF, Leukine)

Thrombopoietin Analogues and Activators
Oprelvekin (IL-11, Neumega)
Eltrombopag (Promacta)
Romiplostim (Nplate)

SELF-ASSESSMENT QUESTIONS

1. A 64-year-old man complains of increasing fatigue and shortness of breath. He was diagnosed with type 2 diabetes 15 years ago, but did not receive treatment until 2 years ago due to his inability to obtain health insurance coverage. Laboratory testing revealed low hemoglobin, glomerular filtration rate, and ferritin and higher than normal creatinine and glucose. The treatment of choice for this man is:
   A. Oral folic acid.
   B. Oral ferrous sulfate.
   C. Subcutaneous epoetin alfa.
   D. Subcutaneous filgrastim.
   E. Oral cyanocobalamin.

2. A 74-year-old woman with breast cancer has been treated for 2 months with cyclophosphamide. She complains of sore throat and chills, and examination reveals an oral ulcer and temperature of 102° F. Laboratory testing indicates low hemoglobin and a low absolute neutrophil count. Treatment for this woman is initiated, allowing her to remain on her chemotherapy regimen. The side effect she is most likely to experience is:
   A. Nausea and vomiting.
   B. Bone pain.
   C. Hemochromatosis.
   D. Hypertension.
   E. Peripheral neuropathy.

3. A 35-year-old woman, undergoing interferon treatment for hepatitis C, presents at the clinic with pinpoint reddish-purple spots on her lower legs and reports that she has been suffering from frequent nose bleeds. Her hemoglobin count indicates anemia. Among the following, which drug would be beneficial to prescribe?
   A. Romiplostim.
   B. Eltrombopag.
   C. Sargramostim.
   D. G-CSF.
   E. Aspirin.

4. Regarding the patient in Question 3, what are concerns during her treatment?
   A. Elevation of hepatic enzymes.
   B. Formation of thromboembolism.
   C. Neutropenia.
   D. Increased incidence of headaches, dizziness, muscle pain, and GI discomfort.
   E. All of the above.

5. A 44-year-old woman has been receiving combination chemotherapy for breast cancer for 3 weeks. In the past 10 days she has noticed that she bruises easily and that her gums are bleeding when she brushes her teeth. A complete blood count is normal with the exception of the platelet count, which is 100×10^3/mcL (normal $130–400 \times 10^3$/mcL). Which of the following drugs could be administered that might allow this patient to continue with her chemotherapy?
   A. Filgrastim
   B. Epoetin alfa
   C. Oprelvekin
   D. Vitamin B12
   E. Ferrous iron

6. Which of the following side effects is most likely to occur in the patient in Question 5?
   A. Diarrhea
   B. Hypertension
   C. Bone pain
   D. Dyspnea
   E. Arthralgia

FURTHER READING

Barreda DR, Hanington PC, Belosevic M. Regulation of myeloid development and function by colony stimulating factors. *Dev Comp Immunol.* 2004; 28(5):509–554.

Hahn D, Esezobor CI, Elserafy N, et al. Short-acting erythropoiesis-stimulating agents for anaemia in predialysis patients. *Cochrane Database Syst Rev.* 2017;(1):CD011690, Jan 9.

Lim VY, Zehentmeier S, Fistonich C, Pereira JP. A Chemoattractant-guided walk through lymphopoiesis: from hematopoietic stem cells to mature B lymphocytes. *Adv Immunol.* 2017;134:47–88. doi:10.1016/bs.ai.2017.02.001.

Songdej N, Rao AK. Hematopoietic transcription factor mutations: important players in inherited platelet defects. *Blood.* 2017;129(21):2873–2881. doi:10.1182/blood-2016-11-709881.

WEBSITES

http://asbmt.org/practice-resources/practice-guidelines
This website is maintained by the American Society for Blood and Marrow Transplantation and presents guidelines for the use of hematopoietic stem cell transplantation for several disorders.

https://www.cdc.gov/mmwr/preview/mmwrhtml/rr4910a1.htm
This website, maintained by the United States Centers for Disease Control and Prevention, has guidelines for preventing opportunistic infections in individuals who have received hematopoietic stem cell transplants.

https://www.fda.gov/Drugs/DrugSafety/ucm200297.htm
This is the United States Food and Drug Administration website containing the latest safety information on the use of ESAs.

Gastrointestinal Disorders and Their Treatment

Walter Prozialeck and Phillip Kopf

MAJOR DRUG CLASSES

Proton pump inhibitors (PPIs)	Laxatives
Histamine (H$_2$) receptor antagonists	Antidiarrheal agents
Antacids	Aminosalicylates
Mucosal protectants	Immunosuppressants
Prostaglandins	Antiemetics
Promotility agents	Antiflatulents

ABBREVIATIONS

5-ASA	5-Aminosalicylic acid
5-HT	5-Hydroxytryptamine (serotonin)
ACh	Acetylcholine
CB	Cannabinoid
CNS	Central nervous system
CTZ	Chemoreceptor trigger zone
CYP	Cytochrome P450
DA	Dopamine
GERD	Gastroesophageal reflux disease
GI	Gastrointestinal
H. pylori	*Helicobacter pylori*
IBD	Inflammatory bowel disease
IBS (IBS-C or IBS-D)	Irritable bowel syndrome (–constipation or –diarrhea)
NK	Neurokinin (substance P)
NSAID	Nonsteroidal antiinflammatory drug
PEG	Polyethylene glycol
PG	Prostaglandin
PPIs	Proton pump inhibitors
PUD	Peptic ulcer disease
TNF-α	Tumor necrosis factor-α

THERAPEUTIC OVERVIEW

The gastrointestinal (GI) system can be viewed as a continuous series of hollow, bag-like, and tubular segments, each with specific physiologic functions, including the storage and digestion of food, absorption of nutrients, secretion of digestive enzymes and mucus, regulation of fluid and electrolyte balance, and the storage and excretion of waste materials. While the specific functions vary along components of the GI tract (esophagus, stomach, small intestine, large intestine), the functions of each segment are regulated by intrinsic nerves of the enteric nervous system (ENS), neural activity of the autonomic (ANS) and central nervous systems (CNS), and an array of hormones. The connections and functions of these systems are summarized in Fig. 71.1.

Drugs are used to treat a wide variety of GI disorders, including peptic ulcer disease (PUD), gastroesophageal reflux disease (GERD), gastroparesis (delayed gastric emptying), constipation, diarrhea, irritable bowel syndrome (IBS), and inflammatory bowel disease (IBD). In each situation, the potential beneficial effects of drugs must be considered carefully against their potential adverse effects.

Pathophysiology

PUD occurs primarily in the upper GI tract (stomach, duodenum, and lower esophagus) at sites where the mucosal epithelium can be exposed to acid and pepsin. Under normal circumstances, there is a balance between the defensive barrier of the GI mucosa and the corrosive actions of acid and pepsin. However, excess acid production or decreased barrier function can overwhelm defense mechanisms to allow ulcers to form in various areas of the GI tract. Contributing factors and causes of PUD can include *Helicobacter pylori (H. pylori)* infection, use of nonsteroidal antiinflammatory drugs (NSAIDs), or stress, especially in patients with chronic illness. **Proton pump inhibitors (PPIs)** are the first-line treatment for these disorders, but patients with *H. pylori* infections require antimicrobial agents to prevent relapse.

GERD is a dysfunctional relaxation of the lower esophageal sphincter that allows the acidic gastric contents to reflux into the esophagus leading to heartburn. If unmanaged, GERD can lead to inflammation of the esophagus (esophagitis), with ulcerations, bleeding, and possibly Barrett esophagus, a precancerous condition. GERD can also cause dental problems, chronic asthma, cough, and laryngitis. GERD is commonly treated using PPIs, **H$_2$ histamine receptor antagonists**, and drugs that increase the tone of the lower esophageal sphincter, such as **dopamine (DA) receptor antagonists**.

Gastroparesis is a delay in gastric emptying that may arise from uncontrolled diabetes, Parkinson's disease, drugs such as the opioids, or other diseases that damage the vagus nerve or interfere with gastric smooth muscle function. Gastroparesis leads to heartburn or GERD, nausea and vomiting, issues controlling blood sugar levels, and bloating. If unmanaged, gastroparesis can lead to the formation of bezoars, solid food masses in the stomach that cause obstruction. Gastroparesis treatment typically involves changes in the diet, as well as **promotility agents** to increase propulsive contractions of the stomach and **antiemetics** to control nausea and vomiting.

Constipation, the abnormally difficult passage of hard or infrequent stools, may arise from many causes, including diet, pregnancy, and drugs (opioids, aluminum-containing antacids, or iron), as well as GI, metabolic, or neurological disorders. While dietary and lifestyle changes, such as increasing fluid and fiber intake or physical exercise, may be sufficient to restore normal bowel habits, often a laxative is necessary. These drugs can effectively treat many forms of constipation.

Diarrhea, the abnormally frequent passage of loose watery feces, usually results from the presence of excessive fluid in the intestinal

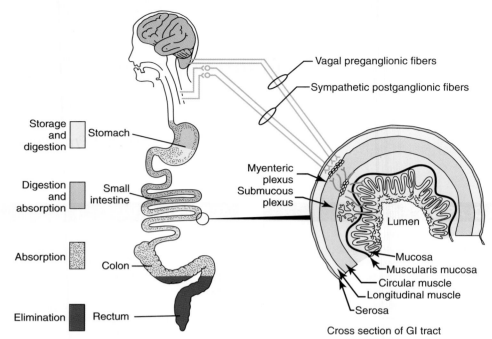

FIG. 71.1 Regulation and Functions of the GI Tract, Depicting the Extrinsic and Intrinsic Autonomic Efferent Innervation of the Wall of the Intestine. The enteric nervous system of the GI tract innervates smooth muscle and mucosa. Efferent and afferent neurons are organized in intramural plexuses; the most prominent plexuses are the myenteric plexus between the longitudinal and circular muscle coats and the submucosal plexus between the circular muscle and the muscularis mucosa.

lumen, generating rapid, high-volume flow that overwhelms the absorptive capacity of the colon, possibly associated with an enteric infection. Diarrhea may also be associated with IBD. Many forms of diarrhea are self-limiting and do not require treatment. However, more severe or chronic diarrhea requires treatment because it can result in serious electrolyte imbalances and morbidity. Diarrhea can often be managed with classic antidiarrheal medications, but antimicrobial or antiinflammatory agents may also be needed. Replacement of fluid and electrolytes is an essential component of treatment.

IBS is a vaguely defined motility disorder affecting the colon that is characterized by concomitant abdominal pain, bloating, gas, and constipation or diarrhea. Due to the idiopathic etiology of IBS, treatment usually involves managing diet and stress and using symptomatic medications, such as antispasmodic agents, for pain and cramping, antiflatulents, and agents that alter bowel function—for example, laxatives or antidiarrheal drugs.

IBD is an inflammatory disorder of all or part of the GI tract and includes ulcerative colitis and Crohn's disease, which are characterized by recurrent acute inflammatory episodes of severe diarrhea, abdominal pain, fatigue, and weight loss. Ulcerative colitis leads to ulcer formation in the colon and rectum, while Crohn's disease involves the large and small intestine or both. GI bleeding may be manifest with both disorders. Although the specific etiology of IBD remains unknown, both genetics and environment appear to play a role in promoting an abnormal immune response. Although there is no cure for IBD, antiinflammatory drugs, such as the aminosalicylates, have been the cornerstone of drug therapy for mild forms of the disease, with glucocorticoids for moderate to severe cases. Antibiotics, antidiarrheals, antispasmodics, and analgesics may also be used. The newer immunomodulators, such as tumor necrosis factor-α (TNF-α) antibodies, antimetabolites, antiintegrin antibodies, and calcineurin inhibitors, have become increasingly important in therapy.

Emesis may be beneficial as a protective mechanism to eliminate potentially toxic substances before they can be absorbed from the GI tract, but it usually appears to serve no beneficial purpose. Although vomiting is usually self-limiting, in some instances it may persist and cause serious morbidity, including fluid and electrolyte imbalances, and aggravate many other health conditions. Nausea and vomiting are caused by multiple factors, such as gastroenteritis, motion sickness and vertigo, pregnancy (morning sickness), or as adverse effects of drugs or radiation treatments. Drugs that modify responses to DA, serotonin (5-HT), histamine, and acetylcholine (ACh), transmitters involved in the sensory and central vomiting reflex sensory and central pathways, are widely used to prevent and treat various types of vomiting.

Drugs used to treat diseases or disturbances of the GI tract are summarized in the Therapeutic Overview Box.

THERAPEUTIC OVERVIEW

Problem	Treatment
Peptic ulcer disease	PPIs, H$_2$ receptor antagonists, sucralfate, misoprostol, microbial agents to eradicate *Helicobacter pylori*
Gastroesophageal reflux disease	PPIs, H$_2$ receptor antagonists, antacids, metoclopramide
Delayed gastric emptying	Promotility agents
Constipation	Laxatives
Diarrhea	Antidiarrheals
Emesis	Antiemetics
IBS	5-HT$_3$ receptor antagonists, intestinal antispasmodics
IBD	Aminosalicylates, TNF-α antibodies, immunosuppressants, corticosteroids

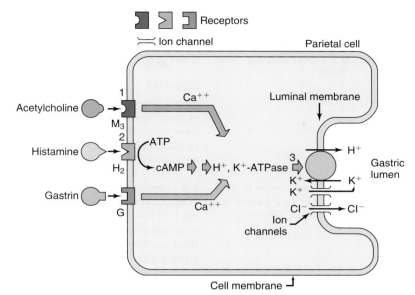

FIG. 71.2 Mechanisms Regulating Secretion of HCl by Gastric Parietal Cell. Receptors for acetylcholine (M_3), histamine (H_2), and gastrin (G) interact when activated by agonists to increase the availability of Ca^{++} and stimulate the H^+, K^+-adenosine triphosphatase (ATPase) of the luminal membrane. Acid secretion can be decreased pharmacologically by blockade of M_3 receptors (1), H_2 receptors (2), or the H^+, K^+-ATPase (3).

MECHANISMS OF ACTION

Gastric Acid Secretion

The secretion of acid by gastric parietal cells is regulated by histamine, ACh, and gastrin (Fig. 71.2), providing several targets for drug actions to decrease secretion. Psychic stimuli, such as the sight and smell of food or the presence of food in the mouth or stomach, activate the vagus nerve, which releases ACh (Chapter 6). Released ACh has a dual effect; it stimulates muscarinic M_3 receptors on parietal cells to increase acid secretion and activates both M_3 and M_1 receptors on enterochromaffin and paracrine cells that increase histamine release. The released histamine stimulates H_2 receptors on parietal cells to further increase acid secretion.

Food in the stomach also raises the antral pH, leading to gastrin release from cells in the antral mucosa. This hormone stimulates gastrin receptors on parietal cells directly to increase acid release. In addition, gastrin causes histamine release from paracrine cells, which stimulates acid production by parietal cells. The final step in the secretion of acid involves activation of the "proton pump," a specialized H^+, K^+-ATPase located at the luminal membrane of the parietal cells.

Antisecretory Drugs, Antacids, Mucosal Protectants, and Prostaglandins

Proton Pump Inhibitors

The **PPIs**, omeprazole, esomeprazole (the S-enantiomer of omeprazole), lansoprazole, dexlansoprazole, pantoprazole, and rabeprazole, share a common mechanism of action to inhibit parietal cell H^+, K^+-ATPase irreversibly, decreasing basal, nocturnal, and food-stimulated gastric acid secretion. The parent drugs are inactive, but under the acidic conditions in the parietal cell are protonated and converted to active compounds that react covalently with cysteine residues in the enzyme. This process prevents the transport of H^+ into the stomach lumen (see Fig. 71.2). Because all secretory stimuli ultimately cause acid production by augmenting the activity of the H^+, K^+-ATPase-dependent transporter, irreversible blockade of this enzyme effectively inhibits this final step to diminish acid secretion efficiently.

TABLE 71.1   Actions of the Antisecretory Drugs, Antacids, Mucosal Protectants, and Prostaglandins

Category	Prototype	Mechanism of Action
Antacids	Magnesium oxide and magnesium hydroxide	Neutralize secreted acid
Anticholinergics	Propantheline	Block muscarinic receptors, decrease acid secretion
Bismuth salts	Bismuth subsalicylate	Topical antibacterial activity
H_2 receptor antagonists	Cimetidine	Block H_2 receptors, decrease acid secretion
Prostaglandins	Misoprostol	Inhibit mucosal prostaglandins, decrease acid secretion
Mucosal protectants	Sucralfate	Protect mucosal barrier
PPIs	Omeprazole	Inhibit H^+, K^+-ATPase, decrease acid secretion

Histamine Receptor Antagonists

The **H_2 receptor antagonists** (cimetidine, famotidine, nizatidine, and ranitidine) are competitive and reversible and decrease basal, nocturnal, and food-stimulated gastric acid secretion (Table 71.1). Although less effective than PPIs, H_2 blockers reduce acid secretion in response to neuronal or hormonal stimulation. The relative antisecretory potencies of compounds in this group vary from cimetidine, the least potent, to famotidine, the most potent, but they are all equally effective when given in equipotent antisecretory doses.

Antacids

Antacids are inorganic bases that act primarily to neutralize hydrochloric acid; they do not decrease acid secretion. The cations (Ca^{++}, Mg^{++}, and

Al^{+++}) react with acid to form soluble chloride salts, followed by reaction with sodium carbonate in the intestinal lumen to form insoluble carbonates. The soluble chloride salts can also react with fatty acid salts in the intestinal lumen to form insoluble soaps. The reactions with Mg^{++} are as follows:

$$Mg(OH)_2 + 2HCl \leftrightarrow MgCl_2 + 2H_2O$$

$$MgCl_2 + Na_2CO_3 \leftrightarrow MgCO_3 + 2NaCl$$

$$MgCl_2 + 2R\text{-}COONa \leftrightarrow Mg(R\text{-}COO)_2 + 2NaCl$$

The poorly soluble carbonates formed precipitate and remain in the bowel followed by excretion in the feces, while the NaCl formed is absorbed. Magnesium has a laxative effect on the bowel, whereas aluminum is constipating.

Mucosal Protectants

Mucosal protectants, such as sucralfate, which is an aluminum salt of sucrose octasulfate, bind electrostatically to positively charged tissue proteins and mucin within the ulcer crater to form a viscous barrier, thereby preventing further damage from the actions of acid and pepsin. Sucralfate also binds bile salts and stimulates the production of mucosal prostaglandins (PGs). Sucralfate does not affect gastric acid secretion; it is used primarily as an alternative to PPIs or H$_2$ antagonists to promote the healing of ulcers.

Prostaglandins

The PGs have several effects on the GI system, including cytoprotection and decreased acid secretion (Chapter 29). Misoprostol is a synthetic PGE$_1$ analogue that increases the secretion of mucus and bicarbonate, enhances mucosal blood flow, and inhibits mucosal cell turnover to enhance mucosal defense. It also directly decreases gastric acid secretion by activating prostanoid receptors on parietal cells.

Drugs Affecting Motility
Promotility Agents

Promotility agents increase contractions in the upper GI tract and facilitate gastric emptying and include cholinomimetic agents that increase ACh, 5-HT$_4$ receptor agonists, DA receptor antagonists, and motilin receptor agonists. Although muscarinic agonists and acetylcholinesterase inhibitors promote smooth muscle contractions and enhance secretions (Chapter 7), these drugs are no longer used because they produce excessive secretions and fail to produce coordinated contractions required for effective gastric emptying. Similarly, drugs that activate 5-HT$_4$ receptors on vagal afferents, such as tegaserod, which increase ACh-mediated contractility and increase gastric emptying, lead to serious adverse vascular effects and are no longer available.

DA receptor antagonists such as metoclopramide promote motility by affecting several types of receptors in the GI tract. DA relaxes the GI system via direct activation of D$_2$ receptors in the lower esophageal sphincter and stomach. DA also activates D$_2$ receptors on postganglionic parasympathetic nerve terminals, inhibiting ACh release from intrinsic myenteric neurons. In addition, metoclopramide stimulates presynaptic excitatory 5-HT$_4$ receptors. As a consequence, metoclopramide increases the tone of the lower esophageal sphincter (important in the therapy of GERD), increases the force of gastric contractions, improves coordination of gastroduodenal contractions, and enhances gastric emptying. Further, metoclopramide is also a highly effective antiemetic agent, an action attributable to blockade of both central D$_2$ and 5-HT$_3$ receptors.

Motilin is a GI tract hormone that participates in the initiation of migrating motor complexes that characterize the fasting motility pattern of the stomach and small intestine. Macrolide antibiotics, such as erythromycin, bind to nerve and muscle motilin receptors to enhance GI contractions and increase gastric emptying. This promotility effect is not related to the antimicrobial activity of these drugs.

Laxatives

Several categories of laxatives (sometimes called evacuants, cathartics, or purgatives) are available, including bulk-forming agents, emollients (stool softeners), lubricants, saline agents, osmotic agents, and stimulants. In addition, two noncategorical agents, lubiprostone and linaclotide, are also effective laxatives.

Bulk-forming laxatives are nonabsorbable cellulose-like materials that resemble dietary fiber. These compounds hydrate in the presence of water and swell to form a pliable soft mass that activates the defecation reflex. As a consequence, intestinal transit time is reduced. It is important to note that many these agents can have a paradoxical antidiarrheal effect resulting from their ability to bind excess water. Common bulk-forming laxatives are psyllium and methylcellulose.

Emollients are ionic detergents that soften feces and permit easier defecation by lowering the surface tension and permitting water to interact more effectively with the solid stool. The most commonly used agent in this category is docusate sodium.

Lubricants, such as mineral oil, are oral nonabsorbable laxatives that act by lubricating the stool to facilitate passage. They may also act on the colonic epithelium to reduce water absorption.

Saline laxatives are inorganic salts, with poorly absorbed cations, such as magnesium, or anions, such as sulfate or phosphate. Saline laxatives draw water into the intestine by osmotic means, resulting in increased GI propulsion and evacuation. Because appreciable amounts of magnesium may be absorbed, these should be avoided in patients with renal insufficiency.

Hyperosmolar agents increase intestinal content osmolarity, leading to accumulation of fluid in the colon. Lactulose and sorbitol, poorly absorbed from the small intestine, undergo bacterial fermentation in the colon to organic acids and CO$_2$. Abdominal bloating and flatulence are common side effects. Polyethylene glycol (PEG) is poorly absorbed but is not metabolized by colonic bacteria. Solutions of PEG with electrolytes are commonly used for bowel cleansing before colonoscopy. PEG without electrolytes may be used daily for chronic constipation.

Stimulant laxatives include anthraquinones such as senna, diphenylmethanes such as bisacodyl, and castor oil. The anthraquinones, converted by colonic bacteria to their pharmacologically active form, act on the intestinal epithelium to increase fluid accumulation in the distal ileum and colon. Bisacodyl has a similar action. Castor oil is hydrolyzed by lipase in the small intestine to ricinoleic acid, to increase intestinal secretion, decrease glucose absorption, and stimulate colonic motor function via release of neurotransmitters from mucosal enterochromaffin cells.

Lubiprostone is a prostanoic acid derivative that stimulates type 2 chloride channel in the small intestine. This resulting increase in chlorine-rich fluid secretions in the intestine softens the stool and increases colonic motility. Linaclotide, a 14–amino acid peptide that activates guanylate cyclase C receptors on the luminal surface of the intestinal epithelium, activates the cystic fibrosis transmembrane conductance regulator ion channel. As with lubiprostone, this activation results in increased intraluminal fluid and accelerated colonic motility.

Antidiarrheal Drugs

Transport of fluid and electrolytes by the intestinal mucosa is regulated by neurons of the enteric nervous system and by the composition of the luminal contents. It is believed that neurons of the submucosal plexus of the intestine terminate near mucosal epithelial cells and act to increase or decrease absorption by villus cells and secretion by crypt cells. Several classes of compounds are available to treat diarrhea, including opioid agonists, 5-HT$_3$ antagonists, antisecretory agents, gel-forming adsorbents, and ion exchange resins.

Opioids act on enteric neurons to decrease secretion and promote fluid reabsorption from the lumen and also act in the CNS to alter extrinsic neural influences on the intestine and promote net absorption of fluid and electrolytes. Opioids decrease propulsive patterns of motility to segmenting patterns, thereby increasing resistance to flow, actions that result in slowed transit through the GI tract, allowing greater time for fluid absorption that may result in drying of the fecal mass. Constipation is a major side effect when these agents are used for pain management. Loperamide and diphenoxylate are specific antidiarrheal agents that do not cross the blood-brain barrier and act locally at neural and smooth muscle sites, primarily in the submucosal plexus, to increase segmenting contractions. Several opioid antagonists are now available to treat and prevent opioid-induced constipation (OIC) and may also be useful in treating postoperative paralytic ileus. The most important of these agents is naloxegol.

When released from enterochromaffin cells in response to stimuli such as food, 5-HT acts distally on 5-HT$_3$ receptors, an action that results in the increased release of ACh, thereby increasing smooth muscle contractions. Thus 5-HT$_3$ **receptor antagonists**, such as alosetron, interfere with peristaltic timing, decreasing motility, and increasing total transit time.

The antisecretory agent **bismuth subsalicylate** has a direct mucosal protective effect, in part, by inhibiting the formation of diarrhea-producing prostaglandins. In addition, it has weak antacid properties and possesses antibacterial properties. This agent has been available as a nonprescription item for many years and is quite effective for the treatment of "heartburn," GI distress, and diarrhea. It is used in some regimens for eradication of *H. pylori* and for prophylaxis and treatment of traveler's diarrhea, but the mechanisms for these therapeutic effects are not well understood. Bismuth subsalicylate also acts as a gel-forming adsorbent.

Gel-forming adsorbents, like the bulk-forming laxatives, are insoluble resins that take up water and swell. The two most common adsorbents are kaolin, which is a form of aluminum silicate, and pectin, which is a citrus fruit extract. The adsorbents increase resistance to flow thereby increasing stool formation.

Cholestyramine is a strong **ion exchange resin** that binds to bile in the GI tract and prevents its reabsorption. It is also known as a bile acid sequestrant. Cholestyramine is not absorbed and, when bound to bile acids, is excreted slowly in the feces.

Aminosalicylates

Sulfasalazine, the prototype aminosalicylate, is a conjugate of 5-aminosalicylic acid (5-ASA) and sulfapyridine linked by a diazo bond. The parent drug passes into the colon unchanged, where colonic bacteria cleave the diazo bond to form 5-ASA (the active moiety) and sulfapyridine. 5-ASA acts locally to interfere with arachidonic acid metabolism, which has a beneficial effect in IBD. Oral preparations include agents coupling 5-ASA with compounds other than sulfapyridine (e.g., balsalazide). Delayed-release pH-dependent enteric-coated tablets and time-dependent enteric-coated granules release 5-ASA in distal small intestine and proximal colon.

Immunosuppressants

Infliximab is a monoclonal antibody against TNF-α. TNF-α is a pro-inflammatory cytokine synthesized by and released from activated immune cells in inflamed mucosa. This cytokine plays a pivotal role in the regulation of immune cell proliferation, the expression of adhesion molecules, and cell death. As a monoclonal antibody, infliximab forms a stable complex with TNF-α on the surface of immune cells, fibroblasts, and epithelial cells to neutralize the activity of the cytokine.

Antiemetics

Nausea and vomiting (emesis) result from a variety of causes. The brainstem contains the chemoreceptor trigger zone (CTZ) located in the area postrema where the blood-brain barrier is essentially absent. Neurons in this brain area contain numerous neurotransmitter receptors, including 5-HT$_3$, D$_2$, H$_1$, cannabinoid (CB), and substance P or neurokinin (NK$_1$) receptors. In addition, the vestibular nuclei of the brainstem also play a role in nausea, particularly motion sickness–induced nausea. Neurons in these sites also express several neurotransmitter receptors that are targets for antiemetic compounds. The antiemetic drugs whose actions are mediated by these receptors are discussed in chapters in this text throughout Sections 2, 3, and 4.

The list of drugs commonly prescribed for nausea and vomiting is quite lengthy. Agents that are not discussed in other chapters in this text include the NK$_1$ receptor antagonists and the 5-HT$_3$ receptor antagonists. **Aprepitant** is a selective NK$_1$ receptor antagonist that acts primarily in the CTZ and is typically used with other medications to prevent nausea and vomiting associated with cancer chemotherapy. Similarly, the 5-HT$_3$ receptor antagonists dolasetron, ondansetron, and granisetron inhibit vagal afferent nerves that activate CNS emetic mechanisms and are also used for the adverse effects accompanying cancer chemotherapy.

Antiflatulents

Simethicone is an antifoaming agent that alters the surface tension of gas bubbles in the stomach and intestines, which facilitates the coalescence and passage of these bubbles via either belching or flatus.

RELATIONSHIP OF MECHANISMS OF ACTION TO CLINICAL RESPONSE

Drugs for Peptic Ulcer Disease and Gastroesophageal Reflux Disease

Drugs that inhibit the proton pump, the PPIs, are very effective and are the drugs of choice for reducing most types of acid hypersecretory disorders, including the Zollinger-Ellison syndrome, and are widely used to decrease the risk of NSAID-induced ulcers. The H$_2$ receptor antagonists are also effective but are now mainly used as alternatives to the PPIs. Both groups of agents relieve the symptoms associated with PUD and GERD and promote ulcer and esophageal healing. The PPIs are typically administered for several days to achieve their full therapeutic effects.

Eradication of *H. pylori*-Associated Ulcers

Administration of single antimicrobial agents is usually not effective in eradicating *H. pylori* due to the development of drug resistance. However, combinations of antibiotics can eradicate the organism and reduce resistance. *H. pylori* organisms have been shown to develop resistance to nitroimidazoles (e.g., metronidazole) and macrolides (e.g., clarithromycin), but resistance to tetracycline and amoxicillin is uncommon. A typical regimen for eradication of *H. pylori* includes two antimicrobial agents and an antisecretory drug. PPIs or H$_2$ blockers are often included to provide symptomatic relief, promote ulcer healing, and increase the sensitivity of the organism to antimicrobial agents. Other agents used include bismuth subsalicylate or bismuth citrate, metronidazole, or a tetracycline. These compounds can be given together or sequentially with oral probiotics to reduce adverse effects. Probiotics contain live non-pathogenic bacteria, including *Bifidobacteria*, found normally in the GI tract, and have been proposed to be beneficial for several GI disorders. Probiotic mechanisms of actions are unknown but are proposed to improve digestion and reduce the growth of pathogenic bacteria.

Antacids

Antacid neutralization provides almost immediate relief of symptoms, but large volumes and frequent dosing are necessary for mucosal healing. Antacids have modest effects on total acid content in the stomach and duodenum, and their neutralizing effects occur for as long as they are present in the stomach. Because of their side effects, disagreeable taste, and poor compliance, antacids are not used as single agents to heal peptic ulcers or esophagitis. They are used primarily for the occasional relief of acid indigestion, epigastric pain, and heartburn.

Mucosal Protectants

Sucralfate heals peptic ulcers as effectively as the H_2 receptor antagonists with a minimum of adverse effects. Because sucralfate has no significant effect on intragastric pH, it is not effective in relieving acid-related symptoms or in healing esophagitis. The use of sucralfate has decreased with the introduction of more effective drugs, such as the PPIs.

Prostaglandins

Misoprostol is used to treat and prevent ulcers induced by NSAID inhibition of cyclooxygenase. Misoprostol exerts both a gastric antisecretory effect and a protective effect on the gastric and duodenal mucosa. Inhibition of prostaglandin production by the NSAIDs results in decreased production of protective mucus and increased histamine-stimulated acid secretion. As a prostaglandin E_1 analogue, misoprostol is effective in reducing the risk of NSAID-induced peptic ulcers.

Promotility Drugs

Promotility drugs are used to increase gastric emptying in the treatment of diabetic gastroparesis and to increase the tone of the lower esophageal sphincter in the management of GERD. Some agents, such as metoclopramide, also exhibit significant antiemetic activity and are used to treat nausea due to general anesthetics, anticancer agents, radiation treatments, and opioids. Tolerance to the promotility effects of metoclopramide may develop and render the drug ineffective.

Antidiarrheal Drugs

The opioid antidiarrheal drugs are remarkably effective in the management of many types of acute diarrhea. Those with CNS activity should be used cautiously because of potential for abuse. The synthetic agent loperamide, which is not a controlled substance, is widely used and is effective for the control of many forms of diarrhea. Opioid antidiarrheal agents should not be used in the symptomatic treatment of diarrhea caused by enteric organisms that penetrate the intestinal epithelium, such as *Shigella* and *Salmonella*.

Bismuth subsalicylate is an effective antidiarrheal agent, especially useful against enterotoxigenic strains of *E. coli*. It is sometimes included for its antimicrobial properties in therapy directed against *H. pylori* and for the prevention of so-called traveler's diarrhea.

Substances that form semisolid gels within the intestinal lumen increase resistance to flow and also increase the firmness of stools. In this context, dietary fiber and the bulk-forming laxatives also have an antidiarrheal effect. Kaolin, a silicate-based clay that forms clay-like gels when hydrated, has minimal efficacy and has been removed from various over-the-counter products, although it is still available in "folk" remedies or via the internet.

Cholestyramine is commonly used to treat diarrhea resulting from bile acid malabsorption. It is also beneficial for the treatment of diarrhea after cholecystectomy and vagotomy.

The 5-HT$_3$ receptor antagonists, such as alosetron, decrease the frequency of bowel movements and improve stool consistency. Abdominal pain and bloating are also reduced in patients with IBS. The 5-HT$_4$ receptor agonists, such as tegaserod and cisapride, increase the frequency of bowel movements and improve stool consistency, but serious adverse cardiovascular effects caused withdrawal in the United States.

Drugs for Irritable Bowel Syndrome

Specific drug treatment for IBS depends on whether the patient is experiencing diarrhea or constipation, termed IBS-D or IBS-C, respectively. Several antimotility compounds are used for IBS-D, including alosetron, rifaximin, and eluxadoline. Alosetron primarily reduces visceral pain and discomfort, with the secondary benefits of decreased frequency of bowel movements and urgency, with bloating usually not improved. Rifaximin is a broad-spectrum antibiotic with a poorly understood mechanism of action; its antimotility effect is likely attributed to its antimicrobial activity in the intestines. Rifaximin modestly improves global IBS symptoms, including bloating. The opioid receptor agent eluxadoline has a beneficial dual action related to both μ-opioid receptor agonist activity to decrease smooth muscle contractility and intestinal secretions and increase rectal sphincter tone and δ-opioid receptor antagonist activity, which may help alleviate abdominal pain. Eluxadoline modestly improves abdominal pain and stool consistency.

Mild constipation and some symptoms of IBS can be treated with bulk-forming laxatives, which increase fecal mass. For these agents to be effective, adequate hydration is essential. Usually, the bulk-forming agents produce beneficial effects within 1 week when used acutely or chronically. Docusate sodium softens feces and facilitates defecation but is less efficacious than bulk-forming agents. The hyperosmolar agents, lubricants, and saline laxatives usually act within a day, whereas stimulant laxatives are effective within hours but may cause abdominal cramping.

Drugs for IBS-C include lubiprostone and linaclotide. Lubiprostone increases spontaneous bowel movements and modestly improves global symptoms of IBS. Linaclotide reduces abdominal pain and increases spontaneous bowel movements. In addition to their uses in the treatment of IBS-related constipation, lubiprostone and linaclotide are also approved for use in the treatment of chronic idiopathic constipation.

Drugs for Inflammatory Bowel Disease

Sulfasalazine and the newer aminosalicylates are effective in treating mild to moderate ulcerative colitis and Crohn's disease. The agents that release 5-ASA in the small intestine are more likely to be effective in patients with ileal involvement. Symptomatic improvement in abdominal pain and diarrhea is seen in approximately 3 weeks, with reduced doses effective in maintaining remission. Topical 5-ASA rectal enemas are effective in treating ulcerative proctitis and proctosigmoiditis.

An infusion of infliximab significantly improves the symptoms of Crohn's disease for up to 12 weeks.

Drugs for Nausea and Vomiting

In general, 5-HT antagonists, which inhibit afferent input from the GI tract and suppress input from CTZ, and DA antagonists, which act mainly on the CTZ, are effective in treating nausea associated with anticancer agents, radiation treatments, general anesthesia, and opioid drugs. Anticholinergics and antihistamines, which affect sensory input from the labyrinth, tend to be more useful in treating nausea associated with motion sickness and vertigo.

Aprepitant is indicated for nausea and vomiting associated with cancer chemotherapy and for postoperative nausea and vomiting. It augments the antiemetic effects of both the 5-HT$_3$ receptor antagonist, ondansetron, and the glucocorticoid dexamethasone and inhibits both acute and delayed emesis associated with cisplatin-induced emesis.

Dronabinol and Δ^9-tetrahydrocannabinol, agonists at CB receptors in the CTZ, are indicated for cancer chemotherapy-associated nausea and vomiting in patients who fail to respond to other conventional treatments. They are also used as appetite stimulants in patients with human immunodeficiency virus.

Antiflatulents

Simethicone alleviates the pain and pressure of bloating by facilitating the passage of gas bubbles in the stomach and intestine. It is also used to treat colic in babies, though clinical trials have not demonstrated efficacy for this usage. It is also included as an ingredient in many laxative and antacid products.

PHARMACOKINETICS

PPIs are available for oral and parenteral administration and must be absorbed and distributed to parietal cells via the circulation. Omeprazole has a low and variable bioavailability that increases with repeated daily dosing, reaching a plateau after 3 to 4 days. The bioavailability of other PPIs is less sensitive to repeated dosing. Because PPIs bind irreversibly to parietal cell H^+, K^+-ATPase, they suppress gastric acid secretion far longer than expected from their short plasma elimination half-lives. Onset of acid inhibition occurs within 1 hour but may require several days of therapy to reach a maximum dosage, and dosage reductions may be necessary in patients with severe liver disease.

H_2 receptor antagonists are available for oral and parenteral administration. They are well absorbed when given orally, but bioavailability is variable. Onset of acid inhibition occurs within 1 hour, lasts from 4–12 hours, and is dose dependent. These drugs are excreted primarily unchanged in the urine; therefore dosage reduction is recommended in patients with impaired renal function.

Antacids have a rapid onset of action, but their neutralizing capacity lasts only approximately 30 minutes on an empty (fasted) stomach. Their rapid onset of action and symptomatic relief may be advantageous in some individuals. If an antacid is taken after a meal, food delays gastric emptying and prolongs the antacid-neutralizing effect for up to 2–3 hours. Calcium-containing antacids may cause acid rebound (i.e., an increase in acid secretion) after their effects wear off.

Sucralfate is available for oral administration, but most is poorly absorbed, with almost all of the drug eliminated in the feces.

Sulfasalazine is only partially absorbed after oral administration and excreted in the bile. The remainder passes unchanged into the colon, where it is hydrolyzed to release 5-ASA and sulfapyridine. Most of the 5-ASA is excreted in the feces. Sulfapyridine is absorbed and metabolized in the liver, and metabolites are excreted in the urine. When given as a pH-dependent enteric-coated tablet or as time-dependent granules, some 5-ASA is released in the small intestine, and absorption is increased. Topical 5-ASA exerts a local antiinflammatory effect and is available as a rectal enema.

The systemic absorption of lubiprostone is minimal after oral administration. The drug undergoes extensive local metabolism in the stomach and jejunum by carbonyl reductase to an active metabolite, which achieves low plasma concentrations.

Linaclotide is administered orally on an empty stomach. Systemic absorption is minimal, and it is metabolized to an active metabolite by carboxypeptidase A in the GI tract.

Aprepitant is well absorbed orally, reaches maximum plasma concentrations within 4 hours, and is highly (95%) bound to plasma proteins. It undergoes extensive metabolism, primarily by cytochrome P450 (CYP) 3A4, and it is a weak to moderate inducer of both CYP3A4 and CYP2C9. Aprepitant is not excreted via the kidneys.

Alosetron is rapidly absorbed after oral administration, reaching peak serum concentration in 1 hour, and is extensively metabolized by the liver with a relatively short half-life of 1.5 hour. Rifaximin is minimally absorbed after oral administration, with over 95% of the drug excreted in the feces unchanged. Eluxadoline reaches peak serum concentrations in 1.5–2 hours after oral administration, with a moderate half-life of 3.5–6 hours. Metabolism is poorly understood at this time.

Simethicone is not absorbed systemically and is excreted in the feces unchanged.

Pharmacokinetic parameters for selected drugs are summarized in Table 71.2.

TABLE 71.2 Selected Pharmacokinetic Parameters

Drug	Route of Administration	Absorption (%)	$t_{1/2}$ (hrs)	Disposition
H_2 Receptor Antagonists				
Cimetidine	Oral, IV	60	2	R (Main), M
Nizatidine	Oral	90	1.5	R (Main), M
Ranitidine	Oral, IV	50	3	R (Main), M
Famotidine	Oral, IV	45	3 R (Main), M	
Proton Pump Inhibitors (PPIs)				
Omeprazole	Oral	40	1	M
Lansoprazole	Oral, IV	85	1.5	M
Rabeprazole	Oral	50	1–2	M
Promotility Agents				
Metoclopramide	Oral, IV, IM	80	2	R (Main), M
Ondansetron	Oral, IV	60	3.5	M
Granisetron	Oral, IV	60	6.2	M
Others				
Sucralfate	Oral	Poor	—	
Diphenoxylate	Oral	90	12	M (Main), B, R
Loperamide	Oral	Poor	11	B (Main), R

B, Biliary excretion; *M*, metabolized; *R*, renal excretion as unchanged drug.

PHARMACOVIGILANCE: ADVERSE EFFECTS AND DRUG INTERACTIONS

Antisecretory Drugs, Antacids, Mucosal Protectants, and Prostaglandins

Proton Pump Inhibitors

The PPIs are well tolerated and have a low incidence of adverse effects. The most common side effect is diarrhea, which appears to be dose related. Like most antisecretory drugs, PPIs increase fasting and post-prandial serum gastrin. The profound effects on acid secretion and the resultant hypergastrinemia in patients taking PPIs have raised concern regarding their long-term use and the potential for causing gastric mucosal hyperplasia and cancer. However, no significant hyperplasia or gastric cancer has been observed in humans taking PPIs for greater than 15 years.

Omeprazole and esomeprazole may interfere with drugs metabolized by hepatic CYP2C (e.g., warfarin, phenytoin, diazepam), but toxicities are uncommon. All PPIs increase intragastric pH and may decrease the bioavailability of drugs that require gastric acidity for absorption. As gastric acid serves as an important barrier to colonization and infection, there is also an increased risk of respiratory and enteric infection. Additionally, gastric acid is also important for the absorption of cyanocobalamin (vitamin B12) and some minerals such as calcium and magnesium. Thus with long-term usage, vitamin B12 deficiency or hypomagnesemia may develop, as well as an increased risk of osteoporosis and fractures.

Histamine Receptor Antagonists

The H_2 receptor antagonists have a low incidence of adverse effects, and the effects that do occur appear unrelated to their blockade of H_2 receptors. The most common side effects, similar for all H_2 receptor antagonists, include headache, diarrhea, constipation, flatulence, and nausea. Dizziness, somnolence, lethargy, agitation, and confusion occur occasionally with these drugs, with transient skin rashes observed in a small number of people. Risk factors include renal impairment and advanced age. Most adverse effects disappear with continued treatment or upon discontinuation of the drug.

A major drug interaction occurs with cimetidine, which is a potent inhibitor of several cytochrome P450 enzymes, including CYP3A4, CYP1A2, CYP2D6, and others. Thus use of cimetidine with drugs metabolized by this system can lead to elevated plasma concentrations and toxic responses to these drugs. In addition, cimetidine, used chronically in high doses, binds to testosterone receptors and exerts antiandrogenic effects that may result in decreased libido, decreased sperm count, impotence, and gynecomastia in men. Famotidine, nizatidine, and ranitidine do not bind substantially to CYP isoenzymes or to testosterone receptors and therefore do not produce these associated problems. All H_2 receptor antagonists increase intragastric pH and, similarly to PPIs, may decrease the bioavailability of drugs that require gastric acidity for absorption.

Antacids

The most common problems encountered in patients taking antacids are constipation (with aluminum-containing antacids) and diarrhea (with magnesium-containing antacids). An acceptable balance in stool frequency and consistency can be achieved by using agents that include mixtures of magnesium and aluminum salts or by alternating doses of magnesium- or aluminum-containing antacids. Ca^{++}, Mg^{++}, and Al^{+++} are usually poorly absorbed, but systemic toxicity can be manifest in patients with renal insufficiency. Calcium salts can produce systemic hypercalcemia with the resultant formation of calculi (milk alkali

syndrome). Aluminum can bind phosphate in the GI lumen and reduce the absorption of phosphate, leading to phosphate deficiency with muscle weakness and reabsorption of bone. Most antacids have been formulated to contain little or no Na^{++}. All antacids increase intragastric pH and, similar to PPIs and H_2 receptor antagonists, may decrease the bioavailability of drugs that require gastric acidity for absorption. Aluminum, magnesium, or calcium-containing antacids may inhibit the absorption of tetracycline antimicrobials and other drugs. Systemic antacids such as $NaHCO_3$ are absorbed into the blood and have the potential to increase blood pH and alkalinize urine.

Mucosal Protectants

Sucralfate is virtually devoid of systemic side effects because it is not readily absorbed. Constipation occurs in a small number of patients and is related to the aluminum salt. Aluminum may also bind dietary phosphate, leading to a phosphate deficiency. Sucralfate may bind to drugs, such as the quinolone antibiotics, warfarin, and phenytoin, and limit their absorption.

Misoprostol leads to frequent diarrhea by promoting secretion of fluid and electrolytes into the bowel lumen and by inhibiting the intestinal segmenting contractions that retard the flow of luminal contents. This is a dose-related effect that often limits use of the drug. Misoprostol also leads to headache and the risk of spontaneous abortion and is contraindicated in pregnancy because it stimulates uterine contractions. It should be used with caution in women of childbearing age.

Bismuth Subsalicylate

Bismuth subsalicylate can cause tinnitus, especially when taken with other salicylates, such as aspirin. It is contraindicated in patients who are allergic to salicylates, and it should not be used in children with influenza or chickenpox because of the risk of Reye syndrome. It will temporarily turn the tongue and stool black.

Drugs Affecting Motility

Promotility Agents

Metoclopramide can induce dystonia or parkinsonian side effects because of its activity as a DA receptor antagonist in the CNS. Central DA blockade can also induce hyperprolactinemia, leading to gynecomastia, galactorrhea, and breast tenderness. Cholinergic agonists produce a variety of side effects typically associated with cholinergic stimulation.

Laxatives

Fiber supplements and lactulose may cause abdominal fullness, bloating, and flatulence due to bacterial degradation of these agents, particularly the natural agents, in the colon. Stimulant and saline laxatives may cause abdominal cramping, watery stools, dehydration, and fluid and electrolyte imbalances. In patients with renal insufficiency or cardiac dysfunction, saline laxatives may cause electrolyte and volume abnormalities. A brown-black pigment (melanosis coli) may develop in the colon of patients taking anthraquinones, but this does not lead to adverse consequences, such as development of colon cancer. Laxatives should never be prescribed for patients with undiagnosed abdominal pain or intestinal obstruction. Because castor oil causes severe intestinal cramping and diarrhea, its use should be avoided. With most laxatives, a major problem with long-term use involves the development of laxative dependence. In this regard, the safest agents for chronic use are the bulk-forming agents and PEG formulations without added electrolytes.

Antidiarrheal Drugs

The adverse effects of the natural opiates (morphine and codeine) and synthetic opioids (loperamide and diphenoxylate) are discussed in Chapter 28. Diphenoxylate crosses the blood-brain barrier poorly under normal conditions and in usual therapeutic doses does not produce CNS side effects. However, in an overdose, it can cause respiratory depression, which can be reversed by naloxone. Diphenoxylate is available in combination with atropine, the latter added to deter abuse. Loperamide does not readily cross the blood-brain barrier and therefore has virtually no CNS effects and a low abuse potential. These agents should be used with caution in patients with IBD because of a slight risk of developing toxic megacolon.

Drugs for Irritable Bowel Syndrome

Constipation is the most common side effect with **alosetron**, which can be severe and require discontinuation. Due to the occurrence of ischemic colitis in a small percentage of patients, alosetron is restricted to use in patients who have not responded to all other forms of conventional therapies. Adverse effects are typically uncommon with **rifaximin**. Constipation, nausea, and abdominal pain occasionally occur with **eluxadoline**. Due to a rare occurrence of pancreatitis, eluxadoline should not be used in patients with a history of pancreatitis or alcohol abuse. Eluxadoline should not be used with other drugs that may reduce GI motility (anticholinergics, opioids, antidiarrheal drugs).

Headache, nausea, and diarrhea are the most common adverse effects of **lubiprostone**. Less frequently, abdominal pain and flatulence may occur. Diarrhea is a very common adverse effect of **linaclotide**. Abdominal pain and flatulence may also occur in some patients. Linaclotide should not be used in patients under the age of 18 due to the occurrence of severe dehydration and death in young rodent trials.

Aminosalicylates

The side effects associated with sulfasalazine include both dose-dependent and dose-independent actions. Dose-dependent effects correlate with sulfapyridine in the blood and include nausea, loss of appetite, headache, malaise, and diarrhea. Dose-independent effects include hypersensitivity reactions typical of sulfonamides. Skin rashes occur occasionally and require that the drug be discontinued. Fever, hemolytic anemia, pulmonary complications, hepatitis, and pancreatitis have been reported. A hypersensitivity reaction has been reported in patients taking 5-ASA dosage forms. Patients allergic to aspirin should not take 5-ASA. The potential for renal damage exists in patients taking high doses of 5-ASA.

Immunosuppressants

During the past 10 years, several severe adverse effects have been reported with the use of infliximab, including acute or delayed infusion reactions, serious infections, leukopenia, and an increased risk of malignancies and autoimmune disorders. Several of these adverse events are thought to be related to the development of antiinfliximab IgG antibody or activation of $\gamma\delta$-T cell proliferation and expansion.

Antiemetics

Adverse effects associated with the use of the 5-HT$_3$ receptor antagonists include constipation or diarrhea, headache, and light-headedness. Adverse effects of antiemetic agents that block DA, histamine, and muscarinic receptors are discussed in the chapters pertaining to these agents.

The adverse effects of the NK$_1$ antagonist aprepitant include fatigue, constipation, diarrhea, anorexia, nausea, and hiccups. Aprepitant induction of CYP3A4 and CYP2D9 may alter the metabolism of both warfarin and tolbutamide with subsequent toxicity because of elevated plasma levels.

Antiflatulents

Simethicone may occasionally cause diarrhea or nausea in some patients, but it is generally free of adverse effects due to a lack of systemic absorption.

CLINICAL PROBLEMS

Antacids
Aluminum salts
  Constipation
  Phosphate depletion
Magnesium salts
  Diarrhea
  Mg^{++} absorption
Sodium salts
  Increased plasma Na$^+$ concentration

Bismuth Subsalicylate
Black tongue and stool
Tinnitus
Risk of Reye's syndrome in children

H$_2$ Receptor Antagonists
Cimetidine
  Interference with metabolism of many drugs
  Antiandrogenic effect—e.g., gynecomastia, impotence, decreased sperm count

Laxatives
Saline
  Mg^{++} absorption
Lubricants (mineral oil)
  Decreased absorption of fat-soluble vitamins
  Pulmonary aspiration
Stimulants
  Abdominal cramping
  Watery diarrhea

Proton Pump Inhibitors (PPIs)
Gastric mucosal hyperplasia

Promotility Drugs
Bethanechol, neostigmine
  Excess GI secretions, cramps, cholinergic stimulation
Metoclopramide
  Parkinsonism and other extrapyramidal effects
  Hyperprolactinemia
  Diarrhea

Prostaglandins
Misoprostol
  Diarrhea
  Uterine stimulation

The adverse effects associated with drugs used for the treatment of GI disorders are summarized in the Clinical Problems Box.

NEW DEVELOPMENTS

With advances in our knowledge, pharmacogenomic factors are being uncovered for GI disorders. In IBD, polymorphisms related to the enzyme caspase have been reported. In addition, variants in immune-related genes that lead to an excessive immune response to normal bacteria have also been identified. In IBS, polymorphisms in genes encoding a variety of neurotransmitter receptors, the 5-HT transporter gene, and genes encoding immunology-related proteins have been implicated. Newer antibodies against TNF-α are in clinical testing for IBD.

Cytokine-based therapies, probiotics, helminth ova therapy, and stem cell transplantation are also under development for IBD. Developing therapies for GERD include new PPI isomers, K^+ competitive acid blockers, and inhibitors of transient lower esophageal sphincter relaxation.

Studies on the use of linaclotide to prevent colorectal cancer continues. Evidence of the role of guanylyl cyclase C as a tumor suppressor in the intestine supports the use of this agent in this preventative strategy. Studies demonstrating the agonist actions of linaclotide on guanylyl cyclase C and the benefit of these actions in the large intestine suggest this ligand alone may not be adequate to prevent colorectal cancer. Studies on this mechanism as a preventative strategy are ongoing, with the necessity of developing such agonists targeting the large intestine highlighted.

CLINICAL RELEVANCE FOR HEALTHCARE PROFESSIONALS

Because many GI drugs are available without a prescription and many individuals may have misconceptions about bowel and digestive functions, it is extremely important that all healthcare professionals understand the basic pharmacology of the major classes of drugs used to treat GI disorders and educate patients about the appropriate use of GI drugs. Digestive and GI disorders can aggravate many health conditions and negatively impact quality of life. An area of particular importance is GERD and other acid reflux conditions that may cause erosion of the teeth and oral lesions. Dentists are often in positions to identify GI disturbances and may recommend or prescribe drugs for specific problems. In addition, dentists often use autonomic and antiemetic drugs in their clinical practice.

TRADE NAMES

In addition to generic and fixed-combination preparations, the following trade-named materials are some of the important compounds available in the United States.

Aminosalicylates
Balsalazide (Colazal)
Mesalamine, 5-ASA (Asacol, Canasa, Lialda, Pentasa, Rowasa)
Sulfasalazine (Azulfidine, Sulfazine)

Antacids
Aluminum hydroxide (AlternaGEL, Amphojel, Dialume)
Aluminum hydroxide/magnesium hydroxide/simethicone (Mylanta)
Calcium carbonate (Tums)
Magaldrate (Lasospan, Lowsium, Maoson, Riopan, Ron Acid)
Magnesium hydroxide (Milk of Magnesia)
Simethicone (Mylicon)

Bismuth Salts
Bismuth subsalicylate (Pepto-Bismol)

Cannabinoid Antagonist Antiemetics
Dronabinol (Marinol)

Dopamine D₂ Receptor Antagonists
Prochlorperazine (Compazine, Compro)

Histamine H₁ Receptor Antagonists
Cyclizine (Marezine)

Histamine H₂ Receptor Antagonists
Cimetidine (Tagamet)
Famotidine (Mylanta, Pepcid)
Nizatidine (Axid)
Ranitidine (Zantac)

Irritable Bowel Syndrome
Alosetron (Lotronex)
Eluxadoline (Viberzi)
Linaclotide (Linzess)
Lubiprostone (Amitiza)
Rifaximin (Xifaxan)

Laxatives
Bisacodyl (Dulcolax)
Castor oil (Emulsoil, Neoloid, Purge)

Docusate (Colace)
Lactulose (Chronulac)
Magnesium hydroxide (milk of magnesia)
Methylcellulose (Citrucel)
Polycarbophil (Fibercon)
Polyethylene glycol
Psyllium (Metamucil)
Senna (Sennakot)

Mucosal Protectants
Sucralfate (Carafate)

Neurokinin NK₁ Antagonist
Aprepitant (Emend)

Opiate Antagonists
Diphenoxylate/atropine (Lomotil, Lonox)
Loperamide (Imodium)

Proton Pump Inhibitors (PPIs)
Dexlansoprazole (Dexilant)
Esomeprazole (Nexium)
Lansoprazole (Prevacid)
Omeprazole (Prilosec)
Pantoprazole (Protonix)
Rabeprazole (Aciphex)

Promotility Agents
Alvimopan (Entereg)
Erythromycin (E-Mycin)
Granisetron (Kytril)
Methylnaltrexone
Metoclopramide (Octamide, Reglan)
Naloxegol (Movantik)

Serotonin 5-HT₃ Antagonists
Alosetron (Lotronex)
Granisetron (Kytril)
Ondansetron (Zofran)

SELF-ASSESSMENT QUESTIONS

1. The promotility and antiemetic effects of metoclopramide are attributed primarily to its ability to:
   A. Antagonize muscarinic receptors.
   B. Inhibit acetylcholinesterase.
   C. Stimulate motilin receptors.
   D. Antagonize D_2 receptors.
   E. Inhibit ACh release.
2. A 62-year-old woman has been taking an aluminum-containing antacid for several years. A serious side effect associated with the long-term use of this preparation includes:
   A. Diarrhea.
   B. Systemic alkalosis.
   C. Phosphate depletion.
   D. Kidney stones.
   E. Dementia.
3. An advertisement for a new laxative preparation states that the product contains a "fecal softener." That agent would most likely be:
   A. Docusate sodium.
   B. Methylcellulose.
   C. Phenolphthalein.
   D. Castor oil.
   E. Bisacodyl.
4. Simethicone is included in many gastrointestinal drug products because of its reputed ability to:
   A. Neutralize stomach acid.
   B. Prevent the formation of gallstones.
   C. Produce a gentle laxative effect.
   D. Prevent the formation of gas bubbles and flatulence.
   E. Enhance the absorption of essential minerals.

FURTHER READING

Camilleri M, Boeckxstaens G. Dietary and pharmacological treatment of abdominal pain in IBS. *Gut.* 2017;66(5):966–974. doi:10.1136/gutjnl-2016-313425. [Epub 2017 Feb 23].

Klem F, Wadhwa A, Prokop LJ, et al. Prevalence, risk factors, and outcomes of irritable bowel syndrome after infectious enteritis: a systematic review and meta-analysis. *Gastroenterology.* 2017;152(5):1042–1054.e1. doi:10.1053/j.gastro.2016.12.039. [Epub 2017 Jan 6].

Ikechi R, Fischer BD, DeSipio J, Phadtare S. Irritable bowel syndrome: clinical manifestations, dietary influences, and management. *Healthcare (Basel).* 2017;5(2):pii: E21:doi:10.3390/healthcare5020021. Apr 26.

Simrén M, Törnblom H, Palsson OS, Whitehead WE. Management of the multiple symptoms of irritable bowel syndrome. *Lancet Gastroenterol Hepatol.* 2017;2(2):112–122. doi:10.1016/S2468-1253(16)30116-9. [Epub 2017 Jan 12].

WEBSITES

http://www.gastro.org/guidelines
This website is maintained by the American Gastroenterological Association and has links to many other resources, including guidelines for the treatment of numerous gastrointestinal disorders.

http://gi.org/acg-institute/evidence-based-reviews/
This website is maintained by the American College of Gastroenterology and has links to evidence-based reviews for gastrointestinal disorders, including irritable bowel syndrome and chronic idiopathic constipation.

http://www.worldgastroenterology.org/guidelines/global-guidelines/irritable-bowel-syndrome-ibs/irritable-bowel-syndrome-ibs-english
This website is maintained by the World Gastroenterology Organisation and has links to many excellent resources, including a global perspective on irritable bowel syndrome.

Pharmacological Treatment of Asthma and COPD

Kirk E. Dineley and Latha Malaiyandi

MAJOR DRUG CLASSES

Glucocorticoids
Antileukotrienes
β₂adrenergic receptor agonists
Muscarinic receptor antagonists
Methylxanthines

ABBREVIATIONS

AHR	Airway hyperresponsiveness
COPD	Chronic obstructive pulmonary disease
CysLT	Cysteinyl leukotrienes
FDA	United States Food and Drug Administration
HDAC	Histone deacetylase
IL	Interleukin
LABA	Long-acting β₂-adrenergic receptor agonist
LT	Leukotriene
MDI	Metered dose inhaler
PDE	Phosphodiesterase
SABA	Short-acting β₂-adrenergic receptor agonist
Th1/2	Type 1 or 2 helper cell

THERAPEUTIC OVERVIEW

Asthma and chronic obstructive pulmonary disease (COPD) are the most prevalent respiratory diseases in the world. In the United States, according to the Centers for Disease Control and Prevention, the mean prevalence of asthma in 2010 was 7% (18.7 million) for adults (>18 years of age) and 8.2% (7 million) for children (under age 18). COPD, which affects primarily those aged 65 years old and older, had a prevalence of 6.4% (15.7 million adults) and was the fourth leading cause of death in the United States in 2014. In addition, asthma-COPD overlap syndrome (ACOS), the diagnosis for individuals exhibiting symptoms characteristic of both asthma and COPD, had a prevalence in the United States of 3.2%. Thus these respiratory disorders represent a major public health burden.

Both asthma and COPD are characterized by airway inflammation and obstruction and breathlessness. Individuals with these conditions exhibit airway limitations that can be measured using spirometry, which involves taking the deepest breath possible and exhaling it as forcefully as possible for as long as possible. Individuals with either asthma or COPD will exhibit a decreased forced expiratory volume (FEV_1) relative to their forced vital capacity (FVC), which can be reversed after inhaling a short-acting bronchodilator such as albuterol.

Asthma

Asthma is characterized by intermittent symptoms, which include wheezing, dyspnea, chest tightness, and cough. Many patients may experience long periods between episodes, but even in a state of apparently normal function, the asthmatic airway shows unusual sensitivity to chemical or physiological stimuli that would not affect a normal airway. This tendency toward bronchoconstriction, known as airway hyperresponsiveness (AHR), is attributed to chronic inflammation as a consequence of immune dysfunction.

The current model of asthma pathogenesis is an immunoglobulin E (IgE)-mediated or class I hypersensitivity (Fig. 72.1). In this scheme, vulnerable individuals become immunologically sensitized to produce IgE specific for various allergens, most notably those from feces of house dust mites and cockroaches, animal dander, mold, and plant pollens. Repeated exposure to the same antigen results in amplified IgE production. When IgE anchored to the mast cell surface cross-links with allergens, cell degranulation occurs, leading to the rapid release of leukotrienes (LTs), prostaglandins, histamine, and other mediators that cause smooth muscle contraction, mucus secretion, and edema. In allergic individuals, the consequences of this early phase can appear rapidly within minutes, and characteristically diminish within an hour or two, before returning several hours later in a more sustained fashion during a late phase.

Immunologically, the late phase is marked by the secretion of cytokines from T helper cells type 2 (Th2), which activate and recruit eosinophils, neutrophils, and other cellular mediators of chronic inflammation. Eosinophil infiltration is central to the development of AHR and long-term airway pathology. If not treated, persistent inflammation eventually causes physical changes or airway remodeling in the form of smooth muscle hypertrophy and hyperplasia, thickening of the basement membrane, and an increased number of blood vessels.

Some agents that provoke asthma are nonallergic and do not rely on antibody production per se. These include drugs such as aspirin, nonsteroidal antiinflammatory drugs (NSAIDs), and opioids; environmental factors including dust, smoke, and fumes; and physiological initiators such as exercise, laughter, and stress. Individuals may be sensitive to only one or a few of these factors, which reinforces the view that asthma represents a family of heterogeneous disorders. In addition, despite the role of allergens in the majority of asthmatics, most acute asthma exacerbations, defined as episodes of breathlessness, wheezing, cough, and chest tightness, are triggered by viral infection and not allergen exposure.

Chronic Obstructive Pulmonary Disease

COPD is marked by airflow limitation, but it differs from asthma in terms of etiology, cellular mediators, treatment, and prognosis. In the

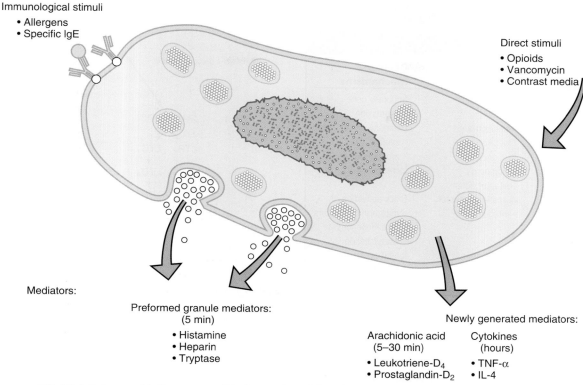

FIG. 72.1 Release of Inflammatory Mediators from Mast Cells. Immunological and direct stimuli lead to the rapid release of preformed mediators such as histamine. The leukotrienes and prostaglandins are synthesized following release of their precursors, while the cytokines are synthesized and released more slowly from mast cells and basophils. *IL-4*, Interleukin-4; *TNF-α*, tumor necrosis factor-α.

United States, the vast majority of COPD has been attributed to cigarette smoking, with occupational risks, such as mining and construction, close behind. About 2%–3% of individuals with COPD in the United States have been found to be deficient in the expression of alpha-1 antitrypsin, a protein that protects the airways from inflammation.

The major cell types involved in COPD immune dysfunction include Th1 cells, cytotoxic T cells, neutrophils, and macrophages. Structural changes include the loss of elasticity and destruction of alveolar walls. Constant breathlessness is a common symptom, especially after minimal exertion.

Drugs used for asthma and COPD either decrease inflammation, produce bronchodilation, or have both actions, summarized in the Therapeutic Overview Box.

THERAPEUTIC OVERVIEW

Antiinflammatory Agents

Glucocorticoids (inhaled or systemic) to inhibit inflammatory gene transcription, thereby suppressing airway hyperreactivity (AHR)

Antileukotrienes to decrease inflammatory signals by inhibiting inflammatory mediator synthesis or antagonizing inflammatory mediator receptors

Methylxanthines at low doses to suppress inflammatory gene transcription

Bronchodilators

Adrenergic β₂-receptor agonists to relax bronchial smooth muscle and decrease microvascular permeability

Muscarinic receptor antagonists to inhibit the bronchoconstrictor effects of endogenous acetylcholine

Methylxanthines at high doses to relax bronchial smooth muscle

---

MECHANISMS OF ACTION

Drugs used for asthma are taken either prophylactically on a regular basis to control symptoms and prevent acute episodes or to reverse the bronchoconstriction typical of acute asthma exacerbation. Inhaled glucocorticoids and, in more serious cases, long-acting β2-adrenergic receptor agonists (LABAs) are used to prevent acute episodes, while short-acting β2-adrenergic receptor agonists (SABAs) are the drugs of choice to treat an acute episode.

Unfortunately, unlike asthma, corticosteroid therapy is of minimal benefit for COPD patients, who have a poor prognosis regardless of treatment. Historically, muscarinic receptor antagonists were the bronchodilators of choice in COPD, but LABAs are also used.

Routine first-line therapies for asthma and COPD are delivered by inhalation, which conveys drug directly to the site of pathology, permits much lower doses than necessary with oral versions of the same drugs, and reduces side effects because smaller amounts of drug are absorbed into the systemic circulation. However, many patients use inhalers incorrectly, diminishing therapeutic benefits by reducing the amount of drug that reaches the airways and increasing side effects because drugs deposited in the mouth and throat are swallowed into the gastrointestinal (GI) tract, where they may be absorbed into the systemic circulation.

Drugs used for asthma and COPD and their mechanisms of action are summarized in Table 72.1.

Glucocorticoids

The pharmacology of the glucocorticoids is presented in Chapter 50. These agents are used to prevent acute asthmatic episodes by suppressing

TABLE 72.1 Mechanisms of Action of Drugs for the Treatment of Asthma and COPD

Therapeutic Benefit	Drug Class	Cellular Mechanisms
Decreased inflammation	Glucocorticoids	Suppress gene expression
	Antileukotrienes	Decrease leukotriene synthesis or antagonize $CysLTR_1$
Bronchodilation	β_2-adrenergic receptor agonists	Increase cAMP
	Muscarinic receptor antagonists	Block activation of muscarinic receptors by endogenous acetylcholine
Decreased inflammation and bronchodilation	Methylxanthines	Inhibit adenosine receptor and increase cAMP

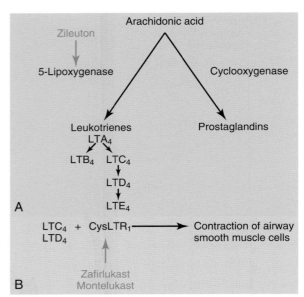

FIG. 72.2 Synthesis and Effects of the Leukotrienes. (A) Leukotrienes are synthesized from arachidonic acid through the action of 5-lipoxygenase. Zileuton inhibits this enzyme, thereby blocking the synthesis of the leukotrienes. (B) The leukotrienes LTC_4 and LTD_4 activate the $CysLTR_1$ to contract smooth muscle cells. Zafirlukast and montelukast are competitive antagonists at this receptor, blocking the action of the leukotrienes.

the expression of proinflammatory genes that are up regulated in asthma and other chronic inflammatory diseases. Corticosteroid-mediated gene inactivation occurs via several mechanisms, the most important of which, in the context of asthma, involves gene silencing through histone deacetylation. Corticosteroids bound to glucocorticoid receptors (GRs) activate histone deacetylase 2 (HDAC2) and inhibit histone acetyltransferases (HAT). The removal of acetyl groups from histone leads to condensed transcriptionally silenced chromatin. Further, glucocorticoids also inhibit the activity of proinflammatory transcription factors, such as nuclear factor-κB (NF-κB) and activator protein-1 (AP-1) and promote the degradation of mRNA transcripts encoding inflammatory proteins, such as granulocyte macrophage–colony stimulating factor (GM-CSF). At higher concentrations, the glucocorticoids increase the transcription of several antiinflammatory genes, including mitogen-activated protein kinase phosphatase-1 (MKP-1).

All of these actions result in a reduction in the number and activity of airway immune mediators, including eosinophils, Th2 lymphocytes, mast cells, macrophages, and dendritic cells, accompanied by reductions in epithelial cell inflammation, endothelial cell permeability, and hyperreactivity of bronchiolar smooth muscle. Some evidence suggests that corticosteroids up regulate adrenergic signaling by increasing the expression and activity of β_2-adrenergic receptors, thus protecting against receptor down regulation hypothesized to mediate tolerance to β_2-receptor agonists, particularly in long-term therapy.

Antileukotrienes

The LTs are synthesized in activated leukocytes by the action of 5-lipoxygenase on arachidonic acid (Chapter 29) to yield the precursor, LTA_4, which is either converted to the dihydroxy LTB_4 or conjugated with glutathione to yield LTC_4. LTC_4 is then exported into the extracellular fluid, where it is converted into LTD_4, which can be further metabolized to LTE_4. LTC_4, LTD_4, and LTE_4 all possess a cysteine residue and are referred to as cysteinyl leukotrienes (CysLTs). The CysLTs are autocrine and paracrine signalers that exert very potent inflammatory and bronchoconstrictive effects (Fig. 72.2); in bronchoprovocation tests, LTs are several orders of magnitude more potent than histamine.

Two cysteinyl LT receptors have been described, $CysLTR_1$ and $CysLTR_2$; both are G-protein–coupled receptors (GPCRs). $CysLTR_1$ is expressed in smooth muscle, mucous glands, eosinophils, and endothelial cells,

and activation by LTC_4 and LTD_4 causes prolonged bronchoconstriction and bronchoreactivity, mucous secretion, vascular leakage, and recruitment of eosinophils and other immune mediators.

Drugs that impede LT signaling are known as the antileukotrienes and consist of agents that inhibit the synthesis of the LTs or antagonize $CysLTR_1$. **Zileuton** is the only currently available inhibitor of 5-lipoxygenase and prevents the formation of LTA_4, while **zafirlukast**, **montelukast**, and **pranlukast** (not available in the United States) are competitive antagonists at $CysLTR_1$ (see Fig. 72.2). Antileukotrienes are used prophylactically to prevent bronchoconstriction; they are not useful for an acute episode.

β_2-Adrenergic Receptor Agonists

The β_2-adrenergic receptor agonists represent the current medications of choice for all types of asthma due to rapid bronchorelaxation with minimal side effects. Although airway smooth muscle does not receive innervation from sympathetic nerves, with adrenergic control of airway diameter limited to catecholamines released from the adrenal medulla, β_2-adrenergic receptors are abundantly expressed throughout bronchiolar smooth muscle. The characteristics of these receptors and their signaling mechanisms are discussed in Chapter 11. Activation of β_2 receptors leads to smooth muscle relaxation via activation of K^+ channels and membrane hyperpolarization, inhibition of the contractile filament machinery, and lowering cytosolic free Ca^{2+}. At the tissue level, these mechanisms produce bronchodilation. Additional beneficial effects may result from activation of these receptors in submucosal glands, which improves mucus secretion in mast cells to inhibit the release of inflammatory mediators and in endothelial cells to reduce leakage from the microvasculature. Both long-acting compounds (commonly referred to as LABAs), such as **salmeterol**, **formoterol**, and **indacaterol**, and short-acting compounds (commonly referred to as SABAs), such as **albuterol**, **bitolterol**, and **pirbuterol**, are available.

Muscarinic Receptor Antagonists

The principal autonomic influence in the normal regulation of bronchomotor tone is parasympathetic (Chapter 6). In chronic inflammatory syndromes, including most cases of COPD and some of asthma, parasympathetic reflexes become overactive and easily triggered, leading to unremitting bronchoconstriction. All five muscarinic receptor subtypes are present in the lung, but cholinergic control of airway smooth muscle is dominated by the M_3 subtype (Chapters 7 and 8). M_3 receptor activation is excitatory, favoring muscle contraction. M_2 muscarinic receptors, located on parasympathetic postganglionic nerve terminals, also play an important role. These autoreceptors dampen acetylcholine release and, when activated, indirectly promote muscle relaxation.

The inhaled muscarinic receptor antagonists include the quaternary compounds ipratropium, tiotropium, and, more recently, aclidinium and umeclidinium. Inhaled antimuscarinics are currently the bronchodilators of choice for the treatment of COPD, and their use in asthma is expanding.

Methylxanthines

Theophylline is a methylxanthine with both bronchodilating and antiinflammatory actions. As a phosphodiesterase (PDE), mainly PDE3, inhibitor, theophylline prevents the catabolism of cAMP and cGMP, leading to the increased intracellular accumulation of these second messengers, which promotes smooth muscle relaxation. Theophylline might also exert a bronchorelaxing effect via antagonism of mast cell adenosine receptors, inhibiting mast cell degranulation and the release of LTs, histamine, and other inflammatory factors. The antiinflammatory action of theophylline, which is achieved at lower concentrations than for bronchodilation, is attributed mainly to increased HDAC activity. As discussed for the glucocorticoids, increased HDAC activity represses the transcription of several genes involved in inflammation. Theophylline also has a negative effect on the number and/or activity of immune mediators, including eosinophils, neutrophils, T lymphocytes, and macrophages. Although the benefits of theophylline closely resemble those derived from corticosteroid therapy, these two drug classes must target distinct pathways because the addition of theophylline to glucocorticoid therapy further reduces inflammation, and theophylline suppresses chronic inflammation in COPD, while corticosteroids often do not.

An additional action of therapeutic importance is the ability of theophylline to improve contraction of the diaphragm, which increases ventilation. The mechanism for this action is unclear but may involve a direct effect on muscle contraction, an indirect effect to decrease muscle fatigue, or stimulation of central respiratory drive.

Monoclonal Antibodies

Monoclonal antibodies directed toward IgE and interleukin-5 (IL-5) have been developed by recombinant technology. Most individuals with asthma or atopy have elevated circulating IgE antibodies. Omalizumab is a humanized monoclonal antibody that binds to the IgE on the surface of mast cells (see Fig. 72.1). Because neither omalizumab nor the omalizumab-IgE complex interacts with cellular antibody receptors, mast cell activation is not provoked.

Mepolizumab and reslizumab are humanized monoclonal antibodies to IL-5, which is a key activator of eosinophils. Both of these antibodies are approved by the United States Food and Drug Administration (FDA) for add-on maintenance treatment of severe eosinophilic asthma.

RELATIONSHIP OF MECHANISMS OF ACTION TO CLINICAL RESPONSE

Asthma

The pharmacological management of asthma typically involves the use of multiple drugs with continuous evaluation and adjustment depending on patient responses. The Global Initiative for Asthma (GINA), which represents a collaborative effort between the United States National Institutes of Health and the World Health Organization, recommends a five-step algorithm that involves increasingly aggressive drug therapy based on the degree of symptom control and the risk of exacerbation.

Adult patients with mild-intermittent asthma should require only infrequent use of a fast-acting "rescue" bronchodilator, the most common of which are short-acting β_2-receptor agonists, such as albuterol. The drug should be used on an occasional basis only, and any patient who requires drug more than two times per week (not including use before exercise), should be considered for add-on controller therapy, usually with low-dose inhaled corticosteroids. Signs of increasing asthma severity include any nocturnal symptoms, daytime symptoms more than twice per week, and any limitation of normal activity; nocturnal symptoms are a serious concern because they are associated with high risk of asthma fatality. Because the benefit-to-risk ratio associated with the use of inhaled corticosteroids is high, experts increasingly recommend starting these agents at any sign of asthma, even for children as young as 6. Attaining full therapeutic benefit from inhaled corticosteroids may require several months of therapy, but some improvements transpire quickly. For instance, AHR and sputum eosinophils can be reduced within a few hours.

Orally administered leukotriene receptor antagonists or low-dose theophylline are alternative controller options, but neither is as reliably effective as inhaled corticosteroids, and theophylline can lead to cardiotoxicity. However, oral drugs may be useful for patients who cannot use an inhaler properly.

For patients requiring more aggressive therapy (moderate asthma by definition), an additional controller, such as the LABA salmeterol, should be considered. Because of the risk of mortality associated with LABA monotherapy (see Pharmacovigilance section), these agents are always given in combination with inhaled corticosteroids. Several inhalable combined preparations are available. For rescue purposes, patients should retain their SABA, but some experts now suggest that patients using formoterol for controller therapy can take advantage of its very rapid onset by using it for rescue purposes, although the FDA warns against using formoterol for this purpose. Alternatives to the use of the combined inhaled corticosteroid-LABA preparations include higher dose inhaled corticosteroid monotherapy and add-on leukotriene receptor antagonists or theophylline.

If symptoms are not adequately controlled, higher doses of the inhaled corticosteroid-LABA preparation are recommended, with the addition of an inhaled muscarinic receptor antagonist such as tiotropium as an alternative add-on treatment for patients age 12 and older who also have a history of exacerbation. Traditionally, antimuscarinics have been regarded as inferior bronchodilators in asthma, but accumulating evidence suggests that they can be as effective as β_2-receptor agonists.

For very severe cases, oral corticosteroid therapy may be required, as they are the most powerful asthma controllers, but their long-term use can cause serious toxicities (Chapter 50). Severe asthma may require antibody therapy with omalizumab, mepolizumab, or reslizumab, the latter two for add-on maintenance treatment of severe asthma in patients with eosinophilic asthma. Omalizumab therapy is reserved for patients age 6 and older who have moderate to severe persistent asthma proven refractory to inhaled corticosteroids. Patients with excessively high circulating IgE levels are not good candidates because it is impossible to reduce IgE to normal levels.

For patients who respond well to a higher level of therapy, demonstrated by good symptom control and no exacerbations for 3 months, "step down" to less aggressive therapy should be considered to identify the minimum amount of pharmacotherapy necessary for asthma control. Stopping inhaled corticosteroid therapy altogether is not recommended for adults due to increased risk of exacerbation.

Chronic Obstructive Pulmonary Disease

As indicated, corticosteroid treatment is of minimal benefit for COPD. The LABAs such as salmeterol and formoterol are typically used, as are muscarinic receptor antagonists. In addition, several ultra-long-acting β_2-receptor agonists have been approved for the treatment of both COPD and asthma, including indacaterol, olodaterol, and vilanterol, the latter available only in a combined formulation.

PHARMACOKINETICS

Corticosteroids

Inhaled corticosteroids are intended for airway delivery and are purposefully designed to limit systemic absorption; thus most inhaled corticosteroids have very low bioavailability. The pharmacokinetics of systemically administered corticosteroids is presented in Chapter 50.

Antileukotrienes

All the antileukotrienes are taken orally and are metabolized extensively by liver enzymes, including cytochrome P450s. Montelukast is taken once daily, whereas zafirlukast is taken twice daily on an empty stomach.

β_2-Adrenergic Receptor Agonists

The β_2 agonists used for respiratory diseases are grouped into categories based on their duration of action. The SABAs, or short-acting agonists, include albuterol and its R isomer levalbuterol and have a duration of about 3–6 hours. When given by a metered-dose inhaler (MDI), 15% improvement in FEV_1 is achieved within 5–10 minutes, and full effect is reached within an hour. Systemic bioavailability with MDI devices is negligible. In nebulized formulations, relatively high doses are needed because large-sized particles are not easily delivered to the airway. This causes a considerable fraction to be swallowed into the GI tract, where about 20% becomes bioavailable. Bronchodilation lasts roughly 3–6 hours with inhaled delivery but is slightly longer with oral administration of immediate-release tablets.

The LABAs, such as salmeterol, produce bronchodilation in 20–40 minutes and lasts ~12 hours. The prolonged action of salmeterol is due mainly to a substituent at the amine nitrogen, which increases lipophilicity and retains the molecule in the smooth muscle membrane near the β_2 receptor. In most patients receiving recommended doses, salmeterol is not detectable in the blood. It is extensively metabolized by several cytochrome P450s, including CYP3A4; less than 5% is excreted unchanged. Typical doses of the drug are so low that drug-drug interactions are exceedingly unlikely.

Muscarinic Receptor Antagonists

All the quaternary antimuscarinics are used as inhalants, and their charged character greatly limits their systemic absorption, minimizing adverse effects. Relative to the inhaled β_2-receptor agonists, the therapeutic effect of muscarinic antagonists is slower in onset and usually takes longer to reach full effect. Ipratropium is a short-acting agent that is taken 3–4 times daily. Tiotropium, aclidinium, umeclidinium, and glycopyrrolate are "long-acting" muscarinic antagonists that can be taken once or twice daily. A comparison of the pharmacokinetics of muscarinic receptor antagonists and β_2-receptor agonists is shown in Table 72.2.

Methylxanthines

Methylxanthines are taken orally. Oral theophylline produces bronchodilation in 15–30 minutes, with an elimination half-life of 3–4 hours in children and 8 hours in adults. Theophylline is metabolized extensively by hepatic enzymes, including CYP1A2. When given by intravenous injection, theophylline produces bronchodilation within a few minutes.

Monoclonal Antibodies

Omalizumab is administered by subcutaneous injection every 2–4 weeks. Because effects require weeks to transpire, trial therapy lasts 3–6 months. For patients who do respond, it is not yet clear how long therapy should continue. Omalizumab-IgE complexes are cleared by the mononuclear phagocyte system of the liver.

PHARMACOVIGILANCE: ADVERSE EFFECTS AND DRUG INTERACTIONS

Glucocorticoids

The likelihood of systemic glucocorticoid toxicity is greatly reduced with inhaled corticosteroids. While high-dose inhaled corticosteroids over extended intervals can sometimes cause hypothalamic-pituitary-adrenal suppression and, possibly, osteoporosis and bone fractures, these effects are a much greater concern following oral administration (Chapter 50).

TABLE 72.2 **Comparison of the Pharmacokinetics of β_2-Adrenergic Receptor Agonists and Muscarinic Receptor Antagonists**

	Receptor Selectivity	Route of Administration	BRONCHODILATOR RESPONSE		
			Onset (min)	Peak (hrs)	Duration (hrs)
β_2-Adrenergic Receptor Agonists					
Epinephrine	None	Inhaled	3–5	–	1–2
		Subcutaneous	6–15	0.5	1–3
Albuterol	β_2	Inhaled	5–10	1–2	4–6
		Oral	15–30	2–3	6–8
Formoterol	β_2	Inhaled	1–3	1–3	8–12
		Oral	20	2–4	5–8
Salmeterol	β_2	Inhaled	15–30	22	12+
Muscarinic Receptor Antagonists					
Ipratropium	None	Inhaled	15–20	1–2	3–6
Tiotropium	$M_{1,3}$	Inhaled	5	1.5–3	24
Umeclidinium	M_3	Inhaled	5–15	2–3	11
For inhaled preparations, values represent averages for administration via both nebulizer and metered dose inhaler (MDI).					

Common side effects associated with inhaled corticosteroids include dysphonia and thrush. Dysphonia likely results from surface irritation, muscle myopathy, and laryngeal superinfection. The incidence varies widely but exceeds 50% in some studies and is more common in female and elderly patients. It is less common with newer MDI formulations that use hydrofluoroalkane propellants instead of chlorofluorocarbons, which have been discontinued. Deposition of corticosteroids in the mouth, pharynx, and larynx also suppresses local immunity, predisposing to candidiasis. Patients should be trained in the best technique of inhaler use and should be encouraged to gargle and spit after every application. The use of MDIs with large-volume spacers appears to reduce the incidence of both dysphonia and thrush. Some patient data suggest that the incidence of thrush with ciclesonide is lower than with fluticasone and other inhaled corticosteroids because ciclesonide is a synthetic corticosteroid prodrug that is activated by esterases in the lung to the pharmacologically active compound desisobutyryl-ciclesonide. Thus when ciclesonide is deposited in the mouth and upper GI tract, it is inactive, thereby avoiding local immunosuppression.

In children, high-dose inhaled corticosteroid treatment is associated with growth deceleration, but this is a minor and temporary effect. Because untreated asthma also causes growth reduction that is probably more severe, the balance of considerations clearly supports inhaled corticosteroid therapy for asthmatic children.

Other side effects associated with systemic glucocorticoid therapy occur rarely, if at all, following inhalation. Estimating the occurrence of cataracts and increased intraocular pressure, psychiatric disturbances such as mood changes, and altered fuel metabolism, including insulin resistance as it relates to inhaled corticosteroid therapy, is difficult because many patients on high-dose therapy will have also received glucocorticoids systemically.

Notably, inhaled glucocorticoid therapy is regarded not only as safe in pregnancy but even necessary because uncontrolled asthma is a known in utero risk. Inhaled glucocorticoids should be used cautiously in patients taking potent inhibitors of CYP3A4, including macrolide antibiotics such as clarithromycin, the "-azole" antifungals such as ketoconazole, and HIV protease inhibitors such as atazanavir and ritonavir.

Antileukotrienes

Patient responses to antileukotrienes are variable, and some evidence suggests that this is influenced by pharmacogenetic factors. Zileuton can elevate liver enzymes and should be used with caution in patients with hepatic impairment. In addition, because zileuton inhibits CYP1A2, dose adjustments may be necessary in patients also receiving theophylline. Mood disorders and behavioral changes have been reported in individuals using antileukotrienes. In patients who also receive oral glucocorticoids, antileukotrienes are associated with eosinophilic granulomatosis with polyangiitis, also known as Churg-Strauss, a potentially fatal multisystem disorder characterized by symptoms of asthma and allergy, vasculitis of the small and medium arteries, and hypereosinophilia. This is very rare and is usually seen in the context of steroid dose reductions.

β₂-Adrenergic Receptor Agonists

Therapy with inhaled β_2-receptor agonists is associated with skeletal muscle tremor, heart palpitations and tachycardia, and nausea and vomiting. In COPD, ventilation-perfusion mismatch can cause pulmonary shunting in which adrenergic-mediated vasodilation reverses the vasoconstriction induced by hypoxia, allowing blood flow to return to poorly ventilated regions. Activation of β_2 receptors in pancreatic beta cells stimulates insulin release, which may account for a reduction in plasma K^+ that usually is not problematic.

The safety of long-term sympathomimetic therapy for asthma has been questioned for decades. Episodes of increased asthma fatalities in the early 1960s and the 1980s were linked to overuse of inhaled β-receptor agonists. In the 1990s, controversy erupted again as epidemiological data suggested that salmeterol and formoterol were associated with a higher frequency of serious events and fatalities, primarily among African-Americans. The FDA responded with a warning for all LABAs, citing "increased risk of severe exacerbation of asthma symptoms, leading to hospitalizations in pediatric and adult patients, as well as death in some patients using LABAs for the treatment of asthma." The reasons behind this suspected toxicity are unclear, but it has been suggested that chronic β_2-receptor agonism causes receptor down regulation, eventually producing an airway unresponsive to rescue therapy. Alternatively, the efficacy of β_2-receptor–mediated bronchodilation may only serve to mask symptoms of progressive airway deterioration. A third hypothesis posits that β_2-receptor agonists themselves are active contributors to the inflammatory process. Some authorities argue that LABAs should not be used at all, while others contend that the statistical risks are too small to merit clinical concern.

Whatever the case, it appears that any potential risks of long-term LABA therapy are mitigated by concurrent inhaled corticosteroid therapy. For this reason, treatment guidelines strongly recommend that patients using LABAs also receive inhaled glucocorticoids or other controller therapy to address underlying inflammation. Numerous combined formulations are available in a single inhaler device. Long-term β_2-receptor agonist therapy is not associated with poorer outcomes in COPD.

Muscarinic Receptor Antagonists

While serious side effects are practically nonexistent with inhaled antimuscarinics, some studies have suggested a higher incidence of cardiac arrhythmia and urinary retention. Patients with preexisting cardiovascular disease or benign prostatic hyperplasia should be evaluated and monitored carefully. In contrast to inhaled sympathomimetics, there are no concerns of either tolerance or worsening inflammation associated with the long-term use of inhaled muscarinic receptor antagonists. These drugs have minimal side effects due to scant absorption from the GI and respiratory tracts.

Methylxanthines

The side effects of theophylline are attributed mainly to PDE inhibition and adenosine receptor antagonism. These effects include headache, nausea, vomiting, GI distress, and tremulousness. Theophylline also stimulates acid secretion and is a weak diuretic. The most serious toxicities result from adenosine receptor blockade in the heart and in the central nervous system, leading to arrhythmias and seizures, respectively. Theophylline triggers catecholamine release from the adrenal medulla, which contributes to tachycardia and arrhythmia, which may also involve adenosine receptor antagonism.

Because theophylline is metabolized primarily by CYP1A2, the concurrent use of other CYP1A2 substrates such as ciprofloxacin, cimetidine, and erythromycin promotes theophylline accumulation and therefore increases the likelihood of toxicity. Smokers usually require higher doses of theophylline because the aromatic hydrocarbons of cigarette smoke induce CYP1A2 expression. Patients who stop smoking while receiving theophylline may require dose reduction. A large body of experience suggests that theophylline is not teratogenic. However, dose reductions are often necessary because theophylline clearance is diminished during pregnancy.

Monoclonal Antibodies

As with all biologics, antibody therapy carries a risk of sensitivity reactions and, rarely, severe anaphylaxis. For these reasons, they should be administered only by healthcare professionals in a medical facility. Also, they should not be administered during acute asthma exacerbation.

NEW DEVELOPMENTS

Investigational approaches that specifically target inflammatory pathways include cytokine inhibitors, new classes of antioxidants, PDE inhibitors, and kinase inhibitors. Pitrakinra (AEROVANT) is a protein-based dual inhibitor of IL-4/IL-13 currently in clinical trials for moderate to severe asthma that is refractory to current controllers. Antioxidants of the nuclear erythroid-2–related factor 2 activator class are in clinical trials for COPD. Clinical trials on the effects of a dual PDE3/4 inhibitor in asthma and COPD were just completed. Inhaled kinase inhibitors of the p38 and NF-κB families are in clinical trials for uncontrolled asthma.

CLINICAL RELEVANCE FOR HEALTHCARE PROFESSIONALS

All healthcare professionals need to be aware of issues facing patients with asthma or COPD. Patient adherence and success using medications are actually very low for several reasons, including the financial cost of a collection of different but necessary medications, the obligation to use medications every day for long periods of time, even when symptoms are not apparent, and the mechanical difficulty of using inhalers. Most patients and even healthcare professionals must be trained to use an inhaler properly. Successful management of these issues requires a high degree of trust and open communication between patient and clinician.

CLINICAL PROBLEMS

Drug Class	Adverse Effects
Corticosteroids	Low doses induce oral candidiasis and dysphonia; high doses cause growth retardation and other systemic effects
Antileukotrienes	Rare hepatotoxicity and eosinophilia
β₂-adrenergic receptor agonists	Tachycardia, tremors
Muscarinic receptor antagonists	Dry mouth
Methylxanthines	Narrow therapeutic index, nausea and vomiting, seizures, cardiac dysrhythmias

TRADE NAMES

In addition to generic preparations, the following trade-named materials are some of the important compounds available in the United States.

β₂-Adrenergic Receptor Agonists
Albuterol (AccuNeb, Proventil, Ventolin)
Bitolterol (Tornalate)
Indacaterol (Arcapta)
Pirbuterol (Maxair)
Formoterol (Foradil, Aerolizer, Perforomist)
Salmeterol (Serevent)

Muscarinic Receptor Antagonists
Ipratropium (Atrovent, Atrovent HFA)
Tiotropium (Spiriva)
Umeclidinium (Incruse)

Glucocorticoids
Beclomethasone (Beclovent, Beconase, Qvar, Vancenase, Vanceril)
Budesonide (Entocort, Rhinocort, Pulmicort)
Ciclesonide (Alvesco)
Flunisolide (AeroBid, Nasalide, Nasarel)
Fluticasone (Cutivate, Flonase, Flovent, Veramyst)
Triamcinolone acetonide (Azmacort)

Methylxanthines
Oxtriphylline (Choledyl)
Theophylline (Slo-bid, Slo-Phyllin, Uniphyl, Theo-24, Theo-Dur)

Antileukotrienes
Montelukast (Singulair)
Zafirlukast (Accolate)
Zileuton (Zyflo CR)

Combinations
Budesonide/formoterol (Symbicort)
Fluticasone/salmeterol (Advair Diskus)

SELF-ASSESSMENT QUESTIONS

1. An 11-year-old boy with bronchial asthma wakes up during the night with difficulty breathing. The most appropriate pharmacological agent to use, which has a rapid onset and will provide quick relief of his problem, is:
   A. Albuterol.
   B. Omalizumab.
   C. Fluticasone.
   D. Ipratropium.
   E. Zafirlukast.

2. A 74-year-old man with a 50-year history of smoking presents to the emergency department with an acute exacerbation of his COPD. Which of the following classes of drugs would be most effective at relieving the bronchoconstrictive component of his disease?
   A. Inhaled β_2-receptor agonists.
   B. Inhaled corticosteroids.
   C. Antileukotrienes.
   D. IgE monoclonal antibodies.
   E. Inhaled muscarinic receptor antagonists.

3. Only about 10%–20% of a typical dose of drug delivered by a metered dose inhaler reaches the lungs; the remainder is swallowed into the gastrointestinal tract, where it may be absorbed to cause systemic effects. Which of the following inhaled drugs avoids this issue because it is selectively bioactivated in the lungs only?
   A. Albuterol.
   B. Formoterol.
   C. Ciclesonide.
   D. Omalizumab.
   E. Montelukast.

4. A patient suddenly experiences an acute asthmatic episode while performing her physical therapy and asks you to get her medication from her bag. When you look inside, there are lots of drugs. Which one should be administered to the patient at this time?
   A. Albuterol inhaler.
   B. Montelukast.
   C. Salmeterol.
   D. Theophylline.
   E. Omalizumab.

5. The bronchodilation that occurs following the use of montelukast is a consequence of:
   A. Antagonism of leukotriene receptors.
   B. Blockade of acetylcholine release.
   C. Increased levels of cAMP.
   D. Deceased levels of IgE.
   E. Antagonism of leukotriene synthesis.

FURTHER READING

Barnes PJ. Severe asthma: advances in current management and future therapy. *J Allergy Clin Immunol.* 2012;129(1):48–59.

Gentry S, Gentry B. Chronic obstructive pulmonary disease: diagnosis and management. *Am Fam Physician.* 2017;95(7):433–441.

Hansbro PM, Kim RY, Starkey MR, et al. Mechanisms and treatments for severe, steroid-resistant allergic airway disease and asthma. *Immunol Rev.* 2017;278(1):41–62.

Wilkinson M, King B, Iyer S, et al. Comparison of a rapid albuterol pathway with a standard pathway for the treatment of children with a moderate to severe asthma exacerbation in the emergency department. *J Asthma.* 2017;26:1–8.

WEBSITES

http://acaai.org/asthma/asthma-treatment
This site is maintained by the American College of Allergy, Asthma, and Immunology and is an excellent resource for both healthcare professionals and patients.

http://ginasthma.org/
This website is maintained by the Global Initiative for Asthma in collaboration with the National Institutes of Health and the World Health Organization and contains guidelines for the management and prevention of asthma.

http://www.lung.org/lung-health-and-diseases/all-diseases.html
This website is maintained by the American Lung Association and gives access to information on all diseases of the lungs with individual links to each disorder.

https://www.nhlbi.nih.gov/
This website is maintained by the National Heart, Lung, and Blood Institute of the National Institutes of Health and is an excellent resource for both asthma and COPD.

https://www.thoracic.org/statements/
This website contains up-to-date information from the American Thoracic Society regarding clinical practice guidelines, policy statements, research areas, and technical standards for thoracic disorders, including asthma and COPD.

The Role of Nutraceuticals and Natural Products

Pamela Potter

MAJOR DRUG CLASSES

Botanicals
Supplements

ABBREVIATIONS

DSHEA	Dietary Supplement Health and Education Act
EPA	United States Environmental Protection Agency
FDA	United States Food and Drug Administration

THERAPEUTIC OVERVIEW

Humans have used plants as medicines since prehistoric times. Plant-based therapeutics have been used and recorded for more than 3000 years, as documented by Egyptian writings, the Chinese Materia Medica, and Ayurvedic medicine. In fact, more than 50% of currently used prescription drugs were originally derived from plants—in particular, antimicrobials and many anticancer drugs.

The term **alternative medicine** is used to describe treatments other than the conventional or mainstream medicine practiced and taught in Western medical institutions. It is also sometimes referred to as "integrative" or "complementary" medicine. The biologically based alternative therapies include botanicals (e.g., herbs) and supplements (including, but not limited to, amino acids, vitamins, and minerals), often referred to as **nutraceuticals**, a term coined in 1989 that refers to any substance considered "a food or part of a food that provides medical or health benefits, including the prevention and/or treatment of a disease."

In a 2012 survey, alternative medicines were used by more than 33% of the population, with the highest rates of use in middle-aged (45–64 years old) individuals with the most education and with private health insurance. The World Health Organization estimates that 80% of people use some form of herbal medication, and estimates indicate that in 2015, Americans spent approximately $13 billion on herbal products and dietary supplements. The reasons underlying the popularity of these products are varied and include dissatisfaction with conventional medicine, the lack of effective treatments for some conditions, the view that alternative therapies are safer or more natural, distrust of pharmaceutical companies, and the idea that alternative medicines focus on causes of illness and are more likely to prevent chronic disease than conventional medicines. Alternative therapies are often sought by individuals with a **holistic** orientation to health who have a chronic condition such as diabetes, pain, or cancer that has not responded to conventional treatment.

The **Dietary Supplement Health and Education Act (DSHEA)**, passed by the United States Congress in 1994, defines a **dietary supplement** as a product to supplement the diet containing a vitamin, mineral, amino acid, herb, or other botanical product, intended for ingestion in the form of a capsule, powder, or extract. Dietary supplements must be labeled with the name and quantity of each ingredient or the total quantity of all ingredients (excluding inert ingredients) in a blend. In addition, products containing herbal or botanical ingredients must state the part of the plant from which the ingredient is derived.

Federal regulations allow various statements on the label of dietary supplements but do not allow claims concerning the use of a dietary supplement to diagnose, prevent, mitigate, treat, or cure a specific disease without sufficient clinical evidence. For example, a product label may not claim that the preparation "cures" diabetes or "treats" cancer unless that claim is evidence based and approved by the United States Food and Drug Administration (FDA). For example, the claim that calcium and vitamin D may reduce the risk of osteoporosis may be used because it has been shown to be valid and has been approved by the FDA. Products can make claims about classical nutrient deficiency diseases, provided the statements disclose the prevalence of the disease in the United States. In addition, if manufacturers want to claim that a supplement has benefits on the "structure or function" of the body or on "well-being," they must substantiate that the statements are truthful and not misleading.

Some of the most commonly used botanical/herbal products and their proposed benefits are shown in the Therapeutic Overview Box. In addition, many of these products are available or can be prepared in different formulations, as shown in Box 73.1.

THERAPEUTIC OVERVIEW

Herbal Products Commonly Used in the United States

Cranberry: treatment of urinary tract infections
Echinacea: treatment of upper respiratory infections
Evening primrose: decreases menopausal symptoms; treatment of arthritis
Feverfew: treatment of migraine headaches; treatment of menstrual cramps
Garlic: treatment of hypertension; lowers cholesterol
Ginger: treatment of nausea and vomiting during pregnancy or chemotherapy
Ginkgo biloba: improves memory
Ginseng: boosts energy; treatment of type II diabetes
Goldenseal: antibacterial properties; treatment of nasal irritation in colds
Green tea: increases energy; promotes weight loss; treatment of atherosclerosis; lowers cholesterol
Saw palmetto: treatment of benign prostatic hyperplasia
Soy, black cohosh: decreases menopausal symptoms
St. John's wort: treatment of depression

BOX 73.3 Herbs Commonly Used for Immunomodulation

Milk thistle	Astragalus root
Echinacea	Licorice
Marigold	Olive leaf
Elderberry	Cat's claw

TABLE 73.1 Herbs and Supplements Proposed to Affect the Central Nervous System

Sedatives	Stimulants	Antidepressants
Kava	Lobelia	St. John's wort
Valerian	Coffee (caffeine)	Kava
Lavender	Green tea	
Chamomile	Tobacco	
Ginger	Ginseng	
Melatonin	Ginkgo biloba	

BOX 73.2 Products Used as Antioxidants or Antiinflammatory Agents

Alpha-lipoic acid	Lutein
Chondroitin	MSM (methylsulfonylmethane)
Cinnamon	Milk thistle (silymarin)
Curcumin (turmeric)	Omega-3 fatty acids (fish oil)
Garlic	Soy (isoflavones, genistein)
Ginkgo biloba	Resveratrol
Glucosamine	Red clover

MECHANISMS OF ACTION

Like other drugs or chemicals, herbal medicines and dietary supplements are presumed to exert their effects on physiological or biological systems. One difference between herbal products and conventional medications is that herbal products often contain large numbers of chemicals, and the activity of each of these is not always known. Further, the interactions between these chemicals may be important in their actions.

Antioxidant and Antiinflammatory Effects

Oxidation of DNA, proteins, carbohydrates, and lipids by reactive oxygen species has been implicated in normal aging and several diseases, including arthritis, cancer, and Alzheimer disease. Oxidative stress occurs when there is an imbalance between free radical generation (by the action of reactive oxygen species) and endogenous antioxidants in cells and tissues. Many herbal products and supplements are used for their potential antioxidant effects (Box 73.2). Among these preparations is the naturally occurring carotenoid lutein, which is known for protecting the health of the eyes and has been shown to decrease the incidence of age-related macular degeneration. In addition, curcumin, which is a component of turmeric, has both antioxidant and antiinflammatory properties, while cinnamon and alpha-lipoic acid, two compounds with antioxidant activity, are also used to reduce blood glucose levels. The amino sugar glucosamine is normally involved in the synthesis of glycosaminoglycans, which contributes to the formation of cartilage, while chondroitin occurs in connective tissue. Thus it is not surprising that glucosamine/chondroitin supplements are often used for the treatment of osteoarthritis. Last, omega-3 fatty acids have been shown

in clinical trials to have antiinflammatory effects and to improve symptoms in patients with arthritis.

Immunomodulation

Some herbals are thought to act by modulating immune function (Box 73.3). Modulation can be indirect via antioxidant effects, or direct, via stimulation of immune cells. Echinacea is perhaps the best-studied herbal product for its ability to enhance T cell activity and has been shown to reduce the duration of upper respiratory infections. Other supplements affect levels of interferon or other cytokines involved in the immune response.

Actions on Neurotransmission

Many plants contain compounds that are used or abused for their psychoactive qualities, usually for sedative, stimulant, or analgesic purposes. These include coffee (caffeine), tobacco (nicotine), coca (cocaine), the opium poppy (opioids), marijuana (cannabinoids), and peyote (mescaline).

Many plant-based compounds affect neurotransmission in the central and peripheral nervous systems by altering activity at neurotransmitter receptors, blocking the uptake of neurotransmitters, stimulating or blocking neurotransmitter release, or altering the enzymatic degradation of neurotransmitters. Thus it is not surprising that many plants, herbs, and supplements are used frequently for their sedative, stimulant, and antidepressant effects (Table 73.1). Indeed, St. John's wort (*Hypericum perforatum*) is a plant that has been used for centuries for mental health conditions, particularly depression, and may inhibit both the reuptake of serotonin and monoamine oxidase activity, mechanisms similar to some prescribed antidepressants (Chapter 17).

Hormonal Actions

Some herbs contain compounds that mimic or block the actions of hormones, particularly estrogen. The phytoestrogens, which are present in some foods, particularly soy, are plant-derived compounds that include isoflavones, coumestans, and lignans. The phytoestrogens have agonist activity in some tissues and antagonist activity in others, in a manner similar to the selective estrogen receptor modulators (Chapter 51). These compounds may protect against the likelihood of breast cancer, depending on dose and usage. The phytoestrogens are frequently used to relieve menopausal symptoms such as hot flashes and night sweats, but clinical studies have not supported efficacy. Evidence has shown, however, that diets high in soy are protective against osteoporosis and heart disease. However, isoflavone is considered an endocrine disruptor by the United States Environmental Protection Agency (EPA) because excessive intake may depress luteinizing hormone levels, leading to secondary depression of estrogen production, which may delay puberty and affect lactation and fertility. The safety and effectiveness of phytoestrogens remains to be determined.

Other botanicals have been proposed to modify hormonal activity in men. Saw palmetto, which has an antiandrogen effect and may block α_1-adrenergic receptors, has been investigated for the treatment of benign prostatic hyperplasia and prostate cancer, but clinical trials have not supported efficacy. Yohimbe, an evergreen tree in western Africa, contains yohimbine, an antagonist at α_2-adrenergic receptors known to increase norepinephrine release by blocking inhibitory presynaptic autoreceptors, thus enhancing sympathetic activity (Chapter 12). Yohimbe bark is sold as a dietary supplement for treating erectile dysfunction, although studies have not supported efficacy. The naturally occurring adrenal hormone that is a precursor of estrogen and testosterone (Chapter 48), dehydroepiandrosterone (DHEA), is often used as a supplement to restore declining levels present in aging. Other herbal products used for their hormonal effects are shown in Box 73.4.

Anticancer Effects

Some herbal products have been suggested to prevent cancer by stimulating the immune system or by antioxidant effects, while others are thought to act by direct toxic effects on neoplastic cells. Several potent conventional cancer treatments (Chapter 68) are derived from plants and other natural products, including taxol from Pacific yew that hyperstabilizes microtubules, and the vinca alkaloids (vincristine, vinblastine) from the Madagascar periwinkle that inhibit microtubule formation, both mechanisms leading to the arrest of cancer cell proliferation. Several other natural products target different postulated anticancer mechanisms, including reversal of multidrug resistance pumps by the flavonoids and inhibition of angiogenesis by shark cartilage.

Herbal products are also used to reduce the adverse effects of conventional chemotherapy and radiation treatments, in addition to alleviating the symptoms associated with cancer. Many patients take large doses of vitamins and antioxidants to boost immune function

---

BOX 73.4 Herbs Used for Hormonal Effects

Menopausal Symptoms
Vasomotor Instability (Hot Flashes)
- Soy, black cohosh, evening primrose, dong quai (angelica)

Mood Disorders
- St. John's wort, valerian

Loss of Libido, Vaginal Dryness, Dyspareunia
- Chasteberry (vitex)
- Ginseng
- Wild yam
- Raspberry leaves

Androgenic Effects
- Saw palmetto
- Yohimbe bark
- Pygeum
- Dehydroepiandrosterone (DHEA)

---

and prevent further neoplastic transformation. Patients believe that, at worst, these supplements can do no harm. However, current research suggests that because conventional cancer therapy frequently depends on oxidative mechanisms, it is possible that antioxidants could interfere with conventional treatments. Also, recent evidence suggests that cancer cell apoptosis is increased by reactive oxygen species, and antioxidants can slow or block this process. The American Institute for Cancer Research has concluded that supplementation with individual or combined antioxidants above levels established by the Institute of Medicine's Dietary Reference Intakes cannot be recommended as either safe or effective. Patients undergoing either chemotherapy or radiation therapy should be advised not to exceed the upper limits for vitamin and mineral supplements and to avoid dietary supplements that contain high levels of antioxidants.

RELATIONSHIP OF MECHANISMS OF ACTION TO CLINICAL RESPONSE

The complex nature of herbal medicines and other natural products creates a major challenge to assessing clinical effectiveness. Evidence to support the efficacy of these agents is minimal at best, due to many confounding factors. First, in the United States, herbal and other dietary supplements do not have to meet the same standards as prescription drugs and over-the-counter medications for proof of safety, effectiveness, and "good manufacturing practices." Second, the active ingredients in many herbs and herbal supplements are unknown. There may be dozens, even hundreds, of such compounds in a single herbal supplement preparation. Published analyses of herbal supplements have reported differences between what is listed on the label and what is actually in the bottle. The term *standardized* on a product label is no guarantee of high product quality because in the United States, there is no legal definition of *standardized* (or *certified* or *verified*) for supplements. Further, some herbal supplements contain metals, unlabeled prescription drugs, microorganisms, or other substances. Thus it is almost impossible to design and conduct evidence-based studies with these preparations to ascertain relationships between mechanisms of action and clinical responses.

PHARMACOKINETICS

In most cases, it is not possible to determine the pharmacokinetics of herbal products because of their complex nature. When the active components are unknown, it is difficult to select the key components to follow in a pharmacokinetic study.

An important issue that needs additional investigation is the interaction of herbal products with other drugs. Drug-herb interactions can occur at the level of absorption, distribution, metabolism, or excretion (Chapter 3), with metabolic interactions receiving the most attention. These interactions are bidirectional, with drugs either interfering with or enhancing the effects of herbs, and herbs or other supplements either interfering with or enhancing the effects (and side effects) of drugs.

Drugs such as cholestyramine, colestipol, and sucralfate may bind to certain herbs, forming an insoluble complex and decreasing the absorption of both substances. Similarly, the absorption of herbs may be adversely affected by drugs that change the pH of the stomach. Antacids, H_2-histamine receptor antagonists, and proton pump inhibitors, such as cimetidine and omeprazole, are used to neutralize, decrease, or inhibit secretion of stomach acid for the treatment of ulcers or gastroesophageal reflux (Chapter 71). With decreased stomach acid, herbs may not be catabolized into components easily absorbable by the intestines. Drugs that affect gastrointestinal motility, such as the opioids, may also affect the absorption of herbs.

Many herbs induce cytochrome P450 enzymes (Chapter 3), leading to increased degradation of concomitantly administered drugs that are metabolized through the same pathways. An herb-drug interaction that has received much attention is the induction of cytochrome CYP3A4 by St. John's wort, used to treat depression. Because cytochrome CYP3A4 is involved in the metabolism of more than half of all prescribed drugs, St. John's wort can decrease the effectiveness of drugs metabolized by this pathway, including oral contraceptives and protease inhibitors used to treat human immunodeficiency virus (HIV). Conversely, drugs that inhibit cytochrome P450s can increase the accumulation of herbs. Examples of drugs that inhibit liver metabolism include, but are not limited to, cimetidine, erythromycin, and ketoconazole.

PHARMACOVIGILANCE: ADVERSE EFFECTS AND DRUG INTERACTIONS

Difficulties in identifying the side effects of herbs arise because the identity of herbal ingredients is largely unknown, most reports are anecdotal, and effects may be attributed to herbs simply because there is no other obvious cause. In addition, herbal products may contain compounds other than those indicated on the label. Because of the numerous compounds in some herbal products, one might expect the potential for side effects to be large. However, a central tenet of herbalism is that complex composition minimizes side effects because of the presence of chemicals that exert the desired effect and other chemicals that antagonize side effects. Unfortunately, these tenets have not been tested in controlled studies. In addition, the potency of an herbal product may be very low compared with that of typical drugs that are administered in the milligram or even microgram range.

Provisions in DSHEA state that the manufacturer is responsible for ensuring that its dietary supplement products are safe before they are marketed. Unlike drug products that must be proven safe and effective for their intended use before marketing (Chapter 5), there are no provisions in the law for the FDA to "approve" dietary supplements for safety or effectiveness before they reach the consumer. Also, unlike manufacturers and distributors of drugs, those of dietary supplements are not currently required by law to record, investigate, or forward to government agencies any reports they receive of injuries or illnesses that may be related to the use of their products. Under DSHEA, once the product is marketed, the FDA has the responsibility to prove that a dietary supplement is "unsafe" before it can take action to restrict its use or remove it from the marketplace.

The pharmacological actions of herbal products can give rise to serious safety concerns. Ephedra was used for many years for weight loss, as a stimulant, and to improve athletic performance. Ephedra posed an interesting dilemma for the current regulatory framework for herbs because it contains ephedrine and other ephedrine-like compounds that, when prepared synthetically, are regulated as drugs. Low doses of ephedrine, an effective decongestant, were present in numerous over-the-counter cold remedies, and the potential adverse effects of ephedrine were well known to include stroke, cardiac arrhythmias, and hyperthermia, caused by its sympathomimetic actions. Because there is no system for reporting adverse events that occur after ingestion of a dietary supplement, the incidence of adverse events linked to ephedra could not be established. However, evidence began to accumulate, and reanalysis of the few clinical studies, in conjunction with the untimely death of a well-known athlete, led the FDA to conclude that ephedra was unsafe, and it was removed from the market in 2004.

A second safety issue is that of contaminants. Because herbs are agricultural products or wild crafted (i.e., gathered in the wild), they can be contaminated with pesticides, herbicides, and soil contaminants such as heavy metals, fungi, and bacteria. In addition, contaminants can be introduced through the manufacturing process, such as solvents used for extraction. The liver toxicity of kava appears to be related to acetone extraction. Whether residual acetone is responsible for this toxicity or whether acetone extracts additional chemicals from the bulk plant material that are not normally present in the teas made by native populations that use kava remains to be determined. However, it is clear that some people who used a commercially available kava extract suffered liver damage, which led the FDA to ban acetone-extracted kava preparations.

A third safety issue is adulteration. Unscrupulous herb dealers and manufacturers of herbal remedies have been known to add pharmaceuticals to their products. Some complex herbal mixtures contain indomethacin, warfarin, and diethylstilbestrol. Because these pharmaceuticals could account for many therapeutic and adverse effects, it is impossible to determine whether the herbal components of a remedy are response for its actions.

A fourth safety issue is misidentification. A pharmacologically active herb may come from only one species of a large genus of plants. Proper identification of the species can often be difficult. One example of this is ginseng. American ginseng is highly sought after for its tonic effects, and the collection of wild American ginseng is strictly controlled to avert decimation of the species. There are other ginseng varieties, according to herbalists, that are much less efficacious but might be advertised and sold as American ginseng in the marketplace. There are essentially no guarantees that the plants identified on the label of an herbal remedy are actually those present. In addition, because herbs are natural products and the chemistry of the plant is determined by growing conditions, including seed stock, considerable variation may exist in the chemical composition of any given batch of herbs. There are no "standards" or methods of certification that are accepted across the industry. When the active ingredients are not known, it is obviously impossible to standardize preparations to achieve a reproducible pharmacological effect. Not only does this make the clinical use of herbs difficult, but it is also a major impediment to research in this area.

Last, the concurrent use of herbs and drugs with similar therapeutic actions creates the risk of pharmacodynamic interactions. The highest risk of clinically significant interactions occurs between herbs and drugs with sympathomimetic, cardiovascular, diuretic, anticoagulant, and antidiabetic effects, as listed in Table 73.2. Some herbs contain salicylates and coumarins, which have antiplatelet activity that may potentiate prescribed anticoagulants. Ginger and ginseng have direct antiplatelet

TABLE 73.2 Drug Interactions of Herbal Products

Drug or Drug Group	Herbal Products
Anticoagulants (e.g., warfarin)	Angelica, Asian ginseng, cranberry, Devil's claw, garlic, ginger, gingko, St. John's wort, willow
Antihypertensive drugs (beta blockers, diuretics)	Asian ginseng, black cohosh, ephedra, bitter orange, evening primrose, garlic, gingko, hawthorn, licorice, St. John's wort
Cardiac drugs	Asian ginseng, ephedra, bitter orange
Antipsychotic drugs	Evening primrose
Corticosteroids	Ephedra, bitter orange, licorice
Antidiabetic agents	Aloe vera, ephedra, gingko, Asian ginseng, milk thistle
Antiretroviral agents	

activity and can potentiate anticoagulant therapy and alter bleeding time. Licorice, consumed as an herbal remedy or as candy, raises blood pressure, and excessive amounts should be avoided in people with hypertension. St. John's wort may potentiate the actions of antidepressants, including serotonin and norepinephrine reuptake inhibitors and monoamine oxidase inhibitors. Additionally, nephrotoxicity and hepatotoxicity can be additive with the concurrent use of drugs and herbs that have similar toxicities. Examples of herbal products with such toxicities are shown in the Clinical Problems Box.

NEW DEVELOPMENTS

Centuries of use have created the impression that herbal remedies are both safe and effective. The challenge to science is to provide controlled, clinical evidence for these claims. Isolation of an active chemical in herbal preparations has sometimes been followed by controlled clinical trials of the active substance. If the trial fails, there is always the caveat that the herbal preparation may require the full spectrum of compounds in the preparation, not just the single ingredient. Similarly, nutraceuticals may function better in the complex environment of the foods from which they have been isolated. Thus it may be useful to investigate complex mixtures of herbs or individually tailored treatment plans with specific dietary changes.

Safety concerns about herbal medicines require well-designed toxicological and pharmacokinetic studies, which could potentially lead to clearer marketing requirements and more stringent monitoring of adverse effects. A requirement that preparations contain the ingredients shown on the label is also a good practice.

Herbal medicine is practiced by a diverse group of alternative medicine providers, including doctors of traditional Chinese medicine, naturopaths, homeopaths, and Ayurvedic practitioners. An expanding trend in healthcare is the concept of complementary or integrative medicine, for which such therapies are combined with conventional Western approaches. More research is needed to determine the advantages (or disadvantages) of these combined, integrated approaches because this trend is being driven by patient demand, as well as evidence for improvements in healthcare and outcomes.

CLINICAL RELEVANCE FOR HEALTHCARE PROFESSIONALS

Healthcare professionals need to be aware of patient use of nutraceutical agents of all types. Use of these agents usually indicates some healthcare issue for the patient for which results of care have been unsatisfactory. Investigation of any issue will allow healthcare providers the opportunity to address the issue and to assure it will not interfere with the delivery of care that is being provided, or considered, for the patient. Additionally, awareness of such agents and their potential use and possible adverse effects can allow healthcare professionals the opportunity to provide input and counseling to patients in this arena. It should be emphasized that most people using alternative medicine do not report such to their physicians or other conventional medical providers, and many conventional medical providers do not readily accept alternative therapeutic approaches. It is imperative that all healthcare professionals question their patients about the use of such preparations and keep an open mind to the possible benefits of such approaches.

SELF-ASSESSMENT QUESTIONS

1. A 42-year-old woman who distrusts conventional medicine and believes strongly in alternatives came down with a bad cough and decided to take which of the following to increase her immune function and relieve her upper respiratory infections?
   A. Kava.
   B. Cayenne.
   C. Echinacea.
   D. Ginger.
   E. Cinnamon.

2. A 54-year-old former athlete began having problems with osteoarthritis. His physician suggested several medications, all of which upset his gastrointestinal system. He went to the local nutrition store seeking an alternative. Which combination would likely have the most benefit?
   A. Glucosamine and chondroitin sulfate.
   B. Ginseng and cinnamon.
   C. Resveratrol and curcumin.
   D. Ginkgo biloba and green tea.
   E. Saw palmetto and garlic.

3. Herbal products are not without side effects. Which of the following correctly matches an herbal product with its major side effect?
   A. Saw palmetto: inhibition of estrogen production.
   B. Echinacea: inhibition of T-cell function.
   C. Curcumin: increased incidence of breast cancer.
   D. Kava: liver damage.

4. A 56-year-old man diagnosed with depression sought an alternative treatment because he heard that conventional antidepressants could lead to impotence. Which of the following alternative preparations may be of help for his mental state?
   A. St. John's wort.
   B. Yohimbe bark.
   C. Omega-3 fatty acids.
   D. Saw palmetto.
   E. Taxol.

5. A 67-year-old man was seen in at an urgent care after cutting his hand on a can. The cut was bleeding far more than would be expected, and the physician assistant who saw him was curious to know if he was on any medication. He said he was taking aspirin, lovastatin, and enalapril, but no other prescription or over the counter drugs. Further questioning revealed that he was taking an herbal product that may have increased his bleeding. What was this product most likely to be?
   A. Saw palmetto
   B. Echinacea
   C. Asian ginseng
   D. Milk thistle
   E. Yohimbe bark

6. A 70-year-old woman who had knee replacement surgery did not recover from anesthesia as quickly as expected. Her current medication list included losartan, hydrochlorothiazide, levothyroxine, and omeprazole. The anesthesiologist suspected that she might have been taking some other medication, and on questioning when she finally awoke, the patient admitted that she was taking something she bought at the health food store for depression but had been too embarrassed to mention it. This was most likely which of the following?
   A. Black cohosh
   B. Asian ginseng
   C. Bitter orange
   D. Evening primrose
   E. St. John's Wort

FURTHER READING

Das L, Bhaumik E, Raychaudhuri U, Chakraborty R. Role of nutraceuticals in human health. *J Food Sci Technol.* 2012;49(2):173–183.

Dias DA, Urban S, Roessner U. A historical overview of natural products in drug discovery. *Metabolites.* 2012;2(2):303–336.

Ji HF, Li XJ, Zhang HY. Natural products and drug discovery. Can thousands of years of ancient medical knowledge lead us to new and powerful drug combinations in the fight against cancer and dementia? *EMBO Rep.* 2009;10(3):194–200.

Li JW, Vederas JC. Drug discovery and natural products: end of an era or an endless frontier? *Science.* 2009;325(5937):161–165.

WEBSITES

http://www.nlm.nih.gov/medlineplus/herbalmedicine.html
This website contains information on herbal medicine from the National Library of Medicine.

https://nccih.nih.gov/
This website is maintained by the National Center for Complementary and Integrative Health of the National Institutes of Health and contains links to information on the uses of alternative medicines, including guidelines.

https://www.mskcc.org/cancer-care/diagnosis-treatment/symptom-management/integrative-medicine/herbs
This website is maintained by the Memorial Sloan Kettering Cancer Center and provides a searchable herbal database on common herbs and other dietary supplements.

http://www.hopkinsmedicine.org/healthlibrary/conditions/complementary_and_alternative_medicine/herbal_medicine_85,P00181/
This website maintained by Johns Hopkins Medicine provides a summary of commonly used herbs and a searchable database.

https://www.consumerlab.com/
This website is maintained by Consumer Lab, which is an independent consumer group that tests herbal products and provides a database of information on product quality and contents.

Essentials of Toxicology

Monica Valentovic and Gary Rankin

TOXICOLOGY OVERVIEW

Every substance is capable of causing harm or injury to humans, depending on the dose and route of exposure. While most individuals think of toxicity or poisoning as unintentional and unwanted adverse reactions to compounds, the intentional use of agents for their lethal or toxic effects has been well documented since the use of hemlock on Socrates, and, unfortunately, continues today.

In assessing toxicity, it is important to understand the most important axiom of toxicology that "the dose makes the poison" because all agents have the potential to produce toxic effects. In addition to dose, several other factors are prime determinants of toxicity, including the form and innate chemical activity of the compound, as well as the duration and route of exposure. Toxic effects are often manifest at the site of absorption—that is, hypersensitivity following dermal exposure or respiratory issues following gaseous exposure. Further, pharmacokinetic parameters may also determine toxicity, with some chemicals leading to toxicity following one route of administration but not after another, such as may occur if the liver inactivates most of the agent by first-pass metabolism.

Toxicity is generally characterized in reference to temporal exposure to a compound. If an agent produces a toxic response following a single exposure, it is referred to as acute toxicity, whereas if toxicity does not manifest until multiple treatments for several days to weeks of exposure, it is referred to as subacute or subchronic toxicity. If effects are apparent after exposure for several months to years, it is referred to as chronic toxicity and typically reflects cumulative damage, such as cirrhosis in alcoholics who have consumed alcohol for several years or pulmonary fibrosis in coal miners.

Toxic substances may be classified as toxicants or toxins. A toxicant is a toxic substance synthesized or introduced into the environment by humans, such as bisphenol A (BPA), while a toxin is defined as a toxic substance present in a natural product, such as bufotoxin or botulinum toxin. Toxic substances may also be classified as environmental agents, biological toxins, or chemical and biological warfare agents. Common environmental agents are listed in Table 74.1, while biological toxins are listed in Table 74.2.

It is impossible to cover all aspects of toxicology in a single chapter. Thus this chapter presents a basic overview of the systemic and organ-specific effects of toxicants and provides specific examples using commonly known toxic compounds.

MECHANISMS OF ACTION

Toxic substances can lead to systemic or specific organ system damage and can induce effects directly on an organ system or cell type and/or indirectly by affecting one group of cells that are critical for the health

of other cells. Although many toxins or toxicants affect a specific target organ, a toxic response in one tissue may have serious effects for other tissues, depending on the characteristics of the agent, as well as those of the individual affected (gender, life stage, overall health, etc.). The primary systemic and organ-specific targets of toxic compounds are listed in the Toxicology Overview Box.

TOXICOLOGY OVERVIEW

Systemic Toxicity

Immunotoxicity	Hypersensitivity, immunosuppression or deficiency, leukemia
Carcinogenicity	Malignancies due to abnormal cell differentiation and proliferation
Developmental	Affects the developing embryo or fetus leading to embryolethality or toxicity and teratogenicity
Genetic	Gene mutations, chromosome aberrations, or aneuploidy/polyploidy that alters DNA
Epigenetic	DNA methylation, histone acetylation, regulation of noncoding RNAs, or other changes in genetic programming

Organ-Specific Toxicity

Hepatotoxicity	Damage to the liver, bile duct, or gallbladder including chemical hepatitis, cholestasis, cirrhosis, or necrosis
Nephrotoxicity	Inability to maintain electrolyte balance and secrete waste, glomerulonephritis, interstitial nephritis, and papillary necrosis
Pulmonary toxicity	Damage to nose, pharynx, larynx, trachea, bronchi, bronchioles, and alveoli leading to inflammation, fibrosis, or pulmonary edema
Cardiotoxicity	Damage to the heart and blood vessels leading to cardiomyopathy, atherosclerosis
Neurotoxicity	Damage to peripheral nerves or brain cells including demyelination, axonopathies, neuronopathies, and other changes leading to frank damage or mental/cognitive disturbances
Reproductive	Damage to male or female systems, infertility
Dermal	Skin lesions, hypersensitivity reactions, skin cancer
Ocular toxicity	Corneal erosion, conjunctivitis, cataracts

TABLE 74.1. Common Environmental Agents

Class	Examples
Dioxins	Polychlorinated dibenzo-p-dioxins (PCDDs), polychlorinated dibenzofurans (PCDFs), dioxin-like polychlorinated biphenyls (PCBs)
Gases	Carbon monoxide (CO), radon, ozone, hydrogen sulfide
Heavy metals	Arsenic, lead, mercury, cadmium, hexavalent chromium
Pesticides	
Fungicides	Zinc dimethyldithiocarbamate, vinclozolin, tricyclazole
Herbicides	Paraquat, glyphosate
Insecticides	Rotenone, malathion, pyrethroids
Rodenticides	Bromethalin, α-naphthylthiourea
Plasticizers	Bisphenol A (BPA), phthalates, and parabens
Volatile organics/ solvents	Benzene, formaldehyde, styrene, trichloroethylene, tetrachloroethylene

TABLE 74.2 Biological Toxins

Toxin	Source
Aflatoxin B$_1$	*Aspergillus flavus*
Anthrax	*Bacillus anthracis*
Botulinum toxin	*Clostridium botulinum*
Bufotoxin	Parotid gland of the cane toad *(Bufo marinus)* and Colorado River toad *(Bufo alvarius)*
Cholera toxin	*Vibrio cholera*
Diphtheria toxin	*Corynebacterium diphtheria*
Pertussis toxin	*Bordetella pertussis*
Ricin (lectin)	Seeds of the castor oil plant *(Ricinus communis)*
Tetanus toxin	*Clostridium tetani*
Tetrodotoxin	Liver and gonads of marine puffer fish of the family Tetraodontiformes *(Tetraodon lineatus, Tetraodon miurus, Tetraodon mbu, Takifugu niphobles, Takifugu pardalis, Takifugu stictonotus)*; saliva of Australian blue-ringed octopuses *(Hapalochlaena maculosa* and *Hapalochlaena lunulata)*

Systemic Toxicity

Immunotoxicity

The immune system recognizes and defends the body against foreign invaders through the production of various cells. A wide variety of toxicants may cause immunosuppression by interfering with cell proliferation, directly destroying immune system components, or distorting normal signaling mechanisms to reduce the immune response. Occupational exposure to the solvent benzene decreases humoral immunity by decreasing levels of complement and immunoglobulins. Further, many aromatic hydrocarbons and phthalates used in the manufacture of numerous products have been shown to disrupt B-cell development and enhance apoptosis. In addition, the polychlorinated biphenyls (PCBs), which were used widely in electrical equipment and were linked with suppression of the immune system, were banned for use in the United States in 1979. Most recently, studies have shown that childhood exposure to perfluorinated compounds, which are used in food packaging and industrial manufacturing, attenuates the effectiveness of several vaccines. Thus many toxicants have immunosuppressive actions and may lead to an increased incidence of bacterial, viral, and parasitic infections.

Carcinogenicity

The development of cancer is a two-stage process involving both the initiation and proliferation of abnormal cells that have a defect in the control mechanisms that govern growth. Some human cancers are believed to be of environmental origin, caused by radiation, viral infection, or chemical exposure. Because cancer may take 20 or more years to develop, cause and effect relationships are difficult to establish. However, many compounds in the environment have been linked to carcinogenicity, including tobacco smoke, heavy metals, gases, and solvents. Cigarette smoke contains many potent cancer-causing chemicals and is a causative factor of lung cancer, while vinyl chloride, benzene, and α-naphthylamine are believed to cause cancer after chronic occupational exposure. Some chemicals interact directly and covalently with DNA, whereas others must be metabolically activated. If cell division occurs before enzymatic repair of the damaged DNA, a permanent mutation is encoded in the genome. Because cellular damage undoubtedly kills some cells in the target tissue, the stimulus for division of adjacent cells is high. The result is a new cell type with altered genotypic and phenotypic properties. Additional mutational events can convert transformed cells to malignant cells.

Developmental Toxicity

Exposure of women or men to some toxins and toxicants can lead to germ cell mutations, which are transmissible, leading to alterations in the fertilized egg, often causing developmental abnormalities in embryos. In addition, if pregnant women are exposed to some toxic agents that cross the placenta, direct teratogenic effects can be produced. Formaldehyde and many other solvents have both embryotoxic and teratogenic effects. One of the most well-known teratogens is thalidomide, which was prescribed for morning sickness during pregnancy in the 1960s and led to thousands of babies born with limb malformations. Unfortunately, the consequences of germ cell mutations are not manifest in the exposed individual and thus are not readily apparent.

Genetic Effects

Genotoxic agents can alter DNA by several mechanisms, including the promotion of chromosomal breakage, modification of the DNA sequence, and changing the number of chromosomes in a cell. The polycyclic aromatic hydrocarbons bind directly to DNA, leading to carcinogenic mutations, while alkylating agents, such as ethylnitrosourea, promote methylation/ethylation of bases, resulting in base mispairings, and sodium azide produces chromosomal breaks. The consequence of these alterations may not be manifest for years, but many of them have been linked to carcinogenesis.

Epigenetic Effects

Knowledge of epigenetic alterations induced by toxicants is an area of research still in its infancy. How toxic agents lead to heritable changes in gene expression without changing DNA sequences represents a very active area of research, with a focus on the effects of toxicants on DNA methylation, histone modifications (acetylation, phosphorylation, and methylation), and the expression of noncoding RNAs (microRNA). BPA has been studied extensively and has been shown to affect both DNA and histone methylation, as well as microRNA expression. Similarly, many heavy metals and pesticides have been shown to alter DNA methylation and histone acetylation. Undoubtedly many, if not all, of these epigenetic changes will be linked to disease etiology.

Organ-Specific Toxicity

It is impossible to present a comprehensive list of agents that adversely affect all organ systems. It is also impossible to enumerate every aspect of each system that is subject to injury. Thus illustrative examples are used for each system.

Hepatotoxicity

The blood supply from the hepatic artery and portal vein expose the liver to toxicants entering from the systemic (e.g., via inhalation) or from the splanchnic (absorbed from the gastrointestinal tract) circulation, respectively. In addition, cytochrome P450s in the liver can activate or inactivate chemicals, thus exposing the liver to high concentrations of toxicants and/or their toxic metabolites. As an example, chloroform is bioactivated by CYP2E1 to phosgene, which is highly toxic and causes hepatonecrosis. Other hepatotoxic agents that are biotransformed to active metabolites include carbon tetrachloride, halogenated benzenes, and several carcinogens (aflatoxin B_1, aromatic amines). All of these agents can produce steatosis, hepatitis, intrahepatic cholestasis, hepatic cancer, or cirrhosis, depending on dose and duration of exposure.

The widespread occurrence of metals in the environment and their numerous industrial and medical uses make them important potential toxicants. Many metals affect specific organs because they have physical similarity to nutritionally essential metals, which are transported by specific proteins expressed by specific organs in the body and function as essential enzyme cofactors. Substitution by a similar but toxic metal may produce enzymatic dysfunction in these organs. The liver represents one such commonly injured organ, along with the kidneys and gastrointestinal tract mucosa. The heavy metal lead is transported by the transport protein for iron and leads to hepatic glycogen depletion, lymphocytic infiltration, and periportal fibrosis that may progress to cirrhosis.

Nephrotoxicity

The kidney is susceptible to injury due to its inherent function and the fact that it receives 25% of cardiac output. The major functions of the kidney are filtration, the regulation of water and electrolyte balance, and the elimination of toxicants. As water is reabsorbed, the concentration of chemicals in the tubule can increase to toxic levels. In some situations, the concentration may exceed the solubility of a chemical and lead to precipitation and obstruction of the affected area. The glomerulus and proximal tubules are highly susceptible to the action of toxicants, while the collecting duct is relatively resistant to injury. The proximal tubules express several cytochrome P450 enzymes, which may explain why this region is so susceptible to chemical injury. For example, carbon tetrachloride and chloroform, two halogenated hydrocarbons that injure the proximal tubule, are biotransformed by cytochrome P450s to highly toxic metabolites. In addition, the proximal tubules are affected by many heavy metals, which may concentrate in proximal tubular epithelial cells or injure vascular endothelial cells, causing renal damage. The kidney can compensate for excessive chemical exposure because it has a reserve mass. Thus tissue injury equal to one entire kidney must occur before loss of function is clinically apparent. The kidney also replaces lost functional capacity by hypertrophy. However, when these mechanisms are insufficient to compensate, toxicant-induced damage will ensue.

Pulmonary Toxicity

Toxic chemicals may affect any part of the pulmonary system, including the nasopharyngeal and tracheobronchial airways and the pulmonary parenchyma (alveoli). Injury results primarily from exposure to agents by inhalation or through circulatory delivery. Gases such as chlorine react with water vapor to produce hydrochloric acid, damaging upper airway mucosal cells, which are also damaged by ammonia and other water-soluble gases. In addition, several gases, including phosgene, xylene, cyanide, chloroform, and other solvents, are well absorbed from the alveoli and can lead to pulmonary edema and acute respiratory distress syndrome.

Particulates, including asbestos, coal dust, and silica, can become trapped in the airway alveoli and can lead to interstitial inflammation, progressing to fibrosis if they are not cleared by the mucociliary apparatus. Although most toxicants gain entry to the pulmonary system through inhalation, some, like the herbicide paraquat, gain access through the circulation. Upon reaching the lungs, paraquat is bioactivated by type II pneumocytes, resulting in pulmonary fibrosis.

Cardiotoxicity

The cardiac system may be affected by toxic substances acting directly on the heart muscle, valves, conduction system, or vasculature, or indirectly by altering the sensitivity of the parasympathetic or sympathetic nervous systems to acetylcholine or norepinephrine, respectively. Alterations at any of these levels can lead to cardiomyopathies, valvular pathologies, arrhythmias, blood pressure abnormalities, vascular disease, or myocardial necrosis. The high energy demands of the heart render it especially susceptible to agents that interfere with oxygen availability, carbohydrate metabolism, or oxidative phosphorylation.

Carbon monoxide (CO) is the leading cause of death by poisoning. CO has more than 200 times higher affinity for hemoglobin than oxygen and shifts the oxyhemoglobin dissociation curve to the left, reducing oxygen release and causing enhanced anaerobic metabolism. Decreased oxygen delivery can lead to severe myocardial ischemia followed by cell death. In addition to CO, other agents that interfere with oxidative phosphorylation include the dinitrophenols, rotenone, and cyanide, all of which decrease the number of functional myocytes.

In addition to effects on cardiac myocytes, toxicants can alter the electrical conduction system of the heart, leading to arrhythmias, including QT interval prolongation. This occurs with arsenic, toxins such as tetrodotoxin and saxitoxin, and solvents such as ethylene glycol, which produces acidosis and hyperkalemia, increasing automaticity. Chloroform and other halogenated hydrocarbons suppress automaticity of the SA node, altering impulse formation. Similarly, Freon sensitizes the myocardium to the effects of the catecholamines, while several pesticides and the nerve gases enhance parasympathetic activity by increasing acetylcholine.

The vasculature is also subject to insult by toxicants. Carbon disulfide (CS_2) is well known to lead to atherosclerosis, even at low concentrations. It may also decrease fibrinolysis and enhance thrombosis.

Lead continues to pose a significant health problem. Industrialization, mining, and leaded gasoline increased environmental lead levels. Indeed, in 2014, levels of lead in the drinking water in Flint, Michigan, were in the toxic range. Lead has prominent effects on the cardiovascular and renal systems. Its accumulation leads to cardiotoxicity manifest by hypertension and altered conduction, precipitating arrhythmias. In addition, lead binds to sulfhydryl groups and inhibits enzymes in the heme biosynthetic pathway, resulting in anemia.

Neurotoxicity

The nervous system is highly susceptible to injury. Toxic substances may affect both the peripheral and central nervous systems at many different levels, all of which impact function. At the most fundamental level, chemicals can affect specific types of cells, such as neurons or glia (astrocytes, microglia, and oligodendrocytes), can alter metabolic processes within these cell types, or can alter communication among cells and circuits. It is often difficult to ascertain whether a toxin or toxicant targets a particular cell type in a specific brain region because an alteration in a single cell type or location typically leads to changes in other cell types and locations.

The vulnerability of the nervous system to insult by environmental toxicants and the relationship between these insults and neurodegenerative diseases such as Parkinson disease, Alzheimer disease, multiple sclerosis, and amyotrophic lateral sclerosis have been suspected for many years. The most compelling evidence is that for Parkinson disease (Chapter 15). Indeed, toxicants such as CO and manganese have been known for many years to lead to parkinsonism, a disorder with symptomatology identical to that of Parkinson disease but with an identifiable etiology. The idea that environmental agents contribute to the development of Parkinson disease began with findings of an association between the incidence of Parkinson disease and the use of paraquat, one of the most commonly used herbicides worldwide. This idea was strengthened by evidence that the neurotoxin 1-methyl-4-phenyl-1,2,3,6-tetrahydropyridine (MPTP) led to pathological alterations in the brain identical to those seen in Parkinson disease. Currently, it is thought that environmental factors such as pesticides, herbicides, and fungicides, as well as industrial solvents and some metals including iron and manganese, may play a significant role in the etiology of sporadic Parkinson disease, likely through actions at the mitochondrial level, leading to oxidative stress and the generation of reactive oxygen species, ultimately resulting in death of nigrostriatal dopaminergic neurons.

In addition to the links between environmental toxins and neuro-degenerative disease, studies have shown that many agents have direct effects on neurons or glia. Agents that interfere with oxidative metabolism, such as cyanide or dinitrophenol, impair neuronal viability, while acrylamide, which can form from sugars during cooking, interferes with axonal transport, depriving nerve terminals of compounds necessary for survival. Nerve terminals themselves are the target of several neurotoxins, such as botulinum toxin and tetrodotoxin.

Lead is particularly toxic to the nervous system, especially in children. Symptoms include anorexia, colicky abdominal pain, and vomiting. If lead exposure continues, children are more likely than adults to develop encephalopathy, manifested by irritability progressing to seizures and coma. Blood lead levels of 10 μg/dL in children are associated with depressed IQ scores and learning disorders.

TOXICANT INTERACTIONS

There are many opportunities for individuals to be exposed multiple times to chemicals in the environment and through their work, and often these exposures are to complex mixtures of undefined chemicals, such as cigarette smoke and hazardous waste. Benzene in petroleum mixtures is a human carcinogen found in air and water. Agricultural chemicals, industrial waste, and incineration by-products also contribute pollutants such as pesticides, polychlorinated biphenyls, dioxins, and polyaromatic hydrocarbons. In addition, there are naturally occurring toxic compounds, including arsenic (in drinking water), methylmercury (in fish), and aflatoxin B_1 (produced by a fungus that grows on corn and peanuts).

In 1984, an explosion in a pesticide factory in Bhopal, India, led to more than 2000 deaths and 10,000 injuries. High concentrations of methylisocyanate, a chemically reactive gas, were released and caused pulmonary damage and death. Continual exposure over long periods of time can also result in accumulation of chemicals to toxic levels, contributing to chronic diseases such as cancer, heart disease, and neurodegenerative disorders. Well-documented examples include rare hepatic angiosarcomas in factory workers exposed to vinyl chloride and asbestos, causing mesothelioma.

Exposure of an individual to multiple compounds can result in toxicant interactions at both the pharmacodynamic and pharmacokinetic levels. Interactions may manifest as additive, synergistic, or antagonistic, depending on the specific agents involved, and can occur between chemicals, between chemicals and receptors, or sequentially in which one compound modifies responses to a second compound. It is critical to understand how exposure to one or more chemicals affects the toxic potential of another chemical.

EMERGING ISSUES

Numerous industrial chemicals are present in our environment, and over 3600 pesticides are available for use throughout the world, with more being synthesized as resistance of susceptible organisms increases. Unfortunately, the health effects of many compounds in our environment are not readily apparent, as it can take generations for a pattern of toxicological effects to become manifest. Long-term monitoring by agencies such as the World Health Organization, the United States Environmental Protection Agency, and the United States Geological Survey is essential. Strategies for the prevention of toxic effects require knowledge of the threshold dose above which chemical toxicity will likely occur. Differences among individuals (age, health status, genetics) also make selection of a single threshold value challenging. Epidemiology studies in exposed and control human populations can yield useful information, but such studies are scarce. Monitoring and "risk assessment" are critical to ensure that public health will be maintained with a high margin of safety.

CLINICAL RELEVANCE FOR HEALTHCARE PROFESSIONALS

It is essential for all healthcare professionals to be aware of basic toxicology principles and the effects of environmental compounds on organ systems. In situations where the cause for an organ system change is not readily apparent, healthcare professionals should question their patients to determine sources of possible toxicity, such as through occupation or travel. Knowledge of this information is critical for an accurate diagnosis and treatment and possible prevention of future occurrences.

SELF-ASSESSMENT QUESTIONS

1. A 56-year-old man who worked in the coal mines for many years was recently diagnosed with pulmonary fibrosis. This is an example of:
   A. Acute toxicity.
   B. Chronic toxicity.
   C. Epigenetic alterations.
   D. Genetic alterations.
   E. Immunotoxicity.

2. Bisphenol A (BPA) exposure can affect both DNA methylation and histone modification. These changes are known as:
   A. Genetic alterations.
   B. Developmental alterations.
   C. Epigenetic alterations.
   D. Cell-specific alterations.
   E. Nonheritable alterations.

3. The leading cause of death by poisoning is due to exposure to:
   A. Benzene.
   B. Chloroform.
   C. Paraquat.
   D. Bisphenol A (BPA).
   E. Carbon monoxide.

4. Which of the following correctly pairs a toxin with an associated abnormality or disease?
   A. Tobacco smoke—cancer.
   B. Formaldehyde—teratogenesis.
   C. Chloroform—hepatic cirrhosis.
   D. Cadmium—nephrotoxicity.
   E. All of the above.

5. The strongest evidence for an association between environmental toxicants and a neurodegenerative disorder exists for which disorder?
   A. Multiple sclerosis.
   B. Alzheimer disease.
   C. Parkinson disease.
   D. Amyotrophic lateral sclerosis.
   E. Myasthenia gravis.

FURTHER READING

Cannon JR, Greenamyre JT. The role of environmental exposures in neurodegeneration and neurodegenerative diseases. *Toxicol Sci.* 2011;124(2):225–250.

Hou L, Zhang X, Wang D, Baccarelli A. Environmental chemical exposures and human epigenetics. *Int J Epidemiol.* 2012;41:79–105.

Younglai EV, Wu YJ, Foster WG. Reproductive toxicology of environmental toxicants: emerging issues and concerns. *Curr Pharm Des.* 2007;13:3005–3019.

WEBSITES

https://www.atsdr.cdc.gov
This website is maintained by the Agency for Toxic Substances and Disease Registry, United States Department of Health and Human Services, and includes the most up-to-date information on hazardous substances.

https://chemm.nlm.nih.gov
This is the Chemical Hazards Emergency Medical Management Site from the United States Department of Health and Human Services and provides information for first responders and other healthcare providers responding to chemical casualties.

https://toxtutor.nlm.nih.gov/
This is a tutorial on key principles of toxicology, maintained by the United States National Library of Medicine.

Therapeutic Considerations for Pregnant, Pediatric, Geriatric, and Obese Individuals

Margaret Nelson and LaToya M. Griffin

THERAPEUTIC OVERVIEW

Pregnant, pediatric, geriatric, and obese individuals represent populations with unique physiological and biochemical characteristics that must be taken into account when considering drug actions. Both pharmacodynamic and pharmacokinetic parameters may be altered, resulting in either decreased or increased drug action, the latter often associated with adverse effects. Physiological alterations associated with pregnant, young, aged, and obese individuals include alterations in total body water, fat, and protein, as well as changes in metabolism and renal function, and are summarized in the Therapeutic Overview Box.

THERAPEUTIC OVERVIEW

Population	Physiological Alterations
Pregnancy	Increased total body water and fat, decreased plasma protein levels, increased renal drug excretion
Neonates and infants	Increased total body water, decreased body fat and plasma protein levels, increased hepatic metabolic capacity, decreased renal drug excretion
Geriatric	Decreased total body water and plasma protein levels, increased body fat, decreased hepatic metabolic capacity and renal drug excretion
Obese	Increased total body water and fat, decreased plasma protein levels, hepatic metabolic capacity and renal drug excretion

RELATIONSHIP OF POPULATION CHARACTERISTICS TO DRUG RESPONSES

The Pregnant Population

Roughly 70% of pregnant women in the United States use at least one or more pharmaceutical agent during pregnancy, and the emergence of serious pregnancy-induced medical conditions like preeclampsia and gestational diabetes often requires pharmacological management. Developing appropriate and safe drug therapy regimens for pregnant women is an exceptionally arduous task due largely in part to the dynamics between the mother and fetus. For example, differences in the acid-base equilibrium between the mother and growing fetus play a role in the extent of fetal exposure to substances consumed by the mother. Further, whereas the primary role of the placenta is to transfer oxygen and nutrients from mother to child, it also serves as a barrier

ABBREVIATIONS

CYP	Cytochrome P450
GFR	Glomerular filtration rate
NSAID	Nonsteroidal antiinflammatory drug
Vd	Volume of distribution

to protect the fetus from potentially harmful xenobiotics to which the mother may be exposed and that do not enter the fetal circulation through passive diffusion.

Pharmacokinetics

Drug absorption may change significantly during pregnancy. The physical transformation that occurs leads to respiratory changes caused by uterine enlargement, which displaces the diaphragm and increases abdominal and rib cage dimensions. Hyperventilation is commonly associated with pregnancy. Additionally, airway smooth muscle tone is altered by increased levels of hormones such as progesterone and prostaglandins E_1 and E_2, leading to bronchodilation, and potentially altering the absorption of inhaled drugs. In addition, intestinal motility and gastric acid secretion are reduced during pregnancy, increasing gastric emptying time and increasing gastric pH, both of which influence the extent to which weak acids and bases undergo ionization and subsequent absorption.

Because total body water increases by 50% during pregnancy, the increased fluid volume may alter the volume of distribution (Vd) of drugs. The increased plasma volume leads to hypoalbuminemia, which can decrease protein-bound drugs and yield greater drug distribution, particularly for hydrophilic drugs. Maternal fat is also increased in pregnancy and may be important for lipophilic agents.

The differential expression and activity of several cytochrome P450 (CYP) enzymes also occur during pregnancy. The activity of CYP2A6, CYP2D6, CYP2C9, and CYP3A4 increase, whereas that for CYP1A2 and CYP2C19 decrease. Thus the metabolism of the anticonvulsant phenytoin, which is a substrate for CYP2C9, and the antihypertensive metoprolol, which is a substrate for CYP2D6, is increased, whereas that for the bronchodilator theophylline, which is a CYP1A2 substrate, is decreased during pregnancy. In addition to alterations in these enzymes, the activity of uridine diphosphate glucuronosyltransferase (UGT) is also altered, with an increase in UGT1A4, leading to an increased clearance of the anticonvulsant lamotrigine during the second and third trimesters.

An increased cardiac output during pregnancy leads to increased organ perfusion, most importantly to the kidneys. Renal blood flow and glomerular filtration rate (GFR) are increased by 50% during pregnancy. Elevated GFR leads to decreased serum creatinine levels and may increase the clearance of drugs that undergo extensive renal elimination, including the psychoactive agent lithium and the cardioactive agents digoxin and atenolol. Although many factors must be considered, increased renal clearance of many drugs during pregnancy is one of the most common and clinically relevant pharmacokinetic changes observed in pregnancy.

Pharmacovigilance: Adverse Effects and Drug Interactions

The most serious concerns during pregnancy are teratogenic consequences and obstetric complications, whereas issues following delivery and during nursing focus on neonatal health and development. Several classes of drugs have a potential impact during these critical periods. For example, if a pregnant patient requires a drug to alleviate pain, the nonsteroidal antiinflammatory drugs (NSAIDs) should not be used early in pregnancy because they increase the risks of miscarriage and malformations. They should also not be used in the third trimester because of an increased risk of premature closure of the fetal ductus arteriosus and oligohydramnios. Fetal and neonatal adverse effects on the brain, kidney, lung, skeleton, gastrointestinal tract, and cardiovascular system have also been reported after prenatal exposure to NSAIDs. Therefore acetaminophen is considered a more appropriate analgesic during pregnancy. NSAIDs should be given during pregnancy only if the maternal benefits outweigh the potential fetal risks, and if they are used, they should be taken at the lowest effective dose and for the shortest duration possible.

Teratogenic effects may result from a primary maternal action that secondarily influences fetal development and may be attributed to altered passage of oxygen and/or nutrients through the placenta, direct actions on differentiation during tissue development, or deficiency of critical nutrients required for development. Several drugs and drug classes are considered teratogenic in humans including but not limited to cytotoxic antineoplastic agents, ethanol, vitamin A derivatives, antipsychotics, antidepressants, and anticonvulsants.

The milk expressed during nursing is comprised predominantly of water, and many drugs can be excreted into breast milk via active transport or, most commonly, passive diffusion. Fetal plasma drug levels correspond with maternal plasma drug concentrations, and thus the milk-to-plasma ratio (M:P) serves as an indicator of the extent of drug secretion into milk. Alcohol is an example of an agent in which M:P approaches 1.0 and should be avoided or limited in the nursing mother. Overall, the benefit of drug therapy versus risk posed to the fetus or nursing infant must be weighed when determining the most appropriate treatment for the pregnant or nursing mother. The underdeveloped metabolic capacity of the infant liver renders neonates and infants especially susceptible to the adverse effects of drugs.

The Pediatric Population

The pediatric population extends from birth until 18 years of age and includes the following groups: preterm (<37 gestational weeks); neonate (birth to 1 month); infant (1 month to 2 years); child (2–12 years); and adolescent (12–18 years). These subpopulations are based upon physiological, biochemical, and compositional differences that accompany pediatric development. Upon birth and throughout the first years of life, changes in body water, fat distribution, and muscle development influence several pharmacokinetic parameters.

Pharmacokinetics

For neonates and infants, drug administration typically involves intramuscular or subcutaneous injections, with absorption primarily affected by blood flow and muscle mass. Within the first days after birth, delayed absorption at the site of injection may be observed due to decreased skeletal muscle blood flow. However, water soluble compounds disperse more readily in neonates due to increased skeletal muscle hydration; neonates and infants have increased epidermal hydration and subcutaneous perfusion relative to adults.

The absorption of orally administered drugs is dictated by changes in gastric acidity during development. In the newborn, gastric pH is neutral and becomes more acidic throughout the infantile period. Normal adult gastric pH values (1.5–3.5) are achieved at approximately 2 years of age. Gastric motility and peristalsis are also delayed during the neonatal and infant phases, which can delay absorption from the gastrointestinal system and increase the time required to reach therapeutic plasma levels.

Neonates and infants often exhibit esophageal reflux, which compromises the efficacy of orally administered drugs; hence, rectal suppositories are often used with drug absorption via the rectal veins. Variability can arise because the depth of suppository insertion determines which veins are exposed to the drug. Drugs exposed to the superior veins undergo first-pass metabolism via the liver whereas drugs absorbed by the inferior and middle rectal veins enter systemic circulation directly.

Drug transport into and out of the brain is compromised in the neonate. Both P-glycoprotein, which transports drugs out of the brain, and the blood-brain barrier, which limits drug entry into the brain, are underdeveloped at this stage, leading to higher drug levels in the central nervous system. This is especially important for mothers who abuse drugs, as compounds such as the opioids or cocaine can readily enter the brain and produce adverse effects.

Throughout child development, body composition changes. During the newborn stage, the body is composed of approximately 80% water, whereas by the end of the first year, it is only 60% water. Thus during the neonatal period, water soluble drugs distribute freely throughout cellular compartments and exhibit a greater Vd. The aminoglycosides, including gentamicin, have an increased Vd in neonates and require a larger dose to reach therapeutic levels. Also, serum albumin and α-1-acid glycoprotein are reduced, resulting in increased plasma levels of unbound drugs, which can contribute to greater efficacy or potential toxicity. By 1 year of age, the capacity of protein binding in pediatric patients is similar to that of adults.

Drug-metabolizing capacity in neonates and infants is reduced due to hepatic immaturity. CYP2E1 and CYP2D6 expression and activity are apparent shortly after birth, whereas CYP3A4, CYP2C9, and CYP2C19 are expressed within the first week of life. CYP1A2 is one of the last enzymes to develop, appearing 1–3 months after birth. Less is known about phase II conjugation enzymes, although their activity does not appear to change significantly during infant development.

Rates and efficiency of drug elimination in neonates are related primarily to kidney maturation. GFR, active tubular secretion, and tubular reabsorption are dictated by renal blood flow and are underdeveloped in newborns. The kidneys develop within the first year, and their associated functional processes reach adult values by 2 years of age. Thus drugs that are excreted primarily via the kidneys require dose reductions to prevent adverse effects.

Pharmacovigilance: Adverse Effects and Drug Interactions

In pediatric patients, body surface area, body composition, and organ development all influence dosing, efficacy, and drug-related toxicities. Most adverse effects can be related to pharmacokinetic parameters.

The Geriatric Population

Over the past century, the average human lifespan has extended well into the late 70s, and in some regions of the world, the average life expectancy is in the 80s. Since humans are living longer and potentially healthier lives, defining the geriatric patient population has become more difficult. Geriatric is usually considered 65 years of age and older and is associated with the development of cardiovascular disease, cancers, and neurodegenerative disorders. A combination of factors can influence the response of older adults to drugs, including alterations in pharmacokinetics, changes in body composition and organ function, increased drug sensitivity, disease, and polypharmacy.

A major pharmacodynamic change observed in aging is a decrease in receptor expression. The down regulation of β-adrenergic receptors in older persons leads to a decrease in responsiveness and sensitivity to β-receptor agonists and antagonists. In contrast, older patients exhibit a greater sensitivity to the sedative effects of certain benzodiazepines including midazolam and flunitrazepam and require smaller doses to achieve therapeutic effects. Several homeostatic mechanisms are also compromised with aging, including a decrease in baroreceptor sensitivity, which can often lead to orthostatic hypotension, particularly in individuals taking antihypertensive medications.

Pharmacokinetics

Compared to young adults, elderly persons have a decrease in total body water and lean muscle mass and an increase in body fat. For water soluble drugs like digoxin, this may result in a decreased Vd and an increased plasma concentration. Thus a reduction in the loading dose of water soluble drugs is encouraged in older patients. In contrast, an increase in body fat increases the Vd and deposition of lipid soluble drugs, leading to a prolonged half-life. Without a concurrent increase in elimination, adverse effects are likely. For example, diazepam is very lipid soluble and has the ability to remain in adipose tissue for an extended period of time. As a result, plasma drug levels should be monitored closely in elderly patients. Since aging predisposes patients to alterations in Vd, careful consideration in dosing is required to minimize adverse effects.

Aged individuals exhibit a decrease in gastric acid secretion and motility that can decrease the rate of drug absorption. Commonly used over-the-counter drugs such as laxatives and antacids can further delay rates of absorption.

Aging is also accompanied by decreased hepatic function and the reduced production of serum albumin, the latter decreasing protein binding and increasing unbound or "free" drug. Warfarin, phenytoin, and tolbutamide exhibit decreased protein binding in the elderly, increasing the risks of adverse or toxic effects. A decrease in liver mass, hepatic blood flow, and activity of hepatic enzymes alter the hepatic metabolism of drugs. Enzymes involved in phase I reactions are reduced in the aged individual, although aging does not appear to alter enzymes involved in phase II metabolism. Thus the metabolism of drugs that utilize phase I enzymes, such as propranolol, verapamil, and opioids, may be delayed in the older patient. In addition, polypharmacy in older patients can potentiate alterations of hepatic metabolism via inhibition or activation of phase I enzymes.

The kidneys are the primary source of drug clearance in the adult body. Thus age-related declines in GFR, active tubular reabsorption, and renal blood flow diminish drug clearance. Furthermore, diseases associated with aging including hypertension and heart failure, which exacerbate renal function, also affect drug clearance. Because an important cause of adverse drug reactions in older adults is drug accumulation, monitoring renal function is paramount to preventing drug toxicities.

Pharmacovigilance: Adverse Effects and Drug Interactions

Polypharmacy is the leading cause of adverse drug reactions and a subsequent cause of hospitalizations and even death in older persons. The trend in the number of medications per individual increases with age, and as such, an increase in the risk for drug-drug interactions is likely. Some patients do not include over-the-counter supplements or herbal therapeutics when listing their current drug regimen as these drugs are not prescribed. However, adverse reactions can manifest from the concomitant use of such agents with prescribed medications. The American Geriatrics Society has set forth Beers Criteria, listing medications that should be avoided in older persons including drug-drug interactions. Some commonly used medications that should be avoided by the elderly are listed in the Clinical Problems Box.

Drug noncompliance is a unique phenomenon observed within the geriatric patient population and is an important factor in successful geriatric therapeutic treatment. A major explanation for noncompliance is the development of overly complicated drug dosing schedules that require patients to take multiple medications at various times throughout the day. In addition, undesirable drug side effects often discourage patients from adhering to their drug therapy regimen. Additional reasons for noncompliance include limited access to pharmacies or medical facilities, forgetfulness, difficulty opening medication bottles, and financial hardship.

The Obese Population

Obesity is a global healthcare issue and presents immense challenges. Obesity in adults aged 20 and older is characterized by a body mass index (BMI) of 30 kg/m^2 or greater. More than one-third of persons in the United States are considered obese. Physiological changes associated with obesity undoubtedly alter drug disposition, leading to significant changes in both drug efficacy and safety. The prevalence of this condition makes dosing adjustments in the obese patient an important issue. The development of appropriate therapeutic dosing schemes for drugs with a narrow therapeutic index in obese patients presents an especially serious concern.

Pharmacokinetics

Obesity is associated with increased gastric emptying, which may cause enhanced absorption of orally administered medications. Additionally, the excessive fat present in obese patients may lead to a number of administration route-specific absorption issues. For example, poor subcutaneous perfusion may also lead to reduced absorption of subcutaneously administered drugs. Generally, obesity is also associated with difficulty administering drugs by either intravenous or intramuscular routes, both resulting in delayed drug presentation to systemic circulation.

Vd is arguably the most important parameter influenced by the physical changes associated with obesity. The mass of body fat (i.e., adipose tissue) per kilogram of body weight is significantly greater in the obese individual. As a result, the Vd of lipophilic drugs is often different in obese persons compared to non-obese persons. Obese individuals also exhibit decreased cardiac output, tissue perfusion, and serum protein levels.

CYP3A4 activity decreases in obesity, leading to the reduced metabolism of erythromycin, cyclosporin, and midazolam. In contrast, CYP2E1 is up regulated in obese patients with nonalcoholic fatty liver disease. This is an important change because CYP2E1 mediates the conversion of acetaminophen to its toxic metabolite N-acetyl-p-benzoquinone imine, thereby increasing the risk of acetaminophen-related hepatotoxicity.

Because of the strong correlation between obesity and nonalcoholic fatty liver disease, hepatic blood flow may be compromised, affecting drug clearance. Reduced clearance has been demonstrated in obese individuals for many commonly used agents including docetaxel, carbamazepine, and midazolam.

Pharmacovigilance: Adverse Effects and Drug Interactions

The ability of lipophilic drugs to become sequestered or stored in fat can result in misleadingly low plasma drug levels, thereby increasing the risk of incorrectly prescribed dosing frequencies, which increases

CLINICAL PROBLEMS

Drug Class (example)	Possible Toxic Manifestations
Tricyclic antidepressants (imipramine)	Cognitive impairment, dry mouth, sedation, orthostatic hypotension
Antihypertensive (prazosin)	Orthostatic hypotension, urinary incontinence
Antihypertensive (clonidine)	Orthostatic hypotension, bradycardia
Antiarrhythmic (amiodarone)	QT prolongation, pulmonary toxicity
Acetylcholinesterase inhibitors (donepezil)	Orthostatic hypotension, bradycardia
Benzodiazepines (diazepam)	Cognitive impairment, delirium, unsteady gait
Sleep medications (eszopiclone, zaleplon, and zolpidem)	Cognitive impairment, delirium, unsteady gait
Aspirin and NSAIDs	Gastrointestinal bleeding, peptic ulcers

NSAIDs, Nonsteroidal antiinflammatory drugs.

the risk of drug-related adverse effects. Currently, obesity-related changes in the distribution of drugs appear to be drug specific and the physicochemical properties of each unique agent must be considered.

Conceivably, decreased liver function due to a reduction in hepatic blood flow may influence the rate and extent of hepatic drug metabolism in obesity. However, observed changes in drug metabolism are highly variable both within and between obese patients. This variability most likely is also attributable to other pathophysiological factors associated with obesity, such as chronic inflammation and diabetes.

New Developments

In 2015, the United States Food and Drug Administration issued standards for drug labeling regarding the use of agents during pregnancy and breastfeeding to provide clinicians with clearer prescribing guidelines for providing care.

Clinical Relevance for Healthcare Professionals

All healthcare professionals may interact with pregnant, pediatric, geriatric, or obese patients and should be aware of basic physiological and biochemical/metabolic alterations present in each of these populations. Awareness of patient medications, both proprietary and over-the-counter, and the actions and adverse effects of these compounds, is important to provide the best and safest care possible.

Pharmacotherapy for all patients presents challenges for healthcare providers. Patients who are members of these special populations present additional challenges that can seem almost insurmountable at times. Clinicians can help minimize noncompliance by consistent patient counseling. It is also critical to educate patients about side effects. An up-to-date health history and periodic reevaluations of current medications (including over-the-counter agents) are necessary to maintain drug compliance in any population.

SELF-ASSESSMENT QUESTIONS

1. Which of the following physiological changes in elderly patients accounts for a small volume of distribution and an increase in the plasma concentration of digoxin?
   A. Increased total body water
   B. Increased activity of hepatic enzymes that facilitate drug metabolism
   C. Decreased total body water
   D. Decreased total body fat
   E. Decreased rate of elimination due to decreased renal function

2. A 32-year-old woman with a history of focal seizures controlled with phenytoin recently became pregnant. Her physician needs to be aware of the fact that:
   A. Her body fat distribution will change.
   B. Her total body water will increase.
   C. Her glomerulation filtration rate will decrease.
   D. Her CYP2C9 will increase.
   E. Her clearance of phenytoin may decrease.

3. The neonatal brain may accumulate toxic levels of drugs because:
   A. Cytochrome P450 enzymes are nonfunctional.
   B. The blood-brain barrier is not fully developed.
   C. The P-glycoprotein transporter is overdeveloped.
   D. Subcutaneous perfusion is nonfunctional.
   E. Gastric motility and peristalsis are delayed.

4. A 72-year-old man was taking a β-adrenergic receptor antagonist to control his hypertension for several years, but it has lost efficacy. A possible reason for this is that:
   A. The sensitivity of these receptors to drug decreases with age.
   B. Gastric acid secretion decreases absorption of the drug.
   C. Increased body fat increases the volume of distribution of the drug.
   D. Increased serum albumin leads to more drug sequestered in the circulation.
   E. Enhanced glomerular filtration clears the drug faster.

5. The most important pharmacokinetic parameter that is altered in the obese individual is:
   A. Clearance.
   B. Metabolism.
   C. Absorption.
   D. Excretion.
   E. Volume of distribution.

FURTHER READING

American Geriatrics Society 2015 Beers Criteria Update Expert Panel. American Geriatrics Society 2015 Updated Beers Criteria for Potentially Inappropriate Medication Use in Older Adults. *J Am Geriatr Soc.* 2015;63(11):2227–2246.

Apovian CM, Aronne LJ, Bessesen DH, et al. Pharmacological management of obesity: an Endocrine Society clinical practice guideline. *J Clin Endocrinol Metab.* 2015;100(2):342–362.

Feghali MN, Mattison DR. Clinical therapeutics in pregnancy. *J Biomed Biotechnol.* 2011;783528. doi:10.1155/2011/783528.

Isoherranen N, Thummel KE. Drug metabolism and transport during pregnancy: how does drug disposition change during pregnancy and what are the mechanisms that cause such changes? *Drug Metab Dispos.* 2013;41(2):256–262.

Ku LC, Smith PB. Dosing in neonates: special considerations in physiology and trial design. *Pediatr Res.* 2015;77(1–1):2–9.

Mangoni AA, Jackson SHD. Age-related changes in pharmacokinetics and pharmacodynamics: basic principles and practical applications. *Br J Pharmacol.* 2003;57(1):6–14.

Wood AJJ, et al. Developmental pharmacology—drug disposition, action, and therapy in infants and children. *N Engl J Med.* 2003;349(12):1157–1167.

WEBSITES

https://www.fda.gov/drugs/developmentapprovalprocess/developmentresources/labeling/ucm093307.htm
This website is maintained by the United States Food and Drug Administration and contains links to many guidelines and sites addressing issues arising during pregnancy and lactation.

http://www.americangeriatrics.org/publications-tools
This website is maintained by the American Geriatrics Society and provides a wealth of information on issues facing the elderly and the healthcare professionals treating them.

https://obesitymedicine.org/
This website is maintained by the Obesity Medicine Association and provides information and links concerning obesity medicine and management.

Appendix

ANSWERS TO SELF-ASSESSMENT QUESTIONS

Chapter 1

No questions

Chapter 2

1. **B.** Binding usually involves multiple weak bonds. It is rarely covalent, is usually stereoselective, and may or may not occur with a high affinity (K_D).
2. **A.** Chronic antagonist exposure will often increase receptor sensitivity. The other answers all refer to decreased receptor sensitivity.
3. **C.** Agonist drugs are specific for various classes of receptors but may not be specific for each receptor subtype within a class.
4. **E.** Intracellular signaling can occur through any of the mechanisms listed.
5. **B.** Based on the information given, one can conclude only that the potencies are different. No conclusions can be made about structure, types of receptors involved, whether they are directly acting agonists, or whether they cause the same extent of relaxation.
6. **D.** The affinity constant describes how well a drug binds to a particular receptor and thus depends on both the drug and the binding site. It is the ratio of the reverse to forward rate constants. The rate of diffusion of drug in the plasma is unrelated to affinity constant.

Chapter 3

1. **D.** Cell membranes are composed of phospholipids; they do not contain DNA. Receptor proteins may be embedded in the membrane.
2. **B.** Tubular reabsorption increases plasma levels of a drug. Biotransformation, plasma protein binding, and renal or biliary excretion all lower plasma drug concentrations.
3. **D.** In general, drugs that have high lipid solubility cross membranes better than those with low lipid solubility. The larger the lipid:water partition coefficient, the greater the lipid solubility.
4. **A.** The percent of the unionized form (HA) of a weak acid would be greatest in an environment with the highest H^+ concentration, which is the lowest pH ($A + H^+ \leftrightarrow HA$).
5. **E.** The Therapeutic Index (TI) of a drug is equal to the ratio of the toxic dose to the therapeutic dose. The larger the TI of a drug, the less potential for adverse or toxic effects.
6. **D.** By definition, the half-life ($t_{1/2}$) of a drug is defined as the time it takes for the concentration of a drug in the circulation to decrease by half.

Chapter 4

1. **A.** Clopidogrel is a prodrug that needs to be activated to be effective. The enzyme responsible is CYP2C19. Individuals who are CYP2C19 poor metabolizers have a reduced ability to activate clopidogrel.

2. **C.** The HLA complex has been linked to drug hypersensitivity reactions including **Stevens-Johnson syndrome** and **toxic epidermal necrolysis.** Several different *HLA* gene polymorphisms have been linked specifically to severe adverse effects for certain drugs including carbamazepine.
3. **B.** The *SLCO1B1* Val174Ala polymorphism can lead to reduced simvastatin transport to the liver, leading to higher simvastatin plasma concentrations and thereby increasing the risk for simvastatin-induced myopathy.
4. **C.** Close to 50% of metastatic melanoma cases have mutations in the v-raf murine sarcoma viral oncogene homolog B (*BRAF*), with the primary mutation resulting in glutamic acid substituted for valine at codon 600, termed V600E. Patients with this mutation respond to the ATP inhibitor vemurafenib.
5. **A.** Patients with nonfunctional *DYPD* variants and treated with 5-FU or capecitabine are at an increased risk for myelosuppression, gastrointestinal toxicities, mucositis, and hand-foot syndrome. They are not at an increased risk for peripheral neuropathy.

Chapter 5

1. **C.** Phase I studies determine safe drug dosages and pharmacokinetics on a small number of human volunteers.
2. **A.** As defined by the DEA, Schedule I drugs, substances, or chemicals are defined as drugs with no currently accepted medical use and a high potential for abuse.
3. **C.** Target validation is an important step in the drug discovery process that provides verification and confidence that modulation of a specific target with the drug will produce a desired therapeutic effect.
4. **B.** The DEA defines a generic drug as identical or bioequivalent to the brand name drug in dosage form, safety, strength, route of administration, quality, performance characteristics, and intended use.
5. **B.** The Latin abbreviation q.i.d. means four times a day.

Chapter 6

1. **B.** The parasympathetic nervous system uses ACh as the neurotransmitter at both ganglia and the neuroeffector junction. Postganglionic parasympathetic neurons are short and located near the organ innervated, preganglionic cell bodies are located in the craniosacral divisions of the spinal cord, and parasympathetic neurons innervating the respiratory system mediate bronchoconstriction.
2. **B.** The neurotransmitter at postganglionic sympathetic neurons is NE. Sympathetic ganglia use ACh as the neurotransmitter and are located primarily in paravertebral chains. Nicotinic receptors are present at all autonomic ganglia.
3. **A.** Nicotinic receptors are ligand-gated ion channels; all the others are GPCRs.
4. **D.** The stimulation of prejunctional α_2 adrenergic receptors on postganglionic sympathetic neurons results in inhibition of NE release.

5. **C.** Activation of the parasympathetic nervous system results in constriction of airway smooth muscle, decreased heart rate, decreased renin secretion, and contraction of the GI tract. The blood vessels do not receive parasympathetic innervation.

Chapter 7

1. **B.** Pilocarpine is a cholinergic agonist that acts on ACh receptors to constrict the pupil.
2. **A.** The patient exhibits typical parasympathetic symptoms with little neuromuscular involvement; consequently the muscarinic antagonist atropine is administered to antagonize the actions of the anticholinesterase insecticide. Atropine is preferred over the quaternary ammonium muscarinic antagonist propantheline because atropine enters the brain.
3. **C.** The respiratory depression that ensues following exposure to this insecticide may lead to death. All other options listed can be managed pharmacologically and are not typically lethal.
4. **D.** Bethanechol activates muscarinic receptors, causing a decrease in heart rate, peripheral vasodilation, and constriction in the airways of the lung. Bethanechol does not activate nicotinic receptors at the neuromuscular junction.
5. **C.** It is likely that these individuals ate mushrooms containing the fungal alkaloid muscarine, which activates muscarinic cholinergic receptors and leads to parasympathomimetic effects including miosis, blurred vision, lacrimation, excessive salivation and bronchial secretions, sweating, bronchoconstriction, bradycardia, abdominal cramping, increased gastric acid secretion, diarrhea, and polyuria. Atropine antagonizes all of these effects and is a useful antidote.

Chapter 8

1. **E.** The adverse effects of muscarinic receptor antagonists include constipation, tachycardia, dry mouth, mydriasis, blurred vision, inhibition of sweating, and urinary retention; thus it is contraindicated in patients with urinary retention.
2. **C.** The symptoms described are all consistent with the ingestion of a muscarinic antagonist such as atropine.
3. **B.** Muscarinic receptor antagonists that do not cross the blood-brain barrier are useful for the treatment of COPD. Among the choices, only ipratropium is such a drug.
4. **D.** The topical application of muscarinic receptor antagonists to a patient with narrow ocular angles can cause acute angle-closure glaucoma and are contraindicated in such patients.
5. **B.** Atropine is a muscarinic receptor antagonist and, as such, will not counteract the effects of the cholinesterase inhibitors at nicotinic receptors that mediate skeletal muscle transmission.

Chapter 9

1. **E.** High doses of nicotine, or prolonged exposure of receptors to agonist, lead to desensitization of nicotinic receptors, which depresses ganglionic transmission.
2. **C.** All studies indicate that agents used in cessation programs are more successful when counseling accompanies drug therapy. Lobeline has not been shown to be effective for smoking cessation.
3. **E.** Neuronal nicotinic receptors in autonomic ganglia, the adrenal gland, the brain, and immune cells are composed of α or α and β subunits. Muscle-type nicotinic receptors are composed of $\alpha 1$, $\beta 1$, δ, and ϵ (γ during development) subunits.

Chapter 10

1. **B.** Genetic variations in butyrylcholinesterase activity resulting in either lower concentrations of normal enzyme or an abnormal enzyme may lead to prolonged actions of succinylcholine and, when administered with halogenated inhalational anesthetics, can precipitate malignant hyperthermia.
2. **C.** Ganglionic blocking agents block the predominant sympathetic or parasympathetic tone of organs and lead to dry mouth, tachycardia, constipation, and urinary retention, as well as excessive hypotension and impotence.
3. **E.** Neuromuscular blockers are useful in several clinical situations when skeletal muscle relaxation can be beneficial, including as a surgical adjunct, for orthopedic procedures, endotracheal intubation, scoping procedures, and electroconvulsive therapy.
4. **A.** Nicotinic receptors at ganglia are neuronal receptors composed of α or α and β subunits, whereas nicotinic receptors at the neuromuscular junction are composed of $\alpha 1$, $\beta 1$, δ, and ϵ (γ during development) subunits. Differences in subunit composition underlie differences in the responses of these receptors to pharmacological agents.

Chapter 11

1. **B.** DA produces complex dose-dependent peripheral actions with low doses relaxing smooth muscle in various vascular beds, including renal, mesenteric, and coronary, due to of D_1 receptor activation; these doses do not activate α_1 or β_1 receptors.
2. **B.** Epinephrine can reduce the bronchospasm associated with anaphylaxis and counter the hypotension of anaphylactic shock by promoting vasoconstriction in some vascular beds and increasing cardiac output.
3. **C.** Dobutamine is used clinically for the short-term management of cardiac decompensation in patients with refractory heart failure (American Heart Association Stage D).

Chapter 12

1. **C.** **Carvedilol** is an $\alpha_1/\beta_1/\beta_2$ receptor antagonist. **Propranolol** is a competitive antagonist at both β_1 and β_2 receptors. In combination with **doxazosin**, which is a selective α_1 receptor antagonist, these drugs will antagonize the same receptors as carvedilol alone.
2. **A.** Phentolamine blocks α_1 and α_2 adrenergic receptors, and thus the effects of epinephrine after phentolamine will reflect effects only by β_1 receptors, most closely resembling the effects of the β_1/β_2 agonist isoproterenol.
3. **B.** Epinephrine-induced renin release is mediated by activation of β_1 receptors. Thus, this action will be blocked by the relatively selective β_1 receptor antagonist metoprolol; the other responses to epinephrine are mediated by different receptor subtypes.

Chapter 13

1. **A.** ACh is the only neurotransmitter whose action is terminated by hydrolysis via the action of acetylcholinesterase; the actions of all the other amine neurotransmitters listed are terminated by reuptake.
2. **A.** All of the biogenic amine neurotransmitters are synthesized in nerve terminals and transported into vesicles by an active process; their concentration in vesicles is 10 to 100 times that in the cytosol.
3. **C.** The long-term administration of agonists leads to a down regulation of receptors in the postsynaptic cell membrane.
4. **C.** Dopaminergic neurons originate in the substantia nigra and hypothalamus; the other types of neurons listed originate in other brain regions.
5. **B.** A high degree of lipophilicity will facilitate the ability of drugs to cross the blood-brain barrier; the other choices would hinder it.
6. **C.** Ethanol, a CNS depressant, produces an initial stage of excitation by reducing the activity of tonically active inhibitory brain systems. It has none of the other effects listed.

Chapter 14

1. **A.** A loss of memory in an elderly individual may represent Alzheimer's disease. Donepezil is an acetylcholinesterase inhibitor that preserves brain acetylcholine, a major neurotransmitter involved in learning and memory thought to decline in Alzheimer's disease. There is no rationale for the use of any other drug listed.

2. **E.** Alzheimer's disease involves the loss of basal forebrain cholinergic neurons, with primary therapy directed at increasing the levels of acetylcholine in the brain.

3. **C.** Early-onset Alzheimer's disease may be linked to mutations in the genes coding for amyloid precursor protein (APP) or presenilins, which are proteins involved in APP processing.

4. **C.** Alzheimer's disease is a progressive neurodegenerative disorder, and thus one would expect to see more atrophy. These is no evidence that drug therapy slows the progression of neuronal loss.

5. **B.** The cognitive benefits of drug therapy vary from individual to individual and, although statistically significant, are clinically modest. Not all patients benefit, and those who do typically show only a slight improvement in abilities.

6. **B.** Galantamine is an acetylcholinesterase inhibitor and a positive allosteric modulator at neuronal nicotinic receptors. Donepezil and rivastigmine only inhibit acetylcholinesterase, and memantine is a glutamate receptor antagonist.

Chapter 15

1. **C.** Carbidopa is a peripheral aromatic amino acid decarboxylase inhibitor that does not cross the BBB and prevents the peripheral metabolism of L-DOPA.

2. **B.** After 5 to 7 years of continued drug treatment, as many as 75% of patients experience L-DOPA–induced dyskinesias, characterized by chorea and dystonia.

3. **B.** Apomorphine is the only injectable drug for use in patients with advanced Parkinson's disease who experience episodes of immobility ("off" times) despite L-DOPA therapy.

4. **C.** Tetrabenazine is a reversible inhibitor of the vesicular monoamine transport 2 (VMAT2) and prevents the uptake of dopamine into vesicles in the presynaptic neuron, leading to dopamine depletion.

Chapter 16

1. **A.** Lithium is filtered by the kidneys, with 95% of an administered dose excreted in the urine in 24 hours. Any drug that interferes with glomerular filtration can increase plasma levels of lithium.

2. **B.** The chronic administration of dopamine receptor antagonists such as haloperidol can lead to an increased density of receptors, which underlies the development of tardive dyskinesia, a drug-induced disorder characterized by abnormal facial movements.

3. **B.** The phenothiazine antipsychotics block muscarinic cholinergic receptors, leading to many anticholinergic effects including dry mouth, urinary retention, and memory impairment.

4. **D.** Clozapine has the potential to produce agranulocytosis, requiring blood cell counts for all patients taking this drug.

5. **E.** Some atypical antipsychotics may temper negative symptoms of schizophrenia as a consequence of their antagonist actions at serotonin receptors.

Chapter 17

1. **B.** The β-adrenergic receptor antagonists such as **propranolol** are useful for the short-term relief of performance anxiety because they suppress sympathetically mediated somatic manifestations of anxiety.

2. **D.** Ketamine is unique in its action as an antidepressant because its intravenous administration tempers suicidal thoughts and depression within a few hours.

3. **C.** All amine reuptake inhibitors have the potential to precipitate serotonin syndrome when used with other agents that also increase serotonin in the brain including many over-the-counter cough preparations containing dextromethorphan. Serotonin syndrome is characterized by fever, chills, diarrhea, myoclonus, tremor, motor weakness, ataxia, and behavioral alterations.

4. **C.** Bupropion is contraindicated for use in any patient with a history of seizures.

5. **A.** Although this woman has been in remission for 2 years, based on her history of alcohol use disorder, it would be unwise to provide a prescription for a benzodiazepine.

Chapter 18

1. **B.** Although the exact pathophysiology of attention deficit hyperactivity disorder is unclear, it is believed to involve suboptimal norepinephrine and dopamine neurotransmission in the frontal lobe.

2. **E.** Common adverse effects associated with the use of the stimulants include headaches, insomnia, anorexia, tic exacerbation, dry mouth, GI upset, weight loss, and reduced growth velocity.

3. **E.** Although atomoxetine is less efficacious than the stimulants for the treatment of attention deficit hyperactivity disorder, it is typically prescribed for children of low weight or stature.

4. **D.** Adverse reactions to guanfacine include hypotension, somnolence, bradycardia, and syncope.

5. **D.** Lisdexamfetamine is a prodrug that is converted to dextroamphetamine by enzymatic hydrolysis by red blood cells.

6. **C.** The effects of the amphetamines are attributed primarily to enhanced dopamine and norepinephrine release.

Chapter 19

1. **E.** Suvorexant is the only agent approved for both sleep-onset and sleep-maintenance insomnia.

2. **D.** The benzodiazepines depress REM sleep, and chronic REM deprivation can lead to psychotic-like behaviors.

3. **A.** **Ramelteon** is the first and only selective melatonin receptor agonist approved for the treatment of insomnia.

4. **E.** The benzodiazepines may lead to CNS depression, dependence, daytime sedation, anterograde amnesia, headache, and dizziness and thus are not ideal drugs for the treatment of insomnia.

5. **A.** Suvorexant blocks orexin neuropeptides from binding to orexin receptors and inhibits arousal signaling.

Chapter 20

1. **C.** Orlistat is the only agent listed whose action is localized to the gastrointestinal tract. All the other agents readily enter the systemic circulation and may adversely affect the cardiovascular system.

2. **A.** The only drug approved for binge-eating disorder is lisdexamfetamine.

3. **D.** Orlistat acts locally within the intestines to reduce the absorption of dietary fat via inhibition of intestinal lipase, which decreases the production of free fatty acids from triglycerides.

4. **C.** Dronabinol, which is used for cachexia, stimulates appetite through agonist actions at the cannabinoid receptor located in both the eating centers in the brain and in the gastrointestinal tract.

5. **C.** Liraglutide is a long-acting GLP-1 receptor agonist approved for both type 2 diabetes and the treatment of obesity.

Chapter 21

1. **E.** The 3-per-second spike and wave activity on the EEG and the clinical presentation are classic for absence seizures. The drug of choice for absence seizures is ethosuximide. Valproic acid also can be used but is not listed as a choice.

2. **B.** Phenytoin is one of few drugs that convert from first-order kinetics to zero-order kinetics in the therapeutic dose range. Therefore it is impossible to estimate a serum concentration based on a direct relationship to dose. When phenytoin becomes zero-order, the serum concentration will be higher than predicted from the dose.

3. **C.** This patient should be treated with antiepileptic drugs because she is having repeated (daily) seizures. The choice of drug is based on her generalized tonic-clonic seizures. Phenytoin and carbamazepine are effective for tonic-clonic seizures, but phenytoin has side effects of hirsutism and coarsening of facial features. Therefore the best choice for this young girl is carbamazepine.

4. **A.** Drugs that block voltage-gated sodium channels such as phenytoin and carbamazepine produce a use- and voltage-dependent blockade, reducing the repetitive firing of neurons and prolonging the inactivated state of the sodium channel. Thus, these drugs would be best for neurons firing with high frequency.

5. **D.** Carbamazepine induces its own metabolism over the first several weeks of treatment. As the patient continues to take the same dose, the half-life shortens and the average plasma concentration falls, possibly below the therapeutic level.

Chapter 22

1. **A.** The most commonly used oral medication to treat spasticity that also enhances GABA activity is **baclofen**, which is an agonist at GABA-B receptors within the brainstem, the dorsal horn of the spinal cord, and other pre- and post-synaptic sites.

2. **C.** Dantrolene binds to the ryanodine receptor 1 in the sarcoplasmic reticulum of skeletal muscle and inhibits the ability of RyR1 to release Ca^{2+}, which is essential for muscle contraction.

3. **E.** There are many limitations to the use of oral spasticity medications of which sedation, drowsiness, and lethargy limit their use.

Chapter 23

1. **E.** Cardiac toxicity, increased caloric intake, and disturbed lipid metabolism caused by alcohol use contribute to cardiovascular disease. Ethanol is metabolized in the liver, and this leads to a myriad of biochemical disturbances via increased NADP and acetaldehyde concentrations. Alcohol is associated with cancer of the larynx and pharynx. Fetal alcohol syndrome (intake of ethanol by the mother during pregnancy) is the leading preventable cause of mental retardation.

2. **A.** Obstructed hepatic venous return increases venous pressure and fluid leakage. Increased osmolality of blood would decrease ascites, and just the opposite happens because of decreased serum protein synthesis by the liver.

3. **D.** The interaction of estrogens may be responsible for the nearly twofold increase in the risk of liver damage in women compared with men.

4. **D.** Disulfiram (via a metabolic product) inhibits high K_m ALDH enzymes in the liver. The mitochondrial enzyme (low K_m enzyme) is inactive in some Asians because of a genetic abnormality. The end result in either case is increased acetaldehyde concentrations in the liver and blood, and a flushing reaction results.

5. **E.** Induction of cytochrome P450 2E1 is independent of ethanol oxidation. When it is present with other substrates for the enzyme, it competes with them for the enzyme, thus inhibiting their metabolism. When ethanol is absent, the increased enzyme content and activity lead to increased metabolic activity.

Chapter 24

1. **C.** The ability of one drug to completely prevent the onset of withdrawal signs and symptoms during abstinence from another drug is evidence of cross-dependence between them.

2. **B.** Several pharmacological classes of abused drugs all share the ability to activate the mesolimbic dopamine reward pathway in the brain.

3. **B.** The withdrawal syndrome from depressant drugs such as alcohol and barbiturates may include severe tremors and convulsions that can be life-threatening.

4. **E.** Alcohol, barbiturates, and benzodiazepines all produce a similar withdrawal syndrome after chronic use, which reflects central nervous system hyperexcitability. They also exhibit cross-dependence to each other.

5. **D.** The unique effects of hallucinogens result from modulation of 5-HT neurotransmission.

Chapter 25

No questions

Chapter 26

1. **B.** None of the other drugs reduces cardiac output significantly at doses usually used, and effects on blood pressure are small compared with those of halothane. Ketamine often increases blood pressure.

2. **E.** All volatile anesthetics and morphine-like opioids decrease the sensitivity of chemoreceptors in the respiratory centers of the brainstem to CO_2, thus blunting the ventilatory response to increases in CO_2 tension in blood and cerebrospinal fluid.

3. **C.** As an ED_{50}, MAC is unaffected by the size of the patient (although it takes longer to anesthetize a large patient than it does a smaller one), the patient's gender, or the length of time over which the anesthetic is administered. Morphine depresses the CNS so that *less* anesthetic is required (i.e., the MAC is lowered). Because of their high basal metabolism, infants have a higher anesthetic requirement than do older patients.

4. **D.** N_2O should be avoided in this patient because the gas diffuses out of the blood into air-filled cavities faster than it leaves those cavities and enters the blood, resulting in increased pressure and distention of enclosed air-filled, nitrogen-containing spaces.

5. **A.** The solubility of the anesthetic, expressed as the blood:gas partition coefficient, determines both the rate of uptake and induction of general anesthesia.

Chapter 27

1. **B.** The mechanism of action of local anesthetics involves blockade of activity-dependent Na^+ channels.

2. **D.** Local anesthetics must cross cell membranes in an unionized form. At an acidic pH, the portion of drug in the unionized form is reduced; thus, local anesthetics are less effective in inflamed or infected tissues that have lower pH than in normal non-inflamed tissues.

3. **D.** Type A subtype δ nerve fibers are the ones affected at the lowest dose and with the earliest onset.

4. **A.** The ester local anesthetics are hydrolyzed by plasma and liver cholinesterases, whereas the amide local anesthetics are metabolized in the liver by cytochrome P450s, followed by hydrolysis.

5. **C.** Methemoglobinemia; this is a specific side effect to benzocaine overdose and an FDA boxed warning is required on products that contain benzocaine.

Chapter 28

1. **D.** All opioid receptors are coupled to an inhibitory G protein, leading to decreased adenyl cyclase, decreased calcium, and increased potassium conductances, resulting in inhibition of neuronal activity.
2. **A.** Activation of μ-opioid receptors leads to respiratory depression, whereas activation of κ receptors does not. Naloxone is an antagonist, and buprenorphine is a mixed agonist with partial agonist activity at μ receptors and antagonist activity at κ and possibly δ receptors.
3. **A.** Naloxone is an opioid receptor antagonist used to reverse overdose. Oxycodone is not used for cough, morphine is a strong agonist for severe pain, naloxone is an antagonist and cannot alleviate cough, and methadone is an agonist used for the treatment of opioid dependence.
4. **A.** The chronic administration of opioids can lead to hyperalgesia, which is an increased sensitivity to pain or enhanced intensity of pain sensations.
5. **C.** Naloxone is used for opioid overdose to compete with the agonist at medullary μ receptors to reverse respiratory depression.

Chapter 29

1. **A.** The symptoms described are classic for aspirin toxicity.
2. **E.** All drugs listed with the exception of acetaminophen are effective antiinflammatory agents; acetaminophen is devoid of this activity.
3. **D.** COX-2 inhibitors can increase the incidence of major cardiovascular events because they prevent the production of PGI_2 in vascular epithelial cells, which inhibits platelet aggregation, but do not affect the synthesis of TXA_2 production by platelets, which promotes aggregation.
4. **B.** Naproxen is an NSAID that inhibits COX and decreases the synthesis of prostaglandins.
5. **D.** The most common side effects produced by the NSAIDs involve the gastrointestinal system and include nausea, dyspepsia, heartburn, and abdominal discomfort. The incidence and severity of these effects are increased by the dose and duration of drug administration, and chronic use may lead to ulceration, bleeding, and gastrointestinal perforation.

Chapter 30

1. **D.** Multiple randomized and controlled clinical studies have demonstrated that the cannabinoids are effective for alleviating both acute and chronic pain. Evidence for the use of these agents for the other indications is inconclusive to date.
2. **E.** The cannabinoids alleviate pain and inflammation through central and peripheral effects on several receptor systems including CB_1 and CB_1 receptors, which are G-protein–coupled receptors, transient receptor potential vanilloid receptor 1 (TRPV1) channels, and peroxisome proliferator-activated receptors (PPARs).
3. **A.** Although not currently approved for the treatment of pain, nabilone is a synthetic THC analogue that has been shown to decrease pain associated with fibromyalgia and may be useful in this situation. Because the patient was tolerant to the opioids, he may be tolerant to CBD, and there is no evidence that dronabinol is efficacious for pain.
4. **E.** All of these mechanisms may serve as targets for drugs to alleviate pain.

Chapter 31

1. **B.** The triptans are highly effective for the short-term treatment of acute migraine attacks and will rapidly decrease the pain and nausea she experienced. The other drugs listed will be ineffective.
2. **B.** The triptans are direct coronary vasoconstrictors and are contraindicated for patients with preexisting cardiovascular disease.
3. **A.** Drugs effective for migraines are believed to exert their effects by activating $5\text{-HT}_{1B}/5\text{-HT}_{1D}/5\text{-HT}_{1F}$ receptors to inhibit the release of CGRP and other peptides implicated in the dilation of intracranial blood vessels, as well as directly constrict blood vessels.
4. **D.** Activation of 5-HT receptors inhibits the release of calcitonin gene–related peptide (CGRP) and substance P, both of which produce inflammation of the pain-sensitive meninges and potently vasodilate affected cranial blood vessels.
5. **A.** Triptans are contraindicated for patients with cardiovascular disease because they are direct coronary vasoconstrictors.
6. **D.** Botulinum toxin is a motor neuron blocker that prevents the release of ACh from neurons at the neuromuscular junction and is used to prevent severe migraines.

Chapter 32

1. **C.** Acute flare-ups of gout are typically treated by colchicine, which decreases the intensity of the inflammatory response to urate crystals by disrupting microtubules. All other drugs listed are used prophylactically to prevent gout.
2. **E.** Probenecid decreases uric acid levels by increasing its renal secretion and can be added to the administration of a xanthine oxidase inhibitor such as allopurinol or febuxostat. Colchicine and NSAIDs are used for flare-ups to decrease inflammation, whereas the recombinant uricase pegloticase is used only for hyperuricemia as a consequence of tumor lysis.
3. **D.** Probenecid inhibits the renal transporter mediating the excretion of some antibiotics including the cephalosporins, and the concomitant use of probenecid with these agents impairs their renal clearance and increases serum levels. Thus, the dose of cephalexin needs to be decreased.
4. **A.** The only other approach available would be to promote the oxidation of uric acid, which can be accomplished with a uricase.

Chapter 33

1. **B.** Cetirizine is specifically approved for perennial allergy. It is approved for ages 2 and older and is available in liquid formulations flavored to appeal to children. Other advantages of second-generation antihistamines include rapid onset of action and once-daily dosing. (Note that Zyrtec-D, a combination of cetirizine and the decongestant pseudoephedrine, is not approved for children under the age of 12.)
2. **B.** The first-generation, "classic" H_1-antihistamines, such as diphenhydramine, readily cross the blood-brain barrier, leading to drowsiness. Fexofenadine and loratadine are second-generation H_1-antihistamines and are largely devoid of CNS effects. Ketotifen and olopatadine are used primarily in ophthalmic drops.
3. **C.** The most important adverse effects associated with the first-generation H_1-antihistamines result from CNS penetration and muscarinic antagonism.
4. **A.** The first-generation H_1-antihistamines readily cross the blood-brain barrier and lead to sedation, whereas the second-generation compounds are largely devoid of CNS effects.
5. **D.** Degranulation of mast cells leads to the early phase response with histamine release causing vasodilation, increased gastrointestinal and mucosal secretions, peristalsis, and bronchoconstriction.

Chapter 34

1. **B.** In addition to being immunosuppressive, glucocorticoids have potent antiinflammatory effects.
2. **D.** Cyclosporine is more selective than other antiproliferative immunosuppressive agents because it specifically inhibits cytokine synthesis in T-lymphocytes.
3. **B.** Cyclosporine can lead to hepatotoxicity and nephrotoxicity but not bone marrow depression.
4. **D.** All of these agents listed have been linked to myelosuppression and/or increased incidence of infection.

Chapter 35

1. **E.** Methotrexate is an antimetabolite that inhibits the synthesis of folic acid. Thus, its side effects can be reduced or eliminated if patients also take folic acid.
2. **D.** The biological and targeted DMARDs are potent inhibitors that cannot be prescribed together because of the high risk for infections, but these agents can be used in combination with a conventional DMARD such as methotrexate to increase effectiveness and decrease some adverse effects.
3. **B.** The biological and targeted DMARDs can lead to the emergence of latent tuberculosis after treatment initiation, and an FDA boxed warning of this risk is present on the labeling.
4. **B.** Infliximab, which is comprised of a mouse Fab antibody portion and a human Fc portion, can generate anti-drug antibodies in up to 40% of patients.

Chapter 36

1. **E.** Activation of the sympathetic nervous system causes all of the effects listed.
2. **B.** Skin is the tissue that is least influenced by the baroreceptor reflex because it is relatively unimportant in such critical physiological processes as maintaining an upright posture.
3. **A.** The nucleus of the tractus solitarius located in the dorsomedial brainstem represents the first central synapse for afferents.
4. **D.** A reduction in arterial pressure activates the baroreceptor reflex, which leads to increased sympathetic nerve activity and decreased vagal nerve activity.
5. **B.** Most blood vessels are innervated by the sympathetic nervous system.

Chapter 37

1. **B.** The preferred drug for the treatment of hypertension during pregnancy is α-methyldopa.
2. **B.** Centrally acting sympatholytic agents are associated with sedation because their primary site of action is in the central nervous system.
3. **C.** Reserpine binds to the vesicular monoamine transporter in both central and peripheral noradrenergic neurons and prevents monoamine accumulation, leading to depletion of the transmitter.
4. **B.** Clonidine possesses a unique activity that renders it useful as adjunctive treatment to produce additional analgesia in patients with severe chronic pain who are inadequately controlled by maximal doses of opioids.
5. **E.** JNC-8 recommends a return to the use of thiazide diuretics for the initiation of treatment for uncomplicated hypertension. This is a change from ACE inhibitors and angiotensin receptor blockers.

Chapter 38

1. **A.** Loop diuretics inhibit the $Na^+/K^+/2Cl$ cotransporter present in the apical cell membrane of the ascending limb of the loop of Henle.
2. **B.** One major adverse effect associated with the use of loop diuretics such as furosemide is hearing loss and vertigo.
3. **E.** Spironolactone is an aldosterone receptor antagonist that is part of the K^+-sparing diuretic family and is responsible for interfering with the exchange of Na^+ and K^+ in favor of retaining K^+.
4. **A.** Thiazide diuretics cause a loss of potassium (hypokalemia), an elevation in plasma glucose (hyperglycemia), and an increase in low-density lipoproteins and triglycerides (hyperlipidemia).
5. **D.** Based upon the recommendations in JNC-8, a patient diagnosed with essential hypertension should begin therapy with a thiazide diuretic because these agents have been shown to reduce hypertension and associated cardiovascular sequelae and are tolerated well in many large clinical studies.

Chapter 39

1. **A.** Lisinopril, eplerenone, and aliskiren all decrease aldosterone signaling. Lisinopril reversibly inhibits the conversion of angiotensin I to angiotensin II, eplerenone is an aldosterone receptor antagonist, and aliskiren binds to renin to prevent the formation of angiotensin I.
2. **C.** First trimester exposure to ACE inhibitors is a teratogenic risk. Therefore, after pregnancy has been established, the use of another antihypertensive agent is mandatory.
3. **C.** Aldosterone increases potassium excretion, and thus blockade of the renin-angiotensin-aldosterone system results in hyperkalemia. Losartan blocks adrenal AT_1 receptors, decreasing aldosterone release, while propranolol inhibits the sympathetic activation of renin release, leading to decreased aldosterone secretion.
4. **A.** The ACE inhibitor lisinopril preserves bradykinin, which has protussive effects and is responsible for the dry cough associated with use of these agents.

Chapter 40

1. **C.** Only the non-dihydropyridines, verapamil and diltiazem, are used for their antiarrhythmic effects.
2. **A.** Dihydropyridines such as amlodipine or clevidipine have the greatest effects in the smooth muscle of the vasculature, but of the two drugs, only amlodipine is used on an outpatient basis. Clevidipine is administered only as an intravenous infusion.
3. **D.** Calcium channel blockers, and especially verapamil, are associated with the development of gingival hyperplasia; good oral hygiene is required when using these agents.
4. **D.** The dihydropyridines such as nifedipine may result in ankle edema due to vasodilation of arteriolar smooth muscle.
5. **D.** The non-dihydropyridines, verapamil and diltiazem, have negative chronotropic, inotropic, and dromotropic effects and would not be beneficial for an individual with congestive heart failure.

Chapter 41

1. **D.** Minoxidil relaxes arterioles through activation of K^+ channels that leads to hyperpolarization.
2. **E.** Sodium nitroprusside directly releases nitric oxide to activate soluble guanylyl cyclase and produce rapid and reversible relaxation of vascular smooth muscle. Chemically the compound contains a number of cyanide moieties that can lead to cyanide/thiocyanate toxicity.
3. **E.** The use of vasodilators leads to all of these adverse effects.
4. **A.** PDE5 inhibitors are contraindicated in patients taking nitroglycerin for angina. Combination administration may cause a substantial and threatening drop in blood pressure.
5. **C.** Benign prostatic hyperplasia (BPH) is a nonmalignant enlargement of the prostate that may cause impaired urethral function, leading to urinary retention. The PDE5 inhibitor tadalafil is

approved for the treatment of BPH and is administered once daily for treatment.

Chapter 42

1. **E.** Current practice guidelines recommend that patients with established coronary heart disease be on a high-intensity statin regimen such as rosuvastatin.
2. **A.** Activation of PPAR-α, which mediates the action of the fibrates, is one of the key drug classes used to treat severe hypertriglyceridemia.
3. **B.** Lomitapide prevents the incorporation of both triglycerides and ApoB-100 into VLDL particles, thereby preventing the assembly of VLDL in hepatocytes.
4. **E.** Ezetimibe can further lower LDL-cholesterol levels and is the only choice that has been demonstrated to further improve clinical outcomes in clinical trials.

Chapter 43

1. **D.** Nitroglycerin dilates the veins, which reduces venous return to the heart, which in turn decreases ventricular filling. The resulting decrease in preload reduces the oxygen requirements of the heart. Nitroglycerin does not increase the blood flow or oxygen supply to the heart. An increase in ventricular filling would increase oxygen demand and result in increased angina pain.
2. **C.** Both nitroglycerin and diltiazem relax vascular smooth muscle through two different mechanisms of action.
3. **C.** Tolerance to the organic nitrates has been proposed to be the result of inactivation of aldehyde dehydrogenase, which converts nitrates and nitrites to NO.
4. **B.** The sublingual route of administration is effective at achieving substantial plasma concentrations with lower doses for agents subject to first-pass metabolism, which occurs in the liver. Drugs taken orally are absorbed and diverted to the liver where many are significantly metabolized.

Chapter 44

1. **C.** Clinical studies have demonstrated clear efficacy of the combination of hydralazine and isosorbide dinitrate for the treatment of heart failure in African Americans who are not adequately treated with RAAS agents or β blockers.
2. **D.** Valsartan is an angiotensin receptor blocking agent, whereas sacubitril inhibits neprilysin.
3. **D.** ACE inhibitors such as lisinopril lead to bradykinin accumulation, which produces a persistent, dry cough that is bothersome enough to decrease patient compliance with drug therapy.
4. **B.** Dobutamine is a relatively selective agonist at β_1-adrenergic receptors.
5. **C.** Milrinone and inamrinone are agents used in refractory heart failure whose mechanism of action involves inhibition of PDE type 3.

Chapter 45

1. **E.** Amiodarone has actions that encompass all four potential mechanism categories.
2. **C.** Esmolol is a β blocker that possesses an extremely short duration of action (10 minutes), which makes it especially useful in emergency situations.
3. **A.** Class 1C agents such as flecainide dissociate from the sodium channel very slowly, leaving a high fraction of sodium channels in the inactivated drug-bound state, which slows conduction.
4. **D.** Intravenous amiodarone is one of many drugs used to treat abnormalities of cardiac rhythm that can produce excessive prolongation of the QT interval.

5. **A.** Adenosine is the drug of choice for the rapid conversion of paroxysmal supraventricular tachycardia.

Chapter 46

1. **C.** In contrast to warfarin, heparin must be given by injection, has a short half-life, and may cause platelet aggregation and thrombocytopenia. It acts by binding to antithrombin, thereby increasing the activity of this serine protease inhibitor.
2. **D.** Warfarin, which can be taken orally, acts by inhibiting vitamin K regeneration, thus preventing the posttranslational modification of clotting factors. Warfarin metabolism is accelerated by barbiturates and other drugs that stimulate the activity of cytochrome P450.
3. **B.** Aspirin and other drugs that inhibit platelet function increase the risk of bleeding in patients receiving other types of anticoagulants.
4. **A.** Aspirin inhibits platelet cyclooxygenase, thereby preventing the formation of TXA_2, a powerful platelet-aggregating agent. Inhibition of platelet aggregation lengthens the bleeding time without affecting the coagulation mechanism.
5. **B.** Heparin is a drug of choice in response to an emergency to produce rapid anticoagulant effects.

Chapter 47

1. **C.** Ferumoxytol is formulated with iron oxide bound to nanoparticles to release more free iron following administration. It can be administered more rapidly than parenteral preparations, completing therapy in a much shorter time frame.
2. **D.** Vitamin B_{12} is necessary to activate folic acid, which is involved in DNA synthesis.
3. **D.** Desmopressin is an ADH analogue that causes release of factor VIII from vascular endothelial cells and can be used to augment the clotting process when needed.
4. **C.** The most common adverse effects associated with oral iron therapy involve the gastrointestinal system.
5. **C.** Oral iron therapy often corrects iron-deficient anemia within 1 to 2 months if there is sufficient GI absorption. The preparation of choice is oral ferrous sulfate.
6. **A.** The most common side effects of oral iron supplementation are gastrointestinal symptoms, which are dose related. Thus, decreasing the dose, or starting with a lower dose and titrating up slowly, may improve these adverse effects.

Chapter 48

No questions

Chapter 49

1. **B.** Desmopressin is preferred because it has a longer half-life than arginine vasopressin, resulting in a longer duration of action.
2. **C.** The pulsatile administration of GnRH has been used successfully to induce ovulation in women with primary hypothalamic amenorrhea, which involves abnormal functioning of the GnRH pulse generator, resulting in inadequate gonadotropin secretion, failure of ovarian follicular development, and amenorrhea. The pulsatile administration of GnRH will release LH and FSH from the pituitary and can compensate for the underlying defect.
3. **A.** Administration of GnRH analogues and antiandrogens are used in treating metastatic hormone-dependent prostate cancer to produce a functional orchiectomy and regression of the cancer.
4. **A.** SRIF analogues bind to pituitary SRIF receptors and block GH secretion. Several studies show that long-acting SRIF analogues are useful as adjunct therapy in acromegaly.
5. **A.** Several GnRH agonists are used to treat idiopathic precocious puberty.

Chapter 50

1. **A.** The 11-hydroxyl group on cortisol conveys maximum activation of the steroid receptor complex and its effect on gene activity.
2. **D.** The addition of a methyl group at position 16 on glucocorticoid, as present in betamethasone and dexamethasone, increases GR activation and virtually eliminates MR activation.
3. **A.** Alternate-day therapy glucocorticoid administration, which involves administration of double the normal daily dose of an intermediate-acting glucocorticoid, such as prednisone, every other day was developed to reduce adverse effects.
4. **C.** Dexamethasone has maximal antiinflammatory activity with little effect on blood pressure, whereas excessive glucocorticoids such as cortisol may lead to hypertension.
5. **E.** A major side effect of the glucocorticoids, especially when given for prolonged periods, involves effects on bone, leading to osteoporosis; children and postmenopausal women are at highest risk.

Chapter 51

1. **A.** Inhibition of aromatase reduces the conversion of androgens to estrogens in peripheral tissues, which has proven useful in the treatment of estrogen-dependent neoplasms.
2. **B.** The conformation of the ER complex after ligand binding is a primary determinant of its ability to alter gene activity. SERMs such as raloxifene are partial agonists or antagonists depending on the conformational changes of the ER complex in different tissues. Differences in tissue distribution of ER subtypes, recruitment of coregulator proteins, and transcriptional activating factors also explain the variability of responses to SERMs.
3. **C.** A medical history of DVT is a contraindication for estrogen use because this significantly increases the risk of recurrence.
4. **B.** The inclusion of a progestin when estrogen is administered to a woman with an intact uterus significantly reduces the risk of endometrial cancer because progestins antagonize estrogen-induced proliferation in the endometrium.
5. **D.** Sequential use of a prostaglandin and oxytocin is preferred for cervical ripening and labor induction. There should be an appropriate interval between administration of these uterine stimulants to minimize adverse effects.
6. **D.** Large doses of ergot alkaloids produce a tonic uterine contraction that controls excessive bleeding. These compounds are usually reserved for use for women who fail to respond to oxytocin or a prostaglandin.

Chapter 52

1. **C.** Finasteride is a competitive inhibitor of the type II 5α-reductase, reducing the formation of dihydrotestosterone from testosterone, thereby decreasing the volume of the prostate.
2. **C.** The androgen receptor antagonist flutamide is used for the treatment of androgen-dependent prostate cancers through negative feedback regulation of testosterone synthesis via the hypothalamic-pituitary axis. Flutamide is also often co-administered with a GnRH agonist to prevent an initial flare of symptoms.
3. **D.** Based on the patient's low testosterone level (normal ranging from 280-1100 ng/dL), hormone replacement therapy with testosterone is warranted.

Chapter 53

1. **E.** The thiazolidinediones, rosiglitazone and pioglitazone, activate the peroxisome proliferator-activated receptor type γ, facilitating glucose utilization for glycerol synthesis and storage of fatty acids as triglycerides, thereby decreasing circulating insulin levels, leading to an increase in insulin sensitivity.
2. **B.** Glulisine is a rapid-acting insulin with a duration of 2 to 4 hours, while glargine insulin is a long-acting agent with a duration of 24 hours. The woman should not increase the dose of either preparation, as she appears to have decreased blood glucose. Further, she cannot omit either preparation. Thus, her best approach would be to decrease her dose of the glulisine prior to any exercise regimen.
3. **D.** The meglitinides, such as repaglinide and nateglinide, promote insulin release by binding to SUR1 of K_{ATP} channels.
4. **D.** An HbA1c of <7% indicates that blood glucose levels are fairly well controlled, and thus one would not want to prescribe any agent that could precipitate hypoglycemic episodes or act at the intestinal level for a short period of time. As a consequence, metformin is indicated.
5. **B.** Miglitol, by delaying glucose absorption, will minimize post-prandial hypoglycemia; the other agents will not.
6. **F.** Sulfonylureas are associated with causing the highest incidence of hypoglycemia among drugs taken orally.

Chapter 54

1. **B.** Hashimoto's disease is a common form of hypothyroidism, which is diagnosed by decreased thyroid hormone, increased TSH, and elevated thyroglobulin antibodies.
2. **A.** Graves' disease is a common form of hyperthyroidism, which is diagnosed by increased thyroid hormone, suppressed TSH, and elevated thyroglobulin antibodies.
3. **B.** Patients who have a history of cardiovascular complications must have their thyroid hormones increased slowly to high normal values to relieve the effects of the increased thyroid hormone levels on their cardiovascular system.
4. **B.** Of these options, only the functioning of the thyroid gland dictates the need and extent of treatment for hypothyroidism.

Chapter 55

1. **E.** The bisphosphonates such as zoledronic acid are used as first-line treatment for osteoporosis.
2. **B.** Etelcalcetide, which is a positive allosteric modulator of calcium-sensing receptors in the parathyroid gland, increases sensitivity to calcium and decreases the concentration of calcium required to suppress parathyroid hormone secretion.
3. **D.** Raloxifene is a selective estrogen receptor modulator that is used to reduce bone loss resulting from postmenopausal osteoporosis; the other agents are not.
4. **D.** The human parathyroid hormone analogue, teriparatide, is capable of both actions at different concentrations.
5. **E.** The second-generation bisphosphonates are released from their association with bone during resorption, which allows them to exert cytotoxic effects on osteoblasts, without inhibiting the attraction of osteoblasts and the recalcification of bone.

Chapter 56

1. **A.** All methicillin-resistant *S. aureus* (MRSA) β-lactams acquire the *mecA* gene, which encodes the PBP2a protein, which has a low affinity for these agents and prevents them from inhibiting cell wall synthesis.
2. **A.** The prophylactic antibiotic should be administered just before the procedure because limiting exposure minimizes the selection of resistant bacteria.
3. **D.** Sulfonamides are known to induce hemolytic anemia in patients deficient in glucose-6-phosphate dehydrogenase.

4. **A.** The β-lactams are cell wall synthesis inhibitors, whereas the aminoglycosides are protein synthesis inhibitors. These agents are synergistic when administered in combination.

5. **D.** The main mechanism of resistance to the tetracyclines involves enhanced drug efflux.

Chapter 57

1. **E.** Patients who have experienced a rash in response to penicillin are at low risk of a serious reaction to other β-lactam antibiotics. However, because the patient is asthmatic and has a documented allergic reaction, all β-lactams should be avoided if possible. Vancomycin is the drug of choice for this patient.

2. **C.** Imipenem binds to brain tissue better than the other β-lactams and is more likely to induce seizures.

3. **C.** The most common cause of bacterial resistance to vancomycin involves an increased number of cell wall binding sites.

4. **A.** Lysis of gram-positive bacteria treated with β-lactams ultimately depends on autolysins, which are normally involved in new cell wall synthesis when cells divide. There are bacteria that lack these autolysins, which are termed "tolerant" because the β-lactams inhibit their growth and division but do not kill them.

5. **C.** When the concentration of meropenem decreases below MIC, the bacteria that have not been killed do not resume growth for another 2 to 4 hours.

Chapter 58

1. **B.** Chloramphenicol can be used to treat bacterial meningitis, but it has pronounced hematological adverse effects including bone marrow depression and aplastic anemia.

2. **D.** The streptogramins bind reversibly to the 50S ribosomal subunit, thereby inhibiting peptide chain elongation.

3. **D.** The aminoglycosides such as gentamicin exhibit a postantibiotic therapeutic effect, with the drug still detectable in the urine after completion of therapy.

4. **A.** Azithromycin is the only macrolide that does not inhibit the cytochrome P450 enzymes and would not lead to a drug-drug interaction with the patient's current medication.

Chapter 59

1. **E.** The symptoms described are characteristic of Stevens-Johnson syndrome, which is a potential adverse effect of the sulfonamides.

2. **D.** First-time urinary tract infections are treated empirically with the combination of trimethoprim/sulfamethoxazole. Cultures should be obtained before initiating therapy in the event the organism is resistant to this treatment.

3. **A.** Fluoroquinolones such as ciprofloxacin are bactericidal agents that interfere with transcription by inhibiting the activity of topoisomerases and DNA gyrase required for the proper replication of DNA.

4. **D.** The synthesis of dihydropteroate synthetase can be modified by a chromosomal mutation or by a plasmid leading to resistance to trimethoprim.

Chapter 60

1. **D.** Rifampin is a potent inducer of the cytochrome P450 enzymes and will result in decreased plasma levels of many drugs, including the oral contraceptives.

2. **E.** All newly diagnosed active cases of tuberculosis are treated initially with four first-line agents: isoniazid, rifampin, pyrazinamide, and ethambutol. Multidrug therapy is required to prevent the development of resistance.

3. **C.** Dapsone may cause hemolytic anemia, particularly in patients deficient in glucose-6-phosphate dehydrogenase.

4. **D.** Isoniazid has multiple mechanisms of action, including inhibition of mycolic acid synthesis.

Chapter 61

1. **D.** Polymyxins are selective for gram-negative bacteria and are not useful against MRSA.

2. **E.** Ceftriaxone is the first line drug for uncomplicated gonococcal infections and is frequently combined with azithromycin or doxycycline to treat chlamydia as well.

3. **B.** Resistance in VRSA and VRE is conferred by acquisition of *van* genes, which remodel the synthesis of peptidoglycan through the production of D-alanine-D-lactate instead of the normal D-alanine-D-alanine, resulting in the destruction of the normal D-alanine-D-alanine precursors to which vancomycin binds. Vancomycin binds D-alanine-D-lactate with a much lower affinity (about 1000-fold) than D-alanine-D-alanine.

4. **E.** The recent emergence of CRE is a major concern for clinical therapy because infections caused by CRE are resistant to most β-lactam antibiotics including the "last-line" carbapenems. Further, the prevalence of CRE infections has increased over the past decade, infections caused by CRE are associated with high mortality rates, and the optimal treatment for CRE infections is still unknown.

5. **C.** When *P. aeruginosa* develops resistance to all other treatment options, the polymyxins (e.g., colistin and polymyxin B) have been used despite their high rate of associated nephrotoxicity and neurotoxicity, the lack of a well-defined optimal dosing regimen for colistin, and a paucity of clinical experience with polymyxin B. These agents are considered the last resort to treat MDR gram-negative bacteria including *P. aeruginosa* because they exhibit good activity against these resistant bacteria.

Chapter 62

1. **B.** Amphotericin B is the only nephrotoxic compound listed; the other drugs listed have minimal effects on kidney function.

2. **B.** The drug of choice for prophylactic therapy against *Cryptococcus neoformans* is fluconazole, and it is often used for maintenance therapy in immunocompromised patients. It is not appropriate for an acute infection, but because of its lower toxicity, it is preferred over amphotericin as a prophylactic drug.

3. **E.** Terbinafine is highly lipophilic and keratophilic, resulting in high concentrations in the stratum corneum, sebum, hair, and nails. The drug may be detected in nails for up to 90 days after treatment is discontinued.

4. **E.** Voriconazole can cause blurred vision and color disturbances, which are transient effects and typically resolve within 30 minutes. The other agents have minimal or no effects on eye function.

5. **D.** Itraconazole and ketoconazole require an acidic environment for dissolution and absorption. The oral absorption of fluconazole and griseofulvin is not influenced by gastric acid, and amphotericin and caspofungin are not oral agents.

Chapter 63

1. **B.** The hypnozoite stage of *P. ovale* and *P. vivax* can form cysts that remain dormant in the liver for extended periods of time and then present as a recurrence of disease. Only primaquine is effective in eradicating this stage.

2. **D.** Primaquine is a well-known cause of hemolysis in persons who have G6PD deficiency. Chloroquine, mefloquine, pyrimethamine, and doxycycline do not cause G6PD deficiency–related hemolysis,

although pyrimethamine can cause anemia by inhibiting human dihydrofolate reductase.

3. **C.** Primaquine is effective against the exoerythrocytic forms of *P. vivax*; the other agents listed are not.

4. **E.** Chloroquine and the combination atovaquone/proguanil are effective in treating the erythrocytic stage of malaria; primaquine is ineffective against this stage.

Chapter 64

1. **C.** The child has an infection of hookworms, commonly acquired through bare feet and also the leading cause of iron-deficiency anemia. Mebendazole is indicated.

2. **E.** The couple has contracted tapeworms from eating undercooked pork. Praziquantel is the drug of choice for treatment.

3. **C.** Permethrin disrupts nerve traffic by interfering with sodium channels and paralyzes the parasite. Malathion is an organophosphate cholinesterase inhibitor, tetracycline is not indicated for the treatment of lice, ivermectin affects the GABA-chloride channels thus disrupting nerve function, and spinosad activates nicotinic receptors and causes neural excitation and involuntary muscle contraction.

4. **A.** Mebendazole or albendazole would be appropriate to treat a pinworm infection, and both work by binding to β-tubulin in susceptible nematodes and inhibiting microtubule assembly, thus decreasing glucose uptake and killing the parasite.

5. **C.** Praziquantel is the recommended treatment for schistosomiasis. The other choices would not be effective against this parasite.

Chapter 65

1. **C.** Famciclovir is indicated for the treatment of both acute herpes zoster virus (shingles) and new and recurrent HSV-1 and HSV-2.

2. **E.** The herpes simplex virus encodes a thymidine kinase that monophosphorylates acyclovir significantly better than does the host cell enzyme. Because acyclovir monophosphate is trapped in cells, it becomes highly concentrated intracellularly.

3. **C.** Oseltamivir is indicated for the treatment of either influenza A or influenza B, whereas amantadine and rimantadine are effective only against influenza A.

4. **C.** The combination of ledipasvir and sofosbuvir, commercially available as Harvoni, has shown great promise in curing hepatitis C infections.

5. **D.** Adefovir produced severe renal toxicity in HIV-positive patients and is now used as adjunctive therapy for hepatitis B.

Chapter 66

1. **B.** Lamivudine and emtricitabine are isomers of the same drug and thus always confer cross resistance to each other. A new effective regimen needs to contain three fully active agents.

2. **A.** Patients with low kidney function and GFR <30 mL/min should not be given any combination agents that contain the TDF formulation of tenofovir.

3. **A.** Tenofovir is the only agent approved for use in the treatment of hepatitis B and HIV infections.

4. **B.** Dolutegravir is the only drug listed here that does not need to be boosted.

5. **E.** Cobicistat is an inhibitor of CYP3A4 and thus will increase plasma levels of the protease inhibitors and integrase strand transfer inhibitors that are metabolized by this enzyme.

Chapter 67

1. **C.** Employing combination therapy with drugs without overlapping toxicities enables the provider to utilize maximally effective, but non-toxic, drug doses.

2. **A.** Adjuvant therapy is administered after surgery/radiation to kill small metastases that may be undetectable clinically.

3. **A.** Unfortunately, there are no drugs that selectively target tumor metastases.

4. **D.** The objective of chemotherapy may be curative to obtain complete remission; adjuvant to improve the chances for a cure or prolong the period of disease-free survival when no detectable cancer is present but subclinical numbers of neoplastic cells are suspected; or debulking to reduce the tumor burden to allow for a more effective surgical removal of the tumor.

Chapter 68

1. **B.** Tumor cells are killed by chemotherapeutic agents according to a first-order process. This means that the same fraction of cells is killed with each drug dose. Therefore, to reduce a tumor burden from 10^{28} cells to 10^4, with a regimen that has a 4 log kill, six courses of therapy are required.

2. **D.** Many chemotherapeutic agents are transported out of tumor cells via a p-glycoprotein transporter. If the transporter is overexpressed, it will affect the transport of multiple drugs, resulting in multidrug resistance.

3. **D.** Mercaptoethane sulfonate-Na$^+$ (MESNA) binds to the toxic metabolite acrolein, rendering it inert.

4. **A.** Cyclophosphamide is converted to the active cytotoxic form by enzymes in the liver.

5. **D.** 5-Fluorouracil is an antimetabolite that is metabolized to 5-FdUMP, which inhibits thymidylate synthase.

6. **B.** Bifunctional alkylating agents such as cyclophosphamide become covalently attached to two different guanines in DNA.

Chapter 69

1. **A.** Anastrazole is an aromatase inhibitor that inhibits the conversion of androstenedione to estrogen.

2. **A.** Through inhibition of vascular endothelial growth factor, bevacizumab can severely impair wound healing and lead to potentially fatal outcomes.

3. **E.** Sunitinib inhibits tyrosine kinase activity associated with both vascular endothelial growth factor and platelet-derived growth factor. It has been approved as an adjuvant agent in the treatment of advanced renal cell carcinoma.

4. **A.** Flutamide binds to intracellular androgen receptors and blocks the binding of testosterone. Testosterone levels will increase in the patient, but the effects are blocked by the presence of the flutamide.

5. **E.** Nivolumab is a monoclonal antibody directed against the PD-L1 protein that suppresses the production and activity of cytotoxic T cells.

Chapter 70

1. **C.** Kidney failure leads to anemia through the decreased production of erythropoietin, requiring replacement therapy with epoetin alfa. The other agents listed will not increase erythropoietin production.

2. **B.** The patient has developed chemotherapy-induced neutropenia and should be treated with granulocyte colony-stimulating factor (filgrastim), which unfortunately leads to bone pain.

3. **B.** Aplastic anemia or thrombocytopenia induced by interferon treatment of hepatitis C is treated with the non-peptide thrombopoietin receptor agonist eltrombopag, which allows patients to continue therapy with interferon and increases platelets and decreases the risk of bleeding.

4. **E.** Eltrombopag may lead to headache, dizziness, myalgia, gastrointestinal discomfort, elevated hepatic enzymes, neutropenia, anemia,

peripheral edema, and dyspnea. Thromboembolism is a potentially severe side effect if platelet levels become excessive.
5. **C.** The patient has developed thrombocytopenia that can be alleviated by oprelvekin, which is recombinant human IL-11.
6. **D.** The side effects of oprelvekin include tachycardia, atrial fibrillation, dyspnea, and anemia.

Chapter 71

1. **D.** Metoclopramide antagonism at D_2 receptors on neurons in the enteric nervous system and in the brainstem mediate its prokinetic and antiemetic effects.
2. **C.** Aluminum can bind phosphate in the gastrointestinal lumen and reduce the absorption of phosphate, leading to phosphate deficiency with muscle weakness and reabsorption of bone.
3. **A.** Docusate sodium is an ionic detergent that softens feces and permits easier defecation by lowering surface tension and permitting water to interact more effectively with the solid stool.
4. **D.** Simethicone is an antifoaming agent that alters the surface tension of gas bubbles in the stomach and intestines, which facilitates the coalescence and passage of these bubbles via either belching or flatus.

Chapter 72

1. **A.** The short-acting β_2-adrenergic receptor agonists such as albuterol represent the current medications of choice for all types of asthma due to rapid bronchorelaxation with minimal side effects.
2. **E.** The bronchoconstrictive component of COPD has been shown to respond better to antimuscarinic agents than β_2-adrenergic selective agonists or any other group of compounds listed.
3. **C.** Ciclesonide is a synthetic corticosteroid prodrug activated by esterases in the lung to the pharmacologically active compound desisobutyryl-ciclesonide.
4. **A.** The SABAs or short-acting β_2-adrenergic receptor agonists, which include albuterol, are the drugs of choice for the fast relief of asthma. When given by a metered-dose inhaler (MDI), 15% improvement in FEV_1 is achieved within 5 to 10 minutes, and full effect is reached within an hour.
5. **A.** Montelukast is a competitive antagonist at the leukotriene receptor $CysLTR_1$.

Chapter 73

1. **C.** Echinacea is an immunomodulator that has been shown in clinical trials to shorten the duration of upper respiratory infections.
2. **A.** The amino sugar glucosamine is normally involved in the synthesis of glycosaminoglycans, which contribute to the formation of cartilage, whereas chondroitin occurs in connective tissue. Thus, it is not surprising that supplements with glucosamine and chondroitin are often used for the treatment of osteoarthritis.
3. **D.** Kava has been shown to cause severe liver toxicity.

4. **D.** St. John's wort has been shown in clinical trials to be somewhat effective in the treatment of mild to moderate depression.
5. **C.** Asian ginseng can potentiate the effects of anticoagulants.
6. **E.** St. John's wort has been shown to decrease recovery from anesthesia.

Chapter 74

1. **B.** Toxicity that becomes manifest after exposure to a compound for several months to years is referred to as chronic toxicity and typically reflects cumulative damage, such as cirrhosis in alcoholics who have consumed alcohol for several years or pulmonary fibrosis in coal miners.
2. **C.** Epigenetic alterations induced by toxicants can lead to heritable changes in gene expression via effects on DNA methylation, histone modifications (acetylation, phosphorylation, and methylation), and the expression of non-coding RNAs (microRNA). BPA has been shown to affect both DNA and histone methylation, as well as microRNA expression.
3. **E.** Carbon monoxide (CO) is the leading cause of death by poisoning.
4. **E.** All of the pairs shown are correct.
5. **C.** The most compelling evidence between environmental toxicants and a neurodegenerative disorder is that for Parkinson's disease. CO and manganese have been known for many years to lead to parkinsonism, and it is thought that environmental factors such as pesticides, herbicides, and fungicides, as well as industrial solvents and some metals including iron and manganese, may play a significant role in the etiology of sporadic Parkinson's disease.

Chapter 75

1. **C.** A major physiological change in elderly persons is a reduction in total body water. As such, the distribution of water-soluble drugs is also decreased. Digoxin, a water-soluble drug, will have a decrease in volume of distribution and exhibit an increase in plasma concentration within the elderly population compared to middle-aged adults.
2. **D.** The differential expression and activity of several cytochrome P450s is altered during pregnancy including that of CYP2C9, which increases during pregnancy. Thus, the metabolism of the anticonvulsant phenytoin, which is a substrate for CYP2C9, would be increased during pregnancy.
3. **B.** Drug transport into and out of the brain is altered in the neonate because the blood-brain barrier and drug transporters are underdeveloped at this stage, leading to higher drug levels in the central nervous system.
4. **A.** A major pharmacodynamic change in aging is a decrease in receptor expression. The down regulation of β-adrenergic receptors in older persons leads to a decrease in responsiveness and sensitivity to β-adrenergic receptor agonists and antagonists.
5. **E.** Volume of distribution is arguably the most important parameter influenced by the physical changes associated with obesity.

Page numbers followed by "*f*" indicate figures, "*t*" indicate tables, and "*b*" indicate boxes.